Bioethics

BLACKWELL PHILOSOPHY ANTHOLOGIES

Each volume in this outstanding series provides an authoritative and comprehensive collection of the essential primary readings from philosophy's main fields of study. Designed to complement the Blackwell Companions to Philosophy series, each volume represents an unparalleled resource in its own right, and will provide the ideal platform for course use.

1 Cottingham: *Western Philosophy: An Anthology* (third edition)
2 Cahoone: *From Modernism to Postmodernism: An* Anthology (expanded second edition)
3 LaFollette: *Ethics in Practice: An Anthology* (fifth edition)
4 Goodin and Pettit: *Contemporary Political Philosophy: An Anthology* (third edition)
5 Eze: *African Philosophy: An Anthology*
6 McNeill and Feldman: *Continental Philosophy: An Anthology*
7 Kim, Korman, and Sosa: *Metaphysics: An Anthology* (second edition)
8 Lycan and Prinz: *Mind and Cognition: An Anthology* (third edition)
9 Schüklenk and Singer: *Bioethics: An Anthology* (fourth edition)
10 Cummins and Cummins: *Minds, Brains, and Computers – The Foundations of Cognitive Science: An Anthology*
11 Sosa, Kim, Fantl, and McGrath: *Epistemology: An Anthology* (second edition)
12 Kearney and Rasmussen: *Continental Aesthetics – Romanticism to Postmodernism: An Anthology*
13 Martinich and Sosa: *Analytic Philosophy: An Anthology* (second edition)
14 Jacquette: *Philosophy of Logic: An Anthology*
15 Jacquette: *Philosophy of Mathematics: An Anthology*
16 Harris, Pratt, and Waters: *American Philosophies: An Anthology*
17 Emmanuel and Goold: *Modern Philosophy – From Descartes to Nietzsche: An Anthology*
18 Scharff and Dusek: *Philosophy of Technology – The Technological Condition: An Anthology* (second edition)
19 Light and Rolston: *Environmental Ethics: An Anthology*
20 Taliaferro and Griffiths: *Philosophy of Religion: An Anthology*
21 Lamarque and Olsen: *Aesthetics and the Philosophy of Art – The Analytic Tradition: An Anthology* (second edition)
22 John and Lopes: *Philosophy of Literature – Contemporary and Classic Readings: An Anthology*
23 Cudd and Andreasen: *Feminist Theory: A Philosophical Anthology*
24 Carroll and Choi: *Philosophy of Film and Motion Pictures: An Anthology*
25 Lange: *Philosophy of Science: An Anthology*
26 Shafer-Landau and Cuneo: *Foundations of Ethics: An Anthology*
27 Curren: *Philosophy of Education: An Anthology*
28 Shafer-Landau: *Ethical Theory: An Anthology* (second edition)
29 Cahn and Meskin: *Aesthetics: A Comprehensive Anthology*
30 McGrew, Alspector-Kelly and Allhoff: *The Philosophy of Science: An Historical Anthology*
31 May: *Philosophy of Law: Classic and Contemporary Readings*
32 Rosenberg and Arp: *Philosophy of Biology: An Anthology*
33 Hetherington: *Metaphysics and Epistemology: A Guided Anthology*
34 Davis: *Contemporary Moral and Social Issues: An Introduction through Original Fiction, Discussion, and Readings*
35 Dancy and Sandis: *Philosophy of Action: An Anthology*
36 Sosa, Fantl, and McGrath: *Contemporary Epistemology: An Anthology*

Bioethics

An Anthology

FOURTH EDITION

Edited by

Udo Schüklenk and Peter Singer

WILEY Blackwell

Registered Office
John Wiley & Sons, Inc., 111 River Street, Hoboken, NJ 07030, USA

Editorial Office
111 River Street, Hoboken, NJ 07030, USA

For details of our global editorial offices, customer services, and more information about Wiley products visit us at www.wiley.com.

Wiley also publishes its books in a variety of electronic formats and by print-on-demand. Some content that appears in standard print versions of this book may not be available in other formats.

Library of Congress Cataloging-in-Publication Data

Names: Schüklenk, Udo, 1964– editor. | Singer, Peter, 1946– editor.
Title: Bioethics : an anthology / edited by Udo Schüklenk, and Peter
    Singer.
Other titles: Bioethics (Kuhse) | Blackwell philosophy anthologies ; 37.
Description: Fourth edition. | Hoboken, NJ : Wiley-Blackwell, 2022. |
    Series: Blackwell philosophy anthologies ; 37 | Includes bibliographical
    references and index.
Identifiers: LCCN 2020032198 (print) | LCCN 2020032199 (ebook) | ISBN
    9781119635116 (paperback) | ISBN 9781119635086 (adobe pdf) | ISBN
    9781119635154 (epub)
Subjects: MESH: Bioethics | Ethics, Medical | Bioethical Issues | Collected
    Work
Classification: LCC R724 (print) | LCC R724 (ebook) | NLM WB 5 | DDC
    174–dc23
LC record available at https://lccn.loc.gov/2020032198
LC ebook record available at https://lccn.loc.gov/2020032199

Cover Design: Wiley
Cover Image: © Imagno/Hulton Fine Art Collection/Getty Images

Set in 10/12pt Bembo by Straive, Pondicherry, India
Printed and bound by CPI Group (UK) Ltd, Croydon, CR0 4YY

C102368_030821

Contents

Acknowledgments   xiii

Introduction   1

Part I   Abortion   9

Introduction   11

1   Abortion and Infanticide   15
Michael Tooley

2   A Defense of Abortion   31
Judith Jarvis Thomson

3   The Wrong of Abortion   42
Patrick Lee and Robert P. George

4   Why Abortion is Immoral   54
Don Marquis

Part II   Issues in Reproduction   67

Introduction   69

Assisted Reproduction   73

5   The McCaughey Septuplets: God's Will or Human Choice?   75
Gregory Pence

6   The Meaning of Synthetic Gametes for Gay and Lesbian People and Bioethics Too   78
Timothy F. Murphy

7   Rights, Interests, and Possible People   85
Derek Parfit

Prenatal Screening, Sex Selection, and Cloning 91

8   Genetics and Reproductive Risk: Can Having Children Be Immoral?   93
    Laura M. Purdy

9   Sex Selection and Preimplantation Genetic Diagnosis   101
    The Ethics Committee of the American Society of Reproductive Medicine

10 Sex Selection and Preimplantation Diagnosis: A Response to the Ethics Committee
    of the American Society of Reproductive Medicine   107
    Julian Savulescu and Edgar Dahl

11 Why We Should Not Permit Embryos to Be Selected as Tissue Donors   110
    David King

12 The Moral Status of Human Cloning: Neo-Lockean Persons versus Human Embryos   115
    Michael Tooley

Part III   Genetic Manipulation 133

Introduction   135

13 Questions about Some Uses of Genetic Engineering   139
    Jonathan Glover

14 The Moral Significance of the Therapy–Enhancement Distinction in Human Genetics   151
    David B. Resnik

15 In Defense of Posthuman Dignity   162
    Nick Bostrom

16 Statement on NIH Funding of Research Using Gene-Editing Technologies in Human Embryos   170
    Francis S. Collins

17 Genome Editing and Assisted Reproduction: Curing Embryos, Society or Prospective Parents?   172
    Giulia Cavaliere

18 Who's Afraid of the Big Bad (Germline Editing) Wolf?   185
    R. Alta Charo

19 An Ethical Pathway for Gene Editing   191
    Julian Savulescu and Peter Singer

Part IV   Life and Death Issues 195

Introduction   197

20 The Sanctity of Life   207
    Jonathan Glover

21 Declaration on Euthanasia   218
    Sacred Congregation for the Doctrine of the Faith

Killing and Letting Die   223

22   Active and Passive Euthanasia   225
James Rachels

23   The Morality of Killing: A Traditional View   230
Germain Grisez and Joseph M. Boyle, Jr.

24   Is Killing No Worse Than Letting Die?   235
Winston Nesbitt

25   Why Killing is Not Always Worse – and Sometimes Better – Than Letting Die   240
Helga Kuhse

26   Moral Fictions and Medical Ethics   244
Franklin G. Miller, Robert D. Truog, and Dan W. Brock

Newborns   255

27   Can a Physician Ever Justifiably Euthanize a Severely Disabled Newborn?   257
Robert M. Sade

28   No to Infant Euthanasia   259
Gilbert Meilaender

29   Physicians Can Justifiably Euthanize Certain Severely Impaired Neonates   262
Udo Schüklenk

30   You Should Not Have Let Your Baby Die   266
Gary Comstock

31   After-Birth Abortion: Why Should the Baby Live?   269
Alberto Giubilini and Francesca Minerva

32   Does a Human Being Gain the Right to Live after He or She is Born?   275
Christopher Kaczor

33   Hard Lessons: Learning from the Charlie Gard Case   280
Dominic Wilkinson and Julian Savulescu

Brain Death   289

34   A Definition of Irreversible Coma   291
Report of the Ad Hoc Committee of the Harvard Medical School to Examine the Definition of Brain Death

35   The Challenge of Brain Death for the Sanctity of Life Ethic   296
Peter Singer

36   The Philosophical Debate   308
The President's Council on Bioethics

37   An Alternative to Brain Death   318
     Jeff McMahan

Advance Directives   323

38   Life Past Reason   325
     Ronald Dworkin

39   Dworkin on Dementia: Elegant Theory, Questionable Policy   333
     Rebecca Dresser

Voluntary Euthanasia and Medically Assisted Suicide   343

40   The Note   345
     Chris Hill

41   When Self-Determination Runs Amok   350
     Daniel Callahan

42   When Abstract Moralizing Runs Amok   356
     John Lachs

43   Physician-Assisted Death and Severe, Treatment-Resistant Depression   361
     Bonnie Steinbock

44   Are Concerns about Irremediableness, Vulnerability, or Competence Sufficient
     to Justify Excluding All Psychiatric Patients from Medical Aid in Dying?   378
     William Rooney, Udo Schüklenk, and Suzanne van de Vathorst

Part V   Resource Allocation   393

Introduction   395

45   In a Pandemic, Should We Save Younger Lives?   399
     Peter Singer and Lucy Winkett

46   The Value of Life   403
     John Harris

47   Bubbles under the Wallpaper: Healthcare Rationing and Discrimination   413
     Nick Beckstead and Toby Ord

48   Rescuing Lives: Can't We Count?   420
     Paul T. Menzel

49   Should Alcoholics Compete Equally for Liver Transplantation?   423
     Alvin H. Moss and Mark Siegler

Part VI Obtaining Organs **431**

Introduction 433

50 Organ Donation and Retrieval: Whose Body is it Anyway? 435
Eike-Henner W. Kluge

51 The Case for Allowing Kidney Sales 439
*Janet Radcliffe-Richards, A. S. Daar, R. D. Guttmann, R. Hoffenberg, I. Kennedy,
M. Lock, R. A. Sells and N. Tilney and for the International Forum Transplant Ethics*

52 Ethical Issues in the Supply and Demand of Kidneys 443
Debra Satz

53 The Survival Lottery 456
John Harris

Part VII Ethical Issues in Research **463**

Introduction 465

Experimentation with Humans **473**

54 Belmont Report: Ethical Principles and Guidelines for the Protection of
Human Subjects of Research 475
National Commission for the Protection of Human Subjects of Biomedical and Behavioral Research

55 Scientific Research is a Moral Duty 483
John Harris

56 Participation in Biomedical Research is an Imperfect Moral Duty: A Response to John Harris 495
Sandra Shapshay and Kenneth D. Pimple

57 Unethical Trials of Interventions to Reduce Perinatal Transmission
of the Human Immunodeficiency Virus in Developing Countries 501
Peter Lurie and Sidney M. Wolfe

58 We're Trying to Help Our Sickest People, Not Exploit Them 507
Danstan Bagenda and Philippa Musoke-Mudido

59 Pandemic Ethics: The Case for Risky Research 510
Peter Singer and Richard Yetter Chappell

Experimentation with Animals **515**

60 Duties towards Animals 517
Immanuel Kant

61 A Utilitarian View 519
Jeremy Bentham

62 The Harmful, Nontherapeutic Use of Animals in Research is Morally Wrong 521
Nathan Nobis

63 The Use of Nonhuman Animals in Biomedical Research 535
Dario L. Ringach

64 Ethical Issues When Modelling Brain Disorders in Non-Human Primates 550
Carolyn P. Neuhaus

Academic Freedom and Research 559

65 On Liberty 561
John Stuart Mill

66 Should Some Knowledge Be Forbidden?: The Case of Cognitive Differences Research 566
Janet A. Kourany

67 Academic Freedom and Race: You Ought Not to Believe What You Think May Be True 575
James R. Flynn

Part VIII Public Health Issues 585

Introduction 587

68 Ethics and Infectious Disease 591
Michael J. Selgelid

69 XDR-TB in South Africa: No Time for Denial or Complacency 602
Jerome Amir Singh, Ross Upshur, and Nesri Padayatchi

70 Clinical Ethics During the Covid-19 Pandemic: Missing the Trees for the Forest 612
Vijayaprasad Gopichandran

71 The Moral Obligation to be Vaccinated: Utilitarianism, Contractualism, and Collective Easy Rescue 620
Alberto Giubilini, Thomas Douglas, and Julian Savulescu

72 Taking Responsibility for Responsibility 638
Neil Levy

Part IX Ethical Issues in the Practice of Healthcare 651

Introduction 653

When do Doctors have a Duty to Treat? 659

73 What Healthcare Professionals Owe Us: Why Their Duty to Treat During a Pandemic
is Contingent on Personal Protective Equipment (PPE) 661
Udo Schüklenk

74 Conscientious Objection in Health Care 667
Mark R. Wicclair

75 Conscientious Objection in Medicine: Accommodation versus Professionalism
and the Public Good 682
Udo Schüklenk

Confidentiality 693

76 Confidentiality in Medicine: A Decrepit Concept 695
Mark Siegler

77 A Defense of Unqualified Medical Confidentiality 699
Kenneth Kipnis

Truth-Telling 713

78 On a Supposed Right to Lie from Altruistic Motives 715
Immanuel Kant

79 Should Doctors Tell the Truth? 717
Joseph Collins

80 On Telling Patients the Truth 724
Roger Higgs

Informed Consent and Patient Autonomy 731

81 On Liberty 733
John Stuart Mill

82 From *Schloendorff v. New York Hospital* 736
Justice Benjamin N. Cardozo

83 Informed Consent: Its History, Meaning, and Present Challenges 737
Tom L. Beauchamp

84 The Doctor–Patient Relationship in Different Cultures 745
Ruth Macklin

85 Transgender Children and the Right to Transition: Medical Ethics When Parents Mean
Well But Cause Harm 758
Maura Priest

86 Amputees by Choice 777
Carl Elliott

87 Rational Desires and the Limitation of Life-Sustaining Treatment 788
Julian Savulescu

Part X   Disability   807

Introduction   809

88   Valuing Disability, Causing Disability   811
     Elizabeth Barnes

89   Is Disability Mere Difference?   829
     Greg Bognar

90   Prenatal Diagnosis and Selective Abortion: A Challenge to Practice and Policy   835
     Adrienne Asch

91   Down Syndrome Screening Isn't about Public Health: It's about Eliminating a Group of People   851
     Renate Lindeman

92   I Would've Aborted a Fetus with Down Syndrome: Women Need that Right   854
     Ruth Marcus

Part XI   Neuroethics   857

Introduction   859

93   Neuroethics: Ethics and the Sciences of the Mind   861
     Neil Levy

94   Engineering Love   867
     Julian Savulescu and Anders Sandberg

95   Unrequited Love Hurts: Should Doctors Treat Broken Hearts?   870
     Francesca Minerva

96   Stimulating Brains, Altering Minds   876
     Walter Glannon

97   Authenticity or Autonomy? When Deep Brain Stimulation Causes a Dilemma 883
     Felicitas Kraemer

98   On the Necessity of Ethical Guidelines for Novel Neurotechnologies   889
     Sara Goering and Rafael Yuste

Index   895

Acknowledgments

The editor and publisher gratefully acknowledge the permission granted to reproduce the copyright material in this book:

1 Michael Tooley, "Abortion and Infanticide," pp. 37–65 from *Philosophy and Public Affairs* 1 (1972). Reproduced with permission of John Wiley & Sons.

2 Judith Jarvis Thomson, "A Defense of Abortion," pp. 47–66 from *Philosophy and Public Affairs* 1: 1 (1971). Reproduced with permission of John Wiley & Sons.

3 Patrick Lee and Robert P. George, "The Wrong of Abortion," pp. 13–26 from Andrew I. Cohen and Christopher Health Wellman (eds.), *Contemporary Debates in Applied Ethics* (Hoboken, NJ: Wiley-Blackwell, 2014). Reproduced with permission of John Wiley & Sons.

4 Don Marquis, "Why Abortion Is Immoral," pp. 183–202 from *Journal of Philosophy* 86: 4 (April 1989). Reproduced with permission of the author and The Journal of Philosophy, Inc.

5 Gregory Pence, "Multiple Gestation and Damaged Babies: God's Will or Human Choice?" This essay draws on "The McCaughey Septuplets: God's Will or Human Choice," pp. 39–43 from Gregory Pence, *Brave New Bioethics* (Lanham, MD: Rowman & Littlefield, 2002). © 2002 Gregory Pence. Reproduced courtesy of Gregory Pence.

6 Timothy Murphy, "The Meaning of Synthetic Gametes for Gay and Lesbian People and Bioethics Too," pp. 762–765 from *Journal of Medical Ethics* 40 (2014). Reproduced with permission of BMJ Publishing Group Ltd.

7 Derek Parfit, "Rights, Interests, and Possible People," pp. 369–375 from Samuel Gorovitz et al. (eds.), *Moral Problems in Medicine* (Englewood Cliffs, NJ: Prentice Hall, 1976). Reproduced courtesy of Derek Parfit.

8 Laura M. Purdy, "Genetics and Reproductive Risk: Can Having Children be Immoral?," pp. 39–49 from *Reproducing Persons: Issues in Feminist Bioethics* (Ithaca, NY: Cornell University Press, 1996). Reproduced with permission of Cornell University Press.

9 The Ethics Committee of the American Society of Reproductive Medicine, "Sex Selection and Preimplantation Genetic Diagnosis," pp. 595–598 from *Fertility and Sterility* 72: 4 (October 1999). Reproduced with permission of Elsevier.

10 Julian Savulescu and Edgar Dahl, "Sex Selection and Preimplantation Diagnosis: A Response to the Ethics Committee of the American Society of Reproductive Medicine," pp. 1879–1880 from *Human Reproduction* 15: 9 (2000). Reproduced with permission of Oxford University Press.

11 David King, "Why We Should Not Permit Embryos to Be Selected as Tissue Donors," pp. 13–16 from *The Bulletin of Medical Ethics* 190 (August 2003). © 2003 RSM Press. Reproduced with permission of the Royal Society of Medicine.

12 Michael Tooley, "The Moral Status of the Cloning of Human Cloning: Neo Lockean Persons Versus Human Embryos." Written for this edition (2021) and reproduced courtesy of Michael Tooley.

13 Jonathan Glover, "Questions about Some Uses of Genetic Engineering," pp. 25–33, 33–36, 42–43, and 45–53 from *What Sort of People Should There Be?* (Harmondsworth: Penguin Books, 1984).

14 David B. Resnik, "The Moral Significance of the Therapy–Enhancement Distinction in Human Genetics," pp. 365–377 from *Cambridge Quarterly of Healthcare Ethics* 9: 3 (Summer 2000) Reproduced with permission of Cambridge University Press.

15 Nick Bostrom, "In Defense of Posthuman Dignity," pp. 202–214 from *Bioethics* 19: 3 (2005). Reproduced with permission of John Wiley & Sons.

16 Francis S. Collins, "Statement on NIH Funding of Research Using Gene-editing Technologies in Human Embryos," https://www.nih.gov/about-nih/who-we-are/nih-director/statements/statement-nih-funding-research-using-gene-editing-technologies-human-embryos. Public domain.

17 Giulia Cavaliere, "Genome Editing and Assisted Reproduction: Curing Embryos, Society or Prospective Parents, pp. 215–225 from *Medicine, Health Care and Philosophy* 21. Springer Nature / CC BY 4.0.

18 R. Alta Charo, "Who's Afraid of the Big Bad (Germline Editing) Wolf?" pp. 93–100 from *Perspectives in Biology and Medicine* 63: 1 (Winter 2020). Reproduced with permission of Johns Hopkins University Press.

19 Julian Savulescu and Peter Singer, "An Ethical Pathway for Gene Editing," pp. 221–222 from *Bioethics* 33: 2 (2019). Reproduced with permission of John Wiley & Sons.

20 Jonathan Glover, "The Sanctity of Life," pp. 39–59 from *Causing Death and Lives* (London: Pelican, 1977).

21 Sacred Congregation for the Doctrine of the Faith, "Declaration on Euthanasia" (Vatican City, 1980). Public domain.

22 James Rachels, "Active and Passive Euthanasia," pp. 78–80 from *New England Journal of Medicine* 292 (1975). © 1975 Massachusetts Medical Society. Reproduced with permission of Massachusetts Medical Society.

23 Germain Grisez and Joseph M. Boyle, Jr., "The Morality of Killing: A Traditional View," pp. 381–419 from *Life and Death with Liberty and Justice: A Contribution to the Euthanasia Debate* (Notre Dame, IN: University of Notre Dame Press, 1971). Reproduced with permission of University of Notre Dame Press.

24 Winston Nesbitt, "Is Killing No Worse Than Letting Die?" pp. 101–105 from *Journal of Applied Philosophy* 12: 1 (1995). Reproduced with permission of John Wiley & Sons.

25 Helga Kuhse, "Why Killing Is Not Always Worse – and Sometimes Better – Than Letting Die," pp. 371–374 from *Cambridge Quarterly of Healthcare* 7: 4 (1998). Reproduced with permission of Cambridge University Press.

26 Franklin G. Miller, Robert D. Truog, and Dan W. Brock, "Moral Fictions and Medical Ethics," pp. 453–460 from *Bioethics* 24: 9 (2010). Reproduced with permission of John Wiley & Sons.

27 Robert M. Sade, "Can a Physician Ever Justifiably Euthanize a Severely Disabled Neonate?" p. 532 from *The Journal of Thoracic and Cardiovascular Surgery* 149 (2015). Reproduced with permission of Elsevier.

28 Gilbert Meilaender, "No to Infant Euthanasia," pp. 533–534 from *The Journal of Thoracic and Cardiovascular Surgery* 149 (2015). Reproduced with permission of Elsevier.

29 Udo Schüklenk, "Physicians Can Justifiably Euthanize Certain Severely Impaired Neonates," pp. 535–537 from *The Journal of Thoracic and Cardiovascular Surgery* 149 (2015). Reproduced with permission of Elsevier.

30 Gary Comstock, "You Should Not Have Let Your Baby Die" from *The New York Times*, July 12, 2017. Reproduced with permission of New York Times / PARS.

31 Alberto Giubilini and Francesa Minerva, "After-Birth Abortion: Why Should the Baby Live?" pp. 261–263 from *Journal of Medical Ethics* 39 (2013). Reproduced with permission of BMJ Publishing Group Ltd.

32 Christopher Kaczor, "Abortion as a Human Rights Violation," pp. 92–98 from Kate Greasley and Christopher Kaczor (eds.), *Abortion Rights: For and Against* (Cambridge: Cambridge University Press, 2018). Reproduced with permission of Cambridge University Press.

33 Dominic Wilkinson and Julian Savulescu, "Hard Lessons: Learning from the Charlie Gard Case," pp. 438–442 from *Journal of Medical Ethics* 44 (2018). Reproduced with permission of BMJ Publishing Group Ltd.

34 Report of the Ad Hoc Committee of the Harvard Medical School to Examine the Definition of Brain Death, "A Definition of Irreversible Coma," pp. 85–88 from *Journal of the American Medical Association* 205: 6 (August 1968).

35 Peter Singer, "The Challenge of Brain Death for the Sanctity of Life Ethic," pp. 153–165 from *Ethics & Bioethics in Central Europe* 8: 3–4 (2018).

36 The President's Council on Bioethics, "The Philosophical Debate," pp. 49–68 from *Controversies in the Determination of Death* (white paper). Washington, D.C., December 2008. Public domain.

37 Jeff McMahan, "Alternative to Brain Death," pp. 47–48 from *Journal of Law, Medicine and Ethics* 34 (2006). Includes only the section "An Alternative Understanding of Brain Death," with some editing to remove references to the earlier section. Reproduced with permission of Sage Publications Ltd.

38 Ronald Dworkin, "Life Past Reason," pp. 218–229 from *Life's Dominion: An Argument about Abortion, Euthanasia, and Individual Freedom* (New York: Knopf, 1993). © 1993 by Ronald Dworkin. Reproduced with permission of Alfred A. Knopf, an imprint of the Knopf Doubleday Publishing Group, a division of Random House LLC. All rights reserved.

39 Rebecca Dresser, "Dworkin on Dementia: Elegant Theory, Questionable Policy," pp. 32–38 from *Hastings Center Report* 25: 6 (November/December 1995). Reproduced with permission of John Wiley & Sons.

40 Chris Hill, "The Note," pp. 9–17 from Helga Kuhse (ed.), *Willing to Listen, Wanting to Die* (Ringwood, Australia: Penguin Books, 1994).

41 Daniel Callahan, "When Self-Determination Runs Amok," pp. 52–55 from *Hastings Center Report* 22: 2 (March/April 1992). Reproduced with permission of John Wiley & Sons.

42 John Lachs, "When Abstract Moralizing Runs Amok," pp. 10–13 from *The Journal of Clinical Ethics* 5: 1 (Spring 1994). Reproduced with permission of The Journal of Clinical Ethics.

43 Bonnie Steinbock, "Physician-Assisted Death and Severe, Treatment-Resistant Depression," pp. 30–42 from *Hastings Center Report* 47: 5 (2017), updated by the author for this edition (2021). Reproduced with permission of John Wiley & Sons.

44 William Rooney, Udo Schüklenk, and Suzanne van de Vathorst, "Are Concerns about Irremediableness, Vulnerability, or Competence Sufficient to Exclude All Psychiatric Patients from Medical Aid in Dying?" pp. 326–343 from *Health Care Analysis* 26 (2018). Reproduced with permission of Springer Nature.

45 Peter Singer and Lucy Winkett, "The Duel: Is It More Important to Save Younger Lives?, *Prospect*, May 4, 2020. Reproduced courtesy of the authors and *Prospect* magazine.

46 John Harris, "The Value of Life," pp. 87–102 from *The Value of Life* (London: Routledge, 1985). © 1985 Routledge. Reproduced with permission of Taylor & Francis Books UK.

47 Nick Beckstead and Toby Ord, "Bubbles under the Wallpaper: Healthcare Rationing and Discrimination," a paper presented to the conference "Valuing Lives" New York University, March 5, 2011, © Nick Beckstead and Toby Ord, reproduced with permission of the authors. The chapter draws on Nick Beckstead and Toby Ord,

"Rationing and Rationality: The Cost of Avoiding Discrimination," pp. 232–239 from N. Eyal et al. (eds.), *Inequalities in Health: Concepts, Measures, and Ethics* (Oxford: Oxford University Press, 2013). Reproduced with permission of Oxford University Press.

48 Paul T. Menzel, "Rescuing Lives: Can't We Count?" pp. 22–23 from *Hastings Center Report* 24: 1 (1994). Reproduced with permission of John Wiley & Sons.

49 Alvin H. Moss and Mark Siegler, "Should Alcoholics Compete Equally for Liver Transplantation?" pp. 1295–1298 from *Journal of the American Medical Association* 265: 10 (1991). © 1991 American Medical Association. All rights reserved.

50 Eike-Henner W. Kluge, "Organ Donation and Retrieval: Whose Body Is It Anyway?" © 1999 Eike-Henner W. Kluge.

51 Janet Radcliffe-Richards et al., "The Case for Allowing Kidney Sales," pp. 1950–1952 from *The Lancet* 351: 9120 (June 27, 1998). Reproduced with permission of Elsevier.

52 Debra Satz, "Ethical Issues in the Supply and Demand of Human Kidneys," pp. 189–206 from *Why Some Things Should Not Be for Sale: The Moral Limits of Markets* (New York: Oxford University Press, 2010). based on an article from *Proceedings of the Aristotelian Society* 2 (2010). Reproduced with permission of Oxford University Press and the Aristotelian Society.

53 John Harris, "The Survival Lottery," pp. 81–87 from *Philosophy* 50 (1975). © 1975 Royal Institute of Philosophy. Reproduced with permission of Cambridge University Press.

54 National Commission for the Protection of Human Subjects of Biomedical and Behavioral Research, U.S. Department of Health, Education and Welfare, "The Belmont Report: Ethical Principles and Guidelines for the Protection of Human Subjects of Research," 1978, pp. 1–20. Public domain.

55 John Harris, "Scientific Research Is a Moral Duty," pp. 242–248 from *Journal of Medical Ethics* 31: 4 (2005). Reproduced with permission of BMJ Publishing Group Ltd.

56 Sandra Shapshay and Kenneth D. Pimple, "Participation in Research Is an Imperfect Moral Duty: A Response to John Harris," pp. 414–417 from *Journal of Medical Ethics* 33 (2007). Reproduced with permission of BMJ Publishing Group Ltd.

57 Peter Lurie and Sidney M. Wolfe, "Unethical Trials of Interventions to Reduce Perinatal Transmission of the Human Immunodeficiency Virus in Developing Countries," pp. 853–856 from *New England Journal of Medicine* 337: 12 (September 1997). © 1997 Massachusetts Medical Society. Reproduced with permission of Massachusetts Medical Society.

58 Danstan Bageda and Philippa Musoke-Mudido, "We're Trying to Help Our Sickest People, Not Exploit Them," from *The Washington Post*, September 28, 1997. © 1997 Washington Post Company. All rights reserved.

59 Richard Yetter Chappell and Peter Singer, "Pandemic Ethics: The Case for Risky Research," pp. 1–8 from *Research Ethics* 16: 3–4 (2020). Reproduced with permission of Sage Publications Ltd.

60 Immanuel Kant, "Duties towards Animals," pp. 239–241 from *Lectures on Ethics*, trans. Louis Infield (London: Methuen, 1930).

61 Jeremy Bentham, "A Utilitarian View," section XVIII, IV from *An Introduction to the Principles of Morals and Legislation*, First published c. 1820. Public domain.

62 Nathan Nobis, "Harmful, Nontherapeutic Use of Animals in Research is Morally Wrong," pp. 297–304 from *American Journal of the Medical Sciences* 342: 4 (October 2011). Reproduced with permission of Elsevier.

63 Dario L. Ringach, "Use of Nonhuman Animals in Biomedical Research," pp. 305–313 from *American Journal of the Medical Sciences* 342: 4 (October 2011). Reproduced with permission of Elsevier.

64 Carolyn P. Neuhaus, "Ethical Issues When Modelling Brain Disorders in Non-Human Primates," pp. 323–327 from *Journal of Medical Ethics* 44. Reproduced with permission of BMJ Publishing Group Ltd.

65 John Stuart Mill, "Of the Liberty of Thought and Discussion" (extract) from *On Liberty*, chapter II. First published 1859. Public domain.

66 Janet A. Kourany, "Should Some Knowledge be Forbidden: The Case of Cognitive Differences Research," pp. 779–790 from *Philosophy of Science* 83 (December 2016). Reproduced with permission of University of Chicago Press.

67 James R. Flynn, "Academic Freedom and Race: You Ought Not to Believe What You Think May Be True," pp. 127–131 from *Journal of Criminal Justice* 59 (2018). Reproduced with permission of Elsevier.

68 Michael J. Selgelid, "Ethics and Infectious Disease," pp. 272–289 from *Bioethics* 19:3 (2005). Reproduced with permission of John Wiley & Sons.

69 Jerome Amir Singh, Ross Upshur, and Nesri Padayatchi, "XDR-TB in South Africa: No Time for Denial or Complacency," PLoS Medicine 4: 1 (2007): e50. © 2007 Singh et al. Open access / CC BY 4.0.

70 Excerpted from Vijayaprasad Gopichandran, "Clinical Ethics During the Covid-19 Pandemic: Missing the Trees for the Forest," pp. 1–5 from *Indian Journal of Medical Ethics* 5: 3 (2020).

71 Alberto Giubilini, Thomas Douglas, and Julian Savulescu, "The Moral Obligation to be Vaccinated: Utilitarianism, Contractualism and Collective Easy Rescue," pp. 547–560 from *Medicine, Health Care and Philosophy* 21 (2018). © 2018 Alberto Giubilini, Thomas Douglas, and Julian Savulescu. Springer Nature /Open access.

72 Neil Levy, "Taking Responsibility for Responsibility," pp. 108–113 from *Public Health Ethics* 12: 2 (July 2019). Oxford University Press / Open access.

73 Udo Schüklenk, "What Healthcare Professionals Owe Us: Why Their Duty to Treat During a Pandemic is Contingent on Personal Protective Equipment (PPE)," pp. 432–435 from *Journal of Medical Ethics* 46: 7 (2020).

74 Mark R. Wicclair, "Conscientious Objection in Health Care," in Hugh LaFollette (ed.), *Ethics in Practice: An Anthology*, Fifth Edition (Hoboken, NJ: Wiley-Blackwell, 2020). Reproduced with permission of John Wiley & Sons.

75 Udo Schüklenk, "Conscientious Objection in Medicine: Accommodation Versus Professionalism and the Public Good," pp. 47–56 from *British Medical Bulletin* 126 (2018).

76 Mark Siegler, "Confidentiality in Medicine: A Decrepit Concept," pp. 1518–1521 from *New England Journal of Medicine* 307: 24 (December 1982). © 1982 Massachusetts Medical Society. Reproduced with permission of Massachusetts Medical Society.

77 Kenneth Kipnis, "A Defense of Unqualified Medical Confidentiality," pp. 7–18 from *American Journal of Bioethics* 6: 2 (2006) Reproduced with permission of Taylor & Francis.

78 Immanuel Kant, "On a Supposed Right to Lie from Altruistic Motives," pp. 361–363 from *Critique of Practical Reason and Other Works on the Theory of Ethics*, 6th edition, trans. T. K. Abbott (London, 1909). Public domain. This essay was first published in a Berlin periodical in 1797.

79 Joseph Collins, "Should Doctors Tell the Truth?" pp. 320–326 from *Harper's Monthly Magazine* 155 (August 1927).

80 Roger Higgs, "On Telling Patients the Truth," pp. 186–202 and 232–233 from Michael Lockwood (ed.), *Moral Dilemmas in Modern Medicine* (Oxford: Oxford University Press, 1985). Reproduced with permission of Oxford University Press.

81 John Stuart Mill, "On Liberty," first published in 1859. Public domain.

82 Justice Benjamin N. Cardozo, Judgment from *Schloendorff* v. *New York Hospital* (1914), p. 526 from Jay Katz (ed.), *Experimentation with Human Beings: The Authority of the Investigator, Subject, Professions, and State in the Human Experimentation Process* (New York: Russell Sage Foundation, 1972). Reproduced with permission of Russell Sage Foundation.

83 om L. Beauchamp, "Informed Consent: Its History, Meaning, and Present Challenges," pp. 515–523 from *Cambridge Quarterly of Health Care Ethics* 20: 4 (2011). © 2011 Royal Institute of Philosophy. Reproduced with permission of Cambridge University Press and Tom L. Beauchamp.

84 Ruth Macklin, "The Doctor–Patient Relationship in Different Cultures," pp. 86–107

from *Against Relativism: Cultural Diversity and the Search of Ethical Universals in Medicine* (New York: Oxford University Press, 1999). © 1999 by Oxford University Press, Inc. Reproduced with permission of Oxford University Press, USA.

85 Maura Priest, "Transgender Children and the Right to Transition: Medical Ethics When Parents Mean Well But Cause Harm," pp. 45–59 from *American Journal of Bioethics* 19 (2019). Reproduced with permission of Taylor & Francis.

86 Carl Elliott, "Amputees by Choice," pp. 208–210, 210–215, 219–223, 227–231, 234–236, 323–326 from *Better Than Well: American Medicine Meets the American Dream* (New York and London: W.W. Norton, 2003). © 2003 by Carl Elliott. Reproduced with permission of W.W. Norton & Company, Inc.

87 Julian Savulescu, "Rational Desires and the Limitation of Life-Sustaining Treatment," pp. 191–222 from *Bioethics* 8: 3 (1994). Reproduced with permission of John Wiley & Sons.

88 Elizabeth Barnes, "Valuing Disability, Causing Disability," pp. 88–113 from *Ethics* 125 (2014). Reproduced with permission of University of Chicago Press.

89 Greg Bognar, "Is Disability Mere Difference," pp. 46–49 from *Journal of Medical Ethics* 42 (2016). Reproduced with permission of BMJ Publishing Group Ltd.

90 Adrienne Asch, "Prenatal Diagnosis and Selective Abortion: A Challenge to Practice and Policy," pp. 1649–1657 from *American Journal of Public Health* 89: 11 (1999). Reproduced with permission of American Public Health Association.

91 Renata Lindeman, "Down Syndrome Screening Isn't About Public Health. It's About Eliminating a Group of People," from *Washington Post*, June 16, 2015. Reproduced courtesy of Renata Lindeman.

92 Ruth Marcus, "I Would've Aborted a Fetus with Down Syndrome: Women Need That Right," *Washington Post*, March 9, 2018. Reproduced with permission of Washington Post / PARS.

93 Neil Levy, "Neuroethics: Ethics and the Sciences of the Mind," pp. 69–74 (extract) from *Philosophy Compass* 4: 10 (2009). Reproduced with permission of John Wiley & Sons.

94 Anders Sandberg and Julian Savulescu, "Love Machine: Engineering Lifelong Romance," pp. 28–29 from *New Scientist* 2864. © 2012 Reed Business Information. Reproduced with permission of Tribune Content Agency.

95 Francesca Minerva, "Unrequited Love Hurts: The Medicalization of Broken Hearts is Therapy, Not Enhancement," pp. 479–485 from *Cambridge Quarterly of Healthcare* Ethics 24: 4 (2015). Reproduced with permission of Cambridge University Press.

96 Walter Glannon, "Stimulating Brains, Altering Minds," pp. 289–292 from *Journal of Medical Ethics* 35 (2009). Reproduced with permission of BMJ Publishing Group Ltd.

97 Felicitas Kramer, "Authenticity or Autonomy? When Deep Brain Stimulation Causes a Dilemma," pp. 757–760 from *Journal of Medical Ethics* 39 (2013). Reproduced with permission of BMJ Publishing Group Ltd.

98 Sara Goering and Rafael Yuste, "On the Necessity of Ethical Guidelines for Novel Neurotechnologies," pp. 882–885 from *Cell* 167 (2016). Reproduced with permission of Elsevier.

Introduction

The term "bioethics" is often mistakenly ascribed to the biologist Van Rensselaer Potter, who used it in the 1970s to describe his proposal that we need an ethic that can incorporate our obligations, not just to other humans, but to the biosphere as a whole.[1] However, a historically correct account should probably give credit for coining the term to Fritz Jahr, a German Protestant pastor, who in 1927 published an article called "Bio-Ethics: A Review of the Ethical Relationships of Humans to Animals and Plants."[2] Jahr tried to establish "bioethics" both as a discipline and as a moral principle. Although the term is still occasionally used in the sense of an ecological ethic, it is now much more commonly used in the narrower sense of the study of ethical issues arising from the biological and medical sciences. So understood, bioethics has become a specialized, although interdisciplinary, area of study. The essays included in this book give an indication of the range of issues which fall within its scope – but it is only an indication. There are many other issues that we simply have not had the space to cover.

Bioethics can be seen as a branch of ethics, or, more specifically, of applied ethics. For this reason some understanding of the nature of ethics is an essential preliminary to any serious study of bioethics. The remainder of this introduction will seek to provide that understanding.

One question about the nature of ethics is especially relevant to bioethics: to what extent is reasoning or argument possible in ethics? Many people assume without much thought that ethics is subjective. The subjectivist holds that what ethical view we take is a matter of opinion or taste that is not amenable to argument. But if ethics were a matter of taste, why would we even attempt to argue about it? If Helen says "I like my coffee sweetened," whereas Paul says "I like my coffee unsweetened," there is not much point in Helen and Paul arguing about it. The two statements do not contradict each other. They can both be true. But if Helen says "Doctors should never assist their patients to die" whereas Paul says "Sometimes doctors should assist their patients to die," then Helen and Paul are disagreeing, and there does seem to be a point in their trying to argue about the issue of physician-assisted suicide.

It seems clear that there is some scope for argument in ethics. If I say "It is always wrong to kill a human being" and "Abortion is not always wrong," then I am committed to denying that abortion kills a human being. Otherwise I have contradicted myself, and in doing so I have not stated a coherent position

Bioethics: An Anthology, Fourth Edition. Edited by Udo Schüklenk and Peter Singer.
Editorial material and organization © 2022 John Wiley & Sons, Inc. Published 2022 by John Wiley & Sons, Inc.

at all. So consistency, at least, is a requirement of any defensible ethical position, and thus sets a limit to the subjectivity of ethical judgments. The requirement of factual accuracy sets another limit. In discussing issues in bioethics, the facts are often complex. But we cannot reach the right ethical decisions unless we are well-informed about the relevant facts. In this respect ethical decisions are unlike decisions of taste. We can enjoy a taste without knowing what we are eating; but if we assume that it is wrong to resuscitate a terminally ill patient against her wishes, then we cannot know whether an instance of resuscitation was morally right or wrong without knowing something about the patient's prognosis and whether the patient has expressed any wishes about being resuscitated. In that sense, there is no equivalent in ethics to the immediacy of taste.

Ethical relativism, sometimes also known as cultural relativism, is one step away from ethical subjectivism, but it also severely limits the scope of ethical argument. The ethical relativist holds that it is not individual attitudes that determine what is right or wrong, but the attitudes of the culture in which one lives. Herodotus tells how Darius, King of Persia, summoned the Greeks from the western shores of his kingdom before him, and asked them how much he would have to pay them to eat their fathers' dead bodies. They were horrified by the idea and said they would not do it for any amount of money, for it was their custom to cremate their dead. Then Darius called upon Indians from the eastern frontiers of his kingdom, and asked them what would make them willing to burn their fathers' bodies. They cried out and asked the King to refrain from mentioning so shocking an act. Herodotus comments that each nation thinks its own customs best. From here it is only a short step to the view that there can be no objective right or wrong, beyond the bounds of one's own culture. This view found increased support in the nineteenth century as Western anthropologists came to know many different cultures, and were impressed by ethical views very different from those that were standardly taken for granted in European society. As a defense against the automatic assumption that Western morality is

superior and should be imposed on "savages," many anthropologists argued that, since morality is relative to culture, no culture can have any basis for regarding its morality as superior to any other culture.

Although the motives with which anthropologists put this view forward were admirable, they may not have appreciated the implications of the position they were taking. The ethical relativist maintains that a statement like "It is good to enslave people from another tribe if they are captured in war" means simply "In my society, the custom is to enslave people from another tribe if they are captured in war." Hence if one member of the society were to question whether it really was good to enslave people in these circumstances, she could be answered simply by demonstrating that this was indeed the custom – for example, by showing that for many generations it had been done after every war in which prisoners were captured. Thus there is no way for moral reformers to say that an accepted custom is wrong – "wrong" just means "in accordance with an accepted custom."

On the other hand, when people from two different cultures disagree about an ethical issue, then according to the ethical relativist there can be no resolution of the disagreement. Indeed, strictly there is no disagreement. If the apparent dispute were over the issue just mentioned, then one person would be saying "In my country it is the custom to enslave people from another tribe if they are captured in war" and the other person would be saying "In my country it is not the custom to allow one human being to enslave another." This is no more a disagreement than such statements as "In my country people greet each other by rubbing noses" and "In my country people greet each other by shaking hands." If ethical relativism is true, then it is impossible to say that one culture is right and the other is wrong. Bearing in mind that some cultures have practiced slavery, or the burning of widows on the funeral pyre of their husbands, this is hard to accept.

A more promising alternative to both ethical subjectivism and cultural relativism is universal prescriptivism, an approach to ethics developed by the Oxford philosopher R. M. Hare. Hare argues that the distinctive property of ethical judgments is that they are universalizable. In saying this, he means that if I make an ethical judgment, I must be prepared to state it in universal terms, and apply it to all relevantly similar situations. By "universal terms" Hare means those terms that do not refer to a particular individual. Thus a proper name cannot be a universal term. If, for example, I were to say "Everyone should do what is in the interests of Kim Kardashian," I would not be making a universal judgment, because I have used a proper name. The same would be true if I were to say that everyone must do what is in *my* interests, because the personal pronoun "my" is here used to refer to a particular individual, myself.

It might seem that ruling out particular terms in this way does not take us very far. After all, one can always describe oneself in universal terms. Perhaps I can't say that everyone should do what is in my interests, but I could say that everyone must do whatever is in the interests of people who . . . and then give a minutely detailed description of myself, including the precise location of all my freckles. The effect would be the same as saying that everyone should do what is in my interests, because there would be no one except me who matches that description. Hare meets this problem by saying that to prescribe an ethical judgment universally means being prepared to prescribe it for all possible circumstances, including hypothetical ones. So if I were to say that everyone should do what is in the interests of a person with a particular pattern of freckles, I must be prepared to prescribe that in the hypothetical situation in which I do not have this pattern of freckles, but someone else does, I should do what is in the interests of that person. Now of course I may *say* that I should do that, since I am confident that I shall never be in such a situation, but this simply means that I am being dishonest. I am not genuinely prescribing the principle universally.

The effect of saying that an ethical judgment must be universalizable for hypothetical as well as actual circumstances is that whenever I make an ethical judgment, I can be challenged to put myself in the position of the parties affected, and see if I would still be able to accept that judgment. Suppose, for example,

that I own a small factory and the cheapest way for me to get rid of some waste is to pour it into a nearby river. I do not take water from this river, but I know that some villagers living downstream do and the waste may make them ill. If I imagine myself in the hypothetical situation of being one of the villagers, rather than the factory-owner, I would not accept that the profits of the factory-owner should outweigh the risk of adverse effects on my health and that of my children. Hence I cannot claim that I am ethically justified in polluting the river.

In this way Hare's approach introduces an element of reasoning in ethical deliberation. For Hare, however, since universalizability is part of the logic of moral language, an amoralist can avoid it by simply avoiding making any ethical judgments. More recently, several prominent moral philosophers, among them Thomas Nagel, T.M. Scanlon, and Derek Parfit have defended the view that we have objective reasons for action. Ethical judgments, in their view, are not statements of fact, but can nevertheless be true or false, in the same way that the truths of logic, or mathematics, are not statements of fact, but can be true or false. It is true, they would argue, that if someone is in agony, and we can relieve that agony, we have a reason for doing so. If we can relieve it at no cost, or a very low cost, to ourselves or anyone else, we will have a conclusive reason for relieving it, and it will be wrong not to do so.

The questions we have been discussing so far are questions *about* ethics, rather than questions *within* ethics. Philosophers call this "metaethics" and distinguish it from "normative ethics" in which we discuss what we ought to do. Normative ethics can also be divided into two parts, ethical theory and applied ethics. As we noted at the beginning of this introduction, bioethics is an area of applied ethics. Ethical theory, on the other hand, deals with broad ethical theories about how we ought to live and act, and we will now outline some of the more important of these theories.

Consequentialism is the view that the rightness of an action depends on its consequences. The best-known form of consequentialism is utilitarianism, developed in the late eighteenth century by Jeremy Bentham and popularized in the nineteenth century by John Stuart Mill. They held that an action is right if it leads to a greater surplus of happiness over misery than any possible alternative, and wrong if it does not. By "greater surplus of happiness," the classical utilitarians had in mind the idea of adding up all the pleasure or happiness that resulted from the action and subtracting from that total all the pain or misery to which the action gave rise. Naturally, in some circumstances, it might be possible only to reduce misery, and then the right action should be understood as the one that will result in less misery than any possible alternative.

The utilitarian view is striking in many ways. It puts forward a single principle that it claims can provide the right answer to all ethical dilemmas, if only we can predict what the consequences of our actions will be. It takes ethics out of the mysterious realm of duties and rules, and bases ethical decisions on something that almost everyone understands and values. Moreover, utilitarianism's single principle is applied universally, without fear or favor. Bentham said: "Each to count for one and none for more than one." By that he meant that the happiness of a peasant counted for as much as that of a noble, and the happiness of an African was no less important than that of a European – a progressive view to take when English ships were engaged in the slave trade.

Some contemporary consequentialists agree with Bentham to the extent that they think the rightness or wrongness of an action must depend on its consequences, but they deny that maximizing net happiness is the only consequence that has intrinsic value. Some of them argue that we should seek to bring about whatever will satisfy the greatest number of desires or preference. This variation, which is known as "preference utilitarianism," does not regard anything as good, except in so far as it is wanted or desired. More intense or strongly held preferences would get more weight than weak preferences. Other consequentialists include independent values, like freedom, justice, and knowledge. They are sometimes referred to as "ideal utilitarians" but it is better to think of them, not as utilitarians at all, but as pluralistic consequentialists (because they hold several independent values, rather than just one).

Consequentialism offers one important answer to the question of how we should decide what is right and what is wrong, but many ethicists reject it. The denial of this view was dramatically presented by Dostoevsky in *The Karamazov Brothers*:

> Imagine that you are charged with building the edifice of human destiny, the ultimate aim of which is to bring people happiness, to give them peace and contentment at last, but that in order to achieve this it is essential and unavoidable to torture just one little speck of creation, that same little child beating her chest with her little fists, and imagine that this edifice has to be erected on her unexpiated tears. Would you agree to be the architect under those conditions? Tell me honestly![3]

The passage suggests that some things are always wrong, no matter what their consequences. This has, for most of Western history, been the prevailing approach to morality, at least at the level of what has been officially taught and approved by the institutions of Church and State. The ten commandments of the Hebrew scriptures served as a model for much of the Christian era, and the Roman Catholic Church built up an elaborate system of morality based on rules to which no exceptions were allowed.

Another example of an ethic of rules is that of Immanuel Kant. Kant's ethic is based on his "Categorical Imperative," which he states in several distinct formulations. One is that we must always act so that we can will the maxim of our action to be a universal law. This can be interpreted as a form of Hare's idea of universalizability, which we have already encountered. Another is that we must always treat other people as ends, never as means. While these formulations of the Categorical Imperative might be applied in various ways, in Kant's hands they lead to inviolable rules, for example, against making promises that we do not intend to keep. Kant also thought that it was always wrong to tell a lie. In response to a critic who suggested that this rule has exceptions, Kant said that it would be wrong to lie even if someone had taken refuge in your house, and a person seeking to murder him came to your door and asked if you knew where he was. Modern Kantians often reject this hardline approach to rules, and claim that Kant's Categorical Imperative did not require him to hold so strictly to the rule against lying.

How would a consequentialist – for example, a classical utilitarian – answer Dostoevsky's challenge? If answering honestly – and if one really could be certain that this was a sure way, and the only way, of bringing lasting happiness to all the people of the world – utilitarians would have to say yes, they would accept the task of being the architect of the happiness of the world at the cost of the child's unexpiated tears. For they would point out that the suffering of that child, wholly undeserved as it is, will be repeated a million fold over the next century, for other children, just as innocent, who are victims of starvation, disease, and brutality. So if this one child must be sacrificed to stop all this suffering then, terrible as it is, the child must be sacrificed.

Fantasy apart, there can be no architect of the happiness of the world. The world is too big and complex a place for that. But we may attempt to bring about less suffering and more happiness, or satisfaction of preferences, for people or sentient beings in specific places and circumstances. Alternatively, we might follow a set of principles or rules – which could be of varying degrees of rigidity or flexibility. Where would such rules come from? Kant tried to deduce them from his Categorical Imperative, which in turn he had reached by insisting that the moral law must be based on formal reason alone, which for him meant the idea of a universal law, without any content from our wants or desires. But the problem with trying to deduce morality from reason alone has always been that it becomes an empty formalism that cannot tell us what to do. To make it practical, it needs to have some additional content, and Kant's own attempts to deduce rules of conduct from his Categorical Imperative are unconvincing.

Others, following Aristotle, have tried to draw on human nature as a source of moral rules. What is good, they say, is what is natural to human beings. They then contend that it is natural and right for us to seek certain goods, such as knowledge, friendship, health,

love, and procreation, and unnatural and wrong for us to act contrary to these goods. This "natural law" ethic is open to criticism on several points. The word "natural" can be used both descriptively and evaluatively, and the two senses are often mixed together so that value judgments may be smuggled in under the guise of a description. The picture of human nature presented by proponents of natural law ethics usually selects only those characteristics of our nature that the proponent considers desirable. The fact that our species, especially its male members, frequently go to war, and are also prone to commit individual acts of violence against others, is no doubt just as much part of our nature as our desire for knowledge, but no natural law theorist therefore views these activities as good. More generally, natural law theory has its origins in an Aristotelian idea of the cosmos, in which everything has a goal or "end," which can be deduced from its nature. The "end" of a knife is to cut; the assumption is that human beings also have an "end," and we will flourish when we live in accordance with the end for which we are suited. But this is a pre-Darwinian view of nature. Since Darwin, we know that we do not exist for any purpose, but are the result of natural selection operating on random mutations over millions of years. Hence there is no reason to believe that living according to nature will produce a harmonious society, let alone the best possible state of affairs for human beings.

Another way in which it has been claimed that we can come to know what moral principles or rules we should follow is through our intuition. In practice this usually means that we adopt conventionally accepted moral principles or rules, perhaps with some adjustments in order to avoid inconsistency or arbitrariness. On this view, a moral theory should, like a scientific theory, try to match the data; and the data that a moral theory must match is provided by our moral intuitions. As in science, if a plausible theory matches most, but not all, of the data, then the anomalous data might be rejected on the grounds that it is more likely that there was an error in the procedures for gathering that particular set of data than that the theory as a whole is mistaken. But ultimately the test of a theory is its ability to explain the data. The problem with applying this model of scientific justification to ethics is that the "data" of our moral intuitions is unreliable, not just at one or two specific points, but as a whole. Here the facts that cultural relativists draw upon are relevant (even if they do not establish that cultural relativism is the correct response to it). Since we know that our intuitions are strongly influenced by such things as culture and religion, they are ill-suited to serve as the fixed points against which an ethical theory must be tested. Even where there is cross-cultural agreement, there may be some aspects of our intuitions on which *all* cultures unjustifiably favor our own interests over those of others. For example, simply because we are all human beings, we may have a systematic bias that leads us to give an unjustifiably low moral status to nonhuman animals. Or, because, in virtually all known human societies, men have taken a greater leadership role than women, the moral intuitions of all societies may not adequately reflect the interests of females.

Some philosophers think that it is a mistake to base ethics on principles or rules. Instead they focus on what it is to be a good person – or, in the case of the problems with which this book is concerned, perhaps on what it is to be a good nurse or doctor or researcher. They seek to describe the virtues that a good person, or a good member of the relevant profession, should possess. Moral education then consists of teaching these virtues and discussing how a virtuous person would act in specific situations. The question is, however, whether we can have a notion of what a virtuous person would do in a specific situation without making a prior decision about what it is right to do. After all, in any particular moral dilemma, different virtues may be applicable, and even a particular virtue will not always give unequivocal guidance. For instance, if a terminally ill patient repeatedly asks a nurse or doctor for assistance in dying, what response best exemplifies the virtues of a healthcare professional? There seems no answer to this question, short of an inquiry into whether it is right or wrong to help a patient in such circumstances to die. But in that case we seem bound, in the end, to come back to discussing such issues as whether it is right to follow

moral rules or principles, or to do what will have the best consequences.

In the late twentieth century, some feminists offered new criticisms of conventional thought about ethics. They argued that the approaches to ethics taken by the influential philosophers of the past – all of whom have been male – give too much emphasis to abstract principles and the role of reason, and give too little attention to personal relationships and the part played by emotion. One outcome of these criticisms has been the development of an "ethic of care," which is not so much a single ethical theory as a cluster of ways of looking at ethics which put an attitude of caring for others at the center, and seek to avoid reliance on abstract ethical principles. The ethic of care has seemed especially applicable to the work of those involved in direct patient care. Not all feminists, however, support this development. Some worry that presenting an ethic of care in opposition to a "male" ethic based on reasoning reflects and reinforces stereotypes of women as more emotional and less rational than men. They also fear that it could lead to women continuing to carry a disproportionate share of the burden of caring for others.

In this discussion of ethics we have not mentioned anything about religion. This may seem odd, in view of the close connection that has often been made between religion and ethics, but it reflects our belief that, despite this historical connection, ethics and religion are fundamentally independent. Logically, ethics is prior to religion. If religious believers wish to say that a deity is good, or praise her or his creation or deeds, they must have a notion of goodness that is independent of their conception of the deity and what she or he does. Otherwise they will be saying that the deity is good, and when asked what they mean by "good," they will have to refer back to the deity, saying perhaps that "good" means "in accordance with the wishes of the deity." In that case, sentences such as "God is good" would be a meaningless tautology. "God is good" could mean no more than "God is in accordance with God's wishes." As we have already seen, there are ideas of what it is for something to be "good" that are not rooted in any religious belief. While religions typically encourage or instruct their followers to obey a particular ethical code, it is obvious that others who do not follow any religion can also think and act ethically.

To say that ethics is independent of religion is not to deny that theologians or other religious believers may have a role to play in bioethics. Religious traditions often have long histories of dealing with ethical dilemmas, and the accumulation of wisdom and experience that they represent can give us valuable insights into particular problems. But these insights should be subject to criticism in the way that any other proposals would be. If in the end we accept them, it is because we have judged them sound, not because they are the utterances of a pope, a rabbi, a mullah, or a holy person.

Ethics is also independent of the law, in the sense that the rightness or wrongness of an act cannot be settled by its legality or illegality. Whether an act is legal or illegal may often be relevant to whether it is right or wrong, because it is arguably wrong to break the law, other things being equal. Many people have thought that this is especially so in a democracy, in which everyone has a say in making the law. Another reason why the fact that an act is illegal may be a reason against doing it is that the legality of an act may affect the consequences that are likely to flow from it. If active voluntary euthanasia is illegal, then doctors who practice it risk going to jail, which will cause them and their families to suffer, and also mean that they will no longer be able to help other patients. This can be a powerful reason for not practicing voluntary euthanasia when it is against the law, but if there is only a very small chance of the offense becoming known, then the weight of this consequentialist reason against breaking the law is reduced accordingly. Whether we have an ethical obligation to obey the law, and, if so, how much weight we should give it, is itself an issue for ethical argument.

Though ethics is independent of the law, in the sense just specified, laws are subject to evaluation from an ethical perspective. Many debates in bioethics focus on questions about what practices should be allowed – for example, should we allow research on stem cells taken from human embryos, sex selection, or cloning? – and committees set up to advise on the ethical, social, and legal aspects of these questions often recommend legislation to prohibit the activity in question, or to allow it to be practiced under some form of regulation. Discussing a question at the level of law and public policy, however, raises somewhat different considerations than a discussion of personal ethics, because the consequences of adopting a public policy generally have much wider ramifications than the consequences of a personal choice. That is why some healthcare professionals feel justified in assisting a terminally ill patient to die, while at the same time opposing the legalization of physician-assisted suicide. Paradoxical as this position may appear – and it is certainly open to criticism – it is not straightforwardly inconsistent.

Many of the essays we have selected reflect the times in which they were written. Since bioethics often comments on developments in fast-moving areas of medicine and the biological sciences, the factual content of articles in bioethics can become obsolete quite rapidly. In preparing this 4th edition, we have taken the opportunity to cover some new issues and to include some more recent writings. Part X, on Disability, is new, as are the section in Part VII on Academic Freedom and Research and the essays in Part IX on Doctors' Duty to Treat. There are new articles in almost every other section as well, on gene editing, the morality of ending the lives of newborns, brain death, the eligibility of mentally ill patients for assisted dying and experiments on humans and on animals, and on public health.

Some authors of articles that have become dated in their facts have kindly updated them especially for this edition. An article may, however, be dated in its facts but make ethical points that are still valid, or worth considering, so we have not excluded older articles for this reason.

Other articles are dated in a different way. During the past few decades we have become more sensitive about the ways in which our language may exclude women, or reflect our prejudices regarding race or sexuality. We see no merit in trying to disguise past practices on such matters (although we have made minor changes to some of the older writings in this anthology, in order to bring the terminology used in line with contemporary usage), so we have not excluded otherwise valuable works in bioethics on these grounds. If they are jarring to the modern reader, that may be a salutary reminder of the extent to which we all are subject to the conventions and prejudices of our times.

Helga Kuhse was a co-editor of the first three editions of this anthology. She has now retired from academic work, and so decided not to join us in co-editing this edition. Nevertheless, her influence remains present, in the articles carried over from earlier editions. We thank her for helping to establish *Bioethics: An Anthology* as a comprehensive and widely used collection of the best articles in the field.

Katherine Carr did a stellar job as the copy-editor of this volume. The number of errors she spotted in previously published peer-reviewed (and presumably copy-edited and proof-read) journal articles is extraordinary.

Last, but not least, we thank two Graduate Students in the Queen's University Department of Philosophy who assisted us in sourcing possible materials for inclusion in the 3rd edition of this text (Nikoo Najand) and in this current edition (Chris Zajner).

Notes

1   See Van Rensselaer Potter, *Bioethics: Bridge to the Future* (Englewood Cliffs, NJ: Prentice-Hall, 1971).

2   Fritz Jahr, Bio-Ethik: Eine Umschau über die ethischen Beziehungen des Menschen zu Tier und Pflanze. *Kosmos. Handweiser für Naturfreunde*, 1927, 24:2–4.

3   *The Karamazov Brothers*, trans. Ignat Avsey (Oxford: Oxford University Press, 1994), vol. I, part 2, bk. 5, ch. 4. First published in 1879.

Part I
Abortion

Introduction

The view that human life has special value is deeply rooted in most people's thinking and no serious ethical theory allows a person to be killed without strong moral justification. Abortions terminate the lives of fetuses. Given that these fetuses are human, and of course innocent of any wrongdoing, it is easy to see why some people consider abortion to be unjustifiable homicide. In some respects fetuses are like persons; but in other respects they are very different. Therefore we need to ask whether they have the same moral status as those human beings we think of as persons.

In the first article in this Part, Michael Tooley provides a challenge to the view that fetuses are persons. In his 1972 landmark article "Abortion and Infanticide," he seeks to articulate and defend an ethically significant criterion that confers personhood and a right to life. To have a right to life, Tooley argues, an entity needs to possess a concept of self, that is, be "capable of desiring to continue existing as a subject of experiences and other mental states." An entity that has this capability is a person, whereas one that lacks it is not. This view has implications that enable us to defend abortion, but also challenge the moral views of most people who accept abortion; for on this view neither fetuses nor newborn infants are persons, whereas some nonhuman animals, such as chimpanzees and elephants, do seem to be persons.

Tooley thus holds that the *potential* to become a person is not sufficient to give fetuses a right to life. Here it is important to take a closer look at the notions of potentiality and capacity. Sleeping persons – unable to exercise the capacity to desire their own continued existence while asleep – are, according to Tooley, still persons because they *possess* the relevant capacity in a sense in which fetuses do not. A person who is asleep was self-conscious before she went to sleep and will be the same self-conscious person when she wakes up; a fetus, on the other hand, has never been awake and self-conscious.

Tooley takes the issue of personhood to be central. Judith Jarvis Thomson, in "A Defense of Abortion" takes a very different approach. For the purposes of her argument, Thomson accepts that the fetus is a person, but argues that *even if* one grants this premise, the conclusion that every person has a right to life – in the sense that would make abortion wrong – does not follow. She then uses an ingenious analogy to support her view that one person's right to life does not always outweigh another person's rights to something less than life. This general view applies, Thomson holds, in the case of pregnancy and abortion. A woman has a right to control her body, and a fetus only has the right to use a woman's body if she has implicitly given it that right. This would be the case if the woman is

Bioethics: An Anthology, Fourth Edition. Edited by Udo Schüklenk and Peter Singer.
Editorial material and organization © 2022 John Wiley & Sons, Inc. Published 2022 by John Wiley & Sons, Inc.

responsible, in some sense of the term, for its presence in her body. In many cases – certainly in the case of a pregnancy resulting from rape, and arguably, if more doubtfully, when contraception has failed – the woman bears little or no responsibility for the presence of the fetus in her body and would thus, according to Thomson, be justified in having an abortion. She would not be killing the fetus unjustly.

Thomson reminds us that any complete assessment of the ethics of abortion must focus not only on the purported rights or interests of fetuses, but also on the rights of women. But her argument has been criticized as incomplete. One of the strongest objections focuses on her narrow understanding of the right to life. It has, for example, been argued that a right to life, properly understood, also entails the provision of positive aid. If this is correct, then Thomson's argument on abortion is inconclusive.

In "The Wrong of Abortion" Patrick Lee and Robert P. George argue that the choice to have an abortion is immoral, in an objective sense. They begin by noting three features of human embryos: their distinctiveness from sperm and egg, their humanness, and their completeness or wholeness. In their view, it follows from this that during an abortion a human being is killed. This human being is at an earlier stage of development than you or I, but is a member of our species nonetheless.

Lee and George reject Tooley's personhood argument. In their view we are not consciousnesses that inhabit human bodies, rather we are continuing living bodily entities, some of which may take years to develop the capacity to reason. Contra Tooley, they think that the right to life belongs to any being with a rational nature, by which they mean, not that the being is actually capable of reasoning, but that it is a being with "the internal resources and active disposition" to develop the higher mental functions that are typically developed by human beings. This implies, of course, that whole human beings have that right, from the moment of conception. They reject Thomson's argument by suggesting that while an unwanted pregnancy may lead to significant inconvenience, this inconvenience pales into insignificance considering that abortion leads to the preventable death of a human being.

In the final article of Part I, Don Marquis adopts yet another approach to explain, as the title of his article indicates, "Why Abortion is Immoral." Like Tooley, and Lee and George, he assumes that the morality of abortion depends on whether or not the fetus is the kind of being whose life it is seriously wrong to end. According to Marquis, abortion is immoral for the same reason that it is wrong to kill you or me – not because the fetus is a person or a potential person, but rather because killing the fetus deprives it of its future. The loss of one's life is one of the greatest losses one can suffer; it deprives the victim of all the projects, experiences, enjoyments and so on that would otherwise have constituted that individual's future. This, Marquis holds, is what makes killing, other things being equal, wrong – regardless of whether one is a fetus, child, or adult.

Marquis argues that his position must not be confused with a sanctity of human life view. It does not, for example, rule out euthanasia. Killing a person who wants to die when she is seriously ill and faces a life of pain and suffering does not deprive that person of a valuable future. Nor is his theory, he claims, speciesist. The view that killing is wrong because it is the loss to the victim of the victim's future is, Marquis points out, straightforwardly incompatible with the view that it is wrong to kill only beings that are biologically human. It would be equally wrong to kill nonhuman animals and species from other planets, if these beings have futures relevantly like ours. Similarly, it would not be wrong to kill a human fetus with a genetic abnormality that precludes any possibility of a life that is worth living.

These features of his theory, Marquis claims, avoid some of the problems faced both by proponents of the sanctity of all human life, and by adherents of a personhood view. Those who deny that fetuses are persons find themselves in the embarrassing position of having to accept that their theory will, in principle, not only allow the killing of fetuses, but also the killing of infants. Opponents of abortion, on the other hand, often rely on what Marquis calls the "invalid inference" that it is wrong to kill fetuses because they are potential persons. But is Marquis' own account really so different from the argument from potential? Does it, like that argument, face the further criticism that such accounts make abortion and contraception equally wrong: if it is wrong to kill a one-cell zygote because doing so deprives the zygote of a valuable future, why is it not equally wrong to deprive an egg and a sperm, still separate but considered jointly, of a valuable future?

1

Abortion and Infanticide

Michael Tooley[1]

This essay deals with the question of the morality of abortion and infanticide. The fundamental ethical objection traditionally advanced against these practices rests on the contention that human fetuses and infants have a right to life. It is this claim which will be the focus of attention here. The basic issue to be discussed, then, is what properties a thing must possess in order to have a serious right to life. My approach will be to set out and defend a basic moral principle specifying a condition an organism must satisfy if it is to have a serious right to life. It will be seen that this condition is not satisfied by human fetuses and infants, and thus that they do not have a right to life. So unless there are other substantial objections to abortion and infanticide, one is forced to conclude that these practices are morally acceptable ones. In contrast, it may turn out that our treatment of adult members of other species – cats, dogs, polar bears – is morally indefensible. For it is quite possible that such animals do possess properties that endow them with a right to life.

I   Abortion and Infanticide

One reason the question of the morality of infanticide is worth examining is that it seems very difficult to formulate a completely satisfactory liberal position on abortion without coming to grips with the infanticide issue. The problem the liberal encounters is essentially that of specifying a cutoff point which is not arbitrary: at what stage in the development of a human being does it cease to be morally permissible to destroy it? It is important to be clear about the difficulty here. The conservative's objection is not that since there is a continuous line of development from a zygote to a newborn baby, one must conclude that if it is seriously wrong to destroy a newborn baby it is also seriously wrong to destroy a zygote or any intermediate stage in the development of a human being. His point is rather that if one says it is wrong to destroy a newborn baby but not a zygote or some intermediate stage in the development of a human being, one should be prepared to point to a *morally relevant* difference

Original publication details: Michael Tooley, "Abortion and Infanticide," pp. 37–65 from *Philosophy and Public Affairs* 1 (1972). Reproduced with permission of John Wiley & Sons.

between a newborn baby and the earlier stage in the development of a human being.

Precisely the same difficulty can, of course, be raised for a person who holds that infanticide is morally permissible. The conservative will ask what morally relevant differences there are between an adult human being and a newborn baby. What makes it morally permissible to destroy a baby, but wrong to kill an adult? So the challenge remains. But I will argue that in this case there is an extremely plausible answer.

Reflecting on the morality of infanticide forces one to face up to this challenge. In the case of abortion a number of events – quickening or viability, for instance – might be taken as cutoff points, and it is easy to overlook the fact that none of these events involves any morally significant change in the developing human. In contrast, if one is going to defend infanticide, one has to get very clear about what makes something a person, what gives something a right to life.

One of the interesting ways in which the abortion issue differs from most other moral issues is that the plausible positions on abortion appear to be extreme positions. For if a human fetus is a person, one is inclined to say that, in general, one would be justified in killing it only to save the life of the mother.[2] Such is the extreme conservative position.[3] On the other hand, if the fetus is not a person, how can it be seriously wrong to destroy it? Why would one need to point to special circumstances to justify such action? The upshot is that there is no room for a moderate position on the issue of abortion such as one finds, for example, in the Model Penal Code recommendations.[4]

Aside from the light it may shed on the abortion question, the issue of infanticide is both interesting and important in its own right. The theoretical interest has been mentioned: it forces one to face up to the question of what makes something a person. The practical importance need not be labored. Most people would prefer to raise children who do not suffer from gross deformities or from severe physical, emotional, or intellectual handicaps. If it could be shown that there is no moral objection to infanticide the

happiness of society could be significantly and justifiably increased.

Infanticide is also of interest because of the strong emotions it arouses. The typical reaction to infanticide is like the reaction to incest or cannibalism, or the reaction of previous generations to masturbation or oral sex. The response, rather than appealing to carefully formulated moral principles, is primarily visceral. When philosophers themselves respond in this way, offering no arguments, and dismissing infanticide out of hand it is reasonable to suspect that one is dealing with a taboo rather than with a rational prohibition.[5] I shall attempt to show that this is in fact the case.

II Terminology: "Person" versus "Human Being"

How is the term "person" to be interpreted? I shall treat the concept of a person as a purely moral concept, free of all descriptive content. Specifically, in my usage the sentence "X is a person" will be synonymous with the sentence "X has a (serious) moral right to life."

This usage diverges slightly from what is perhaps the more common way of interpreting the term "person" when it is employed as a purely moral term, where to say that X is a person is to say that X has rights. If everything that had rights had a right to life, these interpretations would be extensionally equivalent. But I am inclined to think that it does not follow from acceptable moral principles that whatever has any rights at all has a right to life. My reason is this. Given the choice between being killed and being tortured for an hour, most adult humans would surely choose the latter. So it seems plausible to say it is worse to kill an adult human being than it is to torture him for an hour. In contrast, it seems to me that while it is not seriously wrong to kill a newborn kitten, it is seriously wrong to torture one for an hour. This *suggests* that newborn kittens may have a right not to be tortured without having a serious right to life. For it seems to be true that an individual has a right to something whenever it is the case that, if he wants that thing, it would be wrong for others to deprive him of it. Then if it is wrong to inflict a certain sensation upon a kitten if it doesn't want to experience that sensation, it will follow that the kitten has a right not to have sensation inflicted upon it.[6] I shall return to this example later. My point here is merely that it provides some reason for holding that it does not follow from acceptable moral principles that if something has any rights at all, it has a serious right to life.

There has been a tendency in recent discussions of abortion to use expressions such as "person" and "human being" interchangeably. B. A. Brody, for example, refers to the difficulty of determining "whether destroying the foetus constitutes the taking of a human life," and suggests it is very plausible that "the taking of a human life is an action that has bad consequences for him whose life is being taken."[7] When Brody refers to something as a human life he apparently construes this as entailing that the thing is a person. For if every living organism belonging to the species *Homo sapiens* counted as a human life, there would be no difficulty in determining whether a fetus inside a human mother was a human life.

The same tendency is found in Judith Jarvis Thomson's article, which opens with the statement: "Most opposition to abortion relies on the premise that the fetus is a human being, a person, from the moment of conception."[8] The same is true of Roger Wertheimer, who explicitly says: "First off I should note that the expressions 'a human life,' 'a human being,' 'a person' are virtually interchangeable in this context."[9]

The tendency to use expressions like "person" and "human being" interchangeably is an unfortunate one. For one thing, it tends to lend covert support to antiabortionist positions. Given such usage, one who holds a liberal view of abortion is put in the position of maintaining that fetuses, at least up to a certain point, are not human beings. Even philosophers are led astray by this usage. Thus Wertheimer says that "except for monstrosities, every member of our species is indubitably a person, a human being, at the very latest at birth."[10] Is it really *indubitable* that newborn babies are persons? Surely this is a wild contention.

Wertheimer is falling prey to the confusion naturally engendered by the practice of using "person" and "human being" interchangeably. Another example of this is provided by Thomson: "I am inclined to think also that we shall probably have to agree that the fetus has already become a human person well before birth. Indeed, it comes as a surprise when one first learns how early in its life it begins to acquire human characteristics. By the tenth week, for example, it already has a face, arms and legs, fingers and toes; it has internal organs, and brain activity is detectable."[11] But what do such physiological characteristics have to do with the question of whether the organism is a person? Thomson, partly, I think, because of the unfortunate use of terminology, does not even raise this question. As a result she virtually takes it for granted that there are some cases in which abortion is "positively indecent."[12]

There is a second reason why using "person" and "human being" interchangeably is unhappy philosophically. If one says that the dispute between pro- and anti-abortionists centers on whether the fetus is a human, it is natural to conclude that it is essentially a disagreement about certain facts, a disagreement about what properties a fetus possesses. Thus Wertheimer says that "if one insists on using the raggy fact–value distinction, then one ought to say that the dispute is over a matter of fact in the sense in which it is a fact that the Negro slaves were human beings."[13] I shall argue that the two cases are not parallel, and that in the case of abortion what is primarily at stake is what moral principles one should accept. If one says that the central issue between conservatives and liberals in the abortion question is whether the fetus is a person, it is clear that the dispute may be either about what properties a thing must have in order to be a person, in order to have a right to life – a moral question – or about whether a fetus at a given stage of development as a matter of fact possesses the properties in question. The temptation to suppose that the disagreement must be a factual one is removed.

It should now be clear why the common practice of using expressions such as "person" and "human being" interchangeably in discussions of abortion is unfortunate. It would perhaps be best to avoid the term "human" altogether, employing instead some expression that is more naturally interpreted as referring to a certain type of biological organism characterized in physiological terms, such as "member of the species *Homo sapiens*." My own approach will be to use the term "human" only in contexts where it is not philosophically dangerous.

III   The Basic Issue: When is a Member of the Species *Homo sapiens* a Person?

Settling the issue of the morality of abortion and infanticide will involve answering the following questions: What properties must something have to be a person, i.e., to have a serious right to life? At what point in the development of a member of the species *Homo sapiens* does the organism possess the properties that make it a person? The first question raises a moral issue. To answer it is to decide what basic[14] moral principles involving the ascription of a right to life one ought to accept. The second question raises a purely factual issue, since the properties in question are properties of a purely descriptive sort.

Some writers seem quite pessimistic about the possibility of resolving the question of the morality of abortion. Indeed, some have gone so far as to suggest that the question of whether the fetus is a person is in principle unanswerable: "we seem to be stuck with the indeterminateness of the fetus' humanity."[15] An understanding of some of the sources of this pessimism will, I think, help us to tackle the problem. Let us begin by considering the similarity a number of people have noted between the issue of abortion and the issue of Negro slavery. The question here is why it should be more difficult to decide whether abortion and infanticide are acceptable than it was to decide whether slavery was acceptable. The answer seems to be that in the case of slavery there are moral principles of a quite uncontroversial sort that settle the issue. Thus most people would agree to some such principle

as the following: No organism that has experiences, that is capable of thought and of using language, and that has harmed no one, should be made a slave. In the case of abortion, on the other hand, conditions that are generally agreed to be sufficient grounds for ascribing a right to life to something do not suffice to settle the issue. It is easy to specify other, purportedly sufficient conditions that will settle the issue, but no one has been successful in putting forward considerations that will convince others to accept those additional moral principles.

I do not share the general pessimism about the possibility of resolving the issue of abortion and infanticide because I believe it is possible to point to a very plausible moral principle dealing with the question of *necessary* conditions for something's having a right to life, where the conditions in question will provide an answer to the question of the permissibility of abortion and infanticide.

There is a second cause of pessimism that should be noted before proceeding. It is tied up with the fact that the development of an organism is one of gradual and continuous change. Given this continuity, how is one to draw a line at one point and declare it permissible to destroy a member of *Homo sapiens* up to, but not beyond, that point? Won't there be an arbitrariness about any point that is chosen? I will return to this worry shortly. It does not present a serious difficulty once the basic moral principles relevant to the ascription of a right to life to an individual are established.

Let us turn now to the first and most fundamental question: What properties must something have in order to be a person, i.e., to have a serious right to life? The claim I wish to defend is this: An organism possesses a serious right to life only if it possesses the concept of a self as a continuing subject of experiences and other mental states, and believes that it is itself such a continuing entity.

My basic argument in support of this claim, which I will call the self-consciousness requirement, will be clearest, I think, if I first offer a simplified version of the argument, and then consider a modification that seems desirable. The simplified version of my argument is this. To ascribe a right to an individual is to assert something about the prima facie obligations of other individuals to act, or to refrain from acting, in certain ways. However, the obligations in question are conditional ones, being dependent upon the existence of certain desires of the individual to whom the right is ascribed. Thus if an individual asks one to destroy something to which he has a right, one does not violate his right to that thing if one proceeds to destroy it. This suggests the following analysis: "A has a right to X" is roughly synonymous with "If A desires X, then others are under a prima facie obligation to refrain from actions that would deprive him of it."[16]

Although this analysis is initially plausible, there are reasons for thinking it not entirely correct. I will consider these later. Even here, however, some expansion is necessary, since there are features of the concept of a right that are important in the present context, and that ought to be dealt with more explicitly. In particular, it seems to be a conceptual truth that things that lack consciousness, such as ordinary machines, cannot have rights. Does this conceptual truth follow from the above analysis of the concept of a right? The answer depends on how the term "desire" is interpreted. If one adopts a completely behavioristic interpretation of "desire," so that a machine that searches for an electrical outlet in order to get its batteries recharged is described as having a desire to be recharged, then it will not follow from this analysis that objects that lack consciousness cannot have rights. On the other hand, if "desire" is interpreted in such a way that desires are states necessarily standing in some sort of relationship to states of consciousness, it will follow from the analysis that a machine that is not capable of being conscious, and consequently of having desires, cannot have any rights. I think those who defend analyses of the concept of a right along the lines of this one do have in mind an interpretation of the term "desire" that involves reference to something more than behavioral dispositions. However, rather than relying on this, it seems preferable to make such an interpretation explicit. The following analysis is a natural way of doing that: "A has a right to X" is roughly synonymous with "A is the sort of thing that is a subject of experiences and other mental states, A

is capable of desiring X, and if A does desire X, then others are under a prima facie obligation to refrain from actions that would deprive him of it."

The next step in the argument is basically a matter of applying this analysis to the concept of a right to life. Unfortunately the expression "right to life" is not entirely a happy one, since it suggests that the right in question concerns the continued existence of a biological organism. That this is incorrect can be brought out by considering possible ways of violating an individual's right to life. Suppose, for example, that by some technology of the future the brain of an adult human were to be completely reprogrammed, so that the organism wound up with memories (or rather, apparent memories), beliefs, attitudes, and personality traits completely different from those associated with it before it was subjected to reprogramming. In such a case one would surely say that an individual had been destroyed, that an adult human's right to life had been violated, even though no biological organism had been killed. This example shows that the expression "right to life" is misleading, since what one is really concerned about is not just the continued existence of a biological organism, but the right of a subject of experiences and other mental states to continue to exist.

Given this more precise description of the right with which we are here concerned, we are now in a position to apply the analysis of the concept of a right stated above. When we do so we find that the statement "A has a right to continue to exist as a subject of experiences and other mental states" is roughly synonymous with the statement "A is a subject of experiences and other mental states, A is capable of desiring to continue to exist as a subject of experiences and other mental states, and if A does desire to continue to exist as such an entity, then others are under a prima facie obligation not to prevent him from doing so."

The final stage in the argument is simply a matter of asking what must be the case if something is to be capable of having a desire to continue existing as a subject of experiences and other mental states. The basic point here is that the desires a thing can have are limited by the concepts it possesses. For the fundamental way of describing a given desire is as a desire that a certain proposition be true.[17] Then, since one cannot desire that a certain proposition be true unless one understands it, and since one cannot understand it without possessing the concepts involved in it, it follows that the desires one can have are limited by the concepts one possesses. Applying this to the present case results in the conclusion that an entity cannot be the sort of thing that can desire that a subject of experiences and other mental states exist unless it possesses the concept of such a subject. Moreover, an entity cannot desire that it itself *continue* existing as a subject of experiences and other mental states unless it believes that it is now such a subject. This completes the justification of the claim that it is a necessary condition of something's having a serious right to life that it possess the concept of a self as a continuing subject of experiences, and that it believe that it is itself such an entity.

Let us now consider a modification in the above argument that seems desirable. This modification concerns the crucial conceptual claim advanced about the relationship between ascription of rights and ascription of the corresponding desires. Certain situations suggest that there may be exceptions to the claim that if a person doesn't desire something, one cannot violate his right to it. There are three types of situations that call this claim into question: (i) situations in which an individual's desires reflect a state of emotional disturbance; (ii) situations in which a previously conscious individual is temporarily unconscious; (iii) situations in which an individual's desires have been distorted by conditioning or by indoctrination.

As an example of the first, consider a case in which an adult human falls into a state of depression which his psychiatrist recognizes as temporary. While in the state he tells people he wishes he were dead. His psychiatrist, accepting the view that there can be no violation of an individual's right to life unless the individual has a desire to live, decides to let his patient have his way and kills him. Or consider a related case in which one person gives another a drug that produces a state of temporary depression; the recipient expresses a wish that he were dead. The person who administered the drug then kills him. Doesn't

one want to say in both these cases that the agent did something seriously wrong in killing the other person? And isn't the reason the action was seriously wrong in each case the fact that it violated the individual's right to life? If so, the right to life cannot be linked with a desire to live in the way claimed above.

The second set of situations are ones in which an individual is unconscious for some reason – that is, he is sleeping, or drugged, or in a temporary coma. Does an individual in such a state have any desires? People do sometimes say that an unconscious individual wants something, but it might be argued that if such talk is not to be simply false it must be interpreted as actually referring to the desires the individual *would* have if he were now conscious. Consequently, if the analysis of the concept of a right proposed above were correct, it would follow that one does not violate an individual's right if one takes his car, or kills him, while he is asleep.

Finally, consider situations in which an individual's desires have been distorted, either by inculcation of irrational beliefs or by direct conditioning. Thus an individual may permit someone to kill him because he has been convinced that if he allows himself to be sacrificed to the gods he will be gloriously rewarded in a life to come. Or an individual may be enslaved after first having been conditioned to desire a life of slavery. Doesn't one want to say that in the former case an individual's right to life has been violated, and in the latter his right to freedom?

Situations such as these strongly suggest that even if an individual doesn't want something, it is still possible to violate his right to it. Some modification of the earlier account of the concept of a right thus seems in order. The analysis given covers, I believe, the paradigmatic cases of violation of an individual's rights, but there are other, secondary cases where one also wants to say that someone's right has been violated which are not included.

Precisely how the revised analysis should be formulated is unclear. Here it will be sufficient merely to say that, in view of the above, an individual's right to X can be violated not only when he desires X, but also when he *would* now desire X were it not for one of the following: (i) he is in an emotionally unbalanced state; (ii) he is temporarily unconscious; (iii) he has been conditioned to desire the absence of X.

The critical point now is that, even given this extension of the conditions under which an individual's right to something can be violated, it is still true that one's right to something can be violated only when one has the conceptual capability of desiring the thing in question. For example, an individual who would now desire not to be a slave if he weren't emotionally unbalanced, or if he weren't temporarily unconscious, or if he hadn't previously been conditioned to want to be a slave, must possess the concepts involved in the desire not to be a slave. Since it is really only the conceptual capability presupposed by the desire to continue existing as a subject of experiences and other mental states, and not the desire itself, that enters into the above argument, the modification required in the account of the conditions under which an individual's rights can be violated does not undercut my defense of the self-consciousness requirement.[18]

To sum up, my argument has been that having a right to life presupposes that one is capable of desiring to continue existing as a subject of experiences and other mental states. This in turn presupposes both that one has the concept of such a continuing entity and that one believes that one is oneself such an entity. So an entity that lacks such a consciousness of itself as a continuing subject of mental states does not have a right to life.

It would be natural to ask at this point whether satisfaction of this requirement is not only necessary but also sufficient to ensure that a thing has a right to life. I am inclined to an affirmative answer. However, the issue is not urgent in the present context, since as long as the requirement is in fact a necessary one we have the basis of an adequate defense of abortion and infanticide. If an organism must satisfy some other condition before it has a serious right to life, the result will merely be that the interval during which infanticide is morally permissible may be somewhat longer. Although the point at which an organism first achieves self-consciousness and hence the capacity of desiring to continue existing as a subject of experiences and

other mental states may be a theoretically incorrect cutoff point, it is at least a morally safe one: any error it involves is on the side of caution.

IV Some Critical Comments on Alternative Proposals

I now want to compare the line of demarcation I am proposing with the cutoff points traditionally advanced in discussions of abortion. My fundamental claim will be that none of these cutoff points can be defended by appeal to plausible, basic moral principles. The main suggestions as to the point past which it is seriously wrong to destroy something that will develop into an adult member of the species *Homo sapiens* are these: (a) conception; (b) the attainment of human form; (c) the achievement of the ability to move about spontaneously; (d) viability; (e) birth.[19] The corresponding moral principles suggested by these cutoff points are as follows. (1) It is seriously wrong to kill an organism, from a zygote on, that belongs to the species *Homo sapiens*. (2) It is seriously wrong to kill an organism that belongs to *Homo sapiens* and that has achieved human form. (3) It is seriously wrong to kill an organism that is a member of *Homo sapiens* and that is capable of spontaneous movement. (4) It is seriously wrong to kill an organism that belongs to *Homo sapiens* and that is capable of existing outside the womb. (5) It is seriously wrong to kill an organism that is a member of *Homo sapiens* that is no longer in the womb.

My first comment is that it would not do *simply* to omit the reference to membership in the species *Homo sapiens* from the above principles, with the exception of principle (2). For then the principles would be applicable to animals in general, and one would be forced to conclude that it was seriously wrong to abort a cat fetus, or that it was seriously wrong to abort a motile cat fetus, and so on.

The second and crucial comment is that none of the five principles given above can plausibly be viewed as a *basic* moral principle. To accept any of them as such would be akin to accepting as a basic moral principle the proposition that it is morally permissible to enslave black members of the species *Homo sapiens* but not white members. Why should it be seriously wrong to kill an unborn member of the species *Homo sapiens* but not seriously wrong to kill an unborn kitten? Difference in species is not per se a morally relevant difference. If one holds that it is seriously wrong to kill an unborn member of the species *Homo sapiens* but not an unborn kitten, one should be prepared to point to some property that is morally significant and that is possessed by unborn members of *Homo sapiens* but not by unborn kittens. Similarly, such a property must be identified if one believes it seriously wrong to kill unborn members of *Homo sapiens* that have achieved viability but not seriously wrong to kill unborn kittens that have achieved that state.

What property might account for such a difference? That is to say, what *basic* moral principles might a person who accepts one of these five principles appeal to in support of his secondary moral judgment? Why should events such as the achievement of human form, or the achievement of the ability to move about, or the achievement of viability, or birth serve to endow something with a right to life? What the liberal must do is to show that these events involve changes, or are associated with changes, that are morally relevant.

Let us now consider reasons why the events involved in cutoff points (b) through (e) are not morally relevant, beginning with the last two: viability and birth. The fact that an organism is not physiologically dependent upon another organism, or is capable of such physiological independence, is surely irrelevant to whether the organism has a right to life. In defense of this contention, consider a speculative case where a fetus is able to learn a language while in the womb. One would surely not say that the fetus had no right to life until it emerged from the womb, or until it was capable of existing outside the womb. A less speculative example is the case of Siamese twins who have learned to speak. One doesn't want to say that since one of the twins would die were the two to be separated, it therefore has no right to life. Consequently it seems difficult to disagree with the conservative's claim that

an organism which lacks a right to life before birth or before becoming viable cannot acquire this right immediately upon birth or upon becoming viable.

This does not, however, completely rule out viability as a line of demarcation. For instead of defending viability as a cutoff point on the ground that only then does a fetus acquire a right to life, it is possible to argue rather that when one organism is physiologically dependent upon another, the former's right to life may conflict with the latter's right to use its body as it will, and moreover, that the latter's right to do what it wants with its body may often take precedence over the other organism's right to life. Thomson has defended this view: "I am arguing only that having a right to life does not guarantee having either a right to the use of or a right to be allowed continued use of another person's body – even if one needs it for life itself. So the right to life will not serve the opponents of abortion in the very simple and clear way in which they seem to have thought it would."[20] I believe that Thomson is right in contending that philosophers have been altogether too casual in assuming that if one grants the fetus a serious right to life, one must accept a conservative position on abortion.[21] I also think the only defense of viability as a cutoff point which has any hope of success at all is one based on the considerations she advances. I doubt very much, however, that this defense of abortion is ultimately tenable. I think that one can grant even stronger assumptions than those made by Thomson and still argue persuasively for a semiconservative view. What I have in mind is this. Let it be granted, for the sake of argument, that a woman's right to free her body of parasites which will inhibit her freedom of action and possibly impair her health is stronger than the parasite's right to life, and is so even if the parasite has as much right to life as an adult human. One can still argue that abortion ought not to be permitted. For if A's right is stronger than B's, and it is impossible to satisfy both, it does not follow that A's should be satisfied rather than B's. It may be possible to compensate A if his right isn't satisfied, but impossible to compensate B if his right isn't satisfied. In such a case the best thing to do may be to satisfy B's claim and to compensate A. Abortion may be a case in point. If the fetus has a right to life and the right is not satisfied, there is certainly no way the fetus can be compensated. On the other hand, if the woman's right to rid her body of harmful and annoying parasites is not satisfied, she can be compensated. Thus it would seem that the just thing to do would be to prohibit abortion, but to compensate women for the burden of carrying a parasite to term. Then, however, we are back at a (modified) conservative position.[22] Our conclusion must be that it appears unlikely there is any satisfactory defense either of viability or of birth as cutoff points.

Let us now consider the third suggested line of demarcation, the achievement of the power to move about spontaneously. It might be argued that acquiring this power is a morally relevant event on the grounds that there is a connection between the concept of an agent and the concept of a person, and being motile is an indication that a thing is an agent.[23]

It is difficult to respond to this suggestion unless it is made more specific. Given that one's interest here is in defending a certain cutoff point, it is natural to interpret the proposal as suggesting that motility is a necessary condition of an organism's having a right to life. But this won't do, because one certainly wants to ascribe a right to life to adult humans who are completely paralyzed. Maybe the suggestion is rather that motility is a sufficient condition of something's having a right to life. However, it is clear that motility alone is not sufficient, since this would imply that all animals, and also certain machines, have a right to life. Perhaps, then, the most reasonable interpretation of the claim is that motility together with some other property is a sufficient condition of something's having a right to life, where the other property will have to be a property possessed by unborn members of the species *Homo sapiens* but not by unborn members of other familiar species.

The central question, then, is what this other property is. Until one is told, it is very difficult to evaluate either the moral claim that motility together with that property is a sufficient basis for ascribing to an organism a right to life or the factual claim that a motile human fetus possesses that property while a motile fetus belonging to some other species does not. A conservative would presumably reject motility

as a cutoff point by arguing that whether an organism has a right to life depends only upon its potentialities, which are of course not changed by its becoming motile. If, on the other hand, one favors a liberal view of abortion, I think that one can attack this third suggested cutoff point, in its unspecified form, only by determining what properties are necessary, or what properties sufficient, for an individual to have a right to life. Thus I would base my rejection of motility as a cutoff point on my claim, defended above, that a necessary condition of an organism's possessing a right to life is that it conceive of itself as a continuing subject of experiences and other mental states.

The second suggested cutoff point – the development of a recognizably human form – can be dismissed fairly quickly. I have already remarked that membership in a particular species is not itself a morally relevant property. For it is obvious that if we encountered other "rational animals," such as Martians, the fact that their physiological makeup was very different from our own would not be grounds for denying them a right to life.[24] Similarly, it is clear that the development of human form is not in itself a morally relevant event. Nor do there seem to be any grounds for holding that there is some other change, associated with this event, that is morally relevant. The appeal of this second cutoff point is, I think, purely emotional.

The overall conclusion seems to be that it is very difficult to defend the cutoff points traditionally advanced by those who advocate either a moderate or a liberal position on abortion. The reason is that there do not seem to be any basic moral principles one can appeal to in support of the cutoff points in question. We must now consider whether the conservative is any better off.

V   Refutation of the Conservative Position

Many have felt that the conservative's position is more defensible than the liberal's because the conservative can point to the gradual and continuous development of an organism as it changes from a zygote to an adult human being. He is then in a position to argue that it is morally arbitrary for the liberal to draw a line at some point in this continuous process and to say that abortion is permissible before, but not after, that particular point. The liberal's reply would presumably be that the emphasis upon the continuity of the process is misleading. What the conservative is really doing is simply challenging the liberal to specify the properties a thing must have in order to be a person, and to show that the developing organism does acquire the properties at the point selected by the liberal. The liberal may then reply that the difficulty he has meeting this challenge should not be taken as grounds for rejecting his position. For the conservative cannot meet this challenge either; the conservative is equally unable to say what properties something must have if it is to have a right to life.

Although this rejoinder does not dispose of the conservative's argument, it is not without bite. For defenders of the view that abortion is always wrong have failed to face up to the question of the basic moral principles on which their position rests. They have been content to assert the wrongness of killing any organism, from a zygote on, if that organism is a member of the species *Homo sapiens*. But they have overlooked the point that this cannot be an acceptable *basic* moral principle, since difference in species is not in itself a morally relevant difference. The conservative can reply, however, that it is possible to defend his position – but not the liberal's – *without* getting clear about the properties a thing must possess if it is to have a right to life. The conservative's defense will rest upon the following two claims: first, that there is a property, even if one is unable to specify what it is, that (i) is possessed by adult humans, and (ii) endows any organism possessing it with a serious right to life. Second, that if there are properties which satisfy (i) and (ii) above, at least one of those properties will be such that any organism potentially possessing that property has a serious right to life even now, simply by virtue of that potentiality, where an organism possesses a property potentially if it will come to have that property in the normal course of its development. The second

claim – which I shall refer to as the potentiality principle – is critical to the conservative's defense. Because of it he is able to defend his position without deciding what properties a thing must possess in order to have a right to life. It is enough to know that adult members of *Homo sapiens* do have such a right. For then one can conclude that any organism which belongs to the species *Homo sapiens*, from a zygote on, must also have a right to life by virtue of the potentiality principle.

The liberal, by contrast, cannot mount a comparable argument. He cannot defend his position without offering at least a partial answer to the question of what properties a thing must possess in order to have a right to life.

The importance of the potentiality principle, however, goes beyond the fact that it provides support for the conservative's position. If the principle is unacceptable, then so is his position. For if the conservative cannot defend the view that an organism's having certain potentialities is sufficient grounds for ascribing to it a right to life, his claim that a fetus which is a member of *Homo sapiens* has a right to life can be attacked as follows. The reason an adult member of *Homo sapiens* has a right to life, but an infant ape does not, is that there are certain psychological properties which the former possesses and the latter lacks. Now, even if one is unsure exactly what these psychological properties are, it is clear that an organism in the early stages of development from a zygote into an adult member of *Homo sapiens* does not possess these properties. One need merely compare a human fetus with an ape fetus. What mental states does the former enjoy that the latter does not? Surely it is reasonable to hold that there are no significant differences in their respective mental lives – assuming that one wishes to ascribe any mental states at all to such organisms. (Does a zygote have a mental life? Does it have experiences? Or beliefs? Or desires?) There are, of course, physiological differences, but these are not in themselves morally significant. *If* one held that potentialities were relevant to the ascription of a right to life, one could argue that the physiological differences, though not morally significant in themselves, are morally significant by virtue of their causal consequences: they will lead to later psychological differences that are morally relevant, and for this reason the physiological differences are themselves morally significant. But if the potentiality principle is not available, this line of argument cannot be used, and there will then be no differences between a human fetus and an ape fetus that the conservative can use as grounds for ascribing a serious right to life to the former but not to the latter.

It is therefore tempting to conclude that the conservative view of abortion is acceptable if and only if the potentiality principle is acceptable. But to say that the conservative position can be defended if the potentiality principle is acceptable is to assume that the argument is over once it is granted that the fetus has a right to life, and, as was noted above, Thomson has shown that there are serious grounds for questioning this assumption. In any case, the important point here is that the conservative position on abortion is acceptable *only if* the potentiality principle is sound.

One way to attack the potentiality principle is simply to argue in support of the self-consciousness requirement – the claim that only an organism that conceives of itself as a continuing subject of experiences has a right to life. For this requirement, when taken together with the claim that there is at least one property, possessed by adult humans, such that any organism possessing it has a serious right to life, entails the denial of the potentiality principle. Or at least this is so if we add the uncontroversial empirical claim that an organism that will in the normal course of events develop into an adult human does not from the very beginning of its existence possess a concept of a continuing subject of experiences together with a belief that it is itself such an entity.

I think it best, however, to scrutinize the potentiality principle itself, and not to base one's case against it simply on the self-consciousness requirement. Perhaps the first point to note is that the potentiality principle should not be confused with principles such as the following: the value of an object is related to the value of the things into which it can develop. This "valuation principle" is rather vague. There are ways of making it more precise, but we need not consider these here. Suppose now that one were to speak not

of a right to life, but of the value of life. It would then be easy to make the mistake of thinking that the valuation principle was relevant to the potentiality principle – indeed, that it entailed it. But an individual's right to life is not based on the value of his life. To say that the world would be better off if it contained fewer people is not to say that it would be right to achieve such a better world by killing some of the present inhabitants. *If* having a right to life were a matter of a thing's value, then a thing's potentialities, being connected with its expected value, would clearly be relevant to the question of what rights it had. Conversely, once one realizes that a thing's rights are not a matter of its value, I think it becomes clear that an organism's potentialities are irrelevant to the question of whether it has a right to life.

But let us now turn to the task of finding a direct refutation of the potentiality principle. The basic issue is this. Is there any property J which satisfies the following conditions: (1) There is a property K such that any individual possessing property K has a right to life, and there is a scientific law L to the effect that any organism possessing property J will in the normal course of events come to possess property K at some later time. (2) Given the relationship between property J and property K just described, anything possessing property J has a right to life. (3) If property J were not related to property K in the way indicated, it would not be the case that anything possessing property J thereby had a right to life. In short, the question is whether there is a property J that bestows a right to life on an organism *only because* J stands in a certain causal relationship to a second property K, which is such that anything possessing that property *ipso facto* has a right to life.

My argument turns upon the following critical principle: Let C be a causal process that normally leads to outcome E. Let A be an action that initiates process C, and B be an action involving a minimal expenditure of energy that stops process C before outcome E occurs. Assume further that actions A and B do not have any other consequences, and that E is the only morally significant outcome of process C. Then there is no moral difference between intentionally performing action B and intentionally refraining from performing action A, assuming identical motivation in both cases. This principle, which I shall refer to as the moral symmetry principle with respect to action and inaction, would be rejected by some philosophers. They would argue that there is an important distinction to be drawn between "what we owe people in the form of aid and what we owe them in the way of non-interference,"[25] and that the latter, "negative duties," are duties that it is more serious to neglect than the former, "positive" ones. This view arises from an intuitive response to examples such as the following. Even if it is wrong not to send food to starving people in other parts of the world, it is more wrong still to kill someone. And isn't the conclusion, then, that one's obligation to refrain from killing someone is a more serious obligation than one's obligation to save lives?

I want to argue that this is not the correct conclusion. I think it is tempting to draw this conclusion if one fails to consider the motivation that is likely to be associated with the respective actions. If someone performs an action he knows will kill someone else, this will usually be grounds for concluding that he wanted to kill the person in question. In contrast, failing to help someone may indicate only apathy, laziness, selfishness, or an amoral outlook: the fact that a person knowingly allows another to die will not normally be grounds for concluding that he desired that person's death. Someone who knowingly kills another is more likely to be seriously defective from a moral point of view than someone who fails to save another's life.

If we are not to be led to false conclusions by our intuitions about certain cases, we must explicitly assume identical motivations in the two situations. Compare, for example, the following: (1) Jones sees that Smith will be killed by a bomb unless he warns him. Jones's reaction is: "How lucky, it will save me the trouble of killing Smith myself." So Jones allows Smith to be killed by the bomb, even though he could easily have warned him. (2) Jones wants Smith dead, and therefore shoots him. Is one to say there is a significant difference between the wrongness of Jones's behavior in these two cases? Surely not. This shows

the mistake of drawing a distinction between positive duties and negative duties and holding that the latter impose stricter obligations than the former. The difference in our intuitions about situations that involve giving aid to others and corresponding situations that involve not interfering with others is to be explained by reference to probable differences in the motivations operating in the two situations, and not by reference to a distinction between positive and negative duties. For once it is specified that the motivation is the same in the two situations, we realize that inaction is as wrong in the one case as action is in the other.

There is another point that may be relevant. Action involves effort, while inaction usually does not. It usually does not require any effort on my part to refrain from killing someone, but saving someone's life will require an expenditure of energy. One must then ask how large a sacrifice a person is morally required to make to save the life of another. If the sacrifice of time and energy is quite large it may be that one is not morally obliged to save the life of another in that situation. Superficial reflection upon such cases might easily lead us to introduce the distinction between positive and negative duties, but again it is clear that this would be a mistake. The point is not that one has a greater duty to refrain from killing others than to perform positive actions that will save them. It is rather that positive actions require effort, and this means that in deciding what to do a person has to take into account his own right to do what he wants with his life, and not only the other person's right to life. To avoid this confusion, we should confine ourselves to comparisons between situations in which the positive action involves minimal effort.

The moral symmetry principle, as formulated above, explicitly takes these two factors into account. It applies only to pairs of situations in which the motivations are identical and the positive action involves minimal effort. Without these restrictions, the principle would be open to serious objection; with them, it seems perfectly acceptable. For the central objection to it rests on the claim that we must distinguish positive from negative duties and recognize that negative duties impose stronger obligations than positive ones.

I have tried to show how this claim derives from an unsound account of our moral intuitions about certain situations.

My argument against the potentiality principle can now be stated. Suppose at some future time a chemical were to be discovered which when injected into the brain of a kitten would cause the kitten to develop into a cat possessing a brain of the sort possessed by humans, and consequently into a cat having all the psychological capabilities characteristic of adult humans. Such cats would be able to think, to use language, and so on. Now it would surely be morally indefensible in such a situation to ascribe a serious right to life to members of the species *Homo sapiens* without also ascribing it to cats that have undergone such a process of development: there would be no morally significant differences.

Secondly, it would not be seriously wrong to refrain from injecting a newborn kitten with the special chemical, and to kill it instead. The fact that one could initiate a causal process that would transform a kitten into an entity that would eventually possess properties such that anything possessing them *ipso facto* has a serious right to life does not mean that the kitten has a serious right to life even before it has been subjected to the process of injection and transformation. The possibility of transforming kittens into persons will not make it any more wrong to kill newborn kittens than it is now.

Thirdly, in view of the symmetry principle, if it is not seriously wrong to refrain from initiating such a causal process, neither is it seriously wrong to interfere with such a process. Suppose a kitten is accidentally injected with the chemical. As long as it has not yet developed those properties that in themselves endow something with a right to life, there cannot be anything wrong with interfering with the causal process and preventing the development of the properties in question. Such interference might be accomplished either by injecting the kitten with some "neutralizing" chemical or simply by killing it.

But if it is not seriously wrong to destroy an injected kitten which will naturally develop the properties that bestow a right to life, neither can it be seriously wrong

to destroy a member of *Homo sapiens* which lacks such properties, but will naturally come to have them. The potentialities are the same in both cases. The only difference is that in the case of a human fetus the potentialities have been present from the beginning of the organism's development, while in the case of the kitten they have been present only from the time it was injected with the special chemical. This difference in the time at which the potentialities were acquired is a morally irrelevant difference.

It should be emphasized that I am not here assuming that a human fetus does not possess properties which in themselves, and irrespective of their causal relationships to other properties, provide grounds for ascribing a right to life to whatever possesses them. The point is merely that if it is seriously wrong to kill something, the reason cannot be that the thing will later acquire properties that in themselves provide something with a right to life.

Finally, it is reasonable to believe that there are properties possessed by adult members of *Homo sapiens* which establish their right to life, and also that any normal human fetus will come to possess those properties shared by adult humans. But it has just been shown that if it is wrong to kill a human fetus, it cannot be because of its potentialities. One is therefore forced to conclude that the conservative's potentiality principle is false.

In short, anyone who wants to defend the potentiality principle must either argue against the moral symmetry principle or hold that in a world in which kittens could be transformed into "rational animals" it would be seriously wrong to kill newborn kittens. It is hard to believe there is much to be said for the latter moral claim. Consequently one expects the conservative's rejoinder to be directed against the symmetry principle. While I have not attempted to provide a thorough defense of that principle, I have tried to show that what seems to be the most important objection to it — the one that appeals to a distinction between positive and negative duties — is based on a superficial analysis of our moral intuitions. I believe that a more thorough examination of the symmetry principle would show it to be sound. If so, we should reject the potentiality principle, and the conservative position on abortion as well.

VI   Summary and Conclusions

Let us return now to my basic claim, the self-consciousness requirement: An organism possesses a serious right to life only if it possesses the concept of a self as a continuing subject of experiences and other mental states, and believes that it is itself such a continuing entity. My defense of this claim has been twofold. I have offered a direct argument in support of it, and I have tried to show that traditional conservative and liberal views on abortion and infanticide, which involve a rejection of it, are unsound. I now want to mention one final reason why my claim should be accepted. Consider the example mentioned in section II – that of killing, as opposed to torturing, newborn kittens. I suggested there that while in the case of adult humans most people would consider it worse to kill an individual than to torture him for an hour, we do not usually view the killing of a newborn kitten as morally outrageous, although we would regard someone who tortured a newborn kitten for an hour as heinously evil. I pointed out that a possible conclusion that might be drawn from this is that newborn kittens have a right not to be tortured, but do not have a serious right to life. If this is the correct conclusion, how is one to explain it? One merit of the self-consciousness requirement is that it provides an explanation of this situation. The reason a newborn kitten does not have a right to life is explained by the fact that it does not possess the concept of a self. But how is one to explain the kitten's having a right not to be tortured? The answer is that a desire not to suffer pain can be ascribed to something without assuming that it has any concept of a continuing self. For while something that lacks the concept of a self cannot desire that a self not suffer, it can desire that a given sensation not exist. The state desired – the absence of a particular sensation, or of sensations of a certain sort – can be described in a purely phenomenalistic language, and hence without the concept of

a continuing self. So long as the newborn kitten possesses the relevant phenomenal concepts, it can truly be said to desire that a certain sensation not exist. So we can ascribe to it a right not to be tortured even though, since it lacks the concept of a continuing self, we cannot ascribe to it a right to life.

This completes my discussion of the basic moral principles involved in the issue of abortion and infanticide. But I want to comment upon an important factual question, namely, at what point an organism comes to possess the concept of a self as a continuing subject of experiences and other mental states, together with the belief that it is itself such a continuing entity. This is obviously a matter for detailed psychological investigation, but everyday observation makes it perfectly clear, I believe, that a newborn baby does not possess the concept of a continuing self, any more than a newborn kitten possesses such a concept. If so, infanticide during a time interval shortly after birth must be morally acceptable.

But where is the line to be drawn? What is the cutoff point? If one maintained, as some philosophers have, that an individual possesses concepts only if he can express these concepts in language, it would be a matter of everyday observation whether or not a given organism possessed the concept of a continuing self. Infanticide would then be permissible up to the time an organism learned how to use certain expressions. However, I think the claim that acquisition of concepts is dependent on acquisition of language is mistaken. For example, one wants to ascribe mental states of a conceptual sort – such as beliefs and desires – to organisms that are incapable of learning a language. This issue of prelinguistic understanding is clearly outside the scope of this discussion. My point is simply that *if* an organism can acquire concepts without thereby acquiring a way of expressing those concepts linguistically, the question of whether a given organism possesses the concept of a self as a continuing subject of experiences and other mental states, together with the belief that it is itself such a continuing entity, may be a question that requires fairly subtle experimental techniques to answer.

If this view of the matter is roughly correct, there are two worries one is left with at the level of practical moral decisions, one of which may turn out to be deeply disturbing. The lesser worry is where the line is to be drawn in the case of infanticide. It is not troubling because there is no serious need to know the exact point at which a human infant acquires a right to life. For in the vast majority of cases in which infanticide is desirable, its desirability will be apparent within a short time after birth. Since it is virtually certain that an infant at such a stage of its development does not possess the concept of a continuing self, and thus does not possess a serious right to life, there is excellent reason to believe that infanticide is morally permissible in most cases where it is otherwise desirable. The practical moral problem can thus be satisfactorily handled by choosing some period of time, such as a week after birth, as the interval during which infanticide will be permitted. This interval could then be modified once psychologists have established the point at which a human organism comes to believe that it is a continuing subject of experiences and other mental states.

The troubling worry is whether adult animals belonging to species other than *Homo sapiens* may not also possess a serious right to life. For once one says that an organism can possess the concept of a continuing self, together with the belief that it is itself such an entity, without having any way of expressing that concept and that belief linguistically, one has to face up to the question of whether animals may not possess properties that bestow a serious right to life upon them. The suggestion itself is a familiar one, and one that most of us are accustomed to dismiss very casually. The line of thought advanced here suggests that this attitude may turn out to be tragically mistaken. Once one reflects upon the question of the *basic* moral principles involved in the ascription of a right to life to organisms, one may find himself driven to conclude that our everyday treatment of animals is morally indefensible, and that we are in fact murdering innocent persons.

Notes

1 I am grateful to a number of people, particularly the editors of *Philosophy & Public Affairs,* Rodelia Hapke and Walter Kaufmann, for their helpful comments. It should not, of course, be inferred that they share the views expressed in this paper.

2 Judith Jarvis Thomson, in her article "A Defense of Abortion," *Philosophy & Public Affairs,* I, no. I (Fall 1971): 47–66 [see chapter 2 in this volume], has argued with great force and ingenuity that this conclusion is mistaken. I will comment on her argument later in this paper.

3 While this is the position conservatives tend to hold, it is not clear that it is the position they ought to hold. For if the fetus is a person it is far from clear that it is permissible to destroy it to save the mother. Two moral principles lend support to the view that it is the fetus which should live. First, other things being equal, should not one give something to a person who has had less rather than to a person who has had more? The mother has had a chance to live, while the fetus has not. The choice is thus between giving the mother more of an opportunity to enjoy life while giving the fetus none at all and giving the fetus an opportunity to enjoy life while not giving the mother a further opportunity to do so. Surely fairness requires the latter. Secondly, since the fetus has a greater life expectancy than the mother, one is in effect distributing more goods by choosing the life of the fetus over the life of the mother.

The position I am here recommending to the conservative should not be confused with the official Catholic position. The Catholic Church holds that it is seriously wrong to kill a fetus directly even if failure to do so will result in the death of *both* the mother and the fetus. This perverse value judgment is not part of the conservative's position.

4 Section 230.3 of the American Law Institute's *Model Penal Code* (Philadelphia, 1962). There is some interesting, though at times confused, discussion of the proposed code in *Model Penal Code – Tentative Draft No. 9* (Philadelphia, 1959), pp. 146–62.

5   A clear example of such an unwillingness to entertain seriously the possibility that moral judgments widely accepted in one's own society may nevertheless be incorrect is provided by Roger Wertheimer's superficial dismissal of infanticide on pages 69–70 of his article "Understanding the Abortion Argument," *Philosophy & Public Affairs,* I, no. I (Fall 1971): 67–95.

6   Compare the discussion of the concept of a right offered by Richard B. Brandt in his *Ethical Theory* (Englewood Cliffs, NJ, 1959), pp. 434–41. As Brandt points out, some philosophers have maintained that only things that can *claim* rights can have rights. I agree with Brandt's view that "inability to claim does not destroy the right" (p. 440).

7   B. A. Brody, "Abortion and the Law," *Journal of Philosophy,* LXVIII, no. 12 (17 June 1971): 357–69. See pp. 357–8.

8   Thomson, "A Defense of Abortion," p. 47.

9   Wertheimer, "Understanding the Abortion Argument," p. 69.

10 Ibid.

11 Thomson, "A Defense of Abortion," pp. 47–8.

12 Ibid., p. 65.

13 Wertheimer, "Understanding the Abortion Argument," p. 78.

14 A moral principle accepted by a person is *basic for him* if and only if his acceptance of it is not dependent upon any of his (nonmoral) factual beliefs. That is, no change in his factual beliefs would cause him to abandon the principle in question.

15 Wertheimer, "Understanding the Abortion Argument," p. 88.

16 Again, compare the analysis defended by Brandt in *Ethical Theory,* pp. 434–41.

17 In everyday life one often speaks of desiring things, such as an apple or a newspaper. Such talk is elliptical, the context together with one's ordinary beliefs serving to make it clear that one wants to eat the apple and read the newspaper. To say that what one desires is that a certain proposition be true should not be construed as involving any particular ontological commitment. The point is merely that it is sentences such as "John wants it to be the case that he is eating an apple in the next few minutes" that provide a completely explicit description of a person's desires. If one fails to use such sentences

one can be badly misled about what concepts are presupposed by a particular desire.

18 There are, however, situations other than those discussed here which might seem to count against the claim that a person cannot have a right unless he is conceptually capable of having the corresponding desire. Can't a young child, for example, have a right to an estate, even though he may not be conceptually capable of wanting the estate? It is clear that such situations have to be carefully considered if one is to arrive at a satisfactory account of the concept of a right. My inclination is to say that the correct description is not that the child now has a right to the estate, but that he will come to have such a right when he is mature, and that in the meantime no one else has a right to the estate. My reason for saying that the child does not now have a right to the estate is that he cannot now do things with the estate, such as selling it or giving it away that he will be able to do later on.

19 Another frequent suggestion as to the cutoff point not listed here is quickening. I omit it because it seems clear that if abortion after quickening is wrong, its wrongness must be tied up with the motility of the fetus, not with the mother's awareness of the fetus' ability to move about.

20 Thomson, "A Defense of Abortion," p. 56.

21 A good example of a failure to probe this issue is provided by Brody's "Abortion and the Law."

22 Admittedly the modification is a substantial one, since given a society that refused to compensate women, a woman who had an abortion would not be doing anything wrong.

23 Compare Wertheimer's remarks, "Understanding the Abortion Argument," p. 79.

24 This requires qualification. If their central nervous systems were radically different from ours, it might be thought that one would not be justified in ascribing to them mental states of an experiential sort. And then, since it seems to be a conceptual truth that only things having experiential states can have rights, one would be forced to conclude that one was not justified in ascribing any rights to them.

25 Philippa Foot, "The Problem of Abortion and the Doctrine of the Double Effect," *Oxford Review,* 5 (1967): 5–15. See the discussion on pp. 11ff.

2

A Defense of Abortion

Judith Jarvis Thomson[1]

Most opposition to abortion relies on the premise that the fetus is a human being, a person, from the moment of conception. The premise is argued for, but, as I think, not well. Take, for example, the most common argument. We are asked to notice that the development of a human being from conception through birth into childhood is continuous; then it is said that to draw a line, to choose a point in this development and say "before this point the thing is not a person, after this point it is a person" is to make an arbitrary choice, a choice for which in the nature of things no good reason can be given. It is concluded that the fetus is, or anyway that we had better say it is, a person from the moment of conception. But this conclusion does not follow. Similar things might be said about the development of an acorn into an oak tree, and it does not follow that acorns are oak trees, or that we had better say they are. Arguments of this form are sometimes called "slippery slope arguments" – the phrase is perhaps self-explanatory – and it is dismaying that opponents of abortion rely on them so heavily and uncritically.

I am inclined to agree, however, that the prospects for "drawing a line" in the development of the fetus

look dim. I am inclined to think also that we shall probably have to agree that the fetus has already become a human person well before birth. Indeed, it comes as a surprise when one first learns how early in its life it begins to acquire human characteristics. By the tenth week, for example, it already has a face, arms and legs, fingers and toes; it has internal organs, and brain activity is detectable.[2] On the other hand, I think that the premise is false, that the fetus is not a person from the moment of conception. A newly fertilized ovum, a newly implanted clump of cells, is no more a person than an acorn is an oak tree. But I shall not discuss any of this. For it seems to me to be of great interest to ask what happens if, for the sake of argument, we allow the premise. How, precisely, are we supposed to get from there to the conclusion that abortion is morally impermissible? Opponents of abortion commonly spend most of their time establishing that the fetus is a person, and hardly any time explaining the step from there to the impermissibility of abortion. Perhaps they think the step too simple and obvious to require much comment. Or perhaps instead they are simply being economical in argument. Many of

Original publication details: Judith Jarvis Thomson, "A Defense of Abortion," pp. 47–66 from *Philosophy and Public Affairs* 1: 1 (1971). Reproduced with permission of John Wiley & Sons.

Bioethics: An Anthology, Fourth Edition. Edited by Udo Schüklenk and Peter Singer.

those who defend abortion rely on the premise that the fetus is not a person, but only a bit of tissue that will become a person at birth; and why pay out more arguments than you have to? Whatever the explanation, I suggest that the step they take is neither easy nor obvious, that it calls for closer examination than it is commonly given, and that when we do give it this closer examination we shall feel inclined to reject it.

I propose, then, that we grant that the fetus is a person from the moment of conception. How does the argument go from here? Something like this, I take it. Every person has a right to life. So the fetus has a right to life. No doubt the mother has a right to decide what shall happen in and to her body; everyone would grant that. But surely a person's right to life is stronger and more stringent than the mother's right to decide what happens in and to her body, and so outweighs it. So the fetus may not be killed; an abortion may not be performed.

It sounds plausible. But now let me ask you to imagine this. You wake up in the morning and find yourself back to back in bed with an unconscious violinist. A famous unconscious violinist. He has been found to have a fatal kidney ailment, and the Society of Music Lovers has canvassed all the available medical records and found that you alone have the right blood type to help. They have therefore kidnapped you, and last night the violinist's circulatory system was plugged into yours, so that your kidneys can be used to extract poisons from his blood as well as your own. The director of the hospital now tells you, "Look, we're sorry the Society of Music Lovers did this to you – we would never have permitted it if we had known. But still, they did it, and the violinist now is plugged into you. To unplug you would be to kill him. But never mind, it's only for nine months. By then he will have recovered from his ailment, and can safely be unplugged from you." Is it morally incumbent on you to accede to this situation? No doubt it would be very nice of you if you did, a great kindness. But do you *have* to accede to it? What if it were not nine months, but nine years? Or longer still? What if the director of the hospital says, "Tough luck, I agree, but you've

now got to stay in bed, with the violinist plugged into you, for the rest of your life. Because remember this. All persons have a right to life, and violinists are persons. Granted you have a right to decide what happens in and to your body, but a person's right to life outweighs your right to decide what happens in and to your body. So you cannot ever be unplugged from him." I imagine you would regard this as outrageous, which suggests that something really is wrong with that plausible-sounding argument I mentioned a moment ago.

In this case, of course, you were kidnapped; you didn't volunteer for the operation that plugged the violinist into your kidneys. Can those who oppose abortion on the ground I mentioned make an exception for a pregnancy due to rape? Certainly. They can say that persons have a right to life only if they didn't come into existence because of rape; or they can say that all persons have a right to life, but that some have less of a right to life than others, in particular, that those who came into existence because of rape have less. But these statements have a rather unpleasant sound. Surely the question of whether you have a right to life at all, or how much of it you have, shouldn't turn on the question of whether or not you are the product of a rape. And in fact the people who oppose abortion on the ground I mentioned do not make this distinction, and hence do not make an exception in the case of rape.

Nor do they make an exception for a case in which the mother has to spend the nine months of her pregnancy in bed. They would agree that would be a great pity, and hard on the mother; but all the same, all persons have a right to life, the fetus is a person, and so on. I suspect, in fact, that they would not make an exception for a case in which, miraculously enough, the pregnancy went on for nine years, or even the rest of the mother's life.

Some won't even make an exception for a case in which continuation of the pregnancy is likely to shorten the mother's life; they regard abortion as impermissible even to save the mother's life. Such cases are nowadays very rare, and many opponents of abortion do not accept this extreme view. All the same, it is a good place to begin: a number of points of interest come out in respect to it.

1. Let us call the view that abortion is impermissible even to save the mother's life "the extreme view." I want to suggest first that it does not issue from the argument I mentioned earlier without the addition of some fairly powerful premises. Suppose a woman has become pregnant, and now learns that she has a cardiac condition such that she will die if she carries the baby to term. What may be done for her? The fetus, being a person, has a right to life, but as the mother is a person too, so has she a right to life. Presumably they have an equal right to life. How is it supposed to come out that an abortion may not be performed? If mother and child have an equal right to life, shouldn't we perhaps flip a coin? Or should we add to the mother's right to life her right to decide what happens in and to her body, which everybody seems to be ready to grant – the sum of her rights now outweighing the fetus' right to life?

The most familiar argument here is the following. We are told that performing the abortion would be directly killing[3] the child, whereas doing nothing would not be killing the mother, but only letting her die. Moreover, in killing the child, one would be killing an innocent person, for the child has committed no crime, and is not aiming at his mother's death. And then there are a variety of ways in which this might be continued. (1) But as directly killing an innocent person is always and absolutely impermissible, an abortion may not be performed. Or, (2) as directly killing an innocent person is murder, and murder is always and absolutely impermissible, an abortion may not be performed.[4] Or, (3) as one's duty to refrain from directly killing an innocent person is more stringent than one's duty to keep a person from dying, an abortion may not be performed. Or, (4) if one's only options are directly killing an innocent person or letting a person die, one must prefer letting the person die, and thus an abortion may not be performed.[5]

Some people seem to have thought that these are not further premises which must be added if the conclusion is to be reached, but that they follow from the very fact that an innocent person has a right to life.[6] But this seems to me to be a mistake, and perhaps the simplest way to show this is to bring out that while we must certainly grant that innocent persons have a right to life, the theses in (1) through (4) are all false. Take (2), for example. If directly killing an innocent person is murder, and thus is impermissible, then the mother's directly killing the innocent person inside her is murder, and thus is impermissible. But it cannot seriously be thought to be murder if the mother performs an abortion on herself to save her life. It cannot seriously be said that she *must* refrain, that she *must* sit passively by and wait for her death. Let us look again at the case of you and the violinist. There you are, in bed with the violinist, and the director of the hospital says to you, "It's all most distressing, and I deeply sympathize, but you see this is putting an additional strain on your kidneys, and you'll be dead within the month. But you *have* to stay where you are all the same. Because unplugging you would be directly killing an innocent violinist, and that's murder, and that's impermissible." If anything in the world is true, it is that you do not commit murder, you do not do what is impermissible, if you reach around to your back and unplug yourself from that violinist to save your life.

The main focus of attention in writings on abortion has been on what a third party may or may not do in answer to a request from a woman for an abortion. This is in a way understandable. Things being as they are, there isn't much a woman can safely do to abort herself. So the question asked is what a third party may do, and what the mother may do, if it is mentioned at all, is deduced, almost as an afterthought, from what it is concluded that third parties may do. But it seems to me that to treat the matter in this way is to refuse to grant to the mother that very status of person which is so firmly insisted on for the fetus. For we cannot simply read off what a person may do from what a third party may do. Suppose you find yourself trapped in a tiny house with a growing child. I mean a very tiny house, and a rapidly growing child – you are already up against the wall of the house and in a few minutes you'll be crushed to death. The child on the other hand won't be crushed to death; if nothing is done to stop him from growing he'll be hurt, but in the end he'll simply burst open the house and walk out a free man. Now I could well understand it if a bystander were to say, "There's nothing we can do for you. We cannot choose between your life and his, we cannot be the ones to decide who is to live, we cannot intervene." But it cannot be concluded that you too can do nothing, that you cannot attack it to save your life. However innocent the child may be, you do not have to wait passively while it crushes you to death. Perhaps a pregnant woman is vaguely felt to have the status of house, to which we don't allow the right of self-defense. But if the woman houses the child, it should be remembered that she is a person who houses it.

I should perhaps stop to say explicitly that I am not claiming that people have a right to do anything whatever to save their lives. I think, rather, that there are drastic limits to the right of self-defense. If someone threatens you with death unless you torture someone else to death, I think you have not the right, even to save your life, to do so. But the case under consideration here is very different. In our case there are only two people involved, one whose life is threatened, and one who threatens it. Both are innocent: the one who is threatened is not threatened because of any fault, the one who threatens does not threaten because of any fault. For this reason we may feel that we bystanders cannot intervene. But the person threatened can.

In sum, a woman surely can defend her life against the threat to it posed by the unborn child, even if doing so involves its death. And this shows not merely that the theses in (1) through (4) are false; it shows also that the extreme view of abortion is false, and so we need not canvass any other possible ways of arriving at it from the argument I mentioned at the outset.

2. The extreme view could of course be weakened to say that while abortion is permissible to save the mother's life, it may not be performed by a third party, but only by the mother herself. But this cannot be right either. For what we have to keep in mind is that the mother and the unborn child are not like two tenants in a small house which has, by an unfortunate mistake, been rented to both: the mother *owns*

the house. The fact that she does adds to the offensiveness of deducing that the mother can do nothing from the supposition that third parties can do nothing. But it does more than this: it casts a bright light on the supposition that third parties can do nothing. Certainly it lets us see that a third party who says "I cannot choose between you" is fooling himself if he thinks this is impartiality. If Jones has found and fastened on a certain coat, which he needs to keep him from freezing, but which Smith also needs to keep him from freezing, then it is not impartiality that says "I cannot choose between you" when Smith owns the coat. Women have said again and again "This body is *my* body!" and they have reason to feel angry, reason to feel that it has been like shouting into the wind. Smith, after all, is hardly likely to bless us if we say to him, "Of course it's your coat, anybody would grant that it is. But no one may choose between you and Jones who is to have it."

We should really ask what it is that says "no one may choose" in the face of the fact that the body that houses the child is the mother's body. It may be simply a failure to appreciate this fact. But it may be something more interesting, namely the sense that one has a right to refuse to lay hands on people, even where it would be just and fair to do so, even where justice seems to require that somebody do so. Thus justice might call for somebody to get Smith's coat back from Jones, and yet you have a right to refuse to be the one to lay hands on Jones, a right to refuse to do physical violence to him. This, I think, must be granted. But then what should be said is not "no one may choose," but only "*I* cannot choose," and indeed not even this, but "*I* will not *act*," leaving it open that somebody else can or should, and in particular that anyone in a position of authority, with the job of securing people's rights, both can and should. So this is no difficulty. I have not been arguing that any given third party must accede to the mother's request that he perform an abortion to save her life, but only that he may.

I suppose that in some views of human life the mother's body is only on loan to her, the loan not being one which gives her any prior claim to it. One who held this view might well think it impartiality to say "I cannot choose." But I shall simply ignore this possibility. My own view is that if a human being has any just, prior claim to anything at all, he has a just, prior claim to his own body. And perhaps this needn't be argued for here anyway, since, as I mentioned, the arguments against abortion we are looking at do grant that the woman has a right to decide what happens in and to her body.

But although they do grant it, I have tried to show that they do not take seriously what is done in granting it. I suggest the same thing will reappear even more clearly when we turn away from cases in which the mother's life is at stake, and attend, as I propose we now do, to the vastly more common cases in which a woman wants an abortion for some less weighty reason than preserving her own life.

3.   Where the mother's life is not at stake, the argument I mentioned at the outset seems to have a much stronger pull. "Everyone has a right to life, so the unborn person has a right to life." And isn't the child's right to life weightier than anything other than the mother's own right to life, which she might put forward as ground for an abortion?

This argument treats the right to life as if it were unproblematic. It is not, and this seems to me to be precisely the source of the mistake.

For we should now, at long last, ask what it comes to, to have a right to life. In some views having a right to life includes having a right to be given at least the bare minimum one needs for continued life. But suppose that what in fact *is* the bare minimum a man needs for continued life is something he has no right at all to be given? If I am sick unto death, and the only thing that will save my life is the touch of Henry Fonda's cool hand on my fevered brow, then all the same, I have no right to be given the touch of Henry Fonda's cool hand on my fevered brow. It would be frightfully nice of him to fly in from the West Coast to provide it. It would be less nice, though no doubt well meant, if my friends flew out to the West Coast and carried Henry Fonda back with them. But I have no right at all against anybody that he should do this for me. Or again, to return to the story I told earlier, the fact that for continued life that violinist needs

the continued use of your kidneys does not establish that he has a right to be given the continued use of your kidneys. He certainly has no right against you that *you* should give him continued use of your kidneys. For nobody has any right to use your kidneys unless you give him such a right; and nobody has the right against you that you shall give him this right – if you do allow him to do on using your kidneys, this is a kindness on your part, and not something he can claim from you as his due. Nor has he any right against anybody else that *they* should give him continued use of your kidneys. Certainly he had no right against the Society of Music Lovers that they should plug him into you in the first place. And if you now start to unplug yourself, having learned that you will otherwise have to spend nine years in bed with him, there is nobody in the world who must try to prevent you, in order to see to it that he is given something he has a right to be given.

Some people are rather stricter about the right to life. In their view, it does not include the right to be given anything, but amounts to, and only to, the right not to be killed by anybody. But here a related difficulty arises. If everybody is to refrain from killing that violinist, then everybody must refrain from doing a great many different sorts of things. Everybody must refrain from slitting his throat, everybody must refrain from shooting him – and everybody must refrain from unplugging you from him. But does he have a right against everybody that they shall refrain from unplugging you from him? To refrain from doing this is to allow him to continue to use your kidneys. It could be argued that he has a right against us that *we* should allow him to continue to use your kidneys. That is, while he had no right against us that we should give him the use of your kidneys, it might be argued that he anyway has a right against us that we shall not now intervene and deprive him of the use of your kidneys. I shall come back to third-party interventions later. But certainly the violinist has no right against you that *you* shall allow him to continue to use your kidneys. As I said, if you do allow him to use them, it is a kindness on your part, and not something you owe him.

The difficulty I point to here is not peculiar to the right to life. It reappears in connection with all the other natural rights; and it is something which an adequate account of rights must deal with. For present purposes it is enough just to draw attention to it. But I would stress that I am not arguing that people do not have a right to life – quite to the contrary, it seems to me that the primary control we must place on the acceptability of an account of rights is that it should turn out in that account to be a truth that all persons have a right to life. I am arguing only that having a right to life does not guarantee having either a right to be given the use of or a right to be allowed continued use of another person's body – even if one needs it for life itself. So the right to life will not serve the opponents of abortion in the very simple and clear way in which they seem to have thought it would.

4. There is another way to bring out the difficulty. In the most ordinary sort of case, to deprive someone of what he has a right to is to treat him unjustly. Suppose a boy and his small brother are jointly given a box of chocolates for Christmas. If the older boy takes the box and refuses to give his brother any of the chocolates, he is unjust to him, for the brother has been given a right to half of them. But suppose that, having learned that otherwise it means nine years in bed with that violinist, you unplug yourself from him. You surely are not being unjust to him, for you gave him no right to use your kidneys, and no one else can have given him any such right. But we have to notice that in unplugging yourself, you are killing him; and violinists, like everybody else, have a right to life, and thus in the view we were considering just now, the right not to be killed. So here you do what he supposedly has a right you shall not do, but you do not act unjustly to him in doing it.

The emendation which may be made at this point is this: the right to life consists not in the right not to be killed, but rather in the right not to be killed unjustly. This runs a risk of circularity, but never mind: it would enable us to square the fact that the violinist has a right to life with the fact that you do not act unjustly toward him in unplugging yourself, thereby killing him. For if you do not kill him unjustly, you do

not violate his right to life, and so it is no wonder you do him no injustice.

But if this emendation is accepted, the gap in the argument against abortion stares us plainly in the face: it is by no means enough to show that the fetus is a person, and to remind us that all persons have a right to life – we need to be shown also that killing the fetus violates its right to life, i.e., that abortion is unjust killing. And is it?

I suppose we may take it as a datum that in a case of pregnancy due to rape the mother has not given the unborn person a right to the use of her body for food and shelter. Indeed, in what pregnancy could it be supposed that the mother has given the unborn person such a right? It is not as if there were unborn persons drifting about the world, to whom a woman who wants a child says "I invite you in."

But it might be argued that there are other ways one can have acquired a right to the use of another person's body than by having been invited to use it by that person. Suppose a woman voluntarily indulges in intercourse, knowing of the chance it will issue in pregnancy, and then she does become pregnant; is she not in part responsible for the presence, in fact the very existence, of the unborn person inside her? No doubt she did not invite it in. But doesn't her partial responsibility for its being there itself give it a right to the use of her body?[7] If so, then her aborting it would be more like the boy's taking away the chocolates, and less like your unplugging yourself from the violinist – doing so would be depriving it of what it does have a right to, and thus would be doing it an injustice.

And then, too, it might be asked whether or not she can kill it even to save her own life: If she voluntarily called it into existence, how can she now kill it, even in self-defense?

The first thing to be said about this is that it is something new. Opponents of abortion have been so concerned to make out the independence of the fetus, in order to establish that it has a right to life, just as its mother does, that they have tended to overlook the possible support they might gain from making out that the fetus is *dependent* on the mother, in order to establish that she has a special kind of responsibility for it, a responsibility that gives it rights against her which are not possessed by any independent person – such as an ailing violinist who is a stranger to her.

On the other hand, this argument would give the unborn person a right to its mother's body only if her pregnancy resulted from a voluntary act, undertaken in full knowledge of the chance a pregnancy might result from it. It would leave out entirely the unborn person whose existence is due to rape. Pending the availability of some further argument, then, we would be left with the conclusion that unborn persons whose existence is due to rape have no right to the use of their mothers' bodies, and thus that aborting them is not depriving them of anything they have a right to and hence is not unjust killing.

And we should also notice that it is not at all plain that this argument really does go even as far as it purports to. For there are cases and cases, and the details make a difference. If the room is stuffy, and I therefore open a window to air it, and a burglar climbs in, it would be absurd to say, "Ah, now he can stay, she's given him a right to the use of her house – for she is partially responsible for his presence there, having voluntarily done what enabled him to get in, in full knowledge that there are such things as burglars, and that burglars burgle." It would be still more absurd to say this if I had had bars installed outside my windows, precisely to prevent burglars from getting in, and a burglar got in only because of a defect in the bars. It remains equally absurd if we imagine it is not a burglar who climbs in, but an innocent person who blunders or falls in. Again, suppose it were like this: people-seeds drift about in the air like pollen, and if you open your windows, one may drift in and take root in your carpets or upholstery. You don't want children, so you fix up your windows with fine mesh screens, the very best you can buy. As can happen, however, and on very, very rare occasions does happen, one of the screens is defective; and a seed drifts in and takes root. Does the person-plant who now develops have a right to the use of your house? Surely not – despite the fact that you voluntarily opened your windows, you knowingly kept carpets and upholstered furniture, and you knew that screens were sometimes defective. Someone may argue that you are

responsible for its rooting, that it does have a right to your house, because after all you *could* have lived out your life with bare floors and furniture, or with sealed windows and doors. But this won't do – for by the same token anyone can avoid a pregnancy due to rape by having a hysterectomy, or anyway by never leaving home without a (reliable!) army.

It seems to me that the argument we are looking at can establish at most that there are *some* cases in which the unborn person has a right to the use of its mother's body, and therefore *some* cases in which abortion is unjust killing. There is room for much discussion and argument as to precisely which, if any. But I think we should sidestep this issue and leave it open, for at any rate the argument certainly does not establish that all abortion is unjust killing.

5. There is room for yet another argument here, however. We surely must all grant that there may be cases in which it would be morally indecent to detach a person from your body at the cost of his life. Suppose you learn that what the violinist needs is not nine years of your life, but only one hour: all you need do to save his life is to spend one hour in that bed with him. Suppose also that letting him use your kidneys for that one hour would not affect your health in the slightest. Admittedly you were kidnapped. Admittedly you did not give anyone permission to plug him into you. Nevertheless it seems to me plain you *ought* to allow him to use your kidneys for that hour – it would be indecent to refuse.

Again, suppose pregnancy lasted only an hour, and constituted no threat to life or health. And suppose that a woman becomes pregnant as a result of rape. Admittedly she did not voluntarily do anything to bring about the existence of a child. Admittedly she did nothing at all which would give the unborn person a right to the use of her body. All the same it might well be said, as in the newly emended violinist story, that she *ought* to allow it to remain for that hour – that it would be indecent in her to refuse.

Now some people are inclined to use the term "right" in such a way that it follows from the fact that you ought to allow a person to use your body for the hour he needs, that he has a right to use your body for the hour he needs, even though he has not been given that right by any person or act. They may say that it follows also that if you refuse, you act unjustly toward him. This use of the term is perhaps so common that it cannot be called wrong; nevertheless it seems to me to be an unfortunate loosening of what we would do better to keep a tight rein on. Suppose that box of chocolates I mentioned earlier had not been given to both boys jointly, but was given only to the older boy. There he sits, stolidly eating his way through the box, his small brother watching enviously. Here we are likely to say "You ought not to be so mean. You ought to give your brother some of those chocolates." My own view is that it just does not follow from the truth of this that the brother has any right to any of the chocolates. If the boy refuses to give his brother any, he is greedy, stingy, callous – but not unjust. I suppose that the people I have in mind will say it does follow that the brother has a right to some of the chocolates, and thus that the boy does act unjustly if he refuses to give his brother any. But the effect of saying this is to obscure what we should keep distinct, namely the difference between the boy's refusal in this case and the boy's refusal in the earlier case, in which the box was given to both boys jointly, and in which the small brother thus had what was from any point of view clear title to half.

A further objection to so using the term "right" that from the fact that A ought to do a thing for B, it follows that B has a right against A that A do it for him, is that it is going to make the question of whether or not a man has a right to a thing turn on how easy it is to provide him with it; and this seems not merely unfortunate, but morally unacceptable. Take the case of Henry Fonda again. I said earlier that I had no right to the touch of his cool hand on my fevered brow, even though I needed it to save my life. I said it would be frightfully nice of him to fly in from the West Coast to provide me with it, but that I had no right against him that he should do so. But suppose he isn't on the West Coast. Suppose he has only to walk across the room, place a hand briefly on my brow – and lo, my life is saved. Then surely he ought to do it, it would be indecent to refuse. Is it to be said "Ah, well, it follows that in this case she has a right to the touch of his hand on her brow, and so it would be

an injustice in him to refuse"? So that I have a right to it when it is easy for him to provide it, though no right when it's hard? It's rather a shocking idea that anyone's rights should fade away and disappear as it gets harder and harder to accord them to him.

So my own view is that even though you ought to let the violinist use your kidneys for the one hour he needs, we should not conclude that he has a right to do so – we should say that if you refuse, you are, like the boy who owns all the chocolates and will give none away, self-centered and callous, indecent in fact, but not unjust. And similarly, that even supposing a case in which a woman pregnant due to rape ought to allow the unborn person to use her body for the hour he needs, we should not conclude that he has a right to do so; we should conclude that she is self-centered, callous, indecent, but not unjust, if she refuses. The complaints are no less grave; they are just different. However, there is no need to insist on this point. If anyone does wish to deduce "he has a right" from "you ought," then all the same he must surely grant that there are cases in which it is not morally required of you that you allow that violinist to use your kidneys, and in which he does not have a right to use them, and in which you do not do him an injustice if you refuse. And so also for mother and unborn child. Except in such cases as the unborn person has a right to demand it – and we were leaving open the possibility that there may be such cases – nobody is morally *required* to make large sacrifices, of health, of all other interests and concerns, of all other duties and commitments, for nine years, or even for nine months, in order to keep another person alive.

6. We have in fact to distinguish between two kinds of Samaritan: the Good Samaritan and what we might call the Minimally Decent Samaritan. The story of the Good Samaritan, you will remember, goes like this:

A certain man went down from Jerusalem to Jericho, and fell among thieves, which stripped him of his raiment, and wounded him, and departed, leaving him half dead.

And by chance there came down a certain priest that way; and when he saw him, he passed by on the other side.

And likewise a Levite, when he was at the place, came and looked on him, and passed by on the other side.

But a certain Samaritan, as he journeyed, came where he was; and when he saw him he had compassion on him.

And went to him, and bound up his wounds, pouring in oil and wine, and set him on his own beast, and brought him to an inn, and took care of him.

And on the morrow, when he departed, he took out two pence, and gave them to the host, and said unto him, "Take care of him; and whatsoever thou spendest more, when I come again, I will repay thee." (Luke 10: 30–35)

The Good Samaritan went out of his way, at some cost to himself, to help one in need of it. We are not told what the options were, that is, whether or not the priest and the Levite could have helped by doing less than the Good Samaritan did, but assuming they could have, then the fact they did nothing at all shows they were not even Minimally Decent Samaritans, not because they were not Samaritans, but because they were not even minimally decent.

These things are a matter of degree, of course, but there is a difference, and it comes out perhaps most clearly in the story of Kitty Genovese, who, as you will remember, was murdered while thirty-eight people watched or listened, and did nothing at all to help her. A Good Samaritan would have rushed out to give direct assistance against the murderer. Or perhaps we had better allow that it would have been a Splendid Samaritan who did this, on the ground that it would have involved a risk of death for himself. But the thirty-eight not only did not do this, they did not even trouble to pick up a phone to call the police. Minimally Decent Samaritanism would call for doing at least that, and their not having done it was monstrous.

After telling the story of the Good Samaritan, Jesus said "Go, and do thou likewise." Perhaps he meant that we are morally required to act as the Good Samaritan did. Perhaps he was urging people to do more than is morally required of them. At all events it seems plain that it was not morally required of any of the thirty-eight that he rush out to give direct assistance at the risk of his own life, and that it is not morally required of anyone that he give long stretches of his life – nine years or nine months – to sustaining the life of a person who has no special right (we were leaving open the possibility of this) to demand it.

Indeed, with one rather striking class of exceptions, no one in any country in the world is *legally* required to do anywhere near as much as this for anyone else. The class of exceptions is obvious. My main concern here is not the state of the law in respect to abortion, but it is worth drawing attention to the fact that in no state in this country is any man compelled by law to be even a Minimally Decent Samaritan to any person; there is no law under which charges could be brought against the thirty-eight who stood by while Kitty Genovese died. By contrast, in most states in this country women are compelled by law to be not merely Minimally Decent Samaritans, but Good Samaritans to unborn persons inside them. This doesn't by itself settle anything one way or the other, because it may well be argued that there should be laws in this country – as there are in many European countries – compelling at least Minimally Decent Samaritanism.[8] But it does show that there is a gross injustice in the existing state of the law. And it shows also that the groups currently working against liberalization of abortion laws, in fact working toward having it declared unconstitutional for a state to permit abortion, had better start working for the adoption of Good Samaritan laws generally, or earn the charge that they are acting in bad faith.

I should think, myself, that Minimally Decent Samaritan laws would be one thing, Good Samaritan laws quite another, and in fact highly improper. But we are not here concerned with the law. What we should ask is not whether anybody should be compelled by law to be a Good Samaritan, but whether we must accede to a situation in which somebody is being compelled – by nature, perhaps – to be a Good Samaritan. We have, in other words, to look now at third-party interventions. I have been arguing that no person is morally required to make large sacrifices to sustain the life of another who has no right to demand them, and this even where the sacrifices do not include life itself; we are not morally required to be Good Samaritans or anyway Very Good Samaritans to one another. But what if a man cannot extricate himself from such a situation? What if he appeals to us to extricate him? It seems to me plain that there are cases in which we can, cases in which a Good Samaritan would extricate him. There you are, you were kidnapped, and nine years in bed with that violinist lie ahead of you. You have your own life to lead. You are sorry, but you simply cannot see giving up so much of your life to the sustaining of his. You cannot extricate yourself, and ask us to do so. I should have thought that – in light of his having no right to the use of your body – it was obvious that we do not have to accede to your being forced to give up so much. We can do what you ask. There is no injustice to the violinist in our doing so.

7.   Following the lead of the opponents of abortion, I have throughout been speaking of the fetus merely as a person, and what I have been asking is whether or not the argument we began with, which proceeds only from the fetus being a person, really does establish its conclusion. I have argued that it does not.

But of course there are arguments and arguments, and it may be said that I have simply fastened on the wrong one. It may be said that what is important is not merely the fact that the fetus is a person, but that it is a person for whom the woman has a special kind of responsibility issuing from the fact that she is its mother. And it might be argued that all my analogies are therefore irrelevant – for you do not have that special kind of responsibility for that violinist, Henry Fonda does not have that special kind of responsibility for me. And our attention might be drawn to the fact that men and women both *are* compelled by law to provide support for their children.

I have in effect dealt (briefly) with this argument in section 4 above; but a (still briefer) recapitulation now may be in order. Surely we do not have any such "special responsibility" for a person unless we have assumed it, explicitly or implicitly. If a set of parents do not try to prevent pregnancy, do not obtain an abortion, and then at the time of birth of the child do not put it out for adoption, but rather take it home

with them, then they have assumed responsibility for it, they have given it rights, and they cannot *now* withdraw support from it at the cost of its life because they now find it difficult to go on providing for it. But if they have taken all reasonable precautions against having a child, they do not simply by virtue of their biological relationship to the child who comes into existence have a special responsibility for it. They may wish to assume responsibility for it, or they may not wish to. And I am suggesting that if assuming responsibility for it would require large sacrifices, then they may refuse. A Good Samaritan would not refuse – or anyway, a Splendid Samaritan, if the sacrifices that had to be made were enormous. But then so would a Good Samaritan assume responsibility for that violinist; so would Henry Fonda, if he is a Good Samaritan, fly in from the West Coast and assume responsibility for me.

8.   My argument will be found unsatisfactory on two counts by many of those who want to regard abortion as morally permissible. First, while I do argue that abortion is not impermissible, I do not argue that it is always permissible. There may well be cases in which carrying the child to term requires only Minimally Decent Samaritanism of the mother, and this is a standard we must not fall below. I am inclined to think it a merit of my account precisely that it does *not* give a general yes or a general no. It allows for and supports our sense that, for example, a sick and desperately frightened fourteen-year-old schoolgirl, pregnant due to rape, may of *course* choose abortion, and that any law which rules this out is an insane law. And it also allows for and supports our sense that in other cases resort to abortion is even positively indecent. It would be indecent in the woman to request an abortion, and indecent in a doctor to perform it, if she is in her seventh month, and wants the abortion just to avoid the nuisance of postponing a trip abroad. The very fact that the arguments I have been drawing attention to treat all cases of abortion, or even all cases of abortion in which the mother's life is not at stake, as morally on a par ought to have made them suspect at the outset.

Secondly, while I am arguing for the permissibility of abortion in some cases, I am not arguing for the right to secure the death of the unborn child. It is easy to confuse these two things in that up to a certain point in the life of the fetus it is not able to survive outside the mother's body; hence removing it from her body guarantees its death. But they are importantly different. I have argued that you are not morally required to spend nine months in bed, sustaining the life of that violinist; but to say this is by no means to say that if, when you unplug yourself, there is a miracle and he survives, you then have a right to turn round and slit his throat. You may detach yourself even if this costs him his life; you have no right to be guaranteed his death, by some other means, if unplugging yourself does not kill him. There are some people who will feel dissatisfied by this feature of my argument. A woman may be utterly devastated by the thought of a child, a bit of herself, put out for adoption and never seen or heard of again. She may therefore want not merely that the child be detached from her, but more, that it die. Some opponents of abortion are inclined to regard this as beneath contempt – thereby showing insensitivity to what is surely a powerful source of despair. All the same, I agree that the desire for the child's death is not one which anybody may gratify, should it turn out to be possible to detach the child alive.

At this place, however, it should be remembered that we have only been pretending throughout that the fetus is a human being from the moment of conception. A very early abortion is surely not the killing of a person, and so is not dealt with by anything I have said here.

Notes

1   I am very much indebted to James Thomson for discussion, criticism, and many helpful suggestions.

2   Daniel Callahan, *Abortion: Law, Choice and Morality* (New York, 1970), p. 373. This book gives a fascinating survey of the available information on abortion. The Jewish tradition is surveyed in David M. Feldman, *Birth Control in Jewish Law* (New York, 1968), Part 5, the Catholic tradition in John T. Noonan, Jr., "An Almost Absolute Value in History," in *The Morality of Abortion,* ed. John T. Noonan, Jr. (Cambridge, Mass., 1970).

3   The term "direct" in the arguments I refer to is a technical one. Roughly, what is meant by "direct killing" is either killing as an end in itself, or killing as a means to some end, for example, the end of saving someone else's life. See note 6, below, for an example of its use.

4   Cf. *Encyclical Letter of Pope Pius XI on Christian Marriage,* St. Paul Editions (Boston, n.d.), p. 32: "however much we may pity the mother whose health and even life is gravely imperiled in the performance of the duty allotted to her by nature, nevertheless what could ever be a sufficient reason for excusing in any way the direct murder of the innocent? This is precisely what we are dealing with here." Noonan (*The Morality of Abortion,* p. 43) reads this as follows: "What cause can ever avail to excuse in any way the direct killing of the innocent? For it is a question of that."

5   The thesis in (4) is in an interesting way weaker than those in (1), (2), and (3): they rule out abortion even in cases in which both mother *and* child will die if the abortion is not performed. By contrast, one who held the view expressed in (4) could consistently say that one needn't prefer letting two persons die to killing one.

6   Cf. the following passage from Pius XII, *Address to the Italian Catholic Society of Midwives:* "The baby in the maternal breast has the right to life immediately from God – Hence there is no man, no human authority, no science, no medical, eugenic, social, economic or moral 'indication' which can establish or grant a valid juridical ground for a direct deliberate disposition of an innocent human life, that is a disposition which looks to its destruction either as an end or as a means to another end perhaps in itself not illicit. – The baby, still not born, is a man in the same degree and for the same reason as the mother" (quoted in Noonan, *The Morality of Abortion,* p. 45).

7   The need for a discussion of this argument was brought home to me by members of the Society for Ethical and Legal Philosophy, to whom this paper was originally presented.

8   For a discussion of the difficulties involved, and a survey of the European experience with such laws, see *The Good Samaritan and the Law,* ed. James M. Ratcliffe (New York, 1966).

3

The Wrong of Abortion

Patrick Lee and Robert P. George

Much of the public debate about abortion concerns the question whether deliberate feticide ought to be unlawful, at least in most circumstances. We will lay that question aside here in order to focus first on the question: is the choice to have, to perform, or to help procure an abortion morally wrong?

We shall argue that the choice of abortion is objectively immoral. By "objectively" we indicate that we are discussing the choice itself, not the (subjective) guilt or innocence of someone who carries out the choice: someone may act from an erroneous conscience, and if he is not at fault for his error, then he remains subjectively innocent, even if his choice is objectively wrongful.

The first important question to consider is: what is killed in an abortion? It is obvious that some living entity is killed in an abortion. And no one doubts that the moral status of the entity killed is a central (though not the only) question in the abortion debate. We shall approach the issue step by step, first setting forth some (though not all) of the evidence that demonstrates that what is killed in abortion – a human embryo – is indeed a human being, then examining the ethical significance of that point.

Embryos and Fetuses are Complete (though Immature) Human Beings

It will be useful to begin by considering some of the facts of sexual reproduction. The standard embryology texts indicate that in the case of ordinary sexual reproduction the life of an individual human being begins with complete fertilization, which yields a genetically and functionally distinct organism, possessing the resources and active disposition for internally directed development toward human maturity.[1] In normal conception, a sex cell of the father, a sperm, unites with a sex cell of the mother, an ovum. Within the chromosomes of these sex cells are the DNA molecules which constitute the information that guides the development of the new individual brought into being when the sperm and ovum fuse. When fertilization occurs, the 23 chromosomes of the sperm unite with the 23 chromosomes of the ovum. At the end of this process there is produced an entirely new and distinct organism, originally a single cell. This organism, the human embryo, begins to grow by the normal process of cell division – it divides into 2 cells, then

Original publication details: Patrick Lee and Robert P. George, "The Wrong of Abortion," pp. 13–26 from Andrew I. Cohen and Christopher Health Wellman (eds.), *Contemporary Debates in Applied Ethics* (Hoboken, NJ: Wiley-Blackwell, 2014). Reproduced with permission of John Wiley & Sons.

4, 8, 16, and so on (the divisions are not simultaneous, so there is a 3-cell stage, and so on). This embryo gradually develops all of the organs and organ systems necessary for the full functioning of a mature human being. His or her development (sex is determined from the beginning) is very rapid in the first few weeks. For example, as early as eight or ten weeks of gestation, the fetus has a fully formed, beating heart, a complete brain (although not all of its synaptic connections are complete – nor will they be until sometime *after* the child is born), a recognizably human form, and the fetus feels pain, cries, and even sucks his or her thumb.

There are three important points we wish to make about this human embryo. First, it is from the start *distinct* from any cell of the mother or of the father. This is clear because it is growing in its own distinct direction. Its growth is internally directed to its own survival and maturation. Second, the embryo is *human*: it has the genetic makeup characteristic of human beings. Third, and most importantly, the embryo is a *complete* or *whole* organism, though immature. The human embryo, from conception onward, is fully programmed actively to develop himself or herself to the mature stage of a human being, and, *unless prevented by disease or violence, will actually do so, despite possibly significant variation in environment* (in the mother's womb). None of the changes that occur to the embryo after fertilization, for as long as he or she survives, generates a new direction of growth. Rather, *all* of the changes (for example, those involving nutrition and environment) either facilitate or retard the internally directed growth of this persisting individual.

Sometimes it is objected that if we say human embryos are human beings, on the grounds that they have the potential to become mature humans, the same will have to be said of sperm and ova. This objection is untenable. The human embryo is radically unlike the sperm and ova, the sex cells. The sex cells are manifestly not *whole* or *complete* organisms. They are not only genetically but also functionally identifiable as parts of the male or female potential parents. They clearly are destined either to combine with an ovum or sperm or die. Even when they succeed in causing fertilization, they do not survive; rather, their genetic material enters into the composition of a distinct, new organism.

Nor are human embryos comparable to somatic cells (such as skin cells or muscle cells), though some have tried to argue that they are. Like sex cells, a somatic cell is functionally only a part of a larger organism. The human embryo, by contrast, possesses from the beginning the internal resources and active disposition to develop himself or herself to full maturity; all he or she needs is a suitable environment and nutrition. The direction of his or her growth *is not extrinsically determined,* but the embryo is internally directing his or her growth toward full maturity.

So, a human embryo (or fetus) is not something distinct from a human being; he or she is not an individual of any non-human or intermediate species. Rather, an embryo (and fetus) is a human being at a certain (early) stage of development – the embryonic (or fetal) stage. In abortion, what is killed is a human being, a whole living member of the species *homo sapiens,* the same *kind* of entity as you or I, only at an earlier stage of development.

No-Person Arguments: The Dualist Version

Defenders of abortion may adopt different strategies to respond to these points. Most will grant that human embryos or fetuses are human beings. However, they then distinguish "human being" from "person" and claim that embryonic human beings are not (yet) *persons.* They hold that while it is wrong to kill persons, it is not always wrong to kill human beings who are not persons.

Sometimes it is argued that human beings in the embryonic stage are not persons because embryonic human beings do not exercise higher mental capacities or functions. Certain defenders of abortion (and infanticide) have argued that in order to be a person, an entity must be self-aware (Singer, 1993; Tooley, 1983; Warren, 1984). They then claim that, because human embryos and fetuses (and infants) have not yet developed self-awareness, they are not persons.

These defenders of abortion raise the question: Where does one draw the line between those who are subjects of rights and those that are not? A long tradition says that the line should be drawn at *persons*. But what is a person, if not an entity that has self-awareness, rationality, etc.?

This argument is based on a false premise. It implicitly identifies the human person with a consciousness which inhabits (or is somehow associated with) and uses a body; the truth, however, is that we human persons are particular kinds of physical organisms. The argument here under review grants that the human organism comes to be at conception, but claims nevertheless that you or I, the human person, comes to be only much later, say, when self-awareness develops. But if this human organism came to be at one time, but *I* came to be at a later time, it follows that I am one thing and this human organism with which *I* am associated is another thing.

But this is false. We are not consciousnesses that *possess or inhabit* bodies. Rather, we *are* living bodily entities. We can see this by examining the kinds of action that we perform. If a living thing performs bodily actions, then it is a physical organism. Now, those who wish to deny that we are physical organisms think of *themselves,* what each of them refers to as *"I"* as the subject of self-conscious acts of conceptual thought and willing (what many philosophers, ourselves included, would say are non-physical acts). But one can show that this "I" is identical to the subject of physical, bodily actions, and so is a living, bodily being (an organism). Sensation is a bodily action. The act of seeing, for example, is an act that an animal performs with his eye-balls and his optic nerve, just as the act of walking is an act that he performs with his legs. But it is clear in the case of human individuals that it must be the same entity, the same single subject of actions, that performs the act of sensing and that performs the act of understanding. When I know, for example, that "That is a tree," it is by my understanding, or a self-conscious intellectual act, that I apprehend what is meant by "tree,"

apprehending what it is (at least in a general way). But the subject of that proposition, what I refer to by the word "That," is apprehended by sensation or perception. Clearly, it must be the same thing – the same I – which apprehends the predicate and the subject of a unitary judgment.

So, it is the same substantial entity, the same agent, which understands and which senses or perceives. And so what all agree is referred to by the word "I" (namely, the subject of conscious, intellectual acts) is identical with the physical organism which is the subject of bodily actions such as sensing or perceiving. Hence the entity that I am, and the entity that you are – what you and I refer to by the personal pronouns "you" and "I" – is in each case a human, physical organism (but also with nonphysical capacities). Therefore, since you and I are *essentially* physical organisms, *we* came to be when these physical organisms came to be. But, as shown above, the human organism comes to be at conception.[2] Thus you and I came to be at conception; we once were embryos, then fetuses, then infants, just as we were once toddlers, preadolescent children, adolescents, and young adults.

So, how should we use the word "person"? Are human embryos persons or not? People may stipulate different meanings for the word "person," but we think it is clear that what we normally mean by the word "person" is that substantial entity that is referred to by personal pronouns – "I," "you," "she," etc. It follows, we submit, that a person is a distinct subject with the natural capacity to reason and make free choices. That subject, in the case of human beings, is identical with the human organism, and therefore that subject comes to be when the human organism comes to be, even though it will take him or her months and even years to actualize the natural capacities to reason and make free choices, natural capacities which are already present (albeit in radical, i.e. root, form) from the beginning. So it makes no sense to say that the human organism came to be at one point but the person – you or I – came to be at some later point, To have destroyed the human organism that you are or I am even at an early stage of our lives would have been to have killed you or me.

No-Person Arguments: The Evaluative Version

Let us now consider a different argument by which some defenders of abortion seek to deny that human beings in the embryonic and fetal stages are "persons" and, as such, ought not to be killed. Unlike the argument criticized in the previous section, this argument grants that the being who is you or I came to be at conception, but contends that you and I became valuable and bearers of rights only much later, when, for example, we developed the proximate, or immediately exercisable, capacity for self-consciousness. Inasmuch as those who advance this argument concede that you and I once were human embryos, they do not identify the self or the person with a non-physical phenomenon, such as consciousness. They claim, however, that being a person is an accidental attribute. It is an accidental attribute in the way that someone's being a musician or basketball player is an accidental attribute. Just as you come to be at one time, but become a musician or basketball player only much later, so, they say, you and I came to be when the physical organisms we are came to be, but we became persons (beings with a certain type of special value and bearers of basic rights) only at some time later (Dworkin, 1993; Thomson, 1995). Those defenders of abortion whose view we discussed in the previous section disagree with the pro-life position on an ontological issue, that is, on what *kind of entity* the human embryo or fetus is. Those who advance the argument now under review, by contrast, disagree with the pro-life position on an evaluative question.

Judith Thomson argued for this position by comparing the right to life with the right to vote: "If children are allowed to develop normally they will have a right to vote; that does not show that they now have a right to vote" (1995). According to this position, it is true that we once were embryos and fetuses, but in the embryonic and fetal stages of our lives we were not yet valuable in the special way that would qualify us as having a right to life. We acquired that special kind of value and the right to life that comes with it at some point after we came into existence.

We can begin to see the error in this view by considering Thomson's comparison of the right to life with the right to vote. Thomson fails to advert to the fact that some rights vary with respect to place, circumstances, maturity, ability, and other factors, while other rights do not. We recognize that one's right to life does not vary with place, as does one's right to vote. One may have the right to vote in Switzerland, but not in Mexico. Moreover, some rights and entitlements accrue to individuals only at certain times, or in certain places or situations, and others do not. But to have the right to life is to have *moral status at all;* to have the right to life, in other words, is to be the sort of entity that can have rights or entitlements to begin with. And so it is to be expected that *this* right would differ in some fundamental ways from other rights, such as a right to vote.

In particular, it is reasonable to suppose (and we give reasons for this in the next few paragraphs) that having moral status at all, as opposed to having a right to perform a specific action in a specific situation, follows from an entity's being the *type of thing* (or substantial entity) it is. And so, just as one's right to life does not come and go with one's location or situation, so it does not accrue to someone in virtue of an acquired (i.e., accidental) property, capacity, skill, or disposition. Rather, this right belongs to a human being at all times that he or she exists, not just during certain stages of his or her existence, or in certain circumstances, or in virtue of additional, accidental attributes.

Our position is that we human beings have the special kind of value that makes us subjects of rights in virtue of *what* we are, not in virtue of some attribute that we acquire some time after we have come to be. Obviously, defenders of abortion cannot maintain that the accidental attribute required to have the special kind of value we ascribe to "persons" (additional to being a human individual) is an *actual* behavior. They of course do not wish to exclude from personhood people who are asleep or in reversible comas. So, the additional attribute will have to be a capacity or potentiality of some sort.[3] Thus, they will have to concede that sleeping or reversibly comatose human beings will be persons because they have the potentiality or capacity for higher mental functions.

But human embryos and fetuses also possess, albeit in radical form, a capacity or potentiality for such mental functions; human beings possess this radical capacity in virtue of the kind of entity they are, and possess it by coming into being as that kind of entity (viz., a being with a rational nature). Human embryos and fetuses cannot of course *immediately* exercise these capacities. Still, they are related to these capacities differently from, say, how a canine or feline embryo is. They are the kind of being – a natural kind, members of a biological species – which, if not prevented by extrinsic causes, in due course develops by active self-development to the point at which capacities initially possessed in root form become immediately exercisable. (Of course, the capacities in question become immediately exercisable only some months or years after the child's birth.) Each human being comes into existence possessing the internal resources and active disposition to develop the immediately exercisable capacity for higher mental functions. Only the adverse effects on them of other causes will prevent this development.

So, we must distinguish two sorts of capacity or potentiality for higher mental functions that a substantial entity might possess: first, an immediately (or nearly immediately) exercisable capacity to engage in higher mental functions; second, a basic, natural capacity to develop oneself to the point where one does perform such actions. But on what basis can one require the first sort of potentiality – as do proponents of the position under review in this section – which is an accidental attribute, and not just the second? There are three decisive reasons against supposing that the first sort of potentiality is required to qualify an entity as a bearer of the right to life.

First, the developing human being does not reach a level of maturity at which he or she performs a type of mental act that other animals do not perform – even animals such as dogs and cats – until at least several months after birth. A six-week old baby lacks the immediately (or nearly immediately) exercisable capacity to perform characteristically human mental functions. So, if full moral respect were due only to those who possess a nearly immediately exercisable capacity for characteristically human mental functions, it would follow that six-week old infants do not deserve full moral respect. If abortion were morally acceptable on the grounds that the human embryo or fetus lacks such a capacity for characteristically human mental functions, then one would be logically committed to the view that, subject to parental approval, human infants could be disposed of as well.

Second, the difference between these two types of capacity is merely a difference between stages along a continuum. The proximate or nearly immediately exercisable capacity for mental functions is only the development of an underlying potentiality that the human being possesses simply by virtue of the kind of entity it is. The capacities for reasoning, deliberating, and making choices are gradually developed, or brought towards maturation, through gestation, childhood, adolescence, and so on. But the difference between a being that deserves full moral respect and a being that does not (and can therefore legitimately be disposed of as a means of benefiting others) cannot consist only in the fact that, while both have some feature, one has more of it than the other. A mere *quantitative* difference (having more or less of the same feature, such as *the development* of a basic natural capacity) cannot by itself be a justificatory basis for treating different entities in *radically* different ways. Between the ovum and the approaching thousands of sperm, on the one hand, and the embryonic human being, on the other hand, there *is* a clear difference in kind. But between the embryonic human being and that same human being at any later stage of its maturation, there is only a difference in degree.

Note that there *is* a fundamental difference (as we showed above) between the gametes (the sperm and the ovum), on the one hand, and the human embryo and fetus, on the other. When a human being comes to be, a substantial entity that is identical with the entity that will later reason, make free choices, and so on, begins to exist. So, those who propose an accidental characteristic as qualifying an entity as a bearer of the right to life (or as a "person" or being with "moral worth") are *ignoring* a radical difference among groups of beings, and instead fastening onto a mere quantitative difference as the basis for treating different groups in radically different ways. In other words, there are beings a, b, c, d, e, etc. And between a's and b's on the one hand and c's, d's and e's on the other hand, there is a *fundamental difference,* a difference in kind not just in degree. But proponents of the position that being a person is an accidental characteristic ignore that difference and pick out a mere difference in degree between, say, d's and e's, and make that the basis for radically different types of treatment. That violates the most basic canons of justice.

Third, being a whole human being (whether immature or not) is an either/or matter – a thing either is or is not a whole human being. But the acquired qualities that could be proposed as criteria for personhood come in varying and continuous degrees: there is an infinite number of degrees of the *development of* the basic natural capacities for self-consciousness, intelligence, or rationality. So, if human beings were worthy of full moral respect (as subjects of rights) only because of such qualities, and not in virtue of the kind of being they are, then, since such qualities come in varying degrees, no account could be given of why basic rights are not possessed by human beings in varying degrees. The proposition that all human beings are created equal would be relegated to the status of a superstition. For example, if developed self-consciousness bestowed rights, then, since some people are more self-conscious than others (that is, have developed that capacity to a greater extent than others), some people would be greater in dignity than others, and the rights of the superiors would trump those of the inferiors where the interests of the superiors could be advanced at the cost of the inferiors. This conclusion would follow no matter which of the acquired qualities generally proposed as qualifying some human beings (or human beings at some stages) for full respect were selected. Clearly, developed self-consciousness, or desires, or so on, are arbitrarily selected degrees of development of capacities that all human beings possess in (at least) radical form from the coming into existence of the human being until

his or her death. So, it cannot be the case that some human beings and not others possess the special kind of value that qualifies an entity as having a basic right to life, by virtue of a certain degree of development. Rather, human beings possess that kind of value, and therefore that right, in virtue of what (i.e., the kind of being) they are; and *all* human beings – not just some, and certainly not just those who have advanced sufficiently along the developmental path as to be able immediately (or almost immediately) to exercise their capacities for characteristically human mental functions – possess that kind of value and that right.[4]

Since human beings are valuable in the way that qualifies them as having a right to life in virtue of what they are, it follows that they have that right, whatever it entails, from the point at which they come into being – and that point (as shown in our first section) is at conception.

In sum, human beings are valuable (as subjects of rights) in virtue of what they are. But what they are are human physical organisms. Human physical organisms come to be at conception. Therefore, what is intrinsically valuable (as a subject of rights) comes to be at conception.

The Argument that Abortion is Justified as Non-intentional Killing

Some "pro-choice" philosophers have attempted to justify abortion by denying that all abortions are intentional killing. They have granted (at least for the sake of argument) that an unborn human being has a right to life but have then argued that this right does not entail that the child *in utero* is morally entitled to the use of the mother's body for life support. In effect, their argument is that, at least in many cases, abortion is not a case of intentionally killing the child, but a choice not to provide the child with assistance, that is, a choice to expel (or "evict") the child from the womb, despite the likelihood or certainty that expulsion (or "eviction") will result in his or her death (Little, 1999; McDonagh, 1996; Thomson, 1971).

Various analogies have been proposed by people making this argument. The mother's gestating a child has been compared to allowing someone the use of one's kidneys or even to donating an organ. We are not *required* (morally or as a matter of law) to allow someone to use our kidneys, or to donate organs to others, even when they would die without this assistance (and we could survive in good health despite rendering it). Analogously, the argument continues, a woman is not morally required to allow the fetus the use of her body. We shall call this "the bodily rights argument."

It may be objected that a woman has a special responsibility to the child she is carrying, whereas in the cases of withholding assistance to which abortion is compared there is no such special responsibility. Proponents of the bodily rights argument have replied, however, that the mother has not voluntarily assumed responsibility for the child, or a personal relationship with the child, and we have strong responsibilities to others only if we have voluntarily assumed such responsibilities (Thomson, 1971) or have consented to a personal relationship which generates such responsibilities (Little, 1999). True, the mother may have voluntarily performed an act which she knew may result in a child's conception, but that is distinct from consenting to gestate the child if a child is conceived. And so (according to this position) it is not until the woman consents to pregnancy, or perhaps not until the parents consent to care for the child by taking the baby home from the hospital or birthing center, that the full duties of parenthood accrue to the mother (and perhaps the father).

In reply to this argument we wish to make several points. We grant that in some few cases abortion is not intentional killing, but a choice to expel the child, the child's death being an unintended, albeit foreseen and (rightly or wrongly) accepted, side effect. However, these constitute a small minority of abortions. In the vast majority of cases, the death of the child *in utero* is precisely the object of the abortion. In most cases the end sought is to avoid being a parent; but abortion brings that about only by bringing it about that the child dies. Indeed, the attempted abortion would be considered by the woman requesting it and the abortionist performing it to have been *unsuccessful* if the child survives. In most cases abortion *is* intentional killing. Thus, even if the bodily rights argument succeeded, it would justify only a small percentage of abortions.

Still, in some few cases abortion is chosen as a means precisely toward ending the condition of pregnancy, and the woman requesting the termination of her pregnancy would not object if somehow the child survived. A pregnant woman may have less or more serious reasons for seeking the termination of this condition, but if that is her objective, then the child's death resulting from his or her expulsion will be a side effect, rather than the means chosen. For example, an actress may wish not to be pregnant because the pregnancy will change her figure during a time in which she is filming scenes in which having a slender appearance is important; or a woman may dread the discomforts, pains, and difficulties involved in pregnancy. (Of course, in many abortions there may be mixed motives: the parties making the choice may intend both ending the condition of pregnancy and the death of the child.)

Nevertheless, while it is true that in some cases abortion is not intentional killing, it remains misleading to describe it simply as choosing not to provide bodily life support. Rather, it is actively expelling the human embryo or fetus from the womb. There is a significant moral difference between *not doing* something that would assist someone, and *doing* something that causes someone harm, even if that harm is an unintended (but foreseen) side effect. It is more difficult morally to justify the latter than it is the former. Abortion is the *act* of extracting the unborn human being from the womb – an extraction that usually rips him or her to pieces or does him or her violence in some other way.

It is true that in some cases causing death as a side effect is morally permissible. For example, in some cases it is morally right to use force to stop a potentially lethal attack on one's family or country, even if one foresees that the force used will also result in the assailant's death. Similarly, there are instances in which it is permissible to perform an act that one knows or believes will, as a side effect, cause the death of a child *in utero*. For example, if a pregnant woman is discovered to have a cancerous uterus, and this is a proximate danger to the mother's life, it can be morally right to remove the cancerous uterus with the baby in it, even if the child will die as a result. A similar situation can occur in ectopic pregnancies. But in such cases, not only is the child's death a side effect, but the mother's life is in proximate danger. It is worth noting also that in these cases *what is done* (the means) is the correction of a pathology (such as a cancerous uterus, or a ruptured uterine tube). Thus, in such cases, not only the child's death, but also the ending of the pregnancy, are side effects. So, such acts are what traditional casuistry referred to as *indirect or non-intentional,* abortions.

But it is also clear that not every case of causing death as a side effect is morally right. For example, if a man's daughter has a serious respiratory disease and the father is told that his continued smoking in her presence will cause her death, it would obviously be immoral for him to continue the smoking. Similarly, if a man works for a steel company in a city with significant levels of air pollution, and his child has a serious respiratory problem making the air pollution a danger to her life, certainly he should move to another city. He should move, we would say, even if that meant he had to resign a prestigious position or make a significant career change.

In both examples, (a) the parent has a special responsibility to his child, but (b) the act that would cause the child's death would avoid a harm to the parent but cause a significantly worse harm to his child. And so, although the harm done would be a side effect, in both cases the act that caused the death would be an *unjust* act, and morally wrongful *as such*. The special responsibility of parents to their children requires that they *at least* refrain from performing acts that cause terrible harms to their children in order to avoid significantly lesser harms to themselves.

But (a) and (b) also obtain in intentional abortions (that is, those in which the removal of the child is directly sought, rather than the correction of a life-threatening pathology) even though they are not, strictly speaking, intentional killing. First, the mother has a special responsibility to her child, in virtue of being her biological mother (as does the father in virtue of his paternal relationship). The parental relationship itself – not just the voluntary acceptance of that relationship – gives rise to a special responsibility to a child.

Proponents of the bodily rights argument deny this point. Many claim that one has full parental responsibilities only if one has voluntarily assumed them. And so the child, on this view, has a right to care from his or her mother (including gestation) only if the mother has accepted her pregnancy, or perhaps only if the mother (and/or the father?) has in some way voluntarily begun a deep personal relationship with the child (Little, 1999).

But suppose a mother takes her baby home after giving birth, but the only reason she did not get an abortion was that she could not afford one. Or suppose she lives in a society where abortion is not available (perhaps very few physicians are willing to do the grisly deed). She and her husband take the child home only because they had no alternative. Moreover, suppose that in their society people are not waiting in line to adopt a newborn baby. And so the baby is several days old before anything can be done. If they abandon the baby and the baby is found, she will simply be returned to them. In such a case the parents have not voluntarily assumed responsibility; nor have they consented to a personal relationship with the child. But it would surely be wrong for these parents to abandon their baby in the woods (perhaps the only feasible way of ensuring she is not returned), even though the baby's death would be only a side effect. Clearly, we recognize that parents do have a responsibility to make sacrifices for their children, even if they have not voluntar[il]y assumed such responsibilities, or given their consent to the personal relationship with the child.

The bodily rights argument implicitly supposes that we have a primordial right to construct a life simply as we please, and that others have claims on us only very minimally or through our (at least tacit) consent to a certain sort of relationship with them. On the contrary, we are by nature members of communities. Our moral goodness or character consists to a large extent (though not solely) in contributing to the communities of which we are members. We ought to act for our genuine good or flourishing (we take that as a basic ethical principle), but our flourishing involves being in communion with others. And communion with others of itself – even if we find ourselves united with others because of a physical or social relationship which precedes our consent – entails duties or responsibilities. Moreover, the contribution we are morally required to make to others will likely bring each of us some discomfort and pain. This is not to say that we should simply ignore our own good, for the sake of others. Rather, since what (and who) I am is in part constituted by various relationships with others, not all of which are initiated by my will, my genuine good includes the contributions I make to the relationships in which I participate. Thus, the life we constitute by our free choices should be in large part a life of mutual reciprocity with others.

For example, I may wish to cultivate my talent to write and so I may want to spend hours each day reading and writing. Or I may wish to develop my athletic abilities and so I may want to spend hours every day on the baseball field. But if I am a father of minor children, and have an adequate paying job working (say) in a coal mine, then my clear duty is to keep that job. Similarly, if one's girlfriend finds she is pregnant and one is the father, then one might also be morally required to continue one's work in the mine (or mill, factory, warehouse, etc.).

In other words, I have a duty to do something with my life that contributes to the good of the human community, but that general duty becomes specified by my particular situation. It becomes specified by the connection or closeness to me of those who are in need. We acquire special responsibilities toward people, not only by *consenting* to contracts or relationships with them, but also by having various types of union with them. So, we have special responsibilities to those people with whom we are closely united. For example, we have special responsibilities to our parents, and brothers and sisters, even though we did not choose them.

The physical unity or continuity of children to their parents is unique. The child is brought into being out of the bodily unity and bodies of the mother and the father. The mother and the father are in a certain sense prolonged or continued in their offspring. So, there is a natural unity of the mother with her child, and a natural unity of the father with his child. Since we have special responsibilities to those with whom we are closely united, it follows that we in fact do have a special responsibility to our children anterior to our having voluntarily assumed such responsibility or consented to the relationship.[5]

The second point is this: in the types of case we are considering, the harm caused (death) is much worse than the harms avoided (the difficulties in pregnancy). Pregnancy can involve severe impositions, but it is not nearly as bad as death – which is total and irreversible. One needn't make light of the burdens of pregnancy to acknowledge that the harm that is death is in a different category altogether.

The burdens of pregnancy include physical difficulties and the pain of labor, and can include significant financial costs, psychological burdens, and interference with autonomy and the pursuit of other important goals (McDonagh, 1996: ch. 5). These costs are not inconsiderable. Partly for that reason, we owe our mothers gratitude for carrying and giving birth to us. However, where pregnancy does not place a woman's life in jeopardy or threaten grave and lasting damage to her physical health, the harm done to other goods is not total. Moreover, most of the harms involved in pregnancy are not irreversible: pregnancy is a nine-month task – if the woman and man are not in a good position to raise the child, adoption is a possibility. So the difficulties of pregnancy, considered together, are in a different and lesser category than death. Death is not just worse in degree than the difficulties involved in pregnancy; it is worse in kind.

It has been argued, however, that pregnancy can involve a unique type of burden. It has been argued that the *intimacy* involved in pregnancy is such that if the woman must remain pregnant without her consent then there is inflicted on her a unique and serious harm. Just as sex with consent can be a desired experience but sex without consent is a violation of bodily integrity, so (the argument continues) pregnancy involves such a close physical intertwinement with the fetus that not to allow abortion is analogous to rape – it involves an enforced intimacy (Boonin, 2003: 84; Little, 1999: 300–3).

However, this argument is based on a false analogy. Where the pregnancy is unwanted, the baby's "occupying" the mother's womb may involve a harm; but the child is committing no injustice against her. The baby is not forcing himself or herself on the woman, but is simply growing and developing in a way quite natural to him or her. The baby is not performing any action that could in any way be construed as aimed at violating the mother.[6]

It is true that the fulfillment of the duty of a mother to her child (during gestation) is unique and in many cases does involve a great sacrifice. The argument we have presented, however, is that being a mother *does* generate a special responsibility, and that the sacrifice morally required of the mother is less burdensome than the harm that would be done to the child by expelling the child, causing his or her death, to escape that responsibility. Our argument equally

entails responsibilities for the father of the child. His duty does not involve as direct a bodily relationship with the child as the mother's, but it may be equally or even more burdensome. In certain circumstances, his obligation to care for the child (and the child's mother), and especially his obligation to provide financial support, may severely limit his freedom and even require months or, indeed, years, of extremely burdensome physical labor. Historically, many men have rightly seen that their basic responsibility to their family (and country) has entailed risking, and in many cases, losing, their lives. Different people in different circumstances, with different talents, will have different responsibilities. It is no argument against any of these responsibilities to point out their distinctness.

So, the burden of carrying the baby, for all its distinctness, is significantly less than the harm the baby would suffer by being killed; the mother and father have a special responsibility to the child; it follows that intentional abortion (even in the few cases where the baby's death is an unintended but foreseen side effect) is unjust and therefore objectively immoral.

Notes

1 See, for example: Carlson (1994: chs. 2–4); Gilbert (2003: 183–220, 363–90); Larson (2001: chs. 1–2); Moore and Persaud (2003: chs. 1–6); Muller (1997: chs. 1–2); O'Rahilly and Mueller (2000: chs. 3–4).

2 For a discussion of the issues raised by twinning and cloning, see George and Lobo (2002).

3 Some defenders of abortion have seen the damaging implications of this point for their position (Stretton, 2004), and have struggled to find a way around it. There are two leading proposals. The first is to suggest a mean between a capacity and an actual behavior, such as a disposition. But a disposition is just the development or specification of a capacity and so raises the unanswerable question of why just that much development, and not more or less should be required. The second proposal is to assert that the historical fact of someone having exercised a capacity (say, for conceptual thought) confers on her a right to life even if she does not now have the immediately exercisable capacity.

But suppose we have baby Susan who has developed a brain and gained sufficient experience to the point that just now she has the immediately exercisable capacity for conceptual thought, but she has not yet exercised it. Why should she be in a wholly different category than say, baby Mary, who is just like Susan except she did actually have a conceptual thought? Neither proposal can bear the moral weight assigned to it. Both offer criteria that are wholly arbitrary.

4 In arguing against an article by Lee, Dean Stretton claims that the basic natural capacity of rationality also comes in degrees, and that therefore the argument we are presenting against the position that moral worth is based on having some accidental characteristic would apply to our position also (Stretton, 2004). But this is to miss the important distinction between having a basic natural capacity (of which there are no degrees, since one either has it or one doesn't), and the *development of that capacity* (of which there are infinite degrees).

5   David Boonin claims, in reply to this argument – in an earlier and less developed form, presented by Lee (1996: 122) – that it is not clear that it is impermissible for a woman to destroy what is a part of, or a continuation of, herself. He then says that to the extent the unborn human being is united to her in that way, "it would if anything seem that her act is *easier* to justify than if this claim were not true" (2003: 230). But Boonin fails to grasp the point of the argument (perhaps understandably since it was not expressed very clearly in the earlier work he is discussing). The unity of the child to the mother is the basis for this child being related to the woman in a different way from how other children are.

We ought to pursue our own good *and the good of others with whom we are united in various ways*. If that is so, then the closer someone is united to us, the deeper and more extensive our responsibility to the person will be.

6   In some sense being bodily "occupied" when one does not wish to be *is* a harm; however, just as the child does not (as explained in the text), neither does the state inflict this harm on the woman, in circumstances in which the state prohibits abortion. By prohibiting abortion the state would only prevent the woman from performing an act (forcibly detaching the child from her) that would unjustly kill this developing child, who is an innocent party.

References

Boonin, David (2003). *A Defense of Abortion*. New York: Cambridge University Press.

Carlson, Bruce (1994). *Human Embryology and Developmental Biology*. St. Louis, MO: Mosby.

Dworkin, Ronald (1993). *Life's Dominion: An Argument about Abortion, Euthanasia, and Individual Freedom*. New York: Random House.

George, Robert and Lobo, Gòmez (2002). "Personal statement." In *The President's Council on Bioethics, Human Cloning and Human Dignity: The Report of the President's Council on Bioethics*. (2002, pp. 294–306). New York: Public Affairs.

Gilbert, Scott (2003). *Developmental Biology*, 7th edn. Sunderland, MA: Sinnauer Associates.

Larson, William J. (2001). *Human Embryology*, 3rd edn. New York: Churchill Livingstone.

Lee, Patrick (1996). *Abortion and Unborn Human Life*. Washington, DC: Catholic University of America Press.

Little, Margaret Olivia (1999). "Abortion, intimacy, and the duty to gestate." *Ethical Theory and Moral Practice*, 2: 295–312.

McDonagh, Eileen (1996). *Breaking the Abortion Deadlock: From Choice to Consent*. New York: Oxford University Press, 1996.

Moore, Keith, and Persaud, T. V. N. (2003). *The Developing Human, Clinically Oriented Embryology*, 7th edn. New York: W. B. Saunders.

Muller, Werner A. (1997). *Developmental Biology*. New York: Springer Verlag.

O'Rahilly, Ronan, and Mueller, Fabiola (2000). *Human Embryology and Teratology*, 3rd edn. New York: John Wiley & Sons.

Singer, Peter (1993). *Practical Ethics*, 2nd edn. Cambridge: Cambridge University Press.

Stretton, Dean (2004). "Essential properties and the right to life: a response to Lee." *Bioethics*, 18/3: 264–82.

Thomson, Judith Jarvis (1971). "A defense of abortion." *Philosophy and Public Affairs*, 1: 47–66; reprinted, among other places, in Joel Feinberg (ed.) *The Problem of Abortion*, 2nd edn. Belmont, CA: Wadsworth (1984, pp. 173–87).

Thomson, Judith Jarvis (1995). "Abortion." *Boston Review*. Available at [http://bostonreview.net/archives/BR20.3/thomson.php]

Tooley, Michael (1983). *Abortion and Infanticide*. New York: Oxford University Press.

Warren, Mary Ann (1984). "On the moral and legal status of abortion." In Joel Feinberg (ed.) *The Problem of Abortion*, 2nd edn. Belmont, CA: Wadsworth (1984, pp. 102–19).

Further reading

Bailey, Ronald, Lee, Patrick, and George, Robert P. (2001). "Are stem cells babies?" *Reason Online*. Available at https://reason.com/2001/07/11/are-stem-cells-babies/

Beckwith, Francis (1993). *Politically Correct Death: Answering the Arguments for Abortion Rights*. Grand Rapids, MI: Baker.

Beckwith, Francis (2000). *Abortion and the Sanctity of Human Life*. Joplin, MO: College Press.

Chappell, T. D. J. (1998). *Understanding Human Goods: A Theory of Ethics*. Edinburgh: Edinburgh University Press.

Finnis, John (1999). "Abortion and health care ethics." In Helga Kuhse and Peter Singer (eds.), *Bioethics: An Anthology* (pp. 13–20). London: Blackwell.

Finnis, John (2001). "Abortion and cloning: some new evasions." Available at http://lifeissues.net/writers/fin/fin_01aborcloneevasions.html

George, Robert (2001). "We should not kill human embryos – for any reason." In *The Clash of Orthodoxies: Law, Religion, and Morality in Crisis* (pp. 317–23). Wilmington, DL: ISI Books.

Grisez, Germain (1990). "When do people begin?" *Proceedings of the American Catholic Philosophical Quarterly*, 63: 27–47.

Lee, Patrick (2004). "The pro-life argument from substantial identity: A defense." *Bioethics*, 18(3): 249–63.

Marquis, Don (1989). "Why abortion is immoral." *Journal of Philosophy*, 86: 183–202.

Oderberg, David (2000) *Applied Ethics: A Non-Consequentialist Approach*. New York: Oxford University Press.

Pavlischek, Keith (1993). "Abortion logic and paternal responsibilities: One more look at Judith Thomson's 'Defense of abortion'." *Public Affairs Quarterly*, 7: 341–61.

Schwarz, Stephen (1990). *The Moral Question of Abortion*. Chicago: Loyola University Press.

Stone, Jim (1987). "Why potentiality matters." *Journal of Social Philosophy*, 26: 815–30.

Stretton, Dean (2000). "The argument from intrinsic value: A critique." *Bioethics*, 14: 228–39.

4

Why Abortion is Immoral

Don Marquis

The view that abortion is, with rare exceptions, seriously immoral has received little support in the recent philosophical literature. No doubt most philosophers affiliated with secular institutions of higher education believe that the anti-abortion position is either a symptom of irrational religious dogma or a conclusion generated by seriously confused philosophical argument. The purpose of this essay is to undermine this general belief. This essay sets out an argument that purports to show, as well as any argument in ethics can show, that abortion is, except possibly in rare cases, seriously immoral, that it is in the same moral category as killing an innocent adult human being.

The argument is based on a major assumption. Many of the most insightful and careful writers on the ethics of abortion – such as Joel Feinberg, Michael Tooley, Mary Anne Warren, H. Tristram Engelhardt, Jr, L. W. Sumner, John T. Noonan, Jr, and Philip Devine[1] – believe that whether or not abortion is morally permissible stands or falls on whether or not a fetus is the sort of being whose life it is seriously wrong to end. The argument of this essay will assume, but not argue, that they are correct.

Also, this essay will neglect issues of great importance to a complete ethics of abortion. Some anti-abortionists will allow that certain abortions, such as abortion before implantation or abortion when the life of a woman is threatened by a pregnancy or abortion after rape, may be morally permissible. This essay will not explore the casuistry of these hard cases. The purpose of this essay is to develop a general argument for the claim that the overwhelming majority of deliberate abortions are seriously immoral.

I

A sketch of standard anti-abortion and pro-choice arguments exhibits how those arguments possess certain symmetries that explain why partisans of those positions are so convinced of the correctness of their own positions, why they are not successful in convincing their opponents, and why, to others, this issue seems to be unresolvable. An analysis of the nature of this standoff suggests a strategy for surmounting it.

Original publication details: Don Marquis, "Why Abortion Is Immoral," pp. 183–202 from *Journal of Philosophy* 86: 4 (April 1989). Reproduced with permission of the author and The Journal of Philosophy, Inc.

Bioethics: An Anthology, Fourth Edition. Edited by Udo Schüklenk and Peter Singer.

Consider the way a typical anti-abortionist argues. She will argue or assert that life is present from the moment of conception or that fetuses look like babies or that fetuses possess a characteristic such as a genetic code that is both necessary and sufficient for being human. Anti-abortionists seem to believe that (1) the truth of all of these claims is quite obvious, and (2) establishing any of these claims is sufficient to show that abortion is morally akin to murder.

A standard pro-choice strategy exhibits similarities. The pro-choicer will argue or assert that fetuses are not persons or that fetuses are not rational agents or that fetuses are not social beings. Pro-choicers seem to believe that (1) the truth of any of these claims is quite obvious, and (2) establishing any of these claims is sufficient to show that an abortion is not a wrongful killing.

In fact, both the pro-choice and the anti-abortion claims do seem to be true, although the "it looks like a baby" claim is more difficult to establish the earlier the pregnancy. We seem to have a standoff. How can it be resolved?

As everyone who has taken a bit of logic knows, if any of these arguments concerning abortion is a good argument, it requires not only some claim characterizing fetuses, but also some general moral principle that ties a characteristic of fetuses to having or not having the right to life or to some other moral characteristic that will generate the obligation or the lack of obligation not to end the life of a fetus. Accordingly, the arguments of the anti-abortionist and the pro-choicer need a bit of filling in to be regarded as adequate.

Note what each partisan will say. The anti-abortionist will claim that her position is supported by such generally accepted moral principles as "It is always prima facie seriously wrong to take a human life" or "It is always prima facie seriously wrong to end the life of a baby." Since these are generally accepted moral principles, her position is certainly not obviously wrong. The pro-choicer will claim that her position is supported by such plausible moral principles as "Being a person is what gives an individual intrinsic moral worth" or "It is only seriously prima facie wrong to take the life of a member of

the human community." Since these are generally accepted moral principles, the pro-choice position is certainly not obviously wrong. Unfortunately, we have again arrived at a standoff.

Now, how might one deal with this standoff? The standard approach is to try to show how the moral principles of one's opponent lose their plausibility under analysis. It is easy to see how this is possible. On the one hand, the anti-abortionist will defend a moral principle concerning the wrongness of killing which tends to be broad in scope in order that even fetuses at an early stage of pregnancy will fall under it. The problem with broad principles is that they often embrace too much. In this particular instance, the principle "It is always prima facie wrong to take a human life" seems to entail that it is wrong to end the existence of a living human cancer-cell culture, on the grounds that the culture is both living and human. Therefore, it seems that the anti-abortionist's favored principle is too broad.

On the other hand, the pro-choicer wants to find a moral principle concerning the wrongness of killing which tends to be narrow in scope in order that fetuses will *not* fall under it. The problem with narrow principles is that they often do not embrace enough. Hence, the needed principles such as "It is prima facie seriously wrong to kill only persons" or "It is prima facie wrong to kill only rational agents" do not explain why it is wrong to kill infants or young children or the severely retarded or even perhaps the severely mentally ill. Therefore, we seem again to have a standoff. The anti-abortionist charges, not unreasonably, that pro-choice principles concerning killing are too narrow to be acceptable; the pro-choicer charges, not unreasonably, that anti-abortionist principles concerning killing are too broad to be acceptable.

Attempts by both sides to patch up the difficulties in their positions run into further difficulties. The anti-abortionist will try to remove the problem in her position by reformulating her principle concerning killing in terms of human beings. Now we end up with: "It is always prima facie seriously wrong to end the life of a human being." This principle has the advantage of avoiding the problem of the human cancer-cell culture counterexample. But this advantage is purchased at a high price. For although it is clear that a fetus is both human and alive, it is not at all clear that a fetus is a human *being*. There is at least something to be said for the view that something becomes a human being only after a process of development, and that therefore first trimester fetuses and perhaps all fetuses are not yet human beings. Hence, the anti-abortionist, by this move, has merely exchanged one problem for another.[2]

The pro-choicer fares no better. She may attempt to find reasons why killing infants, young children, and the severely retarded is wrong which are independent of her major principle that is supposed to explain the wrongness of taking human life, but which will not also make abortion immoral. This is no easy task. Appeals to social utility will seem satisfactory only to those who resolve not to think of the enormous difficulties with a utilitarian account of the wrongness of killing and the significant social costs of preserving the lives of the unproductive.[3] A pro-choice strategy that extends the definition of "person" to infants or even to young children seems just as arbitrary as an anti-abortion strategy that extends the definition of "human being" to fetuses. Again, we find symmetries in the two positions and we arrive at a standoff.

There are even further problems that reflect symmetries in the two positions. In addition to counterexample problems, or the arbitrary application problems that can be exchanged for them, the standard anti-abortionist principle "It is prima facie seriously wrong to kill a human being," or one of its variants, can be objected to on the grounds of ambiguity. If "human being" is taken to be a *biological* category, then the anti-abortionist is left with the problem of explaining why a merely biological category should make a moral difference. Why, it is asked, is it any more reasonable to base a moral conclusion on the number of chromosomes in one's cells than on the color of one's skin?[4] If "human being," on the other hand, is taken to be a *moral* category, then the claim that a fetus is a human being cannot be taken to be a premise in the anti-abortion argument, for it is precisely what needs to be established. Hence, either the anti-abortionist's

main category is a morally irrelevant, merely biological category, or it is of no use to the anti-abortionist in establishing (noncircularly, of course) that abortion is wrong.

Although this problem with the anti-abortionist position is often noticed, it is less often noticed that the pro-choice position suffers from an analogous problem. The principle "Only persons have the right to life" also suffers from an ambiguity. The term "person" is typically defined in terms of psychological characteristics, although there will certainly be disagreement concerning which characteristics are most important. Supposing that this matter can be settled, the pro-choicer is left with the problem of explaining why *psychological* characteristics should make a *moral* difference. If the pro-choicer should attempt to deal with this problem by claiming that an explanation is not necessary, that in fact we do treat such a cluster of psychological properties as having moral significance, the sharp-witted anti-abortionist should have a ready response. We do treat being both living and human as having moral significance. If it is legitimate for the pro-choicer to demand that the anti-abortionist provide an explanation of the connection between the biological character of being a human being and the wrongness of being killed (even though people accept this connection), then it is legitimate for the anti-abortionist to demand that the pro-choicer provide an explanation of the connection between psychological criteria for being a person and the wrongness of being killed (even though that connection is accepted).[5]

Feinberg has attempted to meet this objection (he calls psychological personhood "commonsense personhood"):

> The characteristics that confer commonsense personhood are not arbitrary bases for rights and duties, such as race, sex or species membership; rather they are traits that make sense out of rights and duties and without which those moral attributes would have no point or function. It is because people are conscious; have a sense of their personal identities; have plans, goals, and projects; experience emotions; are liable to pains, anxieties, and frustrations; can reason and bargain, and so on – it is

because of these attributes that people have values and interests, desires and expectations of their own, including a stake in their own futures, and a personal well-being of a sort we cannot ascribe to unconscious or nonrational beings. Because of their developed capacities they can assume duties and responsibilities and can have and make claims on one another. Only because of their sense of self, their life plans, their value hierarchies, and their stakes in their own futures can they be ascribed fundamental rights. There is nothing arbitrary about these linkages. ("Abortion," p. 270)

The plausible aspects of this attempt should not be taken to obscure its implausible features. There is a great deal to be said for the view that being a psychological person under some description is a necessary condition for having duties. One cannot have a duty unless one is capable of behaving morally, and a being's capability of behaving morally will require having a certain psychology. It is far from obvious, however, that having rights entails consciousness or rationality, as Feinberg suggests. We speak of the rights of the severely retarded or the severely mentally ill, yet some of these persons are not rational. We speak of the rights of the temporarily unconscious. The New Jersey Supreme Court based their decision in the Quinlan case on Karen Ann Quinlan's right to privacy, and she was known to be permanently unconscious at that time. Hence, Feinberg's claim that having rights entails being conscious is, on its face, obviously false.

Of course, it might not make sense to attribute rights to a being that would never in its natural history have certain psychological traits. This modest connection between psychological personhood and moral personhood will create a place for Karen Ann Quinlan and the temporarily unconscious. But then it makes a place for fetuses also. Hence, it does not serve Feinberg's pro-choice purposes. Accordingly, it seems that the pro-choicer will have as much difficulty bridging the gap between psychological personhood and personhood in the moral sense as the anti-abortionist has bridging the gap between being a biological human being and being a human being in the moral sense.

Furthermore, the pro-choicer cannot any more escape her problem by making person a purely moral category than the anti-abortionist could escape by the analogous move. For if person is a moral category, then the pro-choicer is left without the resources for establishing (noncircularly, of course) the claim that a fetus is not a person, which is an essential premise in her argument. Again, we have both a symmetry and a standoff between pro-choice and anti-abortion views.

Passions in the abortion debate run high. There are both plausibilities and difficulties with the standard positions. Accordingly, it is hardly surprising that partisans of either side embrace with fervor the moral generalizations that support the conclusions they preanalytically favor, and reject with disdain the moral generalizations of their opponents as being subject to inescapable difficulties. It is easy to believe that the counterexamples to one's own moral principles are merely temporary difficulties that will dissolve in the wake of further philosophical research, and that the counterexamples to the principles of one's opponents are as straightforward as the contradiction between A and O propositions in traditional logic. This might suggest to an impartial observer (if there are any) that the abortion issue is unresolvable.

There is a way out of this apparent dialectical quandary. The moral generalizations of both sides are not quite correct. The generalizations hold for the most part, for the usual cases. This suggests that they are all accidental generalizations, that the moral claims made by those on both sides of the dispute do not touch on the essence of the matter.

This use of the distinction between essence and accident is not meant to invoke obscure metaphysical categories. Rather, it is intended to reflect the rather atheoretical nature of the abortion discussion. If the generalization a partisan in the abortion dispute adopts were derived from the reason why ending the life of a human being is wrong, then there could not be exceptions to that generalization unless some special case obtains in which there are even more powerful countervailing reasons. Such generalizations would not be merely accidental generalizations; they would point to, or be based upon, the essence of the wrongness of killing, what it is that makes killing wrong. All this suggests that a necessary condition of resolving the abortion controversy is a more theoretical account of the wrongness of killing. After all, if we merely believe, but do not understand, why killing adult human beings such as ourselves is wrong, how could we conceivably show that abortion is either immoral or permissible?

II

In order to develop such an account, we can start from the following unproblematic assumption concerning our own case: it is wrong to kill *us*. Why is it wrong? Some answers can be easily eliminated. It might be said that what makes killing us wrong is that a killing brutalizes the one who kills. But the brutalization consists of being inured to the performance of an act that is hideously immoral; hence, the brutalization does not explain the immorality. It might be said that what makes killing us wrong is the great loss others would experience due to our absence. Although such hubris is understandable, such an explanation does not account for the wrongness of killing hermits, or those whose lives are relatively independent and whose friends find it easy to make new friends.

A more obvious answer is better. What primarily makes killing wrong is neither its effect on the murderer nor its effect on the victim's friends and relatives, but its effect on the victim. The loss of one's life is one of the greatest losses one can suffer. The loss of one's life deprives one of all the experiences, activities, projects, and enjoyments that would otherwise have constituted one's future. Therefore, killing someone is wrong, primarily because the killing inflicts (one of) the greatest possible losses on the victim. To describe this as the loss of life can be misleading, however. The change in my biological state does not by itself make killing me wrong. The effect of the loss of my biological life is the loss to me of all those activities, projects, experiences, and enjoyments which otherwise have constituted my future personal life. These activities, projects, experiences, and enjoyments are

either valuable for their own sakes or are means to something else that is valuable for its own sake. Some parts of my future are not valued by me now, but will come to be valued by me as I grow older and as my values and capacities change. When I am killed, I am deprived both of what I now value which would have been part of my future personal life, but also what I would come to value. Therefore, when I die, I am deprived of all of the value of my future. Inflicting this loss on me is ultimately what makes killing me wrong. This being the case, it would seem that what makes killing *any* adult human being prima facie seriously wrong is the loss of his or her future.[6]

How should this rudimentary theory of the wrongness of killing be evaluated? It cannot be faulted for deriving an 'ought' from an 'is', for it does not. The analysis assumes that killing me (or you, reader) is prima facie seriously wrong. The point of the analysis is to establish which natural property ultimately explains the wrongness of the killing, given that it is wrong. A natural property will ultimately explain the wrongness of killing, only if (1) the explanation fits with our intuitions about the matter and (2) there is no other natural property that provides the basis for a better explanation of the wrongness of killing. This analysis rests on the intuition that what makes killing a particular human or animal wrong is what it does to that particular human or animal. What makes killing wrong is some natural effect or other of the killing. Some would deny this. For instance, a divine-command theorist in ethics would deny it. Surely this denial is, however, one of those features of divine-command theory which renders it so implausible.

The claim that what makes killing wrong is the loss of the victim's future is directly supported by two considerations. In the first place, this theory explains why we regard killing as one of the worst of crimes. Killing is especially wrong, because it deprives the victim of more than perhaps any other crime. In the second place, people with AIDS or cancer who know they are dying believe, of course, that dying is a very bad thing for them. They believe that the loss of a future to them that they would otherwise have experienced is what makes their premature death a very bad thing for them. A better theory of the wrongness of killing would require a different natural property associated with killing which better fits with the attitudes of the dying. What could it be?

The view that what makes killing wrong is the loss to the victim of the value of the victim's future gains additional support when some of its implications are examined. In the first place, it is incompatible with the view that it is wrong to kill only beings who are biologically human. It is possible that there exists a different species from another planet whose members have a future like ours. Since having a future like that is what makes killing someone wrong, this theory entails that it would be wrong to kill members of such a species. Hence, this theory is opposed to the claim that only life that is biologically human has great moral worth, a claim which many anti-abortionists have seemed to adopt. This opposition, which this theory has in common with personhood theories, seems to be a merit of the theory.

In the second place, the claim that the loss of one's future is the wrong-making feature of one's being killed entails the possibility that the futures of some actual nonhuman mammals on our own planet are sufficiently like ours that it is seriously wrong to kill them also. Whether some animals do have the same right to life as human beings depends on adding to the account of the wrongness of killing some additional account of just what it is about my future or the futures of other adult human beings which makes it wrong to kill us. No such additional account will be offered in this essay. Undoubtedly, the provision of such an account would be a very difficult matter. Undoubtedly, any such account would be quite controversial. Hence, it surely should not reflect badly on this sketch of an elementary theory of the wrongness of killing that it is indeterminate with respect to some very difficult issues regarding animal rights.

In the third place, the claim that the loss of one's future is the wrong-making feature of one's being killed does not entail, as sanctity of human life theories do, that active euthanasia is wrong. Persons who are severely and incurably ill, who face a future of pain and despair, and who wish to die will not have

suffered a loss if they are killed. It is, strictly speaking, the value of a human's future which makes killing wrong in this theory. This being so, killing does not necessarily wrong some persons who are sick and dying. Of course, there may be other reasons for a prohibition of active euthanasia, but that is another matter. Sanctity-of-human-life theories seem to hold that active euthanasia is seriously wrong even in an individual case where there seems to be good reason for it independently of public policy considerations. This consequence is most implausible, and it is a plus for the claim that the loss of a future of value is what makes killing wrong that it does not share this consequence.

In the fourth place, the account of the wrongness of killing defended in this essay does straight-forwardly entail that it is prima facie seriously wrong to kill children and infants, for we do presume that they have futures of value. Since we do believe that it is wrong to kill defenseless little babies, it is important that a theory of the wrongness of killing easily account for this. Personhood theories of the wrongness of killing, on the other hand, cannot straightforwardly account for the wrongness of killing infants and young children.[7] Hence, such theories must add special ad hoc accounts of the wrongness of killing the young. The plausibility of such ad hoc theories seems to be a function of how desperately one wants such theories to work. The claim that the primary wrong-making feature of a killing is the loss to the victim of the value of its future accounts for the wrongness of killing young children and infants directly; it makes the wrongness of such acts as obvious as we actually think it is. This is a further merit of this theory. Accordingly, it seems that this value of a future-like-ours theory of the wrongness of killing shares strengths of both sanctity-of-life and personhood accounts while avoiding weaknesses of both. In addition, it meshes with a central intuition concerning what makes killing wrong.

The claim that the primary wrong-making feature of a killing is the loss to the victim of the value of its future has obvious consequences for the ethics of abortion. The future of a standard fetus includes a set of experiences, projects, activities, and such which are identical with the futures of adult human beings and are identical with the futures of young children. Since the reason that is sufficient to explain why it is wrong to kill human beings after the time of birth is a reason that also applies to fetuses, it follows that abortion is prima facie seriously morally wrong.

This argument does not rely on the invalid inference that, since it is wrong to kill persons, it is wrong to kill potential persons also. The category that is morally central to this analysis is the category of having a valuable future like ours; it is not the category of personhood. The argument to the conclusion that abortion is prima facie seriously morally wrong proceeded independently of the notion of person or potential person or any equivalent. Someone may wish to start with this analysis in terms of the value of a human future, conclude that abortion is, except perhaps in rare circumstances, seriously morally wrong, infer that fetuses have the right to life, and then call fetuses "persons" as a result of their having the right to life. Clearly, in this case, the category of person is being used to state the *conclusion* of the analysis rather than to generate the *argument* of the analysis.

The structure of this anti-abortion argument can be both illuminated and defended by comparing it to what appears to be the best argument for the wrongness of the wanton infliction of pain on animals. This latter argument is based on the assumption that it is prima facie wrong to inflict pain on me (or you, reader). What is the natural property associated with the infliction of pain which makes such infliction wrong? The obvious answer seems to be that the infliction of pain causes suffering and that suffering is a misfortune. The suffering caused by the infliction of pain is what makes the wanton infliction of pain on me wrong. The wanton infliction of pain on other adult humans causes suffering. The wanton infliction of pain on animals causes suffering. Since causing suffering is what makes the wanton infliction of pain wrong and since the wanton infliction of pain on animals causes suffering, it follows that the wanton infliction of pain on animals is wrong.

This argument for the wrongness of the wanton infliction of pain on animals shares a number of structural features with the argument for the serious prima facie wrongness of abortion. Both arguments start with an obvious assumption concerning what it is wrong to do to me (or you, reader). Both then look for the characteristic or the consequence of the wrong action which makes the action wrong. Both recognize that the wrong-making feature of these immoral actions is a property of actions sometimes directed at individuals other than postnatal human beings. If the structure of the argument for the wrongness of the wanton infliction of pain on animals is sound, then the structure of the argument for the prima facie serious wrongness of abortion is also sound, for the structure of the two arguments is the same. The structure common to both is the key to the explanation of how the wrongness of abortion can be demonstrated without recourse to the category of person. In neither argument is that category crucial.

This defense of an argument for the wrongness of abortion in terms of a structurally similar argument for the wrongness of the wanton infliction of pain on animals succeeds only if the account regarding animals is the correct account. Is it? In the first place, it seems plausible. In the second place, its major competition is Kant's account. Kant believed that we do not have direct duties to animals at all, because they are not persons. Hence, Kant had to explain and justify the wrongness of inflicting pain on animals on the grounds that "he who is hard in his dealings with animals becomes hard also in his dealing with men."[8] The problem with Kant's account is that there seems to be no reason for accepting this latter claim unless Kant's account is rejected. If the alternative to Kant's account is accepted, then it is easy to understand why someone who is indifferent to inflicting pain on animals is also indifferent to inflicting pain on humans, for one is indifferent to what makes inflicting pain wrong in both cases. But, if Kant's account is accepted, there is no intelligible reason why one who is hard in his dealings with animals (or crabgrass or stones) should also be hard in his dealings with men. After all, men are persons: animals are no more persons than crabgrass or stones. Persons are Kant's crucial moral category. Why, in short, should a Kantian accept the basic claim in Kant's argument?

Hence, Kant's argument for the wrongness of inflicting pain on animals rests on a claim that, in a world of Kantian moral agents, is demonstrably false. Therefore, the alternative analysis, being more plausible anyway, should be accepted. Since this alternative analysis has the same structure as the anti-abortion argument being defended here, we have further support for the argument for the immorality of abortion being defended in this essay.

Of course, this value of a future-like-ours argument, if sound, shows only that abortion is prima facie wrong, not that it is wrong in any and all circumstances. Since the loss of the future to a standard fetus, if killed, is, however, at least as great a loss as the loss of the future to a standard adult human being who is killed, abortion, like ordinary killing, could be justified only by the most compelling reasons. The loss of one's life is almost the greatest misfortune that can happen to one. Presumably abortion could be justified in some circumstances, only if the loss consequent on failing to abort would be at least as great. Accordingly, morally permissible abortions will be rare indeed unless, perhaps, they occur so early in pregnancy that a fetus is not yet definitely an individual. Hence, this argument should be taken as showing that abortion is presumptively very seriously wrong, where the presumption is very strong – as strong as the presumption that killing another adult human being is wrong.

III

How complete an account of the wrongness of killing does the value of a future-like-ours account have to be in order that the wrongness of abortion is a consequence? This account does not have to be an account of the necessary conditions for the wrongness of killing. Some persons in nursing homes may lack valuable human futures, yet it may be wrong to kill them for other reasons. Furthermore, this account does not obviously have to be the sole reason killing is wrong where the victim did have a valuable future. This analysis claims only that, for any killing where the victim did have a valuable future like ours, having

that future by itself is sufficient to create the strong presumption that the killing is seriously wrong.

One way to overturn the value of a future-like-ours argument would be to find some account of the wrongness of killing which is at least as intelligible and which has different implications for the ethics of abortion. Two rival accounts possess at least some degree of plausibility. One account is based on the obvious fact that people value the experience of living and wish for that valuable experience to continue. Therefore, it might be said, what makes killing wrong is the discontinuation of that experience for the victim. Let us call this the *discontinuation account*.[9] Another rival account is based upon the obvious fact that people strongly desire to continue to live. This suggests that what makes killing us so wrong is that it interferes with the fulfillment of a strong and fundamental desire, the fulfillment of which is necessary for the fulfillment of any other desires we might have. Let us call this the *desire account*.[10]

Consider first the desire account as a rival account of the ethics of killing which would provide the basis for rejecting the anti-abortion position. Such an account will have to be stronger than the value of a future-like-ours account of the wrongness of abortion if it is to do the job expected of it. To entail the wrongness of abortion, the value of a future-like-ours account has only to provide a sufficient, but not a necessary, condition for the wrongness of killing. The desire account, on the other hand, must provide us also with a necessary condition for the wrongness of killing in order to generate a pro-choice conclusion on abortion. The reason for this is that presumably the argument from the desire account moves from the claim that what makes killing wrong is interference with a very strong desire to the claim that abortion is not wrong because the fetus lacks a strong desire to live. Obviously, this inference fails if someone's having the desire to live is not a necessary condition of its being wrong to kill that individual.

One problem with the desire account is that we do regard it as seriously wrong to kill persons who have little desire to live or who have no desire to live or, indeed, have a desire not to live. We believe it is seriously wrong to kill the unconscious, the sleeping, those who are tired of life, and those who are suicidal. The value-of-a-human-future account renders standard morality intelligible in these cases; these cases appear to be incompatible with the desire account.

The desire account is subject to a deeper difficulty. We desire life, because we value the goods of this life. The goodness of life is not secondary to our desire for it. If this were not so, the pain of one's own premature death could be done away with merely by an appropriate alteration in the configuration of one's desires. This is absurd. Hence, it would seem that it is the loss of the goods of one's future, not the interference with the fulfillment of a strong desire to live, which accounts ultimately for the wrongness of killing.

It is worth noting that, if the desire account is modified so that it does not provide a necessary, but only a sufficient, condition for the wrongness of killing, the desire account is compatible with the value of a future-like-ours account. The combined accounts will yield an anti-abortion ethic. This suggests that one can retain what is intuitively plausible about the desire account without a challenge to the basic argument of this paper.

It is also worth noting that, if future desires have moral force in a modified desire account of the wrongness of killing, one can find support for an anti-abortion ethic even in the absence of a value of a future-like-ours account. If one decides that a morally relevant property, the possession of which is sufficient to make it wrong to kill some individual, is the desire at some future time to live – one might decide to justify one's refusal to kill suicidal teenagers on these grounds, for example – then, since typical fetuses will have the desire in the future to live, it is wrong to kill typical fetuses. Accordingly, it does not seem that a desire account of the wrongness of killing can provide a justification of a pro-choice ethic of abortion which is nearly as adequate as the value of a human-future justification of an anti-abortion ethic.

The discontinuation account looks more promising as an account of the wrongness of killing. It seems just as intelligible as the value of a future-like-ours account, but it does not justify an anti-abortion position. Obviously, if it is the continuation of one's activities, experiences, and projects, the loss of which makes killing wrong, then it is not wrong to kill fetuses for that reason, for fetuses do not have experiences, activities, and projects to be continued or discontinued. Accordingly, the discontinuation account does not have the anti-abortion consequences that the value of a future-like-ours account has. Yet, it seems as intelligible as the value of a future-like-ours account, for when we think of what would be wrong with our being killed, it does seem as if it is the discontinuation of what makes our lives worthwhile which makes killing us wrong.

Is the discontinuation account just as good an account as the value of a future-like-ours account? The discontinuation account will not be adequate at all, if it does not refer to the *value* of the experience that may be discontinued. One does not want the discontinuation account to make it wrong to kill a patient who begs for death and who is in severe pain that cannot be relieved short of killing. (I leave open the question of whether it is wrong for other reasons.) Accordingly, the discontinuation account must be more than a bare discontinuation account. It must make some reference to the positive value of the patient's experiences. But, by the same token, the value of a future-like-ours account cannot be a bare future account either. Just having a future surely does not itself rule out killing the above patient. This account must make some reference to the value of the patient's future experiences and projects also. Hence, both accounts involve the value of experiences, projects, and activities. So far we still have symmetry between the accounts.

The symmetry fades, however, when we focus on the time period of the value of the experiences, etc., which has moral consequences. Although both accounts leave open the possibility that the patient in our example may be killed, this possibility is left open only in virtue of the utterly bleak future for the patient. It makes no difference whether the patient's immediate past contains intolerable pain, or consists in being in a coma (which we can imagine is a situation of indifference), or consists in a life of value.

If the patient's future is a future of value, we want our account to make it wrong to kill the patient. If the patient's future is intolerable, whatever his or her immediate past, we want our account to allow killing the patient. Obviously, then, it is the value of that patient's future which is doing the work in rendering the morality of killing the patient intelligible.

This being the case, it seems clear that whether one has immediate past experiences or not does no work in the explanation of what makes killing wrong. The addition the discontinuation account makes to the value of a human future account is otiose. Its addition to the value-of-a-future account plays no role at all in rendering intelligible the wrongness of killing. Therefore, it can be discarded with the discontinuation account of which it is a part.

IV

The analysis of the previous section suggests that alternative general accounts of the wrongness of killing are either inadequate or unsuccessful in getting around the anti-abortion consequences of the value of a future-like-ours argument. A different strategy for avoiding these anti-abortion consequences involves limiting the scope of the value of a future argument. More precisely, the strategy involves arguing that fetuses lack a property that is essential for the value-of-a-future argument (or for any anti-abortion argument) to apply to them.

One move of this sort is based upon the claim that a necessary condition of one's future being valuable is that one values it. Value implies a valuer. Given this one might argue that, since fetuses cannot value their futures, their futures are not valuable to them. Hence, it does not seriously wrong them deliberately to end their lives.

This move fails, however, because of some ambiguities. Let us assume that something cannot be of value unless it is valued by someone. This does not entail that my life is of no value unless it is valued by me. I may think, in a period of despair, that my future is of no worth whatsoever, but I may be wrong because others rightly see value – even great value – in it.

Furthermore, my future can be valuable to me even if I do not value it. This is the case when a young person attempts suicide, but is rescued and goes on to significant human achievements. Such young people's futures are ultimately valuable to them, even though such futures do not seem to be valuable to them at the moment of attempted suicide. A fetus's future can be valuable to it in the same way. Accordingly, this attempt to limit the anti-abortion argument fails.

Another similar attempt to reject the anti-abortion position is based on Tooley's claim that an entity cannot possess the right to life unless it has the capacity to desire its continued existence. It follows that, since fetuses lack the conceptual capacity to desire to continue to live, they lack the right to life. Accordingly, Tooley concludes that abortion cannot be seriously prima facie wrong ("Abortion and Infanticide," pp. 46–7 [see chapter 2 in this volume]).

What could be the evidence for Tooley's basic claim? Tooley once argued that individuals have a prima facie right to what they desire and that the lack of the capacity to desire something undercuts the basis of one's right to it (pp. 44–5). This argument plainly will not succeed in the context of the analysis of this essay, however, since the point here is to establish the fetus's right to life on other grounds. Tooley's argument assumes that the right to life cannot be established in general on some basis other than the desire for life. This position was considered and rejected in the preceding section of this paper.

One might attempt to defend Tooley's basic claim on the grounds that, because a fetus cannot apprehend continued life as a benefit, its continued life cannot be a benefit or cannot be something it has a right to or cannot be something that is in its interest. This might be defended in terms of the general proposition that, if an individual is literally incapable of caring about or taking an interest in some X, then one does not have a right to X or X is not a benefit or X is not something that is in one's interest.[11]

Each member of this family of claims seems to be open to objections. As John C. Stevens[12] has pointed out, one may have a right to be treated with a certain medical procedure (because of a health insurance policy one has purchased), even though one cannot conceive of the nature of the procedure. And, as Tooley himself has pointed out, persons who have been indoctrinated, or drugged, or rendered temporarily unconscious may be literally incapable of caring about or taking an interest in something that is in their interest or is something to which they have a right, or is something that benefits them. Hence, the Tooley claim that would restrict the scope of the value of a future-like-ours argument is undermined by counterexamples.[13]

Finally, Paul Bassen[14] has argued that, even though the prospects of an embryo might seem to be a basis for the wrongness of abortion, an embryo cannot be a victim and therefore cannot be wronged. An embryo cannot be a victim, he says, because it lacks sentience. His central argument for this seems to be that, even though plants and the permanently unconscious are alive, they clearly cannot be victims. What is the explanation of this? Bassen claims that the explanation is that their lives consist of mere metabolism and mere metabolism is not enough to ground victimizability. Mentation is required.

The problem with this attempt to establish the absence of victimizability is that both plants and the permanently unconscious clearly lack what Bassen calls "prospects" or what I have called "a future life like ours." Hence, it is surely open to one to argue that the real reason we believe plants and the permanently unconscious cannot be victims is that killing them cannot deprive them of a future life like ours; the real reason is not their absence of present mentation.

Bassen recognizes that his view is subject to this difficulty, and he recognizes that the case of children seems to support this difficulty, for "much of what we do for children is based on prospects." He argues, however, that, in the case of children and in other such cases, "potentiality comes into play only where victimizability has been secured on other grounds" (p. 333).

Bassen's defense of his view is patently question-begging, since what is adequate to secure victimizability is exactly what is at issue. His examples do not support his own view against the thesis of this essay.

Of course, embryos can be victims: when their lives are deliberately terminated, they are deprived of their futures of value, their prospects. This makes them victims, for it directly wrongs them.

The seeming plausibility of Bassen's view stems from the fact that paradigmatic cases of imagining someone as a victim involve empathy, and empathy requires mentation of the victim. The victims of flood, famine, rape, or child abuse are all persons with whom we can empathize. That empathy seems to be part of seeing them as victims.[15]

In spite of the strength of these examples, the attractive intuition that a situation in which there is victimization requires the possibility of empathy is subject to counterexamples. Consider a case that Bassen himself offers: "Posthumous obliteration of an author's work constitutes a misfortune for him only if he had wished his work to endure" (p. 318). The conditions Bassen wishes to impose upon the possibility of being victimized here seem far too strong. Perhaps this author, due to his unrealistic standards of excellence and his low self-esteem, regarded his work as unworthy of survival, even though it possessed genuine literary merit. Destruction of such work would surely victimize its author. In such a case, empathy with the victim concerning the loss is clearly impossible.

Of course, Bassen does not make the possibility of empathy a necessary condition of victimizability; he requires only mentation. Hence, on Bassen's actual view, this author, as I have described him, can be a victim. The problem is that the basic intuition that renders Bassen's view plausible is missing in the author's case. In order to attempt to avoid counterexamples, Bassen has made his thesis too weak to be supported by the intuitions that suggested it.

Even so, the mentation requirement on victimizability is still subject to counterexamples. Suppose a severe accident renders me totally unconscious for a month, after which I recover. Surely killing me while I am unconscious victimizes me, even though I am incapable of mentation during that time. It follows that Bassen's thesis fails. Apparently, attempts to restrict the value of a future-like-ours argument so that fetuses do not fall within its scope do not succeed.

V

In this essay, it has been argued that the correct ethic of the wrongness of killing can be extended to fetal life and used to show that there is a strong presumption that any abortion is morally impermissible. If the ethic of killing adopted here entails, however, that contraception is also seriously immoral, then there would appear to be a difficulty with the analysis of this essay.

But this analysis does not entail that contraception is wrong. Of course, contraception prevents the actualization of a possible future of value. Hence, it follows from the claim that if futures of value should be maximized that contraception is prima facie immoral. This obligation to maximize does not exist, however; furthermore, nothing in the ethics of killing in this paper entails that it does. The ethics of killing in this essay would entail that contraception is wrong only if something were denied a human future of value by contraception. Nothing at all is denied such a future by contraception, however.

Candidates for a subject of harm by contraception fall into four categories: (1) some sperm or other, (2) some ovum or other, (3) a sperm and an ovum separately, and (4) a sperm and an ovum together. Assigning the harm to some sperm is utterly arbitrary, for no reason can be given for making a sperm the subject of harm rather than an ovum. Assigning the harm to some ovum is utterly arbitrary, for no reason can be given for making an ovum the subject of harm rather than a sperm. One might attempt to avoid these problems by insisting that contraception deprives both the sperm and the ovum separately of a valuable future like ours. On this alternative, too many futures are lost. Contraception was supposed to be wrong, because it deprived us of one future of value, not two. One might attempt to avoid this problem by holding that contraception deprives the combination of sperm and ovum of a valuable future like ours. But here the definite article misleads. At the time of contraception, there are hundreds of millions of sperm, one (released) ovum and millions of possible combinations of all of these. There is no actual combination at all. Is the subject of the loss to be a merely possible combination? Which one? This alternative does not yield an actual subject of harm either. Accordingly, the immorality of contraception is not entailed by the loss of a future-like-ours argument simply because there is no nonarbitrarily identifiable subject of the loss in the case of contraception.

VI

The purpose of this essay has been to set out an argument for the serious presumptive wrongness of abortion subject to the assumption that the moral permissibility of abortion stands or falls on the moral status of the fetus. Since a fetus possesses a property, the possession of which in adult human beings is sufficient to make killing an adult human being wrong, abortion is wrong. This way of dealing with the problem of abortion seems superior to other approaches to the ethics of abortion, because it rests on an ethics of killing which is close to self-evident, because the crucial morally relevant property clearly applies to fetuses, and because the argument avoids the usual equivocations on "human life," "human being," or "person." The argument rests neither on religious claims nor on Papal dogma. It is not subject to the objection of "speciesism." Its soundness is compatible with the moral permissibility of euthanasia and contraception. It deals with our intuitions concerning young children.

Finally, this analysis can be viewed as resolving a standard problem – indeed, *the* standard problem – concerning the ethics of abortion. Clearly, it is wrong to kill adult human beings. Clearly, it is not wrong to end the life of some arbitrarily chosen single human cell. Fetuses seem to be like arbitrarily chosen human cells in some respects and like adult humans in other respects. The problem of the ethics of abortion is the problem of determining the fetal property that settles this moral controversy. The thesis of this essay is that the problem of the ethics of abortion, so understood, is solvable.

Notes

1 Feinberg, "Abortion," in *Matters of Life and Death: New Introductory Essays in Moral Philosophy*, Tom Regan, ed. (New York: Random House, 1986), pp. 256–93; Tooley, "*Abortion and Infanticide*," *Philosophy and Public Affairs*, II, 1 (1972): 37–65 [see chapter 1 in this volume], Tooley, *Abortion and Infanticide* (New York: Oxford, 1984); Warren, "*On the Moral and Legal Status of Abortion*," *The Monist*, 1.VII, 1 (1973): 43–61; Engelhardt, "*The Ontology of Abortion*," *Ethics*, I. XXXIV, 3 (1974): 217–34; Sumner, *Abortion and Moral Theory* (Princeton: University Press, 1981); Noonan, "An Almost Absolute Value in History," in *The Morality of Abortion: Legal and Historical Perspectives*, Noonan, ed. (Cambridge: Harvard, 1970); and Devine, *The Ethics of Homicide* (Ithaca: Cornell, 1978).

2 For interesting discussions of this issue, see Warren Quinn, "*Abortion: Identity and Loss*," *Philosophy and Public Affairs*, XIII, 1 (1984): 24–54; and Lawrence C. Becker, "*Human Being: The Boundaries of the Concept*," *Philosophy and Public Affairs*, IV, 4 (1975): 334–59.

3 For example, see my "Ethics and the Elderly: Some Problems," in Stuart Spicker, Kathleen Woodward, and David Van Tassel, eds., *Aging and the Elderly: Humanistic Perspectives in Gerontology* (Atlantic Highlands, NJ: Humanities, 1978), pp. 341–55.

4 See Warren, "On the Moral and Legal Status of Abortion," and Tooley, "Abortion and Infanticide."

5 This seems to be the fatal flaw in Warren's treatment of this issue.

6 I have been most influenced on this matter by Jonathan Glover, *Causing Death and Saving Lives* (New York: Penguin, 1977), ch. 3; and Robert Young, "*What Is So Wrong with Killing People?*" *Philosophy*, LIV, 210 (1979): 515–28.

7 Feinberg, Tooley, Warren, and Engelhardt have all dealt with this problem.

8 Kant, "Duties to Animals and Spirits," in *Lectures on Ethics*, trans. Louis Infeld (New York: Harper, 1963), p. 239.

9 I am indebted to Jack Bricke for raising this objection.

10 Presumably a preference utilitarian would press such an objection. Tooley once suggested that his account has such a theoretical underpinning. See his "Abortion and Infanticide," pp. 44–5.

11 Donald VanDeVeer seems to think this is self-evident. See his "Whither Baby Doe?" in *Matters of Life and Death*, p. 233.

12 "Must the Bearer of a Right Have the Concept of That to Which He Has a Right?" *Ethics*, XCV, 1 (1984): 68–74.

13 See Tooley again in "Abortion and Infanticide," pp. 47–9.

14 "Present Sakes and Future Prospects: The Status of Early Abortion," *Philosophy and Public Affairs*, XI, 4 (1982): 322–6.

15 Note carefully the reasons he gives on the bottom of p. 316.

Part II

Issues in Reproduction

Introduction

Developments in reproductive medicine have, over the past 50 years, presented us with remarkable new options, giving us increasing control over our fertility. Effective contraception and sterilization procedures have separated sex from reproduction, while various infertility treatments, such as in vitro fertilization, have dramatically increased the possibilities for reproduction without sex. Fertile couples are now able to limit and space the number of children they are going to have, while those who were once considered infertile are able to have children.

There are also new opportunities to decide what our children will be like. Prenatal diagnosis of fetuses and testing of in vitro embryos allows prospective parents to decide not to bring a disabled child into the world, even without the use of abortion. (Those who accept the view defended by Patrick Lee and Rober P. George in the previous Part of this *Anthology* will not be mollified by a procedure that still involves the discarding of a viable human embryo.) The same techniques allow parents to select the sex of their child. Cloning and genetic modification of offspring are now possible for several species of mammals, and some think that it is only a matter of time before they take place in humans as well.

A wide range of different issues are covered in this Part of the *Anthology*. Two interrelated clusters of questions, whilst by no means exhaustive of the ethical issues raised, are central to many of the discussions presented here: the limits, if any, to reproductive freedom, and the rights or interests of future children.

Assisted Reproduction

Being unable to have children can be a source of profound grief and great unhappiness. But some widely accepted technologies and procedures for overcoming infertility continue to raise troubling ethical issues. Fertility drugs given to women to enhance the production of eggs can lead to multiple pregnancies. When a woman carries more than one fetus, infants are frequently born prematurely and, if not stillborn, may have to spend long periods in neonatal intensive care. There is also an increased risk of brain damage and other serious disabilities.

In the first article in this Part, Greg Pence ("The McCaughey Septuplets: God's Will or Human Choice?") describes the case of 29-year-old Bobbi McCaughey, whose use of a fertility drug led to her giving birth, in 1996, to seven infants. All survived, but with a range of different disabilities. While aware of the risks, the couple had rejected the idea of selectively aborting a number of the fetuses, saying that whatever happened was "God's will". But, writes Pence, it is difficult to hold God responsible for any children turning out disabled or dead: "If God was clear about anything in this case, it was that the McCaugheys should not have kids. Otherwise, why did He make them infertile?" Rather than being able to claim that God is responsible, Pence argues, those who take fertility drugs should, if necessary, be willing to reduce the number of fetuses "for the good of the children" born.

One outcome of the new reproductive techniques is that they make it easier for same-sex couples to have children who are genetically related to at least one of them.

A few years ago, to discuss the provision of assisted reproduction to same-sex couples would have been pushing the frontiers of what is socially acceptable.

With increasing acceptance of same-sex marriage, and of the rights of same-sex couples to have children, however, the use of assisted reproduction by same-sex couples is increasing, and no longer seems as shocking as it once did. Timothy F. Murphy in "The Meaning of Synthetic Gametes for Gay and Lesbian People and Bioethics too" asks why so many ethical analyses of such technologies still treat same-sex couples' use of them as controversial, while the same questions are not raised when it comes to opposite-sex couples. He responds to arguments defending the view that children ought to be conceived only under certain natural conditions, noting that there is no evidence that children who are conceived by other means are harmed in any way by the conditions of their conception and parentage.

Other authors have argued that anonymous donor gametes are problematic because that option would separate children from their biological parents. David Velleman offers such an account. He thinks that without knowledge of one's genetic parents children would suffer an information deficit in terms of what kind of life they could expect with genes like theirs. Murphy tackles this argument by pointing to the fact that children conceived of the synthetic gametes of a same-sex couple would not actually suffer such an information deficit, and so new technologies

could actually insist in overcoming the disadvantage Velleman is concerned about.

Murphy concludes his analysis by addressing the objection from shared genetics. He rejects the idea that shared genetics is a necessary condition for good parenthood, agreeing instead with Thomas Murray, who argued that what makes for good parenthood is a moral commitment to one's offspring.

When controversial new reproductive possibilities are first mooted, those opposed to the innovation often argue that the children produced by it will be harmed in some way. This argument was used against the introduction of in vitro fertilization, and it was also used against same-sex couples being allowed to have children. So far, such arguments have generally lacked evidence; but in any case, should we accept the assumption that *if* children produced by a new reproductive technique were in some way less well-off than other children, this would be a ground for not permitting the new technique? Derek Parfit offers an argument against this assumption in his article "Rights, Interests, and Possible People." He asks readers to consider the case of a woman who wants to stop taking contraceptive pills in order to have another child. She is told by her doctor that she is suffering from a temporary condition that will result in any child she conceives now having a disability – although one that is still compatible with living a worthwhile life. If she waits three months, on the other hand, she will conceive a normal child. Many people think that if the woman decides not to wait, she will be harming her child. But, Parfit argues, this conclusion does not follow. If the woman were to wait, she would not be having *this* child, but a different child – a child conceived three months later from a different egg and a different sperm. Based on the assumption that the first child, while disabled, has a life worth living, it would thus be difficult to claim that the disabled child has been harmed by having been brought into existence. His life is still better than no life at all.

If Parfit is correct on this point, could it still be claimed that single women and lesbian couples should be denied access to infertility services for the sake of their as-yet-unconceived children? On the face of it, this could be argued only if these children were going to have lives so devoid of happiness and whatever else makes a life worth living that non-existence is preferable to existence. Given that this is an implausible supposition, denying access to infertility services to same-sex couples would prevent the existence of children who would very probably have lived worthwhile lives. We can hardly justify a prohibition on the use of assisted reproduction on the grounds that the prohibition is in the best interests of the children who would be born as a result of that use, if the children would have worthwhile lives, and without the availability of the technique, would not be born at all.

Prenatal Screening, Sex Selection, and Cloning

As our knowledge of genetics expands, prospective parents are increasingly given the opportunity to make use of this knowledge, to prevent the birth of genetically compromised children. Here it is important to note that prevention need not involve abortion or the destruction of preimplantation embryos. At-risk parents can avoid having a disabled child by deciding not to have children, by adopting children, or by using donor gametes or embryos.

Is it wrong to bring severely disabled children into the world, if one could avoid doing so? Laura M. Purdy in "Genetics and Reproductive Risk: Can Having Children be Immoral?" gives an affirmative answer. Rejecting the view "that it is morally permissible to conceive individuals so long as we do not expect them to be so miserable that they wish they were dead," she argues that parents ought to ensure that any children they are going to have, possess "normal health." While she acknowledges that the notion is vague, she takes it to be sufficient to mark out as wrong the bringing into the world of children who are at risk of having serious genetic afflictions, such as Huntington's disease.

The notion that there ought to be a sphere of liberty within which prospective parents are free to make reproductive choices is widely accepted. There is,

however, disagreement as to whether reproductive liberty has limits, and if it does, where these limits ought to be drawn. Take sex selection. Many jurisdictions allow parents to prevent the birth of children affected by certain genetic diseases, but do not allow them to do this for non-medical reasons, such as wanting to balance the sex ratio of their children. In a statement entitled "Sex Selection and Preimplantation Genetic Diagnosis," the Ethics Committee of the American Society of Reproductive Medicine indicates the extent to which it shares the concerns behind such laws. The Committee itself does not believe that non-medical sex selection is so clearly and seriously wrong that it favors the use of the law to prohibit it. Instead, the Committee would stop at discouraging sex selection for non-medical reasons.

Julian Savulescu and Edgar Dahl respond to the Committee's statement in their essay "Sex Selection and Preimplantation Diagnosis." They find its arguments unpersuasive, particularly given that, in Western societies, most people seeking to use sex selection do so not because they value one sex more than the other, but to balance the number of boys and girls in their family.

Those opposing preimplantation genetic diagnosis for the above purpose may, however, have concerns that go beyond the welfare interests of the future child. David King explains "Why We Should Not Permit Embryos to be Selected as Tissue Donors." He believes that the practice objectifies the child and turns it into a mere tool. This contradicts, he says, the basic Kantian ethical principle that human beings must always be treated as ends, and never merely as a means to an end. Even if the future child will be a much-loved member of the family, we ought to resist the temptation to allow the selection of embryos as tissue donors because it is yet another step in the objectification of humans and "and the consequences of doing so are . . . disastrous."

But is the maxim that we must never regard others solely as a means to an end infringed if the tissue-matched child is loved and cherished in its own right, as an end? Kant's maxim provides, as King correctly notes, a plausible account of what is wrong with slavery, but its implication in the present context is far less clear. People generally have children for a variety of reasons: they want a sister for "Ann," a companion for their old age, a son to continue the blood line, and so on. If tissue-matching of embryos to save another child were ruled out by the Kantian maxim, would this not also perhaps rule out many other widely accepted reasons for having children as well?

In allowing tissue-matching of embryos, we are, King holds, proceeding down a slippery slope toward some very bad societal consequences. Critics of this kind of argument might question, however, whether the bad consequences at the bottom of the slope are truly bad, or as bad as they are made out to be. They may also ask whether the slope is really so slippery and if sound laws and public policies would not arrest any possible slide.

For many people reproductive human cloning is one of the bad consequences that lie at the bottom of the slippery slope. When the existence of the sheep "Dolly" (the first mammal to owe its existence to somatic cell nuclear transfer, or cloning) was announced in 1997, there was swift world-wide reaction. People feared that the cloning of humans would

not be far away. Only 24 hours after the world knew of Dolly's existence, a bill outlawing human cloning was announced in New York State, and a few days later, then US President Clinton banned federal funding for research into it.

Michael Tooley examines this issue in "The Moral Status of Human Cloning: Neo-Lockean Persons versus Human Embryos." In earlier editions of this *Anthology*, we included an article by the same author, first published in 1998. In that earlier article, Tooly distinguished between the questions of whether reproductive human cloning is *in principle* morally acceptable and whether it is acceptable *at the present time*, given current scientific knowledge and understanding. He then reached the conclusion that the practice was acceptable in principle, but morally problematic, given the state of knowledge at the time. In this new article, specially written for this volume, Tooley notes more recent research that makes it less likely that cloning from an adult would produce a person with reduced life expectancy. In this and other ways, his conclusion is now more open to the acceptability of human reproductive cloning, both in principle and in practice, than it was in his earlier article.

Assisted Reproduction

5

The McCaughey Septuplets
God's Will or Human Choice?[1]

Gregory Pence

In 1997, American media rejoiced that all seven of the McCaugheys' fetuses made it to birth and seemed healthy. Yet for all the coverage of that story, rarely did the darkerv truth emerge. Call me a curmudgeon, but something is wrong here.

We often over-generalize from well-publicized cases (e.g., after the 1986 Baby M case, some states banned commercial surrogacy). In France since 1982 – where couples sometimes pursue pregnancy with religious zeal because each new baby garners a bonus from the government – use of fertility drugs has increased tenfold the number of triplets and the number of quadruplets, thirtyfold.

Some complain about the costs to society of so many babies in one birth, and true, the gestation, birth, and special care of the septuplets probably cost a cool million dollars. Others complain that the human uterus did not evolve to bear litters and that large multiple births are unnatural. Still others wonder what toll this extraordinary gestation had on mother McCaughey's body and health.

These are important matters, but they strike me as morally secondary. Costs can be absorbed by being spread over millions of payers, and what is unnatural in one era becomes normal in the next (witness anesthesia). And if Mrs McCaughey made an informed choice, she was free to risk injuring her body in childbirth as she saw fit.

Still others wonder if these two parents could really nurture each of the septuplets. Would you want to grow up with one-seventh of the attention you got from your dad? Did the McCaugheys have the time, energy, and money to nourish each child's full potential?

My real concern is about what is best for the children. This couple took the fertility drug Pergonal, conceived seven embryos, refused to reduce any (abort), and then said that any results were "God's will." In doing so, they risked the lives and health of their babies. They took bad odds and hoped that all seven would be healthy. In so doing, they took the risk of having seven disabled, or even seven dead, babies.

Pause a minute and consider the "frame" or background assumptions of how the media presents multiple births: often it's in the language of "miracles," "blessings" and "heroic" parents. But consider my

Original publication details: Gregory Pence, "Multiple Gestation and Damaged Babies: God's Will or Human Choice?" This essay draws on "The McCaughey Septuplets: God's Will or Human Choice," pp. 39–43 from Gregory Pence, *Brave New Bioethics* (Lanham, MD: Rowman & Littlefield, 2002). © 2002 Gregory Pence. Reproduced courtesy of Gregory Pence.

experience once in China during their one-child-only decades: on a public bus, a woman then entered who had just given birth to her second child: the other mothers on the bus quickly shamed her: "How could you be so selfish? Your new child will take food from mine. Why were you so irresponsible?" Imagine what the same women would say to Mrs McCaughey for creating septuplets when she already had one child.

Multiple-birth babies are: usually premature (each may weigh less than two pounds), three times as likely as single babies to be severely handicapped at birth, and often spend months in neonatal intensive care units. In the womb with multiple pregnancies, nutrients and oxygenated blood are scarce (a uterine lifeboat, if you will), so not all the fetuses will likely emerge healthy. To prevent disabilities resulting from deprivation in utero, the American Society for Reproductive Medicine recommends gestating only one embryo at a time.

It seems to me irresponsible to say, as the McCaugheys did, that it would be God's will if any turned out blind, crippled, or dead. If God was clear about anything to them, it was that they should not have kids.

If you take a fertility drug, and if too many embryos conceive, you should be willing to reduce the embryos for the good of the children born. You shouldn't run the risk of severely-disabled kids, and say, if harm happens, that it's "God's will." Be honest and say it's a grave risk you decided to take.

And what about the older sister of the McCaughey septuplets? Was her role in childhood only to help her mother raise the famous septs? Did she have any choice?

In 1985, Mormons Patti and Sam Frustaci conceived septuplets. Informed of the risks of disability and urged to reduce, they refused. Four of their seven babies died, and the three survivors had severe disabilities, including cerebral palsy. The Frustacis then sued their physicians.

In 1996 in England, Mandy Allwood conceived seven embryos at once. Offered a large cash bonus by a tabloid for exclusive rights if all made it to term, Mandy announced she would not reduce any and go for maximal births. As a result, she lost all of them.

I once heard about a case of a multiple pregnancy in West Virginia where the woman refused selective reduction. As a result of taking such a risk, only one child survived and this child was blind, paraplegic, and severely retarded. The physician on the case said that henceforth he would no longer accept women who would not agree to selective reduction. He said he did not get into assisted reproduction to create severely damaged babies, and that, although women have the right to refuse abortion, they would need to find another physician who could accept such terrible outcomes.

Not too many people are interested in long-term follow-up, yet the details that emerge are not encouraging.

At their fourth birthday in 2001, the McCaughey septuplets lagged in development and were not all potty trained. Joel suffered seizures; Nathan has spastic diplegia, a form of cerebral palsy requiring botox injections (to paralyze spastic muscles) and orthopedic braces. Alexis has hypotonic quadriplegia, a cerebral palsy that causes muscle weakness. Nathan could not walk at age seven and had two major surgeries to help him do so. Alexis had an indwelling feeding tube for four years. Although the McCaugheys home-schooled their children, they sent Nathan and Alexis to a school for developmentally challenged children financed by taxpayers.[2]

The Canadian Dionne quintuplets were born in 1934, and although all seemed healthy at birth, only three lived to 2000 (one died at age 20 of an epileptic seizure). Because their selfish parents exploited their fame, the children did not lead happy lives.

Nadya Suleman, aka the "Octomom," of California, 32-years-old in 2009, had six embryos left over from previous in-vitro fertilization treatments; she requested another cycle of IVF to implant them all. Two of the six embryos split into twins, resulting in eight embryos. When sonograms in the first trimester revealed at least five fetuses, Suleman refused reduction. At birth, physicians delivered eight babies. Nadya already had children from previous cycles of IVF, two of whom were disabled.

Kate and Jon Gosselin in Pennsylvania created a family of twin girls (born from insemination of Jon's sperm in 2000) and sextuplets (3 girls and 3 boys). Fertility doctors started the sextuplets by injecting Kate with drugs to stimulate her ovaries (like the McCaughey case) and afterwards, introduced Jon's sperm. Informed of six pregnancies, the Gosselins chose not to reduce, so physicians delivered eight babies by caesarean in 2004.

The 2007 television series *Jon & Kate Plus 8* filmed the controlled chaos of this family of ten glamorized having multiple babies. Shortly after birth, a plastic surgeon did free plastic surgery to correct the distortion of Kate's stomach after gestating six babies.

In 2009, after both Gosselins had extra-marital affairs, they divorced. Thereafter, Jon seemed to abandon his interest in the children. Both Gosselins and Nadya Suleman seemed immature, self-absorbed, and not focused on the best interests of their eight children.

New York City's Major Guiliani was recently on a call-in radio show when an Orthodox Jewish woman with five little babies (three of them identical triplets) said she felt like killing herself because her babies were driving her crazy. Although the Mayor quickly got her help (he was running for re-election), what about all the other parents who don't get the free pampers and cars? In a similar case, Jacqueline Thompson, a black mother of sextuplets, and her husband Linden were living exhausted on the edge in Washington, D. C. until a radio caller publicized their plight.

Some argue that babies born as multiples cannot be harmed because if the mother had reduced to one embryo, the others would not have existed. Isn't it better to exist as a disabled child than not to exist at all? My answer is that we must access morality not only from a consequentialist view but also from other moral perspectives, not just from thinking about harm to children but also from thinking about the motives of parents. Why would any parents deliberately choose a disabled child when they could have a healthy one? Can they universalize not choosing what is the best life for their subsequent children? Wouldn't virtuous parents choose, not what is best for themselves, but what is best for the lives of their children? In the Ethics of Care, wouldn't compassionate parents want the best for their own children?

Someone might here object that choosing only healthy children exhibits prejudice against people with disabilities. I answer that not supporting (or killing) disabled children differs dramatically from not creating them in the first place. Our principles, our moral intuitions, do not support abandoning or terminating babies with severe disabilities, but the same principles and intuitions support not intentionally creating such children.

Overall, in America we are a long way from a philosophically consistent policy on fetal rights and reproductive responsibility. In the *Whitner* case in 1997, the Supreme Court of South Carolina ruled that a pregnant mother can be prosecuted for using cocaine because such usage harms her fetus. In another example, in 2002 the President's Council on Bioethics chaired by Leon Kass said that no child should be originated by cloning because of possible harm to the new baby. Yet the McCaugheys and other parents of multiples take terrible risks of creating disabled children and, when they invoke God's will, are seen as heroes. Something seems akilter here.

Notes

1 This essay originally appeared in the *Birmingham News* 1 December 1997 and was revised by the author for the 4th edition of this anthology.

2 Ann Curry, "After 10 Years, New Adventures for Septuplets," *Dateline*, December 12, 2007. http://www.nbcnews.com/id/22223331/#.USAS0hzB-AE

6

The Meaning of Synthetic Gametes for Gay and Lesbian People and Bioethics Too

Timothy F. Murphy

Researchers have had success in using synthetic gametes – sperm derived from female stem cells and ova derived from male stem cells – to produce live offspring in laboratory animals.[1] The prospects for same-sex couples to have children using only their gametes has been predicted in some of the earliest reports of success in the development of synthetic gametes, and some researchers have mapped this outcome as meaningfully within the range of possibility.[2] Even so, considerable work remains to be done before human beings conceived with synthetic gametes could materialise this way,

Gay and lesbian people do already have children, of course, from opposite-sex relationships, by adoption, through surrogacy arrangements, and – more recently – through various assisted reproductive treatments (ART). As many as six million people in the USA have a gay or lesbian parent.[3] Because of shifting social views, it is likely that many more children of gay and lesbian parents are on the way. For example, the American Society of Reproductive Medicine now counsels its members to offer their services without regard to sexual orientation or marital status.[4] Even

so, two men or two women hoping to have children together cannot expect to share genetic parenthood, although certain symbolic gestures toward shared parenthood are available. For example, one woman might offer ova for fertilisation while her partner gestates the children.[5] Two gay men may blend their sperm prior to insemination when relying on surrogate gestation for a child so that the child's genetics are a matter of chance rather than choice. By contrast with these practices, the use of synthetic gametes – ova derived from males and sperm derived from females – stands poised to offer same-sex couples ways to share full genetic parenthood of their children.

Despite the increasing social acceptance of gay men and lesbians around the world, the prospect of parenthood by homosexual men and women raises suspicion and even outright rejection in some quarters, and these objections carry over to bioethics as well. I want to show examples of these objections in a range of bioethics analysis, and show how synthetic gametes would – paradoxically – disarm key elements of these objections. In doing so, I hope to make the case that it is past time to move past the burdens of proof that

Original publication details: Timothy Murphy, "The Meaning of Synthetic Gametes for Gay and Lesbian People and Bioethics Too," pp. 762–765 from *Journal of Medical Ethics* 40 (2014). Reproduced with permission of BMJ Publishing Group Ltd.

are reflexively invoked in regard to parenthood by gay men and lesbians whenever a novel method of assisted conception surfaces.

Controversial Parenthood

When it comes to same-sex couples turning to synthetic gametes, A. J. Newson and Anna Smajdor say 'new ethical questions' arise, 'such as whether same-sex couples should be able to access this technology to have children who are genetically related to them both'.[6] I fully concede that the prospect of same-sex couples as the genetic parents of children *is* a novel question, but the question of cross-sex gamete production is not any more novel for them than for anyone else. If synthetic gametes become possible, any man or woman can be the source of sperm or ova no matter what kind of relationship they are in. Yet Newson and Smajdor do not treat the use of synthetic gametes for infertile opposite-sex couples as a specifically ethical concern; they certainly do not frame the question of synthetic gametes for opposite-sex couples as a question of access, presumably because they assume these couples to be fit as parents in all the ways that matter. In regard to same-sex couples, Newson and Smajdor go on to ask 'Will a man whose DNA is contained in the egg (used to produce a child) be recognised as a "biological" mother?' (see page 186 from Newson et al.[6]). By contrast, they ask no parallel question of ethics and access for their own example of single men or women who might rely on their own sperm and synthetic ova to produce a child. In any case, why assume that a man whose synthesised ovum is used to produce a child cannot be recognised as the child's mother in a biological sense even as he retains a male identity? After all, one transgender man who gestated his own children expresses no doubts about being the children's father.[7] Techniques of fertility preservation for transgender men and women – preserving gametes prior to body modifications that would otherwise leave people infertile – are likely to increase the ranks of transgender men who are the genetic mothers of their children, and the ranks of

transgender women who are the genetic fathers of their children.[8] Rather than trying to retrofit all parents into mutually exclusive categories of mother and father, why not ask a more searching question, namely whether these categories offer an adequate vocabulary for expressing the relationships progenitors can have with their progeny?

Other discussions also represent the parenthood of gay men and lesbians as ethically controversial. In 2009, a study group of scientists, ethicists, journal editors and lawyers reviewed the science of synthetic gametes and suggested likely uses, some of which they said might require legal and policy oversight. This group indicated that the possibility of using synthetic gametes for reproduction in same-sex couples is unlikely in the future, for genetic reasons related to conception and embryogenesis.[9] Even so, their analysis does not rule out same-sex reproduction as impossible. Perhaps for that reason, the group went on to say 'same-sex reproduction is inarguably a controversial, if highly unlikely, potential end result of this research' (see page 13 from Mathews et al.[9]). The study group, therefore, identifies this kind of reproduction as 'requiring deliberation and possible policy options' (see table 1 from Mathews et al.).

This interpretation of same-sex reproduction as 'inarguably controversial' comes without any supporting rationale. By contrast, the study group did feel obliged to offer a rationale after describing other novel uses of synthetic gametes, such as the in vitro creation of human embryos for research that involves their destruction. The group noted that those practices offend people 'who imbue such embryos with full moral status' (see page 12 from Mathews et al.). By contrast, the idea that two men or two women conceive and raise a child together is represented as self-evidently controversial, requiring no supporting explanation at all.

Interpretations like these treat same-sex couples as a novelty act in bioethics, primarily by suggesting that their moral standing as parents requires levels of moral scrutiny not required of other parents. At the very least, discussions like these still suppose that someone – moral and social authorities – have to function as gatekeepers for homosexual men and women wanting to be parents, as against assuming in advance that any safe and effective treatment for infertility should be presumptively available to any adult, which is the entitlement these commentators confer without qualification on opposite-sex couples, subject only to the constraints of safety and efficacy of the intervention in question.

Protecting Children from Some Possible Parents

As against commentators whose background assumptions throw gay and lesbian parenthood into question, some commentators explicitly reject the idea that same-sex couples should be parents, at least not in any planned or socially approved way. Sometimes these objections focus on the nature of same-sex couples as parents; other times the objections focus on the way in which same-sex couples are able to have children.

As part of her objections to legalising same-sex marriage, Margaret Somerville has argued that giving the right to marry and to found a family 'to same-sex couples necessarily negates the rights of all (sic) children with respect to their biological origins and families, not just those born into same-sex marriage'.[10] She argues that same-sex marriage violates a sexual ecology important to the welfare of children, and undermines a social symbolism essential in the transmission of life. In general, then, society should not endorse gay and lesbian couples having children through, for example, legal recognition of same-sex marriage. Somerville wants society to endorse law and policies that enable children to be children of a woman whom they know as their mother and of a man whom they know as their father, as far as this effect is practically possible. This is not the entirety of her position, though, since she also argues that 'children have a right to be conceived from untampered-with biological origins, a right to be conceived from a natural sperm from one identified, living, adult man and a natural ovum from one identified, living,

adult woman. Society should not be complicit in, that is, should not approve or fund any procedure for the creation of a child, unless the procedure is consistent with the child's right to a natural biological heritage'.[11] This position does not rule out all assisted reproduction, but it would put limits on it, including the use of synthetic gametes by same-sex couples among others.

In one important way, however, synthetic gametes undo Somerville's objections to same-sex couples as parents of children. Relying on synthetic gametes, two men could serve as the genetic parents of a child, one as the source of sperm and the other as the source of ova. A child conceived this way could thus have both genetic parents available to him or her while growing up. Nothing about this circumstance would prevent a child from understanding one parent as its genetic mother and the other as its genetic father, even though both parents are otherwise male. Synthetic gametes give same-sex couples pretty much everything Somerville expects in terms of identifiable, genetic parents who presumptively have as much respect for the transmission of life as anyone else. If what Somerville wants is, however, that every child have available a genetic mother who identifies as a woman and a genetic father who identifies as a man, then synthetic gametes will not satisfy her, but even so, synthetic gametes raise the question of why fatherhood and motherhood must be understood in terms of genetics alone. As mentioned, Somerville defends a second front against parenting by same-sex couples: it is objectionable insofar as it involves any kind of modification of gametes. Synthetic gametes are morally wrong on their face, on this account, as much as for homosexual men and women as for anyone else. Somerville asserts the right of children to be conceived only under certain conditions, but since the children cannot have rights before they do – namely before they exist – the merit of this argument turns on the effects of the modifications in question. Somerville offers no evidence that children of gay and lesbian parents are materially harmed by the conditions of their conception and parentage, over and above being violated in their alleged rights. So long as the welfare of children does not suffer meaningful harm as demonstrated by the social sciences, and I submit that they do not,[12] it is, therefore, hard to see why parenthood by gay men and lesbians should be ruled out in general, or as an effect of synthetic gametes in particular.

Other commentators have also raised variations on the theme of harm that homosexual parents might inflict on their children. Abby Lippman and Stuart A. Newman worry that same-sex couples will see embryos produced with their synthetic and naturally produced gametes as 'assemblages' and feel less responsibility toward them.[13] Giuseppe Testa and John Harris correctly reply to this claim by noting that same-sex couples who expend the time and effort to have children with shared genetics will likely exhibit a strong sense of responsibility and attachment toward the embryos and children in question.[14] Given the moral and social history of suspicion toward homosexuality in general, it is perhaps easy to believe that gay and lesbian parents might have diminished capacities as parents, but the actual evidence shows no such effect, and there is no reason to assume a novel means of conception will change matters.[12]

David Velleman has put some de facto obstacles in the way of gay men and lesbians having children through ARTs. He raises objections to the use of anonymous donor gametes and embryos, saying that children, in general, should not be separated from their biological parents.[15] He holds that access to parents and other relatives, and knowledge about their lives, is a necessary condition of children's development and fulfilment. On this view, one's genetic relatives function as experiments of what one can do in life with genetics like one's own. Without that knowledge, children necessarily suffer a deficit in self-knowledge that is essential to self-formation. It is better, then, that children not be dissociated from their genetic parents and relatives so far as practical. Not all ARTs go forward with anonymous gametes and embryos, of course, but some do, and Velleman's approach raises a bar against any and all parentage by gay men and lesbians that relies on those treatments.

By contrast with anonymous gamete donation, synthetic gametes would give children of same-sex couples what Velleman wants from parental and familial relationships in general. Barring the loss of their parents through death or divorce, children conceived with the natural and synthetic gametes of a gay couple would have available to them genetic relatives on Partner A's side, namely grandparents, aunts and uncles, and other relatives. The children would also have available to them the same gamut of genetic relatives for Partner B. Neither partner, in this case, would function as a genetically identified or socially identified female. Yet, both the parents and their relatives would be available, at least in principle, to the child in providing examples of how to live and how the child might put his or her own similar genetic endowment to work in making choices in life. The same outcome holds for a child of a lesbian couple, conceived with natural and synthetic gametes.

Velleman might try and argue that having two fathers (or two mothers) amounts to a deprivation visited upon the children, but this argument will not succeed because his view does not require any specific content to the lives of genetic relatives, only that their lives and strivings be available to the children as kinds of experimental results of living with a similar genetic endowment. A man who uses ova synthesised from his body to have children is no less an instructional blueprint for living than someone living as a woman who uses her natural ova to have children. In the end, Velleman's arguments about access to genetic parents and relatives lend support to the idea of same-sex couples turning to synthetic gametes to have children. At the very least, the concern about the supposed ill effects of anonymous gamete donation could be bypassed and rendered moot.

Synthetic gametes used by a same-sex couple to produce children also answer a complaint that Daniel Callahan lodges against gamete donation, especially anonymous gamete donation. Callahan argues that people have responsibility for the foreseeable consequences of their autonomous choices.[16] People should not, therefore, take steps to become parents under conditions that disavow all responsibility for the children born with their gametes. Anonymous donation especially, he thinks, sets aside a basic meaning of moral responsibility for the welfare of children conceived with their gametes.

Although Callahan does not mention it, embryo donors should have the same presumptive responsibility too. Same-sex couples who turned to their own natural and synthetic gametes to have children would have no need for donor gametes or embryos, and would, therefore, bypass this entire line of objection; they would not, that is, be complicit in the (alleged) lapses of parental, responsibility because their children involve no parents external to their relationship.

I will mention one last possible objection to the use of synthetic gametes by same-sex couples: that the very desire to have children with shared genetics reflects a dubious understanding of parenthood, namely that one is *only* a parent if one is a genetic parent, that it is genetic relatedness that entitles anyone to the moral status of parenthood. By contrast, some commentators argue that moral commitment creates parenthood, not genetic relatedness, not 'biologism.' For example, Thomas Murray has said 'Genetic parenthood is incidental to parent-child mutuality'. (see page 32 from Murray[17]). From a perspective like this, same-sex couples lack for nothing as parents, and their children lack for nothing as children simply because they might be genetically unrelated in whole or in part. From this perspective, synthetic gametes would only open up same-sex couples to a mistaken view that presently can *only* affect opposite-sex couples: that full genetic relatedness is the morally relevant threshold of parent-child relations. Even if we grant that prospective parents can be mistaken in about the importance of genetics, it is not clear why same-sex couples should be singled out and possibly excluded from the use of synthetic gametes in the name of protecting them from that mistake. Closing off synthetic gametes to same-sex couples would close off an important means by which families, in general, consolidate and express their identities. If the treatment of genetic relatedness as a desideratum in children is tolerated in opposite-sex couples, it is unclear why it should not be tolerated across the spectrum of adults looking to have children in the context of their chosen relationships. In any case, same-sex couples having children via synthetic gametes would represent only a miniscule fraction of the total number of parents looking to have children with their shared genetics. To the extent that 'biologism' is a moral problem, its solution will not be meaningfully advanced by closing off synthetic gametes to gay and lesbian couples. Treating the use of synthetic gametes by gay and lesbian couples as morally suspect would, moreover, leave those couples vulnerable to objections against their use of other ARTs, objections that synthetic gametes silence. In this sense, invoking worries about biologism against gay and lesbian couples seems entirely out of proportion to the nature of the supposed problem, which is hardly remediable by focus on those couples alone.

Conclusions

In some quarters of bioethics, homosexual men and women do not enjoy a strong presumption of equality in regard to social goods and relationships. Some commentators presuppose this inequality in the questions they raise about the prospect of synthetic gametes and the children of same-sex couples, questions that imply burdens of proof that do not apply to others. Other commentators express this view directly in claims that gay and lesbian parenthood compromises the rights and welfare of children, so much so that gay men and lesbians should refrain from having children altogether (according to the more stringent arguments) or should avoid using certain methods to have children (according to the less stringent arguments).

To be fair, some commentators have expressed strong support for the use of synthetic gametes as a way for same-sex couples to have children with shared genetics. Testa and Harris have defended this use on four main fronts: (1) that the idea of 'nature' cannot sustain an argument against it because the 'whole practice of medicine is a comprehensive attempt to frustrate the course of nature', (2) that claims that children are harmed by coming into existence this way cannot be sustained because existence is preferable to non-existence in terms of the value of children's lives to themselves, (3) that ARTs are currently available to homosexual men and women in a way that would make it idiosyncratic to forbid synthetic gametes and (4) that, in any case, the evidence is lacking that children of gay and lesbian parents fare worse than the children of others.[18] Not only do they criticise objections to the use of synthetic gametes as unfounded, but Testa and Harris offer positive arguments in favour of synthetic gametes for gay and lesbian people, for example, by arguing that synthetic gametes would help 'democratise reproduction'. Yet, even here, the defence of gay men and lesbians as parents comes as the conclusion to a long and involved argument, which Testa and Harris concede could have gone on to even greater lengths!

In the early days of bioethics, some commentators analysed homosexuality relative to various theories of disease and health.[19–21] Ironically, many of those early discussions occurred after the interpretation of homosexuality as pathological had already faded in credibility and significance. The UK Wolfenden Report repudiated the view of homosexuality as pathological in 1957, and the American Psychiatric Association followed suit in 1973.[22,23] Bioethics busied itself with this question for some time afterward. Since those discussions, however, most analysts have moved on from questions about the 'pathology' of homosexuality, and focused on questions of healthcare access and equity for gay men and lesbians. Yet some commentators have used synthetic gametes to throw the integrity of homosexual men and women into question again, at least as far as parenthood is concerned. In different ways, Somerville, Velleman and Callahan treat the legitimacy of gay and lesbian parenthood as objectionable. As I have tried to show, however, their very objections can sometimes work in favour of synthetic gametes for same-sex couples, especially by rendering moot worries about the relationships between parents and children.

At this stage of bioethics, though, why should we not assume in an axiomatic way that gay men and lesbians should be respected in their sexual identities, in their relationships in general, and in relationships with their children in particular? How many times must bioethics relitigate parenthood for gay men and lesbians? Questions of ethics do arise in the use of synthetic gametes by same-sex couples, but the most important questions are not about the suitability of same-sex couples as parents or even the welfare of their children. The most important questions involve access and equity. Are prevailing clinical standards – with their framing of infertility in terms of anatomical or physiological deficits involving opposite-sex partners – a hindrance in any way to fertility medicine for same-sex partners? If insurance companies in the USA cover infertility treatments for straight couples, is there any morally compelling reason they should not extend the same benefits to opposite-sex couples, some of whom will be in lawful marriages? Given the historical arc of homosexuality in bioethics, the field may eventually move to embrace these kinds of questions fully, after the novelty of synthetic gametes wears off, and bioethics may yet embrace homosexual men and women as the presumptive equals of everyone else in regard to fitness as parents. The sooner, the better.

References

1   West, F. D., Shirazi R., Mardanpour P., et al. In vitro-derived gametes from stem cells. *Semin Repro Med* 2013; 31:33–8.

2   Den, J. M., Satoh, K., Wang, H., et al. Generation of viable male and female mice from two fathers. *Biol Reprod* 2011; 84:613–18.

3   Gates, G. *LGBT parenting in the United States*. The Williams Institute of UCLA, 2013. https://williamsinstitute.law.ucla.edu/wp-content/uploads/LGBT-Parenting-US-Feb-2013.pdf

4   Ethics Committee of the American Society of Reproductive Medicine. Access to fertility treatments by gay, lesbian, and unmarried people. *Fertil Steril* 2009; 92: 1190–3.

5   Murphy, T. F. Lesbian mothers and genetic choices. *Ethics and Behavior* 1993; 3:220–2.

6   Newson, A. J., and Smajdor, A. C. Artificial gametes: new paths to parenthood? *J Med Ethics* 2005; 31:184–6.

7   Beatie T. *Labor of love: the story of one man's extraordinary pregnancy*. Berkeley, CA: Seal Press, 2008.

8   Murphy, T. F. The ethics of helping transgender men and women have children. *Perspect Biol Med* 2010; 53:46–60.

9   Mathews D. J. H., Donovan, P.J., Harris, J., et al. Pluripotent stem cell-derived gametes: truth and (potential) consequences. *Cell Stem Cell* 2009; 5:11–14.

10 Somerville, M. *The case against 'same-sex marriage'.* Canada: Brief presented to the Standing Committee on Justice and Human Rights, 29 April 2003.

11 Somerville, M. It's all about the children, not selfish adults. *The Australian* 23 July 2011.

12 American Psychological Association Council of Representatives. Sexual orientation, parents, and children. 28 and 30 July 2004. [Updated to Sexual Orientation, Gender Identity (SOGI), Parents and their Children. February 2020. https://www.apa.org/about/policy/resolution-sexual-orientation-parents-children.pdf]

13 Lippman, A., and Newman, S. The ethics of deriving gametes from ES cells [letter]. *Science* 2005;307:515.

14 Testa, G., and Harris, J. Genetics: ethical aspects of ES cell-derived gametes. *Science* 2004; 305:1719.

15 Velleman, J. D. Family history. *Philos Pap* 2005; 34:357–78.

16 Callahan, D. *In search of the good: a life in bioethics.* Cambridge: The MIT Press, 2012.

17 Murray, T. H. Three meanings of parenthood. In: Rothstein, M. A., Murray, T. H., Kaebnick, G., et al. eds. *Genetic ties and the family: the impact of paternity testing on parents and children.* Baltimore: Johns Hopkins University Press, 2005:18–34.

18 Testa, G, and Harris, J. Ethics and synthetic gametes. *Bioethics* 2005; 19:146–66.

19 Boorse, C. On the distinction between disease and illness. *Philos Public Aff* 1975; 5:49–68.

20 Ruse, M. *Homosexuality: a philosophical perspective.* Oxford: Blackwell, 1988.

21 Engelhardt HT. *Foundations of bioethics.* New York: Oxford University Press, 1986.

22 Committee of the Offenses of Homosexuality and Prostitution. *The Wolfenden report.* New York: Stein and Day, 1965.

23 Bayer, R.. *Homosexuality and American psychiatry: the politics of diagnosis.* Princeton: Princeton University Press, 1987.

7

Rights, Interests, and Possible People

Derek Parfit

Do possible people have rights and interests? Professor Hare has argued that they do. I shall claim that, even if they don't, we should often act *as if* they do.

We can start with future people. Suppose that the testing of a nuclear weapon would, through radiation, cause a number of deformities in the people who are born within the next ten years. This would be against the interests of these future people. These people will exist whether or not the weapon is tested, and, if it is, they will be affected for the worse – they will be worse off than they would otherwise have been. We can harm these people though they don't live *now*, just as we can harm foreigners though they don't live *here*.

What about *possible* people? The difference between these and future people can be defined as follows. Suppose that we must act in one of two ways. "Future people" are the people who will exist whichever way we act. "Possible people" are the people who will exist if we act in one way, but who won't exist if we act in the other way. To give the simplest case: if we are wondering whether to have children, the children that we *could* have are possible people.

Do they have rights and interests? Suppose, first, that we decide to have these children. Can this affect their interests? We can obviously rephrase this question so that it no longer asks about possible people. We can ask: can it be in, or be against, an *actual* person's interests to have been conceived? I shall return to this.

Suppose, next, that we decide not to have children. Then these possible people never get conceived. Can *this* affect their interests? Can it, for instance, harm these children?

The normal answer would be "No." Professor Hare takes a different view. We can simplify the example he discussed. We suppose that a child is born with some serious disability or abnormality, which is incurable, and would probably make the child's life, though still worth living, less so than a normal life. We next suppose that unless we perform some operation the child will die; and that, if it does, the parents will have another normal child, whom they wouldn't have if this child lives. The question is, should we operate?

Hare suggests that we should not. He first assumes that we ought to do what is in the best interests of

Original publication details: Derek Parfit, "Rights, Interests, and Possible People," pp. 369–375 from Samuel Gorovitz et al. (eds.), *Moral Problems in Medicine* (Englewood Cliffs, NJ: Prentice Hall, 1976). Reproduced courtesy of Derek Parfit.

all the people concerned. He then claims that among these people is "the next child in the queue" – the normal child whom the parents would later have only if the disabled child dies. The interests of this possible child may, he thinks, "tip the balance." The possible child, unlike the actual child, "has a high prospect of a normal and happy life"; Hare would therefore claim that we do *less* harm to the actual child by failing to save his life than we do to the possible child "by stopping him from being conceived and born."

In this particular case, many would agree with Hare that we shouldn't operate, but for different reasons. They may think that a new-born child is not yet a full person, with rights and interests;[1] or they may doubt whether life with a serious disability would be worth living.

The implications of Hare's view can be better seen in another case. Take a couple who – we assume – live in an age before the world was over-populated, and who are wondering whether to have children. Suppose next that, if they do, their children's lives would probably be well worth living. Then, on Hare's view, if the couple choose not to have these children they would be doing them serious harm. Since there is no over-population, it would seem to follow that their choice is morally wrong. Most of us, I think, would deny this. We believe that there can be nothing wrong in deciding to remain childless. And if we also ask what Hare would count as over-population, his conclusion would again be widely disputed. This is another subject to which I shall return.

What I have called "Hare's view" is that we can harm people by preventing their conception. There are precedents for this view. The Talmud says that when Amram decided not to beget children, he was admonished for denying them the World to Come.[2] But, as Hare admits, his view is unusual. He would argue that it can be justified by an appeal to the logic of moral reasoning.[3] I shall not discuss whether this is so; but instead take a complementary path. I shall assume that we cannot harm those we don't conceive. Even so, I shall argue, it is hard to avoid Hare's conclusions.

The principle with which Hare works is that we should do what is in the best interests of those concerned. Most of us accept some principle of this kind.

We may believe that other principles are often more important; but we accept, as one of our principles, something to do with interests, with preferences, or with happiness and misery. As this list suggests, such a principle can take different forms. We need only look at a single difference. The principle can take what I call an "impersonal" form: for example, it can run

1. We should do what most reduces misery and increases happiness.

It can instead take a "person-affecting" form: for example

2. We should do what harms people the least and benefits them most.

When we can only affect actual people, those who do or will exist, the difference between these forms of the principle makes, in practice, no difference. But when we can affect *who* exists, it can make a great difference.

Return, for instance, to the childless couple in the uncrowded world. According to principle (1) – the "impersonal" principle – they should do what most increases happiness. One of the most effective ways of increasing the quality of happiness is to increase the number of happy people. So the couple ought to have children; their failure to do so is, according to (1), morally wrong.

Most of us would say: "This just shows the absurdity of the impersonal principle. What we ought to do is make people happy, not make happy people. The right principle is (2), the 'person-affecting' principle. If the couple don't have children, there is no-one whom they've harmed, or failed to benefit. That is why they have done nothing wrong."

This reply involves the rejection of Hare's view. It assumes that we cannot harm people by preventing their conception. If we *can*, the childless couple would be doing wrong even on the person-affecting principle.

We can generalize from this example. Most of us hold a person-affecting, not an impersonal, principle. If we reject Hare's view, there are cases where this makes a great practical difference. But if we accept Hare's view, it makes no difference. The person-affecting principle, when combined with Hare's view, leads to the same conclusions as the impersonal principle.

Some of these conclusions are, as I said, striking. I shall now begin to argue towards them. We can avoid these conclusions only if we *both* accept what I shall call "the restriction of our principles to acts which affect people" *and* claim that our acts cannot affect possible people. Hare denies the latter; I shall be denying the former. The person-affecting restriction seems to me, at least in any natural form, unacceptable.

We can start with one of the two questions that I postponed. Can it be in our interests to have been conceived? Can we benefit from receiving life?

If we can, the childless couple are again at fault, even on person-affecting grounds – for if they have children they will be benefitting people, as principle (2) tells them to do.

We might say: "But we can only benefit if we are made better off than we would otherwise have been. This couple's children wouldn't otherwise have been – so they cannot benefit from receiving life." I have doubts about this reasoning. For one thing, it implies that we cannot benefit people if we *save* their lives, for here too they wouldn't otherwise have been. True, there are problems in comparing life with non-existence. But if we assume that a person's life has been well worth living, should we not agree that to have saved this person's life many years ago would be to have done this person a great benefit? And if it can be in a person's interests to have had his life prolonged, even, say, just after it started, why can it not be in his interests to have had it started?

Here is a second problem. If we cannot benefit a person by conceiving him, then we cannot harm him either. But suppose we know that any child whom we could conceive will have an abnormality so severe that it will live for only a few years, will never develop, and will suffer fairly frequent pain. It would seem to be clearly wrong to go ahead, knowingly, and conceive such a child.[4] And the main reason why it would be wrong is that the child will suffer. But if we cannot *harm* a child by giving it a life of this kind, then this reason why the act is wrong cannot be stated in

"person-affecting" terms. We shall have to say, "It is wrong because it increases suffering." We should then be back with half of the impersonal principle; and it will be hard, in consistency, to avoid the other half. (We might perhaps claim that only suffering matters morally – that happiness is morally trivial. But this position, though superficially attractive, collapses when we think it through.)

We have been asking whether the act of conceiving a child can affect this child, for better or worse. If we answer "Yes," the person-affecting restriction makes no difference; principle (2) leads to the same conclusions as principle (1). We may therefore wish to answer "No" – but to this we have found objections.

The problem here can, I think, be solved. We can state the person-affecting principle in a different form:

3. It is wrong to do what, of the alternatives, affects people for the worse.

We interpret (3) so that if people fail to receive possible benefits, they count as affected for the worse. If we adopt principle (3), we can afford to allow that conceiving someone is a case of affecting him. Since failing to receive benefits counts as being affected for the worse, principle (3) still tells us – like principle (2) – to do what benefits people most. But there is one exception. To the one benefit of receiving life (3) – unlike (2) – gives no weight. For when we fail to give this benefit, there isn't an actual person who fails to receive it – who is thus affected for the worse. (I am now assuming, you remember, that we cannot affect possible people.)

Most of us, I claimed, think there is nothing wrong in *not* having children, even if they would have been very happy. But we think that having children who are bound to suffer is wrong. Principle (3) supports this asymmetrical pair of judgments. It supports our view that the Childless Couple did no wrong; but it also supports our view about "wrongful conception" – for the child here is an actual person affected for the worse.

In the move from (2) to (3), a natural principle is revised in a somewhat artificial way. But this revision does not seem to drain the principle of its plausibility.

All the revision does is this. When we are choosing what to do, we are told to aim, not to achieve the outcome where people are better off, but to avoid the outcome where they are worse off. This procedure, adding up the "minuses," seems to be just as general and as plausible as the other, adding up the "pluses." So we are not, in moving to (3), "tailoring" our principles in an *ad-hoc* way. And the justification for the move is that only principle (3) (combined with the assumption that conceiving is affecting) gives support to the asymmetrical judgments that we find plausible.[5]

So far, so good. But I shall now argue that the person-affecting principle needs to be more drastically revised. This *may* drain it of its plausibility.

Consider the following case, which involves two women. The first is one month pregnant, and is told by her doctor that, unless she takes a simple treatment, the child she is carrying will develop a certain disability. We suppose again that life with this disability would probably be worth living, but less so than a normal life. It would obviously be wrong for the mother not to take the treatment, for this will disable her child. And the person-affecting principle tells us that this would be wrong. (Note that we need not assume that a one-month-old foetus is a person, for there *will be* a person whom the woman has affected for the worse.)

We next suppose that there is a second woman, who is about to stop taking contraceptive pills so that she can have another child. She is told that she has a temporary condition such that any child she conceives now will have just the same disability; but that if she waits three months she will then conceive a normal child. It seems clear that it would be wrong for this second woman, by not waiting, to deliberately have a disabled rather than a normal child. And it seems (at least to me) clear that this would be just *as* wrong as it would be for the first woman to deliberately disable her child.

But if the second woman does deliberately have a disabled child, has she harmed him – affected him for the worse? We must first ask: "Could he truly claim, when he grows up, 'If my mother had waited, I would have been born three months later, as a normal child'?" The answer is, "No." If his mother had waited, he would not have been born at all; she would have had

a different child. When I claim this, I need not assume that the time of one's conception, or the particular cells from which one grew, are essential to one's identity. *Perhaps* we can suppose that *I* might have been conceived a year later, if we are supposing that my parents had no child when they in fact had me, but a year later had a child who was exactly or very much *like* me. But in our case the child the woman would have if she waits would be as unlike the child she would have now as any two of her actual children would be likely to be. Given this, we cannot claim that they would have been the same child. (To argue this in another way. Suppose that I am in fact my mother's first child and eldest son. And suppose that things had gone like this: she had no child when I was in fact born, then had a girl, then a boy. Can I claim that I, her first child, would have been that girl? Why not claim that I, her eldest son, would have been that boy? Both claims are equally good, and so, since they cannot both be true, equally bad. So, if she *had* waited before having children, I would not have been born at all.)[6]

The second woman's disabled child is, then, not worse off than he would otherwise have been, for he wouldn't otherwise have been. Might we still claim that in deliberately conceiving a disabled child, the woman harms this child? We might perhaps claim this if the child's life would be not worth living – would be worse than nothing; but we have assumed that it would be worth living. And in this case being disabled is the only way in which this child can receive life. So the case is like that in which a doctor removes a person's limb to save his life. It would not be true, at least in a morally relevant sense, that the doctor harmed this person, or affected him for the worse. We seem bound to say the same about my second woman.

I conclude, then, that if the second woman deliberately conceives a disabled rather than a normal child, she would not be harming this child. The first woman, if she deliberately neglects the treatment, would be harming her child. Notice next that in every other way the two acts are exactly similar. The side-effects on other people should be much the same. These side-effects would provide *some* person-affecting grounds for the claim that the second woman's act would be wrong. But it is obvious that if we judge the two acts on person-affecting principles, the first woman's act must be considerably *more* wrong. In her case, there are not just side-effects – her child is seriously harmed. The second woman's child is *not* harmed. Since this is the only difference between the two acts, the case provides a test for person-affecting principles. The impersonal principle tells us to reduce misery and increase happiness, whether or not people are affected for better or worse. If there is any plausibility in the restriction to acts which affect people, it must be worse to *harm* someone than to cause equivalent unhappiness in a way which harms no-one. The second woman's act must, in other words, be less wrong than the first's. It we think that it is not less wrong, we cannot accept the restriction to acts which affect people.

The acts which I have described are of course unusual. But this does not make them a worse test for the person-affecting restriction. On the contrary, they are unusual because they are designed as a test. The two women's acts are designed to be as similar as they could be, except in one respect. Each woman deliberately brings it about that she has a disabled rather than a normal child. The only difference is that in one case the disabled and the normal child are the same child, while in the other they are not. This is precisely the difference which, on the person-affecting principle, matters. If we think that the two acts would be just as wrong, we cannot believe that it does matter.

Some of you may think that the person-affecting principle survives this test. You may think: "Since the second woman doesn't harm her child, what she does *is* less wrong." But there are other cases where such implications seem harder to accept. Take genetic counseling. We could not advise the dominant carriers of diseases to accept genetic counseling *for the sake of their children*, for if they reject this counseling, and marry other dominant carriers, it will not be true that their children will have been harmed, or affected for the worse. Or again, Dr. Kass has argued that it would be wrong to use certain kinds of artificial fertilization, on the ground that if children are conceived in these ways, rather than in normal ways, they run greater risks of certain deformities.[7] But these particular children cannot be conceived in normal ways. For them, the alternatives are artificial fertilization, or nothing. So we can only claim that we would be harming them, or affecting them for the worse, if the risks of deformities were so great that their lives would probably be not worth living.

When we turn to population policy, the implications become much harder to accept. . . .

[Editorial note: the rest of Parfit's talk is not reprinted here. His more recent thoughts about the problems discussed in this talk, and the larger problems of population policy, will appear in a future issue of the journal, *Philosophy & Public Affairs*, under the title "Overpopulation."]

Notes

1 Cf. Michael Tooley, "Abortion and Infanticide," *Philosophy and Public Affairs*, 2, No. 1 (Fall 1972) [see chapter 1 in this *Anthology*].

2 Quoted in G. Tedeschi, "On Tort Liability for 'Wrongful Life,'" *Israel Law Review*, October 1966, p. 514, footnote 3.

3 The logic he describes in his books, *The Language of Morals*, OUP, 1952, and *Freedom and Reason*, OUP, 1963.

4 For a legal discussion of related issues, see "A Cause of Action for 'Wrongful Life,'" *Minnesota Law Review*, 55, No. 1 (November 1970).

5 This asymmetry is discussed in Jan Narveson's two articles: "Utilitarianism and New Generations," *Mind*, January 1967, and "Moral Problems of Population," *The Monist*, January 1973. I have learned much from both of these.

6 For a different view, take a remark in Gwen Raverat's *Period Piece*, Faber and Faber, 1952, "It is always a fascinating problem to consider who we would have been if our mother (or our father) had married another person."

7 "Making babies – the new biology and the 'old' morality," Leon Kass, *The Public Interest*, Winter, 1972.

Prenatal Screening, Sex Selection, and Cloning

8

Genetics and Reproductive Risk
Can Having Children Be Immoral?

Laura M. Purdy

Is it morally permissible for me to have children? A decision to procreate is surely one of the most significant decisions a person can make. So it would seem that it ought not be made without some moral soul-searching.

There are many reasons why one might hesitate to bring children into this world if one is concerned about their welfare. Some are rather general, such as the deteriorating environment or the prospect of poverty. Others have a narrower focus, such as continuing civil war in one's country or the lack of essential social support for child-rearing in the United States. Still others may be relevant only to individuals at risk of passing harmful diseases to their offspring.

There are many causes of misery in this world, and most of them are unrelated to genetic disease. In the general scheme of things, human misery is most efficiently reduced by concentrating on noxious social and political arrangements. Nonetheless, we should not ignore preventable harm just because it is confined to a relatively small corner of life. So the question arises, Can it be wrong to have a child because of genetic risk factors?[1]

Unsurprisingly, most of the debate about this issue has focused on prenatal screening and abortion: much useful information about a given fetus can be made available by recourse to prenatal testing. This fact has meant that moral questions about reproduction have become entwined with abortion politics, to the detriment of both. The abortion connection has made it especially difficult to think about whether it is wrong to prevent a child from coming into being, because doing so might involve what many people see as wrongful killing; yet there is no necessary link between the two. Clearly, the existence of genetically compromised children can be prevented not only by aborting already existing fetuses but also by preventing conception in the first place.

Worse yet, many discussions simply assume a particular view of abortion without recognizing other possible positions and the difference they make in how people understand the issues. For example, those who object to aborting fetuses with genetic problems often argue that doing so would undermine our conviction that all humans are in some

Original publication details: Laura M. Purdy, "Genetics and Reproductive Risk: Can Having Children be Immoral?," pp. 39–49 from *Reproducing Persons: Issues in Feminist Bioethics* (Ithaca, NY: Cornell University Press, 1996). Reproduced with permission of Cornell University Press.

important sense equal.[2] However, this position rests on the assumption that conception marks the point at which humans are endowed with a right to life. So aborting fetuses with genetic problems looks morally the same as killing "imperfect" people without their consent.

This position raises two separate issues. One pertains to the legitimacy of different views on abortion. Despite the conviction of many abortion activists to the contrary, I believe that ethically respectable views can be found on different sides of the debate, including one that sees fetuses as developing humans without any serious moral claim on continued life. There is no space here to address the details, and doing so would be once again to fall into the trap of letting the abortion question swallow up all others. However, opponents of abortion need to face the fact that many thoughtful individuals do *not* see fetuses as moral persons. It follows that their reasoning process, and hence the implications of their decisions, are radically different from those envisioned by opponents of prenatal screening and abortion. So where the latter see genetic abortion as murdering people who just don't measure up, the former see it as a way to prevent the development of persons who are more likely to live miserable lives, a position consistent with a world-view that values persons equally and holds that each deserves a high-quality life. Some of those who object to genetic abortion appear to be oblivious to these psychological and logical facts. It follows that the nightmare scenarios they paint for us are beside the point: many people simply do not share the assumptions that make them plausible.

How are these points relevant to my discussion? My primary concern here is to argue that conception can sometimes be morally wrong on grounds of genetic risk, although this judgment will not apply to those who accept the moral legitimacy of abortion and are willing to employ prenatal screening and selective abortion. If my case is solid, then those who oppose abortion must be especially careful not to conceive in certain cases, as they are, of course, free

to follow their conscience about abortion. Those like myself who do not see abortion as murder have more ways to prevent birth.

Huntington's Disease

There is always some possibility that reproduction will result in a child with a serious disease or handicap. Genetic counselors can help individuals determine whether they are at unusual risk and, as the Human Genome Project rolls on, their knowledge will increase by quantum leaps. As this knowledge becomes available, I believe we ought to use it to determine whether possible children are at risk *before* they are conceived.

In this chapter I want to defend the thesis that it is morally wrong to reproduce when we know there is a high risk of transmitting a serious disease or defect. This thesis holds that some reproductive acts are wrong, and my argument puts the burden of proof on those who disagree with it to show why its conclusions can be overridden. Hence it denies that people should be free to reproduce mindless of the consequences.[3] However, as moral argument, it should be taken as a proposal for further debate and discussion. It is not, by itself, an argument in favor of legal prohibitions of reproduction.[4]

There is a huge range of genetic diseases. Some are quickly lethal; others kill more slowly, if at all. Some are mainly physical, some mainly mental; others impair both kinds of function. Some interfere tremendously with normal functioning, others less. Some are painful, some are not. There seems to be considerable agreement that rapidly lethal diseases, especially those, such as Tay-Sachs, accompanied by painful deterioration, should be prevented even at the cost of abortion. Conversely, there seems to be substantial agreement that relatively trivial problems, especially cosmetic ones, would not be legitimate grounds for abortion.[5] In short, there are cases ranging from low risk of mild disease or disability to high risk of serious disease or disability. Although it is difficult to decide where the duty to refrain from procreation becomes compelling, I believe that there are some clear cases. I have chosen to focus on Huntington's Disease to illustrate the kinds of concrete issues such decisions entail. However, the arguments are also relevant to many other genetic diseases.[6]

The symptoms of Huntington's Disease usually begin between the ages of 30 and 50:

> Onset is insidious. Personality changes (obstinacy, moodiness, lack of initiative) frequently antedate or accompany the involuntary choreic movements. These usually appear first in the face, neck, and arms, and are jerky, irregular, and stretching in character. Contradictions of the facial muscles result in grimaces; those of the respiratory muscles, lips, and tongue lead to hesitating, explosive speech. Irregular movements of the trunk are present; the gait is shuffling and dancing. Tendon reflexes are increased. . .Some patients display a fatuous euphoria; others are spiteful, irascible, destructive, and violent. Paranoid reactions are common. Poverty of thought and impairment of attention, memory, and judgment occur. As the disease progresses, walking becomes impossible, swallowing difficult, and dementia profound. Suicide is not uncommon.[7]

The illness lasts about fifteen years, terminating in death.

Huntington's Disease is an autosomal dominant disease, meaning it is caused by a single defective gene located on a non-sex chromosome. It is passed from one generation to the next via affected individuals. Each child of such an affected person has a 50 percent risk of inheriting the gene and thus of eventually developing the disease, even if he or she was born before the parent's disease was evident.[8]

Until recently, Huntington's Disease was especially problematic because most affected individuals did not know whether they had the gene for the disease until well into their child-bearing years. So they had to decide about child-bearing before knowing whether they could transmit the disease or not. If, in time, they did not develop symptoms of the disease, then their

children could know they were not at risk for the disease. If unfortunately they did develop symptoms, then each of their children could know there was a 50 percent chance that they too had inherited the gene. In both cases, the children faced a period of prolonged anxiety as to whether they would develop the disease. Then, in the 1980s, thanks in part to an energetic campaign by Nancy Wexler, a genetic marker was found that, in certain circumstances, could tell people with a relatively high degree of probability whether or not they had the gene for the disease.[9] Finally, in March 1993, the defective gene itself was discovered.[10] Now individuals can find out whether they carry the gene for the disease, and prenatal screening can tell us whether a given fetus has inherited it. These technological developments change the moral scene substantially.

How serious are the risks involved in Huntington's Disease? Geneticists often think a 10 percent risk is high.[11] But risk assessment also depends on what is at stake: the worse the possible outcome, the more undesirable an otherwise small risk seems. In medicine, as elsewhere, people may regard the same result quite differently. But for devastating diseases such as Huntington's this part of the judgment should be unproblematic: no one wants a loved one to suffer in this way.[12]

There may still be considerable disagreement about the acceptability of a given risk. So it would be difficult in many circumstances to say how we should respond to a particular risk. Nevertheless, there are good grounds for a conservative approach, for it is reasonable to take special precautions to avoid very bad consequences, even if the risk is small. But the possible consequences here *are* very bad: a child who may inherit Huntington's Disease has a much greater than average chance of being subjected to severe and prolonged suffering. And it is one thing to risk one's own welfare, but quite another to do so for others and without their consent.

Is this judgment about Huntington's Disease really defensible? People appear to have quite different opinions. Optimists argue that a child born into a family afflicted with Huntington's Disease has a reasonable chance of living a satisfactory life. After all, even children born of an afflicted parent still have a 50 percent chance of escaping the disease. And even if afflicted themselves, such people will probably enjoy some thirty years of healthy life before symptoms appear. It is also possible, although not at all likely, that some might not mind the symptoms caused by the disease. Optimists can point to diseased persons who have lived fruitful lives, as well as those who seem genuinely glad to be alive. One is Rick Donohue, a sufferer from the Joseph family disease: "You know, if my mom hadn't had me, I wouldn't be here for the life I have had. So there is a good possibility I will have children."[13] Optimists therefore conclude that it would be a shame if these persons had not lived.

Pessimists concede some of these facts but take a less sanguine view of them. They think a 50 percent risk of serious disease such as Huntington's is appallingly high. They suspect that many children born into afflicted families are liable to spend their youth in dreadful anticipation and fear of the disease. They expect that the disease, if it appears, will be perceived as a tragic and painful end to a blighted life. They point out that Rick Donohue is still young and has not experienced the full horror of his sickness. It is also well-known that some young persons have such a dilated sense of time that they can hardly envision themselves at 30 or 40, so the prospect of pain at that age is unreal to them.[14]

More empirical research on the psychology and life history of suffers and potential sufferers is clearly needed to decide whether optimists or pessimists have a more accurate picture of the experiences of individuals at risk. But given that some will surely realize pessimists' worst fears, it seems unfair to conclude that the pleasures of those who deal best with the situation simply cancel out the suffering of those others when that suffering could be avoided altogether.

I think that these points indicate that the morality of procreation in such situations demands further investigation. I propose to do this by looking first at the position of the possible child, then at that of the potential parent.

Possible Children and Potential Parents

The first task in treating the problem from the child's point of view is to find a way of referring to possible future offspring without seeming to confer some sort of morally significant existence on them. I follow the convention of calling children who might be born in the future but who are not now conceived "possible" children, offspring, individuals, or persons.

Now, what claims about children or possible children are relevant to the morality of child-bearing in the circumstances being considered? Of primary importance is the judgment that we ought to try to provide every child with something like a minimally satisfying life. I am not altogether sure how best to formulate this standard, but I want clearly to reject the view that it is morally permissible to conceive individuals so long as we do not expect them to be so miserable that they wish they were dead.[15] I believe that this kind of moral minimalism is thoroughly unsatisfactory and that not many people would really want to live in a world where it was the prevailing standard. Its lure is that it puts few demands on us, but its price is the scant attention it pays to human well-being.

How might the judgment that we have a duty to try to provide a minimally satisfying life for our children be justified? It could, I think, be derived fairly straightforwardly from either utilitarian or contractarian theories of justice, although there is no space here for discussion of the details. The net result of such analysis would be to conclude that neglecting this duty would create unnecessary unhappiness or unfair disadvantage for some persons.

Of course, this line of reasoning confronts us with the need to spell out what is meant by "minimally satisfying" and what a standard based on this concept would require of us. Conceptions of a minimally satisfying life vary tremendously among societies and also within them. *De rigueur* in some circles are private music lessons and trips to Europe, whereas in others providing eight years of schooling is a major accomplishment. But there is no need to consider this complication at length here because we are concerned only with health as a prerequisite for a minimally satisfying life. Thus, as we draw out what such a standard might require of us, it seems reasonable to retreat to the more limited claim that parents should try to ensure something like normal health for their children. It might be thought that even this moderate claim is unsatisfactory as in some places debilitating conditions are the norm, but one could circumvent this objection by saying that parents ought to try to provide for their children health normal for that culture, even though it may be inadequate if measured by some outside standard.[16] This conservative position would still justify efforts to avoid the birth of children at risk for Huntington's Disease and other serious genetic diseases in virtually all societies.[17]

This view is reinforced by the following considerations. Given that possible children do not presently exist as actual individuals, they do not have a right to be brought into existence, and hence no one is maltreated by measures to avoid the conception of a possible person. Therefore, the conservative course that avoids the conception of those who would not be expected to enjoy a minimally satisfying life is at present the only fair course of action. The alternative is a *laissez-faire* approach that brings into existence the lucky, but only at the expense of the unlucky. Notice that attempting to avoid the creation of the unlucky does not necessarily lead to *fewer* people being brought into being; the question boils down to taking steps to bring those with better prospects into existence, instead of those with worse ones.

I have so far argued that if people with Huntington's Disease are unlikely to live minimally satisfying lives, then those who might pass it on should not have genetically related children. This is consonant with the principle that the greater the danger of serious

problems, the stronger the duty to avoid them. But this principle is in conflict with what people think of as the right to reproduce. How might one decide which should take precedence?

Expecting people to forgo having genetically related children might seem to demand too great a sacrifice of them. But before reaching that conclusion we need to ask what is really at stake. One reason for wanting children is to experience family life, including love, companionship, watching kids grow, sharing their pains and triumphs, and helping to form members of the next generation. Other reasons emphasize the validation of parents as individuals within a continuous family line, children as a source of immortality, or perhaps even the gratification of producing partial replicas of oneself. Children may also be desired in an effort to prove that one is an adult, to try to cement a marriage, or to benefit parents economically.

Are there alternative ways of satisfying these desires? Adoption or new reproductive technologies can fulfill many of them without passing on known genetic defects. Sperm replacement has been available for many years via artificial insemination by donor. More recently, egg donation, sometimes in combination with contract pregnancy,[18] has been used to provide eggs for women who prefer not to use their own. Eventually it may be possible to clone individual humans, although that now seems a long way off. All of these approaches to avoiding the use of particular genetic material are controversial and have generated much debate. I believe that tenable moral versions of each do exist.[19]

None of these methods permits people to extend both genetic lines or realize the desire for immortality or for children who resemble both parents; nor is it clear that such alternatives will necessarily succeed in proving that one is an adult, cementing a marriage, or providing economic benefits. Yet, many people feel these desires strongly. Now, I am sympathetic to William James's dictum regarding desires: "Take any demand, however slight, which any creature, however weak, may make. Ought it not, for its own sole sake be satisfied? If not, prove why not."[20] Thus a world where more desires are satisfied is generally better than one where fewer are. However, not all desires can be legitimately satisfied, because as James suggests, there may be good reasons, such as the conflict of duty and desire, why some should be overruled.

Fortunately, further scrutiny of the situation reveals that there are good reasons why people should attempt with appropriate social support to talk themselves out of the desires in question or to consider novel ways of fulfilling them. Wanting to see the genetic line continued is not particularly rational when it brings a sinister legacy of illness and death. The desire for immortality cannot really be satisfied anyway, and people need to face the fact that what really matters is how they behave in their own lifetimes. And finally, the desire for children who physically resemble one is understandable, but basically narcissistic, and its fulfillment cannot be guaranteed even by normal reproduction. There are other ways of proving one is an adult, and other ways of cementing marriages – and children don't necessarily do either. Children, especially prematurely ill children, may not provide the expected economic benefits anyway. Nongenetically related children may also provide benefits similar to those that would have been provided by genetically related ones, and expected economic benefit is, in many cases, a morally questionable reason for having children.

Before the advent of reliable genetic testing, the options of people in Huntington's families were cruelly limited. On the one hand, they could have children, but at the risk of eventual crippling illness and death for them. On the other, they could refrain from child-bearing, sparing their possible children from significant risk of inheriting this disease, perhaps frustrating intense desires to procreate – only to discover, in some cases, that their sacrifice was unnecessary because they did not develop the disease. Or they could attempt to adopt or try new reproductive approaches.

Reliable genetic testing has opened up new possibilities. Those at risk who wish to have children can get tested. If they test positive, they know their possible children are at risk. Those who are opposed to abortion must be especially careful to avoid conception if

they are to behave responsibly. Those not opposed to abortion can responsibly conceive children, but only if they are willing to test each fetus and abort those who carry the gene. If individuals at risk test negative, they are home free.

What about those who cannot face the test for themselves? They can do prenatal testing and abort fetuses who carry the defective gene. A clearly positive test also implies that the parent is affected, although negative tests do not rule out that possibility. Prenatal testing can thus bring knowledge that enables one to avoid passing the disease to others, but only, in some cases, at the cost of coming to know with certainty that one will indeed develop the disease. This situation raises with peculiar force the question of whether parental responsibility requires people to get tested.

Some people think that we should recognize a right "not to know." It seems to me that such a right could be defended only where ignorance does not put others at serious risk. So if people are prepared to forgo genetically related children, they need not get tested. But if they want genetically related children, then they must do whatever is necessary to ensure that affected babies are not the result. There is, after all, something inconsistent about the claim that one has a right to be shielded from the truth, even if the price is to risk inflicting on one's children the same dread disease one cannot even face in oneself.

In sum, until we can be assured that Huntington's Disease does not prevent people from living a minimally satisfying life, individuals at risk for the disease have a moral duty to try not to bring affected babies into this world. There are now enough options available so that this duty needn't frustrate their reasonable desires. Society has a corresponding duty to facilitate moral behavior on the part of individuals. Such support ranges from the narrow and concrete (such as making sure that medical testing and counseling is available to all) to the more general social environment that guarantees that all pregnancies are voluntary, that pronatalism is eradicated, and that women are treated with respect regardless of the reproductive options they choose.

Notes

1   I focus on genetic considerations, although with the advent of AIDS the scope of the general question here could be expanded. There are two reasons for sticking to this relatively narrow formulation. One is that dealing with a smaller chunk of the problem may help us to think more clearly, while realizing that some conclusions may nonetheless be relevant to the larger problem. The other is the peculiar capacity of some genetic problems to affect ever more individuals in the future.

2   For example, see Leon Kass, "Implications of Prenatal Diagnosis for the Human Right to Life," in *Ethical Issues in Human Genetics*, ed. Bruce Hilton et al. (New York: Plenum, 1973).

3   This is, of course, a very broad thesis. I defend an even broader version in ch. 2 of *Reproducing Persons*, "Loving Future People."

4   Why would we want to resist legal enforcement of every moral conclusion? First, legal action has many costs, costs not necessarily worth paying in particular cases. Second, legal enforcement tends to take the matter out of the realm of debate and treat it as settled. But in many cases, especially where mores or technology are rapidly evolving, we don't want that to happen. Third, legal enforcement would undermine individual freedom and decision-making capacity. In some cases, the ends envisioned are important enough to warrant putting up with these disadvantages.

5   Those who do not see fetuses as moral persons with a right to life may nonetheless hold that abortion is justifiable in these cases. I argue at some length elsewhere that lesser defects can cause great suffering. Once we are clear that there is nothing discriminatory about failing to conceive particular possible individuals, it makes sense, other things being equal, to avoid the prospect of such pain if we can. Naturally, other things rarely are equal. In the first place, many problems go undiscovered until a baby is born. Second, there are often substantial costs associated with screening programs. Third, although women should be encouraged to consider the moral dimensions of routine pregnancy, we do not want it to be so fraught with tension that it becomes a miserable experience. (See ch. 2 of *Reproducing Persons*, "Loving Future People.")

6   It should be noted that failing to conceive a single individual can affect many lives: in 1916, 962 cases could be traced from six seventeenth-century arrivals in America. See Gordon Rattray Taylor, *The Biological Time Bomb* (New York: Penguin, 1968), p. 176.

7   *The Merck Manual* (Rahway, NJ: Merck, 1972), pp. 1363, 1346. We now know that the age of onset and severity of the disease are related to the number of abnormal replications of the glutamine code on the abnormal gene. See Andrew Revkin, "Hunting Down Huntington's," *Discover* (December 1993): 108.

8   Hymie Gordon, "Genetic Counseling," *JAMA*, 217, no. 9 (August 30, 1971): 1346.

9   See Revkin, "Hunting Down Huntington's," 99–108.

10 "Gene for Huntington's Disease Discovered," *Human Genome News*, no. 1 (May 1993): 5.

11 Charles Smith, Susan Holloway, and Alan E. H. Emery, "Individuals at Risk in Families – Genetic Disease," *Journal of Medical Genetics*, 8 (1971): 453.

12 To try to separate the issue of the gravity of the disease from the existence of a given individual, compare this situation with how we would assess a parent who neglected to vaccinate an existing child against a hypothetical viral version of Huntington's.

13 *The New York Times* (September 30, 1975), p. 1. The Joseph family disease is similar to Huntington's Disease except that symptoms start appearing in the twenties. Rick Donohue was in his early twenties at the time he made this statement.

14 I have talked to college students who believe that they will have lived fully and be ready to die at those ages. It is astonishing how one's perspective changes over time and how ages that one once associated with senility and physical collapse come to seem the prime of human life.

15 The view I am rejecting has been forcefully articulated by Derek Parfit, *Reasons and Persons* (Oxford: Clarendon, 1984). For more discussion, see ch. 2 of *Reproducing Persons*, "Loving Future People."

16 I have some qualms about this response, because I fear that some human groups are so badly off that it might still be wrong for them to procreate, even if that would mean great changes in their cultures. But this is a complicated issue that needs to be investigated on its own.

17 Again, a troubling exception might be the isolated Venezuelan group Nancy Wexler found, where, because of inbreeding, a large proportion of the population is affected by Huntington's. See Revkin, "Hunting Down Huntington's."

18 Or surrogacy, as it has been popularly known. I think that "contract pregnancy" is more accurate and more

respectful of women. Eggs can be provided either by a woman who also gestates the fetus or by a third party.

19 The most powerful objections to new reproductive technologies and arrangements concern possible bad consequences for women. However, I do not think that the arguments against them on these grounds have yet shown the dangers to be as great as some believe. So although it is perhaps true that new reproductive technologies and arrangements should not be used lightly, avoiding the conceptions discussed here is well worth the risk. For a series of viewpoints on this issue, including my own "Another Look at Contract Pregnancy" (ch. 12 of *Reproducing Persons*), see Helen B. Holmes, *Issues in Reproductive Technology I: An Anthology* (New York: Garland, 1992).

20 William James, *Essays in Pragmatism*, ed. A. Castell (New York: Hafner, 1948), p. 73.

9

Sex Selection and Preimplantation Genetic Diagnosis

The Ethics Committee of the American Society of Reproductive Medicine

In 1994, the Ethics Committee of the American Society of Reproductive Medicine concluded, although not unanimously, that whereas preimplantation sex selection is appropriate to avoid the birth of children with genetic disorders, it is not acceptable when used solely for nonmedical reasons. Since 1994, the further development of less burdensome and invasive medical technologies for sex selection suggests a need to revisit the complex ethical questions involved.

Background

Interest in sex selection has a long history dating to ancient cultures. Methods have varied from special modes and timing of coitus to the practice of infanticide. Only recently have medical technologies made it possible to attempt sex selection of children before their conception or birth. For example, screening for carriers of X-linked genetic diseases allows potential parents not only to decide whether to have children but also to select the sex of their offspring before pregnancy or before birth.

Among the methods now available for prepregnancy and prebirth sex selection are [1] prefertilization separation of X-bearing from Y-bearing spermatozoa (through a technique that is now available although still investigational for humans), with subsequent selection for artificial insemination or for IVF; [2] preimplantation genetic diagnosis (PGD), followed by the sex selection of embryos for transfer; and [3] prenatal genetic diagnosis, followed by sex-selective abortion. The primary focus of this document is on the second method, sex selection through PGD, although the issues particular to this method overlap with the issues relevant to the others. Preimplantation genetic diagnosis is used with assisted reproductive technologies such as IVF to identify genetic disorders, but it also can provide information regarding the sex of embryos either as a by-product of testing for genetic disorders or when it is done purely for sex selection (Table 9.1).

As the methods of sex selection have varied throughout history, so have the motivations for it. Among the most prominent of motivations historically have been simple desires to bear and raise children of the culturally preferred gender, to ensure

Original publication details: The Ethics Committee of the American Society of Reproductive Medicine, "Sex Selection and Preimplantation Genetic Diagnosis," pp. 595–598 from *Fertility and Sterility* 72: 4 (October 1999). Reproduced with permission of Elsevier.

Table 9.1   Embryo sex identification by preimplantation genetic diagnosis for nonmedical reasons

(a) Patient is undergoing IVF and PGD.
     Patient learns sex identification of embryo as *part of*, or as *a by-product of*, PGD done for other medical reasons.
(b) Patient is undergoing IVF and PGD.
     Patient requests that sex identification be *added to* PGD being done for other medical reasons.
(c) Patient is undergoing IVF, but PGD is not necessary to treatment.
     Patient *requests PGD* solely for the purpose of sex identification.
(d) Patient is not undergoing either IVF or PGD (for the treatment of infertility or any other medical reason).
     Patient *requests IVF and PGD* solely for the purpose of sex identification.

the economic usefulness of offspring within a family, to achieve gender balance among children in a given family, and to determine a gendered birth order. New technologies also have served these aims, but they have raised to prominence the goal of avoiding the birth of children with sex-related genetic disorders.

Whatever its methods or its reasons, sex selection has encountered significant ethical objections throughout its history. Religious traditions and societies in general have responded with concerns varying from moral outrage at infanticide to moral reservations regarding the use of some prebirth methods of diagnosis for the sole purpose of sex selection. More recently, concerns have focused on the dangers of gender discrimination and the perpetuation of gender oppression in contemporary societies.

This document's focus on PGD for sex selection is prompted by the increasing attractiveness of prepregnancy sex selection over prenatal diagnosis and sex-selective abortion, and by the current limited availability of methods of prefertilization sex selection techniques that are both reliable and safe. Although the actual use of PGD for sex selection is still infrequent, its potential use continues to raise important ethical questions.

Central to the controversies over the use of PGD for sex selection, particularly for nonmedical reasons, are

issues of gender discrimination, the appropriateness of expanding control over nonessential characteristics of offspring, and the relative importance of sex selection when weighed against medical and financial burdens to parents and against multiple demands for limited medical resources. In western societies, these concerns inevitably encounter what has become a strong presumption in favor of reproductive choice.

The General Ethical Debate

Arguments for PGD and sex selection make two primary appeals. The first is to the right to reproductive choice on the part of the person or persons who seek to bear a child. Sex selection, it is argued, is a logical extension of this right. The second is an appeal to the important goods to be achieved through this technique and the choices it allows – above all, the medical good of preventing the transmission of sex-linked genetic disorders such as hemophilia A and B, Lesch-Nyhan syndrome, Duchenne-Becker muscular dystrophy, and Hunter syndrome. There also are perceived individual and social goods such as gender balance or distribution in a family with more than one child, parental companionship with a child of one's own gender, and a preferred gender order among one's children. More remotely, it sometimes is argued that PGD and sex selection of embryos for transfer is a lesser evil (medically and ethically) than the alternative of prenatal diagnosis and sex-selected abortion, and even that PGD and sex selection can contribute indirectly to population limitation (i.e., with this technique, parents no longer are compelled to continue to reproduce until they achieve a child of the preferred gender).

Arguments against PGD used for sex selection appeal either to what is considered inherently wrong with sex selection or to the bad consequences that are likely to outweigh the good consequences of its use. Suspicion of sex selection as wrong is lodged in the concerns identified earlier: the potential for inherent gender discrimination, inappropriate control over nonessential characteristics of children, unnecessary medical burdens and costs for parents, and inappropriate and potentially unfair use of limited medical resources for sex selection rather than for more genuine and urgent medical needs. These concerns are closely connected with predictions of negative consequences, such as risk of psychological harm to sex-selected offspring (i.e., by placing on them too high expectations), increased marital conflict over sex-selective decisions, and reinforcement of gender bias in society as a whole. Sometimes the predictions reach to dire consequences such as an overall change in the human sex ratio detrimental to the future of a particular society.

Preimplantation Genetic Diagnosis and Sex Selection: Joining the Particular Issues

The right to reproductive freedom has never been considered an absolute right, certainly not if it is extended to include every sort of decision about reproduction or every demand for positive support in individuals' reproductive decisions. Still, serious reasons (e.g., the likelihood of seriously harmful consequences or the presence of a competing stronger right) must be provided if a limitation on reproductive freedom is to be justified. Hence, the weighing of opposing positions regarding PGD and sex selection depends on an assessment of the strength of the reasons given for and against it.

Preimplantation genetic diagnosis has the potential for serving sex selection in varying categories of cases, each of which raises different medical and ethical questions. Preimplantation genetic diagnosis may be done for disease prevention, or it may be done for any of the other motivations individuals have for determining the sex of their offspring. Moreover, information about the sex of an embryo may be obtained (a) as an essential part of or by-product of PGD performed for other (medical) reasons or (b) through a

test for sex identification that is added to PGD performed for medical reasons. Further, (c) a patient who is undergoing IVF procedures as part of fertility treatment (but whose treatment does not require PGD for medical reasons) may request PGD solely for the purpose of sex selection, and (d) a patient who is fertile (hence, not undergoing IVF as part of treatment) may request IVF and PGD, both solely for the purpose of sex selection. Each of these situations calls for a distinct medical and ethical assessment (Table 9.1).

There presently is little debate over the ethical validity of PGD for sex selection when its aim is to prevent the transmission of sex-linked genetic disease. In this case, sex selection does not prefer one sex over the other for its own supposed value; it does not, therefore, have the potential to contribute as such to gender bias. And when the genetic disorder is severe, efforts to prevent it can hardly be placed in a category of trivializing or instrumentalizing human reproduction. Moreover, prepregnancy sex-selective techniques used for this purpose appear to have a clear claim on limited resources along with other medical procedures that are performed with the goal of eliminating disease and suffering.

It is less easy to eliminate concerns regarding PGD and sex selection when it is aimed at serving social and psychological goals not related to the prevention of disease. It must be recognized, of course, that individuals and couples have wide discretion and liberty in making reproductive choices, even if others object. Yet ethical arguments against sex selection appear to gain strength as the categories of potential cases descend from (a) to (d). For example, desires for family gender balance or birth order, companionship, family economic welfare, and the ready acceptance of offspring who are more "wanted" because their gender is selected may not in every case deserve the charge of unjustified gender bias, but they are vulnerable to it.

Whatever they may mean for an individual or family choice, they also, if fulfilled on a large scale through PGD for sex selection, may contribute to a society's gender stereotyping and overall gender discrimination. On the other hand, if they are expressed and fulfilled only on a small scale and sporadically (as is presently the case), their social implications will be correspondingly limited. Still, they remain vulnerable to the judgment that no matter what their basis, they identify gender as a reason to value one person over another, and they support socially constructed stereotypes of what gender means. In doing so, they not only reinforce possibilities of unfair discrimination, but they may trivialize human reproduction by making it depend on the selection of nonessential features of offspring.

Desired potential social benefits of sex selection also may appear insufficiently significant when weighed against unnecessary bodily burdens and risks for women, and when contrasted with other needs for and claims on medical resources. In particular, many would judge it unreasonable for individuals who do not otherwise need IVF (for the treatment of infertility or prevention of genetic disease) to undertake its burdens and expense solely to select the gender of their offspring. Although individuals may be free to accept such burdens, and although costs may be borne in a way that does not directly violate the rights of others, to encourage PGD for sex selection when it is not medically indicated presents ethical problems.

More remote sorts of consequences of PGD and sex selection, both good and bad, remain too speculative to place seriously in the balance of ethical assessments of the techniques. That is, potential good consequences such as population control, and potential bad consequences such as imbalance in a society's sex ratio, seem too uncertain in their prediction to be determinative of the issues of sex selection. Even if, for example, the current rise in sex selection of offspring in a few countries suggests a correlation between the availability of sex selection methods and the concrete expression of son-preference, there can be no easy transfer of these data to other societies. This does not mean, however, that all concerns for the general social consequences of sex selection techniques regarding general gender discrimination can be dismissed.

The United States is not likely to connect sex selection practices with severe needs to limit population (as

may be the case in other countries). Moreover, gender discrimination is not as deeply intertwined with economic structures in the United States as it may be elsewhere. Nonetheless, ongoing problems with the status of women in the United States make it necessary to take account of concerns for the impact of sex selection on goals of gender equality.

Moreover, the issue of controlling offspring characteristics that are perceived as nonessential cannot be summarily dismissed. Those who argue that offering parental choices of sex selection is taking a major step toward "designing" offspring present concerns that are not unreasonable in a highly technologic culture. Yet it appears precipitous to assume that the possibility of gender choices will lead to a feared radical transformation of the meaning of human reproduction. A "slippery slope" argument seems overdrawn when it is used here. The desire to have some control over the gender of offspring is older than the new technologies that make this possible. This, however, suggests that should otherwise permissible technologies for sex selection be actively promoted for nonmedical reasons — as in (b), (c), and (d) above — their threat to widely valued meanings of human reproduction may call for more serious concern than other speculative and remote negative consequences of PGD and sex selection.

Objections to PGD and sex selection on the grounds of misallocation of resources are more difficult to sustain. Questions of this sort are not so obviously relevant to systems of medical care like the one in the United States. If an individual is able and willing to pay for desired (and medically reasonable) services, there is no direct, easy way to show how any particular set of choices takes away from the right of others to basic care. Yet even here, individual and group decisions do have an impact on the overall deployment of resources for medical care and on the availability of reproductive services.

Although, as already noted, there is little controversy about the seriousness of the need to prevent genetic diseases, it is doubtful that gender preference on the basis of other social and psychological desires should be given as high a priority. The distinction between medical needs and nonmedical desires is particularly relevant if PGD is done solely for sex selection based on nonmedical preferences. The greater the demand on medical resources to achieve PGD for no other reason than sex selection, as in descending order in (b) through (d) above, the more questions surround it regarding its appropriateness for medical practice. If, on the other hand, PGD is done as part of infertility treatment, and the information that allows sex selection is not gained through the additional use of medical resources, it presumably is free of more serious problems of fairness in the allocation of scarce resources and appropriateness to the practice of medicine.

The ethical issues that have emerged in this document's concern for PGD and sex selection are in some ways particular to the uses and consequences of a specific reproductive technology. Their general significance is broader than this, however. For example, the concerns raised here provide at least a framework for an ethical assessment of new techniques for selecting X-bearing or Y-bearing sperm for IUI or IVF (ongoing clinical trial reports of which appeared while this document was being developed). Here, too, sex selection for the purposes of preventing the transmission of genetic diseases does not appear to present ethical problems. However, here also, sex selection for nonmedical reasons, especially if facilitated on a large scale, has the potential to reinforce gender bias in a society, and it may constitute inappropriate use and allocation of medical resources. Finally, although sperm sorting and IUI can entail less burden for parents, questions of the risk to offspring from techniques that involve staining and the use of a laser on sperm DNA remain under investigation.

Recommendations

Of the arguments in favor of PGD and sex selection, only the one based on the prevention of transmittable genetic diseases is strong enough to clearly avoid or override concerns regarding gender equality, acceptance of offspring for themselves and not their inessential characteristics, health risks and burdens for individuals attempting to achieve pregnancy, and equitable use and distribution of medical resources. These concerns remain for PGD and sex selection when it is used to fulfill nonmedical preferences or social and psychological needs. However, because it is not clear in every case that the use of PGD and sex selection for nonmedical reasons entails certainly grave wrongs or sufficiently predictable grave negative consequences, the Committee does not favor its legal prohibition. Nonetheless, the cumulative weight of the arguments against nonmedically motivated sex selection gives cause for serious ethical caution. The Committee's recommendations therefore follow from an effort to respect and to weigh ethical concerns that are sometimes in conflict – namely, the right to reproductive freedom, genuine medical needs and goals, gender equality, and justice in the distribution of medical resources. On the basis of its foregoing ethical analysis, the Committee recommends the following:

1. Preimplantation genetic diagnosis used for sex selection to prevent the transmission of serious genetic disease is ethically acceptable. It is not inherently gender biased, bears little risk of consequences detrimental to individuals or to society, and represents a use of medical resources for reasons of human health.

2. In patients undergoing IVF, PGD used for sex selection for nonmedical reasons – as in (a) through (c) above – holds some risk of gender bias, harm to individuals and society, and inappropriateness in the use and allocation of limited medical resources. Although these risks are lower when sex identification is already part of a by-product of PGD being done for medical reasons (a), they increase when sex identification is added to PGD solely for purposes of sex selection (b) and when PGD is itself initiated solely for sex selection (c). They remain a concern

whenever sex selection is done for nonmedical reasons. Such use of PGD therefore should not be encouraged.

3. The initiation of IVF with PGD solely for sex selection (d) holds even greater risk of unwarranted gender bias, social harm, and the diversion of medical resources from genuine medical need. It therefore should be discouraged.

4. Ethical caution regarding PGD for sex selection calls for study of the consequences of this practice. Such study should include cross-cultural as well as intracultural patterns, ongoing assessment of competing claims for medical resources, and reasonable efforts to discern changes in the level of social responsibility and respect for future generations.

10

Sex Selection and Preimplantation Diagnosis
A Response to the Ethics Committee of the American Society of Reproductive Medicine

Julian Savulescu and Edgar Dahl

Introduction

In its recent statement 'Sex Selection and Preimplantation Genetic Diagnosis', the Ethics Committee of the American Society of Reproductive Medicine concluded that it is ethically appropriate to employ these new reproductive technologies to avoid the birth of children suffering from X-linked genetic disorders (Ethics Committee of the American Society of Reproductive Medicine, 1999 [see chapter 9 in this volume]). However, to use preimplantation genetic diagnosis and sex selection solely for non-medical reasons, the Committee claims, is morally inappropriate. The Committee 'does not favour its legal prohibition', but it strongly advises that sex selection and preimplantation genetic diagnosis for non-medical reasons 'should be discouraged'.

Why does the Ethics Committee think that sex selection and preimplantation genetic diagnosis for non-medical reasons is ethically inappropriate and ought to be discouraged? Although the Committee acknowledges that individuals enjoy procreative liberty and that 'serious reasons must be provided if a limitation on reproductive freedom is to be justified', it claims that the social risks of sex selection outweigh the social benefits. What are these 'social risks' supposed to be?

The reservation against sex selection for non-medical reasons is often based on the assumption that it will invariably lead to a serious distortion of the sex ratio. The Committee has certainly been wise not to rely on this highly speculative objection. According to the available empirical evidence, individuals in Western societies do not have a preference for a particular sex. Most couples still wish to leave the sex of their children 'up to fate'. And those few who would want some control over the gender of their children desire to have a 'balanced family', that is a family with both daughters and sons, most often one daughter and one son (Statham *et al.*, 1993).

While sex selection in the West is unlikely to disturb the sex ratio (Simpson and Carson, 1999), more openly available sex selection would further distort the sex ratio in Asia. The male to female ratio is nearly 1.2 in China and some parts of India. In 1990, there were 100 million women 'missing' as a result of

Original publication details: Julian Savulescu and Edgar Dahl, "Sex Selection and Preimplantation Diagnosis: A Response to the Ethics Committee of the American Society of Reproductive Medicine," pp. 1879–1880 from *Human Reproduction* 15: 9 (2000). Reproduced with permission of Oxford University Press.

Bioethics: An Anthology, Fourth Edition. Edited by Udo Schüklenk and Peter Singer.
Editorial material and organization © 2022 John Wiley & Sons, Inc. Published 2022 by John Wiley & Sons, Inc.

various forms of discrimination (Benagiano and Bianchi, 1999). But some have argued that disturbed sex ratios may not be detrimental to women. Advantages which have been postulated include increase in influence of the rarer gender, reduced population growth and interbreeding of different populations (Sureau, 1999). In a practical sense, sex selection employing preimplantation genetic diagnosis may be preferable to the alternatives. It would be morally preferable to many people to termination of 'wrong sex' pregnancies or female infanticide (Sureau, 1999) and is preferable to increasing population burdens in an attempt to have a child of the desired sex (Simpson and Carson, 1999).

The Committee also does not base its reservation about sex selection on vague 'slippery slope' arguments. The Committee is well aware that it is perfectly possible to draw a legal line between the selection for sex and the selection for other characteristics, such as eye colour, height or intelligence. Thus, if there is consensus that selection for sex is morally acceptable but selection for, let us say, intelligence is not, professional or legislative controls can be employed to allow the former but not the latter. Arguments claiming that sex selection is the initial step down a road that will inevitably lead to the creation of 'designer babies' or a 'new eugenics' are simply invalid.

However, if it is not the fear of a distorted sex ratio or a slide towards eugenics, then, what are the social risks the Committee is referring to? The Committee rests its case against sex selection for non-medical reasons upon four claims. Firstly, sex selection is to be opposed because it identifies 'gender as a reason to value one person over another'. Secondly, it may 'contribute to a society's gender stereotyping and gender discrimination'. Thirdly, because it is 'unreasonable for individuals who do not otherwise need IVF to undertake its burdens and expense solely to select the gender of their offspring'. And fourthly, because it represents a 'misallocation of limited medical resources'.

Consider the first objection. The claim that couples requesting sex selection 'identify gender as a reason to value one person over another' is simply unsound. Couples seeking the service of Gender Clinics are typically in their mid-thirties, have two or three children of the same sex and wish to have at least one child of the opposite sex. Their choice for a child of a particular sex depends entirely upon the sex of the children they already have. If they already have two or three boys they tend to choose a girl, if they already have two or three girls they tend to choose a boy (Fugger et al., 1998). Since their choice is simply based on the gender of already existing children, and not on the absurd assumption that one sex is 'superior' to another, the claim that these couples are making a sexist choice is an unjustified accusation.

The existing data of Gender Clinics also undermine the second objection of the Committee that sex selection for non-medical reasons may 'reinforce gender bias in a society'. Since couples seeking sex selection are almost exclusively motivated by the desire to balance their family and choose girls with the same frequency as boys, it is hard to see how their choices are supposed to contribute to a society's gender discrimination (Khatamee et al., 1989; Liu and Rose, 1995). If these were real concerns, sex selection could be limited to balancing family sex, and only after the first child.

The third objection that it is 'unreasonable' for a woman to undergo a burdensome IVF treatment solely to select the sex of her child smacks suspiciously of medical paternalism. The Committee seems to be aware of this as it tones down its statement in the following sentence, saying that 'individuals may be free to accept such burdens'. Yet, it insists, 'to encourage preimplantation genetic diagnosis for sex selection when it is not medically indicated presents ethical problems.' What ethical problems does it present? Unfortunately, we are not told. More importantly, the issue is not whether preimplantation genetic diagnosis for sex selection is to be 'encouraged', but whether the mere fact that an IVF treatment cycle imposes a burden on a woman is a sufficient reason to 'discourage' her. If a woman is aware of the physical and psychological costs to herself but thinks having a child of a certain sex is worth the trouble, it is an autonomous decision that needs to be respected. After all it is her life and her body. The Committee seems blind to the importance of gender to parents, and that parents are best left to themselves to make decisions about the constitution of their family (Savulescu, 1999).

The Committee did not focus on the physical risks of preimplantation diagnosis to children born and these clearly need to be evaluated in any sex selection procedure (Benagiano and Bianchi, 1999; Simpson and Carson, 1999). Experience so far is encouraging, with several hundred children being born after PGD without apparent detriment. Systematic review is continuing (ESHRE PGD Consortium Steering Committee, 1999).

The fourth and last objection of the Committee is that preimplantation genetic diagnosis for sex selection constitutes 'inappropriate use and allocation of medical resources'. To our knowledge, no-one has so far seriously advocated that the state, i.e. the tax-payer, should subsidize sex selection for non-medical reasons. Again, the Committee seems to be aware of this when it continues: 'If an individual is able and willing to pay for desired services, there is no direct, easy way to show how any particular set of choices takes away from the right of others to basic care.' Nonetheless, it claims: 'Yet even here, individual and group decisions do have an impact on the overall deployment of resources for medical care and on the availability of reproductive services.' The Committee is relentless in its claim that allowing sex selection is a misallocation of resources, repeating itself at least four times on this issue. Since this objection seems to be the most compelling, it would have been helpful to show how a privately paid service for sex selection can possibly deprive the community of its scarce medical resources. If people are permitted to spend their own money on cosmetic surgery without being accused of violating 'the right of others to basic care', it is hard to see why couples willing to spend their own money on sex selection should be treated differently. Moreover, given the burdens, the expense and the low success rate of IVF, it is highly unlikely that preimplantation genetic diagnosis for sex selection will ever become so widespread as to have an 'impact on the overall deployment of resources for medical care and on the availability of reproductive services'.

Thus, when the Committee concludes that preimplantation genetic diagnosis for sex selection poses a 'risk of unwarranted gender bias, social harm, the diversion of medical resources from genuine medical need and should therefore be discouraged', it seems that the boldness of its statement is in conspicuous contrast to the weakness of its arguments.

References

Benagiano, G. and Bianchi, P. (1999). Sex preselection: an aid to couples or a threat to humanity? *Hum. Reprod.*, 14: 868–70.

ESHRE PGD Consortium Steering Committee (1999). ESHRE Preimplantation Genetic Diagnosis (PGD) Consortium: preliminary assessment of data from January 1997 to September 1998. *Hum. Reprod.*, 14: 3138–48.

Ethics Committee of the American Society of Reproductive Medicine (1999). Sex selection and preimplantation genetic diagnosis. *Fertil. Steril.*, 72: 595–8.

Fugger, E. F., Black, S. H., Keyvanfar, K. *et al.* (1998). Births of normal daughters after Microsort sperm separation and intrauterine insemination, in-vitro fertilization, or intracytoplasmic sperm injection. *Hum. Reprod.*, 13: 2367–70.

Khatamee, M. A., Leinberger-Sica, A., Matos, P. *et al.* (1989). Sex preselection in New York City: who chooses which sex and why. *Int. J. Fertil.*, 34: 353–4.

Liu, P. and Rose, A. (1995). Social aspects of >800 couples coming forward for gender selection of their children. *Hum. Reprod.*, 10: 968–971.

Savulescu, J. (1999). Sex selection – the case for. *Med. J. Australia*, 171: 373–5.

Simpson, J. L. and Carson, S.A. (1999). The reproductive option of sex selection. *Hum. Reprod.*, 14: 870–2.

Statham, H., Green, J., Snowdon, C. and France-Dawson, M. (1993). Choice of baby's sex. *Lancet*, 341: 564–5.

Sureau, G. (1999). Gender selection: a crime against humanity or the exercise of a fundamental right? *Hum. Reprod.*, 14: 867–8.

11

Why We Should Not Permit Embryos to Be Selected as Tissue Donors

David King

The announcement of the birth of a son to the Whitaker family, who was selected as an embryo to be a tissue-matched donor for his sick brother, has sparked the usual massive media interest. It seems that the Whitaker family have great public sympathy and support for their use of the technique. As usual, the main voices opposing the use of this technique have been those of the pro-lifers. The predominant view, summarised as: 'What can be wrong with saving the life of a sick child?' demands a proper response, which is not grounded in the belief that embryos possess a right to life.

Children as Things

The main objection to the use of pre-implantation genetic diagnosis (PGD) for this purpose is that it objectifies the child by turning it into a mere tool, and so contradicts the basic ethical principle that we should never use human beings merely as a means to an end (however good that end may be), because they should also be treated as ends in themselves. That

is the basic ethical objection to slavery, for example. In response to this, it is often said that the new child will be loved for himself, and will not be treated by his parents as a mere tool, and this is no doubt true. However, the Whitakers have made it very clear that their primary purpose for conceiving Jamie was to save their other son: this will nearly always be the case for couples in their position. The case against this use of PGD does not depend on fine analysis of each couple's motivations and emotional states, or on how much they succeed in loving their new child despite the reasons for his/her conception, but on the consequences of breaking the ethical rule.

While most people would agree with the ethical principle, many seem to feel that it is a case of abstract principles versus real individual suffering; and because, as is typical in our public discourse, the case is discussed without considering the context, ie. the overall trends promoted by reproductive and biomedical technology, the reasons for concern about objectification seem remote and theoretical. However, I would argue that these cases, far from being special examples, in which we should allow exceptions to

Original publication details: David King, "Why We Should Not Permit Embryos to Be Selected as Tissue Donors," pp. 13–16 from *The Bulletin of Medical Ethics* 190 (August 2003). © 2003 RSM Press. Reproduced with permission of the Royal Society of Medicine.

our principles, are in fact typical examples of the way that reproductive and biomedical technologies objectify human beings. That is why it is so important that we resist the selection of embryos as tissue donors: because these cases significantly advance the objectifying trend, and the consequences of doing so are, in the not-so-long term, disastrous.

Selection of embryos as tissue donors falls squarely into the objectifying trend in two senses: the literal and the ethical. What makes many people very uncomfortable about biomedical technology in general is the way that the relentless march of reductionist science continually turns human beings, at various stages of development, into human organisms, useful sources of biological raw material for spare parts. As science discovers more and more about the workings of the human body, our bodies are seen as no more than machines, with no special moral meaning or dignity, and the pressure to extract various components in order to benefit others becomes ever greater. The problem is the way that this pressure leads to rewriting of ethical rules. Whether it is at the beginning of the lifecycle, with the envisioned creation of cloned embryos purely as sources of stem cells and the proposed extraction of eggs from aborted fetuses for use in IVF, or at the end, with the constant shifting of definitions of death to facilitate 'harvesting' of organs for transplantation, the integrity of human organisms and the ethical rules protecting them seem everywhere under siege from the enthusiasm of biomedical technicians. Only able-bodied post-natal humans seem, for the moment, to be safe.

The creation of babies as sources of tissue, and, as shocking, the co-option of reproduction for reasons other than procreation, push instrumentalisation of human life one step further, and dispose of one more ethical principle. They also set the stage for further steps: how long before we will be told that saving a child this way is the best reason for cloning? And if we can create embryos and children as sources of cells, if it proves necessary, (perhaps because it proves impossible to create the required organs from embryonic stem cells), why not allow the embryos to grow into fetuses and 'harvest' tissues at that stage?

Leaving aside these next steps, many people could benefit medically from matched tissue donation – there is nothing unique about Charlie Whitaker's disease. How will we feel when the tissue recipient is not another child, but an adult, maybe a parent or a more remote family member?

In the reproductive context, objectification has a particular ethical meaning, often summed up in the term 'designer babies'. The increasing technologisation of reproduction, and the use of technology to choose our children's characteristics, tend to make reproduction just another process for producing consumer goods. Although the outputs of this process are undeniably human beings, by choosing their characteristics we turn them into things, just human-designed objects. Conversely, by taking this new power of selection/design over a key part of what constitutes those individuals, we elevate ourselves above them. This is part of what people mean when they talk about playing God. The parent–child relationship becomes a designer–object relationship, rather than one between two fundamentally equal human subjects.

The selection of children as tissue donors is an example of the objectifying trend in techno-reproduction, albeit not a typical one. Here, the child is not selected for characteristics that will 'improve' it, but to benefit another child. In one sense this is more acceptable, since the aim of the procedure is undoubtedly good, and is not motivated by consumerist desires for 'enhancement'. But in another sense it is a more extreme example of objectification, because the primary reason for the child's being is not even to be a child as such, but to be a source of spare parts for another.

As the discussions about how Jamie is likely to feel and be treated have shown, there are immediate consequences of breaking the ethical rule: it is not a matter of 'real suffering versus abstract ethical principles'. Despite all the love that his parents will no doubt give him, how will Jamie feel as he grows up, knowing that he was wanted first for his genes, and only secondly for himself? What if the transplant fails? There is a considerable chance that the cord blood transplant will fail: the next step is bone marrow extraction, which is painful and has risks. It is not hard to see that, having conceived Jamie to save his brother, his parents will feel impelled to submit him to this procedure, and the doctors who might otherwise have counselled them against submitting a young child to this, will feel weakened.

In response to these points, it is suggested that people often have children for bad reasons, and we do nothing about that, so why object to this? In my view this is intellectual laziness of the worst sort. First, two wrongs do not make a right. Secondly, it is precisely this kind of argumentation which always drives us down slippery slopes: 'You've accepted X in the past, so there's no reason for not accepting Y, the next step'. Often the very bioethicists who reject slippery slopes as non-existent, and insist we can always draw a line, are the same people who, when the time for linedrawing arrives, tell us it would be inconsistent to do so. More importantly, we must realise that the availability of technology to change chance and hope into certainty and expectation completely transforms the situation, and the nature of reproduction. While parents may have children for various more or less acceptable social reasons, this use of PGD wrenches procreation from its biological purpose and its social context in a way which objectifies the child in a qualitatively new way – now we have children as medical aids.

In summary, when we look at these cases in their proper context, it is clear that the rule not to use people as mere means to an end (instrumentalising them) is not just a remote theoretical principle. Objectification and instrumentalisation are an inherent feature of reproductive biomedicine, not something that just crops up in occasional cases. Thus we can be quite certain that, if we abandon the principle now, we will see more and worse to follow.

What Kind of Ethics Do We Need?

It is apparent that cases like these pose a challenge not only to our mechanisms for discussion and decision, but to the kind of ethics that underlie the mainstream of debates.

First, it should be clear that the kind of ethics purveyed by the HFEA [Human Fertilisation and Embryology Authority] is not merely grossly inadequate but positively misleading. It is not only that the HFEA is dominated by a philosophy that allows no critique of science itself, or of the direction of medicine. Nor is it that the ethics employed are abstract and have to conform to the discourse rules of bioethics, which forbid historical analysis of social processes, such as the trend of objectification and the forces driving it. The problem is worse: the HFEA cannot even articulate the basic ethical issues at the centre of public concern.

Surveying the HFEA's public statements on the Whitaker case we find two arguments: the potential psychological effect for Jamie, and the risk of PGD to the embryo, which can only be justified if there is benefit to that embryo, i.e. being assured of not suffering from a genetic disorder. The latter argument is the basis of the HFEA's permitting the Hashmi family to undergo embryo selection. Their child Zain suffers from thalassemia, a genetic disease, so they could argue that their primary purpose for PGD was to prevent the new child having thalassemia, and that tissue type selection would add no extra risk to the embryo. The HFEA turned down the Whitakers last year because their son was suffering from a disorder which is not genetic, and there is therefore no case for using PGD to avoid it.

These arguments are pathetically weak and seem almost designed not to stand the test of time and the pressure of public opinion. While it is true that Jamie may be psychologically harmed by the conditions of his coming into being, that harm, of itself (i.e. understood without reference to the objectification inherent in reproductive biomedicine), seems paltry in comparison to the good involved in saving a child. As for the distinction based on whether the child has a genetic or sporadic condition, it is not surprising the public finds it incomprehensible for the HFEA to support publicly the Hashmis one week and turn down the Whitakers the next. The distinction, in a common sense view of the world, is meaningless: to hang the different decisions on it is silly. There is no firm evidence that PGD is harmful and, again, such a risk seems small in comparison to the saving of a life. Either the use of the technique is acceptable in both cases, or in neither.

More importantly, nowhere in the HFEA's public pronouncements can we find any clear reference to the point, which has been at the centre of the public debate, about the Kantian ethical principle of non-instrumentalisation/objectification. Now even the rules of liberal ethics cannot be publicly mentioned. How can this be? The answer is that the HFEA is, by virtue of its own institutional nature, not allowed to use the sort of ethical principles that ordinary people use. It can consider medical benefit and risk and, because it is written into the relevant legislation, the welfare of the child. But for the HFEA, which has legal responsibilities, and exists in a controversial and litigious climate, it is impossible to base its decision even on ethical principles as universally accepted as Kant's, because to do so makes it vulnerable: only benefit, risk and welfare considerations, on a strictly individual case-by-case basis, are legally defensible. (The Whitaker/Hashmi distinction, for example, is not based on any real moral difference between the cases; in the Whitaker case the HFEA overruled its own ethics committee, which wanted to be consistent with its decision on the Hashmis. What dictated the HFEA decision in these cases was the need to stay within the letter of the law, which appears to forbid selection of embryos to benefit another individual. Its calculation was correct, and allowed it to defend its decision in the High Court against a pro-life group's challenge. In effect they made the right decision for the wrong reasons. This is one more example of sensible policy and decision making being tripped up by accidents of drafting of the 1990 HFE Act: it has been comprehensively overtaken by developments in science and technology and needs amending.)

So the result of the HFEA's institutional status is that the key ethical decision-making body in this area is forced to behave as an ethical illiterate, and to operate ethically on the basis of political pragmatism. This will never lead to decisions that are either principled or in the public interest.

What is happening is strikingly reminiscent of the history of genetically modified organisms (GMOs): that experience should be a warning to the government. Throughout the 1990s critics complained that the Advisory Committee on Release to the Environment (ACRE) based judgements about the environmental risk of GMOs on narrow, case-by-case analyses of the direct environmental impact of small-scale experimental trials, without considering wider issues. It did so because of the narrow definition of environmental harm in the 1990 Environmental Protection Act. ACRE was not permitted to consider the impact of GMOs in farming (eg. changes in patterns of pesticide use created by GMO use) which might have large environmental impacts, let alone the wider implications of GMOs. Its members had a narrow range of scientific expertise, with no sociologist, economist or expert in farming and the environment. So it could not address many concerns of environmentalists and other critics, yet it was the main venue of regulatory decisions which, by government dogma, must be 'science-based'. These concerns eventually exploded into direct action and public furore. ACRE was completely overhauled, European law was rewritten, and the government was forced to delay while it mounted farm-scale trials of the impact of GMOs.

The HFEA is in essentially the same position as ACRE in the 1990s. Its legal responsibilities stop it from addressing the public's real concerns, about the trends of objectification, consumerism and eugenics, and where these technologies, step by step, are taking us. As long as HFEA continues to work this way, the head of steam will continue to build, and who knows how it will be released.

Clearly what is needed is an ethical discourse that can articulate and discuss people's real, long-term concerns, and can balance them against the demands of individual cases. Here we see a key distinction from the debate over GMOs, where the pressure for 'progress' was driven by the cold and unsympathetic imperatives of science and the market, with no clear benefit to people. With reproductive technology we risk being overwhelmed by a tidal wave of sentiment about sick children, blinding us to where these decisions are leading. In public discussion of the Whitaker case, many parents said they would do anything to save their sick child. God preserve us from people who will do anything! We must not make public policy, with profound long-term consequences, on the basis of individual families' desperation, however much we may empathise with them.

Ultimately, an adequate ethical discourse needs to reassess the dominant imperative to eliminate all disease and suffering, and the moral blackmail which is wielded at those who dare to suggest that other concerns might have equal importance. For if we fail to do so, we will find, not so far in the future, that the consequences of abandoning principle after principle will be felt not only in terms of a moral vacuum, but in the profound suffering of real human beings, in ways that we can now only begin to imagine.

12

The Moral Status of Human Cloning
Neo-Lockean Persons versus Human Embryos

Michael Tooley

Introduction

Cloning human organisms may have quite different goals. The object may be to produce a human organism that will develop into a normal person. Alternatively, the goal may be to produce a human embryo for scientific research purposes, or as a source of stem cells to be used in medical treatments. Yet another possibility is the creation of a human to serve as a future organ bank for some presently existing person. In this essay, I shall consider whether cloning is or is not morally permissible in each of these three cases.

1 A Crucial Concept: neo-Lockean Persons

1.1 John Locke's concept of a person

In chapter 27 of *An Essay Concerning Human Understanding*, John Locke (1632–1704) discussed the idea of identity, and there he distinguished between the identity of a man – that is, of a human animal – and the identity of a person. As regards the former, Locke's view was as follows:

> This also shows wherein the identity of the same *man* consists: viz. in nothing but a participation of the same continued life, by constantly fleeting particles of matter, in succession vitally united to the same organized body. (chap. 27, para. 6)

As regards the concept of a person, however, Locke offered a very different account:

> . . . to find wherein *personal identity* consists, we must consider what *person* stands for; which I think, is a thinking intelligent being that has reason and reflection and can consider itself as itself, the same thinking thing in different times and places; which it does only by that consciousness which is inseparable from thinking and, as it seems to me, essential to it . . . .. For since consciousness always accompanies thinking, and it is that that makes everyone to be what he calls *self*, and thereby distinguishes himself from all other thinking things: in this alone consists *personal identity*, i.e. the sameness of a rational being. (chap.27, para. 9)

Original publication details: Michael Tooley, "The Moral Status of the Cloning of Human Cloning: Neo Lockean Persons Versus Human Embryos." Written for this edition (2021) and reproduced courtesy of Michael Tooley.

Bioethics: An Anthology, Fourth Edition. Edited by Udo Schüklenk and Peter Singer.

Not all of this is as clear as it could be, and philosophers have offered slightly different interpretations of Locke's concept of personal identity, and thus of his concept of a person. What is crucial here, however, are not the details, but simply that, on Locke's account, a person is an entity that (1) has *conscious* mental states at some times, (2) has *the capacity for thought* at some times, and (3) has thoughts at some times that are *mentally linked* to conscious states at other times.

Locke's concept of a person is clearly very different from his concept of a human animal. It could turn out, of course, that all human animals, at any time, are in fact persons, in Locke's sense. We shall see shortly, however, that there are very strong scientific arguments against that possibility.

1.2   The concept of a neo-Lockean person

I shall sometimes use the expression "neo-Lockean person," and this for three reasons. First of all, as just mentioned, disagreements exist concerning the correct interpretations of the passages where Locke introduces his idea of a person, and no stand need be taken on that issue. Secondly one might want to include in one's concept of a person elements that Locke does not mention, such as desires concerning one's mental states at other times. Thirdly, the term "person" is sometimes used, especially by those who believe that abortion is seriously wrong, in two other, very different ways: sometimes as a purely evaluative term, meaning simply "entity with a right to life," and sometimes as a purely biological expression, meaning "member of the biologically defined species *homo sapiens*." Such uses of the term "person" contain no reference at all to consciousness, or to the capacity for thought, or to any mental states whatsoever. The expression "neo-Lockean person" functions, then, to rule out such interpretations.

Constant use of that expression, however, would become a bit tiresome, so I shall often simply use the term "person," with the understanding that it is always an abbreviation of "neo-Lockean person."

What, then, do I mean by "person"/"neo-Lockean person"? The answer is that a neo-Lockean person is an entity that has, *at least at one time*, a *memory involving a conscious thought about an earlier state of consciousness*. Something that has never enjoyed a single *state of consciousness* is thus not a neo-Lockean person. Similarly, something that has never had *a conscious thought* cannot be a neo-Lockean person. Finally, something that has never had *a memory thought* about an earlier state of consciousness cannot be a neo-Lockean person.

A neo-Lockean person exists, then, when the *consciousness condition*, the *conscious thought* condition, and the *memory thought* conditions are all satisfied.

1.3   Distortions of the concept of a neo-Lockean person

Arguments are rarely offered against the view that only neo-Lockean persons have a right to life, and when offered, they inevitably misrepresent the concept of a neo-Lockean person. A typical example is Christopher Kaczor who, in his book *The Ethics of Abortion*, considers the following possible necessary conditions for existing as a neo-Lockean person at a time: (1) being self-aware at that time; (2) having an immediately exercisable capacity for self-awareness; (3) having functional hardware that is a basis of the capacity for self-awareness; (4) having an active potentiality for reacquiring a capacity for self-awareness; (5) having a passive potentiality for reacquiring the capacity for self-awareness (2014, 31–5).

All of this is a complete failure – or an unwillingness – to recognize what lies at the heart of the concept of a neo-Lockean person, namely, the existence of a memory that, if accessed, will involve a thought about an earlier state of consciousness to which it was causally linked. All of us have some memories, however, that we are able to access at some times, though not at others, and the inability to *access* a memory at a given time does not mean that the memory no longer exists. So none of the conditions that Kaczor mentions are necessary for the continued existence of a neo-Lockean person: as long as the memory exists, the neo-Lockean person exists, and the memory exists as long as the neural basis for it exists.

1.4 Neo-Lockean persons and the right to life

Imagine there are times when you have perceptual experiences and bodily sensations unaccompanied by *any thoughts*. Concerned, you contact your doctor, who tells you of a new virus that temporarily prevents you having any thoughts. Asking about your prognosis, you learn that the temporal gaps between such occurrences will gradually become less and less, until, finally, your ability to have thoughts no longer exists. You ask whether there is any treatment, and are told that there is a drug that, if successful, will completely cure you, but otherwise will kill you.

Consider, now, what it would be like to have sensory experiences and bodily sensations, but to have *no thoughts at all* at any time – no thoughts about your present experiences, no thoughts about what you did in the past, no thoughts when someone speaks to you, no thoughts about anything. What value would you assign to such a life?

Suppose p is the probability that the drug will cure you, and thus $(1 - p)$ the probability that it will kill you. How high does p have to be for you to decide to take the drug at some point before you permanently lose the capacity for thought? The answer to that question will fix the value that a life lacking forever the capacity for thought has for you.

Many people I have talked to about this have said that they would ultimately opt for the drug *regardless of how close to zero the value of p was*. That, however, would imply that the extent to which one values the continued existence of a life with experiences and sensations, but with no capacity for thought, is essentially zero.

The idea is then that it seems plausible to think that there should be a connection between the extent to which people would value such a life and the intrinsic wrongness of killing a person with such a life. If so, the conclusion would be that the wrongness of killing a conscious being permanently lacking the capacity for thought is essentially zero, in which case it would be plausible to conclude that conscious beings *permanently* lacking a capacity for thought, and thus who are not neo-Lockean persons, lack a right to continued existence.

Notice that the conclusion here is that being a neo-Lockean person is a *necessary* condition for having a right to continued existence, and not that it is also a *sufficient* condition, since one might hold, as many philosophers do, that one must also have desires, preferences, or interests in order to have a right to continued existence, and neither Locke's account of a person, nor mine, refers to such mental states. Whether such states are necessary for moral status is a deep and difficult issue in normative ethics, and happily, not one we need not explore here.

2 Cloning to Produce Human Organisms that Will Never Become Persons

2.1 Cloning for medical purposes or scientific research

Embryonic stem cells have proven important for drug discovery and in testing for toxicity, and they also show promise for the treatment of presently incurable diseases, since they can be used to produce different types of cells that can serve to repair damaged tissue (Cerva and Stojkovic, 2007.). To avoid rejection, however, the stems cells should be derived not just from any embryo, but from a clone of the patient.

2.2 Cloning to produce a human organ bank

Here the idea is to clone a human being to produce another human with the same genetic makeup as the original individual, where the human clone will serve as an organ bank, so that if the original individual loses an arm in an accident, or winds up with liver cancer, appropriate spare parts will be available, and no problem of rejection will arise.

If the resulting cloned human being were a person, it would, of course, be wrong to take parts from him or her to repair the damage to the original individual. The idea, however, is that something will be done to the brain of the human that is produced so that the human organism in question *never* has a conscious thought, and thus is not a neo-Lockean person.

2.3   Arguments Against Such Cloning

The objection to cloning that involves the destruction of human embryos is that such entities have a right to life. What support can be offered for the latter claim? There are three important arguments, appealing, respectively, to an immaterial mind or soul, to potentialities, or to a future like ours.

2.3.1   *Appeals to immaterial minds or souls*
Do humans have immaterial minds or souls that are the basis of all their mental states and capacities? The answer is that this is a deeply implausible view, since there are facts about human beings, and other animals, that provide strong evidence for the hypothesis that the categorical basis for all mental states and capacities lies in the brain. First of all, there are extensive correlations between the behavioral capacities of different animals and the neural structures present in their brains. Secondly, the gradual maturation of the brain of a human being is accompanied by a corresponding increase in his or her intellectual capabilities. Thirdly, damage to the brain, due either to external trauma, or to stroke, results in impairment of one's cognitive capacities, and the nature of the impairment is correlated with the part of the brain that was damaged. As I have argued elsewhere (Tooley et al. 2009, 15–19), these facts, and many others, receive a very straightforward explanation given the hypothesis that mental capacities have as their basis appropriate neural circuitry, whereas, on the other hand, they would be both unexplained, and deeply puzzling, if mental capacities had their basis not in the brain, but in some immaterial substance.

2.3.2   *Appeals to potentialities*
Consider fully active potentialities, understood as states of affairs inevitably leading to a certain result in the absence of outside interference, and consider

the thesis that the destruction of a fully active potentiality for the emergence of a neo-Lockean person is seriously wrong. Elsewhere I have offered several arguments against this principle (2009, 42–51). Here is one of the simpler arguments.

Suppose artificial wombs have been perfected, and there is a device containing an unfertilized human egg cell and a human spermatozoon, where if the device is not interfered with, fertilization will result, and the fertilized human egg cell will be transferred to an artificial womb, from which will emerge, in nine months' time, a healthy newborn human. Such a situation involves not merely an "almost active" potentiality for personhood – as in the case of a fertilized human egg cell *on its own* – but, rather, a *fully active potentiality* for personhood. To turn off this device, then, thereby allowing the unfertilized egg cell to die, would involve the destruction of an active potentiality for personhood. Consequently, that action would be seriously wrong if the above, fully active potentiality principle were correct. The action of turning off the device, however, is not morally wrong. Therefore it is not wrong to destroy an active potentiality for personhood.

2.3.3   *The appeal to a future like ours*
One of the most discussed and reprinted papers on abortion is Don Marquis's "Why Abortion is Immoral." In that article, Marquis contends that what makes it wrong to kill something is that thing's having a future like ours.

One objection to this view is that whether something has a future like ours is a matter of that thing's potentialities, so Marquis's view is open to all of the objections that tell against any view that appeals to potentialities.

A second objection involves the idea of the "complete reprogramming" of the mind of a human animal – where all of that human animal's current memories are replaced by totally different, apparent memories, and, similarly, whatever other mental states and traits that may be crucial for personal identity, such as one's personality traits, are also replaced by completely different ones. The neo-Lockean person would not survive such reprogramming, but the human animal would do so, and would have a future like ours. Moreover, if the neo-Lockean person that initially existed had traits making for an unhappy life, whereas the neo-Lockean person who existed after the reprogramming had traits conducive to a very good life, the reprogramming would have enabled the human animal in question to have a *better* future like ours. The question, accordingly, is how Marquis's deprivation account of the wrongness of killing can explain how such complete reprogramming of a human's mind is morally wrong.

My basic claims are then, first, that such "reprogramming" of the mind of a human animal is morally just as wrong as killing a human animal, and secondly, that the wrongness of such reprogramming cannot be explained in terms of depriving *an animal* – as contrasted with a neo-Lockean person – of certain future goods.

2.3.4 Against human organ banks?

The objection to the creation of human organ banks is that, just as in the case of the killing human embryos used either to produce stems cells or for scientific research, one is violating the rights of an individual by damaging its brain. The arguments in support of this claim, however, are the arguments just considered, and found wanting.

3 Cloning to Produce Persons

Let us now turn to the question of whether the use of cloning to produce future persons is in principle morally acceptable or not. In this section, I shall first focus on the question whether such cloning is *intrinsically* wrong. Then I shall consider whether cloning to produce persons is wrong instead *because of its consequences*.

3.1 Is cloning that aims at producing future persons intrinsically wrong?

Let us begin by considering the two lines of argument that Dan Brock (1998, 151–5) thought were crucial.

The first argument appeals to what might initially be described as the right of a person to be a unique individual, but which, in the end, must be characterized instead as the right of a person to a genetically unique nature. The second argument then appeals to the idea that a person has a right to a future that is, in a certain sense, open.

3.1.1 Does a person have a right to a genetically unique nature?

Many people feel that being a unique individual is important, and the basic thrust of this first attempt to show that cloning aimed at producing persons is intrinsically wrong involves the idea that the uniqueness of individuals would be impaired in some way by cloning. In response, I think that one might very well question whether uniqueness is important. If, for example, it turned out that there was, perhaps on some distant planet, a person who was qualitatively identical to oneself, down to the last detail, both physical and psychological, would that really make one's own life less valuable, less worth living?

In thinking about this, it is important to distinguish two different cases: first, the case where the two lives are qualitatively identical due to the operation of deterministic causal laws; secondly, the case where it just happens that both individuals are always in similar situations in which they freely decide upon the same actions, have the same thoughts and feelings, and so on. The second of these scenarios, I suggest, is not troubling. The first, on the other hand, may be, but if it is, is it because there is a person who is qualitatively indistinguishable from oneself, or, rather, because one's life is totally determined?

I am inclined to question, accordingly, the perhaps rather widely held view that uniqueness is important for the value of one's life. Fortunately, however, one need not settle that issue in the present context, since cloning does not produce a person who is qualitatively indistinguishable from the individual who was cloned, for, as is shown by the case of identical twins, two individuals with the same genetic makeup, even when raised within the same family, at the same time, will differ in many respects.

How great are those differences? The result of one study was as follows:

> On average, our questionnaires show that the personality traits of identical twins have a 50 percent correlation. The traits of fraternal twins, by contrast, have a correlation of 25 percent, non-twin siblings a correlation of 11 percent and strangers a correlation of close to zero. (Bouchard, 1995, 54)

Why is the correlation not higher in the case of identical twins? A common answer is that the environment must play a role, and if that is right, it is also natural to think that it must be one's experiences within one's family, during the time that one is maturing, that account for the differences. Judith Rich Harris, however, in her book *The Nurture Assumption*, develops a very strong argument, based on findings by behavioral geneticists, against the view that one's family plays a significant role in the type of person one turns out to be, and she then argues that it is one's peer group that is crucial.

Although Harris makes out a strong case for her view, there is an alternative hypothesis that deserves serious consideration – one suggested by a remark by Steven Pinker in his book, *How the Mind Works*, where he points out that "the genetic assembly instructions for a mental organ do not specify every connection in the brain as if they were a wiring schematic for a Heathkit radio" (1997, 35). Perhaps identical twins, differ, then, because of differences in the wiring of their brains before birth, due to small, more or less accidental events, within their brains at that time.

In any case, regardless of what theory, or combination of theories, is correct, the crucial point is that the personality traits of an individual and his or her clone should, on average, exhibit no more than a 50 percent correlation; moreover, if one thinks that the environment, as normally understood – that is, postnatally – plays an important role, the correlation presumably will generally be even less, given that an individual and his or her clone will typically be raised at different times, and in generations that may differ substantially as regards basic beliefs and fundamental values.

Accordingly, the present argument, if it is to have any chance, must shift from the claim that a person has a right to absolute uniqueness to an appeal to the very different claim that a person has a right to a genetically unique nature. How does the argument fare when thus reformulated?

An initial point worth noticing is that any appeal to a claimed right to a genetically unique nature poses a difficulty for theists: if there is such a right, why has God created a world where identical twins can arise? Many features of the world, of course, are rather surprising if one thinks our world was created by an omnipotent, omniscient, and morally perfect person, so the theist who appeals to a right to a genetically unique nature may simply reply that the presence of twins is just another facet of the general problem of evil. If, however, as I have argued elsewhere (Tooley and Plantinga 2008, 70–150, and 2019, 51–72), evil provides a strong, evidential argument against the existence of God, that response is not very promising.

How can one approach the question of whether persons have a right to a genetically unique nature? Some writers who reject this claim are content to rest with a burden of proof approach. Here the idea is that although it may be that many people think that being a unique individual in the sense of not being *qualitatively identical* with anyone else is an important part of what is valuable about being a person, the idea that persons have a right to a *genetically unique* identity is one that, by contrast, has been introduced only recently. Those who advance the latter claim, therefore, need to offer a *reason* for thinking it is true.

However, one can also offer positive arguments against the claim. One can appeal, for example, to intuitions that one has upon reflection. Thus, one can consider the case of identical twins, and ask oneself whether, upon reflection, one thinks that it would be *prima facie* wrong to reproduce if one somehow knew that doing so would result in identical twins. I think it would be surprising if many people felt that this was so.

Another way of approaching the issue is by appealing to some plausible general theory of rights. Thus, for example, I am inclined to think that rights exist where there are serious, self-regarding interests that deserve to be protected. If some such view is correct, one can then approach the question of whether persons have a right to a genetically unique nature by asking whether there is some serious, self-regarding interest that would be impaired if one were a clone. An initial reason for thinking that this is not so is that the existence of the person from whom one was cloned does not seem to impinge upon one in the way in which being injured, or being prevented from performing some action that harms no one, do: the existence of the other person might well have no impact at all upon one's life.

A second way of thinking about the question of whether there is a right to a genetically unique nature is to consider a scenario in which individuals with the same genetic makeup are very common indeed, and to consider whether such a world would, for example, be inferior to the present world. Imagine, for example, that it is the year 4004 BC, and God is contemplating creating human beings. He has already considered the idea of letting humans come into being via evolution, but has rejected that on the grounds that a lottery approach in such a vital matter as bringing humans into existence seems inappropriate. He also considered creating an original human pair that were genetically distinct, and who would then give rise to humans who would be genetically quite diverse. Upon reflection, however, that idea also seemed flawed, since the random shuffling and mutation of genes would result in individuals who might be physically impaired, or disposed to unpleasant diseases, such as cancer, that would cause them enormous suffering, and lead to premature deaths. In the end, accordingly, the creator decides upon a genetic constitution that is almost the same for everyone, which will not lead to serious physical handicaps and diseases, and which will allow an individual, who makes wise choices, to grow in body, mind and character. God then creates one person with that genetic makeup – call her Eve – and a second individual – Adam – where their only difference is that Adam has an X chromosome, and a funky Y chromosome, whereas Eve has two X chromosomes. The upshot will then be that any descendent

of Adam and Eve will be genetically identical either to Adam or to Eve. That genetic endowment leaves scope, however, for development in different directions, depending upon the choices that individuals freely make.

How would such a world compare with the actual world? One way of thinking about that is by using a variation on an idea introduced by John Rawls in his 1971 book *A Theory of Justice*. Rawls' suggestion was that a just society would be one that it would be rational to choose if one were choosing a society in which to live behind a veil of ignorance, so that one did not know what position one would occupy in that society, or what one's abilities would be. Now apply this idea instead to possible worlds, and consider whether, if one were choosing from behind a Rawlsian veil of ignorance, it would be rational to prefer the actual world, or the alternative world just described.

That is not, perhaps, an easy question, but clearly there would be some significant pluses associated with the alternative world. First, unlike the actual world, one would be assured of a genetic makeup that would not give rise to various unwelcome and life-shortening diseases, or to other debilitating conditions such as depression, schizophrenia, etc. Secondly, inherited traits would be distributed in a completely equitable fashion, so no one would start out, as in the actual world, severely disadvantaged, and facing an enormous uphill battle. Thirdly, aside from the differences between men and women, everyone would be physically the same, so people would differ only with regard to the interests they had chosen to pursue, the beliefs they had formed, and the traits of character they had developed based on choices they had made. There would seem, in short, to be some serious reasons for preferring the alternative world over the actual world.

The third advantage just mentioned points, however, to an obvious *practical* drawback of the alternative world: knowing who was who would be a rather more difficult matter than in the actual world. However, that problem could be dealt with by variants on the above scenario. One variant, for example, would involve having identity of genetic makeup except with regard to the genes that determine the appearance of one's face and hair. Then one could identify individuals in the way one typically does in the actual world.

Given that change, the alternative world would not be one where, gender aside, individuals would be *identical* with respect to genetic makeup. Nevertheless, if this other alternative world would be preferable to the actual world, I think that it still provides an argument against the claim that individuals have a right to a unique genetic makeup. For, first of all, the preferability of this other alternative world strongly suggests that genetic difference, rather than being desirable in itself, is valuable only to the extent that it is needed to facilitate the easy identification of people. Secondly, is it plausible to hold that while genetic *uniqueness* is crucial, an *extremely high degree* of genetic *similarity* would not be troubling? For in the alternative world in question, the degree of genetic similarity between any two individuals would be extraordinarily high. Thirdly, the alternative world is one where the initial structure of one's *brain* is absolutely the same in all individuals. But, then, can one plausibly hold that genetic uniqueness is morally crucial, while conceding that a world in which individuals do not differ from one another with regard to the initial nature of their brains might be better than the actual world? That seems to me implausible.

The upshot is that I think that the three ways mentioned in which the alternative world would be better than the actual world are good grounds for concluding that, all things considered, the alternative world would be better than the actual world. If so, there is good reason to reject the view that genetic uniqueness is morally significant.

3.1.2   The "Open Future" Argument

Brock mentions a second argument for the view that cloning aimed at producing persons is intrinsically wrong (1998, 153–4). The argument is based upon ideas put forward by Joel Feinberg, who speaks of a right to an open future (1980), and by Hans Jonas, who refers to a right to ignorance of a certain sort (1974) – an idea that has since been enthusiastically endorsed by George Annas (1998, 124) – and

the argument is essentially as follows. One's genetic makeup may very well determine to some extent what possibilities are open to one, and thus may constrain the future course of one's life. If no one else has the same genetic makeup, or if someone does, but either one is unaware of that, or else that person is one's contemporary, or someone who is younger, then one will be unable to observe the *previous* course of the life of someone with the same genetic makeup as oneself. But what if one knows of a genetically identical person whose life precedes one's own? Then one could have knowledge that one might well view as showing that certain possibilities were not really open to one, so one would have less of a sense of being able to choose the course of one's life.

To evaluate this argument, one needs to consider *what type of conclusion* one might draw as a result of observing the earlier life of someone with the same genetic makeup as oneself. Suppose that one had observed someone striving very hard, over a long stretch of time, to achieve some goal and failing to get anywhere near it. Perhaps the earlier, genetically identical individual wanted to be the first person to run the marathon in under two hours, and after several years of intense and well-designed training, attention to diet, etc., never got below two and a half hours. Surely one would then be justified in viewing that particular goal as not really open to one. But would that knowledge be a bad thing, as Jonas seems to be suggesting? Would not such knowledge, on the contrary, be valuable, by making it easier to choose goals that one could successfully pursue?

A very different possibility is that, observing the life of the genetically identical individual, one concludes that *no life significantly different from that life* could really be open to one. Then one would certainly feel that one's life was constrained to a very unwelcome extent. That conclusion, however, would be one that is unsupported by the evidence; indeed, one that there is excellent evidence against.

First of all, although identical twins can be very similar in some striking ways, they can also have lives that are quite different. Secondly, as Pinker points out (1997, 35), one's genes do not contain sufficient information to fix the wiring in one's brain, and the differences may be very important with regard to the traits one develops. Thirdly, as was noted earlier, it is a well-established scientific fact that the traits of identical twins display a correlation of only about 50%, so the scope for a different life is very significant – even more so with clones than with identical twins, given that a clone develops inside a different womb, and then is raised by a different family, and belongs to a different peer group. The belief that the course of a clone's life would be seriously constrained is, therefore, not a defensible belief.

In conclusion, then, it seems that this second argument for the view that cloning with the goal of producing persons is intrinsically wrong is unsound.

3.1.3 *Causing psychological distress*
This objection is closely related to the two preceding, violation-of-rights objections, as the idea is that, even if cloning does not violate a person's right to be a unique individual, or to have a unique genetic makeup, or to have an open and unconstrained future, nevertheless, people who are clones may *feel* that their uniqueness is compromised, or that their future is constrained, and this may cause substantial psychological harm.

There is, however, a good reason for viewing this objection as unsound. It emerges once one reflects upon the beliefs in question – namely, the belief that one's uniqueness is compromised by the existence of a clone, or the belief that one's future is constrained if one has knowledge of the existence of a clone. Both beliefs are, as we have seen, false. In addition, however, it also seems plausible that those beliefs would be, in general, irrational, since it is hard to see what grounds one could have for accepting either belief, other than something like genetic determinism – against which, as we have seen, there is conclusive evidence. If, however, the psychological distress would necessarily be due to irrational beliefs, the solution is readily at hand: if cloning that produces persons were allowed, society would need to act to *ensure* that cloned individuals did not acquire an irrational belief in genetic determinism, thereby preventing the distress that might otherwise arise from a false and irrational belief.

Notice, too, what would happen if cloning became a familiar occurrence, and suppose that society had somehow failed to ensure that John, who is a clone, did not acquire the false beliefs in question, and that John has come to feel that he is no longer a unique individual, or that his future is constrained. If Mary is also a clone, she may point out to John that she is different from the person with whom she is genetically identical, and that she has not been constrained by the way the other person lived her life. Would John still persist in his irrational belief? That does not seem likely. Accordingly, distress that might arise in such a case seems unlikely to persist for any significant length of time.

3.1.4 *Failing to treat individuals as ends in themselves*
A fourth objection applies, not to the cloning of persons in general, but to certain cases – such as where parents clone a child who is suffering from some life-threatening condition in order to produce another child who can save the first child's life – and the contention is that such cases involve a failure to treat individuals as ends in themselves. Thus Philip Kitcher, referring to such cases, says that "a lingering concern remains," and he goes on to ask whether such scenarios "can be reconciled with Kant's injunction to 'treat humanity, whether in your own person or in the person of another, always at the same time as an end and never simply as a means'" (1997, 61).

What is one to say about this objection? In thinking about it, it seems important to specify what sacrifices the child being produced will have to make to save his or her sibling. Kitcher, in his formulation, assumes that it will be a kidney transplant, which is a very significant sacrifice indeed, since it may have unhappy consequences for that person in the future. Consequently, I think that Kitcher's case seriously clouds one's thinking about this *general* type of case. Let us suppose, instead, then – as in the non-cloning case to be mentioned later – that the cloned child will instead be the source for a bone marrow transfer that will save the life of a sibling who would otherwise die from leukemia.

In such a case, would there be a violation of Kant's injunction? There could be – if the parents abandoned, or did not really care for the one child, once he or she had provided bone marrow to save the life of the other child. This, however, would surely be a *very* unlikely occurrence. After all, the history of the human race is the history of largely unplanned children, often born into situations where the parents are anything but well off, and yet typically those children are deeply loved by their parents.

In short, though this type of case is by hypothesis one where the parents have a child with a goal in mind that, in itself, has nothing to do with the well-being of *that* child, this is no reason for supposing that they are therefore likely to treat that child merely as a means, and not also as an end in itself. Indeed, surely there is good reason to think, on the contrary, that such a child will be raised in no less loving a way than is normally the case.

3.1.5 *Interfering with personal autonomy*

The final objection – also advanced by Philip Kitcher – is as follows: "If the cloning of human beings is undertaken in the hope of generating a particular kind of person, then cloning is morally repugnant. The repugnance arises not because cloning involves biological tinkering but because it interferes with human autonomy" (1997, 61).

What is one to say about this objection? First, notice that where one's goal is to produce "a particular kind of person," what one is sometimes aiming at is simply a person who will have certain *potentialities*. Parents might, for example, want to have children who would be capable of enjoying intellectual pursuits, or who could enjoy classical music, or the playing of instruments, or who could, if they so chose, excel at various physical activities, such as golf or skiing. The parents would not be forcing the children to engage in such pursuits, so it is hard to see how cloning that is directed at such goals need involve any interference with human autonomy.

Secondly, consider cases where the goal is not to produce a person capable of doing certain things, but a certain sort of person. Perhaps this is the kind of case that Kitcher has in mind when he speaks of interfering with human autonomy. But is it really morally problematic to attempt to create persons with certain dispositions, rather than others? Is it morally wrong, for example, to attempt to produce, via cloning, individuals who will, because of their genetic makeup, be disposed not to suffer from conditions that may cause considerable pain, such as arthritis, or from life-threatening diseases, such as cancer, high blood pressure, strokes, and heart attacks? Or to attempt to produce individuals who will have a cheerful temperament, or who will not be disposed to depression, to anxiety, to schizophrenia, or to Alzheimer's disease?

It seems unlikely that Kitcher, or others, would want to say that producing individuals who will be constitutionally disposed in the ways just indicated is a case of interfering with human autonomy. But then what are the traits such that attempting to create a person with those traits is a case of interfering with human autonomy? Perhaps Kitcher, when he speaks about creating a particular kind of person, is thinking not just of any properties that persons have, but, more narrowly, of such things as personality traits, or traits of character, or the having of certain interests? But again one can ask whether there is anything morally problematic about attempting to create persons with such properties. Some personality traits are desirable, and parents typically encourage their children to develop those traits. Some character traits are virtues, and others are vices, and both parents and society attempt to encourage the acquisition of the former, and to discourage the acquisition of the latter. Finally, many interests – in music, art, mathematics, science, games, physical activities – can add greatly to the quality of one's life, and once again, parents typically expose their children to relevant activities, and help their children to achieve levels of proficiency that will enable them to enjoy those pursuits.

The upshot is that if cloning that aimed at producing people who would be more likely to possess various personality traits, or traits of character, or who would be likely to have certain interests was wrong because it would be interfering with personal autonomy, then the childrearing practices of almost all parents would stand condemned on precisely the same grounds. But such a claim, surely, is deeply counterintuitive.

In addition, however, one need not rest content with an appeal to intuitions here. The same conclusion follows on many high-order moral theories. Suppose, for example, that one is again behind a Rawlsian veil of ignorance, where one is deciding between societies that differ as regards their approaches to the rearing of children. Would it be rational to choose a society where parents did not attempt to encourage their children to develop personality traits that would contribute to the latter's happiness? Or a society where parents did not attempt to instill in their children a disposition to act in ways that are morally right? Or one where parents made no attempt to develop various interests in their children that they believed would add to their lives? It is, I suggest, hard to see how such a choice could be a rational one, given that one would be opting, it would seem, for a society where one would be less likely to have a life that, on average, would be more worth living.

I suggest, therefore, that contrary to what Philip Kitcher has claimed, it is not true that most cloning scenarios are morally repugnant, and that, in particular, there is, in general, nothing morally problematic about aiming at creating a child with specific attributes.

3.2 Consequentialist objections to cloning to produce persons

Let us now turn to the question of whether cloning that aims at the production of neo-Lockean persons might nevertheless be morally problematic because of *undesirable consequences*. I shall consider two arguments in support of this view.

3.2.1 *Cloned persons would have lives less worth living because of reduced life expectancy*

The first argument, and the one that raises a very important issue, deserving serious consideration, involves the question of how cloned individuals will fare when it comes to aging, since it has been suggested that Dolly, who died at the age of six years, may have had a significantly reduced life expectancy by having been developed from the nucleus of a six-year-old sheep. Here is the basis of the worry:

As early as the 1930s investigators took note of pieces of noncoding DNA – DNA that does not give rise to protein – at the ends of each chromosome, which they called telomeres (from the Greek words for "end" and "part"). When the differentiated cells of higher organisms undergo mitosis, the ordinary process of cell division, not all of the DNA in their nuclei is replicated. The enzyme that copies DNA misses a small piece at the ends of each chromosome, and so the chromosomes get slightly shorter each time a cell divides. As long as each telomere remains to buffer its chromosome against the shortening process, mitosis does not bite into any genes (remember that the telomeres are noncoding, much like the leaders at the ends of a reel of film). Eventually, however, the telomeres get so short that they can no longer protect the vital parts of the chromosome. At that point the cell usually stops dividing and dies. (Ronald Hart, Angelo Turturro, and Julian Leakey, 1997, 48)

The question, accordingly, is whether Dolly started life with cells whose chromosomes had telomeres whose length was comparable to those in the cells of a six-year-old sheep. Perhaps not, since it may be that once a nucleus has been transplanted into an egg from which the nucleus has been removed, there is some mechanism that will produce an enzyme – called telomerase – that can create full-length telomeres. The risk, however, is surely a serious one, and provides grounds, in view of the following argument, for holding, not only that one *should not* at this point attempt to produce people by cloning, but also that there should be a temporary legal prohibition on cloning humans where the goal is to produce persons.

The argument rests on what is known as the "non-identity problem," which was the first discussed by Gregory Kavka in his article "The Paradox of Future Individuals" (1981), and then considered at length by Derek Parfit (1984, 351–79). The problem can be raised by comparing two cases:

Mary learns that if she becomes pregnant immediately, her child will suffer from defect X, but still have a life worth living, whereas if she waits three months to become pregnant, she will have a completely normal child. Mary decides not to wait, and gives birth to Johnny.

Jane is pregnant, and learns that unless she takes a certain drug – which has no side effects – she will give birth to a child who will suffer from defect X, but still have a life worth living. Jane decides not to take the drug, and gives birth to Billy.

How does Mary's action compare with Jane's? Most people, I think, initially view the two actions as equally bad. Notice, however, that while Billy can later argue that what Jane did was seriously wrong because he was worse off because of what Jane decided not to do, Johnny cannot argue that what Mary did was seriously wrong because of what Mary did, since Johnny has a life worth living, and had Mary waited, Johnny would not have existed, so Mary has not made Johnny worse off.

If Mary's action is morally as problematic as Jane's, and if it is true that a cloned person will have a significantly lower life expectancy than a person who is not cloned, then we have a serious objection to cloning that aims at producing a person,, unless the cloned person will have a life that is significantly better in other ways, or there is no other way of producing a person in the circumstances that will be satisfactory. The former scenario seems rather unlikely, but this is not so for the second possibility, since there is a type of case, to be discussed shortly, where cloning may very well be morally justified, namely, where parents want to clone one of their children to have a child who can save the first child's life. In an earlier essay on cloning, I failed to consider such possibilities, and thus mistakenly concluded that the possibility of a reduction in life expectancy in the case of cloned individuals provided strong grounds for "a temporary, legal prohibition on the cloning of humans when the goal is to produce persons" (1998, 76).

Subsequent developments, however, provide serious grounds for concluding that the telomere-shortening argument is unsound. First of all, an article by Narumi Ogonuki and others, entitled "Early Death of Mice Cloned from Somatic Cells," says that it appears that, in the case of mice, early deaths resulted, not from shortened telomeres but from some "malfunction in

the immune system" (2002, 253), and the authors also note that

> Telomere shortening is known to be associated with cellular aging. It has recently been reported that, after cloning, telomere length can be restored to its original length by nuclear transfer, implying that the lifespan of clones might not be shortened" (2002, 254).

The most important and detailed scientific publication to date seems to be one by K. D. Sinclair et al. – "Healthy Ageing of Cloned Sheep." In that study, they closely examined "13 cloned sheep aged (7–9 years old), including four from the cell line that gave rise to Dolly" (2016, 1), and there they say that the consensus is that "telomere length is generally restored during nuclear reprogramming" (2016, 7). The concluding paragraph of their article is then as follows:

> In conclusion, although the efficiency of SCNT [somatic-cell nuclear transfer] has improved in recent years, its overall efficiency remains low, with high embryonic and gestational losses compared to natural mating and assisted reproduction. A relatively high proportion of clones also fail to successfully make the transition to extra-uterine life, some harboring congenital defects, such as observed in the kidney. For those clones that survive beyond the perinatal period, however, the emerging consensus, supported by the current data, is that they are healthy and seem to age normally" (2016, 8).

In the light of the above, I believe that there are good grounds for setting aside the telomere-shortening argument against human cloning aimed at producing persons. This is an important conclusion, since if telomere shortening and reduced life expectancy were the case, then one would have a strong argument against cloning where the goal is to produce a person.

3.2.2 The low rate of success objection
Can one then appeal instead to the unreliability of the outcome to argue that there should be a legal ban on human cloning where the goal is to produce a person? That is an ethically difficult question. On

the one hand, with regard to the "high embryonic and gestational losses compared to natural mating and assisted reproduction," it is very doubtful that many women would make an informed choice to run those risks associated with cloning, but if a woman had a very strong desire to produce a cloned individual, or was willing to take part in such an experiment if adequately compensated, then it is hard to see how "embryonic and gestational losses" could justify a legal prohibition.

On the other hand, the situation differs as regards failures "to successfully make the transition to extra-uterine life," since there the crucial issue is whether cloning may lead to the death of a neo-Lockean person. That in turn depends on the answer to the scientific question of *when* developing humans acquire the capacities that are relevant to neo-Lockean person-hood – especially the capacity for thought.

When I surveyed the scientific evidence many years ago (1983, 347–412), it seemed to me that both the psychological and the neurophysiological evidence supported the conclusion that the capacity for thought is only acquired postnatally. It may be that current evidence supports the opposite conclusion, in which case there would be grounds for not allowing human cloning until techniques are improved to eliminate failures "to successfully make the transition to extra-uterine life." Or perhaps we do not yet have a definitive answer to the scientific question, in which case a legal prohibition would be in order until either we do have an answer, or until cloning techniques are appropriately improved.

3.2.3 *Brave New World objections*

Next, there is an objection not frequently encountered in scholarly discussions, but rather common in the popular press, involving scenarios where human beings are cloned in large numbers to serve as slaves, or as enthusiastic soldiers in a dictator's army. Such scenarios, however, seem very implausible. Is it really at all likely that, were cloning to become available, society would for some unknown reason decide that its rejection of slavery had really been a mistake? Or that a dictator who was unable to conscript a sufficient

army from the existing citizenry could induce people to undertake a massive cloning program, in order that, eighteen years or so down the line, he would finally have the army he needed?

3.3 Arguments in favor of cloning to produce persons

If the arguments to show that cloning human persons is intrinsically wrong are, as I have argued, implausible, and if the crucial objection appealing to undesirable consequences can be satisfactorily answered, either now, or in the future, either by an increase in our scientific knowledge or by advances in cloning techniques, are there now, or would there then be, good reasons to move ahead with the cloning of humans where the aim is to bring persons into existence? I shall argue that there are.

The considerations that, other things being equal, support the implementation of cloning aimed at producing persons fall into four main categories: first, there are considerations related to the well-being of the person who is produced via the cloning; secondly, there are cases where those benefited are already existing persons; thirdly, there is a consideration that involves the possibility of benefits to both cloned persons and their parents; finally, there are benefits to society at large, including contributions to important scientific knowledge, and resulting benefits for anyone rearing a child, cloned or otherwise.

3.3.1 *Cloning to avoid the transmission of hereditary diseases*

Inherited diseases fall into various categories, depending on whether they involve a single gene, multiple genes, a chromosomal disorder, or mitochondrial inheritance. If one focuses just on the single gene case, one has, for example, cystic fibrosis, sickle cell anemia, hemochromatosis, and Huntington's disease. If cloning were implemented, then – as John Roberson (1994) and Dan Brock (1998, 146) pointed out – provided that only one of the potential parents had the defective gene, a clone could be made using a cell from the one who does not suffer from the genetic defect, and the result would be a child who was free of the inheritable disease, and also genetically related to one member of the couple – something that many might find preferable to using a donor egg or donor sperm, where the resulting child would involve a genetic contribution from a third party.

3.3.2   Happier and healthier individuals

Secondly, cloning would have the advantage over sexual reproduction that it should make it possible to increase the likelihood that the person created will enjoy a healthier and happier life. For to the extent that one's genetic constitution has a bearing upon how long one is likely to live, upon what diseases, both physical and mental, one is likely to suffer from, and upon whether one will have traits of character or temperament that make for happiness, or, instead, for unhappiness, by cloning a person who has enjoyed a long life, who has remained mentally alert, rather than falling prey to Alzheimer's disease or dementia, who has not suffered from cancer, arthritis, heart attacks, stroke, high blood pressure, etc., and who has exhibited no tendencies to depression or schizophrenia, etc., one is increasing the chances that the individual created will also enjoy a healthy and happy life.

3.3.3   Enabling individuals to have a genetically related child who otherwise could not do so

A third reason for implementing cloning is that it would benefit people who already exist.

3.3.3.1   Infertility

One way, as Dan Brock and others (Eisenberg, 1976; LaBar, 1984; Robertson, 1994) have pointed out, is that "Human cloning would allow women who have no ova or men who have no sperm to produce an offspring that is biologically related to them" (Brock, 1998, 146)." Another advantage, also noted by Brock, is that "Embryos might be cloned, either by nuclear transfer or embryo splitting, in order to increase the number of embryos for implantation and improve the chances of successful conception." (1998, 146).

3.3.3.2   Children for homosexual couples

Many people still believe not only that homosexuality is deeply wrong, but also that homosexual sexual relations should be illegal, and, indeed, severely punished – as had been the case in the United States for many years: "All states had laws against sodomy by 1960" (Mattachine Society, 1964, 1), often with very long maximum terms of imprisonment – and even life imprisonment in the case of one state (GLAPN, 2007, 1). These attitudes were deeply rooted in religious views, especially Christian and Islamic teachings, and the current decline in religious beliefs has been accompanied by a decline in such beliefs about homosexuality (Pew Research Center, 2013).

In the United States, a major turning point was the Supreme Court decision, in 2003 in *Lawrence v. Texas*, that laws against sodomy were unconstitutional, and since then there has been a dramatic change in the attitudes of many Americans on several issues involving homosexuals. Thus, in 2019, a Gallup poll found that 73% of Americans believe that homosexual relations should be legal, while since 2016, over 60% have believed that same-sex marriages should be recognized by law as valid. In addition, by 2019, 75% of Americans believed that homosexual couples should be allowed to adopt children (PPRI, 2019).

Since such views are very widely accepted by philosophers working in ethics, and since the contrary views are generally rooted in religious beliefs, such as those of evangelical Protestants in the United States – beliefs that there are strong arguments against – there are good grounds for concluding that homosexuals should be allowed to adopt children. If so, then another important advantage of implementing the cloning of persons is that, as Philip Kitcher (1997, 61) and others have noted, cloning would seem to be a desirable method of providing a homosexual couple with children that they could raise, since, in the case of a gay couple, each child could be a clone of one person, while in the case of a lesbian couple, every child could, in a sense, be biologically connected with both people:

> A lesbian couple wishes to have a child. Because they would like the child to be biologically connected to each of them, they request that a cell nucleus from one

of them be inserted into an egg from the other, and that the embryo be implanted in the uterus of the woman who donated the egg (1997, 61).[1]

3.3.4 Cloning to save existing persons

Another reason for implementing cloning is suggested by the well-known case of the Ayala parents in California (Grogan, 1990), who decided to have another child in the hope – which turned out to be successful -- that the resulting child would be able to donate bone marrow for a transplant operation that would save the life of their teenage daughter who was suffering from leukemia. If cloning had been possible at the time, a course of action would have been available to them that, unlike having another child in the normal way, would not have been chancy: if they could have cloned the child who was ill, a tissue match would have been certain.

3.3.5 More satisfying childrearing: Individuals with desired traits

Many couples would like to raise children who possess certain traits. In some cases they might prefer to have children who have physical abilities enabling them to perform at a high level in certain sporting activities. Or they might prefer to have children having intellectual capabilities enabling them to enjoy mathematics, or science. Or perhaps they would prefer to have children with traits that would enable them to engage in, and enjoy, various aesthetic pursuits.

Some of the traits that people might like their children to have presumably have a very strong hereditary basis, while others are such as a child, given both the relevant genes, and the right environment, might be more likely to develop. To the extent that the traits in question fall in either of these categories, the production of children via cloning would enable more couples to raise children with traits that they judge to be desirable.

3.3.6 Using self-knowledge to increase the chance that childrearing will go well for both oneself and one's children

There is a second way in which cloning could make childrearing more satisfactory, for both parents and their children, and it emerges if one recalls one's own childhood. Most people, when they do this, remember things that they liked, that contributed to their happiness, and other things that had the opposite effect. These might be ways they were treated by their parents, or, instead, interactions with their peers. The thought, then, is that by raising a child who is a clone of one of the parents, the knowledge the relevant parent has of how he or she was raised, or treated by her or his peers, can enable one both to relate to one's child in a way better attuned to the psychological makeup of the child, and also to have a better sense of peer group interactions that may significantly detract from one's child's happiness. In addition, given the greater psychological similarity existing between the child and one of the parents, that parent will better be able, at any point, to appreciate the child's point of view. So there should be a greater likelihood both that such a couple will find childrearing a more rewarding experience, and that their child will have a happier childhood through being better understood, and from having parents who know how the treatment by one's peers may negatively impact one's happiness.

3.3.7 Benefiting society: Producing people who have the potential for making significant contributions to human well-being

One quite familiar suggestion is that one might benefit mankind by cloning individuals who have made extremely significant contributions to society. In the form that it is usually put, where it is assumed that if, for example, one had been able to clone Albert Einstein, the result would be an individual who would also make some very significant contributions to science, the idea does not seem especially plausible. In the first place, whether an individual will turn out to do highly creative work, rather than being determined simply by his or her genetic makeup, surely depends upon traits whose acquisition is a matter either of the environment in which the individual grows up, or, alternatively, in view of Pinker's point, of the prenatal wiring of that person's brain.

Could it not be argued in response, however – at least if one sets aside the second of those possibilities – that one could control the environment as well, raising a clone of Einstein, for example, in an environment as similar as possible to that in which Einstein was raised? That, of course, might prove difficult. Even if it could be done, however, it is not clear that would be sufficient, since great creative achievements may depend upon things that are to some extent accidental, and whose occurrence is not ensured by the combination of one's genetic makeup, the prenatal wiring of one's brain, and the general kind of environment in which one grows up. Many great mathematicians, for example, have developed an intense interest in numbers at an early age, and even if one leaves aside the prenatal brain-wiring view, **is** there good reason to think that, had one been able to clone Carl Friedrich Gauss, and reared that person in an environment similar to Gauss's, that person would have developed a similar interest in numbers, and gone on to achieve great things in mathematics? Or is it likely that a clone of Einstein, raised in an environment similar to Einstein's, would have wondered, as Einstein did, how the world would appear if one could travel as fast as light, and would then have pondered the questions that fascinated Einstein, and that led ultimately to the development of revolutionary theories in physics?

I am inclined to think, then, that there are problems with the present suggestion in the form in which it is usually put. On the other hand, I'm not convinced that a slightly more modest version cannot be sustained. Consider, for example, the chess-playing Polgár sisters, where the father of three girls succeeded in creating an environment in which all three of his daughters became *very* strong chess players, with one of them – Judit Polgár – becoming the strongest female chess player who has ever lived. Is it not reasonable to think that if one were to make a number of clones of Judit Polgár, and then raised them in an environment very similar to that in which the Polgár sisters were raised, the result would be a number of very strong chess players?

More generally, there is strong evidence of a very significant hereditary basis for intelligence, as Bouchard (1997, 55–6) and many others have argued, and it may well be that the right combination of heredity and environment plays a significant role in the development of other traits that may play a crucial

role in creativity – traits such as extreme persistence, determination, and confidence in one's own abilities. So while the chance that the clone of an outstandingly creative individual will also achieve very great things is perhaps, at least in many areas, not especially high, I think that there is reason for thinking that, given an appropriate environment, the result in a number of areas may well turn out to be an individual who is likely to accomplish things that may benefit society in significant ways.

3.3.8 *furthering scientific knowledge: Psychology, the causes of traits of character, and the rearing of children*

A crucial theoretical task for psychology is the construction of a satisfactory theory to explain the acquisition of traits of character, and central to the development of such a theory is information about the extent to which various traits are (a) inherited, (b) dependent upon aspects of the environment that are controllable, or (c) dependent upon factors, either in the brain, or in the environment, that have a chancy quality. Such knowledge, however, is not just theoretically crucial to psychology. Knowledge of the contributions that are, and are not, made to the individual's development by his or her genetic makeup, by the prenatal state of the individual's brain, by the environment in which he or she matures, and by chance events, will enable one to develop approaches to childrearing that will increase, at least to some extent, the likelihood that one can raise children with desirable traits, and thus people who will have a better chance of realizing their potentials, and of leading happy and satisfying lives. So this knowledge is not merely of great theoretical interest: it is also potentially *very* beneficial to society.

In the attempt to construct an adequate theory of human development, one thing that has been very important, and that has generated considerable information concerning the nature/nurture issue, is the study of identical twins. Complete and fully adequate theories, however, still seem rather remote. Cloning would provide a powerful way of speeding up scientific progress in this area, since society could produce a number of individuals with the same genetic makeup, and then choose adoptive parents who would provide those individuals with good, but significantly different environments, in which to mature. The resulting scientific knowledge, in turn, would hopefully sweep away, in the end, advice of the kinds that are currently being offered to parents – almost all of which, as Judith Rich Harris has convincingly argued (2009, 309–29) – rests on claims against which there is very strong scientific evidence. With that rubbish gone, parents could be provided with scientifically based information about what they can and cannot hope to

achieve in rearing children, and about what things are most likely to be helpful.

Conclusion

I have argued both that there are no sound objections to cloning for scientific research or therapeutic purposes, or to the creation of human organ banks, and also that the cloning of persons is both desirable in various ways and, in principle, morally unproblematic.

Note

1 Although Kitcher mentions this idea as initially attractive, in the end he rejects it, on the grounds that cloning "interferes with human autonomy"

(1997, 61) – a view that I considered, and argued against, in section 3.1.5.

References

Annas, George J. (1998). "Why We Should Ban Human Cloning," *The New England Journal of Medicine,* July 9, 1998.

Bouchard, Thomas J., Jr. (1997). "Whenever the Twain Shall Meet," *The Sciences* 37/5, September/October 1997, 52–7.

Brock, Dan W. (1998). "Cloning Human Beings: An Assessment of the Ethical Issues Pro and Con." In Martha C. Nussbaum and Cass R. Sunstein (eds.), *Clones and Clones,* New York: W. W. Norton and Company.

Cerva, R. P. and Stojkovic, M. (2007). "Human embryonic stem cell derivation and nuclear transfer: impact on regenerative therapeutics and drug discovery," *Clinical Pharmacology & Therapeutics,* 82/3, 310–15.

Eisenberg Leon (1976). "The Outcome as Cause: Predestination and Human Cloning," *The Journal of Medicine and Philosophy,* 1, 318–31.

Feinberg, Joel (1980). "The Child's Right to an Open Future." In W. Aiken and H. LaFollette, *Whose Child? Children's Rights, Parental Authority, and State Power,* Totowa, NJ: Rowan and Littlefield.

Gallop Poll (2019). "Gay and Lesbian Rights", https://news.gallup.com/poll/1651/gay-lesbian-rights.aspx (Accessed January 24, 2020.)

GLAPN (2007). "History of Sodomy Laws," http://www.glapn.org/sodomylaws/history/history.htm (Accessed September 17, 2020).

Grogan, David (1990). "To Save Their Daughter from Leukemia, Abe and Mary Ayala Conceived a Plan-and a Baby, *People,* March 5, 1990. https://people.com/archive/to-save-their-daughter-from-leukemia-abe-and-mary-ayala-conceived-a-plan-and-a-baby-vol-33-no-9/ (Accessed January 24, 2020.)

Harris, Judith Rich (1998). *The Nurture Assumption,* New York: Free Press.

Hart, Ronald, Angelo Turturro, and Julian Leakey, (1997). "Born Again?" *The Sciences* 37/5, September/October 1997, 47–51.

Jonas, Hans (1974). *Philosophical Essay: From Ancient Creed to Technological Man,* Englewood Cliffs, NJ: Prentice-Hall.

Kaczor, Christopher (2014). *The Ethics of Abortion – Women's Rights, Human Life, and the Question of Justice,* 2nd edition, Abingdon-on-Thames: Routledge.

Kavka, Gregory S. (1981). "The Paradox of Future Individuals," *Philosophy & Public Affairs,*" 11:93–112.

Kitcher, Philip (1997). "Whose Self Is It, Anyway?" *The Sciences* 37/5, September/October 1997, 58–62.

LaBar, Martin (1984). "The Pros and Cons of Human Cloning," *Thought* 57: 318–33.

Locke, John. *An Essay Concerning Human Understanding*, (1632–1704)

Marquis, Don (1989). "Why Abortion is Immoral," *Journal of Philosophy*, 86/4, 183–202. (See also Chapter 4 of this *Anthology*).

Mattachine Society Inc., of New York (1964). "Penalties for Sex Offenses in the United States," The New York Public Library Digital Collections. https://digitalcollections.nypl. org/items/67116400-873c-257c-e040-e00a18065646 (Accessed September 17, 2020).

Ogonuki, Narumi, et al (2002). "Early death of mice cloned from somatic cells," *Nature*, 30, 253–4.

Parfit, Derek (1984). *Reasons and Persons*, Oxford: Clarendon Press.

Pew Research Center (2013). "The Global Divide on Homosexuality", https://www.pewresearch.org/global/ 2013/06/04/the-global-divide-on-homosexuality/ (Accessed January 24, 2020.)

Pinker, Steven (1997). *How the Mind Works*. New York: W. W. Norton & Company, Inc.

PPRI (2019). "New Landmark Survey of 50 States Finds Broad Support for LGBT Rights Across the United States," https://www.prri.org/press-release/ new-landmark-survey-of-50-states-finds-broad-support-for-lgbt-rights-across-the-united-states/ (Accessed January 24, 2020.)

Rawls, John (1971). *A Theory of Justice*, Cambridge, MA: Harvard University Press.

Robertson, John A. (1994). "The Question of Human Cloning," *Hastings Center Report* 24, 6–14.

Sinclair, K. D., et al (2016). "Healthy ageing of cloned sheep," *Nature Communications,* 26 July, 2016, 1–10.

Tooley, Michael, and Plantinga, Alvin (2008). *Knowledge of God*, Oxford: Blackwell Publishing.

Tooley, Michael, Wolf-Devine, Celia, Devine, Philip E. and Jaggar, Alison M. (2009). *Abortion: Three Perspectives*, New York: Oxford University Press.

Tooley, Michael (1983). *Abortion and Infanticide*, Oxford: Clarendon Press.

———, (1998). "The Moral Status of the Cloning of Humans," In James Humber and Robert Almeder (eds.), *Biomedical Ethics Reviews: Human Cloning*, Humana Press, Totowa, New Jersey, 65–101.

———, (2019). *The Problem of Evil*, Cambridge: Cambridge University Press.

Part III

Genetic Manipulation

Introduction

Our genes play an important role in what kind of people we are – whether we are, for example, short or tall, healthy or sick, mentally slow or bright; and while there is debate about the extent to which certain characteristics are inherited or the product of our environment, it is difficult to deny that some characteristics at least have a genetic basis. To deny this would, as Jonathan Glover points out in "Questions about Some Uses of Genetic Engineering" amount to thinking "that it is only living in kennels which makes dogs different from cats".

Genetic manipulation, sometimes also referred to as genetic engineering, involves intervening at the genetic level in order to eliminate, modify, or enhance certain genetic traits or conditions. Recent scientific breakthroughs, including the mapping of the human genome, have added significantly to our understanding of our genes, and provide increasing and unprecedented possibilities for control over our genetic destiny. Should we make use of this knowledge, and to which ends? Should we, for example, use genetic manipulation only to prevent serious genetic disorders, or should we also use it for the enhancement of certain traits and characteristics?

The distinction between gene therapy and gene enhancement is not clear-cut. While it might be agreed that increasing the height a boy is expected to reach at maturity from 170 cm to 190 cm is a form of enhancement, what if we are seeking to increase his expected height from 150 cm to 170 cm? The same appears to be true when we are looking at a trait such as intelligence. Increasing a person's IQ by 20 points from 110 to 130 would generally be considered enhancement, but would raising her IQ from 90 to 110 be therapy or of enhancement? The answer ultimately depends, David B. Resnik argues in "The Moral Significance of the Therapy–Enhancement Distinction in Human Genetics," on contested philosophical distinctions, such as the distinctions between health and disease, and normality and abnormality.

Despite some fuzziness at the margins, we do, however, often have a plausible understanding of where the boundary between therapy and enhancement should be drawn. The next question is whether this boundary is morally significant. Again, many people think the answer is "yes." They take the view that gene therapy, as an extension of the conventional goals of medicine, is morally acceptable, while enhancement is morally problematic. But are the arguments in support of the ethical significance of these distinctions sound?

Some people reject positive genetic engineering on the grounds of risk; but is risk – even significant risk – a sufficient reason to rule out all genetic interventions?

Bioethics: An Anthology, Fourth Edition. Edited by Udo Schüklenk and Peter Singer.
Editorial material and organization © 2022 John Wiley & Sons, Inc. Published 2022 by John Wiley & Sons, Inc.

Jonathan Glover argues that the fact that a practice involves risks is not sufficient to show that it is morally wrong, or should be banned. In some cases, the dangers of not proceeding might be greater than the dangers of proceeding selectively and cautiously. Moreover, would considerations of risk be a reason against all positive interventions, or against only some of them? And would it be a reason against positive or enhancing genetic interventions only, or also a reason against therapeutic or negative interventions?

Arguments about risk are important, but do not go to the heart of the objections to genetic engineering. Even if gene therapy could be shown to be relatively safe, one oft-heard objection – that it involves "playing God" – would remain. But this objection, as Glover and others argue, is unpersuasive. Taken literally, it obviously will not appeal to non-believers; and, if understood metaphorically as a prohibition on interfering with "God's creation," that is, with nature, it would seem to rule out not only all genetic engineering (whether positive or negative), but all other medical interventions as well.

A more plausible way of understanding the "playing God" argument might be to see it as an objection to eugenic schemes, where, as Glover puts it, necessarily fallible people with limited horizons are making God-like decisions to improve the human race. Past eugenic programs in Europe (and particularly in Nazi Germany), Great Britain, and the United States continue to cast a dark shadow over contemporary genetics. These programs were widely associated with a variety of often highly questionable coercive government schemes intended to "improve" the gene pool. The question of whether positive genetic engineering is morally acceptable must, however, Glover argues, be separated from the question of whether particular state-controlled eugenic programs are acceptable. One might think that it is wrong for state authorities to decide who should and should not be able to have children, and what these children should be like, but not wrong if individual parents were to make these kinds of reproductive decision themselves.

Those who are most enthusiastic about genetic enhancement call themselves transhumanists to signify that they think it desirable to move beyond the human nature that we have inherited from the long and blind process of evolutionary selection. Nick Bostrom in "In Defense of Posthuman Dignity," defends transhumanism against the criticism that if we change our nature, we will lose our human dignity. Though the idea of human dignity is often invoked, the values behind it are rarely made explicit. Bostrom distinguishes different things that we might mean by "human dignity." He then defends, as the title of his essay indicates, "posthuman dignity" – that is the idea that there is moral worth in seeing human nature as dynamic and changing, and in seeking to make moral progress by improving it.

Francis S. Collins was appointed Director of the United States National Institutes of Health (NIH), one of the world's largest public funders of biomedical research, in 2009. Prior to that, he directed the National Human Genome Research Institute, in which capacity he played a leading role in mapping and sequencing the human genome. In his "Statement on NIH Funding of Research Using Gene-Editing Technologies in Human Embryos," Collins defends NIH's long-standing policy against funding research involving the use of gene-editing technologies in human embryos. As he points out, NIH also does not fund research proposals that alter genes in ways that may be passed on to future generations. Collins notes that some of this research is being done in China, and cites legislation and regulations that exclude the possibility of such research in the US.

Giulia Cavaliere's "Genome Editing and Assisted Reproduction: Curing Embryos, Society or Prospective Parents?" focuses on whether genome editing might be preferable, for ethical reasons, to preimplantation genetic diagnosis (PGD), which is currently in use in several countries, including the United States. Cavaliere evaluates two sets of concerns about the use of genome editing on human embryos or gametes in a clinical setting: safety concerns and ethical objections to introducing changes into the human germline. In this context she cites, and gives reasons for rejecting, the position taken by Francis S. Collins in the statement included in Chapter 16 of this *Anthology*. She then discusses the potential benefits of genome editing, given that it would not be vulnerable to some of the ethical objections to PGD, and could be used in cases where PGD is ineffective.

Cavaliere cautions us to assess thoroughly the safety of genome editing, but she does not find compelling the claim that it is wrong to introduce any modification of the human germline. She argues, however, that societies need an ethical policy for allocating social resources so as to ensure equality of access to assisted reproduction, including assistance that which makes use of genome editing.

R. Alta Charo asks us in her article "Who is Afraid of the Big Bad (Germline Editing) Wolf?" to be wary of unsubstantiated claims about significant dangers associated with human germline editing. She argues that time and again in human history, when biomedical research offered society new technologies and possibilities, there have been dire warnings and predictions about their supposed risks. Among others she mentions the argument that germline editing could turn children into commodities. The same types of arguments were raised historically by opponents of the introduction of, for instance in vitro fertilization (IVF), surrogacy, and PGD. None of these worries turned out to be justified. Charo's concern is that societies might give undue weight to such worries and unnecessarily impede research and the development of new means of reducing the social burden of disease.

In the short article that concludes this Part, Julian Savulescu and Peter Singer discuss a controversial example of gene editing involving two healthy embryos that were allowed to develop into children. He Jiankui, a Chinese biophysicist who has since been sentenced to jail for undertaking this work, claimed to have edited out a gene that produces a protein that permits HIV to enter cells. Savulescu and Singer argue that the experiment was unethical because the risk–benefit ratio did not justify subjecting the children to the currently unreasonable risks associated with human gene editing. They also raise concerns about likely flaws in the process of obtaining informed consent from the future parents of the embryos. But what if, in future, gene editing is possible without the risk of off-target mutations? This paper indicates possible ethical pathways to human germline gene editing.

13

Questions about Some Uses of Genetic Engineering

Jonathan Glover

There is a widespread view that any project for the genetic improvement of the human race ought to be ruled out: that there are fundamental objections of principle. The aim of this discussion is to sort out some of the main objections. It will be argued that our resistance is based on a complex of different values and reasons, none of which is, when examined, adequate to rule out in principle this use of genetic engineering. The debate on human genetic engineering should become like the debate on nuclear power: one in which large possible benefits have to be weighed against big problems and the risk of great disasters. The discussion has not reached this point, partly because the techniques have not yet been developed. But it is also partly because of the blurred vision which fuses together many separate risks and doubts into a fuzzy-outlined opposition in principle.

Avoiding the Debate about Genes and the Environment

In discussing the question of genetic engineering, there is everything to be said for not muddling the issue up with the debate over the relative importance of genes and environment in the development of such characteristics as intelligence. One reason for avoiding that debate is that it arouses even stronger passions than genetic engineering, and so is filled with as much acrimony as argument. But, apart from this fastidiousness, there are other reasons.

The nature–nurture dispute is generally seen as an argument about the relative weight the two factors have in causing differences within the human species: 'IQ is 80 per cent hereditary and 20 per cent environmental' versus 'IQ is 80 per cent environmental and 20 per cent hereditary'. No doubt there is some approximate truth of this type to be found if we consider variations within a given population at a particular time. But it is highly unlikely that there is any such statement which is simply true of human nature regardless of context. To take the extreme case, if we could iron out all environmental differences, any residual variations would be 100 per cent genetic. It is only if we make the highly artificial assumption that different groups at different times all have an identical spread of relevant environmental differences that we

Original publication details: Jonathan Glover, "Questions about Some Uses of Genetic Engineering," pp. 25–33, 33–36, 42–43, and 45–53 from *What Sort of People Should There Be?* (Harmondsworth: Penguin Books, 1984).

can expect to find statements of this kind applying to human nature in general. To say this is not to argue that studies on the question should not be conducted, or are bound to fail. It may well be possible, and useful, to find out the relative weights of the two kinds of factor for a given characteristic among a certain group at a particular time. The point is that any such conclusions lose relevance, not only when environmental differences are stretched out or compressed, but also when genetic differences are. And this last case is what we are considering.

We can avoid this dispute because of its irrelevance. Suppose the genetic engineering proposal were to try to make people less aggressive. On a superficial view, the proposal might be shown to be unrealistic if there were evidence to show that variation in aggressiveness is hardly genetic at all: that it is 95 per cent environmental. (Let us grant, most implausibly, that such a figure turned out to be true for the whole of humanity, regardless of social context.) But all this would show is that, within our species, the distribution of genes relevant to aggression is very uniform. It would show nothing about the likely effects on aggression if we use genetic engineering to give people a different set of genes from those they now have.

In other words, to take genetic engineering seriously, we need take no stand on the relative importance or unimportance of genetic factors in the explanation of the present range of individual differences found in people. We need only the minimal assumption that different genes could give us different characteristics. To deny *that* assumption you need to be the sort of person who thinks it is only living in kennels which makes dogs different from cats.

Methods of Changing the Genetic Composition of Future Generations

There are essentially three ways of altering the genetic composition of future generations. The first is by environmental changes. Discoveries in medicine, the institution of a National Health Service, schemes for poverty relief, agricultural changes, or alterations in the tax position of large families, all alter the selective pressures on genes.[1] It is hard to think of any social change which does not make some difference to who survives or who is born.

The second method is to use eugenic policies aimed at altering breeding patterns or patterns of survival of people with different genes. Eugenic methods are 'environmental' too: the difference is only that the genetic impact is intended. Possible strategies range from various kinds of compulsion (to have more children, fewer children, or no children, or even compulsion over the choice of sexual partner) to the completely voluntary (our present genetic counselling practice of giving prospective parents information about probabilities of their children having various abnormalities).

The third method is genetic engineering: using enzymes to add to or subtract from a stretch of DNA.

Most people are unworried by the fact that a side-effect of an environmental change is to alter the gene pool, at least where the alteration is not for the worse. And even in cases where environmental factors increase the proportion of undesirable genes in the pool, we often accept this. Few people oppose the National Health Service, although setting it up meant that some people with genetic defects, who would have died, have had treatment enabling them to survive and reproduce. On the whole, we accept without qualms that much of what we do has genetic impact. Controversy starts when we think of aiming deliberately at genetic changes, by eugenics or genetic engineering. I want to make some brief remarks about eugenic policies, before suggesting that policies of deliberate intervention are best considered in the context of genetic engineering.

Scepticism has been expressed about whether eugenic policies have any practical chance of success. Medawar has pointed out the importance of genetic polymorphism: the persistence of genetically different types in a population.[2] (Our different blood groups are a familiar example.) For many characteristics, people get a different gene from each parent. So children do not simply repeat parental characteristics. Any simple picture of producing an improved type of person, and then letting the improvement be passed on unchanged, collapses.

But, although polymorphism is a problem for this crudely utopian form of eugenics, it does not show that more modest schemes of improvement must fail. Suppose the best individuals for some quality (say, colour vision) are heterozygous, so that they inherit a gene A from one parent, and a gene B from the other. These ABs will have AAs and BBs among their children, who will be less good than they are. But AAs and BBs may still be better than ACs or ADs, and perhaps much better than CCs or CDs. If this were so, overall improvement could still be brought about by encouraging people whose genes included an A or a B to have more children than those who had only Cs or Ds. The point of taking a quality like colour vision is that it may be genetically fairly simple. Qualities like kindness or intelligence are more likely to depend on the interaction of many genes, but a similar point can be made at a higher level of complexity.

Polymorphism raises a doubt about whether the offspring of the three 'exceptionally intelligent women' fertilized by Dr Shockley or other Nobel prize-winners will have the same IQ as the parents, even apart from environmental variation. But it does not show the inevitable failure of any large-scale attempts to alter human characteristics by varying the relative numbers of children different kinds of people have. Yet any attempt, say, to raise the level of intelligence, would be a very slow affair, taking many generations to make much of an impact. This is one reason for preferring to discuss genetic engineering. For the genetic engineering of human improvements, if it becomes possible, will have an immediate effect, so we will not be guessing which qualities will be desirable dozens of generations later.

There is the view that the genetic-engineering techniques required will not become a practical possibility. Sir Macfarlane Burnet, writing in 1971 about using genetic engineering to cure disorders in people already born, dismissed the possibility of using a virus to carry a new gene to replace a faulty one in cells throughout the body: 'I should be willing to state in any company that the chance of doing this will remain infinitely small to the last syllable of recorded time.'[3] Unless engineering at the stage of sperm cell and egg is easier, this seems a confident dismissal of the topic to be discussed here. More recent work casts doubt on this confidence.[4] So, having mentioned this scepticism, I shall disregard it. We will assume that genetic engineering of people may become possible, and that it is worth discussing. (Sir Macfarlane Burnet's view has not yet been falsified as totally as Rutherford's view about atomic energy. But I hope that the last syllable of recorded time is still some way off.)

The main reason for casting the discussion in terms of genetic engineering rather than eugenics is not a practical one. Many eugenic policies are open to fairly straightforward moral objections, which hide the deeper theoretical issues. Such policies as compulsory sterilization, compulsory abortion, compelling people to pair off in certain ways, or compelling people to have more or fewer children than they would otherwise have, are all open to objection on grounds of overriding people's autonomy. Some are open to objection on grounds of damage to the institution of the family. And the use of discriminatory tax- and child-benefit policies is an intolerable step towards a society of different genetic castes.

Genetic engineering need not involve overriding anyone's autonomy. It need not be forced on parents against their wishes, and the future person being engineered has no views to be overridden. (The view that despite this, it is still objectionable to have one's genetic characteristics decided by others, will be considered later.) Genetic engineering will not damage the family in the obvious ways that compulsory eugenic policies would. Nor need it be encouraged by incentives which create inequalities. Because it avoids these highly visible moral objections, genetic engineering allows us to focus more clearly on other values that are involved.

(To avoid a possible misunderstanding, one point should be added before leaving the topic of eugenics. Saying that some eugenic policies are open to obvious moral objections does not commit me to disapproval of all eugenic policies. In particular, I do not want to be taken to be opposing two kinds of policy. One is genetic counselling: warning people of risks in having children, and perhaps advising them against having them. The other is the introduction of screening-programmes to detect foetal abnormalities, followed by giving the mother the option of abortion where serious defects emerge.)

Let us now turn to the question of what, if anything, we should do in the field of human genetic engineering.

The Positive–Negative Distinction

We are not yet able to cure disorders by genetic engineering. But we do sometimes respond to disorders by adopting eugenic policies, at least in voluntary form. Genetic counselling is one instance, as applied to those thought likely to have such disorders as Huntington's chorea. This is a particularly appalling inherited disorder, involving brain degeneration, leading to mental decline and lack of control over movement. It does not normally come on until middle age, by which time many of its victims would in the normal course of things have had children. Huntington's chorea is caused by a dominant gene, so those who find that one of their parents has it have themselves a 50 per cent chance of developing it. If they do have it, each of their children will in turn have a 50 per cent chance of the disease. The risks are so high and the disorder so bad that the potential parents often decide not to have children, and are often given advice to this effect by doctors and others.

Another eugenic response to disorders is involved in screening-programmes for pregnant women. When tests pick up such defects as Down's syndrome (mongolism) or spina bifida, the mother is given the possibility of an abortion. The screening-programmes are eugenic because part of their point is to reduce the incidence of severe genetic abnormality in the population.

These two eugenic policies come in at different stages: before conception and during pregnancy. For this reason the screening-programme is more controversial, because it raises the issue of abortion. Those who are sympathetic to abortion, and who think it would be good to eliminate these disorders will be sympathetic to the programme. Those who think abortion is no different from killing a fully developed human are obviously likely to oppose the programme. But they are likely to feel that elimination of the disorders would be a good thing, even if not an adequate justification for killing. Unless they also disapprove of contraception, they are likely to support the genetic-counselling policy in the case of Huntington's chorea.

Few people object to the use of eugenic policies to eliminate disorders, unless those policies have additional features which are objectionable. Most of us are resistant to the use of compulsion, and those who oppose abortion will object to screening-programmes. But apart from these other moral objections, we do not object to the use of eugenic policies against disease. We do not object to advising those likely to have Huntington's chorea not to have children, as neither compulsion nor killing is involved. Those of us who take this view have no objection to altering the genetic composition of the next generation, where this alteration consists in reducing the incidence of defects.

If it were possible to use genetic engineering to correct defects, say at the foetal stage, it is hard to see how those of us who are prepared to use the eugenic measures just mentioned could object. In both cases, it would be pure gain. The couple, one of whom may develop Huntington's chorea, can have a child if they want, knowing that any abnormality will be eliminated. Those sympathetic to abortion will agree that cure is preferable. And those opposed to abortion prefer babies to be born without handicap. It is hard to think of any objection to using genetic engineering to eliminate defects, and there is a clear and strong case for its use.

But accepting the case for eliminating genetic mistakes does not entail accepting other uses of genetic engineering. The elimination of defects is often called 'negative' genetic engineering. Going beyond this, to bring about improvements in normal people, is by contrast 'positive' engineering. (The same distinction can be made for eugenics.)

The positive–negative distinction is not in all cases completely sharp. Some conditions are genetic disorders whose identification raises little problem. Huntington's chorea or spina bifida are genetic 'mistakes' in a way that cannot seriously be disputed. But with other conditions, the boundary between a defective state and normality may be more blurred. If there is a genetic disposition towards depressive illness, this seems a defect, whose elimination would be part of negative genetic engineering. Suppose the genetic disposition to depression involves the production of lower levels of an enzyme than are produced in normal people. The negative programme is to correct the genetic fault so that the enzyme level is within the range found in normal people. But suppose that within 'normal' people also there are variations in the enzyme level, which correlate with ordinary differences in tendency to be cheerful or depressed. Is there a sharp boundary between 'clinical' depression and the depression sometimes felt by those diagnosed as 'normal'? Is it clear that a sharp distinction can be drawn between raising someone's enzyme level so that it falls within the normal range and raising someone else's level from the bottom of the normal range to the top?

The positive–negative distinction is sometimes a blurred one, but often we can at least roughly see where it should be drawn. If there is a rough and ready distinction, the question is: how important is it? Should we go on from accepting negative engineering to accepting positive programmes, or should we say that the line between the two is the limit of what is morally acceptable?

There is no doubt that positive programmes arouse the strongest feelings on both sides. On the one hand, many respond to positive genetic engineering or positive eugenics with Professor Tinbergen's thought: 'I find it morally reprehensible and presumptuous for anybody to put himself forward as a judge of the qualities for which we should breed.'

But other people have held just as strongly that positive policies are the way to make the future of mankind better than the past. Many years ago H. J. Muller expressed this hope:

> And so we foresee the history of life divided into three main phases. In the long preparatory phase it was the helpless creature of its environment, and natural selection gradually ground it into human shape. In the second – our own short transitional phase – it reaches out at the immediate environment, shaking, shaping and grinding to suit the form, the requirements, the wishes, and the whims of man. And in the long third phase, it will reach down into the secret places of the great universe of its own nature, and by aid of its ever growing intelligence and co-operation, shape itself into an increasingly sublime creation – a being beside which the mythical divinities of the past will seem more and more ridiculous, and which setting its own marvellous inner powers against the brute Goliath of the suns and the planets, challenges them to contest.[5]

The case for positive engineering is not helped by adopting the tones of the mad scientist in a horror film. But behind the rhetoric is a serious point. If we decide on a positive programme to change our nature, this will be a central moment in our history, and the transformation might be beneficial to a degree we can now scarcely imagine. The question is: how are we to weigh this possibility against Tinbergen's objection, and against other objections and doubts?

For the rest of this discussion, I shall assume that, subject to adequate safeguards against things going wrong, negative genetic engineering is acceptable. The issue is positive engineering. I shall also assume that we can ignore problems about whether positive engineering will be technically possible. Suppose we have the power to choose people's genetic characteristics. Once we have eliminated genetic defects, what, if anything, should we do with this power? [. . .]

The View that Overall Improvement is Unlikely or Impossible

There is one doubt about the workability of schemes of genetic improvement which is so widespread that it would be perverse to ignore it. This is the view that, in any genetic alteration, there are no gains without compensating losses. On this view, if we bring about a genetically based improvement, such as higher intelligence, we are bound to pay a price somewhere else: perhaps the more intelligent people will have less resistance to disease, or will be less physically agile. If correct, this might so undermine the practicability of applying eugenics or genetic engineering that it would be hardly worth discussing the values involved in such programmes.

This view perhaps depends on some idea that natural selection is so efficient that, in terms of gene survival, we must already be as efficient as it is possible to be. If it were possible to push up intelligence without weakening some other part of the system, natural selection would already have done so. But this is a naive version of evolutionary theory. In real evolutionary theory, far from the genetic status quo always being the best possible for a given environment, some mutations turn out to be advantageous, and this is the origin of evolutionary progress. If natural mutations can be beneficial without a compensating loss, why should artificially induced ones not be so too?

It should also be noticed that there are two different ideas of what counts as a gain or a loss. From the point of view of evolutionary progress, gains and losses are simply advantages and disadvantages from the point of view of gene survival. But we are not compelled to take this view. If we could engineer a genetic change in some people which would have the effect of making them musical prodigies but also sterile, this would be a hopeless gene in terms of survival, but this need not force us, or the musical prodigies themselves, to think of the change as for the worse. It depends on how we rate musical ability as against having children, and evolutionary survival does not dictate priorities here.

The view that gains and losses are tied up with each other need not depend on the dogma that natural selection *must* have created the best of all possible sets of genes. A more cautiously empirical version of the claim says there is a tendency for gains to be accompanied by losses. John Maynard Smith, in his paper on 'Eugenics and Utopia',[6] takes this kind of 'broad balance' view and runs it the other way, suggesting, as an argument in defence of medicine, that any loss of genetic resistance to disease is likely to be a good thing: 'The reason for this is that in evolution, as in other fields, one seldom gets something for nothing. Genes which confer disease-resistance are likely to have harmful effects in other ways: this is certainly true of the gene for sickle-cell anaemia and may be a general rule. If so, absence of selection in favour of disease resistance may be eugenic.'

It is important that different characteristics may turn out to be genetically linked in ways we do not yet realize. In our present state of knowledge, engineering for some improvement might easily bring some unpredicted but genetically linked disadvantage. But we do not have to accept that there will in general be a broad balance, so that there is a presumption that any gain will be accompanied by a compensating loss (or Maynard Smith's version that we can expect a compensating gain for any loss). The reason is that what counts as a gain or loss varies in different contexts. Take Maynard Smith's example of sickle-cell anaemia. The reason why sickle-cell anaemia is widespread in Africa is that it is genetically linked with resistance to malaria. Those who are heterozygous (who inherit one sickle-cell gene and one normal gene) are resistant to malaria, while those who are homozygous (whose genes are both sickle-cell) get sickle-cell anaemia. If we use genetic engineering to knock out sickle-cell anaemia where malaria is common, we will pay the price of having more malaria. But when we eradicate malaria, the gain will not involve this loss. Because losses are relative to context, any generalization about the impossibility of overall improvements is dubious.

The Family and Our Descendants

Unlike various compulsory eugenic policies, genetic engineering need not involve any interference with decisions by couples to have children together, or with their decisions about how many children to have. And let us suppose that genetically engineered babies grow in the mother's womb in the normal way, so that her relationship to the child is not threatened in the way it might be if the laboratory or the hospital were substituted for the womb. The cruder threats to family relationships are eliminated.

It may be suggested that there is a more subtle threat. Parents like to identify with their children. We are often pleased to see some of our own characteristics in our children. Perhaps this is partly a kind of vanity, and no doubt sometimes we project on to our children similarities that are not really there. But, when the similarities do exist, they help the parents and children to understand and sympathize with each other. If genetic engineering resulted in children fairly different from their parents, this might make their relationship have problems.

There is something to this objection, but it is easy to exaggerate. Obviously, children who were like Midwich cuckoos, or comic-book Martians, would not be easy to identify with. But genetic engineering need not move in such sudden jerks. The changes would have to be detectable to be worth bringing about, but there seems no reason why large changes in appearance, or an unbridgeable psychological gulf, should be created in any one generation. We bring about environmental changes which make children different from their parents, as when the first generation of children in a remote place are given schooling and made literate. This may cause some problems in families, but it is not usually thought a decisive objection. It is not clear that genetically induced changes of similar magnitude are any more objectionable.

A related objection concerns our attitude to our remoter descendants. We like to think of our descendants stretching on for many generations. Perhaps this is in part an immortality substitute. We hope they will to some extent be like us, and that, if they think of us, they will do so with sympathy and approval. Perhaps these hopes about the future of mankind are relatively unimportant to us. But, even if we mind about them a lot, they are unrealistic in the very long term. Genetic engineering would make our descendants less like us, but this would only speed up the natural rate of change. Natural mutations

and selective pressures make it unlikely that in a few million years our descendants will be physically or mentally much like us. So what genetic engineering threatens here is probably doomed anyway. [. . .]

Risks and Mistakes

[. . .] One of the objections [to genetic engineering] is that serious risks may be involved.

Some of the risks are already part of the public debate because of current work on recombinant DNA. The danger is of producing harmful organisms that would escape from our control. The work obviously should take place, if at all, only with adequate safeguards against such a disaster. The problem is deciding what we should count as adequate safeguards. I have nothing to contribute to this problem here. If it can be dealt with satisfactorily, we will perhaps move on to genetic engineering of people. And this introduces another dimension of risk. We may produce unintended results, either because our techniques turn out to be less finely tuned than we thought, or because different characteristics are found to be genetically linked in unexpected ways.

If we produce a group of people who turn out worse than expected, we will have to live with them. Perhaps we would aim for producing people who were especially imaginative and creative, and only too late find we had produced people who were also very violent and aggressive. This kind of mistake might not only be disastrous, but also very hard to 'correct' in subsequent generations. For when we suggested sterilization to the people we had produced, or else corrective genetic engineering for *their* offspring, we might find them hard to persuade. They might like the way they were, and reject, in characteristically violent fashion, our explanation that they were a mistake.

The possibility of an irreversible disaster is a strong deterrent. It is enough to make some people think we should rule out genetic engineering altogether, and to make others think that, while negative engineering is perhaps acceptable, we should rule out positive engineering. The thought behind this second position is that the benefits from negative engineering are clearer, and that, because its aims are more modest, disastrous mistakes are less likely.

The risk of disasters provides at least a reason for saying that, if we do adopt a policy of human genetic engineering, we ought to do so with extreme caution. We should alter genes only where we have strong reasons for thinking the risk of disaster is very small, and where the benefit is great enough to justify the risk. (The problems of deciding when this is so are familiar from the nuclear power debate.) This 'principle of caution' is less strong than one ruling out all positive engineering, and allows room for the possibility that the dangers may turn out to be very remote, or that greater risks of a different kind are involved in *not* using positive engineering. These possibilities correspond to one view of the facts in the nuclear power debate. Unless with genetic engineering we think we can already rule out such possibilities, the argument from risk provides more justification for the principle of caution than for the stronger ban on all positive engineering. [. . .]

Not Playing God

Suppose we could use genetic engineering to raise the average IQ by fifteen points. (I mention, only to ignore, the boring objection that the average IQ is always by definition 100.) Should we do this? Objectors to positive engineering say we should not. This is not because the present average is preferable to a higher one. We do not think that, if it were naturally fifteen points higher, we ought to bring it down to the present level. The objection is to our playing God by deciding what the level should be.

On one view of the world, the objection is relatively straightforward. On this view, there really is a God, who has a plan for the world which will be disrupted if we stray outside the boundaries assigned to us. (It is *relatively* straightforward: there would still be the problem of knowing where the boundaries came. If genetic engineering disrupts the programme, how do we know that medicine and education do not?)

The objection to playing God has a much wider appeal than to those who literally believe in a divine plan. But, outside such a context, it is unclear what the objection comes to. If we have a Darwinian view, according to which features of our nature have been selected for their contribution to gene survival, it is not blasphemous, or obviously disastrous, to start to control the process in the light of our own values. We may value other qualities in people, in preference to those which have been most conducive to gene survival.

The prohibition on playing God is obscure. If it tells us not to interfere with natural selection at all, this rules out medicine, and most other environmental and social changes. If it only forbids interference with natural selection by the direct alteration of genes, this rules out negative as well as positive genetic engineering. If these interpretations are too restrictive, the ban on positive engineering seems to need some explanation. If we can make positive changes at the environmental level, and negative changes at the genetic level, why should we not make positive changes at the genetic level? What makes this policy, but not the others, objectionably God-like?

Perhaps the most plausible reply to these questions rests on a general objection to any group of people trying to plan too closely what human life should be like. Even if it is hard to distinguish in principle between the use of genetic and environmental means, genetic changes are likely to differ in degree from most environmental ones. Genetic alterations may be more drastic or less reversible, and so they can be seen as the extreme case of an objectionably God-like policy by which some people set out to plan the lives of others.

This objection can be reinforced by imagining the possible results of a programme of positive engineering, where the decisions about the desired improvements were taken by scientists. Judging by the literature written by scientists on this topic, great prominence would be given to intelligence. But can we be sure that enough weight would be given to other desirable qualities? And do things seem better if for scientists we substitute doctors, politicians or civil servants? Or some committee containing businessmen, trade unionists, academics, lawyers and a clergyman?

What seems worrying here is the circumscribing of potential human development. The present genetic lottery throws up a vast range of characteristics, good and bad, in all sorts of combinations. The group of people controlling a positive engineering policy would inevitably have limited horizons, and we are right to worry that the limitations of their outlook might become the boundaries of human variety. The drawbacks would be like those of town-planning or dog-breeding, but with more important consequences.

When the objection to playing God is separated from the idea that intervening in this aspect of the natural world is a kind of blasphemy, it is a protest against a particular group of people, necessarily fallible and limited, taking decisions so important to our future. This protest may be on grounds of the bad consequences, such as loss of variety of people, that would come from the imaginative limits of those taking the decisions. Or it may be an expression of opposition to such concentration of power, perhaps with the thought: 'What right have *they* to decide what kinds of people there should be?' Can these problems be side-stepped?

The Genetic Supermarket

Robert Nozick is critical of the assumption that positive engineering has to involve any centralized decision about desirable qualities: 'Many biologists tend to think the problem is one of *design*, of specifying the best types of persons so that biologists can proceed to produce them. Thus they worry over what sort(s) of person there is to be and who will control this process. They do not tend to think, perhaps because it diminishes the importance of their role, of a system in which they run a "genetic supermarket", meeting the individual specifications (within certain moral limits) of prospective parents. Nor do they think of seeing what limited number of types of persons people's choices would converge upon, if indeed there would

be any such convergence. This supermarket system has the great virtue that it involves no centralized decision fixing the future human type(s).'[7]

This idea of letting parents choose their children's characteristics is in many ways an improvement on decisions being taken by some centralized body. It seems less likely to reduce human variety, and could even increase it, if genetic engineering makes new combinations of characteristics available. (But we should be cautious here. Parental choice is not a guarantee of genetic variety, as the influence of fashion or of shared values might make for a small number of types on which choices would converge.)

To those sympathetic to one kind of liberalism, Nozick's proposal will seem more attractive than centralized decisions. On this approach to politics, it is wrong for the authorities to institutionalize any religious or other outlook as the official one of the society. To a liberal of this kind, a good society is one which tolerates and encourages a wide diversity of ideals of the good life. Anyone with these sympathies will be suspicious of centralized decisons about what sort of people should form the next generation. But some parental decisons would be disturbing. If parents chose characteristics likely to make their children unhappy, or likely to reduce their abilities, we might feel that the children should be protected against this. (Imagine parents belonging to some extreme religious sect, who wanted their children to have a religious symbol as a physical mark on their face, and who wanted them to be unable to read, as a protection against their faith being corrupted.) Those of us who support restrictions protecting children from parental harm after birth (laws against cruelty, and compulsion on parents to allow their children to be educated and to have necessary medical treatment) are likely to support protecting children from being harmed by their parents' genetic choices.

No doubt the boundaries here will be difficult to draw. We already find it difficult to strike a satisfactory balance between protection of children and parental freedom to choose the kind of upbringing their children should have. But it is hard to accept that society should set no limits to the genetic choices parents can make for their children. Nozick recognizes this when he says the genetic supermarket should meet the specifications of parents 'within certain moral limits'. So, if the supermarket came into existence, some centralized policy, even if only the restrictive one of ruling out certain choices harmful to the children, should exist. It would be a political decision where the limits should be set.

There may also be a case for other centralized restrictions on parental choice, as well as those aimed at preventing harm to the individual people being designed. The genetic supermarket might have more oblique bad effects. An imbalance in the ratio between the sexes could result. Or parents might think their children would be more successful if they were more thrusting, competitive and selfish. If enough parents acted on this thought, other parents with different values might feel forced into making similar choices to prevent their own children being too greatly disadvantaged. Unregulated individual decisions could lead to shifts of this kind, with outcomes unwanted by most of those who contribute to them. If a majority favour a roughly equal ratio between the sexes, or a population of relatively uncompetitive people, they may feel justified in supporting restrictions on what parents can choose. (This is an application to the case of genetic engineering of a point familiar in other contexts, that unrestricted individual choices can add up to a total outcome which most people think worse than what would result from some regulation.)

Nozick recognizes that there may be cases of this sort. He considers the case of avoiding a sexual imbalance and says that 'a government could require that genetic manipulation be carried on so as to fit a certain ratio'.[8] He clearly prefers to avoid governmental intervention of this kind, and, while admitting that the desired result would be harder to obtain in a purely libertarian system, suggests possible strategies for doing so. He says: 'Either parents would subscribe to an information service monitoring the recent births and so know which sex was in shorter supply (and hence would be more in demand in later life), thus adjusting their activities, or interested individuals would contribute to a charity that offers bonuses to

maintain the ratios, or the ratio would leave 1:1, with new family and social patterns developing.' The proposals for avoiding the sexual imbalance without central regulation are not reassuring. Information about likely prospects for marriage or sexual partnership might not be decisive for parents' choices. And, since those most likely to be 'interested individuals' would be in the age group being genetically engineered, it is not clear that the charity would be given donations adequate for its job.[9]

If the libertarian methods failed, we would have the choice between allowing a sexual imbalance or imposing some system of social regulation. Those who dislike central decisions favouring one sort of person over others might accept regulation here, on the grounds that neither sex is being given preference: the aim is rough equality of numbers.

But what about the other sort of case, where the working of the genetic supermarket leads to a general change unwelcome to those who contribute to it? Can we defend regulation to prevent a shift towards a more selfish and competitive population as merely being the preservation of a certain ratio between characteristics? Or have we crossed the boundary, and allowed a centralized decision favouring some characteristics over others? The location of the boundary is obscure. One view would be that the sex-ratio case is acceptable because the desired ratio is equality of numbers. On another view, the acceptability derives from the fact that the present ratio is to be preserved. (In this second view, preserving altruism would be acceptable, so long as no attempt was made to raise the proportion of altruistic people in the population. But is *this* boundary an easy one to defend?)

If positive genetic engineering does become a reality, we may be unable to avoid some of the decisions being taken at a social level. Or rather, we could avoid this, but only at what seems an unacceptable cost, either to the particular people being designed, or to their generation as a whole. And, even if the social decisions are only restrictive, it is implausible to claim that they are all quite free of any taint of preference for some characteristics over others. But, although this suggests that we should not be doctrinaire in our support of the liberal view, it does not show that the view has to be abandoned altogether. We may still think that social decisions in favour of one type of person rather than another should be few, even if the consequences of excluding them altogether are unacceptable. A genetic supermarket, modified by some central regulation, may still be better than a system of purely central decisions. The liberal value is not obliterated because it may sometimes be compromised for the sake of other things we care about.

A Mixed System

The genetic supermarket provides a partial answer to the objection about the limited outlook of those who would take the decisions. The choices need not be concentrated in the hands of a small number of people. The genetic supermarket should not operate in a completely unregulated way, and so some centralized decisions would have to be taken about the restrictions that should be imposed. One system that would answer many of the anxieties about centralized decision-making would be to limit the power of the decision-makers to one of veto. They would then only check departures from the natural genetic lottery, and so the power to bring about changes would not be given to them, but spread through the whole population of potential parents. Let us call this combination of parental initiative and central veto a 'mixed system'. If positive genetic engineering does come about, we can imagine the argument between supporters of a mixed system and supporters of other decision-making systems being central to the political theory of the twenty-first century, parallel to the place occupied in the nineteenth and twentieth centuries by the debate over control of the economy.[10]

My own sympathies are with the view that, if positive genetic engineering is introduced, this mixed system is in general likely to be the best one for taking decisions. I do not want to argue for an absolutely inviolable commitment to this, as it could be that some centralized decision for genetic change was the only way of securing a huge benefit or avoiding a

great catastrophe. But, subject to this reservation, the dangers of concentrating the decision-making create a strong presumption in favour of a mixed system rather than one in which initiatives come from the centre. And, if a mixed system was introduced, there would have to be a great deal of political argument over what kinds of restrictions on the supermarket should be imposed. Twenty-first-century elections may be about issues rather deeper than economics.

If this mixed system eliminates the anxiety about genetic changes being introduced by a few powerful people with limited horizons, there is a more general unease which it does not remove. May not the limitations of one generation of parents also prove disastrous? And, underlying this, is the problem of what values parents should appeal to in making their choices. How can we be confident that it is better for one sort of person to be born than another?

Values

The dangers of such decisions, even spread through all prospective parents, seem to me very real. We are swayed by fashion. We do not know the limitations of our own outlook. There are human qualities whose value we may not appreciate. A generation of parents might opt heavily for their children having physical or intellectual abilities and skills. We might leave out a sense of humour. Or we might not notice how important to us is some other quality, such as emotional warmth. So we might not be disturbed in advance by the possible impact of the genetic changes on such a quality. And, without really wanting to do so, we might stumble into producing people with a deep coldness. This possibility seems one of the worst imaginable. It is just one of the many horrors that could be blundered into by our lack of foresight in operating the mixed system. Because such disasters are a real danger, there is a case against positive genetic engineering, even when the changes do not result from centralized decisions. But this case, resting as it does on the risk of disaster, supports a principle of caution rather than a total ban. We have to ask the question whether there are benefits sufficiently great and sufficiently probable to outweigh the risks.

But perhaps the deepest resistance, even to a mixed system, is not based on risks, but on a more general problem about values. Could the parents ever be justified in choosing, according to some set of values, to create one sort of person rather than another?

Is it sometimes better for us to create one sort of person rather than another? We say 'yes' when it is a question of eliminating genetic defects. And we say 'yes' if we think that encouraging some qualities rather than others should be an aim of the upbringing and education we give our children. Any inclination to say 'no' in the context of positive genetic engineering must lay great stress on the two relevant boundaries. The positive–negative boundary is needed to mark off the supposedly unacceptable positive policies from the acceptable elimination of defects. And the genes–environment boundary is needed to mark off positive engineering from acceptable positive aims of educational policies. But it is not clear that confidence in the importance of these boundaries is justified.

The positive–negative boundary may seem a way of avoiding objectionably God-like decisions, on the basis of our own values, as to what sort of people there should be. Saving someone from spina bifida is a lot less controversial than deciding he shall be a good athlete. But the distinction, clear in some cases, is less sharp in others. With emotional states or intellectual functioning, there is an element of convention in where the boundaries of normality are drawn. And, apart from this, there is the problem of explaining why the positive–negative boundary is so much more important with genetic intervention than with environmental methods. We act environmentally to influence people in ways that go far beyond the elimination of medical defects. Homes and schools would be impoverished by attempting to restrict their influence on children to the mere prevention of physical and mental disorder. And if we are right here to cross the positive–negative boundary, encouraging children to ask questions, or to be generous and imaginative, why should crossing the same boundary for the same reasons be ruled out absolutely when the means are genetic?

Notes

1   Chris Graham has suggested to me that it is misleading to say this without emphasizing the painful slowness of this way of changing gene frequencies.

2   *The Future of Man* (The Reith Lectures, 1959), London, 1960, chapter 3; and in 'The Genetic Improvement of Man', in *The Hope of Progress*, London, 1972.

3   *Genes. Dreams and Realities*, London, 1971, p. 81.

4   'Already they have pushed Cline's results further, obtaining transfer between rabbit and mouse, for example, and good expression of the foreign gene in its new host. Some, by transferring the genes into the developing eggs, have managed to get the new genes into every cell in the mouse, including the sex cells; those mice have fathered offspring who also contain the foreign gene.' Jeremy Cherfas: *Man Made Life*, Oxford, 1982, pp. 229–30.

5   *Out of the Night*, New York. 1935. To find a distinguished geneticist talking like this after the Nazi period is not easy.

6   John Maynard Smith: *On Evolution*, Edinburgh, 1972; the article is reprinted from the issue on 'Utopia' of *Daedalus, Journal of the American Academy of Arts and Sciences*, 1965.

7   *Anarchy, State and Utopia*, New York, 1974, p. 315.

8   *Anarchy, State and Utopia*, p. 315.

9   This kind of unworldly innocence is part of the engaging charm of Nozick's dotty and brilliant book.

10 Decision-taking by a central committee (perhaps of a dozen elderly men) can be thought of as a 'Russian' model. The genetic supermarket (perhaps with genotypes being sold by TV commercials) can be thought of as an 'American' model. The mixed system may appeal to Western European social democrats.

14

The Moral Significance of the Therapy–Enhancement Distinction in Human Genetics

David B. Resnik

Introduction

The therapy–enhancement distinction occupies a central place in contemporary discussions of human genetics and has been the subject of much debate.[1–7] At a recent conference on gene therapy policy, scientists predicted that within a few years researchers will develop techniques that can be used to enhance human traits.[8] In thinking about the morality of genetic interventions, many writers have defended somatic gene therapy,[9,10] and some have defended germline gene therapy,[11,12] but only a handful of writers defend genetic enhancement,[13] or even give it a fair hearing.[14–16] The mere mention of genetic enhancement makes many people cringe and brings to mind the Nazi eugenics programs, Aldous Huxley's *Brave New World*, "The X-Files," or the recent movie "Gattaca." Although many people believe that gene therapy has morally legitimate medical uses,[17,18] others regard genetic enhancement as morally problematic or decidedly evil.[19–21]

The purpose of this essay is to examine the moral significance of the therapy–enhancement distinction in human genetics. Is genetic enhancement inherently unethical? Is genetic therapy inherently ethical? I will argue that the distinction does not mark a firm boundary between moral and immoral genetic interventions, and that genetic enhancement is not inherently immoral. To evaluate the acceptability of any particular genetic intervention, one needs to examine the relevant facts in light of moral principles. Some types of genetic therapy are morally acceptable while some types of genetic enhancement are unacceptable. In defending this view, I will discuss and evaluate several different ways of attempting to draw a solid moral line between therapy and enhancement.[22]

Somatic versus Germline Interventions

Before discussing the therapy–enhancement distinction, it is important that we understand another distinction that should inform our discussion, viz. the distinction between somatic and germline interventions.[23,24] Somatic interventions attempt to modify

Original publication details: David B. Resnik, "The Moral Significance of the Therapy–Enhancement Distinction in Human Genetics," pp. 365–377 from *Cambridge Quarterly of Healthcare Ethics* 9: 3 (Summer 2000) Reproduced with permission of Cambridge University Press.

somatic cells, while germline interventions attempt to modify germ cells. The gene therapy clinical trials that have been performed thus far have been on somatic cells. If we combine these two distinctions, we obtain four types of genetic interventions:

1. Somatic genetic therapy (SGT)
2. Germline genetic therapy (GLGT)
3. Somatic genetic enhancement (SGE)
4. Germline genetic enhancement (GLGE)

While I accept the distinction between somatic and germline interventions, it is important to note that even interventions designed to affect somatic cells can also affect germ cells: current SGT trials carry a slight risk of altering germ cells.[25] Even so, one might argue that this is a morally significant distinction because somatic interventions usually affect only the patient, while germline interventions are likely to affect future generations.[26] In any case, the therapy–enhancement distinction encompasses somatic as well as germline interventions, and my discussion of this distinction will include both somatic as well as germline interventions.

The Concepts of Health and Disease

Perhaps the most popular way of thinking about the moral significance of the therapy–enhancement distinction is to argue that the aim of genetic therapy is to treat human diseases while the aim of genetic enhancement is to perform other kinds of interventions, such as altering or "improving" the human body.[27–29] Since genetic therapy serves morally legitimate goals, genetic therapy is morally acceptable; but since genetic enhancement serves morally questionable or illicit goals, genetic enhancement is not morally acceptable.[30–33] I suspect that many people view the distinction and its moral significance in precisely these terms. W. French Anderson states a clear case for the moral significance of genetic enhancement:

On medical and ethical grounds we should draw a line excluding any form of genetic engineering. We should not step over the line that delineates treatment from enhancement.[34]

However, this way of thinking of medical genetics makes at least two questionable assumptions: (1) that we have a clear and uncontroversial account of health and disease, and (2) that the goal of treating diseases is morally legitimate, while other goals are not. To examine these assumptions, we need to take a quick look at discussions about the concepts of health and disease.

The bioethics literature contains a thoughtful debate about the definitions of health and disease and it is not my aim to survey that terrain here.[35,36] However, I will distinguish between two basic approaches to the definition of health, a value-neutral (or descriptive) approach and a value-laden (or normative) one.[37] According to the value-neutral approach, health and disease are descriptive concepts that have an empirical, factual basis in human biology. Boorse defended one of the most influential descriptive approaches to health and disease: a diseased organism lacks the functional abilities of a normal member of its species.[38] To keep his approach value-neutral, Boorse interprets "normal" in statistical terms, i.e., "normal" = "typical." Daniels expands on Boorse's account of disease by suggesting that natural selection can provide an account of species-typical functions: functional abilities are traits that exist in populations because they have contributed to the reproduction and survival of organisms that possessed them.[39] Thus a human with healthy lungs has specific respiratory capacities that are normal in our species, and these capacities have been "designed" by natural selection. A human who lacks these capacities, such as someone with cystic fibrosis or emphysema, has a disease.

According to the value-laden approach, our concepts of health and disease are based on social, moral, and cultural norms. A healthy person is someone who falls within these norms; a diseased person deviates from them. Someone who deviates from species-typical functions could be considered healthy in a society that views that deviation as healthy: although schizophrenia has a biological basis, in some cultures schizophrenics are viewed as "gifted" or "sacred," while in other cultures they are viewed as "mentally ill." Likewise, some cultures view homosexuality as a disease, while others do not.[40–42]

Many different writers have tried to work out variants on these two basic approaches to health and disease, and some have tried to develop compromise views,[43,44] but suffice it to say that the first assumption mentioned above – i.e., that we have a clear and uncontroversial account of health and disease – is questionable.

Even if we lack an uncontroversial account of disease, we could still ask whether either of the two basic approaches would condemn genetic enhancement unconditionally. Consider the descriptive approach first. If statements about disease merely describe deviations from species-typical traits, does it follow that we may perform genetic interventions to treat diseases but not to enhance otherwise healthy people? Since we regard the concept of disease as descriptive, we cannot answer this question without making some normative assumptions. Saying that someone has a disease is like saying that he or she has red hair, is five feet tall, or was born in New York City. These descriptions of that person carry no normative import. Hence the descriptive account of disease, by itself, does not provide us with a way of drawing a solid moral line between therapy and enhancement. For this approach to disease to draw moral boundaries between therapy and enhancement, it needs to be supplemented by a normatively rich account of the rightness of therapy and wrongness of enhancement.

Perhaps the normative approach fares better than the descriptive one. If we accept this view, it follows that therapy has some positive moral value, since therapy is an attempt to treat diseases, which are defined as traits or abilities that do not fall within social or cultural norms. If it is "bad" to have a disease, then we are morally justified in performing interventions that attempt to treat or prevent diseases, since these procedures impart "good" states of being. Thus this normative approach implies that therapy is morally

right. But does it imply that enhancement is morally wrong? The answer to this question depends, in large part, on the scope of the concepts of health and disease. If we hold that the concept of health defines a set of traits and abilities that should be possessed by all members of society and that any deviations are diseases, then any intervention that results in a deviation from these norms would be viewed as immoral. Hence, enhancement would be inherently immoral. But this account of health and disease is way too broad; there must be some morally neutral traits and abilities. If there are no morally neutral traits and abilities, then any person that deviates from health norms is "sick." This view would leave very little room for individual variation, to say nothing of the freedom to choose to deviate from health norms. If we accept a narrower account of health and disease, then we will open up some room for morally acceptable deviations from health norms. But this interpretation implies that enhancement interventions could be morally acceptable, provided that they do not violate other moral norms, such as nonmaleficence, autonomy, utility, and so on. Enhancement would not be inherently wrong, on this view, but the rightness or wrongness of any enhancement procedure would depend on its various factual and normative aspects.

The upshot of this discussion is that neither of the two main approaches to health and disease provides us with solid moral boundaries between genetic enhancement and genetic therapy. One might suggest that we examine alternative approaches, but I doubt that other, more refined theories of health and disease will provide us with a way of drawing sharp moral boundaries between genetic enhancement and genetic therapy. Perhaps we should look at other ways of endowing the distinction with moral significance.

The Goals of Medicine

A slightly different approach to these issues asserts that genetic therapy is on solid moral ground because it promotes the goals of medicine, while genetic enhancement promotes other, morally questionable goals. But what are the goals of medicine? This is not an easy question to answer, since medicine seems to serve a variety of purposes, such as the treatment of disease, the prevention of disease, the promotion of human health and well-being, and the relief of suffering. Many of the so-called goals of medicine, such as the prevention of disease and the promotion of human health, may also be promoted by procedures that we would classify as forms of enhancement.[45] For example, some writers have suggested that we might be able to perform genetic interventions that enhance the human immune system by making it better able to fight diseases, including cancer.[46] Most people would accept the idea that providing children with immunizations against the measles, mumps, and rubella promotes the goals of medicine. If we accept the notion that ordinary, nongenetic enhancement of the immune system promotes the goals of medicine, then shouldn't we also agree that genetic enhancements of the immune system serve the same goals? And what about other forms of healthcare, such as rhinoplasty, liposuction, orthodontics, breast augmentation, hair removal, and hair transplants? If these cosmetic procedures serve medical goals, then cosmetic uses of genetic technology, such as somatic gene therapy for baldness, and germline gene therapy for straight teeth, would also seem to serve medical goals. Finally, consider the procedures that are designed to relieve suffering, such as pain control and anesthesia. If we can develop drugs to promote these goals, then why not develop genetic procedures to meet similar objectives? It is not beyond the realm of possibility that we could use genetic therapy to induce the body to produce endorphins. Many forms of enhancement may serve medical goals. Once again, the therapy-enhancement distinction appears not to set any firm moral boundaries in genetic medicine.

One might attempt to avoid this problem by narrowly construing the goals of medicine: the goals of medicine are to treat and prevent diseases in human beings. Other uses of medical technology do not serve the goals of medicine. There are two problems with this response. First, it assumes that we agree on the goals of medicine and the definitions of health and

disease. Second, even if we could agree that medicine's goals are to treat and prevent diseases and we can define "health" and "disease," why would it be immoral to use medical technology and science for nonmedical purposes? If a medical procedure, such as mastectomy, is developed for therapeutic purposes, what is wrong with using that procedure for "nonmedical" purposes, such as breast reduction surgery in men with overdeveloped breasts? Admittedly, there are many morally troubling nonmedical uses of medical science and technology, such as the use of steroids by athletes and the use of laxatives by anorexics, but these morally troubling uses of medicine are morally troubling because they violate various moral principles or values, such as fairness and nonmaleficence, not because they are nonmedical uses of medicine.

One might argue that those who use medical science and technology for nonmedical purposes violate medicine's professional norms, but this point only applies to those who consider themselves to be medical professionals. If a procedure violates medical norms, it is medically unethical, but this does not mean that the procedure is unethical outside of the context of medical care. For example, the American Medical Association holds that it is unethical for physicians to assist the state in executions, but this policy does not constitute an unconditional argument against capital punishment. To make the case against capital punishment, one must appeal to wider moral and political norms. Hence the goals of medicine also do not set a morally sharp dividing line between genetic therapy and enhancement.

Our Humanness

One might try to draw moral boundaries between genetic therapy and genetic enhancement by arguing that genetic enhancement is inherently immoral because it changes the human form. Genetic therapy only attempts to restore or safeguard our humanness, while enhancement changes those very features that make us human. Although GLGE and GLGT can more profoundly change human traits than SGE and SGT, both technologies can alter our humanness (or our humanity). To explore these issues in depth, we need to answer two questions: (1) What traits or abilities make us human? and (2) Why would it be wrong to change those traits or abilities? Philosophers have proposed answers to the first question ever since Aristotle defined man as "the rational animal." A thorough answer to the question of defining our humanness takes us way beyond the scope of this essay, but I will offer the reader a brief perspective.[47]

If we have learned anything from the abortion debate, we have learned that it is not at all easy to specify necessary and sufficient conditions for a thing to be human. Humanness is best understood as a cluster concept in that it can be equated with a list of characteristics but not with a set of necessary and sufficient conditions.[48] Some of these characteristics include:

a. physical traits and abilities, such as an opposable thumb, bipedalism, etc.
b. psychosocial traits and abilities, such as cognition, language, emotional responses, sociality, etc.
c. phylogenetic traits, such as membership in the biological species *Homo sapiens*.

The beings that we call "human" possess many of these traits and abilities, even though some humans have more of these traits and abilities than others. For example, a newborn and an adult have many of the same physical and phylogenetic traits and abilities, even though the adult has more psychosocial traits and abilities. For my purposes, I do not need to say which of these traits and abilities are more "central" to the concept of humanness, since I am not defending a definition that provides necessary or sufficient conditions.

The question I would like to explore in more depth concerns the wrongness of changing those traits that make us human. Would it be inherently wrong to alter the human form? This question presupposes the pragmatically prior question, Can we alter the human form? The answer to this question depends on two factors: (1) the definition of our humanness; and (2)

our scientific and technological abilities. According to the definition I assume in this essay, it is possible to alter the human form, since the human form consists of a collection of physiological, psychosocial, and phylogenetic traits and abilities, which can be changed in principle.[49] Although we lacked the ability to change the traits that constitute our humanness at one time, advances in science and technology have given us the ability to change human traits. Since we have good reasons to believe that we can change our humanness, we can now ask whether we should do so.

Most moral theories, with the notable exception of the natural law approach, imply that there is nothing inherently wrong with changing the human form. For the purposes of this essay, I will not examine all of these moral theories here but will only briefly mention two very different perspectives on morality that reach similar conclusions. According to utilitarianism, an action or policy that alters our humanness could be morally right or it could be morally wrong, depending on the consequences of that action or policy. If genetic enhancement produces a greater balance of good/bad consequences, then enhancement would be morally acceptable. For example, genetic interventions that enhance the human immune system might be morally acceptable, but interventions that result in harmful mutations would be unacceptable. Kantians would object to attempts to alter our humanness if those attempts violate human dignity and autonomy. Some, but not all, genetic interventions could threaten our dignity and autonomy. For example, using SGT to promote hair growth should pose no threat to human dignity and autonomy (if informed consent is not violated), but using GLGE to create a race of "slaves" or "freaks" would pose a dire threat to dignity and autonomy. The main point here is that most moral theories would hold that there is nothing inherently wrong with changing our humanness; the moral rightness or wrongness of such attempts depends on their relation to other moral concerns, such as utility, autonomy, natural rights, virtue, etc.[50]

However, the natural law approach to morality could be interpreted as implying that tampering with the human form is inherently wrong. This argument assumes that the human form has inherent worth and that any changes to that form defile or destroy its worth. The human form is morally sacred and should not be altered.[51] For example, one might hold that a great painting, such as the "Mona Lisa," has inherent worth and it should therefore be left as it is; to change the "Mona Lisa" is to destroy it. Or perhaps one might argue that it would be wrong to change the formula for "Coke" or the plot of "Hamlet." But what is inherently wrong with changing the human form?

One argument that changing the human form is inherently wrong is that natural selection has "designed" us to have specific traits, and that any attempt to change those traits would be a foolhardy and vain intervention in nature's wisdom. It has taken thousands of years of adaptation for the human species to evolve into its present form. How can we possibly improve on nature's perfection? We are more likely to make a major blunder or mistake with human genetic engineering than to make an important advance.[52] Human genetic engineering is likely to produce harmful mutations, gross abnormalities, Frankenstein monsters, etc.[53] There are two problems with this neo-Darwinian view. First, it is Panglossian and naïve: natural selection is not perfect – nature makes mistakes all the time. We possess many traits, such as the appendix, that serve no useful function. There are some traits that we could add, such as enhancements to the immune system, that could be very useful. Though we should not underestimate nature's wisdom and our ignorance, it is simply false that nature has made us perfect with no room for change or improvement.[54] Second, the argument overestimates human ignorance and carelessness. The history of medical technology allows us to see that while we have had many failures in altering the human form, such as Nazi eugenics programs, we have also had some successes, such as artificial limbs and eyeglasses. Although we should exhibit extreme care, discretion, and circumspection in all genetic interventions, not all changes we make in the human form will result in natural disasters.

A second argument approaches the issue from a theological perspective. According to this view, God, not natural selection, has designed us to have specific traits. Hence any human attempt to change those traits would be a foolish (and arrogant) challenge to God's wisdom. Those who attempt to "play God" by changing human nature commit the mortal sin of hubris. One obvious difficulty with this argument is that it is not likely to convince nonbelievers, but let us set aside that problem and engage in some speculative theology. The question we need to ask in response to this argument is, Would God not want us to change human traits? Changes we can now make to human traits could promote human welfare and justice. Why would God allow us to have this power and not use it? Of course, God would not want us to use our power to increase human suffering or injustice, but why would He not want us to use this power for good purposes? Although several well-known theologians have taken a strong stance against human genetic engineering,[55] religious denominations are not united in their opposition to genetic engineering.[56] For example, the National Council of Churches adopted a resolution that the effort to use genetics to improve on nature is not inherently wrong, and the Council later stated that God has given men and women powers of co-creation, though these powers should be used with care.[57,58]

Regardless of whether one accepts the views of a particular church, it is not at all clear that a theologically based natural law theory provides us with good reasons for thinking that it is inherently wrong to change the human form. One could accept a theologically based approach to morality that leaves some room for human beings to alter the human form, provided that we exhibit wisdom, care, and restraint in changing our form.[59] Some changes (e.g., those that result in suffering or injustice) are morally wrong, but other changes (e.g., those that promote happiness or justice) are morally acceptable.

The Rights of the Unborn

Another way of arguing that at least some forms of genetic enhancement are inherently wrong is to claim that GLGE and GLGT violate the rights of unborn children.[60] These procedures are often said to violate the rights of unborn children because they:

a. are experimental procedures that violate the informed consent of unborn children;[61]
b. deny unborn children the right to have a germline that has not been genetically manipulated;[62] or
c. deny unborn children a right to an open future.[63]

All of these arguments make the morally controversial assumption that unborn children have rights. I will not challenge this assertion here.[64] Even if one assumes that unborn children have rights, it still does not follow that GLGE or GLGT violate those rights.

Let's consider (a) first. GLGT and GLGE do not violate the unborn child's right to informed consent because this right can be exercised by competent adults acting in the child's best interests. We allow proxy consent as a legitimate way of exercising informed consent for many procedures that can profoundly affect the welfare of children, such as fetal surgery and experimental surgery on newborns to repair congenital defects. If it makes sense to use proxy consent in these kinds of experiments, then it should also make sense to use proxy consent for other types of experiments, such as GLGT or GLGE, provided that these experiments can be shown to be in the best interests of unborn children.[65]

(b) is a very esoteric position. What kind of right is the "right to have a genome that has not been genetically manipulated"? Most writers conceive of rights in terms of interests: rights function to protect the interests of individuals.[66] Interests are needs and benefits that most people require to have a fulfilling life, such as freedom, health, education, self-esteem, and so on. So do unborn children have an interest in being born with a genome that has not been manipulated? If such an interest exists, then it is highly unusual and certainly not universal. Children whose parents hold specific religious or philosophical doctrines that forbid germline manipulation may have an interest in being born with an unadulterated genome, but other children will not have this interest. For most children, being born with a genome that predisposes them

to health and a wide range of opportunities is more important than being born with a genome that has not been manipulated.

This brings us to argument (c). A right to an "open future" is a right to make one's own choices and life plans on reaching adulthood.[67] Parents who excessively impose their own choices, values, and life plans on their children may violate this right. For example, parents who decide to have a son castrated in order to make sure that he becomes a good singer close off many choices and plans that he could have made as an adult, e.g., having children through natural means. The right to an open future is by no means an unusual or esoteric right, since almost all children have the interests that this right protects, e.g., freedom of choice, freedom of opportunity, etc. But even if we admit this much, does it follow that GLGT or GLGE constitute an inherent violation of this right? I don't think so. While some uses of genetic technology could be regarded as an overbearing imposition of parental values on children, other uses of GLGT and GLGE may augment a child's right to an open future. If parents use GLGE to enhance a child's immune system, then they could be increasing his opportunities to an open future by helping him fight diseases, which can limit opportunities. On the other hand, parents who attempt to produce an eight-foot-tall child in order to make her into a basketball player probably are violating her right to an open future by imposing their choices on her life.

However, there is not a sharp distinction between violating a child's right to an open future and being a responsible parent.[68] We readily accept the idea that parents should try to raise children who are healthy, intelligent, responsible, and happy, and we endorse various parental attempts to promote these values, such as private education, athletics, SAT preparation, and so on. Parents that act in the best interests of the children and have hope for their future are simply being good parents. But when does this healthy and responsible concern for a child's future interfere with the child's right to choose his own values and life plans? This is not an easy question to answer. In any case, this quandary supports my claim that GLGT and

GLGE do not inherently violate a child's right to an open future. Some uses of these technologies might have this effect; others might not. The upshot of this section is that we have once again debunked several arguments that might be construed as proving that genetic enhancement is inherently wrong. It may be wrong under some circumstances, but not in others.

Eugenics

Some have attacked GLGT and GLGE on the grounds that they constitute a form of eugenics, an attempt to control the human gene pool.[69] Is eugenics inherently wrong? To understand this question, we can distinguish between positive and negative eugenics: positive eugenics attempts to increase the number of favorable or desirable genes in the human gene pool, while negative eugenics attempts to reduce the number of undesirable or harmful genes, e.g., genes that cause genetic diseases. We should also distinguish between state-sponsored and parental eugenics: under state-sponsored eugenics programs the government attempts to control the human gene pool; in parental eugenics parents exert control over the gene pool through their reproductive choices.[70]

Parental eugenics occurs every time people select mates or sperm or egg donors. Most people do not find this kind of eugenics to be as troubling as the state-sponsored eugenics programs envisioned by Aldous Huxley or implemented by Nazi Germany. Indeed, one might argue that this kind of eugenics is a morally acceptable exercise of parental rights.[71] Moreover, most parents do not make their reproductive choices with the sole aim of controlling the human gene pool; any effects these choices have on the gene pool are unintended consequences of parental actions. As long as we accept the idea that parents should be allowed to make some choices that affect the composition of the human gene pool, then parental eugenics is not inherently wrong.

But what about state-sponsored eugenics? One might argue that state-sponsored eugenics programs, such as involuntary sterilization of the mentally

disabled or mandatory genetic screening, are morally wrong because they:

a. constitute unjustifiable violations of individual liberty and privacy;
b. are a form of genetic discrimination;
c. can have adverse evolutionary consequences by reducing genetic diversity; and
d. can lead us down a slippery slope toward increased racial and ethnic hatred, bias, and genocide.

Although these arguments do not prove that all forms of state-sponsored eugenics are morally wrong, they place a strong burden of proof on those who defend these programs. It is not my aim to explore state-sponsored eugenics in depth here.[72] However, even if we assume that state-sponsored eugenics is inherently wrong, this still only proves that some forms of GLGE or GLGT are inherently wrong. There is nothing inherently wrong with parental choices to use GLGE or GLGT to help children achieve health, freedom, and other values. Thus arguments that appeal to our concerns about eugenics do not prove that genetic enhancement is inherently wrong. Some forms of genetic enhancement, e.g., state-sponsored eugenics, are wrong, others are not.

Conclusion: The Significance of the Distinction

Two decades ago, James Rachels challenged the moral significance of the active–passive euthanasia distinction in a widely anthologized essay.[73] This paper has attempted to perform a similar debunking of the therapy–enhancement distinction in human genetics. It has considered and rejected a variety of different ways of arguing that the therapy–enhancement distinction in human genetics marks a solid, moral boundary. Genetic enhancement is not inherently immoral nor is genetic therapy inherently moral. Some forms of enhancement are immoral, others are not; likewise, some types of therapy are immoral, others are not. The implication of this view is that we should not use the therapy–enhancement distinction as our moral compass in human genetics. In evaluating the ethical aspects of any particular genetic intervention, we should ask not whether it is therapy or enhancement but whether the intervention poses significant risks, offers significant benefits, violates or promotes human dignity, is just or unjust, and so on.

Having said this much, I think some forms of enhancement can be morally justified, provided that they can be shown to be safe and effective. For example, using genetic technology to protect people against diseases could be justified on the grounds that it benefits patients. I think one can even justify the use of genetics for cosmetic purposes in terms of benefits to patients. We can also view some forms of genetic therapy as unacceptable (at present) because they pose unjustifiable risks to patients or future generations. For example, all forms of GLGT and some types of SGT, such as a procedure for fighting cancer at the genetic level, are too risky, given our current scientific and technical limitations. In any case, the moral assessment of these procedures depends on considerations of probable benefits and harms (as well as other moral qualities), not on their classification as "therapy" or "enhancement."

So what is the significance of the therapy–enhancement distinction? What role should it play in thinking about the ethics of human genetics? Can it guide public policy? The most I can say in favor of the distinction is that it defines moral zones without any sharp boundaries. The significance of the distinction may lie in its ability to address our fears and hopes: we hope that genetic therapy will help us treat diseases and improve human health, but we fear that genetic enhancement will lead us down a slippery slope toward a variety of undesirable consequences, such as discrimination, bias, eugenics, injustice, biomedical harms, and so on.[74] Genetic enhancement will probably always dwell in the shadow of the slippery slope argument, while genetic therapy will probably always bask in the glory of modern medicine. Our hopes and fears may or may not be warranted; only time will tell. In the meantime, even if the therapy–enhancement distinction does not draw any solid moral boundaries, we need to be aware of the distinction in public dialogues about genetics. In these dialogues, it may be useful to address the fears of enhancement and the hopes of therapy while attempting to grapple with the realities of the genetic revolution.

Notes

1 Juengst E. Can enhancement be distinguished from prevention in genetic medicine? *Journal of Medicine and Philosophy* 1997; 22: 125–42.

2 Holtug N. Altering humans – the case for and against human gene therapy. *Cambridge Quarterly of Healthcare Ethics* 1997; 6: 157–74.

3 Berger E., and Gert B. Genetic disorders and the ethical status of germ-line gene therapy. *Journal of Medicine and Philosophy* 1991; 16: 667–83.

4 Anderson W. Human gene therapy: scientific and ethical considerations. *Journal of Medicine and Philosophy* 1985; 10: 275–91.

5 Anderson W. Human gene therapy: why draw a line? *Journal of Medicine and Philosophy* 1989; 14: 81–93.

6 Anderson W. Genetics and human malleability. *Hastings Center Report* 1990; 20(1): 21–4.

7 McGee G. *The Perfect Baby*. Lanham, MD: Rowman and Littlefield, 1997.

8 Vogel G. Genetic enhancement: from science fiction to ethics quandary. *Science* 1997; 277: 1753–4.

9 See note 4, Anderson 1985.

10 Fowler G, Juengst E, and Zimmerman B. Germ-line gene therapy and the clinical ethos of medical genetics. *Theoretical Medicine* 1989; 19: 151–7.

11 See note 3, Berger and Gert 1991.

12 Zimmerman B. Human germ-line gene therapy: the case for its development and use. *Journal of Medicine and Philosophy* 1991; 16: 593–612.

13 Glover J. *What Sort of People Should There Be?* New York: Penguin Books, 1984.

14 See note 7, McGee 1997.

15 Resnik D. Debunking the slippery slope argument against human germ line gene therapy. *Journal of Medicine and Philosophy* 1993; 19: 23–40.

16 Resnik D. Genetic engineering and social justice: a Rawlsian approach. *Social Theory and Practice* 1997; 23(3): 427–48.

17   See note 3, Berger and Gert 1991.

18   See note 4, Anderson 1985.

19   See note 6, Anderson 1990.

20   Rifkin J. *Algeny*. New York: Viking Press, 1983.

21   Ramsey P. *Fabricated Man: The Ethics of Genetic Control*. New Haven: Yale University Press, 1970.

22   It is not my aim in this essay to argue that there is no distinction between therapy and enhancement; I am only attempting to question the moral significance of the distinction. If it turns out that there is not a tenable distinction between therapy and enhancement, so much the worse for the moral significance of this distinction. For the purpose of this essay I will define "enhancement" as a medical intervention that has goals other than therapeutic ones. There may be many types of enhancement on this view. Some forms of enhancement, such as a circumcision, can have therapeutic aims as well, e.g., preventing urinary tract infections. Some forms of therapy, such as heart transplantation, could have enhancement effects, e.g., a person could acquire an above average heart. Some interventions, such as preventative medicine, could straddle the line between enhancement and therapy. For further discussion, see note 1, Juengst 1997.

23   See note 4, Anderson 1985.

24   Suzuki D and Knudtson P. *Genethics*. Cambridge, Mass: Harvard University Press, 1989.

25   Resnik D, Langer P, and Steinkraus H. *Human Germline Gene Therapy: Scientific, Ethical, and Political Issues*. Austin, Texas: RG Landes, 1999.

26   See note 24, Suzuki and Knudtson 1989.

27   See note 5, Anderson 1989.

28   See note 6, Anderson 1990.

29   Baird P. Altering human genes: social, ethical, and legal implications. *Perspectives in Biology and Medicine* 1994; 37: 566–75.

30   In the current debate in bioethics, several writers have attempted to use the concepts of health and disease to distinguish between genetic therapy and genetic enhancement.

31   See note 1, Juengst 1997.

32   See note 3, Berger and Gert 1991.

33   See note 5, Anderson 1989.

34   See note 6, Anderson 1990: 24.

35   Caplan A. The concepts of health, illness, and disease. In: Veatch R, ed. *Medical Ethics*, 2nd ed. Sudbury, Mass: Jones and Bartlett, 1997: 57–74.

36   Khushf G. Expanding the horizon of reflection on health and disease. *Journal of Medicine and Philosophy* 1995; 1–4.

37   Some writers distinguish between relativist and nonrelativist accounts; some others distinguish between biological and social accounts. But the basic insight is the same: the concepts of health and disease are normative or descriptive.

38   Boorse C. Health as a theoretical concept. *Philosophy of Science* 1977; 44: 542–73.

39   Daniels N. *Just Health Care*. Cambridge: Cambridge University Press, 1985.

40   Sigerist H. *Civilization and Disease*. Chicago: University of Chicago Press, 1943.

41   Pellegrino E.D., and Thomasma D.C. *For the Patient's Good*. New York: Oxford University Press, 1988.

42   For an overview of the normative approach, see Caplan A. *Moral Matters*. New York: John Wiley and Sons, 1995.

43   Culver C. and Gert B. *Philosophy in Medicine*. New York: Oxford University Press, 1982.

44   Lennox J. Health as an objective value. *Journal of Medicine and Philosophy* 1995; 20: 501–11.

45   See note 44, Lennox 1995.

46   Culver K. The current status of gene therapy research. *The Genetic Resource* 1993; 7: 5–10.

47   See note 25, Resnik, Langer, and Steinkraus 1999.

48   English J. Abortion and the concept of a person. *Canadian Journal of Philosophy* 1975; 5(2): 233–43.

49   It is possible to define "human" in such a way that it is logically impossible to change our humanness. If we stipulate that possession of a single property is a necessary and sufficient condition for being human, then any changes we make in that property would result in people that are not human. For example, we can define "triangle" = "three-sided object." If we make an object that has four sides, it is not an altered triangle; it is not a triangle at all. For a definition of humanness that would seem to imply that it is difficult (though not impossible) to alter our humanness, see Anderson W. Genetic engineering and our humanness. *Human Gene Therapy* 1994; 5: 755–60.

50   See note 25, Resnik, Langer, and Steinkraus 1999.

51   For the purposes of this essay, I will not attribute this view to any particular author, since I think it deserves consideration on its own merit. For writers who come close to defending this view, see note 8, Vogel 1997, as well as Kass L. *Toward a More Natural Science*. New York: Free Press, 1985.

52   See note 20, Rifkin 1983.

53   These arguments do not address genetic enhancement per se, since they also apply to GLGT and they do not apply to SGT or SGE.

54 See note 25, Resnik, Langer, and Steinkraus 1999.

55 See note 21, Ramsey 1970.

56 Cole-Turner R. Genes, religion, and society: the developing views of the churches. *Science and Engineering Ethics* 1997; 3(3): 273–88.

57 National Council of Churches. *Human Life and the New Genetics*. New York: National Council of Churches of Christ in the USA, 1980.

58 National Council of Churches. *Genetic Engineering: Social and Ethical Consequences*. New York: National Council of Churches of Christ in the U.S.A., 1983.

59 Peters T. *Playing God?: Genetic Determinism and Human Freedom*. New York: Routledge, 1997.

60 For further discussion see Buchanan A, Brock D. *Deciding for Others*. Cambridge: Cambridge University Press, 1989.

61 Lappé M. Ethical issues in manipulating the human germ line. *Journal of Medicine and Philosophy* 1991; 16:621–39.

62 Commission of the European Community. *Adopting a Specific Research and Technological Development Programme in the Field of Health*. Brussels: Commission of the European Community, 1989.

63 Davis D. Genetic dilemmas and the child's right to an open future. *Hastings Center Report* 1997; 27(2): 7–15.

64 These arguments do not constitute an objection to SGT or SGE.

65 See note 25, Resnik, Langer, and Steinkraus 1999.

66 Feinberg J. *Social Philosophy*. Englewood Cliffs, NJ: Prentice-Hall, 1973.

67 Feinberg J. The child's right to an open future. In: Aiken W. and Lafollette H. eds. *Whose Child? Children's Rights, Parental Authority, and State Power*. Totowa, NJ: Littlefield, Adam, 1980: 124–53.

68 See note 7, McGee 1997.

69 For further discussion of eugenics, see Paul D. *Controlling Human Heredity: 1865 to the Present*. Atlantic Highlands, N.J.: Humanities Press International, 1995.

70 Kitcher P. *The Lives to Come*. New York: Simon and Schuster, 1997.

71 Robertson J. *Children of Choice*. Princeton, N.J.: Princeton University Press, 1994.

72 For further discussion, see Parens E. Taking behavioral genetics seriously. *Hastings Center Report* 1996; 26(4): 13–18.

73 Rachels J. Active and passive euthanasia. *New England Journal of Medicine* 1975; 292(2): 78–80.

74 See note 15, Resnik 1993.

15

In Defense of Posthuman Dignity

Nick Bostrom

Transhumanists vs. Bioconservatives

Transhumanism is a loosely defined movement that has developed gradually over the past two decades, and can be viewed as an outgrowth of secular humanism and the Enlightenment. It holds that current human nature is improvable through the use of applied science and other rational methods, which may make it possible to increase human health-span, extend our intellectual and physical capacities, and give us increased control over our own mental states and moods.[1] Technologies of concern include not only current ones, like genetic engineering and information technology, but also anticipated future developments such as fully immersive virtual reality, machine-phase nanotechnology, and artificial intelligence.

Transhumanists promote the view that human enhancement technologies should be made widely available, and that individuals should have broad discretion over which of these technologies to apply to themselves (morphological freedom), and that parents should normally get to decide which reproductive technologies to use when having children (reproductive freedom).[2] Transhumanists believe that, while there are hazards that need to be identified and avoided, human enhancement technologies will offer enormous potential for deeply valuable and humanly beneficial uses. Ultimately, it is possible that such enhancements may make us, or our descendants, 'posthuman', beings who may have indefinite health-spans, much greater intellectual faculties than any current human being – and perhaps entirely new sensibilities or modalities – as well as the ability to control their own emotions. The wisest approach *vis-à-vis* these prospects, argue transhumanists, is to embrace technological progress, while strongly defending human rights and individual choice, and taking action specifically against concrete threats, such as military or terrorist abuse of bioweapons, and against unwanted environmental or social side-effects.

In opposition to this transhumanist view stands a bioconservative camp that argues against the use of technology to modify human nature. Prominent bioconservative writers include Leon Kass, Francis Fukuyama, George Annas, Wesley Smith, Jeremy

Original publication details: Nick Bostrom, "In Defense of Posthuman Dignity," pp. 202–214 from *Bioethics* 19: 3 (2005). Reproduced with permission of John Wiley & Sons.

Rifkin, and Bill McKibben. One of the central concerns of the bioconservatives is that human enhancement technologies might be 'dehumanizing'. The worry, which has been variously expressed, is that these technologies might undermine our human dignity or inadvertently erode something that is deeply valuable about being human but that is difficult to put into words or to factor into a cost-benefit analysis. In some cases (for example, Leon Kass) the unease seems to derive from religious or crypto-religious sentiments, whereas for others (for example, Francis Fukuyama) it stems from secular grounds. The best approach, these bioconservatives argue, is to implement global bans on swathes of promising human enhancement technologies to forestall a slide down a slippery slope towards an ultimately debased, posthuman state.

While any brief description necessarily skirts significant nuances that differentiate between the writers within the two camps, I believe the above characterization nevertheless highlights a principal fault line in one of the great debates of our times: how we should look at the future of humankind and whether we should attempt to use technology to make ourselves 'more than human'. This paper will distinguish two common fears about the posthuman and argue that they are partly unfounded and that, to the extent that they correspond to real risks, there are better responses than trying to implement broad bans on technology. I will make some remarks on the concept of dignity, which bioconservatives believe to be imperiled by coming human enhancement technologies, and suggest that we need to recognize that not only humans in their current form, but posthumans too could have dignity.

Two Fears about the Posthuman

The prospect of posthumanity is feared for at least two reasons. One is that the state of being posthuman might in itself be degrading, so that by becoming posthuman we might be harming ourselves. Another is that posthumans might pose a threat to 'ordinary' humans. (I shall set aside a third possible reason, that the development of posthumans might offend some supernatural being.)

The most prominent bioethicist to focus on the first fear is Leon Kass:

> Most of the given bestowals of nature have their given species-specified natures: they are each and all of a given *sort*. Cockroaches and humans are equally bestowed but differently natured. To turn a man into a cockroach – as we don't need Kafka to show us – would be dehumanizing. To try to turn a man into more than a man might be so as well. We need more than generalized appreciation for nature's gifts. We need a particular regard and respect for the special gift that is our own given nature . . .[3]

Transhumanists counter that nature's gifts are sometimes poisoned and should not always be accepted. Cancer, malaria, dementia, aging, starvation, unnecessary suffering, and cognitive shortcomings are all among the presents that we would wisely refuse. Our own species-specified natures are a rich source of much of the thoroughly unrespectable and unacceptable – susceptibility for disease, murder, rape, genocide, cheating, torture, racism. The horrors of nature in general, and of our own nature in particular, are so well documented[4] that it is astonishing that somebody as distinguished as Leon Kass should still in this day and age be tempted to rely on the natural as a guide as to what is desirable or normatively right. We should be grateful that our ancestors were not swept away by the Kassian sentiment, or we would still be picking lice off each other's backs. Rather than deferring to the natural order, transhumanists maintain that we can legitimately reform ourselves and our natures in accordance with humane values and personal aspirations.

If one rejects nature as a general criterion of the good, as most thoughtful people nowadays do, one can of course still acknowledge that particular ways of modifying human nature would be debasing. Not all change is progress. Not even all well-intentioned technological intervention in human nature would be on balance beneficial. Kass goes far beyond these truisms, however, when he declares that utter dehumanization lies in store for us as the inevitable result of our obtaining technical mastery over our own nature:

> The final technical conquest of his own nature would almost certainly leave mankind utterly enfeebled. This form of mastery would be identical with utter dehumanization. Read Huxley's *Brave New World*, read C. S. Lewis's *Abolition of Man*, read Nietzsche's account of the last man, and then read the newspapers. Homogenization, mediocrity, pacification, drug-induced contentment, debasement of taste, souls without loves and longings – these are the inevitable results of making the essence of human nature the last project of technical mastery. In his moment of triumph, Promethean man will become a contented cow.[5]

The fictional inhabitants of *Brave New World*, to pick the best known of Kass's examples, are admittedly short on dignity (in at least one sense of the word). But the claim that this is the *inevitable* consequence of our obtaining technological mastery over human nature is exceedingly pessimistic – and unsupported – if understood as a futuristic prediction, and false if construed as a claim about metaphysical necessity.

There are many things wrong with the fictional society that Huxley described. It is static, totalitarian, caste-bound; its culture is a wasteland. The brave new worlders themselves are a dehumanized and undignified lot. Yet posthumans they are not. Their capacities are not super-human but in many respects substantially inferior to our own. Their life expectancy and physique are quite normal, but their intellectual, emotional, moral, and spiritual faculties are stunted. The majority of the brave new worlders have various degrees of engineered mental retardation. And everyone, save the ten world controllers (along with a miscellany of primitives and social outcasts who are confined to fenced preservations or isolated islands), are barred or discouraged from developing individuality, independent thinking, and initiative, and are conditioned not to desire these traits in the first place. *Brave New World* is not a tale of human enhancement gone amok, but is rather a tragedy of technology and

social engineering being deliberately used to cripple moral and intellectual capacities – the exact antithesis of the transhumanist proposal.

Transhumanists argue that the best way to avoid a *Brave New World* is by vigorously defending morphological and reproductive freedoms against any would-be world controllers. History has shown the dangers in letting governments curtail these freedoms. The last century's government-sponsored coercive eugenics programs, once favored by both the left and the right, have been thoroughly discredited. Because people are likely to differ profoundly in their attitudes towards human enhancement technologies, it is crucial that no single solution be imposed on everyone from above, but that individuals get to consult their own consciences as to what is right for themselves and their families. Information, public debate, and education are the appropriate means by which to encourage others to make wise choices, not a global ban on a broad range of potentially beneficial medical and other enhancement options.

The second fear is that there might be an eruption of violence between unaugmented humans and posthumans. George Annas, Lori Andrews, and Rosario Isasi have argued that we should view human cloning and all inheritable genetic modifications as 'crimes against humanity' in order to reduce the probability that a posthuman species will arise, on grounds that such a species would pose an existential threat to the old human species:

> The new species, or 'posthuman,' will likely view the old 'normal' humans as inferior, even savages, and fit for slavery or slaughter. The normals, on the other hand, may see the posthumans as a threat and if they can, may engage in a preemptive strike by killing the posthumans before they themselves are killed or enslaved by them. It is ultimately this predictable potential for genocide that makes species-altering experiments potential weapons of mass destruction, and makes the unaccountable genetic engineer a potential bioterrorist.[6]

There is no denying that bioterrorism and unaccountable genetic engineers developing increasingly potent weapons of mass destruction pose a serious threat to our civilization. But using the rhetoric of bioterrorism and weapons of mass destruction to cast aspersions on therapeutic uses of biotechnology to improve health, longevity, and other human capacities is unhelpful. The issues are quite distinct. Reasonable people can be in favor of strict regulation of bioweapons, while promoting beneficial medical uses of genetics and other human enhancement technologies, including inheritable and 'species-altering' modifications.

Human society is always at risk of some group deciding to view another group of humans as being fit for slavery or slaughter. To counteract such tendencies, modern societies have created laws and institutions, and endowed them with powers of enforcement, that act to prevent groups of citizens from enslaving or slaughtering one another. The efficacy of these institutions does not depend on all citizens having equal capacities. Modern, peaceful societies can have large numbers of people with diminished physical or mental capacities along with many other people who may be exceptionally physically strong or healthy or intellectually talented in various ways. Adding people with technologically enhanced capacities to this already broad distribution of ability would not need to rip society apart or trigger genocide or enslavement.

The assumption that inheritable genetic modifications or other human enhancement technologies would lead to two distinct and separate species should also be questioned. It seems much more likely that there would be a continuum of differently modified or enhanced individuals, which would overlap with the continuum of as-yet unenhanced humans. The scenario in which 'the enhanced' form a pact and then attack 'the naturals' makes for exciting science fiction, but is not necessarily the most plausible outcome. Even today, the segment containing the tallest ninety percent of the population could, in principle, get together and kill or enslave the shorter decile. That this does not happen suggests that a well-organized society can hold together even if it contains many possible coalitions of people sharing some attribute

such that, if they ganged up, they would be capable of exterminating the rest.

To note that the extreme case of a war between humans and posthumans is not the most likely scenario is not to say that there are no legitimate social concerns about the steps that may take us closer to posthumanity. Inequity, discrimination, and stigmatization – against, or on behalf of, modified people – could become serious issues. Transhumanists would argue that these (potential) social problems call for social remedies. One example of how contemporary technology can change important aspects of someone's identity is sex reassignment. The experiences of transsexuals show that Western culture still has work to do in becoming more accepting of diversity. This is a task that we can begin to tackle today by fostering a climate of tolerance and acceptance towards those who are different from ourselves. Painting alarmist pictures of the threat from future technologically modified people, or hurling preemptive condemnations of their necessarily debased nature, is not the best way to go about it.

What about the hypothetical case in which someone intends to create, or turn themselves into, a being of such radically enhanced capacities that a single one or a small group of such individuals would be capable of taking over the planet? This is clearly not a situation that is likely to arise in the imminent future, but one can imagine that, perhaps in a few decades, the prospective creation of superintelligent machines could raise this kind of concern. The would-be creator of a new life form with such surpassing capabilities would have an obligation to ensure that the proposed being is free from psychopathic tendencies and, more generally, that it has humane inclinations. For example, a future artificial intelligence programmer should be required to make a strong case that launching a purportedly human-friendly superintelligence would be safer than the alternative. Again, however, this (currently) science fiction scenario must be clearly distinguished from our present situation and our more immediate concern with taking effective steps towards incrementally improving human capacities and health-span.

Is Human Dignity Incompatible with Posthuman Dignity?

Human dignity is sometimes invoked as a polemical substitute for clear ideas. This is not to say that there are no important moral issues relating to dignity, but it does mean that there is a need to define what one has in mind when one uses the term. Here, we shall consider two different senses of dignity:

1. Dignity as moral status, in particular the inalienable right to be treated with a basic level of respect.
2. Dignity as the quality of being worthy or honorable; worthiness, worth, nobleness, excellence.[7]

On both these definitions, dignity is something that a posthuman could possess. Francis Fukuyama, however, seems to deny this and warns that giving up on the idea that dignity is unique to human beings – defined as those possessing a mysterious essential human quality he calls 'Factor X'[8] – would invite disaster:

> Denial of the concept of human dignity – that is, of the idea that there is something unique about the human race that entitles every member of the species to a higher moral status than the rest of the natural world – leads us down a very perilous path. We may be compelled ultimately to take this path, but we should do so only with our eyes open. Nietzsche is a much better guide to what lies down that road than the legions of bioethicists and casual academic Darwinians that today are prone to give us moral advice on this subject.[9]

What appears to worry Fukuyama is that introducing new kinds of enhanced person into the world might cause some individuals (perhaps infants, or the mentally handicapped, or unenhanced humans in general) to lose some of the moral status that they currently possess, and that a fundamental precondition of liberal democracy, the principle of equal dignity for all, would be destroyed.

The underlying intuition seems to be that instead of the famed 'expanding moral circle', what we have is more like an oval, whose shape we can change but whose area must remain constant. Thankfully, this purported conservation law of moral recognition lacks empirical support. The set of individuals accorded full moral status by Western societies has actually increased, to include men without property or noble descent, women, and non-white peoples. It would seem feasible to extend this set further to include future posthumans, or, for that matter, some of the higher primates or human–animal chimaeras, should such be created – and to do so without causing any compensating shrinkage in another direction. (The moral status of problematic borderline cases, such as foetuses or late-stage Alzheimer patients, or the brain-dead, should perhaps be decided separately from the issue of technologically modified humans or novel artificial life forms.) Our own role in this process need not be that of passive bystanders. We can work to create more inclusive social structures that accord appropriate moral recognition and legal rights to all who need them, be they male or female, black or white, flesh or silicon.

Dignity in the second sense, as referring to a special excellence or moral worthiness, is something that current human beings possess to widely differing degrees. Some excel far more than others do. Some are morally admirable; others are base and vicious. There is no reason for supposing that posthuman beings could not also have dignity in this second sense. They may even be able to attain higher levels of moral and other excellence than any of us humans. The fictional brave new worlders, who were subhuman rather than posthuman, would have scored low on this kind of dignity, and partly for that reason they would be awful role models for us to emulate. But surely we can create more uplifting and appealing visions of what we may aspire to become. There may be some who would transform themselves into degraded posthumans – but then some people today do not live very worthy human lives. This is regrettable, but the fact that some people make bad choices is not generally a sufficient ground for rescinding people's right to choose. And legitimate countermeasures are available: education, encouragement, persuasion, social and cultural reform. These, not a blanket prohibition of all posthuman ways of being, are the measures to which those bothered by the prospect of debased posthumans should resort. A liberal democracy should normally permit incursions into morphological and reproductive freedoms only in cases where somebody is abusing these freedoms to harm another person.

The principle that parents should have broad discretion to decide on genetic enhancements for their children has been attacked on the grounds that this form of reproductive freedom would constitute a kind of parental tyranny that would undermine the child's dignity and capacity for autonomous choice; for instance, by Hans Jonas:

> Technological mastered nature now again includes man who (up to now) had, in technology, set himself against it as its master . . . But whose power is this – and over whom or over what? Obviously the power of those living today over those coming after them, who will be the defenseless other side of prior choices made by the planners of today. The other side of the power of today is the future bondage of the living to the dead.[10]

Jonas is relying on the assumption that our descendants, who will presumably be far more technologically advanced than we are, would nevertheless be defenseless against our machinations to expand their capacities. This is almost certainly incorrect. If, for some inscrutable reason, they decided that they would prefer to be less intelligent, less healthy, and lead shorter lives, they would not lack the means to achieve these objectives and frustrate our designs.

In any case, if the alternative to parental choice in determining the basic capacities of new people is entrusting the child's welfare to nature, that is blind chance, then the decision should be easy. Had Mother Nature been a real parent, she would have been in jail for child abuse and murder. And transhumanists can accept, of course, that just as society may in exceptional circumstances override parental autonomy, such as in cases of neglect or abuse, so too may society impose regulations to protect the child-to-be from genuinely harmful genetic interventions – but not because they represent choice rather than chance.

Jürgen Habermas, in a recent work, echoes Jonas' concern and worries that even the mere *knowledge* of having been intentionally made by another could have ruinous consequences:

> We cannot rule out that knowledge of one's own hereditary features as programmed may prove to restrict the choice of an individual's life, and to undermine the essentially symmetrical relations between free and equal human beings.[11]

A transhumanist could reply that it would be a mistake for an individual to believe that she has no choice over her own life just because some (or all) of her genes were selected by her parents. She would, in fact, have as much choice as if her genetic constitution had been selected by chance. It could even be that she would enjoy significantly *more* choice and autonomy in her life, if the modifications were such as to expand her basic capability set. Being healthy, smarter, having a wide range of talents, or possessing greater powers of self-control are blessings that tend to open more life paths than they block.

Even if there were a possibility that some genetically-modified individuals might fail to grasp these points and thus might feel oppressed by their knowledge of their origin, that would be a risk to be weighed against the risks incurred by having an unmodified genome, risks that can be extremely grave. If safe and effective alternatives were available, it would be irresponsible to risk starting someone off in life with the misfortune of congenitally diminished basic capacities or an elevated susceptibility to disease.

Why We Need Posthuman Dignity

Similarly ominous forecasts were made in the seventies about the severe psychological damage that children conceived through in vitro; fertilization would suffer upon learning that they originated from a test tube – a prediction that turned out to be entirely false. It is hard to avoid the impression that some bias or philosophical prejudice is responsible for the readiness with which many bioconservatives seize on even the flimsiest of empirical justifications for banning human enhancement technologies of certain types but not others. Suppose it turned out that playing Mozart to pregnant mothers improved the child's subsequent musical talent. Nobody would argue for a ban on Mozart-in-the-womb on grounds that we cannot rule out that some psychological woe might befall the child once she discovers that her facility with the violin had been prenatally 'programmed' by her parents. Yet when, for example, it comes to genetic enhancements, eminent bioconservative writers often put forward arguments that are not so very different from this parody as weighty, if not conclusive, objections. To transhumanists, this looks like doublethink. How can it be that to bioconservatives almost any anticipated downside, predicted perhaps on the basis of the shakiest pop-psychological theory, so readily achieves that status of deep philosophical insight and knockdown objection against the transhumanist project?

Perhaps a part of the answer can be found in the different attitudes that transhumanists and bioconservatives have towards posthuman dignity. Bioconservatives tend to deny posthuman dignity and view posthumanity as a threat to human dignity. They are therefore tempted to look for ways to denigrate interventions that are thought to be pointing in the direction of more radical future modifications that may eventually lead to the emergence of those detestable posthumans. But unless this fundamental opposition to the posthuman is openly declared as a premise of their argument, this then forces them to use a double standard of assessment whenever particular cases are considered in isolation: for example, one standard for germ-line genetic interventions and another for improvements in maternal nutrition (an intervention presumably not seen as heralding a posthuman era).

Transhumanists, by contrast, see human and posthuman dignity as compatible and complementary. They insist that dignity, in its modern sense, consists in what we are and what we have the potential to become, not in our pedigree or our causal origin. What we are is not a function solely of our DNA but also of our technological and social context. Human nature in this broader sense is dynamic, partially human-made, and improvable. Our current extended phenotypes (and the lives that we lead) are markedly different from those of our hunter-gatherer ancestors. We read and write, we wear clothes, we live in cities, we earn money and buy food from the supermarket, we call people on the telephone, watch television, read newspapers, drive cars, file taxes, vote in national elections, women give birth in hospitals, life-expectancy is three times longer than in the Pleistocene, we know that the Earth is round and that stars are large gas clouds lit from inside by nuclear fusion, and that the universe is approximately 13.7 billion years old and enormously big. In the eyes of a hunter-gatherer, we might already appear 'posthuman'. Yet these radical extensions of human capabilities – some of them biological, others external – have not divested us of moral status or dehumanized us in the sense of making us generally unworthy and base. Similarly, should we or our descendants one day succeed in becoming what relative to current standards we may refer to as posthuman, this need not entail a loss dignity either.

From the transhumanist standpoint, there is no need to behave as if there were a deep moral difference between technological and other means of enhancing human lives. By defending posthuman dignity we promote a more inclusive and humane ethics, one that will embrace future technologically modified people as well as humans of the contemporary kind. We also remove a distortive double standard from the field of our moral vision, allowing us to perceive more clearly the opportunities that exist for further human progress.[12]

Notes

1   N. Bostrom. 2003. The Transhumanist FAQ, v. 2.1. *World Transhumanist Association*.

2   N. Bostrom. Human Genetic Enhancements: A Transhumanist Perspective. *Journal of Value Inquiry*, Vol. 37, No. 4, pp. 493–506.

3   L. Kass. Ageless Bodies, Happy Souls: Biotechnology and the Pursuit of Perfection. *The New Atlantis* 2003; 1.

4   See e.g. J. Glover. 2001. *Humanity: A Moral History of the Twentieth Century*. New Haven. Yale University Press.

5   L. Kass. 2002. *Life, Liberty, and Defense of Dignity: The Challenge for Bioethics*. San Francisco. Encounter Books: p. 48.

6   G. Annas, L. Andrews and R. Isasi. Protecting the Endangered Human: Toward an International Treaty Prohibiting Cloning and Inheritable Alterations. *American Journal of Law and Medicine* 2002; 28, 2&3: p. 162.

7   J. A. Simpson and E. Weiner, eds. 1989. *The Oxford English Dictionary, 2nd ed*. Oxford. Oxford University Press.

8   F. Fukuyama. 2002. *Our Posthuman Future: Consequences of the Biotechnology Revolution*. New York. Farrar, Strauss and Giroux, p. 149.

9   Fukuyama, *Our Posthuman Future*, p. 160.

10 H. Jonas. 1985. *Technik, Medizin und Ethik: Zur Praxis des Prinzips Verantwortung*. Frankfurt am Main. Suhrkamp.

11 J. Habermas. 2003. *The Future of Human Nature*. Oxford. Blackwell, p. 23.

12 For their comments I am grateful to Heather Bradshaw, John Brooke, Aubrey de Grey, Robin Hanson, Matthew Liao, Julian Savulescu, Eliezer Yudkowsky, Nick Zangwill, and to the audiences at the Ian Ramsey Center seminar of June 6th in Oxford 2003, the Transvision 2003 conference at Yale, and the 2003 European Science Foundation Workshop on Science and Human Values, where earlier versions of this paper were presented, and to two anonymous referees.

16

Statement on NIH Funding of Research Using Gene-Editing Technologies in Human Embryos

Francis S. Collins

Genomic editing is an area of research seeking to modify genes of living organisms to improve our understanding of gene function and advance potential therapeutic applications to correct genetic abnormalities. Researchers in China have recently described their experiments in a nonviable human embryo to modify the gene responsible for a potentially fatal blood disorder using a gene-editing technology called CRISPR/Cas9.

Genomic editing is already widely studied in a variety of organisms. For example, CRISPR/Cas9 has greatly shortened the time it takes to produce knock-out mouse models of disease, enabling researchers to study more easily the underlying genetic causes of those diseases. This technology is also being used to develop the next generation of antimicrobials, which can specifically target harmful strains of bacteria and viruses. In the first clinical application of genomic editing, a related genome editing technique (using a zinc finger nuclease) was used to create HIV-1 resistance in human immune cells, bringing HIV viral load down to undetectable levels in at least one individual. All of these examples of research using genomic editing technologies can and are being funded by NIH [National Institutes of Health].

However, NIH will not fund any use of gene-editing technologies in human embryos. The concept of altering the human germline in embryos for clinical purposes has been debated over many years from many different perspectives, and has been viewed almost universally as a line that should not be crossed. Advances in technology have given us an elegant new way of carrying out genome editing, but the strong arguments against engaging in this activity remain. These include the serious and unquantifiable safety issues, ethical issues presented by altering the germline in a way that affects the next generation without their consent, and a current lack of compelling medical applications justifying the use of CRISPR/Cas9 in embryos.

Practically, there are multiple existing legislative and regulatory prohibitions against this kind of work. The Dickey-Wicker amendment prohibits the use of appropriated funds for the creation of human embryos for research purposes or for research in which human embryos are destroyed (H.R. 2880, Sec. 128).

Original publication details: Francis S. Collins, "Statement on NIH Funding of Research Using Gene-editing Technologies in Human Embryos," https://www.nih.gov/about-nih/who-we-are/nih-director/statements/statement-nih-funding-research-using-gene-editing-technologies-human-embryos. Public domain.

Furthermore, the NIH Guidelines state that the Recombinant DNA Advisory Committee, *". . .will not at present entertain proposals for germ line alteration"*. It is also important to note the role of the U.S. Food and Drug Administration (FDA) in this arena, which applies not only to federally funded research, but to any research in the U.S. The Public Health Service Act and the Federal Food, Drug, and Cosmetic Act give the FDA the authority to regulate cell and gene therapy products as biological products and/or drugs, which would include oversight of human germline modification. During development, biological products may be used in humans only if an investigational new drug application is in effect (21 CFR Part 312).

NIH will continue to support a wide range of innovations in biomedical research, but will do so in a fashion that reflects well-established scientific and ethical principles.

17

Genome Editing and Assisted Reproduction

Curing Embryos, Society or Prospective Parents?

Giulia Cavaliere

Introduction: Genetic Diseases, Genome Editing and Existing Alternatives

Different reproductive options are available for couples or individuals at risk of transmitting genetic diseases to their offspring who wish to have children. In this paper, I explore ethical and social questions raised by the use of genome editing into the context of assisted reproduction and, in particular, as a potential alternative to preimplantation genetic diagnosis (PGD).

Some of the reproductive options available to this group of individuals include refraining from having genetically related children and/or using technologies to reduce or avoid the risk of transmission. The first set of options includes adopting existing children or turning to third-party reproduction (i.e. relying on a gamete donor). Adoption is currently legal in many European countries, but eligibility criteria vary. For instance, in some countries, access to this practice is limited to married heterosexual couples (e.g. Italy),

while other countries have wider access criteria and allow same-sex couples (e.g. the Netherlands and the United Kingdom) and single parents (e.g. France and the United Kingdom) to adopt. In addition, other criteria such as marital status and age play a role in the decision to grant adoption.

Another possibility to avoid transmission of genetic diseases is for individuals to have partly genetically-related children and to seek gamete donors. This is commonly referred to as third-party reproduction, which allows couples to have children who are genetically related to a donor and to the unaffected individual in the couple. Third-party reproduction is currently only legal in some countries (e.g. the United Kingdom, the Netherlands and Spain) and usually restricted to heterosexual couples. Moreover, the state only subsidises IVF with donor gametes in a few countries (Gianaroli et al. 2016).

Alternatively, prospective parents at risk of transmitting genetic conditions to their offspring can seek to procreate with the aid of assisted reproductive technologies (ARTs) and preimplantation screening technologies (such as PGD), which would allow them

Original publication details: Giulia Cavaliere, "Genome Editing and Assisted Reproduction: Curing Embryos, Society or Prospective Parents, pp. 215–225 from *Medicine, Health Care and Philosophy* 21. Springer Nature / CC BY 4.0.

to have genetically related children free from the condition that affects them (or one of them). PGD allows the testing of embryos created with IVF for genetic abnormalities prior to their transfer in utero. This technology is currently legal in many European countries (Gianaroli et al. 2016), but in some countries it remains restricted to so-called 'serious' conditions (e.g. in Italy and Germany), and in others is completely banned (e.g. in Poland and Switzerland; Biondi 2013; Gianaroli et al. 2016). Across Europe, eligibility criteria vary. In the United Kingdom, for instance, the Human Fertilisation and Embryology Authority (HFEA) periodically revises and updates the lists of conditions that are eligible for screening with PGD. Other countries, such as Germany and Italy, recently approved the use of PGD, but access to this practice remains restricted to a very limited number of severe, early onset conditions (Biondi 2013; Gianaroli et al. 2016).

PGD and Assisted Reproduction

Where PGD is legal, it is typically used in cases where both prospective parents are carriers of an autosomal recessive mutation. These mutations are responsible for the occurrence of autosomal recessive monogenic diseases (i.e. diseases caused by a mutation in a single gene) such as cystic fibrosis and sickle cells anaemia.[1] When both prospective parents are carriers of such mutations, future offspring have a 1 in 4 chance of inheriting the mutated gene and developing an autosomal recessive disease, while they have a 1 in 2 chance of inheriting one abnormal gene and thus becoming healthy carriers. PGD allows the testing and selection of embryos created through IVF to transfer in utero those that are either free from the abnormal gene related to the prospective parents' condition (or that are carriers of such mutated gene when no mutation-free embryo is obtained). PGD is also effective in cases where one of the prospective parents is heterozygous for an autosomal dominant mutation, meaning that they carry two different variants of a gene. Autosomal dominant mutations are responsible for the occurrence of diseases such as Huntington's

and neurofibromatosis type 1. Future offspring have a 1 in 2 chance of developing autosomal dominant diseases even if only one of the prospective parents is affected, because it is possible that the embryo would carry the 'good' genetic variant from both parents. If the embryo inherited the disease-causing variant from only one parent, however, the resulting child would be affected by the disease.

It could be the case that none of the embryos created through IVF is free from the undesirable genetic mutation. For instance, when one of the prospective parents is homozygous for a dominant genetic disorder, the risk of transmission to offspring is as high as 100%, and hence no mutation-free embryos can be obtained. In addition, when prospective parents are both heterozygous for a dominant genetic disorder, the risk of transmission is as high as 75%, hence the chances of finding mutation-free embryos significantly low. Another case where PGD is not effective is when both parents are homozygous for a recessive genetic disorder, meaning that they both carry two variants of the disease-causing gene (Nuffield Council on Bioethics 2016; Vassena et al. 2016). In such cases, genome editing could represent an alternative to PGD and a new reproductive option for some prospective parents: mutations potentially leading to monogenic diseases would be corrected in embryos created with IVF prior to the transfer in utero or directly onto prospective parents' gametes prior to fertilisation. Lastly, gene editing could replace PGD for women at risk of transmitting mitochondrial diseases as mitochondrial DNA mutations present in oocytes[2] could be corrected in the embryo (Vassena et al. 2016).

In the following section, I briefly present the debate on genome editing technologies applied to human embryos and I show how these technologies could be used as an alternative to PGD for the aforementioned cases where PGD is not effective. In [the] "Assisted reproduction and PGD, or assisted reproduction and CRISPR?" section, I present the moral reasons in favour of and against introducing genome editing as an alternative to PGD. In particular, I present arguments in favour of using genome editing instead of, or as an alternative to, PGD, and argue that some of the moral arguments against PGD would not be applicable to genome editing. I conclude, ad interim, that such arguments offer a *prima facie* case in favour of introducing genome editing as a new reproductive option, given that safety concerns are thoroughly assessed. In [the] "Curing embryos, society or prospective parents?" section, I turn to other arguments on the ethics of introducing genome editing as a new reproductive option and argue that there are additional questions that need to be carefully addressed. I conclude that introducing genome editing in the context of assisted reproduction would have some benefits, but that concerns regarding the equality of access to assisted reproduction and the allocation of scarce resources should be addressed beforehand.

CRISPR and Assisted Reproduction

Gene-editing technologies have been around for over a decade. Zinc finger nucleases (ZFNs) and transcription activator-like effector nucleases (TALENs), two gene-editing technologies, were discovered in 2005 and 2010 respectively (Nuffield Council on Bioethics 2016). ZFNs and TALENS are relatively precise techniques, but have the disadvantage that they need engineered proteins to target specific sequences of the DNA, a procedure that requires time and resources (Nuffield Council on Bioethics 2016).

A new gene editing technique sparked debate early in 2015 due to its application on non-viable human embryos by a group of Chinese scientists (Baltimore et al. 2015; Lanphier and Urnov 2015). The technique in question is CRISPR/Cas9, an RNA-guided tool composed of two parts: clustered regularly interspaced short palindromic repeat (CRISPR) and CRISPR-associated protein 9 (Cas9). CRISPR/Cas9 makes use of a naturally occurring defence mechanism that bacteria use to avoid harmful infections caused by pathogenic organisms (e.g. viruses). The RNA tool (CRISPR) functions as a guide for the Cas proteins to target specific parts of the genome, which are

subsequently cut by the Cas proteins. These cut strands can be exploited to modify the nucleotide sequence of DNA and to insert genes at the cut site. The application of this technique to human embryos and human gametes (i.e. oocytes and sperm cells) has been widely criticised for a number of issues, but chiefly for its potential to introduce *inheritable changes* in the human genome (germline modification). Indeed, the issue of germline modification has catalysed the attention of many scientists and ethicists (Brokowski et al. 2015; Lander 2015; Lanphier and Urnov 2015).

This paper focuses on PGD and CRISPR[3] applications to the field of assisted reproduction. In particular, it focuses on CRISPR as a potential alternative to PGD. CRISPR could represent a tool to avoid the occurrence of genetic diseases in future children through the modification of the genetic makeup of embryos created with IVF from couples with a known risk of transmitting such genetic diseases. Since using CRISPR on early embryos could give to prospective parents who are either affected by monogenic diseases or who are carriers of them a chance to avoid the transmission of these diseases to their offspring, this particular application of CRISPR can be considered a new reproductive option for parents who want to have genetically related children.

Assisted Reproduction and PGD, or Assisted Reproduction and CRISPR?

Research on human embryos with CRISPR technology is still at an early stage and only [a] few experiments have been carried out thus far (Vassena et al. 2016). Despite this, the issue of allowing clinical research has been discussed recently (Gyngell et al. 2016; Vassena et al. 2016; Reyes and Lanner 2017). The two main precautionary reasons that have been advanced against clinical applications of genome editing on human embryos or gamete cells are concerns regarding introducing changes in the human germline and safety questions. Many scholars and members of the public consider germline modifications unethical and a "line that should not be crossed" (Collins 2015; for a discussion of this claim, see: Camporesi and Cavaliere 2016). The worry is that edited embryos will pass their edited genome on to future generations, thus introducing changes in humanity's gene pool. While it is of fundamental moral importance to consider the impact of present actions that could potentially have an impact on future generations, it seems reductive to limit these precautionary reflections to changes introduced with genome editing technologies on reproductive cells and embryos. In particular, those who worry about germline modifications via CRISPR and other genome editing technologies maintain that there is something exceptional in changes introduced *technologically* in our genomes via genome editing (and indirectly into the genomes of our offspring). The worry about germline modification encompasses a number of concerns, including the view that the human genome should be preserved intact as a "common heritage of our humanity" (cf. UNESCO statement against cloning, UNESCO 1997); the view that would be ethically problematic to change the germline of future generations "without their consent" (Collins 2015); and concerns regarding the safety of the technique not only for the child born thanks to its aid, but also for the child's children (more about this below and in [the] "Reproductive autonomy, child welfare and the interests of society" section). This first view misrepresents partially the natural history of humankind and how past and present humanly introduced innovations shape future generations (Buchanan 2011; Harris 1992). The introduction of agriculture, for instance, played a role not only in shaping our environment, but has fundamentally changed our genomes. The same could be said about technologies such as literacy and numeracy, which laid the foundations for technological innovations that have significantly changed us (Buchanan 2008, 2011). In other words, from a moral point of view, it seems irrelevant which *means* are used and whether inheritable changes are introduced with genome editing technologies or caused by other technological innovations, unless one is able to show the

moral exceptionality of using genome editing technologies (Harris 2010). In addition to this, focusing solely on technical means to introduce changes the human gene pool overlooks how other policies (such as those dealing with greenhouse gas mitigation), innovations (such as those in the field of agriculture) and human habits could have similar effects (i.e. introduce changes in the gene pool) with potentially much more serious consequences (Dupras et al. 2014). The view that emphasises the need to ask the consent of future generations, as argued by Harris (2016), fails to state how such consent could be obtained. Most procreative decisions affect future generations, but it is unclear how and why the consent of future offspring should be obtained prior to act (Harris 2016).

The other argument against allowing genome editing for clinical uses is concern for the safety of future offspring (and of this offspring's offspring). At this stage, safety is indeed an issue and the efficiency of genome editing on embryos remains low, with mosaic embryos (i.e. embryos that have abnormal numbers of chromosomes in certain cells resulting in genetically different cells coexisting in the same organism) being the main known drawback of these technologies (Vassena et al. 2016). Despite this, some studies have proven the feasibility of gene editing in animals (Heo et al. 2014; Shao et al. 2014; Yoshimi et al. 2014; Zou et al. 2015), even though the efficiency of genetically modifying zygotes with Cas9 ranges between 0.5 and 40% (Araki and Ishii 2014). In addition, a recent study demonstrated the feasibility of preventing the onset of a genetic disorder such as cataract development (Wu et al. 2013) and the injection of Cas9 into primate zygotes led to the birth of genetically modified offspring (Liu et al. 2014; Niu et al. 2014).

The Case for Genome Editing: Two Sets of Arguments

There are two sets of arguments for introducing CRISPR and other gene editing technologies into the clinic, provided that safety concerns are properly addressed. In this section I first outline the first group of arguments, which concerns the benefits of genome editing for future children (and their children too) and for prospective parents (Gyngell et al. 2016; Reyes and Lanner 2017). In the following section, I present additional reasons why genome editing could be a morally preferable alternative to PGD: genome editing would not be subjected to some of the critiques moved against PGD.

The moral reasons that ground the case for PGD (the welfare of future children and the reproductive autonomy of prospective parents; Pennings et al. 2007; Buchanan et al. 2001; Harris 1992) can be extended to defend the clinical use of genome editing in reproduction. It is widely accepted that reproductive autonomy and respect for parental discretion in reproduction are values worth defending[4] (Buchanan et al. 2001; Harris 1992; Robertson 1996). With respect to reproductive autonomy, genome editing would be comparatively better than PGD: it would offer an alternative to this technology for those aforementioned cases where PGD is not effective or for prospective parents who wish to increase their chances of having mutation-free embryos. In this sense, genome editing could be said to enhance reproductive autonomy. With respect to the welfare of the child, the case in favour of genome editing seems *prima facie* stronger than the case in favour of PGD. Unlike the latter technology, whereby embryos implanted can be carriers of the parents' mutated gene, genome editing would allow modification of the genetic makeup of embryos who would consequently develop into mutation-free offspring. In other words, genome editing would prevent the occurrence of genetic diseases in future generations, while PGD can sometimes only prevent the occurrence of genetic diseases in the child that develops from the implanted embryo (Gyngell et al. 2016).

There are, however, other arguments in favour of preferring genome editing to PGD. PGD is a contested practice as its scopes are not therapeutic (i.e. PGD does not *treat* embryos) but rather selective (i.e. PGD selects the embryos that should be transferred in utero. Asch and Barlevy 2012; Parens and Asch 2003). PGD as a means to select embryos that

have a decreased risk of developing into a child with a genetic condition is seen as ethically troubling for two reasons: firstly, because it goes against the traditional ends of medicine and 'selects out' rather than 'cures' persons affected by genetic conditions (MacKellar and Bechtel 2014), and secondly, because decisions on which embryos should be selected are said to embody value judgements regarding people living with certain disabilities (Knoppers et al. 2006; Parens and Asch 2003), a critique of screening technologies that became known as the 'expressivist argument' or 'expressivist objection' (Buchanan 1996; Shakespeare 2006).

Selection versus Therapy

PGD (at the moment) and CRISPR (potentially in the future) are two technologies that enable similar ends: in both cases, these technologies increase the chances of giving parents genetically related offspring unaffected by specific genetic conditions. Despite the similarity of the outcomes (i.e. healthy child), the means used are rather different. PGD is a form of genetic testing that allows screening for abnormalities in early embryos and to subsequently implant only those with a decreased risk of developing a certain condition. Instead, CRISPR and other gene editing technologies are tools for gene therapy that allow the modification of embryos or of gamete cells in order to avoid the occurrence of certain conditions in the future child (and in future generations).

Following this distinction of means, there is a sense that while PGD entails the *selection* of embryos, CRISPR is more akin to *therapy*. At this point, however, it is important to note that CRISPR and other genome editing technologies can be considered both therapeutic and non-strictly-therapeutic (or, following Wrigley et al. "pre-emptively therapeutic"; Wrigley et al. 2015, p. 636). I am not trying to violate Aristotle's principle of non-contradiction on the impossibility that contradictory assertions can be both true at the same time here. What I mean is rather that whether these technologies are therapeutic depends on what sort of factual and moral considerations are taken into account. If the focus is on the prospective parents, then CRISPR can be considered therapeutic in some instances because it could be a solution (or a treatment?) for those couples who would not otherwise be able to conceive children that are related to them and that are free from the risk of developing (or have a decreased risk to develop) the condition that affects them.

If the focus is on the future children, we have two possible interpretations: following the view that equates embryos with persons, CRISPR *is* therapeutic because it treats the embryos (i.e. it treats persons), whereas PGD is selective because it selects in/out the embryos (i.e. it selects out persons). If, however, we are more inclined to think of embryos as beings with the *potential* to develop into persons (i.e. potentiality view, arguably a more widely shared position), then CRISPR is not straightforwardly therapeutic, because there is no person to be treated at the moment that we use the technology.[5] Despite this remark, I argue that there is a sense whereby genome editing can still be considered therapeutic, or, as mentioned above, pre-emptively therapeutic. In order to assess whether CRISPR can be considered pre-emptively therapeutic, it is necessary to determine whether embryo X (i.e. the embryo that exists prior to the application of CRISPR) is identical to newborn X+ about 9 months (i.e. the child that is born after the application of CRISPR on embryo X). This assessment matters for the ethical debate on PGD and genome editing because if these two entities (embryo X and newborn X+ about 9 months) are identical, *then* PGD would be more problematic than CRISPR as the first would be a selective technology, whereas the second would be a therapeutic technology. A brief explanation of the question of identity is needed before proceeding with the discussion on PGD and CRISPR and the ethics thereof. Currently, ethicists and philosophers involved in the debate on reproductive genetic technologies seem to be divided on whether genome editing technologies applied to embryos are identity-affecting technologies or not, as this largely depends on the circumstances taken into account.[6] When I say "identity-affecting"

I refer to the idea of numerical identity and to the metaphysical problem of determining how we can rightly refer to one and the same person in any different set of circumstances, despite the changes that the person undergoes over time. Thus, for instance, there is numerical identity between a person X and a person Y only if person X and Y are the same person. To put it simply, I am numerically identical to the person that is writing this paper at the moment. The challenge of any account of numerical identity is then to explain what determines the entity that we in fact are despite the changes that we undergo over time. In this sense, if I grow taller or if I lose an eye due to an accident, I am still numerically identical to the entity I was before having that accident or when I was shorter. This is the case because changes such as losing an eye or growing taller are largely considered *contingent* to numerical identity, namely they do not change the entity that I am.

Returning to genome editing, those who do not subscribe to the embryos as persons view can view the technology in two different ways. The contentious matter is whether applying CRISPR on embryo X creates a numerically different entity (call it embryo Z, that will eventually develop into person Z) or it just leads to a numerically identical entity (call it embryo X⋆, that will eventually develop into person X⋆) in the same sense that applying gene therapy on adult X does not create a different adult Z, but only leads to a numerically identical adult X⋆. While in the first case genome editing would be considered an identity-affecting technology (i.e. a technology that by virtue of its use creates an entirely new entity), in the second case it would amount to a non-identity-affecting technology.[7] Following the first interpretation, CRISPR cannot be considered a therapy as, by virtue of its use on an embryo, it determines the kind of person that is brought into being rather than pre-emptively curing the same pre-person. On the contrary, if we are inclined to follow the second interpretation, then CRISPR is therapeutic as it pre-emptively cures an embryo that will develop into a numerically identical child that does not have the genetic condition that is consciously avoided.[8] It is only in this second sense that it is possible to say that if the genome of an embryo affected by a certain genetic condition is modified and this condition eradicated, then this embryo will develop into a numerically identical child who, had CRISPR not been used, would have been affected by a genetic disease. As a consequence, even if one does not subscribe to the embryo-as-persons view, *there is a sense* whereby genome editing can be considered at least *more similar* to therapy than to selection: genome editing would be a pre-emptive treatment for the genetic disease that is caused by the genetic mutation at the embryonic stage.

If the second interpretation about genome editing being non-identity-affecting is embraced, then both the teleological objection (i.e. PGD is morally problematic because it does not fall within the traditional ends of medicine) and the selective attitudes objection (i.e. PGD is morally problematic because it promotes selective and discriminatory attitudes) seem to be less applicable to the use of genome editing on embryos to prevent the occurrence of certain conditions in future children. As explained above, editing the genome of embryos can be considered pre-emptively therapeutic and thus falls within (or at least closer to) the traditional ends of medicine. From this, it also follows that it would be problematic to consider such practice as selective or discriminatory: disability scholars would have to condemn all the interventions aimed at treating genetic diseases (Barnes 2014).

These clarifications have normative implications, namely that, once the safety of editing the genome of human embryos is carefully assessed, the latter technology should be considered preferable to PGD. In the next section, I will outline some additional questions that need to be addressed and explain why preferring CRISPR over PGD is not completely cost-free.

Curing Embryos, Society or Prospective Parents?

In the previous sections, two main questions have remained unaddressed. One question is on the value and meaning of genetic parenthood. Another, albeit related, question concerns the ethics of existing alternatives. I explore these two questions in this last section and conclude that they provide at least some *prima facie* moral reasons for carefully considering the introduction of a new reproductive option when similar options are already available.

A peculiar feature of assisted reproductive technologies such as PGD, and possibly genome editing, is that they are often offered to prospective parents who are affected by a genetic condition in order to conceive (or increase their chances of conceiving) healthy offspring. It is in this sense that these technologies represent a *solution* for those prospective parents whose *problem* is the impossibility of having a *genetically related* and *healthy* child; or at least healthier than the child that would otherwise be brought into the world had these technologies not be employed. As explained in the first section of this paper, there are other options than PGD to increase the chances of having healthy children, but they entail refraining from having genetically related children (for one individual in the couple or, in the case of adoption, both parties). Reproductive technologies such as PGD and genome editing convey the interests of different groups: the prospective parents, the future offspring and the society where these offspring will grow and thrive. Despite the importance of all three stakeholders, their interests are not granted equal importance: the welfare of future children and the reproductive autonomy of the prospective parents are usually considered of greater moral importance than the aggregate interests of society in having healthy members, respecting competing values on assisted reproduction, and limiting the use of certain technologies against a backdrop of scarce resources. This is what I define as the received view on the ethics of assisted reproductive technologies. An ethical assessment of whether introducing new technologies in the context of reproduction should thus consider these three aspects (with the aforementioned prioritisation in mind) in turn.

Reproductive autonomy, child welfare and the interests of society

Genome editing, at first sight, seems to score high on the reproductive autonomy and welfare of the child fronts: unlike PGD, it allows for more conditions to be corrected and the reduction of the occurrence of certain genetic conditions in future generations; it also increases the reproductive autonomy of the parents by offering not only one more possibility in the geneticists tool-box, but also by allowing those couples for whom PGD is not always successful to have biologically related, healthy offspring. So far so good. Or maybe not? The idea that more choice leads to greater freedom has been challenged (Dworkin 1982; Rose 1999; Rothman 1985). More options can also translate into more uncertainties, and greater perceived and actual responsibilities for the prospective parents (Dworkin 1982). In this sense, introducing genome editing into the clinic as an alternative to PGD may be detrimental for the very same prospective parents that it is designed for. While genome editing may be more routinely employed in the future, some issues will likely remain. These issues include, for instance, reflections upon which conditions should be eligible for the use of genome editing and whether parents who fail to employ the most efficient technology available could be considered morally responsible (Rothman 1985).

What about the welfare of the future child? The empirical question of whether safety concerns will be put to rest and genome editing will ever be *safe enough* to represent a concrete alternative to PGD divides scholars (Harris 2016). The reasons for this are twofold: first, no one knows the answer to such questions *yet*. Secondly, this empirical question is strongly influenced by the value judgements of scientists, ethicists, policy-makers and the public on the degree of certainty required to move forward. Hence, even without denying that such empirical questions will be eventually be put to rest, it is still important to note that a consensus on the question of safety will be hard to reach due to the competing values at stake in stakeholders' assessments. Those taking a precautionary

stance concerning technological development will favour existing technologies over the newly discovered, while those who are generally in favour of technological development will be ready to accept a higher degree of risk in the name of such progress and of the potential benefits that it may yield. With respect to the safety and the welfare of the future child, whether genome editing really represents a better option than PGD will thus divide scholars, scientists and the public (and, as exemplified by the debate on embryo-applications of CRISPR, already does). A decision on whether to allow genome editing will thus have to rest not only on a thorough assessment of the safety of the techniques, but also on a democratic process that takes into account such differing views and values (Cavaliere 2017; Jasanoff et al. 2015; Kitcher 2001). The ethical assessment of new techniques ought to not only rest on a cost/benefit analysis, but also on an evaluation of existing alternatives, including those that do not rely on biomedical means. In other words, whether genome editing really represents a worthy alternative to existing options (such as PGD) depends on the extent to which the welfare of the future child can be put at risk to allow couples to have a genetically related child. Regulators and ethicists that argue in favour of eventually replacing PGD with genome editing, and couples for whom PGD does not represent an option, will have to consider whether reproductive autonomy should trump questions on the welfare of the child in light of uncertainty.

Lastly, what role should societal interests and views play in the decision over whether genome editing should replace PGD? There are different ways in which assisted reproductive technologies and procreative decisions more generally impinge on society. Procreative decisions influence the *type* and the *number* of people that will be created. They allow new consumers, producers, workers, mothers, fathers, etc. to come into existence. We live in an increasingly interlinked world and the aggregate effects of individual decisions affect a wider range of people than ever before (Singer 2004). There are historical reasons why third parties' interventions in procreation are looked at with suspicion, and the shadow of eugenics seems to extend over any discussion regarding reproductive technologies and their governance (Paul 1992). Despite these worries, the regulation of new reproductive technologies will be influenced by governments' policies, which in turn will reflect the interests of society and societal views on emerging reproductive technologies. Regarding the governance of genome editing technologies and their potential use in the context of assisted reproduction, the interests of society might play a role in two main ways: the first is whether genome editing is ethically acceptable for a large segment of society (Kitcher 2001), and second, related, is whether existing alternatives warrant the introduction of a new practice and the clinical research necessary to safely implement it. Almost every new technology introduced or discussed for potential introduction in reproduction seems to stir controversies. The recent debates on genome editing (Camporesi and Cavaliere 2016), mitochondrial replacement techniques (Appleby 2015) and 'older' debates on PGD (Scott 2006) are just a few instances of these controversies. However, once certain uses are constrained and lines drawn (for instance between therapeutic and enhancing uses), these technologies have been approved and, at least in certain countries, accepted by large swaths of the population. Thus, even if genome editing will be met with controversies and will encounter resistance, it does not *prima facie* translate into the need for banning any research involving it. On the contrary, this should translate into support for a democratic and deliberative approach to the governance of technological innovation (Jasanoff et al. 2015) and into the respecting of competing moral views on these issues (Cavaliere 2017).

Societal interests and the costs of introducing genome editing in the context of assisted reproduction

At this point, there is, however, there is one last thing to consider, which concerns the aforementioned interests of society and how they should and could play a role

in the ethical assessment of introducing genome editing in the context of assisted reproduction. While it is true that genome editing could open up new reproductive possibilities for certain couples (i.e. enhance reproductive autonomy) and provide heritable benefits to their future offspring (i.e. considerations regarding the welfare of future child), these benefits ought to be balanced against the costs of introducing a new reproductive technology. These costs include the investment of public resources, considering both the scarcity of such resources and the existence of available alternatives. Emanuel et al. (2000) argue that for clinical research to be ethical, among other requirements, it needs to have social value, namely it should be directed at "a diagnostic and therapeutic intervention that could lead to improvements in health and well-being" (Emanuel et al. 2000). Being of social value is an ethical requirement for clinical research to go forward precisely because it operates in a context of scarce resources. From this it follows that if the social value of a technology is limited, then the investment of public resources for the development and implementation of such technology may be unethical (Rulli 2016b). The proposed clinical research (in this case that needed in order to implement genome editing as an alternative to PGD) needs to be evaluated on two levels: absolute and relative. The absolute level is settled once the proposed research is expected to bring about improvements to health and well-being. The relative level, however, needs more: the proposed research (and the improvements to health and well-being thereof) needs to be compared both with other potential uses of those scarce resources and with existing alternatives to bring about similar improvements to health and well-being. Two of the criteria that are often employed to assess whether to invest resources in certain clinical research and whether it will bring about significant improvements to health and well-being are the severity of the condition and the number of individuals that it affects (Rulli 2016b). If we consider these two criteria, the benefits of the introduction of genome editing as a new reproductive option are arguably minor and thus may not warrant the investment of public resources. The number of cases for which PGD is not an option, as mentioned in the first section, is limited. In addition, considering the importance of taking into account future children's welfare, the unresolved questions concerning safety seem to indicate that health improvements may not be so significant. An obvious critique to this is the following: clinical research is aimed at improving techniques in order to achieve significant benefits for future children. This is certainly correct and we would not enjoy the benefits of many technologies and drugs if it was not for clinical research. But again: resources are limited and not all research can be publicly funded.

Returning to the relative level to evaluate clinical research, it is important to consider that improvements in the health and well-being of future children can also be achieved by looking at alternative solutions, for instance third party reproduction or adoption. For those limited number of parents for whom PGD is not an option, the choice is not between genome editing and a sick child. The choice is much wider than that. This does not mean that the choice of adopting or relying on third party reproduction comes without a cost, or that prospective parents' wishes should be neglected. It only means that there are other interests at stake and that there are other strategies than developing new technologies to tackle health needs.

These considerations do not lead to the conclusion that public interest (in the form of a prudent use of resources) should be prioritised over prospective parents' reproductive autonomy and future offspring's welfare. On the contrary, the received view, namely the view that considers the interests of these two groups as more morally relevant than those of society, ought to be taken as the default position. But this position should not prevent us from seeking alternatives. Perfecting existing technologies such as PGD, and possibly widening the criteria of access to adoption or third party reproduction, would be a less costly and possibly quicker strategy to grant future children's welfare while at the same time respecting prospective parents' wishes. Making existing technologies and practices available via broader state funding schemes would allow their use by larger swaths of the population.

Conclusions: Context Matters

In this article, I have analysed the moral case for introducing genome editing as an alternative to PGD. I have presented the reasons in favour and the two main arguments against this possibility, namely safety and germline modifications. After presenting some of the available data on the safety of CRISPR, I have argued that concerns with germline modifications do not represent a compelling argument against the introduction of genome editing into the clinic. I have then turned to arguments in favour of genome editing and concluded that there seems to be a *prima facie* case in favour of starting clinical research with CRISPR. In the last section, I have focused on the moral reasons that are normally taken into account in debates on reproductive technologies, namely the welfare of future children, the reproductive autonomy of the parents and the interests of society. I have showed that a closer look at genome editing in light of these moral reasons seems to generate some additional reasons for caution in accepting genome editing as a new reproductive option. These reasons may entail shifting from funding new resources, such as CRISPR, and advocating for its introduction in the name of values such as reproductive autonomy and the welfare of future children, to focusing on widening the criteria of access to existing options and possibly re-thinking resource allocation and state funding of assisted reproduction. This paper does not attempt to provide decisive arguments in favour of or against the introduction of CRISPR as a new reproductive option. As many have argued, it may be too soon to have a conclusive assessment of this possibility, if only for the dearth of empirical data regarding its safety and feasibility. Rather, this paper offers a basis to begin a discussion on the ethics of introducing genome editing as an alternative to PGD and stresses the need to consider that scientific research does not happen in a vacuum where the soundest theoretical argument wins. Rather, it happens in a context where resources are limited, where genetic parenthood is an important value cherished by many, and where technical solutions are often given preference over other strategies.

References

Appleby, John B. 2015. The ethical challenges of the clinical introduction of mitochondrial replacement techniques. *Medicine, Health Care and Philosophy* 18 (4): 501–14.

Araki, Motoko, and Tetsuya Ishii. 2014. International regulatory landscape and integration of corrective genome editing into in vitro; fertilization. *Reproductive Biology and Endocrinology* 12 (1): 1–12.

Asch, Adrienne, and Dorit Barlevy. 2012. Disability and genetics: A disability critique of pre-natal testing and pre-implantation genetic diagnosis (PGD). In *Encyclopaedia of life science, eLS*. Chichester: Wiley.

Baltimore, David, Paul Berg, Michael Botchan, Dana Carroll, R. Alta Charo, George Church, Jacob E. Corn, et al. 2015. A prudent path forward for genomic engineering and germline gene modification. *Science* 348 (6230): 36–8.

Barnes, Elizabeth. 2014. Valuing disability, causing disability. *Ethics* 125 (1): 88–113.

Biondi, Stefano. 2013. Access to medical-assisted reproduction and PGD in Italian law: A deadly blow to an illiberal statute? Commentary to the European Court on Human Rights's decision Costa and Pavan v Italy (ECtHR, 28 August 2012, App. 54270/2010). *Medical Law Review* 21 (3): 474–86.

Brokowski, Carolyn, Marya Pollack, and Robert Pollack. 2015. Cutting eugenics out of CRISPR-Cas9. *Ethics in Biology, Engineering and Medicine: An International Journal* 6 (3–4): 263–79.

Buchanan, Allen. 1996. Choosing who will be disabled: Genetic intervention and the morality of inclusion. *Social Philosophy and Policy* 13 (2): 18–46.

Buchanan, Allen. 2008. Enhancement and the ethics of development. *Kennedy Institute of Ethics Journal* 18 (1): 1–34.

Buchanan, Allen. 2011. *Beyond humanity?: The ethics of biomedical enhancement*. Oxford: Oxford University Press.

Buchanan, Allen, Dan W. Brock, Norman Daniels, and Daniel Wikler. 2001. *From chance to choice: Genetics and justice*. Cambridge: Cambridge University Press.

Camporesi, Silvia, and Giulia Cavaliere. 2016. Emerging ethical perspectives in the clustered regularly interspaced short palindromic repeats genome-editing debate. *Personalized Medicine* 13 (6): 575–586.

Cavaliere, Giulia. 2017. A 14-day limit for bioethics: The debate over human embryo research. *BMC Medical Ethics* 18 (1): 38.

Collins, Francis S. 2015. Statement on the NIH funding of research using gene-editing technologies in human embryos. National Institute of Health (NIH) http://www.nih.gov/about-nih/who-we-are/nih-director/statements/statement-nih-funding-research-using-gene-editing-technologies-human-embryos. Accessed 12 July 2017.

Dupras, Charles, Vardit Ravitsky, and Bryn Williams-Jones. 2014. Epigenetics and the environment in bioethics. *Bioethics* 28 (7): 327–34.

Dworkin, Gerald. 1982. Is more choice better than less? *Midwest Studies in Philosophy* 7 (1): 47–61.

Emanuel, Ezekiel J., David Wendler, and Christine Grady. 2000. What makes clinical research ethical? *JAMA* 283 (20): 2701–11.

Gianaroli, Luca, Anna Pia Ferraretti, Maria Cristina Magli, and Serena Sgargi. 2016. Current regulatory arrangements for assisted conception treatment in European countries. *European Journal of Obstetrics & Gynecology and Reproductive Biology* 207: 211–13.

Gyngell Christopher, Thomas, Douglas, and Julian, Savulescu. 2016. The ethics of germline gene editing. *Journal of Applied Philosophy* 34 (3): 1–16.

Harris, John. 1992. *Wonderwoman & superman: Ethics & human biotechnology*. Oxford: Oxford University Press.

Harris, John. 2010. *Enhancing evolution: The ethical case for making better people*. Princeton: Princeton University Press.

Harris, John. 2016. Germline modification and the burden of human existence. *Cambridge Quarterly of Healthcare Ethics* 25 (1): 6–18.

Heo, Young Tae, Xiaoyuan Quan, Yong Nan Xu, Soonbong Baek, Hwan Choi, Nam-Hyung Kim, and Jongpil Kim. 2014. CRISPR/Cas9 nuclease-mediated gene knock-in in bovine-induced pluripotent cells. *Stem Cells and Development* 24 (3): 393–402.

Hyun, Insoo, Amy Wilkerson, and Josephine Johnston. 2016. Embryology policy: Revisit the 14-day rule. *Nature* 533 (7602): 169–71.

Jasanoff, Sheila, J. Benjamin Hurlbut, and Krishanu Saha. 2015. CRISPR democracy: Gene editing and the need for inclusive deliberation. *Issues in Science and Technology* 32 (1): 37–49.

Kitcher, Philip. 2001. *Science, truth and democracy*. New York: Oxford University Press.

Knoppers, Bartha M., Sylvie Bordet, and Rosario M. Isasi. 2006. Preimplantation genetic diagnosis: An overview of socio-ethical and legal considerations. *Annual Review of Genomics and Human Genetics* 7: 201–21.

Lander, Eric S. 2015. Brave new genome. *New England Journal of Medicine* 373 (1): 5–8.

Lanphier, Edward, and Fyodor Urnov. 2015. Don't edit the human germ line. *Nature* 519 (7544): 410.

Liao, S. Matthew. 2017. Do mitochondrial replacement techniques affect qualitative or numerical identity? *Bioethics* 31 (1): 20–6.

Liu, Yunhong, Xiaoyan Lv, Ruizhi Tan, Tianming Liu, Tielin Chen, Mi Li, and Yuhang Liu, et al. 2014. A modified TALEN-based strategy for rapidly and efficiently generating knockout mice for kidney development studies. *PLoS ONE* 9 (1): e84893.

MacKellar, Calum, and Christopher Bechtel. 2014. *The ethics of the new eugenics*. New York: Berghahn Books.

McMahan, Jeff. 2006. Is prenatal genetic screening unjustly discriminatory? *Virtual Mentor* 8 (1): 50–2.

Niu, Jingwen, Bin Zhang, and Hu Chen. 2014. Applications of TALENs and CRISPR/Cas9 in human cells and their potentials for gene therapy. *Molecular Biotechnology* 56 (8): 681–8.

Nuffield Council on Bioethics. 2016. *Genome editing: An ethical review*. London: Nuffield Council on Bioethics.

Palacios-González, César. 2017. Are there moral differences between maternal spindle transfer and pronuclear transfer? Medicine, Health Care and Philosophy. doi:10.1007/s11019-017-9772-3.

Parens, Erik, and Adrienne Asch. 2003. Disability rights critique of prenatal genetic testing: Reflections and recommendations. *Mental Retardation and Developmental Disabilities Research Reviews* 9 (1): 40–7.

Parfit, Derek. 1984. *Reasons and persons*. Oxford: Oxford University Press.

Paul, Diane B. 1992. Eugenic anxieties, social realities, and political choices. *Social Research* 59 (3): 663–83.

Pennings, Guido, Guido de Wert, Francoise Shenfield, Jacques Cohen, Basil Tarlatzis, and Paul Devroey. 2007. ESHRE Task Force on Ethics and Law 13: The welfare of the child in medically assisted reproduction. *Human Reproduction* 22 (10): 2585–8.

Reyes, Alvaro P., and Fredrik Lanner. 2017. Towards a CRISPR view of early human development: Applications, limitations and ethical concerns of genome editing in human embryos. *Development* (Cambridge, England) 144 (1): 3–7.

Robertson, John A. 1996. *Children of choice: Freedom and the new reproductive technologies*. Princeton: Princeton University Press.

Rose, Nikolas. 1999. *Powers of freedom: Reframing political thought*. Cambridge: Cambridge University Press.

Rothman, Barbara Katz. 1985. The products of conception: The social context of reproductive choices. *Journal of medical ethics* 11 (4): 188–95.

Rulli, Tina. 2016a. The mitochondrial replacement 'therapy' myth. Bioethics. doi:10.1111/bioe.12332.

Rulli, Tina. 2016b. What is the value of three-parent IVF? *Hastings Center Report* 46 (4): 38–47.

Scott, Rosamund. 2006. Choosing between possible lives: Legal and ethical issues in preimplantation genetic diagnosis. *Oxford Journal of Legal Studies* 26 (1): 153–78.

Shakespeare, Tom. 2006. *Disability rights and wrongs*. New York: Routledge.

Shao, Yanjiao, Yuting Guan, Liren Wang, Zhongwei Qiu, Meizhen Liu, Yuting Chen, and Lijuan Wu, et al. 2014. CRISPR/Cas-mediated genome editing in the rat via direct injection of one-cell embryos. *Nature Protocols* 9 (10): 2493–512.

Singer, Peter. 2004. *One world. The ethics of globalization*. New Haven: Yale University Press.

Sparrow, Robert. 2008. Genes, identity and the expressivist critique. In *The sorting society*, eds. Loane Skene, and Janna Thompson, 111–32. Cambridge: Cambridge University Press.

UNESCO International Bioethics Committee (IBC). 1997. *Universal declaration on the human genome and human rights*. Paris: UNESCO.

Vassena, Rita, Björn Heindryckx, Peco, R., Guido Pennings, Raya, A., Sermon, K., and Veiga, A. 2016. Genome engineering through CRISPR/Cas9 technology in the human germline and pluripotent stem cells. *Human Reproduction Update* 22 (4): 411–19.

Wrigley, Anthony, Stephen Wilkinson, and John B. Appleby. 2015. Mitochondrial replacement: Ethics and identity. *Bioethics* 29 (9): 631–8.

Wu, Yuxuan, Dan Liang, Yinghua Wang, Meizhu Bai, Wei Tang, Shiming Bao, Zhiqiang Yan, Dangsheng Li, and Jinsong Li. 2013. Correction of a genetic disease in mouse via use of CRISPR-Cas9. *Cell Stem Cell* 13 (6): 659–62.

Yoshimi, K., Kaneko, T., Voigt, B., and Mashimo, T. 2014. Allele-specific genome editing and correction of disease-associated phenotypes in rats using the CRISPR–Cas platform. *Nature Communications* 5: 4240.

Zou, Qingjian, Xiaomin Wang, Yunzhong Liu, Zhen Ouyang, Haibin Long, Shu Wei, and Jige Xin, et al. 2015. Generation of gene-target dogs using CRISPR/Cas9 system. *Journal of Molecular Cell Biology* 7 (6): 580–3.

Notes

1 Autosomal recessive diseases develop when an individual has two copies of an abnormal gene.

2 Currently, the United Kingdom is the only country that has allowed mitochondrial DNA replacement techniques. Such techniques represent the only existing method for couples where one member is affected by a mitochondrial condition to have genetically related children.

3 The arguments made for CRISPR can be extended also to other future genome editing technologies. Throughout the paper, I use CRISPR and genome editing or gene editing technologies interchangeably.

4 At least when it is about medical conditions, but this is the case in question, so I will not enter into a discussion on so-called cosmetic traits and enhancement.

5 This observation is conditional as it relies on the interpretation of therapy as a practice that can only be defined as such if there is a *person* to be treated (Rulli 2016a).

6 I refer here to the debate on mitochondrial replacement techniques (MRTs) and not strictly on genome editing with CRISPR, as few commentators have dealt specifically with the question of whether genome editing is identity-affecting (for two examples, see: Gyngell et al. 2016; Liao 2017). One of the two techniques for the replacement of faulty mitochondrial DNA, pronuclear transfer (PNT), arguably represents the most similar case to genome editing as, unlike the other technique for the replacement of mitochondrial DNA (maternal spindle transfer – MST), it is applied after the oocytes has been fertilised. The contention, in the case of PNT, is whether this technique is identity-affecting or not, and commentators have presented differing views on this matter (Liao 2017; Palacios-González 2017; Rulli 2016a; Wrigley et al. 2015). While I am aware that PNT and CRISPR are two distinct technologies, PNT arguably represents the most similar case to genome editing as both CRISPR and PNT are applied *after* fertilisation. Hence, other things being equal, arguments concerning whether PNT is identity-affecting or not can also be considered valid in discussions on whether CRISPR is identity-affecting. It must be noted however, that those who explicitly referred to genome editing maintained that it is *not* identity-affecting (Gyngell et al. 2016; Liao 2017). Interestingly, authors who speculatively consider the possibility of using gene therapy on human

embryos before the availability of CRISPR are also divided on this issue (Buchanan 1996; McMahan 2006; Sparrow 2008).

7 Despite some challenges, the biological origin (or gametic origin) that a person has is widely considered a necessary condition of what determines the human being that we are. This is well explained by philosopher Derek Parfit's 'Origin View' (or gametic essentialism): "each person has this necessary property: that of having grown from the particular pair of cells from which this person in fact grew" (Parfit 1984, p. 353). In other words, the fact that two gametes came together and generated me is, under this view, considered a necessary condition of my identity: I am the entity that I am by virtue of my gametic origin. Now, this is linked to the discussion of treatment and selection because a technology such as PGD is identity-affecting. In other words, using PGD causes a numerically different person to come into being, namely a different person than the person that would have come into being had PGD not been used. In the case of genome editing, since the intervention takes place *after* fertilisation, the gametic origin of the genetically modified embryo and the gametic origin of the non-genetically modified embryos are identical. In other words, these two embryos are numerically identical. The contention, however, is that gametic origin is only a necessary and not sufficient condition for having a specific identity. Thus, whether genome editing technologies applied to zygotes/embryos cause a different person to come into being or not remains an open question. If they do, then such technologies cannot be considered therapeutic because a different person comes into being due to the use of genome editing. If they do not, they can be considered therapeutic.

8 If genome editing is employed before the 14th day after fertilisation (as it is required by embryos research regulations in the United Kingdom and in many other countries, Hyun et al. 2016), the embryo could still cleave into two (i.e. twinning). In this case, the children that could potentially develop from such embryo will be two. However, twinning occurs spontaneously and it is not influenced by the use of genome editing on the embryo. As a consequence, the use of the technique does not directly affect the numerical identity of the future child/children as it is not the direct causation of the embryo splitting.

18

Who's Afraid of the Big Bad (Germline Editing) Wolf?

R. Alta Charo

The surprise announcement in November 2018 that a Chinese researcher had implanted and brought to term two gene-edited embryos, resulting in the birth of twin girls, had the effect of galvanizing a debate that goes back decades (Begley 2018; Evans 2002; Kevles 1985). Should we make heritable changes in our children's DNA? Until recently, this was hypothetical only, and the easy response was to say it is too uncertain and too unnecessary to be tolerated. Suddenly, however, the possibility that there might be real uses for mitochondrial DNA replacement or for germline editing has led to a more nuanced debate, ranging from calls to double-down on prohibiting this technology to discussions of how to permit it for a limited range of conditions, under strict oversight (Baltimore et al. 2015; NAS 2017; UNESCO 2015). Often lacking in this debate has been an effort to look back at debates surrounding earlier advances in reproductive technologies, most of which have been accompanied by fears of eugenics, the loss of human dignity, and the disruption of parent-child relationships. While these advances have each had pockets of abusive uses, they have been integrated into modern life without bringing about wholesale destruction of society.

A true prohibition of germline editing already exists in a number of countries, by virtue of their signatures to an international instrument. A number of international efforts focus on human rights, including the Universal Declaration of Human Rights, the International Covenant on Civil and Political Rights, the International Covenant on Economic, Social and Cultural Rights, the Convention on the Rights of the Child, the Convention for the Protection of Human Rights and Fundamental Freedoms, and the European Social Charter. But it is the 1997 Council of Europe's Convention for the Protection of Human Rights and Dignity of the Human Being with Regard to the Application of Biology and Medicine, better known as the Oviedo Convention, that was written specifically to address the intersection of human rights and biomedical developments, and aimed to protect the "dignity and identity of all human beings" (Council of Europe 1997).

Article 13 reads: "An intervention seeking to modify the human genome may only be undertaken for

Original publication details: R. Alta Charo, "Who's Afraid of the Big Bad (Germline Editing) Wolf?" pp. 93–100 from *Perspectives in Biology and Medicine* 63: 1 (Winter 2020). Reproduced with permission of Johns Hopkins University Press.

preventive, diagnostic or therapeutic purposes and *only if its aim is not to introduce any modification in the genome of any descendants*" (emphasis added). In other words, even if done with the best of intentions, to ward off devastating – even lethal– conditions, the Convention admits of no alterations that are meant to affect descendants, though this position has not been without its critics (Council of Europe 2017; Cyngell, Douglas, and Savulescu 2017; De Wert et al. 2018; Hasson 2018).

Debates around germline editing focus on multiple concerns. With regard to physical harm to individuals living in the future, this involves a risk-benefit analysis that is complicated by the multigenerational potential of the change (Baylis 2018; Rubeis and Steger 2018). This alone introduces questions about the stability and durability of the alteration, its effect under future (presumably different) environments, and the ever-increasing number of generations between the person affected and the person initially giving consent.

A different objection goes directly to how we understand autonomy. As noted in the July 2018 report by the UK Nuffield Council, one might argue that "choosing someone else's genetic endowment . . . offends against the essential dignity and nature of the person as a free and independent human being." In essence, this argument is that germline editing interferes with a child's "right to an open future" (Feinberg 1980, 1992). But one response has been not only that parents make many momentous decisions affecting their children's lives, but that the acceptability of parental choices rests on whether they serve to expand or narrow a child's prospects, and whether the changes were made for the welfare of the future child, such as preventing serious disease and disability (NAS 2017; Nuffield Council 2018). Of course, it should be noted that many in the deaf community and the community of little people would not define those conditions as disabilities, but rather as varieties of the human community. But this is the exception, and other groups with shared disabilities have not refused the designation, although they often argue the degree of impairment is as much a function of social and physical context as it is anything intrinsic to the body.

Other concerns about germline editing revolve around fear that it will lead to intolerance of imperfection, turning children into commodities rather than the subjects of parental love, and that it will result in stigmatization of those who are disabled (Thiessen 2018). These concerns are not unfamiliar. They have been raised repeatedly with each new advance in reproductive technologies, whether prenatal screening, gamete donation, IVF, surrogacy, preimplantation diagnosis, and cloning. Germline editing is simply the latest rehearsal of what are fundamentally the same concerns around intolerance for diversity or imperfection.

By the 1970s, amniocentesis had entered clinical care and was used to screen early second trimester fetuses for chromosomal abnormalities such as triploidy associated with Down syndrome (Cowan 1993). The prospect of abortion being used to eliminate the birth of children with this and other chromosomal conditions sparked widespread discussion about the value that persons with disabilities find in their own lives, about the prospect of nongovernmental eugenics (even absent government influence, a pattern of common decision-making among individuals), and about whether the ability to avoid the birth of children with these conditions would affect the way parents regard all children and lead to "commodification" of children that undermined their status as a gift or a blessing. But while the rate of births with Down syndrome has been dramatically affected in some places, the overall number of these births has continued to be substantial and, if anything, acceptance of people with Down's has only increased in the intervening years (Guralnick, Connor, and Hammond 1995; Hocutt 1996; Kasari et al. 1999; Mansfield, Hopfer, and Marteau 1999; Natoli et al. 2012).

The 1980s saw the rising use of artificial insemination, with its associated public fears that women would flock toward the "Genius Bank" for "superior sperm." This did not happen, and reportedly no more than a few dozen children were born from this source. Surveys show that most people simply want donors who will resemble the nongenetic rearing parent (Klock and Maier 1991; Nielsen, Pedersen, and Lauritsen 1995; Nijs 1982; Scheib, Raboy, and Shaver 1998).

That decade was also the era of surrogate motherhood and in vitro; fertilization, two reproductive techniques that were, again, predicted to undermine parent-child relationships. in vitro; fertilization (IVF), by which eggs are fertilized in a laboratory and grown until ready for transfer to a woman who will gestate them until birth, was viewed as unnatural, yet parent-child relations have not in fact been harmed. While surrogacy has had a problematic history, it is due not to the loss of parental love but rather to the effects of wealth inequality, which has led some to worry about exploitation of low-income women, in the US and elsewhere (Markens 2007). This is particularly true when IVF is used in conjunction with surrogacy, as in these cases the rearing couple uses their own gametes and the pregnant woman has no genetic relationship with the child she bears, so her own physical and genetic characteristics may be of little concern to the rearing couple (Johnson v Calvert, 851 P.2d 776 (Cal. 1993)).

The one area where problems have seemed most acute is egg donation. An overly deterministic view of genetics led some rearing couples to seek egg donors who had high standardized test scores or were students at elite universities, with exaggerated payments as inducements. While there is little evidence of long-term physical harm from ovulation stimulation, especially when done only once, it still poses some risk to healthy young women. But here, again, despite many articles discussing the phenomenon, evidence of the practice has been anecdotal, and it is not clear how widespread it became (Almeling 2007).

In the 1990s, the next development to stir controversy was preimplantation genetic diagnosis, whereby in vitro; embryos could be biopsied and those with known deleterious mutations left unused. Debates surrounding appropriate use of PGD focused on two fears. First, there was concern that parents would use the technique for ever more trivial reasons and finally push society toward the commodification of children and intolerance of imperfection that had been predicted with each of the previous reproductive

technology advances (Greely 2016). Here too, however, experience showed that the expense and inconvenience of IVF, plus the limited range of conditions that could be reliably identified, meant that its use was largely restricted to serious or lethal conditions And the Americans with Disabilities Act (ADA) led to tremendous progress toward making workplaces, homes, and public facilities accessible so that those with disabilities would no longer be isolated from the wider community.

The second fear, however, was that it might be used for sex selection, which in turn was viewed by some as reification of sex differences that had undergirded centuries of discrimination against girls and women. Sex selection had been possible with amniocentesis since the 1970s, but the prospect of selective abortion deterred many people in the US. In PGD, however, there was the chance to do sex selection without an abortion. But again, only very highly motivated people have been willing to undergo the expense and inconvenience of IVF simply to ensure the birth of a child of one sex or the other (Macklin 2010; Steinbock 2002).

Later in the 1990s, the prospect of human cloning led to a flurry of efforts to ban what was seen as an immoral or dangerous procedure. But the public showed little appetite to pursue it for human purposes, despite some high profile (and rather silly) claims about its success – all of which proved to be fraudulent. Nonetheless, both the Oviedo Convention and a host of state laws in the US and national policies abroad have adopted criminal penalties for attempting this.

As we entered the 21st century, attention turned to mitochondrial replacement, a technique that would be useful for women whose eggs carried mitochondrial DNA known to cause a wide variety of health problems. PGD provided no solution, so for those who wished to maintain a genetic connection to their offspring, one solution was to use donated, healthy mitochondria. A number of attempts were made over the course of two decades, beginning in 1996 (Wolf, Mitalipov, and Mitalipov 2015). By 2016, several dozen children around the world had been born following conception using this technique, though with varying (and arguably inadequate) attention to longterm followup and transparency in data reporting and sharing (IOM 2016; Kula 2016).

Mitochondrial replacement entered the realm of transgenerational genetic modification, as the altered eggs would result in offspring who, if they were girls, would carry that donated mitochondrial DNA in their own eggs and pass it down to the next generation, and the next, and the next. The Oviedo Convention appeared to prohibit this. Critics worried that this would become a sought-after technology for older women, including those with no known mitochondrial disease, in the hope it would enhance their fertility. It is too early to know if this dire prediction will come true, but based on past experience, the risks and discomfort (to say nothing of the expense) associated with this technology will limit its users to those with a compelling need. In addition, a recent study suggests the technique is not particularly successful at increasing the chance of conception for older women (Mazur et al. 2019). For the moment, such a procedure has been rendered de facto illegal in the US, by virtue of a federal budgetary provision that precludes FDA review of a request to begin clinical trials involving the technique (Kaiser 2019), and the UK remains the only country with explicit regulations governing permitted indications (HFEA 2015).

In sum, as we approach the end of the first quarter-century of the new millennium, there has been a half century of experience with new technologies predicted to alter human relations and give people a power that they would inevitably abuse, but which did not in fact result in these dystopian futures. Despite this, the same predictions are made about germline editing.

The debates around germline editing continue, but the science remains in preliminary stages, and there is still time to take a close look at why and how these earlier reproductive technologies spread, what their limiting factors were, and how such factors might help in formulating better predictions for the range and scale of use one might expect for germline editing. For example, IVF was originally developed to circumvent blocked fallopian tubes, but its use rapidly expanded to encompass idiopathic infertility, male sub-fecundity (in conjunction with intracytoplasmic sperm injection), egg donation, and gestational surrogacy. But given the expense, discomfort, and risks of IVF, it did not expand to populations able to conceive through intercourse without significant fear of passing on a serious genetic condition but who (as was feared and predicted at the time) would want to use PGD to screen for conditions that do not seriously impair health. At most, there was some small uptake that involved screening for later-onset cancers. How much this has been due to the lack of motivating reasons to undergo IVF versus the limits of PGD screening would be quite relevant if one wished to extrapolate to probable patterns of germline use.

Another worthwhile effort would be to calculate the number of people who might be interested in germline editing. Primarily this would be the very small number of people for whom PGD is not an option, such as those couples where one parent is homozygous for a dominant mutation such as Huntington's. Secondarily it might be couples for whom the number of available embryos following PGD is quite small. Who are these people, and are their numbers (and their marital patterns) sufficient to raise the spectre of exacerbating inequities or creating a genetically superior caste of society, as is feared by some? A peculiar aspect of the germline editing debate has been the assertion, on the one hand, that it could be banned, as very few people actually need it, and the assertion, on the other hand, that it will become sufficiently popular to have a global effect on humanity's own genome.

In the debates surrounding the use of genome editing for germline alteration, one of the frequently raised concerns is its possible effect on human evolution. Given the need to do IVF, it would seem unlikely to become a sufficiently prominent part of human reproduction to have any evolutionary effects in the foreseeable future, even if its substantial technical, regulatory, logistical, and economic barriers could be overcome. More likely to become a part of our lives would be genome editing that lacks transgenerational effects, such as somatic editing at the fetal or postnatal stages, or − even more limited in its effects – epigenetic editing for transient alterations. It is for this reason that the ongoing effort by the World Health Organization to develop guidance for global governance of genome editing will focus not only on germline changes but on the broader range of uses (WHO 2018). More distantly related to the subject of this essay, genome editing may become a potent addition to the already extensive arsenal of tools available to create – and defend against – biological weapons.

As germline editing moves from science fiction to laboratory to (perhaps) the clinic, good governance will always begin with good facts.

References

Almeling, R. 2007. "Selling Genes, Selling Gender: Egg Agencies, Sperm Banks, and the Medical Market in Genetic Material." *Am Soc Rev* 72 (3): 319–40.

Baltimore, D., et al. 2015. "A Prudent Path Forward for Genomic Engineering and Germline Gene Modification." *Science* 348 (6230): 36–8.

Baylis, F. 2018. "Counterpoint: The Potential Harms of Human Gene Editing Using CRISPR-Cas9." *Clin Chem* 64: 489–91.

Begley, S. 2018. "Amid Uproar, Chinese Scientist Defends Creating Gene-Edited Babies." *STAT News,* Sept. 28.

Council of Europe. 1997. *Convention for the Protection of Human Rights and Dignity of the Human Being with Regard to the Application of Biology and Medicine.* Strasbourg: Council of Europe. https://www.coe.int/en/web/bioethics/oviedo-convention.

Council of Europe. Parliamentary Assembly. 2017. "Recommendation 2115." https://assembly.coe.int/nw/xml/XRef/Xref-XML2HTML-en.asp?fileid=24228&lang=en.

Cowan, R. 1993. "Aspects of the History of Prenatal Diagnosis." *Fetal Diagn Ther* 8 (suppl. 1): 10–17.

Cyngell, C., T. Douglas, and J. Savulescu. 2017. "The Ethics of Germline Gene Editing." *J Appl Philos* 34 (4): 498–513.

De Wert, G., et al. 2018. "Human Germline Gene Editing: Recommendations of ESHG and ESHRE." *Hum Reprod Open* 1 (1): hox025.

Evans, J. 2002. *Playing God? Human Genetic Engineering and the Rationalization of Public Bioethical Debate.* Chicago: University of Chicago Press.

Feinberg, J. 1980. "The Child's Right to an Open Future." In *Whose Child? Children's Rights, Parental Authority, and State Power,* ed. W. Aiken and H. LaFollette, 124–53. Totowa, NJ: Rowman & Littlefield.

Feinberg, J. 1992. *Freedom and Fulfillment.* Princeton: Princeton University Press.

Greely, H. 2016. *The End of Sex and the Future of Human Reproduction.* Cambridge: Harvard University Press.

Guralnick, M., R. Connor, and M. Hammond. 1995. "Parent Perspectives of Peer Relationships and Friendships in Integrated and Specialized Programs." *Am J Ment Retard* 99: 457–76.

Hasson, K. 2018. "UK's Nuffield Council Releases Report on Human Genome Editing." *Bio Political Times,* Aug. 2.

Hocutt, A. 1996. "Effectiveness of Special Education: Is Placement the Critical Factor?" *Future Child* 6: 77–102.

Human Fertilisation and Embryology Authority (HFEA). 2015. "Human Fertilisation and Embryology (Mitochondrial Donation) Regulations." http://www.legislation.gov.uk/uksi/2015/572/contents/made.

Institute of Medicine (IOM). 2016. *Mitochondrial Replacement Techniques: Ethical, Social, and Policy Considerations.* Washington, DC: National Academies Press.

Kaiser, J. 2019. "Update: House Spending Panel Restores U.S. Ban on Gene-Edited Babies." *Science,* June 5. DOI: 10.1126/science.aay1607.

Kasari, C., et al. 1999. "Parental Perspectives on Inclusion: Effects of Autism and Down Syndrome." *J Autism Dev Disord* 29: 297–305.

Kevles, D. 1985. *In the Name of Eugenics: Genetics and the Uses of Human Heredity.* Berkeley: University of California Press.

Klock, S., and D. Maier. 1991. "Psychological Factors Related to Donor Insemination." *Fertil Steril* 56: 489–95.

Kula, S. 2016. "Three-Parent Children Are Already Here." *Slate,* Feb. 18.

Macklin, R. 2010. "The Ethics of Sex Selection and Family Balancing." *Semin Reprod Med* 28 (4): 315–21.

Markens, S. 2007. *Surrogate Motherhood and the Politics of Reproduction.* Berkeley: University of California Press.

Mazur, P. et al. 2019. "P-221 Mitochondrial Replacement Therapy Give No Benefits to Patients of Advanced Maternal Age." Paper presented at American Society for Reproductive Medicine (ASRM) Scientific Conference and Expo, Philadelphia, Oct. 14–16. https://asrm.confex.com/asrm/2019/meetingapp.cgi/Paper/2347.

Mansfield, C., S. Hopfer, and T. Marteau. 1999. "Termination Rates After Prenatal Diagnosis of Down Syndrome, Spina Bifida, Anencephaly, and Turner and Klinefelter Syndromes: A Systematic Literature Review. European Concerted Action: DADA (Decision-Making After the Diagnosis of a Fetal Abnormality)." *Prenat Diagn* 19 (9): 808–12.

National Academies of Sciences, Engineering and Medicine (NAS). 2017. *Human Genome Editing: Science, Ethics, and Governance.* Washington, DC: National Academies Press.

Natoli, J., et al. 2012. "Prenatal Diagnosis of Down Syndrome: A Systematic Review of Termination Rates (1995–2011)." *Prenat Diagn* 32 (2): 142–53.

Nielsen, A, B. Pedersen, and J. Lauritsen. 1995. "Psychosocial Aspects of Donor Insemination: Attitudes and Opinions of Danish and Swedish Donor Insemination Patients to Psychosocial Information Being Supplied to Offspring and Relatives." *Acta Obstet Gynecol Scand* 74: 45–50.

Nijs, P. 1982. "Aspects médico-psychologiques de l'insémination artificielle." *Jus Medicum (Acta Fourth World Congress on Medical Law)* 69–81.

Nuffield Council on Bioethics. 2018. *Genome Editing and Human Reproduction.* London: Nuffield Council. http://nuffieldbioethics.org/wp-content/uploads/ Genome-editing-and-human-reproduction-FINAL-website.pdf.

Rubeis, G., and F. Steger. 2018. "Risks and Benefits of Human Germline Genome Editing: An Ethical Analysis." *Asian Bioethics Rev* 10: 133.

Scheib, J., B. Raboy, and P. Shaver. 1998. "Selection of Sperm Donors: Recipients' Criteria and Donor Attributes That Predict Choice." *Fertil Steril* 70 (suppl. 1): S279.

Steinbock, B. 2002. "Sex Selection: Not Obviously Wrong." *Hastings Cent Rep* 32 (1): 23–8.

Thiessen, M. 2018. "Gene Editing Is Here: It's an Enormous Threat." *Washington Post,* Nov. 29.

UNESCO. 2015. "UNESCO Panel of Experts Calls for Ban on 'Editing' of Human DNA to Avoid Unethical Tampering with Hereditary Traits." UNESCO. https:// en.unesco.org/news/unesco-panel-experts-calls-ban-editing-human-dna-avoid-unethical-tampering-hereditary-traits.

Wolf, D., N. Mitalipov, and S. Mitalipov. 2015. "Mitochondrial Replacement Therapy in Reproductive Medicine." *Trends Molec Med* 21 (2): 68–76.

World Health Organization (WHO). 2018. "Announcement of Expert Panel." WHO. https://www.who.int/ethics/topics/human-genome-editing/en/.

19

An Ethical Pathway for Gene Editing

Julian Savulescu and Peter Singer

Ethics is the study of what we ought to do; science is the study of how the world works. Ethics is essential to scientific research in defining the concepts we use (such as the concept of 'medical need'), deciding which questions are worth addressing, and what we may do to sentient beings in research.

The central importance of ethics to science is exquisitely illustrated by the recent gene editing of two healthy embryos by the Chinese biophysicist He Jiankui, resulting in the birth of baby girls born in November 2018, Lulu and Nana. A second pregnancy is underway with a different couple. To make the babies resistant to human immunodeficiency virus (HIV), He edited out a gene (CCR5) that produces a protein which allows HIV to enter cells. One girl has both copies of the gene modified (and may be resistant to HIV), while the other has only one (making her still susceptible to HIV).[1]

He Jiankui invited couples to take part in this experiment where the father was HIV positive and the mother HIV negative. He offered free in vitro; fertilization (IVF) with sperm washing to avoid transmission of HIV. He also offered medical insurance, expenses and treatment capped at 280,000 RMB/ CNY, equivalent to around $40,000. The package includes health insurance for the baby for an unspecified period. Medical expenses and compensation arising from any harm caused by the research were capped at 50,000 RMB/CNY ($7000 USD).[2] He says this was from his own pocket.[3] Although the parents were offered the choice of having either gene-edited or -unedited embryos transferred, it is not clear whether they understood that editing was not necessary to protect their child from HIV, nor what pressure they felt under. There has been valid criticism of the process of obtaining informed consent.[4] The information was complex and probably unintelligible to lay people.

The most basic ethical constraint on research involving humans is that it should not expose participants to unreasonable risk.[5] Risks should be the minimum necessary to answer the scientific question, and the expected benefits should be proportionate to expected harms.[6] While the Declaration of Helsinki states that research involving incompetent participants must be 'minimal risk and minimal burden',[7] this is

Original publication details: Julian Savulescu and Peter Singer, "An Ethical Pathway for Gene Editing," pp. 221–222 from *Bioethics* 33: 2 (2019). Reproduced with permission of John Wiley & Sons.

most plausibly interpreted as minimal *overall* risk or burden, where expected benefits match or outweigh expected harms. After all, children are exposed to trials of new toxic chemotherapeutic agents with significant risks.

In deciding whether a risk is reasonable, it is important to evaluate not only the probability of achieving a benefit, but also the extent of the benefit in question. A greater expected benefit is worth greater risk than a smaller expected benefit. Avoiding HIV is certainly a benefit, but the probability that Lulu and Nana would have contracted HIV is low. In contrast, the unknown effects of the editing could cost them a normal life.

Given our ignorance of the full ramifications of changing a gene, what could justify taking the risk of a gene-editing trial in humans? The answer is, if the embryo had a catastrophic single gene disorder. Several genetic disorders, such as BRAT 1, JAM3 and PHGDH, are lethal in the neonatal period, so for embryos with them, gene editing is potentially life-saving.[8] There is a risk of off-target mutations, but the expected harm of such mutations is arguably no worse than the fate of the unedited embryos.

The geneticist George Church has defended He's research on the grounds that HIV is a public health problem for which there is no cure or vaccine.[9] Church is right to the extent that there is no problem in principle with editing out the CCR5 gene in the future. What he fails to take into account, however, is that Lulu and Nana are being used, at great risk, and without proportionate benefit, when there are more ethical experimental designs that would meet the need for greater knowledge of the effects of editing genes.

At the conference at which He presented his experiment, George Daley, the Dean of Harvard Medical School, indicated that Huntington's disease or Tay–Sachs disease might be suitable targets for gene editing.[10] It is not clear whether Daley is endorsing these as first-in-human trials. Huntington's disease is very different to Tay–Sachs disease. Babies with Tay–Sachs disease die in the first few years of life; people with Huntington's disease have around 40 good years. Hence Tay–Sachs disease is a better candidate for early

trials, as babies with that condition have less to lose. This mirrors the rationale for experimenting with gene therapy on babies with a lethal form of ornithine transcarbamylase (OTC) deficiency rather than on adults with a mild form, such as Jesse Gelsinger who lost his life in a badly designed gene therapy trial in 1999.[11]

He Jiankui's trial was unethical, not because it involved gene editing, but because it failed to conform to the basic values and principles that govern all research involving human participants.

Further into the future, if gene editing can be done without off-target mutations, it could be used to address genetic dispositions to common diseases, such as diabetes or cardiovascular disease. These involve tens or hundreds of genes. In principle, gene editing could be used to modify many genes accurately. Gene editing has been successfully employed to remove 62 porcine endogenous retroviruses from a kidney cell line.[12]

It is notable that the first human gene-edited babies were enhanced to have resistance to a disease, not to treat an existing disease. In future, perhaps gene editing will be used to engineer super-resistance to infectious threats.

At the Second International Summit on Human Genome Editing, where He revealed his research, the National Academies of Science, Engineering and Medicine called for a 'translational pathway to human germ line gene editing'. In our view, to be ethically justifiable, such a 'translational pathway' should be: catastrophic single gene disorders (like Tay–Sachs disease), then severe single gene disorders (like Huntington's disease), then reduction in the genetic contribution to common diseases (like diabetes and cardiovascular disease), then enhanced immunity and perhaps even delaying ageing.

Should the translational pathway extend to enhancing normal traits, such as intelligence? This has been the subject of almost 20 years of debate.[13] One approach to enhancement has been to ban it. Many jurisdictions, including most in Europe and Australia ban pre-implantation genetic diagnosis (PGD) for non-disease traits. However, one US company recently announced the use of polygenic risk scores for low normal intelligence in PGD. They admitted the same techniques could be used to predict high normal intelligence and believe such a step is inevitable.[14]

Further into the future, gene editing could be used for enhancement of the genetic contribution to general intelligence. China is currently funding research that is trying to unravel the genetics of high intelligence.[15] Perhaps the best we can hope for is harm reduction and a regulated market to make important enhancements, such as resistance to disease or the enhancement of intelligence (should it ever be possible), part of a basic healthcare plan so that the benefits of gene editing are distributed equally.

Notes

1   Marchione, M. (2018). Chinese researcher claims first gene-edited babies. *AP News*. Retrieved from https://www.apnews.com/4997bb7aa36c45449b488e19ac83e86d. Accessed Jan. 16, 2019.

2   He, J. *Informed consent. Version: Female 3.0.* Retrieved from http://www.sustc-genome.org.cn. Accessed Nov. 26, 2018.

3   Lucas, L., & Liu, N. (2018, Nov. 28). Chinese scientist defends controversial gene-editing experiment. *Financial Times*. Retrieved from https://www.ft.com/content/766c4824-f2f6-11e8-ae55-df4bf40f9d0d. Accessed Dec 10, 2018.

4   Schaefer, G. O. (2018). Rogue science strikes again: The case of the first gene-edited babies. *The Conversation*.

5   Savulescu, J., & Hope, T. (2010). Ethics of research. In J. Skorupski (Ed.), *The Routledge companion to ethics* (pp. 781–795). Abingdon, UK: Routledge.

6   World Medical Association. (2013). Declaration of Helsinki Ethical principles for medical research involving human subjects. *Journal of the American Medical Association, 310*(20), 2191–4, Paragraphs 16 and 17.

7   World Medical Association. (2013). Declaration of Helsinki Ethical principles for medical research involving human subjects. *Journal of the American Medical Association, 310*(20), 2191–4, Paragraph 28.

8   Thanks to Zornitza Stark for examples.

9   Cohen, J. (2018). 'I feel an obligation to be balanced.' Noted biologist comes to defense of gene editing babies. *Science*. Retrieved from http://www.sciencemag.org/news/2018/11/i-feel-obligation-be-balanced-noted-biologist-comes-defense-gene-editing-babies.

10 Cyranoski, D. (2018). CRISPR-baby scientist fails to satisfy critics. *Nature, 564*(7734), 13–14.

11 Savulescu, J. (2001). Harm, ethics committees and the gene therapy death. *Journal of medical ethics, 27*(3), 148–50.

12 Yang, L., Güell, M., Niu, D., George, H., Lesha, E., Grishin, D., . . . Church, G. (2015). Genome-wide inactivation of porcine endogenous retrovirus or other sequences in the pig genome endogenous retroviruses (PERVs). *Science, 350*, 1101–4.

13 Kass, L. (2003). Beyond therapy: Biotechnology and the pursuit of human improvement. *The President's Council on Bioethics*. Retrieved from https://bioethicsarchive.georgetown.edu/pcbe/background/kasspaper.html; Savulescu, J., & Bostrom, N. (2009). *Human enhancement*. Oxford, UK: Oxford University Press.

14 Wilson, C. (2018, Nov). Exclusive: A new test can predict IVF embryos' risk of having a low IQ. *New Scientist*. Retrieved from https://www.newscientist.com/article/mg24032041-900-exclusive-a-new-test-can-predict-ivf-embryos-risk-of-having-a-low-iq/.

15 Yong, E. (2013). Chinese project probes the genetics of genius. *Nature, 497*, 297–9. Retrieved from https://www.nature.com/news/chinese-project-probes-the-genetics-of-genius-1.12985.

Part IV

Life and Death Issues

Introduction

It is widely believed that it is wrong to kill an innocent person, but there are great variations in people's beliefs as to whether this rule is absolute, without any exceptions, or if not, what those exceptions are. This diversity of views also characterizes the contributions to this *Anthology*.

When discussing issues related to the wrongness of killing, two clusters of questions immediately present themselves:

1. To *whom* does the prohibition of killing apply? To *all* human beings? To *only* human beings? An answer to these questions is central to discussions of abortion (see Part I of this volume), the ethics of experimenting on nonhuman animals (see Part VII) and, in the present Part to the ethical issues raised by the birth of seriously ill or premature infants, by the concept of brain death, and by the use of advance directives.

2. When is a decision that leads to death wrong? Is there, for example, a morally relevant difference between killing a person and deliberately not saving her? Is it morally wrong to kill a person, when the person is suffering from an incurable disease, and asks for help in dying? Must doctors always prolong their patients' lives by all possible means, or are there times when the quality of a patient's life is so poor that it would be wrong for doctors not to allow, or perhaps even help, the patient die?

Jonathan Glover sets the scene in "The Sanctity of Life" by asking when and why killing is directly wrong. He rejects the view that all human life has sanctity, or is intrinsically or absolutely valuable, and instead develops the concept of a "life worth living." What makes killing directly wrong, he holds, is that it destroys a life that is worth living. Views based on the concept of a "life worth living" do not rule out all killings; they would in principle permit the taking of lives that are *not* worth living. This might, for example, be the case when a terminally ill and suffering patient asks his doctor to end his life, or when a patient has irreversibly lost all consciousness.

The idea that we may be justified in ending the lives of some human beings because the quality of their lives is so poor is contrary to the traditional Roman Catholic position, espoused in the "Declaration on Euthanasia." On this view, *all* innocent human lives, regardless of their quality or kind, have sanctity and must never intentionally be cut short. As the *Declaration* states:

> . . .nothing and no one can in any way permit the killing of an innocent human being, whether a fetus or an

Bioethics: An Anthology, Fourth Edition. Edited by Udo Schüklenk and Peter Singer.
Editorial material and organization © 2022 John Wiley & Sons, Inc. Published 2022 by John Wiley & Sons, Inc.

embryo, an infant or an adult, an old person, or one suffering from an incurable disease, or a person who is dying.

While the *Declaration* thus absolutely prohibits killing, it does not impose an absolute duty to prevent the death of innocent human beings. This applies also to the practice of medicine. While doctors must not practice "euthanasia," they are, under certain circumstances, permitted to allow their patients to die. But is there a conceptually and morally sound way of distinguishing between killing and letting die, and between doctors practicing "euthanasia" and making deliberate decisions not to keep patients alive despite the ready availability of the means to do so?

Killing and Letting Die

In attempting to draw a distinction between killing and allowing to die (often also referred to as the distinction between "active" and "passive euthanasia"), writers typically invoke a number of further distinctions, such as those between

- acts and omissions,
- ordinary and extraordinary (or burdensome) means of treatment; and
- intending death and merely foreseeing death.

In his influential 1975 article "Active and Passive Euthanasia," James Rachels argues that there is, other things being equal, no moral difference between active and passive euthanasia, or between doing something that leads to death and doing nothing to prevent death. To show this, Rachels asks readers to consider two cases that are identical in all relevant respects, except that one is a case of killing and one a case of letting die. Rachels argues that the two cases are morally on a par, and that the same is true of active and passive euthanasia in the practice of medicine: the mere difference between killing a patient and letting a patient die is in itself morally irrelevant.

Not everyone accepts Rachels' implicit assumption that the killing/letting die distinction rests on the distinction between actions and omissions, or between "doing something" and "doing nothing." Germain Grisez and Joseph M. Boyle, Jr ("The Morality of Killing: A Traditional View") hold that what distinguishes killing from letting die is the agent's intention. An agent kills, they argue, when she directly intends death; she allows to die when she merely foresees that the patient will die as a consequence of another morally permissible action or omission. On this view, then, some omissions intended to lead to death can amount to killings. If one *aims* at death, that is, if one commits oneself to a project that includes a person's death, then one kills, even if the project is carried out by way of an omission. If, on the other hand, one does not aim at death, but rather commits oneself to some other morally good or at least morally indifferent project, then a foreseen death could be a case of letting die, and not a case of impermissible killing.

On this view all intentional killings of innocent human beings are wrong; but not every case in which death is an outcome of someone's action or omission involves moral wrongdoing. Just as martyrs may lay down their lives for a higher good, so patients may reasonably reject "extraordinary treatment" (treatment that is experimental, risky, or unduly burdensome or costly, or disproportionate to the benefit it brings), without thereby committing an act of suicide; and doctors may withdraw or withhold life-prolonging treatment, or administer life-shortening palliative care, without thereby intending to kill these patients.

Winston Nesbitt asks: "Is Killing No Worse Than Letting Die?" and agrees with both Grisez and Boyle, and with Rachels, that some omissions that result in death are the moral equivalent of killings. But, he argues, a person who is prepared to kill someone for personal gain poses a greater threat to other members of society than a person who is merely prepared, for the same reason, to let someone die. The person who is prepared to "let die" may not save me when my life is in danger, but "is no more dangerous than an incapacitated person, or for that matter, a rock or a tree." If a person is prepared to kill, however, I must also fear some positive attempts on my life. This shows, Nesbitt concludes, that killing is indeed worse than letting die.

Helga Kuhse, in "Why Killing is Not Always Worse – And Sometimes Better – Than Letting Die" grants, for the sake of the argument, that we should be more concerned by the presence of people who are prepared to kill for personal gain, than by the presence of people who are merely prepared to let die for personal gain. But, she argues, it does not follow from this that killing is always worse than letting die. That judgment should be reversed when agents are not seeking to benefit themselves, but to benefit others, as would be the case in euthanasia. Doctors sometimes allow their patients to die because death is assumed to be a benefit, from the patient's point of view. And if death is, in these cases, a benefit, rather than a harm, then active euthanasia will not be worse, and might be better, than passive euthanasia. Should we feel threatened by doctors who are not only prepared to let die, but also prepared to kill? No, says Kuhse: "We should be comforted by their presence."

In the final contribution on the killing/letting die distinction, Franklin G. Miller, Robert D. Truog, and Dan W. Brock explore the role of moral fictions in sustaining the idea that a physician who brings about a patient's death by withdrawing a ventilator, at the patient's request, acts both legally and ethically, whereas a physician who gives a lethal injection, again at the request of the patient, acts contrary both to ethics and to the law (in almost all countries). These fictions operate in regard to such central issues as the nature of the act, the causal role played by the physician, and the physician's intention. Exposing these fictions shows, according to Miller, Truog, and Brock, that on the issue of killing and letting die, conventional medical ethics is "radically mistaken."

Newborns

Some infants are born with severe disabilities; others are born prematurely, at the margin of viability. Should the lives of these babies always be prolonged, or are there grounds – such as the baby's best interests – for sometimes allowing or helping an infant to die?

In the first of a series of three articles that form a mini-symposium on this issue, Robert M. Sade

describes in "Can a Physician Ever Justifiably Euthanize a Severely Disabled Newborn?" the case of an ill-fated newborn suffering from heterotaxy syndrome involving a complex heart malformation. The attending doctors and the parents struggle with the different treatment options: surgery, medical treatment without surgery, mere comfort care, or active euthanasia. Gilbert Meilaender in his response article "No to Infant Euthanasia" urges doctors – and parents – to never abandon such newborns, no matter how small their odds of survival, and no matter how low their quality of life. In line with the Roman Catholic Church's views in its *Declaration on Euthanasia* he concedes that sometimes maximizing care can mean ceasing to struggle against death, but he is opposed to actively bringing about that death by means of euthanasia. Meilaender invokes, among his arguments, the acts and omissions distinction that James Rachels discusses in his article in this Section. Udo Schüklenk responds to Meilaender and argues for a quite different conclusion in "Physicians Can Justifiably Euthanize Certain Severely Impaired Neonates". In his view it is ethically defensible to euthanize a newborn infant if its continued existence would not be a net benefit to it. Unlike Meilaender, who is a proponent of the Sanctity of Life Doctrine in Medicine, Schüklenk argues that quality of life consideration should be the relevant decision-making criterion in cases such as that described in Sade's scenario.

Philosophy professor Gary Comstock, in a widely read *New York Times* column, offers a vivid account of the death of his son Sam, a newborn who has trisomy 18. Sam's brain cannot regulate his lungs, and there is no realistic possibility that he will ever be able to breathe on his own. Sam was born because his mother was opposed to abortion on theological and moral grounds, and so amniocentesis, which could have provided information about his condition, was not performed, given that she would not have chosen an abortion in any case. Comstock describes how his son died, and his subsequent thoughts about what he did.

"After-Birth Abortion: Why Should the Baby Live?" caused a global outcry when it was published in the *Journal of Medical Ethics* in 2012. Alberto Giubilini and

Francesca Minerva argue that infanticide is morally defensible even in newborns without serious disability. Their argument starts from the acknowledgment that in most jurisdictions abortion is accepted for reasons unrelated to fetal health. Following Tooley's line of reasoning (in his article included as Chapter 1 in Part I of this *Anthology*) they argue that fetuses and newborns are not persons, and their potential to become persons is morally irrelevant. In their view someone is not harmed by being prevented from becoming a person. They conclude that the interests of actual persons override those of potential persons, and so in cases where abortion would be permissible, infanticide is also permissible.

Christopher Kaczor tackles Giubilini and Minerva's analysis head-on in "Does a Human Being Gain the Right to Live after He or She Is Born?" taken from his "Abortion as a Human Rights Violation." He argues that Giubilini and Minerva wrongly equate "harm" with morally "wrong," when it is arguable that wrong can be done even if no harm is incurred by anyone. "A failed assassination attempt may harm no one, but the target is wronged regardless." Kaczor also objects to making John Locke's definition of personhood (a variety of which is also defended by Michael Tooley in his article in Part I) a necessary condition for a right to life.

In the last article in this section Dominic Wilkinson and Julian Savulescu discuss lessons they think society ought to learn from a high-profile case in the UK, that of Charlie Gard. Charlie was born in summer 2016, seemingly healthy. After a few weeks he had to be admitted to hospital where he was diagnosed with a rare severe mitrochondrial disorder that rapidly progresses and results in death in infancy. A conflict arose between the attending medical specialists at London's Great Ormond Hospital, and his parents. His parents wanted the newborn to receive an experimental therapy that the doctors were initially willing to provide, but then refused to do so when the newborn deteriorated so rapidly that in their best judgment such a therapy would have been futile. After much publicity and interventions from such figures as US President Donald Trump and Pope Francis, the conflict between doctors and parents was litigated in a European human rights court as well as in various UK courts.

Wilkinson and Savulescu focus their analysis on various policy-related questions including when the use of experimental treatments would be ethically defensible, how such cases should be handled in public healthcare systems where resources are limited, whether the parents should have been permitted to travel with the child to a jurisdiction where professionals were willing to continue treatment, and if they should have been permitted, who should have paid for that.

Brain Death

Before the development of sophisticated means of life-support, people were assumed to be dead when their hearts stopped beating and they were no longer breathing. The advent of respirators complicated matters. With the help of these machines, breathing and heartbeat can be sustained indefinitely, even if the patient is completely unresponsive and all electrical activity of the brain has ceased. But if their brains had irreversibly ceased to function, was there any point in maintaining these vital functions for patients who were taking up hospital beds and other scarce resources?

In 1967, while many hospital directors were becoming concerned about this situation, the dramatic news broke of the world's first heart transplant, performed by Dr Christiaan Barnard in South Africa. The prospect of preserving lives by transplanting hearts raised questions about when a vital organ like the heart may be removed for transplantation. If the transplant team have to wait until the heart has stopped beating, it is likely to suffer damage and be less suitable for transplantation.

These concerns led the Dean of the Harvard Medical School to appoint an Ad Hoc Committee to Examine the Definition of Brain Death. The Committee's report, "A Definition of Irreversible Coma," was published in 1968 and led to the widespread acceptance of what has become popularly known as "brain death" – that is, the permanent loss of all brain function – as an additional criterion of death, alongside the traditional criterion. Almost every country in the world now treats patients as dead if either the heartbeat and the circulation of the blood have ceased, or the brain has irreversibly ceased to function, as determined by standard medical tests.

This acceptance means, as Peter Singer notes in "The Challenge of Brain Death for the Sanctity of Life Ethic," that patients can be declared dead when their hearts are beating and their blood is circulating. Once patients have met the legal criterion for death, further medical support can be withdrawn, and, subject only to the consent of the family or the prior consent of the now-dead patients, their hearts and other organs can be cut out of their bodies and given to strangers.

Every year thousands of patients are pronounced dead on the basis of the concept of brain death. One would therefore hope that this concept has a strong, clear and consistent rationale; but it is difficult to find such a rationale in the chapter included here from "Controversies in the Determination of Death," a White Paper issued by the President's Council of Bioethics, and the most recent high-level US government document discussing this question. The chapter begins by observing that the question of whether a human being whose brain has irreversibly ceased to function – which the council refers to as "total brain failure" – is dead is not a scientific question of fact, but a philosophical question.

Next the Council examines the view that there is no sound biological justification for today's use of total brain failure as a criterion of death. It refers to the work of Dr Alan Shewmon, perhaps the foremost medical critic of the view that brain death is the death of the human being. Shewmon's observations of patients who have *correctly* been tested and found to meet the tests for brain death challenged what had been the standard philosophical rationale for regarding the death of the brain as the death of the human organism: the claim that once the brain is dead, there is no longer an integrated human organism. The Council accepts that Shewmon's evidence

shows that this rationale is no longer tenable. Instead of accepting, as Shewmon does, the conclusion that brain death is not the death of the human organism, however, the Council then seeks, and finds, an alternative rationale. We suggest that in assessing how convincing the Council's rationale for retaining brain death is, the reader refer to Section V of Singer's previously mentioned article, Chapter 35 in this Part.

Although Singer is a supporter of abortion and euthanasia, he is a strong critic of the view that brain death is the death of the human organism. He argues that the brain death criterion is a convenient fiction, readily accepted, because of its practical benefits for organ transplantation and for making the best use of our limited medical resources. (The discussion of moral fictions in the article by Miller, Truog, and Brock, Chapter 26 in this Part of the *Anthology*, is relevant here.) This does not mean that he thinks it is wrong to transplant organs from someone whose brain has irreversibly ceased to function. His view is, rather, that in accepting the fiction of "brain death" we are, in effect, abandoning the traditional ethic of the sanctity of human life. We should face the facts: we are cutting hearts out of innocent living human beings to give them to strangers. This is not wrong. It is justified because once people's brains have irreversibly ceased to function they will never recover consciousness. Hence their continued life is of no benefit to them, whereas their hearts can preserve the lives of other people who can have many years of worthwhile life ahead of them.

Jeff McMahan offers a different way of answering the question: "When do we die?" He turns the focus to another philosophical question: "What are we"? He gives two reasons for thinking that we are *not* human organisms, and argues that we are minds. On this basis he defends a view that the President's Council of Bioethics briefly considers, and rejects, in the opening pages of the chapter included in this *Anthology* the view that there are "two deaths," the death of the person, or conscious mind, and the death of the organism. Both Singer and McMahan therefore challenge the standard idea of brain death. They do so in different ways, but their conclusions are similar to the extent that they both justify removing organs from living human organisms, as long as consciousness has been irreversibly lost.

Advance Directives

Today there is widespread agreement that competent and informed patients have the right to refuse unwanted medical treatment, including life-sustaining treatment. Many people also assume that this right can be extended into the future by way of advance directives, such as "living wills" or proxy directives. Living wills allow people, while they are still competent, to stipulate that, should they one day become incompetent, they do not wish to receive certain treatments; and proxy directives allow for the appointment of an agent or "proxy", to make treatment decisions for the incompetent patient, should this situation occur.

Advance directives seem attractive. Medicine is continually increasing its capacity to prolong life, but cannot always restore functioning and well-being. Many people regard such diminished lives as undesirable. Moreover, given that death is often preceded by a period of mental incapacity, advance directives seem to offer a relatively simple and, many people think, morally defensible way of guiding medical decision-making, in accordance with the formerly competent person's values and beliefs.

But, as Ronald Dworkin points out, in "Life Past Reason," there is a possible problem: the interests of the formerly competent person may not be identical with the interests of the now incompetent patient. Dworkin focuses his discussion on the case of "Margo", who was suffering from advanced Alzheimer's disease. Although Margo was no longer able to make medical decisions for herself, she was in the words of one of her carers "one of the happiest people" he had ever known. If Margo, whilst still competent, had stipulated that her life should not be sustained (or that it should be actively terminated) should she ever become permanently incompetent, then, Dworkin argues, a seemingly happy life would be lost if her carers complied with her wishes.

This raises the question of whether decision-making should (always) be based on a person's earlier decision, or whether it should be based on the interests of the incompetent patient she has become.

Dworkin argues for the "precedence of autonomy" – that is, the view that a competent or autonomous person's interest in controlling her life ought to take precedence over any interests the future incompetent individual might have. Rebecca Dresser responds, in "Dworkin on Dementia: Elegant Theory, Questionable Policy," that the precedence Dworkin urges we give to autonomy must face a philosophical challenge posed by the psychological view of personal identity. On this view, psychological continuity is a *necessary* condition of personal identity. This presupposes that for Margo at, say, 70, to be the same person as Margo at 80, there must be sufficient psychological continuity (exemplified by memories, intentions, beliefs, desires, and so on) between the formerly competent person and the now incompetent patient. If these psychological links become very weak or are absent, as often will be the case in advanced Alzheimer's disease, there are grounds for claiming that the severely demented patient is not the same person as the author of the advance directive. Why then should the earlier Margo have the moral authority to control what happens to the demented Margo later on?

Voluntary Euthanasia and Medically Assisted Suicide

Few topics in bioethics have received as much consistent public attention during the last four decades as voluntary euthanasia and medically assisted suicide. Does a person who is incurably ill, who suffers much and wants to die, have the right to bring her life to an end, and is it proper for others to help her in this quest?

Different philosophers and cultures have given very different answers to this question. Some have condemned suicide and voluntary euthanasia – even in the face of great suffering – as cowardly and wrong, while others have praised a self-chosen death as courageous and as an expression of our ultimate freedom and dignity. The pre-Christian philosopher Seneca, for example, was among those who thought it was better to choose one's own death than to live with vastly diminished capacities. As he put it:

> I will not abandon old age, if old age preserves me intact as regards the better part of myself; but if old age begins to shatter my mind, and to pull its various faculties to pieces, if it leaves me not life, but only the breath of life, I shall rush out of a house that is crumbling and tottering. I shall not avoid illness by seeking death, as long as the illness is curable and does not impede my soul. I shall not lay violent hands upon myself just because I am in pain; for death under such circumstances is defeat. But if I find out that the pain must always be endured, I shall depart, not because of the pain, but because it will be a hindrance to me as regards all my reasons for living.[1]

Today, incurable illness, the loss of one's faculties, and unrelievable pain and suffering are still the basis of many requests for voluntary euthanasia and medically assisted suicide. But since the advent of Christianity, suicide has widely been regarded as intrinsically wrong. Life began to be seen not as our own to be disposed of when we choose, but as a gift from God, which only He has the right to reclaim. While this has been the prevailing attitude in Western societies for hundreds of years, it is not universally shared. Many people – Christians and non-Christians alike – take the view that in the face of incurable illness and suffering, assisted suicide and voluntary euthanasia can be rational and morally defensible choices. Chris Hill took this view after he became a paraplegic. As he describes in "The Note," he had been, before his accident, a great traveller and adventurer, who loved skiing, diving, dancing, and sex. After his accident, he was paralysed from the chest down, doubly incontinent, sexless, "a talking head mounted on a bloody wheelchair." His unwillingness to involve others in an act that might cause them to be charged with the criminal offence of assisting suicide meant that, as his doctor later wrote, he died alone in a deserted parking lot.[2]

Some people accept that suicide, without the assistance of others, can sometimes be a morally defensible choice, but, they argue, voluntary euthanasia is quite a different matter because it involves others in the life-ending act. Daniel Callahan appears to share this view. In "When Self-Determination Runs Amok," he writes that euthanasia requires two people, and "a complicit society to make it acceptable." To counter the argument that doctors are already providing euthanasia when they discontinue life-support, Callahan argues that there is a moral difference between stopping life support on the one hand and "more active forms of killing, such as lethal injection," on the other. In stopping life-support, doctors are not causing death, he holds; they are not killing the patient; rather it is the disease that kills the patient. This issue is, of course, more thoroughly discussed in the earlier essays in this Part that we have grouped under the heading "Killing and Letting Die."

Callahan holds that the provision of voluntary euthanasia is incompatible with the aims of medicine. Often people will commit suicide or request euthanasia not only because they are ill, but also and predominantly because they find life oppressive, empty, or meaningless. But, he argues, it is "not medicine's place" to deal with the anguish we may feel when contemplating the human condition.

John Lachs disagrees. In "When Abstract Moralizing Runs Amok," he accuses Callahan of relying more on intuitional guideposts than on argument. But, Lachs holds, intuitions are inherently problematical. Rather than constituting an expression of eternal moral truths, they may simply echo traditional views that have not been subjected to much critical scrutiny.

Callahan also makes a slippery slope argument against the acceptance of voluntary euthanasia and supports this argument by referring to what he believed to be happening in the Netherlands. When Callahan wrote his article, in 1992, Dutch courts had ruled that doctors who carried out euthanasia in accordance with guidelines set by the Royal Dutch Medical Association should not be convicted of a crime; nevertheless the statute law that made euthanasia a crime still existed, and there was little data available to throw light on the consequences of permitting or prohibiting voluntary euthanasia. The Dutch Parliament legalized voluntary euthanasia in 2002. The situation in the Netherlands has now been studied thoroughly, and there are also studies from Belgium (which has also legalized voluntary euthanasia) and the US states of Oregon and Washington, which have legalized physician assistance in dying. Other studies in countries like Australia and New Zealand, where, at the time the studies were carried out, euthanasia and physician assistance in dying were illegal, allow comparisons of medical practice under different legal situations. These studies provide a good basis for assessing factual claims about the consequences of legalizing or not legalizing voluntary euthanasia and physician assistance in dying.[3]

Since the first edition of this *Anthology* was published more than two decades ago the global situation with regard to voluntary euthanasia and medically assisted suicide has changed radically. The number of jurisdictions where a medically assisted death is legally available in some form or shape has grown significantly from initially the Netherlands and Switzerland to include at the time of writing Belgium, Luxembourg, Colombia, Canada, New Zealand, Spain, Portugal and several states in Australia and the United States. In none of the jurisdictions that have made medically assisted dying available are significant efforts under way to criminalize the practice again. New ethical questions have emerged, most prominent among them whether legally binding advance directives (as discussed in the Dworkin and Dresser articles, Chapters 38 and 39 in this Part) should be made available to patients concerned about losing decisional capacity. Also under discussion today is the question of who should be eligible for assisted dying. While typically access is limited to decisionally capable dying adult patients, a small number of jurisdictions include among those eligible mature minors, as well as patients suffering from severe intractable mental health issues. The final two articles in this Section offer conflicting points of view on the question of whether decisionally capable patients suffering from intractable psychiatric illnesses should be eligible for assisted dying.

Bonnie Steinbock in her article "Physician-Assisted Death and Severe, Treatment-Resistant Depression"

discusses sound ethical reasons that could justify including decisionally capable patients suffering from intractable severe depression among those eligible to receive medical aid in dying. Steinbock describes what she considers slippery slope type cases that have occurred in permissive jurisdictions like the Netherlands and Belgium. She thinks that this ought to give pause for thought in legislators who are considering similar regulatory regimes. She also argues that the number of patients who would be eligible would likely be so small that it might not justify introducing potentially risky permissive regulatory regimes. Steinbock ends with a note of caution to policy makers, suggesting that jurisdictions that are in the process of introducing medical aid in dying should be "moving slowly to expand eligibility criteria when and if that is warranted."

William Rooney and his co-authors, in their article "Are Concerns About Irremediableness, Vulnerability, or Competence Sufficient to Justify Excluding All Psychiatric Patients from Medical Aid in Dying?", tackle what they consider to be the strongest reasons against giving such patients access to assisted dying. Among these reasons is the question of whether a disease that is intractable today would necessarily remain irremediable during a patient's biological life-span, the issue of whether psychiatric patients are so vulnerable that they require protections against abuse that might occur if medically assisted dying was available to them, and last but not least the reliability of decisional capacity assessments in psychiatric patients.

Unlike Steinbock, Rooney and co-authors conclude that a more permissive regime can operate at a defensible societal cost. That there is a possible cost, in terms of uncontroversially undesirable cases of assisted dying – they do not deny; but they also point out that refusing decisionally capable mentally ill patients access to assisted dying is not cost-neutral because it can mean that they must endure decades of unbearable suffering. Hence Rooney and his colleagues argue for stringent access restrictions but reject the view that we should refuse all psychiatric patients, regardless of individual circumstances, access to medically assisted dying.

Notes

1 Seneca, "58th Letter to Lucilius," trans. R. M. Gummere, in T. E. Page et al. (eds) *Seneca: Ad Lucilium Epistulae Morales*, vol. I, Heinemann: London, 1961, p. 409.

2 George Quittner, "Some thoughts on the life and death of Chris Hill," in Helga Kuhse (ed.) *Willing to Listen – Wanting to Die*. Ringwood, Vic: Penguin, 1994, p. 20

3 See e.g. P. J. van der Maas, G. van der Wal, I. Haverkate et al: "Euthanasia, physician assisted suicide, and other medical practices involving the end of life in the Netherlands, 1990–1995," *New England Journal of Medicine*, 1996, Vol. 335, pp. 1699–705; H. Kuhse, P. Singer, P. Baume, et al., "End-of-Life Decisions in Australian Medical Practice," *Medical Journal of Australia*, 1997, Vol. 166, pp. 191–6; Luc Deliens, Freddy Mortier, Johan Bilsen et al: "End-of-life decisions in medical practice in Flanders, Belgium: A nationwide survey", 2000, Vol. 356, pp. 1806–11; Kay Mitchell and R. Glynn Owens: "National survey of medical decisions at end of life made by New Zealand general practitioners", *British Medical Journal*, 2003, Vol. 327, pp. 202–3; Bregje D. Onwuteaka-Philipsen, Agnes van der Heide, Dirk Koper et al: "Euthanasia and other end-of-life decisions in the Netherlands in 1990, 1995, and 2001", *The Lancet*, 2003, Vol. 362, pp. 395–9. For official reports on the application of Oregon's Death with Dignity Act, see: http://public.health.oregon.gov/ProviderPartnerResources/EvaluationResearch/DeathwithDignityAct

20

The Sanctity of Life

Jonathan Glover

I cannot but have reverence for all that is called life. I cannot avoid compassion for all that is called life. That is the beginning and foundation of morality.

Albert Schweitzer, *Reverence for Life*

To persons who are not murderers, concentration camp administrators, or dreamers of sadistic fantasies, the inviolability of human life seems to be so self-evident that it might appear pointless to inquire into it. To inquire into it is embarrassing as well because, once raised, the question seems to commit us to beliefs we do not wish to espouse and to confront us with contradictions which seem to deny what is self-evident.

Edward Shils, 'The Sanctity of Life', in D. H. Labby, *Life or Death: Ethics and Options*, 1968

Most of us think it is wrong to kill people. Some think it is wrong in all circumstances, while others think that in special circumstances (say, in a just war or in self-defence) some killing may be justified. But even those who do not think killing is always wrong normally think that a special justification is needed. The assumption is that killing can at best only be justified to avoid a greater evil.

It is not obvious to many people what the answer is to the question '*Why* is killing wrong?' It is not clear whether the wrongness of killing should be treated as a kind of moral axiom, or whether it can be explained by appealing to some more fundamental principle or set of principles. One very common view is that some principle of the sanctity of life has to be included among the ultimate principles of any acceptable moral system.

In order to evaluate the view that life is sacred, it is necessary to distinguish between two different kinds of objection to killing: direct objections and those based on side-effects.

Original publication details: Jonathan Glover, "The Sanctity of Life," pp. 39–59 from *Causing Death and Lives* (London: Pelican, 1977).

Bioethics: An Anthology, Fourth Edition. Edited by Udo Schüklenk and Peter Singer.

1   Direct Objections and Side-Effects

Direct objections to killing are those that relate solely to the person killed. Side-effects of killings are effects on people other than the one killed. Many of the possible reasons for not killing someone appeal to side-effects. (To call them 'side-effects' is not to imply that they must be less important than the direct objections.) When a man dies or is killed, his parents, wife, children or friends may be made sad. His family may always have a less happy atmosphere and very likely less money to spend. The fatherless children may grow up to be less secure and confident than they would have been. The community loses whatever good contribution the man might otherwise have made to it. Also, an act of killing may help weaken the general reluctance to take life or else be thought to do so. Either way, it may do a bit to undermine everyone's sense of security.

Most people would probably give some weight to these side-effects in explaining the wrongness of killing, but would say that they are not the whole story, or even the main part of it. People who say this hold that there are direct objections to killing, independent of effects on others. This view can be brought out by an imaginary case in which an act of killing would have no harmful side-effects.

Suppose I am in prison, and have an incurable disease from which I shall very soon die. The man who shares my cell is bound to stay in prison for the rest of his life, as society thinks he is too dangerous to let out. He has no friends, and all his relations are dead. I have a poison that I could put in his food without him knowing it and that would kill him without being detectable. Everyone else would think he died from natural causes.

In this case, the objections to killing that are based on side-effects collapse. No one will be sad or deprived. The community will not miss his contribution. People will not feel insecure, as no one will know a murder has been committed. And even the possible argument based on one murder possibly weakening my own reluctance to take life in future carries no weight here, since I shall die before having opportunity for further killing. It might even be argued that consideration of side-effects tips the balance positively in favour of killing this man, since the cost of his food and shelter is a net loss to the community.

Those of us who feel that in this case we cannot accept that killing the man would be either morally right or morally neutral must hold that killing is at least sometimes wrong for reasons independent of side-effects. One version of this view that killing is directly wrong is the doctrine of the sanctity of life. To state this doctrine in an acceptable way is harder than it might at first seem.

2   Stating the Principle of the Sanctity of Life

The first difficulty is a minor one. We do not want to state the principle in such a way that it must have overriding authority over other considerations. To say 'taking life is always wrong' commits us to absolute pacifism. But clearly a pacifist and a non-pacifist can share the view that killing is in itself an evil. They need only differ over when, if ever, killing is permissible to avoid other evils. A better approximation is 'taking life is directly wrong', where the word 'directly' simply indicates that the wrongness is independent of effects on other people. But even this will not quite do. For, while someone who believes in the sanctity of life must hold that killing is directly wrong, not everyone who thinks that killing is sometimes or always directly wrong has to hold that life is sacred. (It is possible to believe that killing is directly wrong only where the person does not want to die or where the years of which he is deprived would have been happy ones. These objections to killing have nothing to do with side-effects and yet do not place value on life merely for its own sake.) The best formulation seems to be 'taking life is intrinsically wrong'.

There is another problem about what counts as 'life'. Does this include animals? When we think of higher animals, we may want to say 'yes', even if we want to give animal life less weight than human life.

But do we want to count it wrong to tread on an ant or kill a mosquito? And, even if we are prepared to treat all animal life as sacred, there are problems about plant life. Plants are living things. Is weeding the garden wrong? Let us avoid these difficulties for the moment by stating the principle in terms of human life. When we have become clearer about the reasons for thinking it wrong to kill people, we will be better placed to see whether the same reasons should make us respect animal or plant life as well. So, to start with, we have the principle: 'taking human life is intrinsically wrong'.

Can any explanation be given of the belief that taking human life is intrinsically wrong? Someone who simply says that this principle is an axiom of his moral system, and refuses to give any further explanation, cannot be 'refuted' unless his system is made inconsistent by the inclusion of this principle. (And, even then, he might choose to give up other beliefs rather than this one.) The strategy of this chapter will be to try to cast doubt on the acceptability of this principle by looking at the sort of explanation that might be given by a supporter who was prepared to enter into some discussion of it. My aim will be to suggest that the doctrine of the sanctity of life is not acceptable, but that there is embedded in it a moral view we should retain. We should reject the view that taking human life is *intrinsically* wrong, but retain the view that it is normally *directly* wrong: that most acts of killing people would be wrong in the absence of harmful side-effects.

The concept of human life itself raises notorious boundary problems. When does it begin? Is an eight-month fetus already a living human being? How about a newly fertilized egg? These questions need discussing, but it seems preferable to decide first on the central problem of why we value human life, and on that basis to draw its exact boundaries, rather than to stipulate the boundaries arbitrarily in advance. But there is another boundary problem that can be discussed first, as it leads us straight into the central issue about the sanctity of life. This boundary problem is about someone fallen irreversibly into a coma: does he still count as a living human being? (It

may be said that what is important is not the status of 'human being', but of 'person'. In this chapter I write as though human beings are automatically persons. [. . .])

3 The Boundary between Life and Death

It was once common to decide that someone was dead because, among other things, his heart had stopped beating. But now it is well known that people can sometimes be revived from this state, so some other criterion has to be used. Two candidates sometimes proposed are that 'death' should be defined in terms of the irreversible loss of all electrical activity in the brain or that it should be defined in terms of irreversible loss of consciousness.

Of these two definitions, the one in terms of irreversible loss of consciousness is preferable. There is no point in considering the electrical activity unless one holds the (surely correct) view that it is a necessary condition of the person being conscious. It seems better to define 'death' in terms of irreversible loss of consciousness itself, since it is from this alone that our interest in the electrical activity derives. This is reinforced by the fact that, while loss of all brain activity guarantees loss of consciousness, the converse does not hold. People incurably in a vegetable state normally have some electrical activity in some parts of the brain. To define 'death' in terms of irreversible loss of consciousness is not to deny that our best evidence for this may often be continued absence of electrical activity. And, when we understand more about the neurophysiological basis of consciousness, we may reach the stage of being able to judge conclusively from the state of his brain whether or not someone has irreversibly lost consciousness.

An argument sometimes used in favour of the definition in terms of irreversible loss of consciousness is that it avoids some of the problems that nowadays arise for adherents of more traditional criteria. Glanville Williams[1] has discussed a hypothetical case that might raise legal difficulties. Suppose a man's heart stops beating and, just as the doctor is about to revive him, the man's heir plunges a dagger into his breast. Glanville Williams wonders if this would count as murder or merely as illegal interference with a corpse. If, to avoid complications, we assume that there was a reasonable expectation that the man would otherwise have been revived, the question is one of the boundary between life and death. Making irreversible loss of consciousness the boundary has the advantage, over more traditional criteria, of making the heir's act one of murder.

It may be objected that, in ordinary language, it makes sense to say of someone that he is irreversibly comatose but still alive. This must be admitted. The proposed account of death is a piece of conceptual revision, motivated by the belief that, for such purposes as deciding whether or not to switch off a respirator, the irreversibly comatose and the traditionally 'dead' are on a par. Those who reject this belief will want to reject the 'irreversible loss of consciousness' account of death. And, if they do reject it, they are not forced to revert to traditional views that give a paradoxical answer to the Glanville Williams case. It would be possible to have two tests that must be passed before someone is counted as dead, involving respiratory and circulatory activities stopping *and* brain damage sufficient to make loss of consciousness irreversible. Let us call this the 'double-test' view.

In giving an account of 'death', how should we choose between irreversible loss of consciousness and the double-test view? If we are worried about doctors being wrong in their diagnosis of irreversible loss of consciousness, the double-test view would in practice give an additional safeguard against the respirator being switched off too early. But that is a rather oblique reason, even if of some practical importance. If detecting irreversible loss of consciousness posed no practical problem, how would we then choose between the two views? Appeals to traditional usage are of no value, for what is in question is a proposal for conceptual reform. The only way of choosing is to decide whether or not we attach any value to the preservation of someone irreversibly comatose. Do

we value 'life' even if unconscious, or do we value life only as a vehicle for consciousness? Our attitude to the doctrine of the sanctity of life very much depends on our answer to this question.

4 'Being Alive Is Intrinsically Valuable'

Someone who thinks that taking life is intrinsically wrong may explain this by saying that the state of being alive is itself intrinsically valuable. This claim barely rises to the level of an argument for the sanctity of life, for it simply asserts that there is value in what the taking of life takes away.

Against such a view, cases are sometimes cited of people who are either very miserable or in great pain, without any hope of cure. Might such people not be better off dead? But this could be admitted without giving up the view that life is intrinsically valuable. We could say that life has value, but that not being desperately miserable can have even more value.

I have no way of refuting someone who holds that being alive, even though unconscious, is intrinsically valuable. But it is a view that will seem unattractive to those of us who, in our own case, see a life of permanent coma as in no way preferable to death. From the subjective point of view, there is nothing to choose between the two. Schopenhauer saw this clearly when he said of the destruction of the body:

> But actually we feel this destruction only in the evils of illness or of old age; on the other hand, for the *subject*, death itself consists merely in the moment when consciousness vanishes, since the activity of the brain ceases. The extension of the stoppage to all the other parts of the organism which follows this is really already an event after death. Therefore, in a subjective respect, death concerns only consciousness.[2]

Those of us who think that the direct objections to killing have to do with death considered from the standpoint of the person killed will find it natural to regard life as being of value only as a necessary condition of consciousness. For permanently coma-tose existence is subjectively indistinguishable from death, and unlikely often to be thought intrinsically preferable to it by people thinking of their own future.

5 'Being Conscious Is Intrinsically Valuable'

The believer in the sanctity of life may accept that being alive is only of instrumental value and say that it is consciousness that is intrinsically valuable. In mak-ing this claim, he still differs from someone who only values consciousness because it is necessary for hap-piness. Before we can assess this belief in the intrinsic value of being conscious, it is necessary to distinguish between two different ways in which we may talk about consciousness. Sometimes we talk about 'mere' consciousness and sometimes we talk about what might be called 'a high level of consciousness'.

'Mere' consciousness consists simply in awareness or the having of experiences. When I am awake, I am aware of my environment. I have a stream of conscious-ness that comes abruptly to a halt if I faint or fades out when I go to sleep (until I have dreams). There are large philosophical problems about the meaning of claims of this kind, which need not be discussed here. I shall assume that we all at some level understand what it is to have experiences, or a stream of consciousness.

But this use of 'consciousness' should be distin-guished from another, perhaps metaphorical, use of the word. We sometimes say that men are at a higher level of consciousness than animals, or else that few, if any, peasants are likely to have as highly devel-oped a consciousness as Proust. It is not clear exactly what these claims come to, nor that the comparison between men and animals is of the same sort as the comparison between peasants and Proust. But perhaps what underlies such comparisons is an attempt to talk about a person's experiences in terms of the extent to which they are rich, varied, complex or subtle, or the extent to which they involve emotional responses, as well as various kind of awareness. Again, it is not

necessary to discuss here the analysis of the meaning of these claims. It is enough if it is clear that to place value on 'mere' consciousness is different from valu-ing it for its richness and variety. I shall assume that the claim that being conscious is intrinsically good is a claim about 'mere' consciousness, rather than about a high level of consciousness.

If one is sceptical about the intrinsic value of 'mere' consciousness, as against that of a high level of con-sciousness, it is hard to see what consideration can be mentioned in its favour. The advocate of this view might ask us to perform a thought experiment of a kind that G. E. Moore would perhaps have liked. We might be asked to imagine two universes, identical except that one contained a being aware of its envi-ronment and the other did not. It may be suggested that the universe containing the conscious being would be intrinsically better.

But such a thought experiment seems unconvinc-ing. There is the familiar difficulty that, confronted with a choice so abstract and remote, it may be hard to feel any preference at all. And, since we are deal-ing with 'mere' consciousness rather than with a high level of consciousness, it is necessary to postulate that the conscious being has no emotional responses. It cannot be pleased or sorry or in pain; it cannot be interested or bored; it is merely aware of its environ-ment. Views may well differ here, but, if I could be brought to take part in this thought experiment at all, I should probably express indifference between the two universes. The only grounds I might have for pre-ferring the universe with the conscious being would be some hope that it might evolve into some more interesting level of consciousness. But to choose on these grounds is not to assign any intrinsic value to 'mere' consciousness.

The belief that the sole reason why it is directly wrong to take human life is the intrinsic value of 'mere' consciousness runs into a problem concerning animals. Many of us place a special value on human life as against animal life. Yet animals, or at least the higher ones, seem no less aware of their surround-ings than we are. Suppose there is a flood and I am faced with the choice of either saving a man's life or else saving the life of a cow. Even if all side-effects were left out of account, failure to save the man seems worse than failure to save the cow. The person who believes that the sanctity of life rests solely on the value of 'mere' consciousness is faced with a dilemma. Either he must accept that the life of the cow and the life of the man are in themselves of equal value, or he must give reasons for thinking that cows are less conscious than men or else not conscious at all.

It is hard to defend the view that, while I have good grounds for thinking that other people are conscious, I do not have adequate reasons for thinking that animals are conscious. Humans and animals in many ways respond similarly to their surroundings. Humans have abilities that other animals do not, such as the ability to speak or to do highly abstract reasoning, but it is not only in virtue of these abilities that we say people are conscious. And there is no neurophysiological evidence that suggests that humans alone can have experiences.

The alternative claim is that animals are less conscious than we are. The view that 'mere' consciousness is a matter of degree is attractive when considered in relation to animals. The philosophical literature about our knowledge of other minds is strikingly silent and unhelpful about the animal boundaries of consciousness. How far back down the evolutionary scale does consciousness extend? What kind and degree of complexity must a nervous system exhibit to be the vehicle of experiences? What kind and degree of complexity of behaviour counts as the manifestation of consciousness? At least with our present ignorance of the physiological basis of human consciousness, any clear-cut boundaries of consciousness, drawn between one kind of animal and another, have an air of arbitrariness. For this reason it is attractive to suggest that consciousness is a matter of degree, not stopping abruptly, but fading away slowly as one descends the evolutionary scale.

But the belief that 'mere' consciousness is a matter of degree is obscure as well as attractive. Is it even an intelligible view?

There are two ways in which talk of degrees of consciousness can be made clearer. One is by explaining it in terms of the presence or absence of whole 'dimensions' of consciousness. This is the way in which a blind man is less conscious of his environment than a normal man. (Though, if his other senses have developed unusual acuity, he will in other respects be more conscious than a normal man.) But if a lower degree of consciousness consists either in the absence of a whole dimension such as sight, or in senses with lower acuity than those of men, it is not plausible to say that animals are all less conscious than we are. Dogs seem to have all the dimensions of consciousness that we do. It is true that they often see less well, but on the other hand their sense of smell is better than ours. If the sanctity of life were solely dependent on degree of consciousness interpreted this way, we often could not justify giving human life priority over animal life. We might also be committed to giving the life of a normal dog priority over the life of a blind man.

The other way in which we talk of degrees of 'mere' consciousness comes up in such contexts as waking up and falling asleep. There is a sleepy state in which we can be unaware of words that are softly spoken, but aware of any noise that is loud or sharp. But this again fails to separate men from animals. For animals are often alert in a way that is quite unlike the drowsiness of a man not fully awake.

Whether or not 'mere' consciousness fades away lower down on the evolutionary scale (and the idea of a sharp boundary *does* seem implausible), there seems at least no reason to regard the 'higher' animals as less aware of the environment than ourselves. (It is not being suggested that animals are only at the level of 'mere' consciousness, though no doubt they are less far above it than most of us.) If the whole basis of the ban on killing were the intrinsic value of mere consciousness, killing higher animals would be as bad as killing humans.

It would be possible to continue to hold mere consciousness to be of intrinsic value, and either to supplement this principle with others or else to abandon the priority given to human life. But when the principle is distinguished from different ones that would place a value on higher levels of consciousness, it has so little intuitive appeal that we may suspect its attractiveness to depend on the distinction not being made. If, in your own case, you would opt for a state never rising above mere consciousness, in preference to death, have you purged the illegitimate assumption that you would take an interest in what you would be aware of?

6 'Being Human Is Intrinsically Valuable'

It is worth mentioning that the objection to taking human life should not rest on what is sometimes called 'speciesism': human life being treated as having a special priority over animal life *simply* because it is human. The analogy is with racism, in its purest form, according to which people of a certain race ought to be treated differently *simply* because of their membership of that race, without any argument referring to special features of that race being given. This is objectionable partly because of its moral arbitrariness: unless some relevant empirical characteristics can be cited, there can be no argument for such discrimination. Those concerned to reform our treatment of animals point out that speciesism exhibits the same arbitrariness. It is not in itself sufficient argument for treating a creature less well to say simply that it is not a member of our species. An adequate justification must cite relevant differences between the species. We still have the question of what features of a life are of intrinsic value.

7 The Concept of a 'Life Worth Living'

I have suggested that, in destroying life or mere consciousness, we are not destroying anything intrinsically valuable. These states only matter because they are necessary for other things that matter in themselves. If a list could be made of all the things that are valuable for their own sake, these things would be the ingredients of a 'life worth living'.

One objection to the idea of judging that a life is worth living is that this seems to imply the possibility of comparing being alive and being dead. And, as Wittgenstein said, 'Death is not an event in life: we do not live to experience death.'

But we can have a preference for being alive over being dead, or for being conscious over being unconscious, without needing to make any 'comparisons' between these states. We prefer to be anaesthetized for a painful operation; queuing for a bus in the rain at midnight, we wish we were at home asleep; but for the most part we prefer to be awake and experience our life as it goes by. These preferences do not depend on any view about 'what it is like' being unconscious, and our preference for life does not depend on beliefs about 'what it is like' being dead. It is rather that we treat being dead or unconscious as nothing, and then decide whether a stretch of experience is better or worse than nothing. And this claim, that life of a certain sort is better than nothing, is an expression of our preference.

Any list of the ingredients of a worthwhile life would obviously be disputable. Most people might agree on many items, but many others could be endlessly argued over. It might be agreed that a happy life is worth living, but people do not agree on what happiness is. And some things that make life worth living may only debatably be to do with happiness. (Aristotle:[3] 'And so they tell us that Anaxagoras answered a man who was raising problems of this sort and asking why one should choose rather to be born than not – "for the sake of viewing the heavens and the whole order of the universe".')

A life worth living should not be confused with a morally virtuous life. Moral virtues such as honesty or a sense of fairness can belong to someone whose life is relatively bleak and empty. Music may enrich someone's life, or the death of a friend impoverish it, without him growing more or less virtuous.

I shall not try to say what sorts of things do make life worth living. (Temporary loss of a sense of the absurd led me to try to do so. But, apart from the disputability of any such list, I found that the ideal life suggested always sounded ridiculous.) I shall assume that a life worth living has more to it than mere consciousness. It should be possible to explain the wrongness of killing partly in terms of the destruction of a life worth living, without presupposing more than minimal agreement as to exactly what makes life worthwhile.

I shall assume that, where someone's life is worth living, this is a good reason for holding that it would be directly wrong to kill him. This is what can be extracted from the doctrine of the sanctity of life by someone who accepts the criticisms made here of that view. If life is worth preserving only because it is the vehicle for consciousness, and consciousness is of value only because it is necessary for something else, then that 'something else' is the heart of this particular objection to killing. It is what is meant by a 'life worth living' or a 'worthwhile life'.

The idea of dividing people's lives into ones that are worth living and ones that are not is likely to seem both presumptuous and dangerous. As well as seeming to indicate an arrogant willingness to pass godlike judgements on other people's lives, it may remind people of the Nazi policy of killing patients in mental hospitals. But there is really nothing godlike in such a judgement. It is not a moral judgement we are making, if we think that someone's life is so empty and unhappy as to be not worth living. It results from an attempt (obviously an extremely fallible one) to see his life from his own point of view and to see what he gets out of it. It must also be stressed that no suggestion is being made that it automatically becomes right to kill people whose lives we think are not worth living. It is only being argued that, if someone's life is worth living, this is *one* reason why it is directly wrong to kill him.

someone has a worthwhile life involves thinking from his point of view, rather than thinking of his contribution to the lives of other people.

This proposal would commit us to believing that a person cannot want to end his life if it is worth living, and that he cannot want to prolong his life where it is not worth living. But these beliefs are both doubtful. In a passing mood of depression, someone who normally gets a lot out of life may want to kill himself. And someone who thinks he will go to hell may wish to prolong his present life, however miserable he is. The frying pan may be worse than nothing but better than the fire. And some people, while not believing in hell, simply fear death. They may wish they had never been born, but still not want to die.

For these reasons, someone's own desire to live or die is not a conclusive indication of whether or not he has a life worth living. And, equally obviously, with people who clearly do have lives worth living, the relative strength of their desires to live is not a reliable indicator of how worthwhile they find their lives. Someone whose hopes are often disappointed may cling to life as tenaciously as the happiest person in the world.

If we are to make these judgements, we cannot escape appealing to our own independent beliefs about what sorts of things enrich or impoverish people's lives. But, when this has been said, it should be emphasized that, when the question arises whether someone's life is worth living at all, his own views will normally be evidence of an overwhelmingly powerful kind. Our assessments of what other people get out of their lives are so fallible that only a monster of self-confidence would feel no qualms about correcting the judgement of the person whose life is in question.

8   Is the Desire to Live the Criterion of a Worthwhile Life?

It might be thought that a conclusive test of whether or not someone's life is worth living is whether or not he wants to go on living. The attractiveness of this idea comes partly from the fact that the question whether

9   Length of Life

The upshot of this discussion is that one reason why it is wrong to kill is that it is wrong to destroy a life which is worth living.

This can be seen in a slightly different perspective when we remember that we must all die one day, so that killing and life-saving are interventions that alter length of life by bringing forward or postponing the date of death. An extreme statement of this perspective is to be found in St Augustine's *City of God*:

> There is no one, it goes without saying, who is not nearer to death this year than he was last year, nearer tomorrow than today, today than yesterday, who will not by and by be nearer than he is at the moment, or is not nearer at the present time than he was a little while ago. Any space of time that we live through leaves us with so much less time to live, and the remainder decreases with every passing day; so that the whole of our lifetime is nothing but a race towards death, in which no one is allowed the slightest pause or any slackening of the pace. All are driven on at the same speed, and hurried along the same road to the same goal. The man whose life was short passed his days as swiftly as the longer-lived; moments of equal length rushed by for both of them at equal speed, though one was farther than the other from the goal to which both were hastening at the same rate.

The objection to killing made here is that it is wrong to shorten a worthwhile life. Why is a longer-lasting worthwhile life a better thing than an equally worthwhile but briefer life? Some people, thinking about their own lives, consider length of life very desirable, while others consider the number of years they have is of no importance at all, the quality of their lives being all that matters.

There is an argument (echoed in Sartre's short story *Le Mur*) used by Marcus Aurelius in support of the view that length of life is unimportant:

> If a god were to tell you 'Tomorrow, or at least the day after, you will be dead', you would not, unless the most abject of men, be greatly solicitous whether it was to be the later day rather than the morrow, for what is the difference between them? In the same way, do not reckon if of great moment whether it will come years and years hence, or tomorrow.[4]

This argument is unconvincing. From the fact that some small differences are below the threshold of mattering to us, it does not follow that all differences are insignificant. If someone steals all your money except either a penny or twopence, you will not mind much which he has left you with. It does not follow that the difference between riches and poverty is trivial.

There are at least two good reasons why a longer life can be thought better than a short one. One is that the quality of life is not altogether independent of its length: many plans and projects would not be worth undertaking without a good chance of time for their fulfilment. The other reason is that, other things being equal, more of a good thing is always better than less of it. This does not entail such absurd consequences as that an enjoyable play gets better as it gets longer, without limit. The point of the phrase 'other things being equal' is to allow for waning of interest and for the claims of other activities. So, unless life begins to pall, it is not in any way unreasonable to want more of it and to place a value on the prolonging of other people's worthwhile lives.

This suggests an answer to a traditional scepticism about whether people are harmed by being killed. This scepticism is stated in its most extreme form by Socrates in the *Apology*: 'Now if there is no consciousness, but only a dreamless sleep, death must be a marvellous gain.' There is clearly some exaggeration here. Death is not a dreamless sleep, but something we can treat as on a par with it. There is the doubtful suggestion that people would normally prefer a dreamless sleep to their waking lives. But, stripped of these exaggerations, there remains the valid point that being dead is not a state we experience, and so cannot be unpleasant. It was this that led Lucretius to think that the fear of death was confused:

> If the future holds travail and anguish in store, the self must be in existence, when that time comes, in order to experience it. But from this fate we are redeemed by death, which denies existence to the self that might have suffered these tribulations.

He reinforced this by a comparison with the time before birth:

> Look back at the eternity that passed before we were born, and mark how utterly it counts to us as nothing. This is a mirror that nature holds up to us, in which

we may see the time that shall be after we are dead. Is there anything terrifying in the sight – anything depressing. . .?[5]

Lucretius is right that being dead is not itself a misfortune, but this does not show that it is irrational to want not to die, nor that killing someone does him no harm. For, while I will not be miserable when dead, I am happy while alive, and it is not confused to want more of a good thing rather than less of it.

Bernard Williams has suggested that a reply to Lucretius of this kind does not commit us to wanting to be immortal.[6] He argues that immortality is either inconceivable or terrible. Either desires and satisfactions change so much that it is not clear that the immortal person will still be *me*, or else they are limited by my character and will start to seem pointlessly boring: 'A man at arms can get cramp from standing too long at his post, but sentry-duty can after all be necessary. But the threat of monotony in eternal activities could not be dealt with in that way, by regarding immortal boredom as an unavoidable ache derived from standing ceaselessly at one's post.' It is true that the reply to Lucretius does not commit us to desiring immortality. But I am not convinced that someone with a fairly constant character *need* eventually become intolerably bored, so long as they can watch the world continue to unfold and go on asking new questions and thinking, and so long as there are other people to share their feelings and thoughts with. Given the company of the right people, I would be glad of the chance to sample a few million years and see how it went.

10   The 'No Trade-Off' View

In stating the principle of the sanctity of life, it seemed important not to suggest that it always took priority over other values: 'taking human life is intrinsically wrong', not 'taking human life is always wrong'. The same point holds for the acceptable principle that we have tried to extract from the sanctity of life view: 'it is wrong to destroy a life which is worth living'.

There is a tacit 'other things being equal' clause. For we can hold this view while thinking that the avoidance of other things even worse may sometimes have to take priority. We can have this objection to killing without being absolute pacifists.

The alternative, which may be called the 'no trade-off' view, gives an infinite value to not killing people (whose lives are worthwhile) compared to anything else. This may be because the *act* of killing seems infinitely appalling, which is an implausible view when we think of other horrendous acts, such as torturing. Or it may be because infinite value is set on worthwhile life itself. If this second alternative is chosen, it commits us to giving the saving of life overriding priority over all other social objectives. A piece of life-saving equipment is to be preferred to any amount of better housing, better schools or higher standard of living. Neither of these versions of the no trade-off view seems particularly attractive when the implications are clear.

11   The Social Effects of Abandoning the Sanctity of Life

Sometimes the doctrine of the sanctity of life is defended in an oblique way. The social implications of widespread abandonment of the view that taking human life is intrinsically wrong are said to be so appalling that, whatever its defects, the doctrine should not be criticized.

It must be faced that there is always a real possibility of producing a society where an indifference to the lives of at least some groups of people has terrible results. The sort of attitude is exhibited clearly in some passages from letters sent by the I.G. Farben chemical trust to the camp at Auschwitz.[7]

> In contemplation of experiments with a new soporific drug, we would appreciate your procuring for us a number of women. . .We received your answer but consider the price of 200 marks a woman excessive. We propose

to pay not more than 170 marks a head. If agreeable, we will take possession of the women. We need approximately 150. . .Received the order of 150 women. Despite their emaciated condition, they were found satisfactory. We shall keep you posted on developments concerning this experiment. . .The tests were made. All subjects died. We shall contact you shortly on the subject of a new load.

If criticism of the doctrine of the sanctity of life made even a small contribution to developing such attitudes, that would be an overwhelming reason for not making any criticism. But the views to be argued for here in no way give support to these attitudes. (It is the first and most elementary test to be passed by an adequate account of the morality of killing that it should not fail to condemn them.) It is a thesis of this book that conventional moral views about killing are often intellectually unsatisfactory. The attempt to replace the unsatisfactory parts of a moral outlook may even result in something less likely to be eroded.

References

1   Glanville Williams, *The Sanctity of Life and the Criminal Law* (London, 1958), ch. 1.
2   Arthur Schopenhauer, *The World as Will and Representation*, translated by E. J. F. Payne (New York, 1969), Book 4, section 54.
3   *Eudemian Ethics*, 1216 a 11.
4   Marcus Aurelius, *Meditations*, trans. M. Staniforth (Harmondsworth, 1964).
5   Lucretius, *The Nature of the Universe*, trans. R. E. Latham (Harmondsworth, 1951).
6   Bernard Williams, 'The Makropulos Case', in *Problems of the Self* (Cambridge, 1973).
7   Bruno Bettelheim, *The Informed Heart* (London, 1961), ch. 6.

21

Declaration on Euthanasia

Sacred Congregation for the Doctrine of the Faith

The Congregation considers it opportune to set forth the Church's teaching on euthanasia.

It is indeed true that, in this sphere of teaching, the recent popes have explained the principles, and these retain their full force;[1] but the progress of medical science in recent years has brought to the fore new aspects of the question of euthanasia, and these aspects call for further elucidation on the ethical level.

In modern society, in which even the fundamental values of human life are often called into question, cultural change exercises an influence upon the way of looking at suffering and death; moreover, medicine has increased its capacity to cure and to prolong life in particular circumstances, which sometimes give rise to moral problems. Thus people living in this situation experience no little anxiety about the meaning of advanced old age and death. They also begin to wonder whether they have the right to obtain for themselves or their fellowmen an "easy death", which would shorten suffering and which seems to them more in harmony with human dignity.

A number of Episcopal Conferences have raised questions on this subject with the Sacred Congregation for the Doctrine of the Faith. The Congregation, having sought the opinion of experts on the various aspects of euthanasia, now wishes to respond to the Bishops' questions with the present Declaration, in order to help them to give correct teaching to the faithful entrusted to their care, and to offer them elements for reflection that they can present to the civil authorities with regard to this very serious matter. . .

It is hoped that this Declaration will meet with the approval of many people of good will, who, philosophical or ideological differences notwithstanding, have nevertheless a lively awareness of the rights of the human person. These rights have often in fact been proclaimed in recent years through declarations issued by International Congresses;[2] and since it is a question here of fundamental rights inherent in every human person, it is obviously wrong to have recourse to arguments from political pluralism or religious freedom in order to deny the universal value of those rights.

I   The Value of Human Life

Human life is the basis of all goods, and is the necessary source and condition of every human activity

Original publication details: Sacred Congregation for the Doctrine of the Faith, "Declaration on Euthanasia" (Vatican City, 1980). Public domain.

and of all society. Most people regard life as something sacred and hold that no one may dispose of it at will, but believers see in life something greater, namely a gift of God's love, which they are called upon to preserve and make fruitful. And it is this latter consideration that gives rise to the following consequences:

1. No one can make an attempt on the life of an innocent person without opposing God's love for that person, without violating a fundamental right, and therefore without committing a crime of the utmost gravity.[3]
2. Everyone has the duty to lead his or her life in accordance with God's plan. That life is entrusted to the individual as a good that must bear fruit already here on earth, but that finds its full perfection only in eternal life.
3. Intentionally causing one's own death, or suicide, is therefore equally as wrong as murder; such an action on the part of a person is to be considered as a rejection of God's sovereignty and loving plan. Furthermore, suicide is also often a refusal of love for self, the denial of the natural instinct to live, a flight from the duties of justice and charity owed to one's neighbour, to various communities or to the whole of society – although, as is generally recognized, at times there are psychological factors present that can diminish responsibility or even completely remove it.

However, one must clearly distinguish suicide from that sacrifice of one's life whereby for a higher cause, such as God's glory, the salvation of souls or the service of one's brethren, a person offers his or her own life or puts it in danger (cf. *Jn* 15: 14).

II   Euthanasia

In order that the question of euthanasia can be properly dealt with, it is first necessary to define the words used.

Etymologically speaking, in ancient times *euthanasia* meant an *easy death* without severe suffering. Today one no longer thinks of this original meaning of the word, but rather of some intervention of medicine whereby the sufferings of sickness or of the final agony are reduced, sometimes also with the danger of suppressing life prematurely. Ultimately, the word *euthanasia* is used in a more particular sense to mean "mercy killing", for the purpose of putting an end to extreme suffering, or saving abnormal babies, the mentally ill or the incurably sick from the prolongation, perhaps for many years, of a miserable life, which could impose too heavy a burden on their families or on society.

It is therefore necessary to state clearly in what sense the word is used in the present document.

By euthanasia is understood an action or an omission which of itself or by intention causes death, in order that all suffering may in this way be eliminated. Euthanasia's terms of reference, therefore, are to be found in the intention of the will and in the methods used.

It is necessary to state firmly once more that nothing and no one can in any way permit the killing of an innocent human being, whether a fetus or an embryo, an infant or an adult, an old person, or one suffering from an incurable disease, or a person who is dying. Furthermore, no one is permitted to ask for this act of killing, either for himself or herself or for another person entrusted to his or her care, nor can he or she consent to it, either explicitly or implicitly. Nor can any authority legitimately recommend or permit such an action. For it is a question of the violation of the divine law, an offence against the dignity of the human person, a crime against life, and an attack on humanity.

It may happen that, by reason of prolonged and barely tolerable pain, for deeply personal or other reasons, people may be led to believe that they can legitimately ask for death or obtain it for others. Although in these cases the guilt of the individual may be reduced or completely absent, nevertheless the error of judgement into which the conscience falls, perhaps in good faith, does not change the nature of this act of killing, which will always be in itself something to be rejected. The pleas of gravely ill people who sometimes ask for death are not to be understood as implying a true desire for euthanasia; in fact it is almost always a case of an anguished plea for help and love.

What a sick person needs, besides medical care, is love, the human and supernatural warmth with which the sick person can and ought to be surrounded by all those close to him or her, parents and children, doctors and nurses.

III   The Meaning of Suffering for Christians and the Use of Painkillers

Death does not always come in dramatic circumstances after barely tolerable sufferings. Nor do we have to think only of extreme cases. Numerous testimonies which confirm one another lead one to the conclusion that nature itself has made provision to render more bearable at the moment of death separations that would be terribly painful to a person in full health. Hence it is that a prolonged illness, advanced old age, or a state of loneliness or neglect can bring about psychological conditions that facilitate the acceptance of death.

Nevertheless the fact remains that death, often preceded or accompanied by severe and prolonged suffering, is something which naturally causes people anguish.

Physical suffering is certainly an unavoidable element of the human condition; on the biological level, it constitutes a warning of which no one denies the usefulness; but, since it affects the human psychological makeup, it often exceeds its own biological usefulness and so can become so severe as to cause the desire to remove it at any cost.

According to Christian teaching, however, suffering, especially suffering during the last moments of life, has a special place in God's saving plan; it is in fact a sharing in Christ's Passion and a union with the redeeming sacrifice which he offered in obedience to the Father's will. Therefore one must not be surprised if some Christians prefer to moderate their use of painkillers, in order to accept voluntarily at least a part of their sufferings and thus associate themselves in a conscious way with the sufferings of Christ crucified (cf. *Mt* 27: 34). Nevertheless it would be imprudent to

impose a heroic way of acting as a general rule. On the contrary, human and Christian prudence suggest for the majority of sick people the use of medicines capable of alleviating or suppressing pain, even though these may cause as a secondary effect semiconsciousness and reduced lucidity. As for those who are not in a state to express themselves, one can reasonably presume that they wish to take these painkillers, and have them administered according to the doctor's advice.

But the intensive use of painkillers is not without difficulties, because the phenomenon of habituation generally makes it necessary to increase their dosage in order to maintain their efficacy. At this point it is fitting to recall a declaration by Pius XII, which retains its full force; in answer to a group of doctors who had put the question: "Is the suppression of pain and consciousness by the use of narcotics. . .permitted by religion and morality to the doctor and the patient (even at the approach of death and if one foresees that the use of narcotics will shorten life)?" the Pope said: "If no other means exist, and if, in the given circumstances, this does not prevent the carrying out of other religious and moral duties: Yes."[4] In this case, of course, death is in no way intended or sought, even if the risk of it is reasonably taken; the intention is simply to relieve pain effectively, using for this purpose painkillers available to medicine.

However, painkillers that cause unconsciousness need special consideration. For a person not only has to be able to satisfy his or her moral duties and family obligations; he or she also has to prepare himself or herself with full consciousness for meeting Christ. Thus Pius XII warns: "It is not right to deprive the dying person of consciousness without a serious reason."[5]

IV   Due Proportion in the Use of Remedies

Today it is very important to protect, at the moment of death, both the dignity of the human person and the Christian concept of life, against a technological attitude that threatens to become an abuse. Thus, some people speak of a "right to die", which is an expression that does not mean the right to procure death either by one's own hand or by means of someone else, as one pleases, but rather the right to die peacefully with human and Christian dignity. From this point of view, the use of therapeutic means can sometimes pose problems.

In numerous cases, the complexity of the situation can be such as to cause doubts about the way ethical principles should be applied. In the final analysis, it pertains to the conscience either of the sick person, or of those qualified to speak in the sick person's name, or of the doctors, to decide, in the light of moral obligations and of the various aspects of the case.

Everyone has the duty to care for his or her own health or to seek such care from others. Those whose task it is to care for the sick must do so conscientiously and administer the remedies that seem necessary or useful.

However, is it necessary in all circumstances to have recourse to all possible remedies?

In the past, moralists replied that one is never obliged to use "extraordinary" means. This reply, which as a principle still holds good, is perhaps less clear today, by reason of the imprecision of the term and the rapid progress made in the treatment of sickness. Thus some people prefer to speak of "proportionate" and "disproportionate" means. In any case, it will be possible to make a correct judgement as to the means by studying the type of treatment to be used, its degree of complexity or risk, its cost and the possibilities of using it, and comparing these elements with the result that can be expected, taking into account the state of the sick person and his or her physical and moral resources.

In order to facilitate the application of these general principles, the following clarifications can be added:

– If there are no other sufficient remedies, it is permitted, with the patient's consent, to have recourse to the means provided by the most advanced medical techniques, even if these means are still at the experimental stage and are not without a certain risk. By accepting them, the patient can even show generosity in the service of humanity.

– It is also permitted, with the patient's consent, to interrupt these means, where the results fall short of expectations. But for such a decision to be made, account will have to be taken of the reasonable wishes of the patient and the patient's family, as also of the advice of the doctors who are specially competent in the matter. The latter may in particular judge that the investment in instruments and personnel is disproportionate to the results foreseen; they may also judge that the techniques applied impose on the patient strain or suffering out of proportion with the benefits which he or she may gain from such techniques.

– It is also permissible to make do with the normal means that medicine can offer. Therefore one cannot impose on anyone the obligation to have recourse to a technique which is already in use but which carries a risk or is burdensome. Such a refusal is not the equivalent of suicide; on the contrary, it should be considered as an acceptance of the human condition, or a wish to avoid the application of a medical procedure disproportionate to the results that can be expected, or a desire not to impose excessive expense on the family or the community.

– When inevitable death is imminent in spite of the means used, it is permitted in conscience to take the decision to refuse forms of treatment that would only secure a precarious and burdensome prolongation of life, so long as the normal care due to the sick person in similar cases is not interrupted. In such circumstances the doctor has no reason to reproach himself with failing to help the person in danger.

Conclusion

The norms contained in the present Declaration are inspired by a profound desire to serve people in accordance with the plan of the Creator. Life is a gift of God, and on the other hand death is unavoidable; it is necessary therefore that we, without in any way hastening the hour of death, should be able to accept it with full responsibility and dignity. It is true that death marks the end of our earthly existence, but at the same time it opens the door to immortal life. Therefore all must prepare themselves for this event in the light of human values, and Christians even more so in the light of faith.

As for those who work in the medical profession, they ought to neglect no means of making all their skill available to the sick and the dying; but they should also remember how much more necessary it is to provide them with the comfort of boundless kindness and heartfelt charity. Such service to people is also service to Christ the Lord, who said: "As you did it to one of the least of these my brethren, you did it to me" (*Mt* 25: 40).

At the audience granted to the undersigned Prefect, His Holiness Pope John Paul II approved this Declaration, *adopted at the ordinary meeting of the Sacred Congregation for the Doctrine of the Faith, and ordered its publication.*

Rome, the Sacred Congregation for the Doctrine of the Faith, 5 May 1980.

Franjo Card. Šeper
Prefect

✠ Jérôme Hamer, O. P.
Tit. Archbishop of Lorium
Secretary

Notes

1   Pius XII, *Address to those attending the Congress of the International Union of Catholic Women's Leagues*, 11 September 1947: *AAS* 39 (1947), p. 483; *Address to the Italian Catholic Union of Midwives*, 29 October 1951: *AAS* 43 (1951), pp. 835–54; *Speech to the members of the International Office of military medicine documentation*, 19 October 1953: *AAS* 45 (1953), pp. 744–54; *Address to those taking part in the IXth Congress of the Italian Anaesthesiological Society*, 24 February 1957: *AAS* 49 (1957), pp. 146; cf. also *Address on "reanimation"*, 24 November 1957: *AAS* 49 (1957), pp. 1027–33; Paul. VI, *Address to the members of the United Nations Special Committee on Apartheid*, 22 May 1974: *AAS* 66 (1974), p. 346; John Paul II: *Address to the Bishops of the United States of America*, 5 October 1979: *AAS* 71 (1979), p. 1225.

2   One thinks especially of Recommendation 779 (1976) on the rights of the sick and dying, of the Parliamentary Assembly of the Council of Europe at its XXVIIth Ordinary Session; cf. Sipeca, no. 1 (March 1977), pp. 14–15.

3   We leave aside completely the problems of the death penalty and of war, which involve specific considerations that do not concern the present subject.

4   Pius XII, *Address of 24 February 1957: AAS* 49 (1957), p. 147.

5   Pius XII, ibid., p. 145; cf. *Address of 9 September 1958: AAS* 50 (1958), p. 694.

Killing and Letting Die

22

Active and Passive Euthanasia

James Rachels

The traditional distinction between active and passive euthanasia requires critical analysis. The conventional doctrine is that there is such an important moral difference between the two that, although the latter is sometimes permissible, the former is always forbidden. This doctrine may be challenged for several reasons. First of all, active euthanasia is in many cases more humane than passive euthanasia. Secondly, the conventional doctrine leads to decisions concerning life and death on irrelevant grounds. Thirdly, the doctrine rests on a distinction between killing and letting die that itself has no moral importance. Fourthly, the most common arguments in favor of the doctrine are invalid. I therefore suggest that the American Medical Association policy statement that endorses this doctrine is unsound.

The distinction between active and passive euthanasia is thought to be crucial for medical ethics. The idea is that it is permissible, at least in some cases, to withhold treatment and allow a patient to die, but it is never permissible to take any direct action designed to kill the patient. This doctrine seems to be accepted by most doctors, and it is endorsed in a statement adopted by the House of Delegates of the American Medical Association on December 4, 1973.

> The intentional termination of the life of one human being by another – mercy killing – is contrary to that for which the medical profession stands and is contrary to the policy of the American Medical Association.
>
> The cessation of the employment of extraordinary means to prolong the life of the body when there is irrefutable evidence that biological death is imminent is the decision of the patient and/or his immediate family. The advice and judgment of the physician should be freely available to the patient and/or his immediate family.

However, a strong case can be made against this doctrine. In what follows I will set out some of the relevant arguments, and urge doctors to reconsider their views on this matter.

To begin with a familiar type of situation, a patient who is dying of incurable cancer of the throat is in terrible pain, which can no longer be satisfactorily alleviated. He is certain to die within a few days, even if present treatment is continued, but he does not

Original publication details: James Rachels, "Active and Passive Euthanasia," pp. 78–80 from *New England Journal of Medicine* 292 (1975).
© 1975 Massachusetts Medical Society. Reproduced with permission of Massachusetts Medical Society.

Bioethics: An Anthology, Fourth Edition. Edited by Udo Schüklenk and Peter Singer.
Editorial material and organization © 2022 John Wiley & Sons, Inc. Published 2022 by John Wiley & Sons, Inc.

want to go on living for those days since the pain is unbearable. So he asks the doctor for an end to it, and his family joins in the request.

Suppose the doctor agrees to withhold treatment, as the conventional doctrine says he may. The justification for his doing so is that the patient is in terrible agony, and since he is going to die anyway, it would be wrong to prolong his suffering needlessly. But now notice this. If one simply withholds treatment, it may take the patient longer to die, and so he may suffer more than he would if more direct action were taken and a lethal injection given. This fact provides strong reason for thinking that, once the initial decision not to prolong his agony has been made, active euthanasia is actually preferable to passive euthanasia, rather than the reverse. To say otherwise is to endorse the option that leads to more suffering rather than less, and is contrary to the humanitarian impulse that prompts the decision not to prolong his life in the first place.

Part of my point is that the process of being "allowed to die" can be relatively slow and painful, whereas being given a lethal injection is relatively quick and painless. Let me give a different sort of example. In the United States about one in 600 babies is born with Down's syndrome. Most of these babies are otherwise healthy – that is, with only the usual pediatric care, they will proceed to an otherwise normal infancy. Some, however, are born with congenital defects such as intestinal obstructions that require operations if they are to live. Sometimes, the parents and the doctor will decide not to operate, and let the infant die. Anthony Shaw describes what happens then:

> When surgery is denied [the doctor] must try to keep the infant from suffering while natural forces sap the baby's life away. As a surgeon whose natural inclination is to use the scalpel to fight off death, standing by and watching a salvageable baby die is the most emotionally exhausting experience I know. It is easy at a conference, in a theoretical discussion, to decide that such infants should be allowed to die. It is altogether different to stand by in the nursery and watch as dehydration and infection wither a tiny being over hours and days. This is a terrible ordeal for me and the hospital staff – much more so than for the parents who never set foot in the nursery.[1]

I can understand why some people are opposed to all euthanasia, and insist that such infants must be allowed to live. I think I can also understand why other people favor destroying these babies quickly and painlessly. But why should anyone favor letting "dehydration and infection wither a tiny being over hours and days?" The doctrine that says that a baby may be allowed to dehydrate and wither, but may not be given an injection that would end its life without suffering, seems so patently cruel as to require no further refutation. The strong language is not intended to offend, but only to put the point in the clearest possible way.

My second argument is that the conventional doctrine leads to decisions concerning life and death made on irrelevant grounds.

Consider again the case of the infants with Down's syndrome who need operations for congenital defects unrelated to the syndrome to live. Sometimes, there is no operation, and the baby dies, but when there is no such defect, the baby lives on. Now, an operation such as that to remove an intestinal obstruction is not prohibitively difficult. The reason why such operations are not performed in these cases is, clearly, that the child has Down's syndrome and the parents and doctor judge that because of that fact it is better for the child to die.

But notice that this situation is absurd, no matter what view one takes of the lives and potentials of such babies. If the life of such an infant is worth preserving, what does it matter if it needs a simple operation? Or, if one thinks it better that such a baby should not live on, what difference does it make that it happens to have an unobstructed intestinal tract? In either case, the matter of life and death is being decided on irrelevant grounds. It is the Down's syndrome, and not the intestines, that is the issue. The matter should be decided, if at all, on that basis, and not be allowed to depend on the essentially irrelevant question of whether the intestinal tract is blocked.

What makes this situation possible, of course, is the idea that when there is an intestinal blockage, one can "let the baby die," but when there is no such defect there is nothing that can be done, for one must not "kill" it. The fact that this idea leads to such results as deciding life or death on irrelevant grounds is another good reason why the doctrine should be rejected.

One reason why so many people think that there is an important moral difference between active and passive euthanasia is that they think killing someone is morally worse than letting someone die. But is it? Is killing, in itself, worse than letting die? To investigate this issue, two cases may be considered that are exactly alike except that one involves killing whereas the other involves letting someone die. Then, it can be asked whether this difference makes any difference to the moral assessments. It is important that the cases be exactly alike, except for this one difference, since otherwise one cannot be confident that it is this difference and not some other that accounts for any variation in the assessments of the two cases. So, let us consider this pair of cases:

In the first. Smith stands to gain a large inheritance if anything should happen to his six-year-old cousin. One evening while the child is taking his bath. Smith sneaks into the bathroom and drowns the child, and then arranges things so that it will look like an accident.

In the second. Jones also stands to gain if anything should happen to his six-year-old cousin. Like Smith, Jones sneaks in planning to drown the child in his bath. However, just as he enters the bathroom Jones sees the child slip and hit his head, and fall face down in the water. Jones is delighted: he stands by, ready to push the child's head back under if it is necessary, but it is not necessary. With only a little thrashing about, the child drowns all by himself, "accidentally," as Jones watches and does nothing.

Now Smith killed the child, whereas Jones "merely" let the child die. That is the only difference between them. Did either man behave better, from a moral point of view? If the difference between killing and letting die were in itself a morally important matter, one should say that Jones's behavior was less reprehensible than Smith's. But does one really want to say that? I think not. In the first place, both men acted from the same motive, personal gain, and both had exactly the same end in view when they acted. It may be inferred

from Smith's conduct that he is a bad man, although that judgment may be withdrawn or modified if certain further facts are learned about him – for example, that he is mentally deranged. But would not the very same thing be inferred about Jones from his conduct? And would not the same further considerations also be relevant to any modification of this judgement? Moreover, suppose Jones pleaded, in his own defense. "After all, I didn't do anything except just stand there and watch the child drown. I didn't kill him: I only let him die." Again, if letting die were in itself less bad than killing, this defense should have at least some weight. But it does not. Such a "defense" can only be regarded as a grotesque perversion of moral reasoning. Morally speaking, it is no defense at all.

Now, it may be pointed out, quite properly, that the cases of euthanasia with which doctors are concerned are not like this at all. They do not involve personal gain or the destruction of normal healthy children. Doctors are concerned only with cases in which the patient's life is of no further use to him, or in which the patient's life has become or will soon become a terrible burden. However, the point is the same in these cases: the bare difference between killing and letting die does not, in itself, make a moral difference. If a doctor lets a patient die, for humane reasons, he is in the same moral position as if he had given the patient a lethal injection for humane reasons. If his decision was wrong – if, for example, the patient's illness was in fact curable – the decision would be equally regrettable no matter which method was used to carry it out. And if the doctor's decision was the right one, the method used is not in itself important.

The AMA policy statement isolates the crucial issue very well: the crucial issue is "the intentional termination of the life of one human being by another." But after identifying this issue, and forbidding "mercy killing," the statement goes on to deny that the cessation of treatment is the intentional termination of a life. This is where the mistake comes in, for what is the cessation of treatment, in these circumstances, if it is not "the intentional termination of the life of one human being by another?" Of course it is exactly that, and if it were not, there would be no point to it.

Many people will find this judgment hard to accept. One reason, I think, is that it is very easy to conflate the question of whether killing is, in itself, worse than letting die, with the very different question of whether most actual cases of killing are more reprehensible than most actual cases of letting die. Most actual cases of killing are clearly terrible (think, for example, of all the murders reported in the newspapers), and one hears of such cases every day. On the other hand, one hardly ever hears of a case of letting die, except for the actions of doctors who are motivated by humanitarian reasons. So one learns to think of killing in a much worse light than of letting die. But this does not mean that there is something about killing that makes it in itself worse than letting die, for it is not the bare difference between killing and letting die that makes the difference in these cases. Rather, the other factors – the murderer's motive of personal gain, for example, contrasted with the doctor's humanitarian motivation – account for different reactions to the different cases.

I have argued that killing is not in itself any worse than letting die: if my contention is right, it follows that active euthanasia is not any worse than passive euthanasia. What arguments can be given on the other side? The most common. I believe, is the following:

"The important difference between active and passive euthanasia is that, in passive euthanasia, the doctor does not do anything to bring about the patient's death. The doctor does nothing, and the patient dies of whatever ills already afflict him. In active euthanasia, however, the doctor does something to bring about the patient's death: he kills him. The doctor who gives the patient with cancer a lethal injection has himself caused his patient's death: whereas if he merely ceases treatment, the cancer is the cause of the death."

A number of points need to be made here. The first is that it is not exactly correct to say that in passive euthanasia the doctor does nothing, for he does do one thing that is very important: he lets the patient die. "Letting someone die" is certainly different, in some respects, from other types of action – mainly in that it is a kind of action that one may perform by way of not performing certain other actions. For example, one may let a patient die by way of not giving medication, just as one may insult someone by way of not shaking his hand. But for any purpose of moral assessment, it is a type of action nonetheless. The decision to let a patient die is subject to moral appraisal in the same way that a decision to kill him would be subject to moral appraisal: it may be assessed as wise or unwise, compassionate or sadistic, right or wrong. If a doctor deliberately let a patient die who was suffering from a routinely curable illness, the doctor would certainly be to blame for what he had done, just as he would be to blame if he had needlessly killed the patient. Charges against him would then be appropriate. If so, it would be no defense at all for him to insist that he didn't "do anything." He would have done something very serious indeed, for he let his patient die.

Fixing the cause of death may be very important from a legal point of view, for it may determine whether criminal charges are brought against the doctor. But I do not think that this notion can be used to show a moral difference between active and passive euthanasia. The reason why it is considered bad to be the cause of someone's death is that death is regarded as a great evil – and so it is. However, if it has been decided that euthanasia – even passive euthanasia – is desirable in a given case, it has also been decided that in this instance death is no greater an evil than the patient's continued existence. And if this is true, the usual reason for not wanting to be the cause of someone's death simply does not apply.

Finally, doctors may think that all of this is only of academic interest – the sort of thing that philosophers may worry about but that has no practical bearing on their own work. After all, doctors must be concerned about the legal consequences of what they do, and active euthanasia is clearly forbidden by the law. But even so, doctors should also be concerned with the fact that the law is forcing upon them a moral doctrine that may well be indefensible, and has a considerable effect on their practices. Of course, most doctors are not now in the position of being coerced in this matter, for they do not regard themselves as merely going along with what the law requires. Rather, in statements such as the AMA policy statement that I have quoted, they are endorsing this doctrine as a central point of medical ethics. In that statement, active euthanasia is condemned not merely as illegal but as "contrary to that for which the medical profession stands," whereas passive euthanasia is approved. However, the preceding considerations suggest that there is really no moral difference between the two, considered in themselves (there may be important moral differences in some cases in their *consequences*, but, as I pointed out, these differences may make active euthanasia, and not passive euthanasia, the morally preferable option). So, whereas doctors may have to discriminate between active and passive euthanasia to satisfy the law, they should not do any more than that. In particular, they should not give the distinction any added authority and weight by writing it into official statements of medical ethics.

Reference

1   A. Shaw 'Doctor, Do We Have a Choice?' *New York Times Magazine*. January 30, 1972, p. 54.

23

The Morality of Killing
A Traditional View

Germain Grisez and Joseph M. Boyle, Jr.

The Morality of Killing

In the strict sense one kills a person when, having considered bringing about a person's death as something one could do, one commits oneself to doing it by adopting this proposal instead of some alternative and by undertaking to execute it. By definition killing in the strict sense is an action contrary to the good of life. The adoption of a proposal to bring about someone's death is incompatible with respect for this good. Thus every act which is an act of killing in the strict sense is immoral. No additional circumstance or condition can remove this immorality.

This definition and moral characterization of killing in the strict sense make no distinction between intent to kill, attempt to kill, and the consummation of the undertaking by successful execution. These distinctions, which are legally significant, are morally irrelevant. If one commits oneself to realizing a certain state of affairs, by the commitment one constitutes oneself as a certain type of person. If one commits oneself to killing a person, one constitutes oneself a murderer. This remains true even if one is prevented

from attempting to execute one's purpose – for example, if someone else kills the intended victim first. Even more obviously it remains true if one attempts to execute one's purpose but fails – for example, if one shoots to kill but misses the intended victim.

Although everything which is an act of killing in the strict sense is immoral, not every deadly deed is an act of killing in this sense. As we have explained, some deadly deeds carry out a consciously projected design, but the performance is not the execution of a proposal adopted by the actor's choice to bring about the death of a human individual. The examples of the enraged wife and the dutiful soldier belong here. In what follows we call this type of performance a "deadly deed" to distinguish it from a killing in the strict sense.

Finally, there are other cases of causing death, such as some killing in self-defense, which are neither killing in the strict sense nor deadly deeds as here defined. The proposal adopted or the consciously projected design carried out by persons defending themselves might not extend beyond incapacitating the attacker, but this can result in the attacker's death if the only

Original publication details: Germain Grisez and Joseph M. Boyle, Jr., "The Morality of Killing: A Traditional View," pp. 381–419 from *Life and Death with Liberty and Justice: A Contribution to the Euthanasia Debate* (Notre Dame, IN: University of Notre Dame Press, 1971). Reproduced with permission of University of Notre Dame Press.

available and adequate means to incapacitate the attacker also will result in mortal wounds. . .

We turn now to the consideration of cases in which one brings about one's own death. Even in ordinary language some ethically significant distinctions are made in speaking of this, for one does not call "suicide" all cases in which someone causes his or her own death. Most people who consider suicide immoral do not class martyrs and heroes as suicides, since "suicide" suggests an act of killing oneself. Yet not all who commit suicide do a moral act of killing in the strict sense.

In cases in which suicide is an act of killing in the strict sense the proposal to kill oneself is among the proposals one considers in deliberation, and this proposal is adopted by choice as preferable to alternatives. For example, a person who for some reason is suffering greatly might think: "I wish I no longer had to suffer as I am suffering. If I were dead, my suffering would be at an end. But I am not likely to die soon. I could kill myself. But I fear death and what might follow after it. I could put up with my misery and perhaps find some other way out." One thinking in this way is deliberating. In saying "I could kill myself" suicide is proposed. If this proposal is adopted, one's moral act is killing in the strict sense. As in other instances this act is incompatible with the basic good of human life, and it cannot morally be justified, regardless of what else might be the case.

One can propose to kill oneself without saying to oneself "I could kill myself." One might say something which one would accept as equivalent in meaning: "I could destroy myself," "I could rub myself out," or something of the sort. Again, one might say something which one would admit amounts to "I could kill myself" although not equivalent in meaning to it, such as "I could shoot myself," when what one has in mind is shooting oneself in the head and thereby causing death, not merely shooting oneself to cause a wound. . .

There are still other cases in which individuals contribute to the causation of their own deaths by acts which are morally significant but which in no way execute proposals which are properly suicidal.

Typical martyrs lay down their lives. The death could be avoided if the martyr were willing to do something believed wrong or to leave unfulfilled some duty which is accepted as compelling. But the martyr refuses to avoid death by compromise or evasion of duty. Such persons do only what they believe to be morally required; the consequent loss of their own lives is willingly accepted by martyrs, neither sought nor chosen as a means to anything.

The martyr reasons somewhat as follows: "I would like to please everyone and to stay alive. But they are demanding of me that I do what I believe to be wrong or that I omit doing what I believe to be my sacred mission. They threaten me with death if I do not meet their demands. But if I were to comply with their threat, I would be doing evil in order that the good of saving my life might follow from it. This I may not do. Therefore, I must stand as long as I can in accord with my conscience, even though they are likely to kill me or torture me into submission."

Someone who does not understand the martyr's reasoning is likely to consider the martyr a suicide. But martyrs who reason thus do not propose to bring about their own deaths. The martyr bears witness to a profound commitment, first of all before the persecutors themselves. The latter can and in the martyr's view should accept this testimony and approve the rightness of the commitment. The martyr's refusal to give in does not bring about the persecutor's act of killing; the martyr only fails to win over the persecutor and to forestall the deadly deed. . .

Of course, we hold that suicide which is killing in the strict sense is necessarily immoral simply because it violates the basic good of human life. One who deliberately chooses to end his or her own life constitutes by this commitment a self-murderous self. But considerations which tell against even nonsuicidal acts which bring about a person's own death also argue against the moral justifiability of suicidal acts, which execute a proposal to destroy one's own life.

Considering matters from a moral point of view and from the side of the one whose life is to be ended, voluntary euthanasia is not significantly different from other cases of suicide. The proposal is to bring about death as a means to ending suffering. This proposal, if adopted and executed, is an instance of killing in the strict sense. It can never be morally justified.

Of course, a person who is in severe pain and who seeks death to escape it is likely to have mitigated responsibility or even to be drawn into acceptance without a deliberate choice, just as is the case with others whose suffering drives them to a deadly deed against themselves.

However, if an individual plans to seek euthanasia and arranges for it well in advance of the time of suffering, then the possibility that the demand for death is not an expression of deliberate choice is greatly lessened. The conditions which from the point of view of proponents of euthanasia are optimum for making a decision about the matter are precisely the conditions in which the decision is likely to be a morally unjustifiable act of killing in the strict sense.

Considering voluntary euthanasia from the point of view of the person who would carry out the killing, matters seem no better from a moral viewpoint. The performance can hardly fail to be an execution of a deliberate choice; the one carrying out the killing can hardly be driven to it, nor can anyone in the present culture accept the duty unquestioningly. . .

Nonvoluntary euthanasia also clearly proposes death as a treatment of choice. The act hardly can fail to be killing in the strict sense. And in addition to the violation of the good of life, the rights of those to be killed also will be violated – for example, by denial to them of equal protection of the laws. Nonvoluntary euthanasia would violate both life and justice. . .

The preceding treatment has been concerned with instances in which people bring about death by an outward performance. We now turn to a consideration of cases in which individuals refuse treatment for themselves or others, or withhold treatment, or fail or neglect to give it. To apply the moral theory which we articulated to such cases we must first say something about omissions.

If people act when they carry out a proposal which they have adopted by choice, certain cases of outward nonperformance must count as human actions. One can adopt a proposal and carry it out by deliberately not causing or preventing something which one could cause or prevent. One's choice not to cause or prevent something can be a way of realizing a state of affairs one considers somehow desirable. For example, one might adopt the proposal to protest against a government policy permitting the use of public funds for abortion by not paying certain taxes. In this case one aims to realize a desired state of affairs by means of nonconformance with the demands of the law. The nonconformance need involve no outward performance at all.

Omissions of this type – those in which one undertakes to realize a proposed state of affairs by not causing or preventing something – are very important for understanding the morality of withholding treatment from dying patients, refusing treatment proposed for oneself, and in general letting people die.

It clearly is possible to kill in the strict sense by deliberately letting someone die. If one adopts the proposal to bring about a person's death and realizes this proposal by not behaving as one otherwise would behave, then one is committed to the state of affairs which includes the person's death. This commitment, although carried out by a nonperformance, is morally speaking an act of killing. It involves the adoption and execution of a proposal contrary to the basic good of human life. Thus, any case in which one chooses the proposal that a person die and on this basis allows the person to die is necessarily immoral.

For example, if a child is born suffering from various defects and if the physicians and parents decide that the child, the family, and society will all be better off if the burdens entailed by the child's continued life are forestalled by its death, and if they therefore adopt the proposal not to perform a simple operation, which otherwise would be done, so that the child will die, then the parents and physicians morally speaking kill the child – "kill" in the strict sense clarified at the beginning of this chapter. The fact that there is no blood spilled, no poison injected, that the death certificate can honestly show that the child has died from complications arising from its defective condition – none of this is morally relevant. The moral act is no different from any other moral act of murder.

The same thing will be true in every instance in which a judgement is made that someone – whether oneself or another – would be better off dead, the proposal to bring about death by not causing or preventing something is considered and adopted, and this proposal is executed by outward nonperformance of behavior which one otherwise might have attempted. . .

Michael Tooley and others also have criticized those who hold that there is a significant moral difference between killing a person and letting the person die. Their criticism is that if one considers a case of killing and a case of letting die between which there is no difference except that in the one the death is brought about by a performance which causes it while in the other it is brought about by not causing or preventing something, then there is no moral difference between the two cases.

We agree. Both actions are killing in the strict sense; neither can ever be moral. However, not every instance in which someone deliberately lets another die is an action shaped by the proposal that the person whose death is accepted should die or die sooner than would otherwise be the case. We turn now to the consideration of such deliberate omissions which, considered from a moral point of view, are not acts of killing.

The fundamental point about these omissions is that one can omit to do some good or prevent some evil without adopting any proposal which either is opposed to the good or embraces (as means) the evil whose occurrence one accepts. This possibility is most obviously instantiated when one must forgo doing a certain good or preventing a certain evil because one has a duty, incompatible with doing the good or preventing the evil, to do some other good or prevent some other evil.

For example, in an emergency situation in which many people are seriously injured and the medical resources – including time and personnel – are limited, those making decisions must choose to treat some and put off the treatment of others, perhaps with fatal consequences to those not treated first. The nontreatment of those who are not treated is deliberate; even

their deaths might be foreseen as an inevitable consequence and knowingly accepted when the decision to treat others is made. Yet plainly the nontreatment of those who are not treated need involve no proposal that these people should die or die more quickly than they otherwise would. Provided there is no partiality or other breach of faith with those not treated, the execution of a proposal to save others does not embrace the death of those who die, and no immorality is done. . .

There is another type of reason for forgoing doing good which involves no disrespect for the good which would be realized by the action. One might notice that doing the action good in itself will in fact bring about many undesirable consequences. And one might choose not to adopt the proposal to do the good in order to avoid accepting these various bad consequences. This situation is exemplified in a very important way in many instances in which potentially life-prolonging treatment is refused, withheld, or withdrawn – even in the case of a patient who is not dying – because of the expected disadvantages of accepting, carrying out, or continuing treatment. . .

We have articulated grounds on which someone might reasonably consider treatment undesirable: if the treatment is experimental or risky, if it would be painful or otherwise experienced negatively, if it would interfere with activities or experiences the patient might otherwise enjoy, if it would conflict with some moral or religious principle to which the patient adheres, if it would be psychologically repugnant to the patient, or if the financial or other impact of the treatment upon other persons would constitute a compelling reason to refuse treatment.

The moral legitimacy of refusing treatment in some cases on some such grounds certainly was part of what Pius XII was indicating by his famous distinction between ordinary and extraordinary means of treatment. The Pope defined "extraordinary means" as ones which involve a "great burden," and he allowed that one could morally forgo the use of extraordinary means. The conception of extraordinary means clearly is abused, however, when the proposal is to bring about death by the omission of treatment, and the difficulties of the treatment are pointed to by way of rationalizing the murderous act. If it is decided that a person would be better off dead and that treatment which would be given to another will be withheld because of the poor quality of the life to be preserved, then the focus in decision is not upon the means and its disadvantageous consequences. Rather, what is feared is that the means would be effective, that life would be preserved, and that the life itself and its consequences would be a burden.

Moreover, even when treatment is refused, withheld, or withdrawn because of an objection to the means – and without the adopting of a proposal to bring about death – there still can be a serious moral failing.

A person who refuses lifesaving or life-prolonging treatment, not on a suicidal proposal but because of great repugnance for the treatment itself, might have an obligation to maintain life longer in order to fulfill duties toward others.

For example, someone on dialysis might wish to give up the treatment because of the difficulties it involves, and some persons in this situation could discontinue treatment and accept death without moral fault. But a parent with children in need of continued care, a professional person with grave responsibilities, and many other persons who can prolong their lives at considerable sacrifice to themselves are morally bound to do so, even by this extraordinary means, because they have accepted duties which others are entitled to have fulfilled, and persons who love the goods as one ought will faithfully fulfill duties toward others at considerable cost to themselves.

Similarly, if one refuses, withholds, or withdraws lifesaving or life-prolonging treatment for another because of the grave burdens entailed by such treatment, the burdens must be grave indeed. This is especially clear in cases in which the patient is not dying – for example, cases of defective infants. One must be quite sure, at the least, that with no suicidal proposal one would in the patient's place not wish the treatment. Otherwise, one accepts moral responsibility for a very grave wrong toward the patient.

24

Is Killing No Worse Than Letting Die?

Winston Nesbitt

I want in this paper to consider a kind of argument sometimes produced against the thesis that it is worse to kill someone (that is, to deliberately take action that results in another's death) than merely to allow someone to die (that is, deliberately to fail to take steps which were available and which would have saved another's life). Let us, for brevity's sake, refer to this as the 'difference thesis', since it implies that there is a moral difference between killing and letting die.

One approach commonly taken by opponents of the difference thesis is to produce examples of cases in which an agent does not kill, but merely lets someone die, and yet would be generally agreed to be just as morally reprehensible as if he had killed. This kind of appeal to common intuitions might seem an unsatisfactory way of approaching the issue. It has been argued[1] that what stance one takes concerning the difference thesis will depend on the ethical theory one holds, so that we cannot decide what stance is correct independently of deciding what is the correct moral theory. I do not, however, wish to object to the approach in question on these grounds. It may be true that different moral theories dictate different stances concerning the difference thesis, so that a theoretically satisfactory defence or refutation of the thesis requires a satisfactory defence of a theory which entails its soundness or unsoundness. However, the issue of its soundness or otherwise is a vital one in the attempt to decide some pressing moral questions,[2] and we cannot wait for a demonstration of the correct moral theory before taking up any kind of position with regard to it. Moreover, decisions on moral questions directly affecting practice are rarely derived from ethical first principles, but are usually based at some level on common intuitions, and it is arguable that at least where the question is one of public policy, this is as it should be.

2

It might seem at first glance a simple matter to show at least that common moral intuitions favour the difference thesis. Compare, to take an example of John Ladd's,[3] the case in which I push someone who I know cannot swim into a river, thereby killing her,

Original publication details: Winston Nesbitt, "Is Killing No Worse Than Letting Die?" pp. 101–105 from *Journal of Applied Philosophy* 12: 1 (1995). Reproduced with permission of John Wiley & Sons.

Bioethics: An Anthology, Fourth Edition. Edited by Udo Schüklenk and Peter Singer.

with that in which I come across someone drowning and fail to rescue her, although I am able to do so, thereby letting her die. Wouldn't most of us agree that my behaviour is morally worse in the first case?

However, it would be generally agreed by those involved in the debate that nothing of importance for our issue, not even concerning common opinion, can be learned through considering such an example. As Ladd points out, without being told any more about the cases mentioned, we are inclined to assume that there are other morally relevant differences between them, because there usually would be. We assume, for example, some malicious motive in the case of killing, but perhaps only fear or indifference in the case of failing to save. James Rachels and Michael Tooley, both of whom argue against the difference thesis, make similar points,[4] as does Raziel Abelson, in a paper defending the thesis.[5] Tooley, for example, notes that as well as differences in motives, there are also certain other morally relevant differences between typical acts of killing and typical acts of failing to save which may make us judge them differently. Typically, saving someone requires more effort than refraining from killing someone. Again, an act of killing necessarily results in someone's death, but an act of failing to save does not – someone else may come to the rescue. Factors such as these, it is suggested, may account for our tendency to judge failure to save (i.e., letting die) less harshly than killing. Tooley concludes that if one wishes to appeal to intuitions here, 'one must be careful to confine one's attention to pairs of cases that do not differ in these, or other significant respects.'[6]

Accordingly, efforts are made by opponents of the difference thesis to produce pairs of cases which do not differ in morally significant respects (other than in one being a case of killing while the other is a case of letting die or failing to save). In fact, at least the major part of the case mounted by Rachels and Tooley against the difference thesis consists of the production of such examples. It is suggested that when we compare a case of killing with one which differs from it *only* in being a case of letting die, we will agree that either agent is as culpable as the other; and this is then taken to show that any inclination we ordinarily

have to think killing worse than letting die is attributable to our tending, illegitimately, to think of typical cases of killing and of letting die, which differ in other morally relevant respects. I want now to examine the kind of example usually produced in these contexts.

3

I will begin with the examples produced by James Rachels in the article mentioned earlier, which is fast becoming one of the most frequently reprinted articles in the area.[7] Although the article has been the subject of a good deal of discussion, as far as I know the points which I will make concerning it have not been previously made. Rachels asks us to compare the following two cases. The first is that of Smith, who will gain a large inheritance should his six-year-old nephew die. With this in mind, Smith one evening sneaks into the bathroom where his nephew is taking a bath, and drowns him. The other case, that of Jones, is identical, except that as Jones is about to drown his nephew, the child slips, hits his head, and falls, face down and unconscious, into the bath-water. Jones, delighted at his good fortune, watches as his nephew drowns.

Rachels assumes that we will readily agree that Smith, who kills his nephew, is no worse, morally speaking, than Jones, who merely lets his nephew die. Do we really want to say, he asks, that either behaves better from the moral point of view than the other? It would, he suggests, be a 'grotesque perversion of moral reasoning' for Jones to argue, 'After all, I didn't do anything except just stand and watch the child drown. I didn't kill him; I only let him die.'[8] Yet, Rachels says, if letting die were in itself less bad than killing, this defence would carry some weight.

There is little doubt that Rachels is correct in taking it that we will agree that Smith behaves no worse in his examples than does Jones. Before we are persuaded by this that killing someone is in itself morally no worse than letting someone die, though, we need to consider the examples more closely. We concede that Jones, who merely let his nephew die, is just as reprehensible as Smith, who killed his nephew. Let us ask, however, just what is the ground of our judgement of the agent in each case. In the case of Smith, this seems to be adequately captured by saying that Smith drowned his nephew for motives of personal gain. But can we say that the grounds on which we judge Jones to be reprehensible, and just as reprehensible as Smith, are that he let his nephew drown for motives of personal gain? I suggest not – for this neglects to mention a crucial fact about Jones, namely that he was fully prepared to kill his nephew, and would have done so had it proved necessary. It would be generally accepted, I think, quite independently of the present debate, that someone who is fully prepared to perform a reprehensible action, in the expectation of certain circumstances, but does not do so because the expected circumstances do not eventuate, is just as reprehensible as someone who actually performs that action in those circumstances. Now this alone is sufficient to account for our judging Jones as harshly as Smith. He was fully prepared to do what Smith did, and would have done so if circumstances had not turned out differently from those in Smith's case. Thus, though we may agree that he is just as reprehensible as Smith, this cannot be taken as showing that his letting his nephew die is as reprehensible as Smith's killing his nephew – for we would have judged him just as harshly, given what he was prepared to do, even if he had not let his nephew die. To make this clear, suppose that we modify Jones' story along the following lines – as before, he sneaks into the bathroom while his nephew is bathing, with the intention of drowning the child in his bath. This time, however, just before he can seize the child, *he* slips and hits his head on the bath, knocking himself unconscious. By the time he regains consciousness, the child, unaware of his intentions, has called his parents, and the opportunity is gone. Here, Jones neither kills his nephew *nor* lets him die – yet I think it would be agreed that given his preparedness to kill the child for personal gain, he is as reprehensible as Smith.

The examples produced by Michael Tooley, in the book referred to earlier, suffer the same defect as those produced by Rachels. Tooley asks us to consider the following pair of scenarios, as it happens also featuring Smith and Jones. In the first, Jones is about to shoot Smith when he sees that Smith will be killed by a bomb unless Jones warns him, as he easily can. Jones does not warn him, and he is killed by the bomb – i.e., Jones lets Smith die. In the other, Jones wants Smith dead, and shoots him – i.e., he kills Smith.

Tooley elsewhere[9] produces this further example: two sons are looking forward to the death of their wealthy father, and decide independently to poison him. One puts poison in his father's whiskey, and is discovered doing so by the other, who was just about to do the same. The latter then allows his father to drink the poisoned whiskey, and refrains from giving him the antidote, which he happens to possess.

Tooley is confident that we will agree that in each pair of cases, the agent who kills is morally no worse than the one who lets die. It will be clear, however, that his examples are open to criticisms parallel to those just produced against Rachels. To take first the case where Jones is saved the trouble of killing Smith by the fortunate circumstance of a bomb's being about to explode near the latter: it is true that we judge Jones to be just as reprehensible as if he had killed Smith, but since he was fully prepared to kill him had he not been saved the trouble by the bomb, we would make the same judgement even if he had neither killed Smith nor let him die (even if, say, no bomb had been present, but Smith suffered a massive and timely heart attack). As for the example of the like-minded sons, here too the son who didn't kill was prepared to do so, and given this, would be as reprehensible as the other even if he had not let his father die (if, say, he did not happen to possess the antidote, and so was powerless to save him).

Let us try to spell out more clearly just where the examples produced by Rachels and Tooley fail. What both writers overlook is that what determines whether someone is reprehensible or not is not simply what he in fact does, but what he is prepared to do, perhaps as revealed by what he in fact does. Thus, while Rachels is correct in taking it that we will be inclined to judge Smith and Jones in his examples equally harshly, this is not surprising, since both are judged reprehensible for precisely the same reason, namely that they were fully prepared to kill for motives of personal gain. The same, of course, is true of Tooley's examples. In each example he gives of an agent who lets another die, the agent is fully prepared to kill (though in the event, he is spared the necessity). In their efforts to ensure that the members of each pair of cases they produce do not differ in any morally relevant respect (except that one is a case of killing and the other of letting die), Rachels and Tooley make them *too* similar – not only do Rachels' Smith and Jones, for example, have identical motives, but both are guilty of the same moral offence.

4

Given the foregoing account of the failings of the examples produced by Rachels and Tooley, what modifications do they require if they are to be legitimately used to gauge our attitudes towards killing and letting die, respectively? Let us again concentrate on Rachels' examples. Clearly, if his argument is to avoid the defect pointed out, we must stipulate that though Jones was prepared to let his nephew die once he saw that this would happen unless he intervened, he was not prepared to kill the child. The story will now go something like this: Jones stands to gain considerably from his nephew's death, as before, but he is not prepared to kill him for this reason. However, he happens to be on hand when his nephew slips, hits his head, and falls face down in the bath. Remembering that he will profit from the child's death, he allows him to drown. We need, however, to make a further stipulation, regarding the explanation of Jones' not being prepared to kill his nephew. It cannot be that he fears untoward consequences for himself, such as detection and punishment, or that he is too lazy to choose such an active course, or that the idea simply had not occurred to him. I think it would be common ground in the debate that if the only explanation of his not being prepared to kill his nephew was one of these kinds, he would be morally no better than Smith, who differed only in being more daring, or

more energetic, whether or not fate then happened to offer him the opportunity to let his nephew die instead. In that case, we must suppose that the reason Jones is prepared to let his nephew die, but not to kill him, is a moral one – not intervening to save the child, he holds, is one thing, but actually bringing about his death is another, and altogether beyond the pale.

I suggest, then, that the case with which we must compare that of Smith is this: Jones happens to be on hand when his nephew slips, hits his head, and falls unconscious into his bath-water. It is clear to Jones that the child will drown if he does not intervene. He remembers that the child's death would be greatly to his advantage, and does not intervene. Though he is prepared to let the child die, however, and in fact does so, he would not have been prepared to kill him, because, as he might put it, wicked though he is, he draws the line at killing for gain.

I am not entirely sure what the general opinion would be here as to the relative reprehensibility of Smith and Jones. I can only report my own, which is that Smith's behaviour is indeed morally worse than that of Jones. What I do want to insist on, however, is that, for the reasons I have given, we cannot take our reactions to the examples provided by Rachels and Tooley as an indication of our intuitions concerning the relative heinousness of killing and of letting die.

So far, we have restricted ourselves to discussion of common intuitions on our question, and made no attempt to argue for any particular answer. I will conclude by pointing out that, given the fairly common view that the *raison d'être* of morality is to make it possible for people to live together in reasonable peace and security, it is not difficult to provide a rationale for the intuition that in our modified version of Rachels' examples, Jones is less reprehensible than Smith. For it is clearly preferable to have Jones-like persons around rather than Smith-like ones. We are not threatened by the former – such a person will not save me if my life should be in danger, but in this he is no more dangerous than an incapacitated person, or for that matter, a rock or tree (in fact he may be better, for he *might* save me as long as he doesn't think he will profit from my death). Smith-like persons, however, *are* a threat – if such a person should come to believe that she will benefit sufficiently from my death, then not only must I expect no help from her if my life happens to be in danger, but I must fear positive attempts on my life. In that case, given the view mentioned of the point of morality, people prepared to behave as Smith does are clearly of greater concern from the moral point of view than those prepared only to behave as Jones does; which is to say that killing is indeed morally worse than letting die.

Notes

1   See, for example, John Chandler (1990), 'Killing and letting die – putting the debate in context', *Australasian Journal of Philosophy*, 68, no. 4, pp. 420–31.

2   It underlies, or is often claimed to underlie, for example, the Roman Catholic position on certain issues in the abortion debate, and the view that while 'passive' euthanasia may sometimes be permissible, 'active' euthanasia never is. It also seems involved in the common view that even if it is wrong to fail to give aid to the starving of the world, thereby letting them die, it is not as wrong as dropping bombs on them, thereby killing them.

3   John Ladd (1985), 'Positive and negative euthanasia' in James E. White (ed.), *Contemporary Moral Problems* (St Paul: West Publishing Co), pp. 58–68.

4   James Rachels (1979), 'Active and passive euthanasia,' in James Rachels (ed.), *Moral Problems* (New York: Harper and Row), pp. 490–7; Michael Tooley (1983), *Abortion and Infanticide* (Oxford: Clarendon Press), pp. 187–8. [See Chapters 22 and 1, respectively, in this *Anthology*.]

5   Raziel Abelson (1982), 'There is a moral difference,' in Raziel Abelson and Marie-Louise Friquegnon (eds.), *Ethics for Modern Life* (New York: St Martin's Press), pp. 73–83.

6   Tooley, *Abortion and Infanticide*, p. 189.

7   Rachels, 'Active and passive euthanasia'.

8   Ibid., p. 494.

9   Michael Tooley (1980), 'An irrelevant consideration: killing and letting die' in Bonnie Steinbock (ed.), *Killing and Letting Die* (Englewood Cliffs, NJ: Prentice-Hall), pp. 56–62.

25

Why Killing is Not Always Worse – and Sometimes Better – Than Letting Die

Helga Kuhse

I

The conventional assumption is that killing a person is worse than allowing her to die. Beginning with James Rachels' famous article "Active and Passive Euthanasia", first published in the *New England Journal of Medicine* in 1975[1] this "difference thesis"[2] has been challenged by producing pairs of cases in which an agent who lets someone die would generally be judged to be no less reprehensible than an agent who kills. In a recent article, Winston Nesbitt argues that these pairs of cases typically contain a crucial common feature which will indeed make *these* cases of letting die the same as killing.[3] Once this crucial feature is removed, he holds, these cases will support, rather than undermine, the difference view.

Winston Nesbitt's argument in support of the difference thesis rests on a number of contestable assumptions. In briefly retracing his argument, I shall leave these assumptions unchallenged, to show then that *even if* we accept these assumptions, Nesbitt's conclusion – that killing is worse than letting die – does not follow.

It will be adequate, for our purposes, to focus on just one of the paired examples discussed by Nesbitt: James Rachels' case of the "nasty uncles".[4] The first case involves Smith, who will gain a large inheritance should his six-year-old nephew die. One evening, Smith sneaks into the bathroom where his nephew is taking a bath, and drowns him. The second case, that of Jones, is exactly like the first case, except that as Jones is about to drown his nephew, the child slips, hits his head, and falls, face down and unconscious, into the water. Jones is delighted, and stands by as his nephew drowns.

In these examples, both men were motivated by personal gain, and both were aiming at the child's death. The only relevant difference between the cases is that Smith killed the child, whereas Jones allowed the child to die. But that difference, Rachels claims, is not morally relevant in itself, and the difference thesis is false.

Nesbitt agrees with Rachels that these examples support the common intuition that Jones is no less reprehensible than Smith, and that there is, in these cases, no difference between killing and allowing to

Original publication details: Helga Kuhse, "Why Killing Is Not Always Worse – and Sometimes Better – Than Letting Die," pp. 371–374 from *Cambridge Quarterly of Healthcare* 7: 4 (1998). Reproduced with permission of Cambridge University Press.

die. The reason is, Nesbitt holds, that both agents were prepared to kill, for the sake of personal gain. After all, Jones was no less prepared to kill than Smith was – except that an accident (the child slipping, hitting his head and falling face down in the water) obviated the need for Jones to act on his intention. "[W]hat determines whether someone is reprehensible or not", Nesbitt holds, "is not what he in fact does but what he is prepared to do, perhaps as revealed by what he in fact does" (p. 104).

This entails, Nesbitt continues, that Rachels' examples cannot show that the difference thesis is false. Both cases contain the morally relevant feature that the agent was *prepared* to kill. To test the difference thesis, this common feature must be removed. We must assume that Jones believes the difference thesis to be true, and that he was prepared to let his nephew die, but, unlike Smith, was not prepared to kill the child (p. 104). In this case, Nesbitt holds, we might indeed want to judge Smith more reprehensible than Jones.

It is this difference, the difference between an agent being prepared to kill and an agent merely being prepared to let die, that is, according to Nesbitt, morally significant – at least if we accept the widely held view that "the *raison d'être* of morality is to make it possible for people to live together in reasonable peace and security" (p. 105).

We are not threatened, Nesbitt concludes his argument, if a person is prepared to allow another to die, but is not prepared to kill. Such a person "will not save me if my life should be in danger, but in this he is no more dangerous than an incapacitated person, or for that matter, a rock or a tree". A person who is prepared to kill, on the other hand, *is* a threat.

> If such a person should come to believe that she will benefit sufficiently from my death, then not only must I expect no help from her if my life happens to be in danger, but I must fear positive attempts on my life. In that case, given the view mentioned of the point of morality, people prepared to behave as Smith does are clearly of greater concern from the moral point of view than those prepared only to behave as Jones does; which is to say that killing is indeed morally worse than letting die. (p. 105)

II

Let us accept that Nesbitt is correct and that we should indeed be more concerned by the presence of Smith-type persons than by Jones-type persons. But what does this show? Does it show, as Nesbitt holds, that "killing is indeed morally worse than letting die", or does it show that it is worse if agents, who are motivated by personal gain, are not merely content to stand by as "nature" bestows some good on them, but are also prepared to intervene in the course of nature, to achieve their ends?

There is an illegitimate conflation in Winston Nesbitt's argument between the rightness and wrongness of actions, and the goodness and badness of agents.[5] We might thus agree that it is a bad thing for individuals to be motivated by personal gain, rather than by, say, the common good, and that it is *worse*, other things being equal, if such an agent is not only prepared to "let death happen", but to "make death happen".[6] But this is not, of course, the same as showing that killing is worse than letting die. Killing may be worse than letting die in these cases, and better than letting die in others.

Consider the following case, similar to a case that came before the Swedish courts some years ago:

> A truck driver and his co-driver had an accident on a lonely stretch of road. The truck caught fire and the driver was trapped in the wreckage of the cabin. The co-driver struggled to free him, but could not do so. The driver, by now burning, pleaded with his colleague – an experienced shooter – to take a rifle, which was stowed in a box on the back of the truck, and shoot him. The co-driver took the rifle and shot his colleague.

Was what the co-driver did morally reprehensible? Did he act wrongly? Students who are presented with this case will generally answer both questions in the negative. The reason for their intuitions is not hard to find. In this case, the agent was not motivated by personal gain, but by compassion. He acted not to benefit himself, but to benefit another. Should we feel threatened by such agents? Hardly. We should be comforted by their presence. Conversely, however, we should feel threatened, or at least abandoned, if we were surrounded by agents who believed in the difference thesis and behaved like "an incapacitated person, or. . .a rock or a tree", who would "let us die" when we sincerely wanted someone "to make us die".

Not only does Nesbitt conflate the distinction between agents and actions, he also implicitly assumes that death is always and everywhere an evil. If this view is already challenged by the above example, it has been utterly rejected in the practice of medicine by patients and doctors alike. Patients and doctors do not believe that life is always a good and will, in many cases, deliberately choose a shorter life over a longer one. Terminally or incurably ill patients standardly refuse life-sustaining treatment, and doctors allow these patients to die, for the patients' good. To put it slightly differently, while death is normally an evil, and to kill a person (or to let her die when we could save her) is harming her, this is not the case when continued life presents an intolerable burden to the person whose life it is. In short, then, doctors who are "letting" a patient die, for the patient's good, are benefiting rather than harming the patient – they are practising what is often called "passive euthanasia".

If patients can, however, be benefited by being "let die", because death is a good, then they can also be benefited by being killed – by the doctor practising "active euthanasia". Indeed, in some cases, active euthanasia will be preferable, from the patient's point of view, to passive euthanasia: being "let die" may involve unwanted protracted pain and suffering for the patient, and fail to give her the dignified death she wants. Moreover, there are patients for whom death would be a good, but who do not need life support, and whom the doctor cannot let die. This means that a doctor who is merely prepared to "let die", but not to "make die", is, once again, like an incapacitated person, a rock or a tree, who, while not preventing good befalling some patients, will merely stand by and do nothing to make the good happen for others.[7]

If the *raison d'être* of morality is to allow people to live together in relative peace and security, what kind of motivation would we like doctors to have, and what kinds of action would we like them to perform? Clearly, we would like them to be motivated to primarily seek *our* good, rather than their own; to keep us alive, if this is in our best interests, and to "let" us die, or to "make" us die, when either one of these actions serves us best. If this is correct, the difference thesis is false. Killing is not always worse than letting die. Sometimes it is morally better.

III

James Rachels had devised the case of "the nasty uncles" to demonstrate that there is no intrinsic moral difference between killing and letting die, or active and passive euthanasia. Now, if Nesbitt is right, Rachels' example of the "nasty uncles" fails to show that the difference thesis is false. If I am right, however, Nesbitt in turn fails to establish the truth of the difference thesis. While he has shown that killing is sometimes worse than letting die, I have shown that killing is sometimes better than letting die.

This has clear implications for the public debate over (voluntary) euthanasia. Nesbitt accepts that the truth or falsity of the difference thesis may ultimately depend on the truth of the moral theory that underpins it. But, he says, "we cannot wait for a demonstration of the correct moral theory" before we attempt to make decisions on pressing moral questions, such as "active" or "passive" euthanasia (or killing a patient and letting her die). Rather, answers to practical public-policy questions are rarely derived from first ethical principles, but are, quite properly, based on common intuitions (p. 101, n. 2).

Acceptance of Nesbitt's "common intuition" view would lead one to question the contemporary blanket public-policy distinction between active and passive euthanasia: while doctors are typically permitted, by law, to "let" patients die, at the patients' request, they are almost everywhere prohibited from "making" them die. In countries like Australia, Britain and the United States, recognition of people's common intuitions would, however, lead one to the view that not only passive, but also active voluntary euthanasia should be allowed.[8]

Far from establishing the truth of the difference thesis, Winston Nesbitt has undermined the very thesis he set out support. Not only is active euthanasia no worse than passive euthanasia, and sometimes morally better; his argument also lends support to the view that public policies should allow some forms of active euthanasia.

Notes

1 Rachels, J. 'Active and Passive Euthanasia', *New England Journal of Medicine* (9 January, 1975): 78–80. [See Chapter 22 in this *Anthology*.]

2 See note 3; Nesbitt, p. 101.

3 Nesbitt, W. 'Is Killing No Worse Than Letting Die?' *Journal of Applied Philosophy*, 12 (1) (1995): 101–6.

4 See note 2.

5 Kuhse, H. *The Sanctity of Life Doctrine in Medicine – A Critique* (Oxford: Clarendon Press, 1987), pp. 88–90, 142, 148, 158–63. See also 'Frankena W. McCormick and the Traditional Distinction' in R. McCormick and P. Ramsey (eds), *Doing Evil to Achieve Good* (Chicago: Loyola University Press, 1978).

6 Walton, D. *On Defining Death* (Montreal: McGill–Queens University Press, 1979), pp. 118–20; Kuhse (see note 5), pp. 79–81.

7 Here it is, of course, important to not confuse the distinction between killing and letting die, or between "making happen" and "letting happen" with the distinction between actions and omissions. In distinction from a tree or a rock, an agent may act to "let happen" – for example, by telling the nurse not to attach the patient to a respirator, or by turning the respirator off. See note 5, Kuhse, chs 2 and 3.

8 Opinion polls in these countries have consistently shown strong public support for active voluntary euthanasia. For the opinions of some groups of health-care professionals see, for example, Heilig, S., 'The SFMS Euthanasia Survey: Results and Analyses', *San Francisco Medicine* (May, 1988): 24–6, 34; Ward, B. J., 'Attitudes among NHS Doctors to Requests for Euthanasia', *BMJ*, 308 (1995): 1332–4; Baume P. and O'Malley, E., 'Euthanasia: Attitudes and Practices of Medical Practitioners', *Medical Journal of Australia*, 161 (1994): 137–44; Kuhse, H. and Singer, P., 'Voluntary Euthanasia and the Nurse: an Australian Survey', *International Journal of Nursing Studies*, 30(4) (1993): 311–22.

26

Moral Fictions and Medical Ethics

Franklin G. Miller, Robert D. Truog, and Dan W. Brock

John and Sam are motorcycle enthusiasts. At age 50 both of them have serious accidents that leave them quadriplegic and dependent on a ventilator to breathe. Two years after the accident John remains ventilator-dependent, whereas Sam has regained the capacity to breathe spontaneously and has been weaned off his ventilator. During the third year after their accidents, both John and Sam find their lives intolerable; they don't want to go on living because of their complete dependence on others for the activities of daily life and the associated absence of privacy. John requests to be admitted to the hospital where he was treated after the accident, in order to have his home ventilator withdrawn and receive the palliative care he needs to die peacefully. Hospital clinicians are initially reluctant to honor John's request but agree to do so after being persuaded that he is a competent decision-maker who has thought carefully about his situation. Sam requests his physician to administer a lethal dose of medication so that he can die a swift and dignified death. Although Sam's physician is sympathetic to his request, he refuses to comply with it because active euthanasia, even with consent, is contrary to the law and medical ethics.

Why are the normative responses to these two patient requests so different within the prevailing stance of medical ethics? John's decision to die by stopping treatment is not considered suicide, despite the fact that he is not terminally ill and has the potential to live at least 10 years while being maintained on a ventilator. Rather, it is understood as a refusal of burdensome or unwanted treatment. Because it is not suicide, the assistance of physicians and nurses in agreeing to withdraw the ventilator is not assisted suicide. In stopping the ventilator they are omitting to continue life-sustaining treatment; they are not performing voluntary active euthanasia. Instead, their conduct is sometimes described as 'passive euthanasia.' They do not kill John, but merely allow him to die from his underlying spinal cord injury and inability to breathe spontaneously. They do not (and must not) intend to cause John's death, but do and must respect his right to refuse treatment. John's medical condition, not the ventilator withdrawal, is considered the cause of death. Accordingly, the clinicians agreeing to stop John's ventilator are not morally responsible for a death-causing act. Their conduct is morally

Original publication details: Franklin G. Miller, Robert D. Truog, and Dan W. Brock, "Moral Fictions and Medical Ethics," pp. 453–460 from *Bioethics* 24: 9 (2010). Reproduced with permission of John Wiley & Sons.

permissible; indeed, it is (arguably) morally obligatory, as competent patients have a right to refuse unwanted medical treatment. Refusing to honor patients' refusals of medical treatment amounts to battery under the common law; and patients have a constitutional right to refuse medical treatment, endorsed by the US Supreme Court in the Cruzan case.[1]

In contrast, Sam is asking for help in causing his death; hence, his request can be understood as suicidal. If what he does is not committing suicide, it is because the final act that causes death, when a physician accedes to Sam's request, is performed by the physician. This act is characterized as (voluntary) active euthanasia. Clearly, a physician deliberately administering a known lethal dose of medication would be intending to cause the patient's death, and thus would be morally responsible for killing the patient. Such conduct is morally forbidden in prevailing medical ethics throughout the world and is treated legally as criminal homicide, except in the Netherlands and Belgium.

In this article we challenge the standard assessment within medical ethics of withdrawing life-sustaining treatment [WLST] and voluntary active euthanasia [VAE]. The major points in our ethical analysis are not original, as both we and other commentators have made similar points about the lack of a cogent basis for treating withdrawing life-sustaining treatment as fundamentally different from assisted suicide and active euthanasia, from an ethical perspective.[2] Yet standard medical ethics and the law have remained impervious to this critique. We suggest that the concept of *moral fictions*, as applied to the contrasting characterization of the cases of John and Sam, can help exhibit concretely how and why the conventional moral conceptualization is radically mistaken.

The Concept of Moral Fictions

Fictions are commonplace in the law, but they have received scant attention in medical ethics. Fictions are false statements; but not all false statements are fictions. Fictions are *motivated* false statements, endorsed in order

to uphold a position felt to be important.[3] (By stressing the motivated character of moral fictions, we do not suggest that the motivation to endorse false beliefs is always conscious.) For those critics who do not share the motivation – the commitment to the position in question – fictions appear to be patently false or confused. Moral fictions are false statements endorsed to uphold cherished or entrenched moral positions in the face of conduct that is in tension with these established moral positions. Professionals are uncomfortable with the thought that they may be practising unethically. Especially when routine practices, viewed candidly, appear to conflict with established norms, there is a strong incentive to construe these practices in a way that removes the conflict. Moral fictions serve this purpose. In other words, moral fictions can be understood as a tool for counteracting a form of cognitive dissonance[4] – specifically, the cognitive dissonance constituted by the inconsistency between routine practices and prevailing norms.

Viewed without the confabulations of moral fictions, accepted end-of-life practices patently conflict with standard medical ethics. The moral fictions relating to end-of-life decisions are motivated to make morally challenging medical practices, such as withdrawing life-sustaining treatment and providing pain-relieving medication at the risk of hastening death, consistent with the norm that doctors must not kill, or assist in killing, patients. We shall argue that the underlying fault that the moral fictions conceal lies not in accepted practices, which are justified, but in established norms that cannot withstand critical scrutiny.

Two types of moral fictions are on display in the standard assessment of John's request to withdraw life-sustaining treatment (see Table 26.1). First, as we demonstrate below, the description of withdrawing life-sustaining treatment involves a series of motivated false factual statements. These include false statements about the nature of the patient's request, the nature of the act that clinicians are asked to perform in this case, the causal relationship between the act of treatment withdrawal and the patient's death, and the intention of physicians who accede to such requests. Second,

Table 26.1 Comparing end-of-life decisions
Consider two cases: (1) ventilator-dependent quadriplegic requests withdrawal of ventilator (WLST); (2) quadriplegic, who has regained spontaneous breathing and weaning from ventilator, requests lethal dose of medication (VAE)

Status quo		
	WLST	VAE
Is the doctor causing death?	No	Yes
Is it an active intervention?	No	Yes
Is the doctor intending death?	No	Yes
Does the doctor kill the patient?	No	Yes
Is it suicide?	No	Maybe
Is it assisted suicide	No	Maybe
Is the doctor morally responsible for death?	No	Yes
Is it permitted morally?	Yes	No
Is it legal?	Yes	No

Without moral fictions		
	WLST	VAE
Is the doctor causing death?	Yes	Yes
Is it an active intervention?	Yes	Yes
Is the doctor intending death?	Sometimes Yes, sometimes No	Yes
Does the doctor kill the patient?	Yes	Yes
Is it suicide?	Yes	Yes
Is it assisted suicide?	Yes	Yes
Is the doctor morally responsible for death?	Yes	Yes
Is it permitted morally?	Yes	Yes
Is/should it be legal?	Yes	Open question

there are erroneous moral judgments based on these mistaken factual claims: judgments about moral responsibility and moral permissibility. When shorn of these moral fictions, the differential moral assessment of complying with the patient requests of John and Sam is undermined.

Appeal to fictions in moral discourse does not entail deliberate fabrication, lying, or deception. Most people who espouse moral fictions believe them (in good faith) to be true. Moreover, because these fictions are culturally entrenched, even when

their falsity or invalidity is exposed, not everyone will agree that a given proposition counts as a moral fiction. Moral fictions, according to our analysis, differ from legal fictions in that the latter are never believed to be literally true propositions. For example, the legal doctrines that a corporation is a person, or that persons who are absent and unaccounted for are considered dead after a period of seven years, are not taken as true statements of fact. Rather, the law treats corporations *as if* they are persons and missing persons as if they are dead. Those who appeal to moral fictions, however, typically assert them with confidence as literally true.

Exposing the Moral Fictions

Suicide

If we think of suicide literally as aiming at and causing one's own death, then both John and Sam are making suicidal requests. There is a difference between the situations of John and Sam, which might be thought relevant to whether their respective requests are suicidal. John has a burdensome life-sustaining treatment and Sam does not. Might John's aim be to stop the burden of the ventilator but not to end his life? Assuming, however, that it is the pervasive paralysis and associated burdens that are driving John's judgment that his life is not worth living, then his decision to seek withdrawal of life-sustaining treatment does not stem from the mere fact that he needs the assistance of a burdensome mechanical ventilator to breathe. For the sake of this analysis, we make the reasonable supposition that he would be no less interested in ending his life if he were in the same condition as Sam, who is able to breathe spontaneously.

To be sure, the description of suicide for these two cases might be resisted because neither patient is directly capable of causing his own death and each is seeking the help of others to do so. Yet both John and Sam are aiming at death, for only death in their eyes will free them from a condition that they find intolerable; and it is their request for help in dying that sets in motion the causal chain leading to death when clinicians comply with their requests.

Another reason to resist the use of 'suicide' in these cases is that suicide is thought typically to reflect irrational conduct, driven by depression or psychosis. Both John and Sam find their lives no longer worth living in the light of the disabilities caused by spinal cord injury. Some may disagree with their personal quality-of-life assessments, but it is difficult to see their aim to end their lives as irrational, especially in the case of individuals who have completed rehabilitation and had ample time to adjust to a life with paralysis below the neck. The concept of rational suicide is not incoherent, unless one stipulates dogmatically (thus begging the question) that it is always irrational to opt for death, no matter what the circumstances. Hence, we conclude that it is a moral fiction to assert that the requests of either John or Sam are not suicidal.

Suppose we concede that John and Sam are seeking suicide. It would seem natural to infer that both are requesting assisted suicide; for they need the help of someone else to realize their wish to die. Nevertheless, from a conceptual perspective it might be insisted that regardless of the suicidal nature of the requests of John and Sam, clinicians who accede to these requests are not engaging in assisted suicide because the immediate death-causing act is performed by the physician, not the patient. As a matter of linguistic stipulation there is no objection to this stance. Yet we see no reason why some life-terminating acts (including the cases of John and Sam) cannot be legitimately described as both assisted suicide and active euthanasia; even though others can only be described as one or the other: prescribing a lethal dose of medication ingested by a patient is assisted suicide, not active euthanasia; whereas giving a lethal dose of medication to an incompetent patient, who has not voluntarily requested to end her life, is active non-voluntary euthanasia, not assisted suicide. In any case, the standard assessment in medical ethics of compliance with John's request rejects the label of 'assisted suicide' because of moral fictions concerning causation and intention that we discuss below.

Causation

How should we think about the act of an attending physician who complies with John's request to stop his ventilator? According to conventional medical ethics, the withdrawal of life-sustaining therapy allows the patient to die from his underlying spinal cord injury and inability to breathe spontaneously; it is an omission of treatment, not an act that causes the patient's death.[5] We contend that this familiar account flies in the face of a candid look at the facts. Now at 50 years of age, John has the potential to live for a decade or more supported by continued mechanical ventilation and personal care. What explains his death following withdrawal of mechanical ventilation is not the course of his spinal cord injury but the act of turning off the ventilator. It is the proximate cause of death. Moreover, disconnecting the ventilator without his consent would be homicide. The very same act of stopping treatment that causes death in the latter case of homicide is performed by a clinician with John's consent.[6] The consent makes the difference between homicide and legitimate treatment withdrawal, but this ethical and legal difference has nothing to do with the cause of the patient's death, which is the same in both cases.

Withdrawing life-sustaining treatment, when followed shortly by the patient's death, is a life-terminating intervention. Indeed, the very fact that mechanical ventilation can sustain life for those patients incapable of breathing on their own implies that stopping mechanical ventilation will end the life of these patients. In other words, the power to sustain life by technological means goes hand-in-hand with the power to end life when these means are withheld or withdrawn. This characterization of medical practice in the case of life-sustaining therapy is an obvious application of our common sense understanding of causation,[7] which is obscured by the moral fictions embraced by conventional medical ethics. To be sure, John's inability to breathe on his own is part of the causal explanation for why he dies after his ventilator is stopped. If Sam happened to be attached temporarily to a ventilator, he most likely would not die if the ventilator were stopped. But in John's case, the withdrawal of the ventilator contributes causally to his death precisely because had it not been withdrawn he would continue living, probably for a substantial period of time. The withdrawal of the ventilator is what results in John's dying at the time and in the manner that he does. Hence, we conclude that it is a fiction to describe John's death following withdrawal of the ventilator as merely allowing him to die and not causing his death.

This fiction about causation is closely tied to another fiction about killing. The ordinary common sense notion of A killing B is that A performs an action that causes B's death. The moral fiction that John's physician does not cause his death by removing the ventilator seems also to imply that he does not kill John. And if he does not kill John, then what he must do is allow John to die of his underlying disease. The conceptual picture in this view is that John has a lethal condition, his inability to breathe on his own, that the ventilator is keeping that lethal condition from proceeding to John's death, and so when the physician removes the ventilator in doing so he merely allows John's lethal disease process to proceed unimpeded to his death. The moral fiction about causation is thus closely related to another moral fiction about the difference between killing and allowing to die and, more specifically, about whether stopping the ventilator is killing or allowing to die.

It is important to correct a widespread misconception about the use of 'killing' to describe the death-causing act of withdrawing life-sustaining treatment. In the medical context, 'killing' is commonly understood as meaning the unjustified taking of life, despite the fact that we recognize that in other contexts, such as self-defence, killing can be justified. Accordingly, it seems jarring to describe withdrawing life support as killing. We understand 'killing' in medicine, however, to mean causing death, which may or may not be morally justified, depending on the circumstances.

Intention

Withdrawing life-sustaining treatment is considered legally permitted and ethically justified when it is based on a valid refusal of treatment by a competent patient or by an authorized surrogate decision-maker, based on the prior preferences of the patient or a sound judgment about the patient's best interest. In medical ethics, however, according to the conventional view, it is unethical for physicians to intend to cause death. To square these two potentially conflicting positions, the moral fiction is endorsed that whenever clinicians justifiably withdraw life support, they do not intend to cause death. We have argued above that withdrawal of a ventilator, as in the case of John, causes death. Is it credible that physicians never do, nor should, intend to cause death when they justifiably withdraw life support? In John's case, his plan is to end his life by withdrawing the ventilator, as he has decided that it is no longer worth continuing to live with the profound disability caused by his spinal cord injury. A clinician who views John's plan as reasonable given his circumstances, values, and preferences and is prepared to help by withdrawing his ventilator, intends not only to respect John's autonomous choice but to cause death in order to realize his plan. If this account is resisted, it is owing to the moral fiction that it is always unethical for clinicians to intend the death of their patients.

Recent empirical evidence indicates that many physicians, at least in Europe, acknowledge an intention to cause death when withdrawing life support. A large-scale survey of end-of-life decisions in six European countries (Belgium, Denmark, Italy, the Netherlands, Sweden, and Switzerland) demonstrated that a majority of physicians reported an explicit intention to hasten death when mechanical respiration (66%) and dialysis (69%) were withdrawn.[8] (Intending to hasten death is the same as intending to cause death, as hastening death causes death to occur earlier than it otherwise would.) Discussing their findings, the authors state that '[t]he data presented in this paper clearly show that the view that withholding or withdrawing treatment means allowing patients to die, even though not intending them to do so, is untenable from an empirical point of view.' Additionally, they observe that 'in the context of withholding and withdraw-ing treatment there is a great divergence between the traditional moral rule and today's medical practice'.

We do not claim, however, that whenever life-sustaining treatment is withdrawn clinicians necessar-ily intend to cause death. Certainly, if the intention is to determine whether the patient can be weaned from a ventilator, as in the earlier care of Sam, there is no such intent. Additionally, in the case of immi-nently dying patients who are likely to die in a short period of time regardless of continued life-sustaining treatment, the intention of clinicians often may be to remove a burdensome and unwanted impediment to a peaceful death, foreseeing that doing so is likely to hasten death.

Moral responsibility

Once the fictions are exposed, underlying conven-tional descriptions of causality and intention with respect to withdrawing life-sustaining treatment, it becomes clear that denying the moral responsibility of clinicians for the death of the patient in John's case is also a fiction. It is important to understand what is meant by 'moral responsibility'. We are mor-ally responsible for acts that can be attributed to us, whether right or wrong.[9] Specifically, a clinician is morally responsible for causing a patient's death by withdrawing a ventilator when this life-terminat-ing act can be attributed from a moral perspective to the clinician. Is causing the death something that the physician did voluntarily and knowingly, so that it can be attributed to him? We are morally respon-sible for what we intend to do, or do knowingly, or do negligently. It follows that clinicians are responsi-ble for causing the death of patients by withdrawing life support, regardless of whether one agrees with our claim that death is intended in many, but not necessarily all, of these cases. Moral responsibility for causing death does not equate to culpability for wrong-doing, unless it is presumed that it is always wrong to do so. Death-causing treatment withdraw-als can be right or wrong acts depending on the

circumstances, including critically the informed con-sent of competent patients or legally authorized sur-rogate decision-makers.

In withdrawing life-sustaining treatment, responsi-bility for causing death is shared by patients or surro-gates and clinicians. Indeed, the primary responsibility rests with the patient, or surrogate deciding on behalf of the patient. This prior authorization for treatment withdrawal is a morally necessary condition for clini-cians (justifiably) taking responsibility for withdraw-ing life support and thus for causing the death that ensues.

Differential moral assessment

Finally, we come to the differential moral evaluation of voluntary active euthanasia by means of a requested lethal injection in the case of Sam and a withdrawal of mechanical ventilation in response to the request/ treatment refusal of John. If these cases don't vary with respect to the physician's role in the causation of death, intention to cause death, and moral responsibil-ity for causing death, and the patients provide valid consent, then it is puzzling to regard physician con-duct in acceding to John's request as morally permis-sible but morally forbidden in the case of Sam. This differential judgment presupposes that there is some morally relevant characteristic that makes withdraw-ing life-sustaining treatment permissible but admin-istering a lethal dose of medication impermissible, which also constitutes a moral fiction.

To reject this differential moral judgment does not imply that there are no morally significant differences, either in evaluating the acts themselves or for public policy, between withdrawing life-sustaining treatment from a competent patient and voluntary active eutha-nasia by means of injecting patients with a lethal dose of medication.[10] Patients have both a moral and a legal claim-right to stop unwanted life-sustaining treatment, which physicians and health care institutions are obli-gated to respect. The validity of this right is not con-tingent on clinicians endorsing the patient's reasons for treatment refusal. The right to refuse treatment, how-ever, is not the same as the right to receive whatever treatment is demanded by a patient or a surrogate. Even if voluntary euthanasia is regarded as ethically legitimate, as in the Netherlands and Belgium, a physician may legitimately refuse a competent patient's request for a lethal dose of medication in some circumstances. However, the moral judgment that we are concerned with here is whether it is legitimate ethically in some circumstances (setting aside issues of legality) for a physician to comply willingly with a competent patient's voluntary and resolute request for a lethal injection. Voluntary active euthanasia is akin to abortion in this respect. Patients arguably have a moral liberty-right of noninterference by others with their physician's voluntary compliance with a valid request for abortion or active euthanasia, not a claim-right to receive an abortion or lethal injection upon demand from an objecting and unwilling physician.[11]

There are psychological differences between stopping life-sustaining treatment and administering a lethal injection, just as there are psychological differences between withholding and withdrawing life-sustaining treatment. When the moral fictions surrounding withdrawal of life-sustaining treatment are exposed, it doesn't follow that the psychological differences vanish. Giving a patient a lethal injection feels different from turning off a ventilator. The absence of any necessary difference in intention, causation of death, and moral responsibility doesn't make this feeling go away. Some commentators argue that there is a difference in the impact on professional integrity between these two ways of causing a patient's death.[12] Active euthanasia uses the ordinary tools of medicine – a syringe filled with drugs – to cause a patient's death. Stopping life-sustaining treatment withdraws the technological tools of medicine, resulting in a patient's death. We fail to see how this amounts to any meaningful difference in what it is permitted for a physician to do.

It might be objected that the reluctance of physicians to perform active euthanasia should be respected because there is no need for patients who choose to end their lives to receive physician assistance. Instead they can find other ways to kill themselves, including stopping eating and drinking.[13] Of course, the fact that there is a permissible alternative to active euthanasia does not show that active euthanasia is in itself morally wrong. The major difficulty with stopping eating and drinking is that it can take a considerable period of time to die in this way, lasting up to two weeks or more. Moreover, the option of stopping eating and drinking is not only open to someone like Sam who is not on life support, but also to John, who is. If it is problematic for physicians to assist Sam in requesting death by lethal injection, why is it not problematic to assist John by stopping his ventilator? In both cases patients are seeking a swift and peaceful death with physician assistance, and there is no relevant difference between these means of assisted death with respect to causation and moral responsibility for the patient's death. When the moral fictions underlying the stance of prevailing medical ethics to withdrawing life-sustaining treatment are exposed, the difference in attitudes of clinicians with respect to these two ways of complying with patient requests for assisted death is seen to lack rational support.

The Moral Work of Moral Fictions

Moral fictions, being motivated beliefs, serve a purpose. The moral fictions we have reviewed here uphold the traditional norm of medical ethics that doctors must not kill or intend their patients' deaths; and they are needed to square medical practice with the prevailing law, which treats intentional causing of death as criminal homicide, with exceptions such as self-defence, capital punishment, and just war. Bioethics scholars can expose and decry these moral fictions, as sins against commitment to the truth and as grounding erroneous moral judgments. But clinicians, ethics consultants, and teachers of clinical ethics cannot so easily escape the grip of these moral fictions. For the legitimate practice of withdrawing life-sustaining treatment *appears* to depend on upholding these moral fictions in view of the law and prevailing medical ethics.

With respect to the law, it is relatively easy to see these moral fictions as fictions that need to be endorsed in order to make medical practice consistent with the law. They can be understood essentially as legal fictions. We can look at withdrawing life-sustaining treatment *as if* it is not suicide or assisted suicide; as if it is passive euthanasia and merely allowing to die; as if it does not cause death; as if death necessarily is not intended. Therefore, physicians are not legally responsible for causing the death of their patients and not guilty of homicide when they withdraw life-sustaining treatment. Furthermore, the fiction about suicide permits the families of patients who decide to stop life-sustaining treatment to receive life insurance payments, which may be precluded if the death is officially denominated as suicide. Perhaps more important, it permits patients and families who are morally opposed to suicide to accept the withdrawal of life-sustaining treatment.

From a moral perspective, however, embracing these moral fictions is problematic. The *as if* approach doesn't work comfortably with respect to bona fide moral judgments. The teacher of medical ethics can attempt to teach end-of-life decision-making without moral fictions, pointing out how a candid appraisal of the facts and associated moral judgments conflict with prevailing medical ethics, and why it is better from a moral perspective (and in an ideal world) to abandon the fictions. But what message does this send to clinicians and trainees who have been socialized into a profession that owes allegiance to the norm that doctors must not kill patients? There is a risk that physicians will balk at medical ethics without moral fictions, becoming reluctant to engage patients and family members in conversations about stopping life-sustaining treatment and resistant to patient or family requests to do so. The moral progress with respect to the use of life-sustaining treatment that has developed since the 1970s might be imperiled. On the other hand, the extent to which patients, families, and/or clinicians already recognize these beliefs to be fictions – even if not fully consciously and explicitly – may contribute to unease or reluctance about withdrawing life-sustaining treatment, which could be reduced by greater clarity.

Abandoning the Moral Fictions

We do not claim that there is an easy response to this quandary, in part because of uncertainty about what the effects would be of abandoning these moral fictions. One way to reduce the tension between exposing moral fictions and practising ethically within the prevailing legal and moral status quo is to emphasize the principles that justify compliance with requests to withdraw life-sustaining treatment and the provision of needed palliative care: respecting patient self-determination and promoting patient well-being.[14] It must be emphasized that causing death is not necessarily harmful and can be good for patients, depending on their situation. The intentions of patients and physicians with respect to causing death and what counts as causing death have nothing to do, in themselves, with whether withdrawing of life-sustaining treatment can be justified by appeal to these principles. The entrenched but ethically dubious norm that doctors must not kill can be surrendered without abandoning the traditional norm of doing no harm to patients (that is not compensated by proportional patient benefit). More specifically, the unqualified prohibition on doctors killing patients (i.e. intentionally causing the death of patients) should be replaced by the norm that doctors should not kill without valid consent, either from competent patients or authorized surrogate decision-makers. There is no way, however, to adopt this strategy of eschewing moral fictions without giving up the differential moral judgment that withdrawing life-sustaining treatment, but not voluntary active euthanasia, is permissible.

It remains an open question, which we do not attempt to address here, whether there are legitimate grounds as a matter of policy and law for continuing to prohibit assisted suicide and active euthanasia. It is possible that the potential for abuse that accompanies legalization of physician-assisted death justifies continuing to prohibit these practices. In one respect, there is an inherently greater potential for abuse in active euthanasia, because any person can be killed by lethal injection, whereas withdrawing life-sustaining treatment can only kill those who are on life support and need it to continue living. Although careful oversight of decisions to undertake active euthanasia can minimize abuses, the absence of abuse can never be guaranteed.[15] To put this in perspective, however, we need to recognize that our currently accepted practices of withdrawing life-sustaining treatment also have the potential for abuse, especially in the case of incompetent patients. With the rare exception of disputed cases reviewed by the courts, decisions to withdraw life support are made without standard procedures to assess the decisions of patients and surrogate decision-makers and without formal oversight. Hence, there is no way to know the extent of abuse that our society has been prepared to tolerate in recognizing the right to refuse life-sustaining treatment. It is an empirical issue, on which there is little evidence, whether expanding the scope of legitimate, legally permissible death-causing acts by clinicians would foster intolerable abuses that could not be obviated by reasonable regulatory procedures.

In view of moral discomfort with the idea of doctors killing patients, is it clear that we should give up the moral fictions that permeate conventional medical ethics relating to end-of-life decisions? Perhaps the truth is unbearable and facing it will produce worse consequences than indulging in fictions about our accepted end-of-life practices.[16] If we knew that facing the truth about these practices would create a backlash, with the result that suffering patients are made worse off, then tolerating these moral fictions would seem desirable. A problem, however, is that once a moral fiction is seen for what it is, it is difficult to continue to pass the fiction off as the truth. Moreover, we don't know that abandoning these moral fictions will set back moral progress or plunge us down the slippery slope. It may be best to proceed gradually in abandoning the moral fictions relating to end-of-life practices, tolerating some measure of obfuscation along the way. However, medical ethics that is shot through with fictions is unstable and likely to be transformed over time as the reality of end-of-life practices is exposed.

In theory, the moral work done by the moral fictions in the ethics of end-of-life decisions is expendable. Nothing need be lost from a moral perspective in abandoning these moral fictions, and much is to be gained in honesty, moral clarity, and professional integrity. The transition, however, from the moral status quo to a landscape of medical ethics without moral fictions will demand a cultural transformation within the practice of medicine and medical ethics.

Notes

1   A. Meisel. The Legal Consensus about Forgoing Life-Sustaining Treatment: Its Status and Prospects. *Kennedy Inst Ethics J* 1992; 2: 309–45; N.L. Cantor. Twenty-Five Years after *Quinlan*: A Review of the Jurisprudence of Death and Dying. *J Law Med Ethics* 2001; 29: 182–96.

2   J. Rachels. 1986. *The End of Life*. New York: Oxford University Press; P. Singer. 1994. *Rethinking Life and Death: The Collapse of Our Traditional Ethics*. New York: St. Martin's Press; D. Brock. 1993. *Life and Death*. New York: Cambridge University Press.

3   G. Calabresi and P. Bobbitt. 1978. *Tragic Choices*. New York: W.W. Norton.

4   C. Tavris and E. Aronson. 2007. *Mistakes Were Made: (But Not by Me)*. Orlando, FL: Harcourt: 13–20.

5   E.D. Pellegrino. Doctors Must Not Kill. *J Clin Ethics* 1992; 3: 95–102; D. Callahan. 1993. *The Troubled Dream of Life*. Washington DC: Georgetown University Press: 158–72; B. Brody. 2003. *Taking Issue*. Washington DC: Georgetown University Press: 158–72.

6   Brock, *Life and Death*, pp. 208–13.

7   H.L.A. Hart and T. Honore. 1985. *Causation in the Law*, 2nd edn. New York: Oxford University Press.

8   G. Bosshard et al. Intentionally Hastening Death by Withholding or Withdrawing Treatment. *Wiener Klinische Wochenschrift* 2006; 118: 322–6.

9 T. Scanlon. 1998. *What We Owe to Each Other.* Cambridge, MA: Harvard University Press: 248–51.

10 F.G. Miller, J.J. Fins and L. Snyder. Assisted Suicide Compared with Refusal of Treatment: A Valid Distinction? *Ann Intern Med* 2000; 132: 470–5.

11 R. Dworkin et al. 1998. The Philosopher's Brief. In *Physician-Assisted Suicide.* M.P. Battin, R. Rhodes and A. Silvers, eds. New York: Routledge.

12 W. Gaylin et al. Doctors Must Not Kill. *JAMA* 1988; 259: 2139–40; L.R. Kass. Neither for Love nor Money: Why Doctors Must Not Kill. *Public Interest* 1989; 94: 25–46.

13 J.L. Bernat, B. Gert and R.P. Mogielnicki. Patient Refusal of Hydration and Nutrition: An Alternative to Physician-Assisted Suicide or Voluntary Active Euthanasia. *Arch Intern Med* 1993; 153: 2723–8.

14 Brock, *Life and Death*, pp. 205–8.

15 F.G. Miller et al. Regulating Physician-Assisted Death. *N Engl J Med* 1994; 331: 119–23.

16 D. Brock. Truth or Consequences: The Role of Philosophers in Policy-Making. In Brock, *Life and Death*, pp. 408–16.

Newborns

27

Can a Physician Ever Justifiably Euthanize a Severely Disabled Newborn?

Robert M. Sade

Physician-assisted suicide (PAS) has been legalized in eight states of the United States – California, Colorado, Hawai'i, Maine, New Jersey, Oregon, Vermont, and Washington – and the District of Columbia; it has been judicially sanctioned in Montana.[1] PAS is illegal in the remaining 41 states, but 18 states are currently (2019–2020) considering legalization bills.[2] No state is considering legalizing euthanasia, but it is now legal in at least four countries: Belgium, Colombia, Luxembourg, and The Netherlands (it might also be legal in Canada and Japan, but the law is ambiguous in those countries).[3]

In assisted suicide, the assister is passively involved in causing death; in euthanasia, one person actively causes the death of another for the purpose of relieving pain and suffering. Although euthanasia is illegal in all US states, some believe it is only a matter of time before euthanasia is legalized, particularly in states where PAS has already been adopted.

Euthanasia of children has not been legitimate under any national legal code, but in The Netherlands, a specific process guides selection of children under the age of 12 years who could be candidates for euthanasia – the Groningen Protocol, developed in 2004, which is not a law, but public prosecutors deem it acceptable under certain guidelines.[4,5] The Belgium Parliament recently modified its 2002 Act on Euthanasia to include not only adults, but also children under the age of 18 years.[6]

Assisted suicide and euthanasia have profound implications for the way we view the relationship among physicians, other professionals, health care, and death; the implications are especially serious for medical ethics. The Cardiothoracic Ethics Forum invited two outstanding philosophers to explore some of these issues; they are both well-known for their scholarly positions in defense of opposing viewpoints regarding the acceptability of euthanasia. Their debate at the 94th Annual Meeting of the American Association for Thoracic Surgery focused on a hypothetical case involving euthanasia of a newborn infant.

The Case of the Ill-fated Newborn

A full-term newborn infant is noted to turn blue while feeding a few hours after birth. Evaluation by a pediatric cardiologist reveals heterotaxy syndrome

Original publication details: Robert M. Sade, "Can a Physician Ever Justifiably Euthanize a Severely Disabled Neonate?" p. 532 from *The Journal of Thoracic and Cardiovascular Surgery* 149 (2015). Reproduced with permission of Elsevier.

(polysplenia) with a group of extremely complex heart malformations that result in complete mixing of blood flow to the body and to the lungs. The cardiologist meets with the parents, explains the diagnosis, and outlines four alternative courses: surgical treatment, medical treatment, comfort care with feeding, and euthanasia.

Surgical treatment will require at least three risky heart operations before age five years. If the three or more operations are successful, the child might survive his teenage years. Additionally, he has impaired splenic function, which exposes him to increased threat of infections, and is at risk for intestinal obstruction, which would require one or more abdominal operations.

Medical therapy for heart failure without surgery would not reverse his inevitably declining condition, and at best would allow him to survive into early childhood.

With *feeding and comfort care only*, the baby would be expected to become progressively disabled and would most likely die within a year.

Euthanasia at this point would prevent future suffering. It is an option only because the state in which they reside has had a long-time policy allowing physician-assisted suicide and recently amended the law to allow euthanasia under circumstances such as this.

The parents consider this information and discuss it with other family members, close friends, and their spiritual advisor before making their decision. At the cardiologist's next visit, they tell him that if they had known about this problem, they would have terminated the pregnancy because they do not wish their child to have a poor quality of life. Of the four available options, they believe euthanasia is the most humane. Should the physician help them in this way?

References

1   Death With Dignity Acts. Available at https://www. deathwithdignity.org/learn/death-with-dignity-acts. Accessed August 14, 2019.

2   Take Action in Your State. Available at https://www. deathwithdignity.org/take-action/. Accessed August 14, 2019.

3   Euthanasia & Physician-Assisted Suicide (PAS) around the World. Legal Status in 28 Countries from Australia to Uruguay. Available at https://euthanasia.procon. org/view.resource.php?resourceID=000136. Accessed August 14, 2019.

4   Verhagen E., Sauer P.J.J. The Groningen Protocol – Euthanasia in Severely Ill Newborns. *New England Journal of Medicine* 2005; 352: 959–62.

5   Verhagen A. A. The Groningen Protocol for Newborn Euthanasia; Which Way did the Slippery Slope Tilt? *Journal of Medical Ethics* 2013 May; 39(5): 293–5.

6   Siegel A. M., Sisti, D. A., Caplan, A. L. Pediatric Euthanasia in Belgium: Disturbing Developments. *JAMA* 2014 May 21; 311(19): 1963–4.

28

No to Infant Euthanasia

Gilbert Meilaender

Although I am not a physician, and although there is surely much about the medical complexities of this case that I do not fully understand, it is clear even to me that this baby is likely to have a short, perhaps very short, life even under the best of circumstances and with the best medical care. What follows from that? What follows, I want to suggest, is that it is our obligation to seek for this little boy a death we can live with; a death that does not undermine our equal dignity but that cares for his life and honors his time among us from first to last.

Faced with the sadness and suffering of such a case, and forced to confront the limits of our own expertise and ability to help, we are tempted to turn in either of 2 directions, which seem at first sight to be complete opposites but which in fact are closely related kin.[1] We are tempted either to struggle with all our power and technical skill against death, never giving up that fight until have we nothing left to do and must admit defeat, or we are tempted to decide to intentionally cause death, solving the problem of suffering by eliminating the sufferer.

However different these 2 approaches may seem on the surface, each is a form of abandonment. Neither constitutes care for this child, and our obligation is precisely to maximize care. I will outline briefly 3 kinds of wisdom (moral, political, and medical) that should invite us always to care and never to kill in cases of this sort.

First, deeply embedded in our moral tradition is the distinction between, on the one hand, allowing someone to die, and, on the other hand, intentionally causing death. For this child with heterotaxy syndrome and for many others, both young and old, who face life-threatening illness, maximizing care will sometimes mean ceasing to struggle against death. Medical treatments may rightly be withdrawn if they are either useless or excessively burdensome. Perhaps in the case of this little boy they are both; I do not know for sure. Perhaps even well-trained physicians, if they are honest with themselves, will not always know for sure. Anyone who simply plunges forward, certain that he knows which possible treatment approach is best, needs to learn to live with a little more fear and trembling.

Original publication details: Gilbert Meilaender, "No to Infant Euthanasia," pp. 533–534 from *The Journal of Thoracic and Cardiovascular Surgery* 149 (2015). Reproduced with permission of Elsevier.

Still, we can be clear that no one should be subjected to useless treatment and that no one need suffer any and all possibly life-saving or life-prolonging treatments, however burdensome they may be. That much can be clear, even if we do not always know how best to evaluate the facts of a particular case. The questions we should ask ourselves are questions about what is medically indicated, what is medically best for the child: Will a treatment benefit the life this child has? Is a treatment excessively burdensome to the life of this child? These questions are a little different from others we may be tempted to ask ourselves: Is it a benefit to have this life? Is this life a burden?

The latter questions distance us from the one who needs our care. They invite us not just to allow this child to die but to embrace his death as a good at which we aim; that is, to take into our character a willingness intentionally to kill the innocent. That would be to think of ourselves not as fellow human beings and fellow sufferers with this child but, instead, as people who are fit to exercise a kind of ultimate authority over the life of another. We often speak of the need for compassion when we think about such troubling cases, but we do not always pay close attention to what the word actually means and what it asks of us: that we suffer with the one who needs our care, entering as best we can into his suffering, not distancing ourselves from him as if we were not equals in dignity. Indeed, a readiness not to distance themselves from their patients has been deeply embedded in physicians' professional practice.

Second there is also a tradition of political wisdom that instructs us always to care and never to kill in cases such as the one we are considering. In recent decades, as the issue of euthanasia has become more widely debated in North American societies, supporters have regularly appealed to 2 sorts of warrants. One is compassion for the suffering, about which I have already said something. The other is autonomy or self-determination. The "whose life is it anyway?" question has great appeal for us. If for decades I have been making important decisions about the course my life should take, why, some may ask, should I not also decide at some point that the game is no longer worth the candle?

Opponents of euthanasia have argued that these warrants turn out to reinforce each other in ways that would in time expand the class of candidates for euthanasia.[2] After all, if compassionate relief of suffering is so important, we may be hard pressed to understand why it should be available only to those who are autonomous and self-determining. When now we find our political communities beginning to consider whether we should euthanize a child such as the one in this case, we do well to remember the critics who argued that such expansion was inevitable. Once a society begins to blur the line that distinguishes allowing to die from killing, it can become very difficult in law and in practice to limit the permission to take life. And that, in turn, can undermine our commitment to human equality.

The danger to equality arises from 2 angles, both that of the person who seeks euthanasia or, as in the case of this child, for whom it is desired, and that of the person who offers it. If I seek to give ultimate authority over my life to others, I become something less than their equal. I join what John Locke called the "inferior ranks of Creatures," and I make my person an object to be possessed and controlled by others.[3] And the same is true when I give such authority over this child's life to others. Likewise, the person who carries out the euthanizing deed pulls rank and, in effect, exercises a more-than-human authority over the life of one who is, in fact, his moral and political equal. For us to try to exercise such authority is to pretend to be what we in truth are not: something other than beings of equal dignity. And that would be to lose one of the greatest achievements of our political tradition: an affirmation of equal dignity laboriously gained at great cost over centuries.

Third, in a setting such as this meeting, we should certainly remind ourselves of the medical wisdom that teaches physicians always to care and never to kill. After all, although the background to our deliberations is the general question of whether it is morally or politically wise for a society to endorse euthanasia, the actual question we face is narrower and more pointed. How did the case end? What did it ask us? The question is: "Should the physician help them in this way?"

I have been arguing that we should not agree to euthanize this baby. I have not tried to decide which of the alternatives to euthanasia is most choice worthy. Perhaps we should provide comfort care only; perhaps we should not embark on a series of surgeries that will probably give at best a couple decades of life. Or, on the other hand, perhaps we should not assume that a couple of decades even of medically burdened life is an unacceptable choice. After all, each moment of life is equidistant from eternity. Your thinking, your doing, your caring, and your loving are all important in this moment even if you will not wake up tomorrow. Hence, although we should choose life for this child, I am not sure which of the available life choices would really maximize care for him.

But I do know that if we never attempt any of those life choices, if we simply sweep such children off our doorstep every morning with euthanasia, medicine will never learn better ways to help them and others like them. That may not be the best way to understand the vocation that is yours.

In any case, if we do not sweep such children off our doorstep, and whatever course we decide maximizes our care for them, it is certain that genuinely compassionate and caring physicians themselves bear heavy burdens here. I do not underrate those burdens. Nevertheless, your burdens are inextricably connected with your good fortune.

For it is your good fortune to have found in medicine work that can be genuinely worthwhile, as you seek to impart at least a small measure of wholeness (healing and health) to your patients. But, of course, in giving yourselves to this work you risk, as William F. May once put it, drowning in the sea of human need in which you swim daily. That may tempt you, as it could tempt any of us, to try to eliminate suffering by eliminating the sufferer. We are tempted to "avoid ties to the perishing," lest they drag us down with them.[4]

Faced with that temptation, physicians may understandably take refuge in a kind of managerial competence, using their technical skills to manage death. Still, good medical care does not forget that all patients must sooner or later die. The task of the physician is to accompany them on the way to that death, neither abandoning them by imposing treatments that are useless or excessively burdensome, nor abandoning them by deliberately aiming at their death. Neither of those seemingly opposite but, in reality, related forms of abandonment can constitute a medical success story. Our goal as physicians, as citizens, as parents of suffering children, and as patients or potential patients ourselves should be to affirm life even in the midst of death, and to commit ourselves to helping to shape a death we can live with.

References

1 Ramsey P. *The Patient as Person*. New Haven, Conn, and London, UK: Yale University Press, 1970: 144–57.

2 Callahan D. *The Troubled Dream of Life*. New York: Simon & Schuster, 1993: 107–12.

3 Locke J. *Two Treatises of Government*. New York: New American Library, 1965: 311.

4 May W. F. *The Physician's Covenant*. 2nd ed. Louisville, KY: Westminster John Knox Press, 2000: 137.

29

Physicians Can Justifiably Euthanize Certain Severely Impaired Neonates

Udo Schüklenk

Clinicians in a scenario involving a neonate with heterotaxy syndrome would not have included euthanasia as an option for the parents had they believed surgical procedures would likely be successful and permit the infant to live a reasonably healthy life.

Legislators in the jurisdiction where the case scenario played out concluded that there are circumstances where infanticide is morally acceptable. They legislated that physician-assisted death be made available in their jurisdiction for certain severely impaired neonates, including apparently the infant under consideration. A majority of practicing neonatologists in Europe concurs that intensive care is only acceptable if it will result not merely in the survival of an infant but also in an acceptable future quality of life.[1] In the United States the President's Commission for the Study of Ethical Problems in Medicine and Biomedical and Behavioral Research also concluded that there can be conditions sufficiently serious "that continued existence would not be a net benefit to the infant."[2]

There appear to be some cases, then, where continuing existence is not in a severely impaired neonate's best interest. Terminating its life, based on parent choice, seems a prima facie reasonable option.

Discussion

Infants lack decision-making capacity

What makes cases such as this morally circumspect in the eyes of many is that, unlike with competent adults, a neonate has no occurrent capacity to express his reflective wishes. There are no reflective wishes, not even a reflective interest in continuing existence. Adults facing this infant's life prospects might well decide to ask for assisted dying. They would have been able to gather relevant information and make up their minds on whether or not they would want to live that kind of life. This option is unavailable to the neonate. His parents should be the ones making this difficult decision.

Sanctity of life versus quality of life

What is controversial is whether there can be legitimate circumstances where the life of a severely impaired

Original publication details: Udo Schüklenk, "Physicians Can Justifiably Euthanize Certain Severely Impaired Neonates," pp. 535–537 from *The Journal of Thoracic and Cardiovascular Surgery* 149 (2015). Reproduced with permission of Elsevier.

neonate may be actively terminated. For most Christian ethicists this question is relatively easily settled: Human life from the moment of conception is of infinite value, and whereas we are not obliged to go to however-defined extraordinary length to keep such a severely impaired neonate alive, we must not actively end its life. This view has been challenged by many prominent secular ethicists.[3] They propose an alternative approach to what is also known as the sanctity-of-life doctrine in medicine.[4] In their view we should replace the sanctity-of-life doctrine with a quality-of-life ethic.[5]

Quality-of-life ethic and infanticide

A quality-of-life ethic requires us to focus on a neonate's current and future quality of life as relevant decision-making criteria. We would ask questions such as: Does this baby have the capacity for development to an extent that will allow him or her to have a life and not merely be alive?[6] If we reach the conclusion that it would not, we would have reason to conclude that his life is not worth living. Prolonging his life would not be in the infant's best interest. Importantly, in addressing this question we ought to look at the infant's current and future life prospects as well as we can from his own point of view. We are asking questions such as, What is he getting out of his life now and what would he get out of his life if the proposed surgery was successful? Would it be worth it to him?

An objection could be made that we cannot know with certainty what is in such a severely disabled infant's best interest. The President's Commission emphasized that infants have well-being interests, including experiencing pleasure rather than pain and suffering, very much like we do. If we face a situation where an infant's current and future life prospects involve overwhelming pain and suffering we would have a good reason to proactively end his life. The neonate in our case has no capacity or desire to exist now or in the future. In morally important ways his developmental state is closer to that of a fetus than to that of a person like you and me. The parents should be able to freely decide on what would amount to postnatal abortion.

Quality-of-life ethic and terminal sedation

An objection could be made on the basis that if we are fundamentally concerned about quality of life, why couldn't we decide to forgo the life-prolonging medical interventions and provide instead terminal sedation to the infant? This would permit those opposed to assisted dying to claim that a natural death would occur. In this scenario little or no pain would be experienced by the infant.

The logic behind this solution is based on an unsound kind of reasoning; namely, St Thomas Aquinas' doctrine-of-the-double-effect.[7] The doctrine states that if you undertake an action where you intend to achieve something desirable (alleviate suffering) and in the process something undesirable occurs (death), you are ethically in the clear as long as you did not intend for the foreseeable death to occur. Typically today a proportionality condition is attached to the doctrine. That is, the undesirable unintended consequence must not outweigh the desirable intended outcome. This is not a plausible account of moral responsibility. We are morally responsible for foreseeable consequences of our actions, whether we intend for those consequences to occur or not. The outcome of this action is no different to an outcome whereby someone proactively terminated the life of a neonate. The doctrine permits doctors to do the right thing – while claiming somewhat disingenuously that they did not quite mean for the foreseeable death to occur. There appears to be some psychological comfort that the doctrine offers to clinicians, but that does not make it any more plausible.

The other reason why this course of action appears to be popular with doctors has to do with another doctrine, the so-called acts and omission doctrine. It holds that there is a moral difference between actively killing a patient and omitting to keep a patient alive. It permits those who have not brought about the death of a patient by actively killing him but by omitting to keep him alive, to feel better about their chosen course of action. However, in our case this distinction isn't plausible either. Here the deliberate omission to act to keep the patient alive leads foreseeably to the death of the patient. The outcome between not acting and omitting to act is exactly the same – except omitting to act delays the inevitable for no good reason.

From a quality-of-life ethic point of view terminal sedation could prima facie be an acceptable option, were it not for the following issues.

Parental and health care professionals' interests matter

If doctors were to terminally sedate the infant he would not suffer any longer, so why terminate his life proactively? Why then should doctors provide assisted dying on the parents' request?

They should do so because the parents and attending health care professionals' interests matter in morally relevant ways. The unnecessarily prolonged dying of their infant son would extend a severely distressing situation for the parents. They would have to witness the deterioration of their infant son over a period of days, possibly weeks. Some of the attending health care professionals would undoubtedly also find it psychologically difficult to watch the child die foreseeably an unnecessarily slow death. What we ought to enter into the equation are the interests of those involved in the care of the infant. Given that a terminally sedated infant would have no surviving interests to speak of, the interests of these other parties matter. If his prolonged dying is harmful to them, a further quality-of-life based argument in favor of terminating the infant's life is established.

Resource allocation justice

The question of whether it would be a wise allocation of scarce health care resources to undertake the proposed surgical procedures invariably arises in circumstances such as this. Continuing life-prolonging care for the infant would be futile, it would constitute a waste of scarce health care resources. Health care resources ought to be deployed where they can actually benefit patients by improving their quality of life. This cannot be achieved in the scenario under consideration.

Slippery slope concerns

Prenatal testing renders the need for infanticide exceedingly rare. For an indication of how rare such cases are it is worthwhile to look at published evidence from The Netherlands where involuntary euthanasia for severely impaired neonates is legally available. Of about 200,000 children born in The Netherlands on an annual basis only very few newborns saw their lives ended by this means (4 in total between 1995 and 2005, none between 2005 and 2010).[8] A larger number of impaired neonates' lives are ended by a combination of withdrawing or withholding treatment. Withdrawing treatment almost always entails the withdrawal of artificial nutrition and hydration. These cases still number below 300, decreasing from 299 in 1995 to 177 in 2010. The permissibility of infanticide in The Netherlands has not led that country down a slippery slope to an ever-increasing number of killed impaired neonates. Apparently the doctrine of the double-effect is alive and well even in The Netherlands.

Unfair discrimination against the disabled?

Does such a policy unfairly discriminate against the disabled? That does not appear to be the case. Assisted dying for impaired infants is not available in all cases of disability. Assisted dying is available only in circumstances where continuing medical care would be futile. The available evidence suggests that that is where clinicians and parents draw the line when it comes to infanticide.

Human dignity

Opponents of infanticide under the circumstances described in our scenario often argue that such a course of action would violate human dignity. This is not the place to elaborate in-depth on this subject, but arguably such claims are question-begging; they typically assume the truth of what they need to demonstrate.[9] Human dignity has no clear, universally agreed-upon meaning. A quality-of-life proponent could just as well argue that respect for human dignity demands that the infant's life be terminated on compassionate grounds. Human dignity is mostly a rhetorical cloak for other – more controversial – ideologic convictions. Incidentally, this applies to other types of nonarguments, too. For instance, opponents of infanticide frequently ask whether we would want to live in a society that permitted such a course of action. Proponents could simply reply affirmatively. We would be better served to avoid this kind of rhetoric in public and professional discourse altogether.

Conclusions

Once we have concluded that death is what is in the best interest of the infant, it is unreasonable not to bring about this death as painlessly and as much controlled in terms of timing by the parents as is feasible.

The author thanks Suzanne van de Vathorst, MD, Erasmus Medical Centre, The Netherlands, for critical comments on an earlier draft of this paper as well as for assistance with one of the references.

References

1 Verhagen E., and Sauer, P. J. The Groningen Protocol – euthanasia in severely ill newborns. *N Engl J Med*. 2005; 352: 959–62.

2 President's Commission for the Study of Ethical Problems in Medicine and Biomedical and Behavioral Research. Deciding to forego life-sustaining treatment a report on the ethical, medical, and legal issues in treatment decisions. Available at: https://bioethicsarchive.georgetown.edu/pcbe/reports/past_commissions/deciding_to_forego_tx.pdf. Accessed May 1, 2014.

3 Kuhse, H. *The sanctity-of-life-doctrine in medicine: a critique*. Oxford: Oxford University Press, 1987.

4 Singer, P. *Rethinking life and death*. Melbourne, Australia: Text, 1994.

5 Tooley, M. *Abortion and infanticide*. Oxford: Oxford University Press, 1983. [See also Chapter 1 in this *Anthology*.]

6 Rachels, J. *The end of life*. Oxford: Oxford University Press, 1986.

7 Uniacke, S. The doctrine of the double-effect. In: Ashcroft, R.E., Dawson, A., Draper, H., and McMillan, J.R., eds. *Principles of health care ethics*. 2nd ed. Chichester: Wiley, 2007: 263–8.

8 van de Vathorst S, Gevers JKM, van der Heide A, Bolt LLE, Cate K. Evaluatie: Regeling centrale deskundigen-commissie late zwangerschapsafbreking in een categorie-2 geval en levensbeëindiging bij pasgeborenen [in Dutch]. Available at: http://www.zonmw.nl/uploads/tx_vipublicaties/Evaluatie_Rdc_zalpdef.pdf. Accessed May 1, 2014.

9 Schüklenk, U., van Delden, J.J., Downie, J., McLean, S.A., Upshur, R., and Weinstock, D. End-of-life decision-making in Canada: the report by the Royal Society of Canada Expert Panel on End-of-Life Decision-Making. *Bioethics*. 2011; 25(Suppl 1): 38–44.

30

You Should Not Have Let Your Baby Die

Gary Comstock

Sam, your newborn son, has been suffocating in your arms for the past 15 minutes. You're as certain as you can be that he is going to die in the next 15. He was born two days ago with "trisomy 18," a disease that proved no obstacle to his cementing himself immediately and forevermore as the love of your life. Your wife has already composed his own lullaby, "Sam, Sam, the Little Man." But she and you and your three other children have spent the past 24 hours learning about the incredible uphill battle Sam faces.

"Trisomy" means "three chromosomes." Each cell in your son's body should have a healthy pair of the chromosomes scientists call No. 18. The unkind twists of the genetic lottery have given him instead a crippling threesome.

Sam was born breech in an emergency procedure in Mary Greeley Hospital, in Ames, Iowa. You and your wife accepted the attending physician's advice to Life Flight him immediately in a helicopter to the Infant Intensive Care Unit at the Iowa City Hospitals. You were told that Sam could not breathe on his own, although no one ever asked whether you approved his being hooked up to a ventilator. You overheard the emergency personnel relaying in medicalese the reasons for the flight to Iowa City: microcephaly, low-set ears, flat midface, short stature, proximally placed thumb and potentially abnormal male genitalia. All signs, you have since learned, of genetic abnormality, and indicators that he will be, as a friend puts it — choking on the words — "mentally retarded."

Not all people with trisomy 18 have problems. The literature reports a dozen cases of individuals living for 10 years, and SOFT, a trisomy 18 support group, lists even more living into their 20s and 30s. Those with the conditions known as mosaicism and translocation of the 18 chromosome may live relatively long and happy lives, bring joy to their parents, siblings and friends, and be relatively free of adverse symptoms. But there is a wide range of disorders associated with trisomy, and for those with Sam's symptoms, life expectancy is brutally short.

Sam's case is classified as one of the worst. His brain cannot regulate his lungs. He grew successfully in your wife's body and came to term because her blood provided him with oxygen. Now that his mother can no longer breathe for him, there is, the genetic

Original publication details: Gary Comstock, "You Should Not Have Let Your Baby Die" from *The New York Times*, July 12, 2017. Reproduced with permission of New York Times/PARS.

Bioethics: An Anthology, Fourth Edition. Edited by Udo Schüklenk and Peter Singer.

counselor gently tells you, little chance that he will ever breathe on his own.

Some 1,100 infants are born annually in this country with trisomy 18. Many of them die of heart failure or apnea, irregular breathing that stops temporarily. Sam cannot breathe on his own at all. In an era of less technologically sophisticated medicine, your wife suggests, Sam would have died at birth? Yes. Even with today's respirators, cardiac support equipment and antibiotics, nearly 30 percent will die in the first month; 90 percent will die before their first birthday. Of those who survive, most will have radical cognitive limitations, a condition the most recent revision of the Diagnostic and Statistical Manual of Mental Disorders refers to as "profound intellectual disability."

How do you know? You pose the question to Sam's geneticist, a kindly man in his mid-40s. He measures his response. He has an MD and a PhD, and has worked with trisomy infants for 15 years. You like him. You hear in his voice the ring of years of medical practice, scientific research and practical wisdom. You see in his eyes the face of a father. Well, he says, as to the diagnosis of the genetic problem, the results of chromosome analysis are accurate 99.9 percent of the time. As for the prognosis? Unfortunately, Sam seems to have a version of trisomy 18 that makes it impossible for his brain to successfully stimulate and coordinate the activities of the respiratory tract.

Are you sure? What would happen if you removed that air hose taped to his face? Have you tried it? Yes, once, for a few seconds. His lungs showed no signs of beginning to operate on their own. It would be inhumane to experiment on him by leaving the tube out for any longer period of time. He cannot breathe.

But couldn't that change? Yes. Some trisomy 18 babies in Sam's condition eventually improve to the point at which they no longer need the respirator. Some leave the hospital and begin to respond to their parents' affection. But a majority never leave the hospital, never respond to the presence of others and die while still connected to the respirator.

What are the choices? Some parents choose to use all possible means of continuing their child's life in the hope that their child will beat the odds and eventually overcome problems. Others choose to let the children die to spare the babies the pain of the ordeal.

Forget the statistics and what others do or don't do. We would like to know what our Sam's chances are for reaching the point where his life is valuable to him. But there is no answer to that question. No one can tell you whether your son's life is worth living from his perspective, or yours. We cannot say whether your son will ever breathe on his own or look at you. We can say only that the literature suggests the odds are stacked heavily against him.

You and your wife had no warning during the pregnancy that the child might be genetically abnormal. You were offered the services of amniocentesis, a test that may have revealed his condition. You and your wife refused to have genetic testing done on the fetus because your wife opposes abortion on theological and moral grounds. Knowing ahead of time that the child was genetically abnormal would not have provided any useful information. Genetic testing is done to allow parents the choice to abort fetuses with severe problems. But your wife would never abort her baby, so there was no point in having the tests performed.

The two of you have support in deciding to let your baby die: your wife's best friend from church, her mother and sister from 2,000 miles away, your own mother and father, your two brothers and sister, and every member of their families, gathered from 300 miles away. They help you think through the decision to remove the air tube. They squirm with you, hesitating to give their opinions. In the end, they express support for your decision. Your brother calls it "courageous."

There seems to you both a difference between killing your baby and letting him die. You are letting Sam die. Your father gathers the family, nearly 20 adults and children, in the room. You hold hands, collectively sing a psalm, weep through Grandpa's prayer. Everyone leaves. Your wife tries to sing Sam's lullaby to him, one last time, *goodbye, Sam*, but her voice fails her. She hands him to you. She cannot bear to go through it. Your brother and mother have offered to sit with you, but you decide it is something you must do alone. Just you and Sam.

The nurse comes in, mute. You look at him, sleeping. He seems at peace. You nod your head. She gently pulls the tube. It slides out quickly, as though he were helping to expel it. Without his lifeline, he does not move. A minute later, his eyes open. It is the first time you have seen them. His head jerks slightly forward. He does not cry. He gasps silently for breath. His eyes close. You almost yell for the nurse, to beg her to put it back in. To keep from doing so, you pray, arguing with God that letting him die is best for him. After five minutes, his face pales, then turns a sickly purple. His tiny chest convulses irregularly in an unsuccessful attempt to draw air into the lungs. After 20 minutes, he lies still. His fingers turn gray.

Thirty minutes. There are no visible signs of life. You rock his limp body as tears fall on the blue blanket. You wonder what sort of beast you are. Forty-five minutes. Grandma looks in, ashen faced, seeing in a glance that it is over. Shortly your wife appears. She immediately takes her son's body in her arms and coddles him. She sits there with him for three hours.

You should not have let your baby die. You should have killed him.

This thought occurs to you years later, thinking about the gruesome struggle of his last 20 minutes. You are not sure whether it makes sense to talk about his life, because he never seemed to have the things that make a life: thoughts, wants, desires, interests, memories, a future. But supposing that he had thoughts, his strongest thought during those last minutes certainly appeared to be: "This hurts. Can't someone help it stop?" He didn't know your name, but if he had, he would have said: "Daddy? Please. *Now*."

It seems the medical community has few options to offer parents of newborns likely to die. We can leave our babies on respirators and hope for the best. Or remove the hose and watch the child die a tortured death. Shouldn't we have another choice? Shouldn't we be allowed the swift humane option afforded the owners of dogs, a lethal dose of a painkiller?

For years you repress the thought. Then, early one morning, remembering again those last minutes, you realize that the repugnant has become reasonable. The unthinkable has become the right, the good. Painlessly. Quickly. With the assistance of a trained physician.

You should have killed your baby.

31

After-Birth Abortion

Why Should the Baby Live?

Alberto Giubilini and Francesca Minerva

Introduction

Severe abnormalities of the fetus and risks for the physical and/or psychological health of the woman are often cited as valid reasons for abortion. Sometimes the two reasons are connected, such as when a woman claims that a disabled child would represent a risk to her mental health. However, having a child can itself be an unbearable burden for the psychological health of the woman or for her already existing children,[1] regardless of the condition of the fetus. This could happen in the case of a woman who loses her partner after she finds out that she is pregnant and therefore feels she will not be able to take care of the possible child by herself.

A serious philosophical problem arises when the same conditions that would have justified abortion become known after birth. In such cases, we need to assess facts in order to decide whether the same arguments that apply to killing a human fetus can also be consistently applied to killing a newborn human.

Such an issue arises, for example, when an abnormality has not been detected during pregnancy or occurs during delivery. Perinatal asphyxia, for instance, may cause severe brain damage and result in severe mental and/or physical impairments comparable with those for which a woman could request an abortion. Moreover, abnormalities are not always, or cannot always be, diagnosed through prenatal screening even if they have a genetic origin. This is more likely to happen when the disease is not hereditary but is the result of genetic mutations occurring in the gametes of a healthy parent. One example is the case of Treacher-Collins syndrome (TCS), a condition that affects 1 in every 10,000 births causing facial deformity and related physiological failures, in particular potentially life-threatening respiratory problems. Usually those affected by TCS are not mentally impaired and they are therefore fully aware of their condition, of being different from other people and of all the problems their pathology entails. Many parents would choose to have an abortion if they find out, through genetic prenatal testing, that their fetus is affected by TCS. However, genetic prenatal tests for TCS are usually taken only if there is a family history of the disease. Sometimes, though, the disease is

Original publication details: Alberto Giubilini and Francesa Minerva, "After-Birth Abortion: Why Should the Baby Live?" pp. 261–263 from *Journal of Medical Ethics* 39 (2013). Reproduced with permission of BMJ Publishing Group Ltd.

caused by a gene mutation that intervenes in the gametes of a healthy member of the couple. Moreover, tests for TCS are quite expensive and it takes several weeks to get the result. Considering that it is a very rare pathology, we can understand why women are not usually tested for this disorder.

However, such rare and severe pathologies are not the only ones that are likely to remain undetected until delivery; even more common congenital diseases that women are usually tested for could fail to be detected. An examination of 18 European registries reveals that between 2005 and 2009 only the 64% of Down's syndrome cases were diagnosed through prenatal testing.[2] This percentage indicates that, considering only the European areas under examination, about 1,700 infants were born with Down's syndrome without parents being aware of it before birth. Once these children are born, there is no choice for the parents but to keep the child, which sometimes is exactly what they would not have done if the disease had been diagnosed before birth.

Abortion and After-Birth Abortion

Euthanasia in infants has been proposed by philosophers[3] for children with severe abnormalities whose lives can be expected to be not worth living and who are experiencing unbearable suffering.

Also medical professionals have recognised the need for guidelines about cases in which death seems to be in the best interest of the child. In The Netherlands, for instance, the Groningen Protocol (2002) allows to actively terminate the life of 'infants with a hopeless prognosis who experience what parents and medical experts deem to be unbearable suffering'.[4]

Although it is reasonable to predict that living with a very severe condition is against the best interest of the newborn, it is hard to find definitive arguments to the effect that life with certain pathologies is not worth living, even when those pathologies would constitute acceptable reasons for abortion. It might be maintained that 'even allowing for the more optimistic assessments of the potential of Down's syndrome children, this

potential cannot be said to be equal to that of a normal child'.[3] But, in fact, people with Down's syndrome, as well as people affected by many other severe disabilities, are often reported to be happy.[5]

Nonetheless, to bring up such children might be an unbearable burden on the family and on society as a whole, when the state economically provides for their care. On these grounds, the fact that a fetus has the potential to become a person who will have an (at least) acceptable life is no reason for prohibiting abortion. Therefore, we argue that, when circumstances occur *after birth* such that they would have justified abortion, what we call *after-birth abortion* should be permissible.

In spite of the oxymoron in the expression, we propose to call this practice 'after-birth abortion', rather than 'infanticide', to emphasise that the moral status of the individual killed is comparable with that of a fetus (on which 'abortions' in the traditional sense are performed) rather than to that of a child. Therefore, we claim that killing a newborn could be ethically permissible in all the circumstances where abortion would be. Such circumstances include cases where the newborn has the potential to have an (at least) acceptable life, but the well-being of the family is at risk. Accordingly, a second terminological specification is that we call such a practice 'after-birth abortion' rather than 'euthanasia' because the best interest of the one who dies is not necessarily the primary criterion for the choice, contrary to what happens in the case of euthanasia.

Failing to bring a new person into existence cannot be compared with the wrong caused by procuring the death of an existing person. The reason is that, unlike the case of death of an existing person, failing to bring a new person into existence does not prevent anyone from accomplishing any of *her* future aims. However, this consideration entails a much stronger idea than the one according to which severely disabled children should be euthanised. If the death of a newborn is not wrongful to her on the grounds that she cannot have formed any aim that she is prevented from accomplishing, then it should also be permissible to practise an after-birth abortion on a healthy newborn too, given that she has not formed any aim yet.

There are two reasons which, taken together, justify this claim:

1. The moral status of an infant is equivalent to that of a fetus, that is, neither can be considered a 'person' in a morally relevant sense.
2. It is not possible to damage a newborn by preventing her from developing the potentiality to become a person in the morally relevant sense.

We are going to justify these two points in the following two sections.

The Newborn and the Fetus are Morally Equivalent

The moral status of an infant is equivalent to that of a fetus in the sense that both lack those properties that justify the attribution of a right to life to an individual.

Both a fetus and a newborn certainly are human beings and potential persons, but neither is a 'person' in the sense of 'subject of a moral right to life'. We take 'person' to mean an individual who is capable of attributing to her own existence some (at least) basic value such that being deprived of this existence represents a loss to her. This means that many non-human animals and intellectually disabled human individuals are persons, but that all the individuals who are not in the condition of attributing any value to their own existence are not persons. Merely being human is not in itself a reason for ascribing someone a right to life. Indeed, many humans are not considered subjects of a right to life: spare embryos where research on embryo stem cells is permitted, fetuses where abortion is permitted, criminals where capital punishment is legal.

Our point here is that, although it is hard to exactly determine when a subject starts or ceases to be a 'person', a necessary condition for a subject to have a right to X is that she is harmed by a decision to deprive her of X. There are many ways in which an individual can be harmed, and not all of them require that she values or is even aware of what she is deprived of. A person might be 'harmed' when someone steals from her the winning lottery ticket even if she will never find out that her ticket was the winning one. Or a person might be 'harmed' if something were done to her at the stage of fetus which affects for the worse her quality of life as a person (eg, her mother took drugs during pregnancy), even if she is not aware of it. However, in such cases we are talking about a person who is at least *in the condition* to value the different situation she would have found herself in if she had not been harmed. And such a condition depends on the level of her mental development,[6] which in turn determines whether or not she is a 'person'.

Those who are only capable of experiencing pain and pleasure (like perhaps fetuses and certainly newborns) have a right not to be inflicted pain. If, in addition to experiencing pain and pleasure, an individual is capable of making any aims (like actual human and non-human persons), she is harmed if she is prevented from accomplishing her aims by being killed. Now, hardly can a newborn be said to have aims, as the future we imagine for it is merely a projection of our minds on its potential lives. It might start having expectations and develop a minimum level of self-awareness at a very early stage, but not in the first days or few weeks after birth. On the other hand, not only aims but also well-developed plans are concepts that certainly apply to those people (parents, siblings, society) who could be negatively or positively affected by the birth of that child. Therefore, the rights and interests of the actual people involved should represent the prevailing consideration in a decision about abortion and after-birth abortion.

It is true that a particular moral status can be attached to a non-person by virtue of the value an actual person (eg, the mother) attributes to it. However, this 'subjective' account of the moral status of a newborn does not debunk our previous argument. Let us imagine that a woman is pregnant with two identical twins who are affected by genetic disorders. In order to cure one of the embryos the woman is given the option to use the other twin to develop a therapy. If she agrees, she attributes to the first embryo the status of 'future child' and to the other one the status of a mere means to cure the 'future child'. However, the different moral status does not spring from the fact that the first one is a 'person' and the other is not, which would be non-sense, given that they are identical. Rather, the different moral statuses only depends on the particular value the woman projects on them. However, such a projection is exactly what does not occur when a newborn becomes a burden to its family.

The Fetus and the Newborn are Potential Persons

Although fetuses and newborns are not persons, they are potential persons because they can develop, thanks to their own biological mechanisms, those properties which will make them 'persons' in the sense of 'subjects of a moral right to life': that is, the point at which they will be able to make aims and appreciate their own life.

It might be claimed that someone is harmed because she is prevented from becoming a person capable of appreciating her own being alive. Thus, for example, one might say that we would have been harmed if our mothers had chosen to have an abortion while they were pregnant with us[7] or if they had killed us as soon as we were born. However, whereas you can benefit someone by bringing her into existence (if her life is worth living), it makes no sense to say that someone is harmed by being prevented from becoming an actual person. The reason is that, by virtue of our definition of the concept of 'harm' in the previous section, in order for a harm to occur, it is necessary that someone is in the condition of experiencing that harm.

If a potential person, like a fetus and a newborn, does not become an actual person, like you and us, then there is neither an actual nor a future person who can be harmed, which means that there is no harm at all. So, if you ask one of us if we would have been harmed, had our parents decided to kill us when we were fetuses or newborns, our answer is 'no', because they would have harmed someone who does not exist (the 'us' whom you are asking the question), which means no one. And if no one is harmed, then no harm occurred.

A consequence of this position is that the interests of actual people over-ride the interest of merely potential

people to become actual ones. This does not mean that the interests of actual people always over-ride *any* right of future generations, as we should certainly consider the well-being of people who will inhabit the planet in the future. Our focus is on the right to become a particular person, and not on the right to have a good life once someone will have started to be a person. In other words, we are talking about particular individuals who might or might not become particular persons depending on our choice, and not about those who will certainly exist in the future but whose identity does not depend on what we choose now.

The alleged right of individuals (such as fetuses and newborns) to develop their potentiality, which someone defends,[8] is over-ridden by the interests of actual people (parents, family, society) to pursue their own well-being because, as we have just argued, merely potential people cannot be harmed by not being brought into existence. Actual people's well-being could be threatened by the new (even if healthy) child requiring energy, money and care which the family might happen to be in short supply of. Sometimes this situation can be prevented through an abortion, but in some other cases this is not possible. In these cases, since non-persons have no moral rights to life, there are no reasons for banning after-birth abortions. We might still have moral duties towards future generations in spite of these future people not existing yet. But because we take it for granted that such people *will* exist (*whoever* they will be), we must treat them as *actual* persons of the future. This argument, however, does not apply to this particular newborn or infant, because we are not justified in taking it for granted that she will exist as a person in the future. Whether she will exist is exactly what our choice is about.

Adoption as an Alternative to After-Birth Abortion?

A possible objection to our argument is that after-birth abortion should be practised just on potential people who could never have a life worth living.[9] Accordingly, healthy and potentially happy people should be given up for adoption if the family cannot raise them up. Why should we kill a healthy newborn when giving it up for adoption would not breach anyone's right but possibly increase the happiness of people involved (adopters and adoptee)?

Our reply is the following. We have previously discussed the argument from potentiality, showing that it is not strong enough to outweigh the consideration of the interests of actual people. Indeed, however weak the interests of actual people can be, they will always trump the alleged interest of potential people to become actual ones, because this latter interest amounts to zero. On this perspective, the interests of the actual people involved matter, and among these interests, we also need to consider the interests of the mother who might suffer psychological distress from giving her child up for adoption. Birthmothers are often reported to experience serious psychological problems due to the inability to elaborate their loss and to cope with their grief.[10] It is true that grief and sense of loss may accompany both abortion and after-birth abortion as well as adoption, but we cannot assume that for the birthmother the latter is the least traumatic. For example, 'those who grieve a death must accept the irreversibility of the loss, but natural mothers often dream that their child will return to them. This makes it difficult to accept the reality of the loss because they can never be quite sure whether or not it is irreversible'.[11]

We are not suggesting that these are definitive reasons against adoption as a valid alternative to after-birth abortion. Much depends on circumstances and psychological reactions. What we are suggesting is that, if interests of actual people should prevail, then after-birth abortion should be considered a permissible option for women who would be damaged by giving up their newborns for adoption.

Conclusions

If criteria such as the costs (social, psychological, economic) for the potential parents are good enough reasons for having an abortion even when the fetus is healthy, if the moral status of the newborn is the same as that of the foetus and if neither has any moral value by virtue of being a potential person, then the same reasons which justify abortion should also justify the killing of the potential person when it is at the stage of a newborn.

Two considerations need to be added.

First, we do not put forward any claim about the moment at which after-birth abortion would no longer be permissible, and we do not think that in fact more than a few days would be necessary for doctors to detect any abnormality in the child. In cases where the after-birth abortion were requested for non-medical reasons, we do not suggest any threshold, as it depends on the neurological development of newborns, which is something neurologists and psychologists would be able to assess.

Second, we do not claim that after-birth abortions are good alternatives to abortion. Abortions at an early stage are the best option, for both psychological and physical reasons. However, if a disease has not been detected during the pregnancy, if something went wrong during the delivery, or if economical, social or psychological circumstances change such that taking care of the offspring becomes an unbearable burden on someone, then people should be given the chance of not being forced to do something they cannot afford.

References

1   *Abortion Act*. London: Stationery Office, 1967.
2   European Surveillance of Congenital Anomalies. *EUROCAT Database*. http://www.eurocat-network. eu/Prenatalscreeninganddiagnosis/prenataldetection rates (data uploaded 27 Oct 2011), (accessed 11 Nov 2011).

3   Kuhse, H. and Singer, P. *Should the Baby Live? The Problem of Handicapped Infants*. Oxford: Oxford University Press, 1985: 143.
4   Verhagen, E. and Sauer, P. The Groningen Protocol – euthanasia in severely ill newborns. *N Engl J Med* 2005; 10: 959–62.

5   Alderson, P. Down's Syndrome: cost, quality and the value of life. *Soc Sci Med* 2001; 5: 627–38.

6   Tooley, M. Abortion and infanticide. *Philos Public Aff* 1972; 1: 37–65. [See Chapter 1 in this *Anthology*.]

7   Hare, R. M. Abortion and the golden rule. In: Hare, R.M., ed. *Essays on Bioethics*. New York: Oxford University Press, 1993: 147–67.

8   Hare, R. M. A Kantian approach to abortion. In: Hare, R.M., ed. *Essays on Bioethics*. New York: Oxford University Press, 1993: 168–84.

9   Hare, R. M. The abnormal child. Moral dilemmas of doctors and parents. In: Hare, R.M., ed. *Essays on Bioethics*. New York: Oxford University Press, 1993: 185–91.

10   Condon, J. Psychological disability in women who relinquish a baby for adoption. *Med J Aust* 1986; 144: 117–19.

11   Robinson, E. Grief associated with the loss of children to adoption. In: *Separation, reunion, reconciliation: Proceedings from The Sixth Australian Conference on Adoption*. Stones Corner, Brisbane: Benson J, for Committee of the Conference, 1997: 268–93, 278.

32

Does a Human Being Gain the Right to Live after He or She is Born?

Christopher Kaczor

The most famous recent article about abortion is Alberto Giubilini and Francesca Minerva's "After-Birth Abortion: Why Should the Baby Live?" (2013; see also Chapter 31 in this *Anthology*). Following a standard line of argument, the authors distinguish between a "person" and a "human being" as terms with a technical sense in this discussion. A person is a being with moral worth, with basic rights, with equal status in the moral community. A human being is a member of the species *Homo sapiens*, a biological category, an organism of the same species as Hillary Clinton.

Simply to be a human being is not, on their view, sufficient for having a right to life, as acceptance of embryonic research, abortion prior to birth, and capital punishment indicate. To have the right to live, what counts is not being a *human being* but being a *person*.

Giubilini and Minerva point out that the same conditions that advocates of abortion say justify abortion may also exist after birth. Before birth, someone may seek an abortion because of poverty, but loss of job or dramatic reversal of economic fortune may also take place after birth. Abortions may be sought because the

man who impregnated the woman is a cad. But after a baby is born, a woman may discover that the father is cheating on her or otherwise is an unfit partner. Abortion may be sought because of fetal anomaly, but some infants become disabled in the process of being born, while the disability of others is discovered only after birth. Giubilini and Minerva suggest that, "when circumstances occur after birth such that they would have justified abortion, what we call after-birth abortion should be permissible" (Giubilini and Minerva 2013, 2). Killing newborn human beings is permissible whenever abortion would be permissible. Their argument is that there are no morally significant differences between a newborn and a fetal human being in utero, neither one is a "person" in the moral sense of the term. So, if abortion is ethically permissible, then post-birth abortion is also ethically permissible.

Giubilini and Minerva hold, "Both a fetus and a newborn certainly are human beings and potential persons, but neither is a 'person' in the sense of 'subject of a moral right to life'" (2013, 2). What then is a person? "We take 'person' to mean an individual who

Original publication details: Christopher Kaczor, "Abortion as a Human Rights Violation," pp. 92–98 from Kate Greasley and Christopher Kaczor (eds.), *Abortion Rights: For and Against* (Cambridge: Cambridge University Press, 2018). Reproduced with permission of Cambridge University Press.

Bioethics: An Anthology, Fourth Edition. Edited by Udo Schüklenk and Peter Singer.

is capable of attributing to her own existence some (at least) basic value such that being deprived of this existence represents a loss to her" (2013, 2). Now a newborn baby does not know that he or she exists, and so cannot attribute value to his or her existence. If a person does not exist even after birth, a fortiori there is no person at any time during gestation. Yes, it is true that the newborn is a potential person, that is, a being with the intrinsic orientation to develop into a person who values her own existence just as we do. But a potential person does not have the rights of an actual person, even as a potential president does not have the rights of an actual president.

But, they imagine someone objecting, isn't a newborn (or a human fetus) harmed by being destroyed and losing life? They reply that "it makes no sense to say that someone is harmed by being prevented from becoming an actual person. The reason is that, by virtue of our definition of the concept of 'harm' in the previous section, in order for a harm to occur, it is necessary that someone is in the condition of experiencing that harm" or being capable of experiencing the harm. They continue:

> So, if you ask one of us if we would have been harmed, had our parents decided to kill us when we were fetuses or newborns, our answer is "no," because they would have harmed someone who does not exist (the "us" whom you are asking the question), which means no one. And if no one is harmed, then no harm occurred.
>
> (2013, 3)

The interests of actual people (parents, family, society) override the nonexistent interests of potential people (newborns, prenatal human beings). The financial expense and personal burden of infants can detrimentally affect the interests of actual people. So, killing a newborn is morally permissible. "In these cases, since non-persons have no moral rights to life, there are no reasons for banning after-birth abortions" (2013, 3). Some people may wish to place unwanted infants in families by adoption, just as some women with unwanted pregnancies arrange to do, but this choice may be difficult or unwanted and should not abolish the choice of ending the life of the unwanted infant.

Giubilini and Minerva's argument can now be summarized. If we accept the principle that abortion is ethically permissible in certain social, economic, or psychological circumstances, then consistency demands that in similar circumstances post-birth abortion also be accepted. The same reasons that justify abortion of the human being prior to birth also justify killing a newborn after birth. Since in neither case does killing destroy a "person," both pre-birth and post-birth abortion is ethically acceptable and should also be legally acceptable.

Giubilini and Minerva decline to state at what moment after-birth abortion becomes ethically wrong. But psychologists indicate that self-awareness in children typically begins around two years of age (Rochat 2003, 718). Since you cannot *value* your own existence until you are *aware* that you exist, if these psychologists are correct, then post-birth abortion is permissible until around two years of age. Until human beings become aware of their own existence, they cannot take an *interest* in their continued existence. So, if Giubilini and Minerva's account is correct, infanticide is ethically permissible and should also be legally permitted until the child is around two years old (unless the child is intellectually disabled, in which case the right to live would arise even later or never arise at all in cases of severe intellectual disability).

If their conclusion is unacceptable, then something is wrong with Giubilini and Minerva's argument. Indeed, I believe their argument is riddled with questionable assumptions and false assertions. Giubilini and Minerva assume that killing a human being is wrong because the human being *desires, takes an interest in,* or *values* their continued existence and not being killed. But suicidal human beings (such as those who are deeply depressed, addicted to drugs, or brainwashed cult followers) do not desire their continued existence, but it would still be wrong to kill them. In fact, we desire things (like continued living) because we (rightly or wrongly) think that such things are good. So, what is relevant in determining whether someone has been wronged is not simply whether they were deprived of something they *desired* but also whether they were deprived of something *good*. After all, no one thinks it is wrong to deprive the suicide bomber of the explosive vest he desires in order to kill judge, jury, and everyone else in a courtroom. What we desire can be insane, tyrannical, unjust, uninformed, sexist, or racist. What is relevant ethically is not undermining someone's desires but undermining someone's good.

Moreover, Giubilini and Minerva assume "harm" is possible only if someone *experiences* (or is capable of experiencing) it as a harm. However, the lobotomy of a normal person may so damage the brain that the person does not experience the loss of brain power as a harm. Likewise, someone rendered permanently unconscious is harmed, but does not experience her condition as a harm and is not capable of experiencing her condition as a harm. Imagine a killing that is totally unexpected and instantaneous, like getting incinerated in a surprise nuclear blast by terrorists. In this kind of killing, unless we assume that people consciously survive their own deaths (which Giubilini and Minerva surely reject), the victims do not *experience* their death as harm, since they do not *experience* anything at or after death. So mass murder (as long as it is unanticipated and instantaneous) does not wrong the victims killed.

Giubilini and Minerva assume that no one has been *wronged* if no one has been *harmed*. This assumption is false because a wrong can be done even if no one is harmed. A failed assassination attempt may harm no one, but the target is wronged nonetheless. Malicious slander of someone's reputation (even if no one believes it) wrongs the person slandered.

Another questionable assumption of Giubilini and Minerva's view is its implicit body–self dualism. On their view, "you" are your aims, desires, awareness. Your body (the organism that was born and that your mother had in her womb) is not you. A human organism – not you – was born, and then months later "you" began to exist, when your thoughts, desires, and self-awareness began. If this view were true, you would not have a birthday, since you actually arose around two years after the human organism that you make use of was born.

The problematic nature of body–self dualism is illustrated by considering the case of twin three-year-old girls. Let's call them Sophia and Madison. The girls survive a car crash, but both have memory loss. Sophia will eventually recover most of her memories, but Madison will never recover hers. If the right to live depends on psychological connections, to kill Sophia is seriously wrong, but to kill Madison is not. The identical twins have radically different moral statuses because one will recover a few memories and the other will not. This is hard to believe. Moreover, the car accident both destroyed a person (Madison before her crash) and led to the creation of a new person (Madison after her crash). This is very hard to believe. It is much easier to believe that there is just one individual person (Madison) who survived her crash but was injured as a result of her crash. Indeed, this is what everyone not in the grip of a theory called body–self dualism believes.

If we accept body–self dualism, then one individual human being may in fact be several persons. Consider someone who suffers from dissociative identity disorder, formerly called multiple personality disorder. One individual human being may be both Dr Jekyll and Mr Hyde, with two sets of memories, desires, and loci of conscious awareness. Sometimes people suffering from dissociative identity disorder report not just two but sixteen different sets of identities. Each "alter" has his or her own memories, desires, and conscious awareness. If body–self dualism is correct, one human being with dissociative identity disorder is actually sixteen persons, and every person has a right to live. Thus, to kill one human being with dissociative identity disorder is to murder sixteen people. This is implausible.

Let's suppose a psychiatrist invents a breakthrough serum that completely and permanently cures dissociative identity disorder. Within one hour of injection into the back of the head just above the spinal column, the human being who had sixteen different personalities has only one personality. If body–self dualism is correct, administering the injection destroys fifteen persons. It is very hard to believe that the psychiatrist curing multiple personality disorder is not a compassionate healer but rather a mass murderer. (For more challenges to this assumption of Giubilini and Minerva, see Lee and George, *Body–Self Dualism*).

Some defenders of post-birth abortion appeal to John Locke's definition of a person, namely, a being with (1) an awareness of his or her own existence (2) over time and in different places with (3) the capacity to have wants and (4) plans for the future (Singer 1994, 218). A newborn baby (let alone a prenatal human being) does not satisfy these conditions, so post-birth abortion does not destroy anyone with a right to live.

No one disputes that Locke's conditions are *sufficient* for being a person, but why should we think of these conditions as *necessary* for the right to live? Picking out sufficient conditions for personhood is fairly easy. Everyone who can read *Leaves of Grass* or calculate the interior angles of a triangle is a person. But it does not follow that those who cannot appreciate Walt Whitman or Euclid's proofs do not have a right to live.

Why does Locke think of a person in this way? For Locke, on at least one plausible interpretation (Waldron 2002), our rights arise from our duties. According to Locke, we have a duty to obey God, a duty that we cannot discharge if others kill us or interfere with us, so we also have a right to life and liberty. Everyone who has the same capacity to act as a moral agent has equivalent duties to us, and therefore equal rights to us. The theological basis for Locke's view is a basis that I suspect many defenders of abortion (as well as many critics) would not accept.

But even if we were to strip away Locke's theological basis, and redefine Locke's person as a being that can discharge his or her duties (whether or not the moral obligation comes from God), this basis too proves problematic. Although there are a few defenders of post-birth abortion, no one defends the idea that *only* those who can act as moral agents discharging their duties merit respect as persons. If the right to live is enjoyed only by those who can act ethically, then the right to live arises only when a human being can be held morally accountable, namely, at the "age of reason" usually thought to be around seven or eight years of age. So, the basis for Locke's view of personhood is implausible, both as originally formulated theologically and as reformulated nontheologically. Unless we are provided another basis for thinking that all persons must have self-awareness etc., we have no reason for thinking Locke provides the necessary conditions for personhood.

Other aspects of the Lockean definition of a person are also problematic. Is self-awareness really necessary for personhood? *Actual* self-awareness cannot be necessary, unless we suppose that the right to live vanishes and reappears whenever someone loses consciousness in sleep. Nor is the *immediately exercisable* capacity for self-awareness necessary for basic rights, since no one thinks that a normal adult who is heavily sedated may be killed, yet such adults do not have an immediately exercisable capacity for self-awareness. Maybe the "mental hardware" or *current neural architecture* (or something functionally equivalent) that enables self-awareness (Savulescu 2002) is what is necessary for the right to live. But consider someone who has been in a car accident with temporary swelling of the brain that makes self-awareness temporarily impossible. The current neural architecture of such a swollen brain is incapable of self-awareness, but it is difficult to believe that such people in temporary comas have lost their right to live.

One proposed solution to the temporary coma case is to think of the right to live as a right that once attained with initial consciousness is retained for the rest of the being's life. However, this would mean that a human being in a permanent coma, a persistent vegetative state, maintains a right to live, which many defenders of abortion do not believe. Moreover, it is unclear why someone who attained self-awareness briefly and then lost it merits more protection than someone just about to attain self-awareness and who will have it for a long life. Why should an individual who had self-awareness once and never will again deserve more protection than another individual who will (if not killed) enjoy a full lifetime of self-awareness?

References

Giubilini, A. and Minerva, F. 2013. After-Birth Abortion: Why Should the Baby Live?" *J Med Ethics*, *39*: 261–3. [Chapter 31 in this *Anthology*.]

Lee, P. and George, R. P. 2007. *Body–Self Dualism in Contemporary Ethics and Politics*. Cambridge: Cambridge University Press.

Rochat, P. 2003. Five Levels of Self-Awareness as They Unfold early in Life. *Conscious and Cognition*, *12*(4), 717–31.

Savulescu, J. 2002. Abortion, Embryo Destruction and the Future of Value Argument. *Journal of Medical Ethics*, *25*(3), 133–5.

Singer, P. 1994. Rethinking Life and Death: The Collapse of Our Traditional Ethics. New York: St. Martin's Press.

Waldron, J. 2002. *God, Locke and Equality: Christian Foundations of Locke's Political Thought*. Cambridge: Cambridge University Press.

33

Hard Lessons

Learning from the Charlie Gard Case

Dominic Wilkinson and Julian Savulescu

On 24 July 2017, the long-running, deeply tragic and emotionally fraught case of Charlie Gard reached its sad conclusion (box 1). Following further medical assessment of the infant, Charlie's parents and doctors finally reached agreement that continuing medical treatment was not in Charlie's best interests. Life support was subsequently withdrawn and Charlie died on 28 July 2017.

Over the course of multiple hearings at different levels of courts in both London and Strasbourg, the Charlie Gard case has raised a number of vexed ethical questions (box 2). The important role of practical ethics in cases like this is to help clarify the key concepts, identify central ethical questions, separate them from questions of scientific fact, and subject arguments to critical scrutiny. The authors have disagreed about the right course of action for Charlie Gard,[1,2] but we agree on the key ethical principles as well as the role of ethical analysis and the importance of robust and informed debate. Ethics is not about personal opinion, but about argument, reasons and rational reflection. While the lasting ramifications of the case for medical treatment decisions in children are yet to become apparent, we here outline some of the potential lessons.

Parents' Role In Decision-Making for Children: We Need to Clarify Harm

Much of the media attention in the Gard case has focused on the rights of parents in decision-making for children, and whether the intervention of the courts in this case means that doctors frequently overrule parents in the UK. However, cases of intractable disagreement like this are the exception rather than the rule. In the majority of cases in the UK, as elsewhere,[3] parents and doctors reach decisions together through a process of shared decision-making. However, there have to be limits. Parents should not be allowed to make decisions that carry a significant risk of serious harm to a child. That includes refusing treatments of likely benefit for a child, or demanding treatments that impose a significant burden without

Original publication details: Dominic Wilkinson and Julian Savulescu, "Hard Lessons: Learning from the Charlie Gard Case," pp. 438–442 from *Journal of Medical Ethics* 44 (2018). Reproduced with permission of BMJ Publishing Group Ltd.

Box 1   Case summary and timeline[21–23]

Charlie Gard was born at full term, apparently healthy, in August 2016. At a few weeks of age his parents noticed early signs of muscle weakness. At 2 months of age, he was admitted to Great Ormond Street Hospital (GOSH) with poor feeding, failure to thrive and respiratory failure. He was admitted to intensive care, where investigations led to the diagnosis of a rare severe mitochondrial disorder – infantile onset encephalomyopathic mitochondrial DNA depletion syndrome (MDDS).

The specific genetic form of MDDS in Charlie Gard (RRM2B) had previously been reported in approximately 15 infants, with typical clinical features including early onset, rapid progression and death in infancy.[24] By that point, Charlie was paralysed and unable to breathe without respiratory support. He was found to have congenital deafness, and his heart, liver and kidneys were affected by the disorder. Doctors felt that Charlie's prognosis was extremely poor.

In early 2017, Charlie's parents identified an experimental treatment, previously used in a different form of MDDS, which they hoped might benefit Charlie. In mouse models of a myopathic form of MDDS (TK2), early supplementation with deoxypryrimidine nucleosides apparently bypasses the genetic defect and leads to a reduction in the biochemical defect and in the severity of the clinical phenotype.[25,26] Doctors at GOSH initially planned to use nucleoside treatment in Charlie, but in January he developed evidence of electrical seizures, and clinicians became convinced that treatment, both continued intensive care and the requested

nucleoside therapy, would be futile. A US physician involved in the nucleoside research offered to provide treatment, and Charlie's parents raised funds for him to travel to the USA.

However, doctors at GOSH were not happy with Charlie being transferred overseas for treatment. They applied to the Family Division of the High Court on 28 February for permission to withdraw life support and to provide palliative care. Charlie's parents opposed this plan. On 11 April, Justice Francis ruled in favour of the hospital. Charlie's family appealed, and the decision was reviewed (and upheld) in the Court of Appeal (23 May), Supreme Court (8 June) and European Court of Human Rights (20 June). At that stage, all avenues of legal appeal had been exhausted, and plans were made to withdraw medical treatment.

Following widespread public and media attention, including statements of support by President Trump and Pope Francis, a number of international medical and scientific experts came forward offering treatment and presenting apparently new evidence of allegedly increased chance of benefit from nucleoside treatment. On 10 July, GOSH elected to bring this evidence back to the High Court. The court arranged for the US mitochondrial specialist to review Charlie in London. Following a multi-disciplinary meeting and new evidence of the severity of Charlie's illness including the results of a full body MRI, on 24 July his parents accepted that further treatment could not help him and withdrew their application to the court.

---

benefit. The challenge, of course, and here there needs to be much more work, is in defining what constitutes a sufficient level or chance of harm to justify overruling parents.[4] Charlie would have had to potentially undergo some months of pain and discomfort from continued intensive care,[1] however, the doctors at Great Ormond Street Hospital indicated that they

felt that his neurological damage was so great that he was 'beyond experience'.[5] If that were truly the case, then it is not clear that acquiescing to parental request for treatment would have actually constituted significant harm (although it would also, almost certainly, mean that treatment would have had no chance at all of securing the improvement they desired). We have both disagreed about whether this harm threshold was reached, and consequently whether Charlie's parents' request should have been granted.[1,2]

Decisions for Adults Versus Decisions for Children: Allow Adults to Choose Treatment for Themselves even if Suboptimal

While there has been intense debate about whether or not requested treatment should be provided to Charlie Gard, it is important not to extrapolate from this case to decisions about medical treatment in adults. The ethical and legal basis for decisions in competent (or formerly competent) adults is different from that in children. If Charlie had been a young adult who had made clear his wishes to be kept alive on a ventilator, and to receive experimental treatment (even if there was a low chance of benefiting), then it should certainly have been provided.[6] For public health systems, it is important to manage fairly the limited healthcare resources we have. However, adult patients should be allowed to access cost-equivalent treatment alternatives, even if they would be inferior to the usually recommended standard of care.[7]

Experimental Treatment: We Should Have A Lower Threshold For Allowing Access Where Patients Have No Other Options, And Allow Earlier Innovative Treatment

Faced with certain death without treatment, Charlie's parents sought, and found, an experimental treatment that could conceivably benefit him. This treatment had not been tried in any previous patients with Charlie's illness, and on that basis was rejected as offering no known benefit. However, this suggests

a Catch-22: new treatments can only be tried if there is evidence from previous patients, but that evidence can only be acquired by trying it.

Moreover, Charlie was only one of four patients in the world with this condition. Large trials could not be performed and animal models could not be developed in time to help Charlie.

Novel experimental treatments are sometimes tried first in patients with lesser forms of an illness, or in healthy patients. However, that approach is arguably mistaken as such patients have little to gain and may have much to lose.[8] At least in some circumstances, novel treatments can only be tried on extremely sick patients first. Indeed, the ethical calculus is potentially inverted: patients like Charlie arguably have everything to gain and nothing to lose.

There are three potential lessons here. First, that there should be a low threshold for allowing innovative therapies in patients who have exhausted all other conventional medical therapies and otherwise will die. Second, that experimental treatments should potentially be embarked upon *without delay*.[9] In Charlie's case, it is ironic that delayed decision-making means that he could have received nucleoside treatment months ago, and by the time the case was finally concluded in court it would have been possible to assess if it had led to any improvement, or not. Third, there are of course limits to aggressively offering experimental treatment, particularly where the side effects of treatment may make it highly likely not to be in the individual's interests. Where the side effects are uncertain, it may be better to allow a time-limited trial of the therapy with a plan to actively withdraw treatment if side effects are significant or if there is no benefit after a suitable period.

The Role of Resources: We Need to Talk about Limited Resources

Even if it were not harmful, treatment (whether experimental therapy or life support in intensive care) should not be provided if it is excessively costly and would mean denying other patients their slice of the limited healthcare pie. This issue of limited healthcare resources does not apply directly in the Gard case as Charlie's parents had raised funds independently for him to travel to the USA for treatment.[1,2] It was not considered by the court. The Gard decision should not be seen therefore (contrary to the claims of some US politicians) as the decision of a single payer health system that is explicitly rationing treatment.

However, as noted by US paediatric intensivist Robert Truog, concern about finite health resources is legitimate even if parents or insurers pay for treatment.[10] It is relevant even in the USA (and perhaps especially in the USA).[11] Tertiary healthcare facilities, such as those that offered treatment to Charlie, are a result of community investment in medical research, medical education and medical care. The community has a stake in how those facilities are used, and in ensuring that they are used wisely (ie, with at least some plausible prospect of benefit).[10]

Furthermore, there is a deep resource-related paradox at the heart of this case, as in other cases of disputed, possibly futile treatment. While there is potential uncertainty about whether or not treatment would have been in Charlie's best interests, there is no uncertainty about resources. Continued intensive care in this case, in the face of a very low probability of improvement and high costs of treatment, represents an unreasonable and unfair use of limited healthcare resources. However, in an effort to adjudicate the difficult ethical question of the benefits and burdens of treatment for Charlie, treatment was prolonged at public expense for months. In that time, it is virtually certain that some children were denied transfer to the highly specialised intensive care unit at Great Ormond Street Hospital because of lack of capacity. It is virtually certain that in that time some elective (but vital) surgery was delayed. Because of concern for the well-being of other children needing the vital resource of the intensive care unit, it may have been better to allow the parents to take Charlie overseas months ago. Indeed, even if we accept that that would have been contrary to Charlie's best interests, it may have been a lesser harm overall.

However, resources have not been part of the central ethical debate for Charlie, and that is fundamentally because there is no clear process for clinicians to make resource-based decisions about provision of intensive care for patients. There is also no legal mechanism for courts to adjudicate on the issue of resources where there is a dispute.

The Role of the Courts: We Need a Fair, Expedient Way of Resolving Disputes

Parents cannot have a final say in medical decisions for children, but nor can doctors. Just as in every other area of life, where there is a dispute that cannot be resolved between two parties about an important issue, there needs to be a fair and impartial process for arbitration. In the UK, as in most other countries, the court serves that role. However, the court process is not perfect. It is adversarial, and can potentially make the ideal solution (agreement between parents and doctors) harder to achieve. It is costly. And it is potentially lengthy. In this case, the series of appeals has led to the worst of possible outcomes. Charlie Gard received months of intensive care that health professionals felt was contrary to his interests and doing more harm than good. But he did not receive the desired nucleoside treatment that his parents desired. Nobody has got the outcome that they wanted.

Is there an alternative? Because of the formidable epistemic and normative challenges in determining when treatment is futile,[12] one solution in some jurisdictions has been to focus on developing a fair and legally supported due process for decision-making.[13,14] There are two key components to this process that could and arguably should be adopted in the UK for future disputes about treatment. The first is the establishment of a process of case review by an independent ethics review panel where physicians feel that continued treatment would be futile. That panel would be able to reach decisions about withholding or withdrawing treatment without the lengthy process of adjudicating and appealing evident in the Gard case. Importantly, we suggest that it would be important for such a panel to include ethical expertise and to consider (where relevant) inviting ethical experts as well as medical experts to inform decisions. It would require a wide range of clinical and scientific opinion to get the facts clear but also to make clear the level of uncertainty about the facts. The second is to allow families to secure desired treatment if they are able to identify alternative healthcare providers who are prepared and able to provide treatment. One limit to that may be the location of alternative providers.

Ethical Decisions versus Clinical Decisions: Allow and Support Reasonable Disagreement

Much of the debate in the courtroom in the Gard case has been around medical evidence and factual claims, particularly about the reversibility of brain damage and the scientific plausibility of the experimental treatment (box 2). However, the decision in this case, and in other similar cases, is not a 'clinical decision'. It cannot be settled by questions of medical fact or scientific evidence alone.

Indeed, one of the striking (though not unique) features of this case is the presence of divergent expert testimony, and disagreement between key witnesses on whether treatment could help Charlie and whether it should be provided.

In court cases, one approach to witnesses who disagree about key facts is to assess the credibility of the witnesses and assign different weights to their testimony. Yet where the central question is value based and ethical, rather than scientific, consensus may be impossible. In those situations, dissensus may be just as important to note as consensus.[15] Where there is reasonable disagreement between experts about medical treatment, we should usually allow patients (or their surrogates) to decide. In the Charlie Gard case, there was just such disagreement, with experts in New York and Rome initially willing to provide the requested treatment. That provided a powerful (though not irrefutable) argument in favour of allowing continued

intensive care and nucleoside treatment. One vexed question is whether the disagreement in this case represented 'reasonable' disagreement.[16] Those offering treatment need to be able to provide clear and coherent reasons for doing so, to demonstrate understanding of the specific clinical circumstances, and to demonstrate willingness to revise their view in the face of changing facts.

Medical Tourism: Allow Families to Travel Unless Illegal or Risks Significant Harm

None of the medical experts in the UK who reviewed Charlie felt that the requested treatment would be in his best interests. However, experts in the USA and Italy offered to provide treatment.

On the face of it, stopping patients from undertaking medical tourism appears to violate two important freedoms – the freedom to travel and the freedom to make decisions about medical treatment. There might be reasons for a country not to provide a particular treatment option, for example because it is unaffordable within a public healthcare system, or because doctors in that country do not approve of it, or lack experience or expertise in providing it, but usually patients should not be prevented from accessing treatment overseas.

However, particularly for children, there are a range of situations where it might be problematic for parents to travel to access controversial treatment.[17] It is not acceptable for parents to bypass laws that are designed to protect children from harm by taking them out of the country (eg, to obtain female circumcision).

Where treatment options are contentious, but not illegal (and perhaps experimental treatment falls into this category), decisions to allow travel may need to be considered on a case-by-case basis. On the one hand, health professionals should arguably respect reasonable disagreement. On the other, they have a professional and legal duty to report cases if they suspect that parents' plans to take a child out of the country risk significant harm.

Box 2   Some of the key factual and ethical questions arising from the Charlie Gard case

Factual questions

- What was Charlie's level of awareness/cognition?
- How much did he experience pain/suffer from intensive care?
- Can suffering from intensive care be alleviated completely/partly by sedation/analgesia?
- What was the chance of improvement in Charlie's encephalopathy or myopathy?
- How long would treatment need to be provided to determine if he had any improvement?
- What is the best function that he could achieve with treatment?
- Could he be ventilator independent with treatment?
- How long could he live with continued life-sustaining treatment?

Ethical questions
What is the right thing to do?

- Would it be in Charlie's best interests to receive continued intensive care and nucleoside treatment?
- Would life for Charlie in his impaired state be a life worth living?
- Should we judge this based on subjective or objective accounts of well-being?
- In the best-case scenario (with maximum realistic improvement from nucleoside treatment), would his life be worth living?
- Should the interests of parents be taken into account?

- Should, and if so when should treatment be denied on the basis of limited public healthcare resources?

How should decisions be made?

- When should parents' requests for medical treatment be overruled?
- Should parents be permitted to consent to untested or extremely uncertain experimental treatment if a child would certainly die without it?
- What constitutes 'significant harm' to justify overruling parents?
- If parents are able to pay for treatment, should that change the permissibility of continuing/providing treatment?
- How should decisions about allocation of resources be made for individual patients?
- How should diverging views about medical facts be taken into account?
- Does it matter if those diverging views come from health professionals in different countries?
- How should diverging views about normative issues (eg, life worth living, parental rights) be taken into account?
- Should parents be free to take their child overseas for medical treatment unavailable in their home country?
- Should decisions be made through the courts, or in some extra-judicial process?

Challenging Normative and Conceptual Issues: Need for Further Ethical Analysis

The central question about providing desired treatment or withdrawing and allowing Charlie to die is irreducibly normative. Because of that, it is important to be clear about some of the key value questions and concepts at stake. For example, in the initial court ruling, Judge Francis referred to Charlie's interest in maintaining his dignity, and the significance of allowing him to 'die with dignity'. Yet it was not clear what independent ethical role dignity played in the ethical evaluation of treatment. Dignity is a deeply contested concept in medical ethics.[18,19] There were clearly different views between parents and professionals about whether it would be consistent with Charlie's dignity to continue intensive care.

Another fundamental issue is what counts as sufficient benefit to prolong life. The concept of a 'life worth living' is highly controversial, yet it remains at the heart of this case, and other cases.[2] For adults, it is possible to rely to a degree on subjective accounts of well-being, since adults can report on their experience of pain or pleasure. It is also possible (in at least some cases) to draw on their evaluations of what is or would be a sufficient benefit to provide life-prolonging treatment. However, for young children, and others who are not and have never been able to express their wishes or preferences, a subjective account is either meaningless or misleading. The alternative is an objective account of a life worth living that is robust and clear enough to be applied to contested cases, and also respects reasonable disagreement about value and values. That alternative remains to be established.

Reflective Equilibrium, Reasons and Evidence: Need for Humility and Transparency

How should value judgements be made? Philosopher John Rawls described a process of reflective equilibrium. This involves developing principles (such as the best interests principle and those of distributive justice) and concepts (such as well-being and a life worth living), but crucially revising these in line with intuitions about specific cases, such as Charlie's. This process is what judges engage in but judges, or doctors, are not necessarily or exclusively ethical experts.

Rawls described the qualities of people who should be engaged in reflective equilibrium. They should be knowledgeable about the relevant facts. Importantly, they should be 'reasonable': (1) being willing to use inductive logic, (2) being disposed to find reasons for and against a solution, (3) having an open mind, (4) making a conscientious effort to overcome their intellectual, emotional and moral prejudices. Lastly, they are to have 'sympathetic knowledge. . . of those human interests which, by conflicting in particular cases, give rise to the need to make a moral decision'.[20]

When a decision is arrived at, the decision together with its reasons and evidence needs to be made clear to those involved, and, in high-profile public cases, to the public at large.

In decisions about life support for a critically ill child, those who have to make the decision, whether they are parents, health professionals or high court judges, should aspire to the above qualities and engage in reflective equilibrium. However, perhaps the most distinctive feature of the Charlie Gard case is the way that this decision has been shared in real time with a massive national and international audience. Tens of thousands, perhaps hundreds of thousands, of people have been reading, thinking, and venturing opinions on the core questions and value judgements at stake.

Given the emotional and intellectual involvement of so many people in this profound and profoundly difficult decision, it is salient to remember Rawls' other key lesson about value judgements: participants in reflective equilibrium should display epistemic and normative humility, that is a calibrated confidence in their knowledge of empirical and moral truth.

As the sad case of Charlie Gard comes to a close, it is sobering but vital to step back from our own personal views on the case, and to remember that we can all get it wrong.

References

1   Wilkinson, D. Beyond resources: denying parental requests for futile treatment. *Lancet* 2017; 389: 1866–7.

2   Savulescu, J. Is it in Charlie Gard's best interest to die? *Lancet* 2017; 389: 1868–9.

3   Verhagen, A.A., de Vos, M., Dorscheidt, J.H., et al. Conflicts about end-of-life decisions in NICUs in the Netherlands. *Pediatrics* 2009; 124:e112–e119.

4   Nair, T., Savulescu, J., Everett, J., et al. Settling for second best: when should doctors agree to parental demands for suboptimal medical treatment? *J Med Ethics* 2017; 43:831–40.

5   Great Ormond Street Hospital for Children. Latest statement on Charlie Gard. 2017. https://www.gosh.nhs.uk/news/latest-press-releases/latest-statement-charlie-gard

6   Wilkinson, D. Burke, Briggs and Wills: why we should not fear the judgment in Charlie Gard: Practical Ethics blog. 2017. http://blog.practicalethics.ox.ac.uk/2017/07/burke-briggs-and-wills-why-we-should-not-fear-the-judgment-in-charlie-gard/

7   Wilkinson, D., and Savulescu, J. Cost-equivalence and pluralism in publicly-funded health-care systems. *Health Care Anal.* Published Online First: 6 Jan 2017. doi:10.1007/ s10728-016-0337-z.

8   Savulescu J. Harm, ethics committees and the gene therapy death. *J Med Ethics* 2001; 27: 148–50.

9   Savulescu J. The moral of the case of Charlie Gard: give dying patients experimental treatment . . . early. *Practical Ethics [blog]*, 5 Jul 2017. http://blog.practicalethics.ox.ac.uk/2017/07/the-moral-of-the-case-of-charlie-gard-give-dying-patients-experimental-treatment-early/.

10   Truog, R.D. The United Kingdom sets limits on experimental treatments: the case of Charlie Gard. *JAMA* 2017; 318: 1001–2.

11   Camosy, C. *Too expensive to treat? Finitude, tragedy and the neonatal ICU.* Grand Rapids, Michigan: Eerdmans, 2010.

12   Wilkinson, D. Futility. *The International Encyclopedia of Ethics,* Wiley, 2017.

13   Stewart, C. Futility determination as a process: problems with medical sovereignty, legal issues and the strengths and weakness of the procedural approach. *J Bioeth Inq* 2011; 8: 155–63.

14   Fine, R.L. and Mayo, T.W. Resolution of futility by due process: early experience with the Texas Advance Directives Act. *Ann Intern Med* 2003; 138: 743–6.

15   Wilkinson, D., Truog R., Savulescu J. In favour of medical dissensus: Why We should agree to disagree about end-of-life decisions. *Bioethics* 2016; 30: 109–18.

16   Wilkinson, D. and Savulescu J. Agreement and disagreement about experimental treatment: the Charlie Gard appeal: Practical Ethics blog. 2017. http://blog.practicalethics.ox.ac.uk/2017/05/agreement-and-disagreement-about-experimental-treatment-the-charlie-gard-appeal/

17   Wilkinson, D. Medical tourism for controversial treatment options: Practical Ethics blog. 2017. http://blog.practicalethics.ox.ac.uk/2017/07/medical-tourism-for-controversial-treatment-options/

18   Macklin, R. Dignity is a useless concept. *BMJ* 2003; 327: 1419–20.

19   Killmister, S. Dignity: not such a useless concept. *J Med Ethics* 2010; 36: 160–4.

20   Rawls, J. Outline of a decision procedure for ethics. *Philos Rev* 1951; 60: 177–97.

21   Dyer, C. and Law, D.C. Law, ethics, and emotion: the Charlie Gard case. *BMJ* 2017; 358: j3152.

22   Francis J. Decision and short reasons to be released to the media in the case of Charlie Gard: Judiciary of England and Wales. 2017. https://www.judiciary.gov.uk/wp-content/uploads/2017/04/gard-press-summary-20170411.pdf (accessed 27 Apr 17).

23   *Great Ormond Street Hospital -v- Yates and Gard*: EWHC 1909 (Fam), 2017.

24   El-Hattab, A.W. and Scaglia F. Mitochondrial DNA depletion syndromes: review and updates of genetic basis, manifestations, and therapeutic options. *Neurotherapeutics* 2013; 10: 186–98.

25   Garone, C., Garcia-Diaz, B., Emmanuele, V., et al. Deoxypyrimidine monophosphate bypass therapy for thymidine kinase 2 deficiency. *EMBO Mol Med* 2014; 6:1016–27.

26   Lopez-Gomez, C., Levy, R.J., Sanchez-Quintero, M.J., et al. Deoxycytidine and deoxythymidine treatment for thymidine kinase 2 deficiency. *Ann Neurol* 2017; 81: 641–52.

Brain Death

34

A Definition of Irreversible Coma

Report of the Ad Hoc Committee of the Harvard Medical School to Examine the Definition of Brain Death

Our primary purpose is to define irreversible coma as a new criterion for death. There are two reasons why there is need for a definition: (1) Improvements in resuscitative and supportive measures have led to increased efforts to save those who are desperately injured. Sometimes these efforts have only partial success so that the result is an individual whose heart continues to beat but whose brain is irreversibly damaged. The burden is great on patients who suffer permanent loss of intellect, on their families, on the hospitals, and on those in need of hospital beds already occupied by these comatose patients. (2) Obsolete criteria for the definition of death can lead to controversy in obtaining organs for transplantation.

Irreversible coma has many causes, but *we are concerned here only with those comatose individuals who have no discernible central nervous system activity*. If the characteristics can be defined in satisfactory terms, translatable into action – and we believe this is possible – then several problems will either disappear or will become more readily soluble.

More than medical problems are present. There are moral, ethical, religious, and legal issues. Adequate definition here will prepare the way for better insight into all of these matters as well as for better law than is currently applicable.

Characteristics of Irreversible Coma

An organ, brain or other, that no longer functions and has no possibility of functioning again is for all practical purposes dead. Our first problem is to determine the characteristics of a *permanently* nonfunctioning brain.

A patient in this state appears to be in deep coma. The condition can be satisfactorily diagnosed by points 1, 2, and 3 to follow. The electroencephalogram (point 4) provides confirmatory data, and when available it should be utilized. In situations where for one reason or another electro-encephalographic monitoring is not available, the absence of cerebral function has to be determined by purely clinical signs, to be described, or by absence of circulation as judged by standstill of blood in the retinal vessels, or by absence of cardiac activity.

Original publication details: Report of the Ad Hoc Committee of the Harvard Medical School to Examine the Definition of Brain Death, "A Definition of Irreversible Coma," pp. 85–88 from *Journal of the American Medical Association* 205: 6 (August 1968).

Unreceptivity and Unresponsitivity. – There is a total unawareness to externally applied stimuli and inner need and complete unresponsiveness – our definition of irreversible coma. Even the most intensely painful stimuli evoke no vocal or other response, not even a groan, withdrawal of a limb, or quickening of respiration.

1. *No Movements or Breathing.* – Observations covering a period of at least one hour by physicians is adequate to satisfy the criteria of no spontaneous muscular movements or spontaneous respiration or response to stimuli such as pain, touch, sound, or light. After the patient is on a mechanical respirator, the total absence of spontaneous breathing may be established by turning off the respirator for three minutes and observing whether there is any effort on the part of the subject to breathe spontaneously. (The respirator may be turned off for this time provided that at the start of the trial period the patient's carbon dioxide tension is within the normal range, and provided also that the patient had been breathing room air for at least 10 minutes prior to the trial.)

2. *No Reflexes.* – Irreversible coma with abolition of central nervous system activity is evidenced in part by the absence of elicitable reflexes. The pupil will be fixed and dilated and will not respond to a direct source of bright light. Since the establishment of a fixed, dilated pupil is clear-cut in clinical practice, there should be no uncertainty as to its presence. Ocular movement (to head turning and to irrigation of the ears with ice water) and blinking are absent. There is no evidence of postural activity (decerebrate or other). Swallowing, yawning, vocalization are in abeyance. Corneal and pharyngeal reflexes are absent.

3. As a rule the stretch of tendon reflexes cannot be elicited; i.e., tapping the tendons of the biceps, triceps, and pronator muscles, quadriceps and gastrocnemius muscles with the reflex hammer elicits no contraction of the respective muscles. Plantar or noxious stimulation gives no response.

4. *Flat Electroencephalogram.* – Of great confirmatory value is the flat or isoelectric EEG. We must assume that the electrodes have been properly applied, that the apparatus is functioning normally, and that the personnel in charge is competent. We consider it prudent to have one channel of the apparatus used for an electrocardiogram. This channel will monitor the ECG so that, if it appears in the electroencephalographic leads because of high resistance, it can be readily identified. It also establishes the presence of the active heart in the absence of the EEG. We recommend that another channel be used for a noncephalic lead. This will pick up space-borne or vibration-borne artifacts and identify them. The simplest form of such a monitoring noncephalic electrode has two leads over the dorsum of the hand, preferably the right hand, so the ECG will be minimal or absent. Since one of the requirements of this state is that there be no muscle activity, these two dorsal hand electrodes will not be bothered by muscle artifact. The apparatus should be run at standard gains 10µv/mm, 50 µv/5mm. Also it should be isoelectric at double this standard gain which is 5µv/mm or 25µv/5mm. At least ten full minutes of recording are desirable, but twice that would be better.

It is also suggested that the gains at some point be opened to their full amplitude for a brief period (5 to 100 seconds) to see what is going on. Usually in an intensive care unit artifacts will dominate the picture, but these are readily identifiable. There shall be no electroencephalographic response to noise or to pinch.

All of the above tests shall be repeated at least 24 hours later with no change.

The validity of such data as indications of irreversible cerebral damage depends on the exclusion of two conditions: hypothermia (temperature below 90°F [32.2°C]) or central nervous system depressants, such as barbiturates.

Other Procedures

The patient's condition can be determined only by a physician. When the patient is hopelessly damaged as defined above, the family and all colleagues who have participated in major decisions concerning the patient, and all nurses involved, should be so informed. Death is to be declared and *then* the respirator turned off. The decision to do this and the responsibility for it are to be taken by the physician-in-charge, in consultation with one or more physicians who have been directly involved in the case. It is unsound and undesirable to force the family to make the decision.

Legal commentary

The legal system of the United States is greatly in need of the kind of analysis and recommendations for medical procedures in cases of irreversible brain damage as described. At present, the law of the United States, in all 50 states and in the federal courts, treats the question of human death as a question of fact to be decided in every case. When any doubt exists, the courts seek medical expert testimony concerning the time of death of the particular individual involved. However, the law makes the assumption that the medical criteria for determining death are settled and not in doubt among physicians. Furthermore, the law assumes that the traditional method among physicians for determination of death is to ascertain the absence of all vital signs. To this extent, *Black's Law Dictionary* (4th edition, 1951) defines death as

> The cessation of life; the ceasing to exist; *defined by physicians* as a total stoppage of the circulation of the blood, and a cessation of the animal and vital functions consequent thereupon, such as respiration, pulsation, etc. [italics added]

In the few modern court decisions involving a definition of death, the courts have used the concept of the total cessation of all vital signs. Two cases are worthy of examination. Both involved the issue of which one of two persons died first.

In *Thomas vs Anderson* (96 Cal App 2d 371, 211 P 2d 478) a California District Court of Appeal in 1950 said, "In the instant case the question as to which of the two men died first was a question of fact for the determination of the trial court. . ."

The appellate court cited and quoted in full the definition of death from *Black's Law Dictionary* and concluded, "death occurs precisely when life ceases and does not occur until the heart stops beating and respiration ends. Death is not a continuous event and is an event that takes place at a precise time."

The other case is *Smith vs Smith* (229 Ark, 579, 317 SW 2d 275) decided in 1958 by the Supreme Court of Arkansas. In this case the two people were husband and wife involved in an auto accident. The husband was found dead at the scene of the accident. The wife was taken to the hospital unconscious. It is alleged that she "remained in coma due to brain injury" and died at the hospital 17 days later. The petitioner in court tried to argue that the two people died simultaneously. The judge writing the opinion said the petition contained a "quite unusual and unique allegation." It was quoted as follows:

> That the said Hugh Smith and his wife, Lucy Coleman Smith, were in an automobile accident on the 19th day of April, 1957, said accident being instantly fatal to each of them at the same time, although the doctors maintained a vain hope of survival and made every effort to revive and resuscitate said Lucy Coleman Smith until May 6th, 1957, when it was finally determined by the attending physicians that their hope of resuscitation and possible restoration of human life to the said Lucy Coleman Smith was entirely vain, and
>
> That as a matter of modern medical science, your petitioner alleges and states, and will offer the Court competent proof that the said Hugh Smith, deceased, and said Lucy Coleman Smith, deceased, lost their power to will at the same instant, and that their demise as earthly human beings occurred at the same time in said automobile accident, neither of them ever regaining any consciousness whatsoever.

The court dismissed the petition as a *matter of law*. The court quoted *Black's* definition of death and concluded,

> Admittedly, this condition did not exist, and as a matter of fact, it would be too much of a strain of credulity for us to believe any evidence offered to the effect that Mrs. Smith was dead, scientifically or otherwise, unless the conditions set out in the definition existed.

Later in the opinion the court said, "Likewise, we take judicial notice that one breathing, though unconscious, is not dead."

"Judicial notice" of this definition of death means that the court did not consider that definition open to serious controversy; it considered the question as settled in responsible scientific and medical circles. The judge thus makes proof of uncontroverted facts unnecessary so as to prevent prolonging the trial with unnecessary proof and also to prevent fraud being committed upon the court by quasi "scientists" being called into court to controvert settled scientific principles at a price. Here, the Arkansas Supreme Court considered the definition of death to be a settled, scientific, biological fact. It refused to consider the plaintiff's offer of evidence that "modern medical science" might say otherwise. In simplified form, the above is the state of the law in the United States concerning the definition of death.

In this report, however, we suggest that responsible medical opinion is ready to adopt new criteria for pronouncing death to have occurred in an individual sustaining irreversible coma as a result of permanent brain damage. If this position is adopted by the medical community, it can form the basis for change in the current legal concept of death. No statutory change in the law should be necessary since the law treats this question essentially as one of fact to be determined by physicians. The only circumstance in which it would be necessary that legislation be offered in the various states to define "death" by law would be in the event that great controversy were engendered surrounding the subject and physicians were unable to agree on the new medical criteria.

It is recommended as a part of these procedures that judgement of the existence of these criteria is solely a medical issue. It is suggested that the physician in charge of the patient consult with one or more other physicians directly involved in the case before the patient is declared dead on the basis of these criteria. In this way, the responsibility is shared over a wider range of medical opinion, thus providing an important degree of protection against later questions which might be raised about the particular case. It is

further suggested that the decision to declare the person dead, and then to turn off the respirator, be made by physicians not involved in any later effort to transplant organs or tissue from the deceased individual. This is advisable in order to avoid any appearance of self-interest by the physicians involved.

It should be emphasized that we recommend the patient be declared dead before any effort is made to take him off a respirator, if he is then on a respirator. This declaration should not be delayed until he has been taken off the respirator and all artificially stimulated signs have ceased. The reason for this recommendation is that in our judgement it will provide a greater degree of legal protection to those involved. Otherwise, the physicians would be turning off the respirator on a person who is, under the present strict, technical application of law, still alive.

Comment

Irreversible coma can have various causes: cardiac arrest; asphyxia with respiratory arrest; massive brain damage; intracranial lesions, neoplastic or vascular. It can be produced by other encephalopathic states such as the metabolic derangements associated, for example, with uremia. Respiratory failure and impaired circulation underlie all of these conditions. They result in hypoxia and ischemia of the brain.

From ancient times down to the recent past it was clear that, when the respiration and heart stopped, the brain would die in a few minutes; so the obvious criterion of no heart beat as synonymous with death was sufficiently accurate. In those times the heart was considered to be the central organ of the body; it is not surprising that its failure marked the onset of death. This is no longer valid when modern resuscitative and supportive measures are used. These improved activities can now restore "life" as judged by the ancient standards of persistent respiration and continuing heart beat. This can be the case even when there is not the remotest possibility of an individual recovering consciousness following massive brain damage. In other situations "life" can be maintained only by means of artificial respiration and electrical stimulation of the heart beat, or in temporarily bypassing the heart, or, in conjunction with these things, reducing with cold the body's oxygen requirement.

In an address, "The Prolongation of Life," (1957),[1] Pope Pius XII raised many questions; some conclusions stand out: (1) In a deeply unconscious individual vital functions may be maintained over a prolonged period only by extraordinary means. Verification of the moment of death can be determined, if at all, only by a physician. Some have suggested that the moment of death is the moment when irreparable and overwhelming brain damage occurs. Pius XII acknowledged that it is not "within the competence of the Church" to determine this. (2) It is incumbent on the physician to take all reasonable, ordinary means of restoring the spontaneous vital functions and consciousness, and to employ such extraordinary means as are available to him to this end. It is not obligatory, however, to continue to use extraordinary means indefinitely in hopeless cases. "But normally one is held to use only ordinary means – according to circumstances of persons, places, times, and cultures – that is to say, means that do not involve any grave burden for oneself or another." It is the church's view that a time comes when resuscitative efforts should stop and death be unopposed.

Summary

The neurological impairment to which the terms "brain death syndrome" and "irreversible coma" have become attached indicates diffuse disease. Function is abolished at cerebral, brain-stem, and often spinal levels. This should be evident in all cases from clinical examination alone. Cerebral, cortical, and thalamic involvement are indicated by a complete absence of receptivity of all forms of sensory stimulation and a lack of response to stimuli and to inner need. The term "coma" is used to designate this state of unreceptivity and unresponsitivity. But there is always coincident paralysis of brain-stem and basal ganglionic mechanisms as manifested by an abolition of all postural reflexes, including induced decerebrate postures; a complete paralysis of respiration; widely dilated, fixed pupils; paralysis of ocular movements; swallowing; phonation; face and tongue muscles. Involvement of spinal cord, which is less constant, is reflected usually in loss of tendon reflex and all flexor withdrawal or nocifensive reflexes. Of the brain-stem–spinal mechanisms which are conserved for a time, the vasomotor reflexes are the most persistent, and they are responsible in part for the paradoxical state of retained cardiovascular function, which is to some extent independent of nervous control, in the face of widespread disorder of cerebrum, brain stem, and spinal cord.

Neurological assessment gains in reliability if the aforementioned neurological signs persist over a period of time, with the additional safeguards that there is no accompanying hypothermia or evidence of drug intoxication. If either of the latter two conditions exist, interpretation of the neurological state should await the return of body temperature to normal level and elimination of the intoxicating agent. Under any other circumstances, repeated examinations over a period of 24 hours or longer should be required in order to obtain evidence of the irreversibility of the condition.

Reference

1   Pius XII: The Prolongation of Life. *Pope Speaks*, 4 (1958): 393–8.

35

The Challenge of Brain Death for the Sanctity of Life Ethic

Peter Singer

I   Introduction

In 1968, *Black's Law Dictionary* defined death as follows:

> The cessation of life; the ceasing to exist; defined by physicians as a total stoppage of the circulation of the blood, and a cessation of the animal and vital functions consequent thereupon, such as respiration, pulsation, etc.

Twenty years later, most of the world had accepted, with surprisingly little controversy, a new way in which one could be dead, even if one's heart was beating, one's blood was circulating, and "animal and vital functions", including having a pulse, continued. That new way was defined in terms of the irreversible cessation of all functions of the entire brain, including the brain stem. One reason why this view gained acceptance without controversy was that the new definition was generally presented as an improved scientific understanding of the nature of death, and not as taking a new stance on an ethical issue. This was consistent with an oft-cited statement made by Pope Pius

XII at a conference of anaesthesiologists, held in 1957, at a time when ventilators were beginning to be used. Pius XII was asked how a doctor should determine that a patient on a ventilator is dead. He reiterated the Church's view that death occurred when the soul separated from the body; but, aware that this was not of great practical help to the doctors in his audience, he added: "It remains for the doctor, and especially the anaesthesiologist, to give a clear and precise definition of 'death' and 'the moment of death' of a patient who passes away in a state of unconsciousness" (The prolongation of life, 1957, p. 396).

Over the thirty years since brain death became widely accepted as a criterion of death, a few bioethicists and physicians have raised questions about it, but public discussions have been rare. More recently, the case of Jahi McMath has raised new questions about brain death, and especially about the standard diagnostic guidelines for diagnosing brain death. In 2013, at the age of 13, Jahi underwent what should have been a routine tonsillectomy in a California hospital. After the operation she bled excessively, and the bleeding was not stopped. Jahi was placed on a

Original publication details: Peter Singer, "The Challenge of Brain Death for the Sanctity of Life Ethic," pp. 153–165 from *Ethics & Bioethics in Central Europe 8*: 3–4 (2018).

ventilator, and two days later, declared brain-dead. A social worker urged her family to take her off the ventilator, and to consider donating her organs. Her mother, Nailah McMath, did not understand how she could be dead when her skin was still warm and she was occasionally moving her arms, ankles and hips – movements that the hospital doctors said were only a spinal reflex. In any case, the family insisted on first finding out what had happened to her before taking her off the ventilator. (The family is African American, and suspected that a white patient would have received better care.) A lawyer agreed to take their case on a pro bono basis.

The coroner issued a death certificate for Jahi, but the family, using funds raised online, took what was then officially a corpse, and flew it (or her), attached to a portable ventilator, to New Jersey, where state law forbids hospitals from treating a patient with a beating heart as dead if the family has religious objections to brain death. Nailah, a Christian, said she did have such objections. Jahi was admitted to St Peter's University Hospital, a Roman Catholic hospital in New Brunswick.

In newspapers and on television, leading American bioethicists criticized both the family's actions and the hospital's decision to admit Jahi. Lawrence McCullough said the hospital's decision was "crazy". Art Caplan managed to say both "Keeping her on a ventilator amounts to desecration of a body" and "There isn't any likelihood that she's gonna [sic] survive very long". Robert Truog, on the other hand, was troubled by criticisms of the family, subsequently telling Rachel Aviv of the *New Yorker*: "I think that the bioethics community felt this need to support the traditional understanding of brain death, to the point that they were really treating the family with disdain, and I felt terrible about that" (Aviv, 2018).

After eight months at St Peter's, Jahi was discharged from hospital: the diagnosis on the discharge was brain death. But her family had not given up. They rented a nearby apartment where, for nearly four years, she remained on a ventilator and was fed through a tube. Her condition remained stable for nearly four years, but then she suffered further medical complications.

Her heart stopped and she was declared dead in the traditional way, which her family accepted.

During the years Jahi was on a ventilator, her family engaged a malpractice attorney, and sued the California hospital where the tonsillectomy was performed. If that suit had come to trial, whether Jahi was really dead would have been a central issue, because under Californian law, damages awarded in medical malpractice suits involving children who die cannot exceed $250,000. There is no limit on damages when patients survive (Aviv, 2018). After Jahi's death, however, the case was settled for an undisclosed amount.

The first aim of this article is to update my earlier writings in which I argued that there are good reasons for rejecting the prevailing view of brain death.[1] A second aim is to show that rejecting brain death raises the stakes in the debate between those who believe in the sanctity of human life, and those who hold that the quality of a life must affect its value. I also take account of a new issue raised by the Jahi McMath case. I conclude by pointing to possible ways forward.

II The Origins of the New Definition of Death

The first step towards the development of a new definition of death can be traced to Henry Beecher, a distinguished professor of medicine at Harvard University and chair of a committee that oversaw the ethics of experimentation on human beings. In 1967 he wrote to Robert Ebert, Dean of the Harvard Medical School, proposing that the committee should take up the issue of the definition of death. This idea had emerged, he told Ebert, from conversations with Joseph Murray, a surgeon at Massachusetts General Hospital and a pioneer in kidney transplantation. The need for further consideration of the definition of death arose, Beecher wrote, from the fact that "[E] very major hospital has patients stacked up waiting for suitable donors".[2] The issue gained added urgency when Dr Christiaan Barnard carried out the world's first heart transplant. Shortly thereafter Ebert set up the Harvard Brain Death Committee, under Beecher's chairmanship. It published its report in the *Journal of the American Medical Association* in August 1968. The report began as follows:

> "Our primary purpose is to define irreversible coma as a new criterion for death. There are two reasons why there is a need for a definition: (1) Improvements in resuscitative and supportive measures have led to increased efforts to save those who are desperately injured. Sometimes these efforts have only partial success so that the result is an individual whose heart continues to beat but whose brain is irreversibly damaged. The burden is great on patients who suffer permanent loss of intellect, on their families, on the hospitals, and on those in need of hospital beds already occupied by these comatose patients. (2) Obsolete criteria for the definition of death can lead to controversy in obtaining organs for transplantation" (Report, 1968, p. 337).

Nowhere in the Harvard committee's final report does the committee claim that the new definition of death reflects some scientific discoveries about, or improved scientific understanding of, the nature of death. It was, instead, because the committee saw the status quo as imposing great burdens on various people and institutions affected by it, including preventing the proper use of the "life-saving potential" of the organs of people in "irreversible coma" that the committee recommended the new definition of death. But the judgment that it is good to avoid these burdens, and to ensure that organs can be used, is an ethical judgment, not a scientific one.

The Harvard committee's report was influential. In the decade following its publication, a number of US states changed their legal definition of death so that, if tests showed that the brain had ceased to function, patients could be declared dead, despite the fact that their hearts were still beating, and their blood circulating. That meant that a patient with a beating heart but no brain function might be declared dead in one state, but if moved to another state would legally be alive.

In 1981 the United States President's Commission for the Study of Ethical Problems in Medicine took up the problem of the definition of death. Its report, *Defining Death,* recommended uniform legislation that would enable people to be declared dead if tests established the irreversible cessation of all brain function (President's Commission, 1981). The report was endorsed by the American Medical Association, and subsequently every state and territory of the US adopted legislation recognizing that a person whose brain has irreversibly ceased to function is dead.

III   Death as the Irreversible Loss of Integrated Organic Functioning

A proponent of the view that brain death really is death might argue that the Harvard committee made the right recommendation for the wrong reasons. What reasons, other than the various benefits mentioned by the committee, would there be for holding that the death of the brain really is the death of the whole human being? A typical answer is that the introduction of modern methods of intensive care has exposed a certain vagueness in the concept of death, and a new account is needed to clear this up. The question is what that new account should be.

The President's Commission said that brain death is the death of the human organism because without brain function, the body is no longer an integrated whole, but just a collection of cells and organs. In this they were following two prominent Roman Catholic bioethicists, Germain Grisez and Joseph Boyle, who, in *Life and Death with Liberty and Justice,* had argued that death is to be understood in theoretical terms as "the permanent termination of the integrated functioning characteristic of a living body as a whole. . ." (Grisez & Boyle, 1979, p. 77; Lamb, 1985).

Since *Defining Death* was published, however, it has become clear that integrated organic functioning can persist despite the irreversible cessation of all brain functions. Already in 1998, a literature search conducted by Alan Shewmon, then professor of paediatric neurology at the University of California, Los Angeles, Medical School, found 175 cases of brain dead patients "surviving" for at least one week, 80 for at least two weeks, 44 for at least four weeks, 20 for at least two months, and seven for at least six months.

These were all cases in which there was a formal diagnosis of brain death made by a physician, usually including at least one neurologist or neurosurgeon. Shewmon notes that many examples are of "unequivocal BD [brain death] confirmed by multiple clinical examinations, EEGs, intracranial blood flow, and necropsy findings" (Shewmon, 1998a, pp. 1538–45; Shewmon, 1999, pp. 1369–72). Moreover in many of these cases, treatment was eventually withdrawn. The number of patients "surviving" for long periods would have been greater still if treatment had been maintained in all cases. As Shewmon says, the diagnosis of brain death is nearly always "a self-fulfilling prophecy" as it is followed by organ harvesting or the discontinuation of support. Occasionally, however, a family will insist on support being maintained even after a diagnosis of brain death, as Jahi McMath's mother did. Another such case has been described by Shewmon. A patient, known as "TK" contracted a form of meningitis at the age of four and was declared dead. Shewmon visited him when he was 18 years old. He described the case as follows:

"Cerebral edema was so extreme that the cranial sutures split. Multiple EEGs have been isoelectric, and no spontaneous respirations or brain-stem reflexes have been observed over the past 14 1/2 years. Multimodality evoked potentials revealed no intracranial peaks, magnetic resonance angiography disclosed no intracranial blood flow, and neuroimaging showed the entire cranial cavity to be filled with disorganised membranes, proteinaceous fluids and ghost-like outlines of the former brain" (Shewmon, 1998a, p. 1543).

Shewmon examined TK and documented everything photographically. He concluded: "There is no question that he became "brain-dead" at age 4; neither is there any question that he is still alive at age 18 1/2". TK "lived" – if that is the right word – at home on a ventilator, fed by a gastrostomy tube. His heart continued to beat for another six years after Shewmon wrote the account just quoted. During the 20 years he was without brain function, he grew, overcame infections, and healed wounds (Shewmon, 1998b, pp. 125–45; Repetinger, 2006, pp. 591–5).

In cases like TK exhaustive tests have shown that the brain no longer exists, and there can be no brain function at all. Such cases force us to reconsider the assumption on which Grisez and Boyle, as well as the President's Commission, rely for their acceptance of brain death: that a functioning brain is a necessary condition for an integrated organism. Instead, Shewmon concludes: "The body's integrative unity derives from mutual interaction among its parts, not from a top-down imposition of one "critical organ" upon an otherwise mere bag of organs and tissues" (Shewmon, 2001, pp. 457–78; Shewmon, 2012, pp. 423–494). How this is possible, and what parts are interacting to maintain this integrative unity, is an interesting scientific question, but is beyond the scope of this paper.

The development of Shewmon's own views is worth a short digression. A Roman Catholic, in 1989 he presented a defence of a version of "whole-brain death" to the Pontifical Academy of Sciences. Subsequently he rejected all brain-based formulations of death. In this he is joined by another leading Roman Catholic scholar in this area, John Finnis, Professor of Law at the University of Oxford, and by the former archbishop of Cologne, Joachim Cardinal Meisner, who in 1994 declared that "the identification of brain death with death of the person is from a Christian point of view no longer justifiable".[3]

Once it became clear that a human organism can, with the aid of a ventilator and good nursing care, continue to function for months or even years after the irreversible cessation of all brain function, the view that this irreversible cessation is equivalent to the death of the human being was on shaky ground. We can see this in the case of patients with a high spinal cord injury that leaves the patient paralysed below the injury and unable to breathe on his or her own. Although the brain has not lost all functions, it has lost its integrative function, because it can no longer communicate with the body below the injury. Yet patients with such an injury are still conscious. It would be absurd to say that because the brain has lost its integrative function, a fully conscious patient is dead.

IV   What do the Standard Tests for Brain Death Show?

More recently, Shewmon has added another complication to the discussion. He examined Jahi McMath, and also watched videos taken by her family in which she appears to respond, with a frequency Shewmon says is highly unlikely to be chance, to spoken requests to raise a finger or make other movements. His conclusion is that at the time when Jahi was declared dead, she did fulfil the requirements of brain death, but "[W]ith the passage of time, her brain has recovered the ability to generate electrical activity, in parallel with its recovery of ability to respond to commands". Jahi was therefore at the time of Shewmon's statement, in his view, "an extremely disabled but very much alive teenage girl" (Aviv, 2018). Brain death is defined as the *irreversible* cessation of all brain functions, so it is logically impossible for Jahi to have been dead in accordance with this definition, and for her brain to then recover some function. If her brain now has some function, she was never brain dead.

Shewmon knows this, of course, so when he says that Jahi fulfilled the requirements of brain death, he must mean that when Jahi was declared dead, the tests standardly used to establish brain death were correctly carried out, and yielded the readings standardly taken to mean that all brain functions have irreversibly ceased. If that is the case, however, it shows that the standard tests are not a completely reliable indicator of brain death. Shewmon believes that Jahi was probably in a minimally conscious state, as a result of a condition known as global ischemic penumbra, in which intracranial blood flow is too low to support synaptic function, but is just sufficient to prevent the death of the cells. At present, the standard tests for blood flow used to diagnose brain death are not sensitive enough to distinguish this low level of blood flow from no flow at all (Shewmon, 2018).

If Shewmon is right about this, it would seem that we have a choice. One option is to devise new tests with the requisite sensitivity and use them instead of the now-standard tests in the guidelines for diagnosing brain death, so that they are able to detect global ischemic penumbra, and possibly other conditions from which the brain can recover some function but which are not detected by the standard tests. This may not be as simple as it sounds. According to Shewmon:

> "[T]he "accepted medical standards" do not include ruling out GIP as a confounding factor. . . and there is no way to rule it out in a given case short of actual measurement of blood flow in every part of the brain, for which no practical test exists (an area ripe for urgent clinical research)" (Shewmon, 2018, p. 169).

Under the present legal definition of death, however, unless we can develop such a test, there is a risk that every removal of a heart from a patient who has been declared to be brain dead is, legally speaking, murder.

The other option is therefore to return to the traditional definition of death, and cease to remove organs from patients with beating hearts. I will now turn to the deliberations of President George W. Bush's Council on Bioethics, which considered this possibility.

V   President George W. Bush's Council on Bioethics Enters the Debate

In 2008, the President's Council on Bioethics, a conservative-leaning body appointed by President George W. Bush to replace its more liberal predecessor, took up the question of brain death, noting controversy about the view that "total brain failure" (as the Council refers to brain death) is the death of the human being. On the basis of evidence from Shewmon and others, the Council rejected the view that total brain failure means the end of an integrated organism. It might therefore seem that the Council must reject brain death itself. After all, Shewmon concluded, as the Council correctly notes, that to hold that the condition of the brain determines the death of the organism is a mistake (President's Council on

Bioethics, pp. 54–5). Nevertheless, the Council did not recommend a return to the traditional view that death occurs when the heart stops beating and the blood ceases to circulate. Instead a majority of its members found a new rationale for supporting the view that brain death is the death of the organism. The majority proposed that we take note of the fact that living organisms "engage in commerce with the surrounding world" (President's Council on Bioethics, p. 60). The "commerce" on which the majority focused most attention, and regarded as most critical, is breathing:

"As a vital sign, the spontaneous action of breathing can and must be distinguished from the technologically supported, passive condition of being ventilated (i.e., of having one's "breathing" replaced by a mechanical ventilator). The natural work of breathing, even apart from consciousness or self-awareness, is itself a sure sign that the organism as a whole is doing the work that constitutes – and preserves – it as a whole. In contrast, artificial, non-spontaneous breathing produced by a machine is not such a sign. It does not signify an activity of the organism as a whole. It is not driven by felt need, and the exchange of gases that it effects is neither an achievement of the organism nor a sign of its genuine vitality" (President's Council on Bioethics, p. 63).

The idea that spontaneous breathing could be used as a criterion for deciding whether someone is dead or alive faces several objections; most obviously, many patients placed on ventilators have lost the ability to breathe spontaneously. They will, after an interval, regain it, and walk out of hospital. The Council is aware of this, of course, and sees only the *irreversible* loss of the capacity as a sign of death but people with a high spinal cord injury may have irreversibly lost the ability to breathe spontaneously, and yet be fully conscious. Again, the Council acknowledges this, and adds that "other vital capacities might still be present". The report continues:

"For example, patients with spinal cord injuries may be permanently apneic or unable to breathe without ventilatory support and yet retain full or partial possession of their conscious faculties. Just as much as striving

to breathe, signs of consciousness are incontrovertible evidence that a living organism, a patient, is alive" (President's Council on Bioethics, p. 63).

The Council therefore decides, though with some dissenting members, to stay with brain death, not because this signifies the death of the integrated organism, but because "total brain failure" indicates the irreversible absence of both spontaneous breathing and consciousness.

This is a desperate attempt to reach a much-desired conclusion. Let's first see why the Council was so keen to preserve the definition of death in terms of brain death, and then see why its attempt to do so fails.

The Council's report contemplates the possible conclusion that brain death is not the death of the organism, and that consequently we need to return to defining death in terms of the cessation of heartbeat and circulation of the blood. What practical difference would this make? There are two possible ways of responding to this situation. One is that we preserve the rule that organs may only be taken from dead donors, and therefore do not take organs from donors whose hearts are still beating, even if their brains have irreversibly ceased to function. Because some organs, including the liver and the heart itself, are subject to rapid damage once the heart stops, this is likely to mean that significantly fewer people would benefit from organ transplants, and many lives now saved would be lost. In addition, the Council expresses concern that the need to certify a patient as dead as soon as possible after the heart stops beating would have an adverse impact on the care of dying patients whose hearts stop, but perhaps could be resuscitated. In other words, if we combine the traditional definition of death with a world in which transplants can save lives, we will introduce a new tension between making absolutely certain that the patient is dead, and saving the lives of other patients.

The other possible way of responding to the return to the traditional definition of death is to draw on the present criteria for ascertaining total brain failure in order to determine, not that a patient is dead, but that the patient is eligible to be an organ donor. Such patients would be eligible because (and here I use my own words, not those of the Council) their lives are over, not as organisms, but as conscious beings. They will never again experience anything. In these very specific circumstances, continuing their lives beyond this point is of no further benefit to them. (Singer, 1995; Miller & Truog, 2011).

The Council is aware of the attractions of this view. It requires no questionable arguments defending a new concept of death, and it does not force us to reject or significantly hamper the practice of organ donation. Nevertheless, the Council finds this view unacceptable on ethical grounds:

> "[T]his solution is deeply disturbing, for it embraces the idea that a living human being may be used merely as a means for another human being's ends, losing his or her own life in the process. For good reason, many recoil from the thought that it would be permissible to end one life in order to obtain body parts needed by another. . . abandoning the "dead donor rule" would entail dismantling the moral foundations of the practice of organ donation" (President's Council on Bioethics, p. 17).

In short, the Council knows that if organs cannot ethically be removed from donors with beating hearts, then many people whose lives could be saved by organ transplants will die; but the Council nevertheless believes that it is ethically unacceptable to remove vital organs from living human beings in order to benefit others. No wonder that most members of the Council were desperate to find a basis for retaining a definition of death that includes total brain failure.

A strong desire to reach a pre-determined conclusion often leads to poor reasoning. That applies to the Council's stance that the absence of spontaneous breathing is a sign of death – except when it isn't, for example when there is consciousness in the absence of spontaneous breathing. This addition to the initial selection of the absence of spontaneous breathing reveals that the Council has been forced to patch together from disparate elements its account of the difference between life and death. As Albert Garth Thomas, an anaesthesiologist with qualifications in

philosophy, notes in his discussion of the Council's report, this conjunction "marks their analysis as *ad hoc* and unconvincing". Thomas also points out that "[J]ust how one would understand spontaneous respiration as the epitome of human life is difficult to grasp". That's because breathing is no more crucial to our normal lives than many other functions, such as those of the kidneys, liver, and pancreas (Thomas, 2012, p. 106). These organs too could be described as "engaged in commerce with the surrounding world" and they can continue to operate spontaneously after spontaneous breathing has ceased. Why is their spontaneous operation not enough to show that a patient is alive?

As we have seen, the Council sought to avoid a return to the traditional definition of death. It rejected, not unanimously but by a majority, the alternative of abandoning the "dead donor rule" on the grounds that this would "dismantle" the moral foundations of the practice of organ donation. That is not so; at most, it would amend the moral foundations of that practice, and even that claim presupposes that these moral foundations have the Kantian basis described in the passage quoted above. Historically speaking, this presupposition is highly dubious. As we saw earlier, the moral foundations of the initial stimulus for the change in the definition of death, and thereby for the development of the modern practice of organ transplantation, seems to have been much closer to utilitarian principles than to Kantian ones.

One might, of course, accept, as a matter of historical fact, that the Harvard committee was thinking upon broadly utilitarian lines, and yet deplore this, and seek to persuade current practitioners that the only defensible moral foundation of the practice is Kantian. The more significant question, however, is whether the Kantian objection to using living, but irreversibly brain-dead human beings as organ donors, is valid. In my view, it is not. Whatever Kant may have meant by his famous statement that we should treat others "never merely as a means to an end, but always at the same time as an end", the principle is plainly indefensible unless it includes, in the idea of treating someone "merely as a means" the proviso that the person did not freely and voluntarily consent to being so used. Otherwise, why is not mailing a letter wrongly using as mere means the people who collect, sort and deliver the mail? The standard Kantian answer to this obvious objection is that postal employees freely consent to do their work. Hence the work is an end, for them, and there is no wrong-doing in mailing a letter; but organ donors also consent, prior to their death, at least in countries that have "opt-in" systems of donation, as the United States does. It is also arguable that in "opt-out" systems, people who do not opt out are giving implicit consent, as long as the opportunity to opt out is well-known to everyone and easily accessible.

It might be said that under either opt-in or opt-out systems, donors consent for their organs to be taken after their death, but if we abandon the dead donor rule, the organs will be taken when they are not dead. If that is the concern, then the problem that the President's Council finds so morally fundamental could easily be overcome. All that is necessary is to rephrase the question potential donors are asked, so that they are asked to consent to organs being taken after irreversible total brain failure, with no hope of any recovery of consciousness. We could then see what proportion of those currently willing to be organ donors would continue to be willing to donate under the new conditions. My hope is that this change would not cause a significant drop in the number of donors, as long as they were accurately informed about the irreversible nature of the condition that they would be have to be in before they could be considered as a donor, and the degree of confidence with which that condition could be diagnosed.

VI The significance of irreversible unconsciousness

We have seen that the Harvard committee thought that people in an "irreversible coma" should be regarded as dead. We have also noted the reasons the Harvard committee gave for this change. It was, in large part, because of the good consequences that would flow from this change, for the families of the

person in the irreversible coma, for the hospitals, and for the potential organ recipients. All of these reasons apply not only to patients whose brains have totally and irreversibly ceased to function, but also to patients who have irreversibly lost all capacity for consciousness. Why then did the Harvard committee limit its concern to those with no brain activity at all?

One reason may be that in 1968, the only form of "irreversible coma" that could be reliably diagnosed – with no possibility of a patient being declared dead and then "waking up" – was that in which there was no discernible brain activity at all. Another possible reason for the committee redefining death to cover only those with no brain activity at all is that if the ventilator is removed from such patients, they stop breathing and so will soon be dead by anyone's standard. People in a persistent vegetative state, on the other hand, continue to breathe without mechanical assistance. So if the Harvard committee had included in its definition of death people who are in an irreversible coma but still have some brain activity, they would have been suggesting that people could be buried while they are still breathing.

Technology has, in many cases, eliminated the first of these reasons. Admittedly, in some cases of patients in a long-term persistent vegetative state, we still lack any completely reliable means of saying when recovery is impossible. In other cases, however, new forms of brain imaging can establish that parts of the brain necessary for consciousness have ceased to exist, and hence that consciousness cannot return. This would be the case, for example, if there has been no blood flow to the cortex for so long that the entire cortex had turned to liquid. The brain stem may still be functioning, however, so the problem of declaring patients dead when they are breathing spontaneously remains. This condition would be visible on a scan, and would also serve to ensure that the patient was not even in a minimally conscious state, as Jahi McMath appears to have been.

Several writers have urged that the solution to the present unsatisfactory state of the definition of death is to draw on our improved diagnostic abilities to move on to a definition of death in terms of the irreversible loss of consciousness. Among those defending this view are Michael Green and Daniel Wikler, John Lizza, Calixto Machado, Jeff McMahan, and Robert Veatch (see for example: Engelhardt, 1975, pp. 587–90; Veatch, 1975, pp. 13–30; Green & Wikler, 1980, pp. 105–33; Machado, 1995; McMahan, 1995, pp. 91–126; Lizza, 2018, pp. 1–19).

The significance of consciousness, and its link with the brain, answers the fundamental question – "why the brain?" – that supporters of the whole brain death criterion have never been able to answer satisfactorily. The death of the whole brain is the end of everything that matters about a person's life, but so too is the death of those parts of the brain necessary for consciousness. So the definition of death in terms of the irreversible loss of consciousness means that the criterion for death is the irreversible cessation of function of what is variously referred to as the cortex, the cerebral hemispheres, or the cerebrum. To avoid the need to define this more precisely, I shall use the expression "the higher brain" to refer to whatever parts of the brain are necessary for consciousness.

We have already seen that even total brain failure is not the same as the death of the organism. Given that, it is obviously going to be difficult to argue that an irreversible loss of consciousness is equivalent to the death of the human organism. Warm, breathing human beings, with their hearts beating and their blood circulating, are not dead, whether the breathing is spontaneous or mechanically assisted. "Dead" is a term applied much more widely than human beings, or conscious beings, or beings with brains. An oyster has no brain at all, let alone a higher brain, yet oysters are alive, and they can die.

Jeff McMahan's defence of the higher brain account of the death of human beings is more philosophically sophisticated than most, and worth our attention for that reason. McMahan takes his cue from Mark Johnston's assertion that we are not "essentially human organisms" (Johnston, 1987, pp. 75–6) and uses this claim to distinguish the death of the person from the death of the organism. Our survival as persons, McMahan claims, requires "continuity of mind", and so our continued existence, for all practical purposes, "requires the preservation of various mental powers or capacities in the areas of the brain in which consciousness and mental activity occur" (McMahan, 1995, p. 111; Green & Wikler, 1980). Thus, unlike organisms without minds, we can die while our body is still alive. McMahan recognises that the category of "organisms with minds" is not limited to the human species, nor applicable to all members of that species. A dog may die while its body is still living, and an anencephalic human infant is a living human organism without a mind. On this view, the grieving family of the warm, breathing body in the hospital ward are right to think that they are not facing a dead body. But they are also right if they understand that the person they loved is gone forever. In McMahan's terms, that person is dead.

VII   The Centrality of Ethics

McMahan's proposal has the merit of not denying that human organisms die in the same sense that plants die. Hence it does less violence to the common conception of death than other defences of a move to a higher brain definition of death. His view helps us to conceptualise what is going on when the higher brain has been destroyed and the body continues to live, but he acknowledges that it does not resolve the ethical questions. Is it wrong to cut the heart out of an anencephalic infant, which is a living human organism but can never be a person? Or out of an irreversibly unconscious human organism who has been, but can never again be, a person?

The existence, over the past three or four decades, of the definition of death in terms of brain death has, quite literally, made it possible for Christians to get away with what would, under the earlier traditional definition of death, have been murder – and without abandoning their support for the sanctity of all human life. Moreover, if brain death is not the death of the human organism, it is hard to see how defenders of the equal value of all human life can support the removal of ventilators from brain-dead patients with beating hearts. Roman Catholic teaching holds that extraordinary treatment is not obligatory when it imposes a disproportionate burden on the patient or others – disproportionate, that is, in terms of the benefits gained. This doctrine allows Christians to discontinue extraordinary means of life-support that are burdensome to a patient or demand scarce medical resources, and the burden on the patient or the use of resources is disproportionate to the benefit that will be achieved. This may be the case when the patient is suffering and will, in any case, live for only a short time, or when the medical resources could save other patients who will live much longer. Now consider a brain-dead human being who, like TK, could live another 10 or 15 years, cared for at home by his family at relatively modest cost. In what way are the measures taken to keep him alive disproportionate to the benefit of an extra 10 years of life? There is no suffering. Admittedly, there is also no joy nor any other experiences at all but to say that the extension of human life is not a significant benefit because it brings no conscious experiences of any sort, and therefore the life of the human being need not be prolonged, is to invoke an explicit quality-of-life judgment as the basis for discontinuing treatment. That is in direct contradiction to the words of Pope John Paul II in *Evangelium Vitae*: "As far as the right to life is concerned, every innocent human being is absolutely equal to all others. . ." For those who take this view, if brain dead human beings can be kept alive for many years without the use of scarce medical resources, the distinction between "ordinary" and "extraordinary" or between "proportionate" and "disproportionate" means of care cannot be used to justify withdrawing medical support from them.[4]

If, on the other hand, we reject the view that all human life is of equal value, we have another ethical option. We could accept the traditional conception of death – thus agreeing, in effect, with Shewmon and Finnis on this question – but reject their ethical view that it is always wrong intentionally to end the life of an innocent human being. We could then regard it as justifiable to remove organs for transplantation, when there has been an irreversible loss of consciousness, as long as the donor gave the appropriate consent,

applicable to this situation. We would then achieve the same practical outcome as we would achieve by redefining death in terms of the irreversible loss of consciousness. To return to the language used by the Harvard committee, we would be able to relieve the burden on families, hospitals and those in need of hospital beds, not only when the patient's brain has wholly ceased to function, but also when the patient's higher brain has irreversibly ceased to function. We would be able to do this without having had to finesse the definition of death in order to achieve our objective. Last, but by no means least, we would have made our ethical judgments transparent, thus advancing public understanding of the issues involved rather than obscuring it.

The most troubling objection to this approach is a practical one: no matter how logically compelling the proposal may be, it may seem to be such a radical ethical change that it stands no chance of success. After all, it is a head-on challenge to the traditional doctrine of the sanctity of all human life. Better, some will say, to do our best to push back the extent of that doctrine's reach, than to hurl ourselves vainly against its citadel. Better, in other words, to maintain the belief that brain death really is death, and indeed to try to go beyond whole brain death, by arguing that we die when we irreversibly lose consciousness. Otherwise, we risk denting the public confidence in brain death. That could lead to fewer people giving consent for the removal of organs – their own or those of their loved ones – when brain death is diagnosed, and that would mean that fewer lives could be saved by organ transplantation.

VIII   Conclusion

We are left with two options that preserve and extend the possibility of organ transplantation without using anyone without their consent, or violating anyone's human rights. We could hold that conscious beings die when they irreversibly lose consciousness, and that this, and not the death of the organism, is what makes permissible the removal of organs from a consenting donor.

Alternatively, we could return to the traditional definition of death in terms of the cessation of heartbeat and the stoppage of the circulation of the blood, but hold that it is not wrong to remove organs from living human beings who have irreversibly lost consciousness, and have consented to the donation of their vital organs in such circumstances. Both of these options avoid the misconceptions involved in the view that organs can only be taken from dead human organisms, and that the test of death for a donor with a beating heart is the irreversible loss of all brain function.

I will not here attempt to choose between these two options, for they converge on the crucial point:

the existence of a living human organism is not a sufficient reason for ruling out the removal of vital organs from that organism. There is, however, one remaining problem; both of these options require that we establish that the patient has irreversibly lost consciousness. In the light of the Jahi McMath case, that may not be simple, given that we would not want to wait, in every case, for the liquefaction of the cortex in order to establish it. Such a delay would come at a high price, both in financial and human terms. Nevertheless, this is a technical problem. If solving it became a requirement of continuing organ transplants from beating heart donors, I assume that a solution would soon be found.

Notes

1 See especially *Rethinking Life and Death* (Singer, 1995).
2 Henry Beecher to Robert Ebert, 30 October 1967 (Rothman, 1991, pp. 160–1). 155
3 John Finnis expressed his view in unpublished comments on a paper I gave to the Philosophy Society, Oxford University, 14 May 1998; for Joachim Cardinal Meisner, see "Erklärung des Erzbischofs von Köln zum beabsichtigten Transplanationsgesetz" [Declaration of the Archbishop of Cologne on the proposed transplantation

law], September 27, 1996, *PEK Pressedienst*, 1996, Erklärung nr. 316, cited by Gerhard Wolf, "Strafbarkeit von Organentnahmen für Transplantationen?" In: Jan Joerden, (ed.): *Der Mensch und seine Behandlung in der Medizin*. Berlin: Springer, 1999, p. 301, n. 91.
4 For a critique of attempts by Catholic ethicists to appeal to these distinctions as a way of avoiding explicit quality-of-life judgments, see *The Sanctity-of-Life Doctrine in Medicine: A Critique* (Kuhse, 1987).

References

Aviv, R. (2018): What does it mean to die? In: *New Yorker*, February 5.

Beecher, H. (1967): Henry Beecher to Robert Ebert. In: D. Rothman (1991): *Strangers at the Bedside*. New York: Basic books, pp. 160–1.

Engelhardt, T., Jr. (1975): Defining death: A philosophical problem for medicine and law. In: *American Review of Respiratory Disease*, 112(5), pp. 587–90.

Green, M. & Wikler, D. (1980): Brain Death and Personal Identity. In: *Philosophy and Public Affairs*, 9(2), pp. 105–133.

Grizez, G. & Boyle, J. (1979): *Life and Death with Liberty and Justice*. Notre Dame: University of Notre Dame Press.

Johnston, M. (1987): Human beings. In: *Journal of Philosophy*, 84(2), pp. 59–83.

Kuhse, H. (1987): *The Sanctity-of-Life Doctrine in Medicine: A Critique*. Oxford: Oxford University Press.

Lamb, D. (1985): *Death, Brain Death and Ethics*. London: Croom Helm.

Lizza, J. (2018): Defining Death: Beyond Biology. In: *Diametros*, 55, pp. 1–19.

Machado, C. (1995): A New Definition of Death Based on the Basic Mechanism of Consciousness Generation in Human Beings. In: C. Machado (ed.): *Brain Death: Proceedings of the Second International Symposium on Brain Death*. Amsterdam: Elsevier, pp. 57–66.

McMahan, J. (1995): The Metaphysics of Brain Death. In: *Bioethics*, 9(2), pp. 91–126.

Miller, F. & Truog, R. (2011): *Death, Dying, and Organ Transplantation*. New York: Oxford University Press.

President's Commission for the Study of Ethical Problems in Medicine (1981): *Defining Death: A Report on the Medical, Legal and Ethical Issues in the Determination of Death*. Washington: U.S. Government Printing Office.

President's Council on Bioethics (2008): *Controversies in the Determination of Death*. Washington, [online] [Retrieved August 30, 2018]. Available at: https://bioethicsarchive. georgetown.edu/pcbe/reports/death/

Repetinger, S. (2006): Long Survival Following Bacterial Meningitis-Associated Brain Destruction. In: *Journal of Child Neurology*, 21(7), pp. 591–5.

Report of the Ad Hoc Committee of the Harvard Medical School (1968): A Definition of Irreversible Coma. In: *Journal of the American Medical Association*, 205(6), pp. 337–40.

Shewmon, D. A. (1998a): Chronic 'Brain Death': Meta-Analysis and Conceptual Consequences. In: *Neurology*, 51(6), pp. 1538–45.

Shewmon, D. A. (1998b): 'Brain-stem Death', 'Brain Death' and Death: A critical re-evaluation of the purported equivalence. In: *Issues in Law & Medicine*, 14(2), pp. 125–45.

Shewmon, D. A. (1999): Chronic 'Brain Death': Meta-Analysis and Conceptual Consequences [response to letters]. In: *Neurology*, 53(6), pp. 1369–72.

Shewmon, D. A. (2001): The Brain and Somatic Integration: Insights into the standard biological rationale for equating 'brain death' with death. In: *Journal of Medicine and Philosophy*, 26(5), pp. 457–78.

Shewmon, D. A. (2012): You Only Die Once: Why brain death is not the death of a human being. In: *Communio*, 39(2), pp. 423–94.

Shewmon, D. A. (2018): Truly Reconciling the Case of Jahi McMath. In: *Neurocritical Care*, 29(2), pp. 165–70.

Singer, P. (1995): *Rethinking life and death*. Oxford: Oxford University Press.

The Prolongation of Life: An Address of Pope Pius Xii to International Congress of Anaesthesiologists (1957): In: *The Pope speaks*, p. 396.

Thomas, A. G. (2012): Continuing the Definition of Death Debate: The Report of the President's Council on Bioethics on Controversies in the Definition of Death. In: *Bioethics*, 26(2), pp. 101–7.

Veatch, R. (1975): The Whole-Brain-Oriented Concept Of Death: An outmoded philosophical formulation. In: *Journal of Thanatology*, 3(1), pp. 13–30.

36

The Philosophical Debate

The President's Council on Bioethics

Why do we describe the central question of this inquiry as a *philosophical* question? We do so, in part, because this question cannot be settled by appealing exclusively to clinical or pathophysiological facts. Those facts were our focus in [. . .] previous chapters in which we sought to clarify important features of "total brain failure," a condition diagnosed in a well-defined subset of comatose, ventilator-dependent patients. As a condition, it is the terminus of a course of pathophysiological events, the effects of which account for certain clinically observable signs (all manifestations of an incapacitated brainstem) and for confirmatory results obtained through selected imaging tests. A patient diagnosed with this condition will never recover brain-dependent functions, including the capacity to breathe and the capacity to exhibit even minimal signs of conscious life. If the patient is sustained with life-supporting technologies, this condition need not lead immediately to somatic disintegration or failure of other organ systems. These facts are all crucial to answering the question, *Is a human being with total brain failure dead?* But determining the significance of these facts

presents challenges for philosophical analysis and interpretation.

In this chapter, we set forth and explore two positions on this philosophical question. One position rejects the widely accepted consensus that the current neurological standard is an ethically valid one for determining death. The other position defends the consensus, taking the challenges posed in recent years as opportunities to strengthen the philosophical rationale for the neurological standard.

At the outset, it is important to note what is common to these two opposing positions. *First, both reject the idea that death should be treated merely as a legal construct or as a matter of social agreement.* Instead, both embrace the idea that a standard for determining death must be defensible on biological as well as philosophical grounds. That is to say, both positions respect the *biological reality* of death. At some point, after all, certainty that a body is no longer a living whole *is* attainable. The impressive technological advances of the last several decades have done nothing to alter the reality of death, even if they have complicated the task of judging whether and when death

Original publication details: The President's Council on Bioethics, "The Philosophical Debate," pp. 49–68 from *Controversies in the Determination of Death* (white paper). Washington, D.C., December 2008. Public domain.

has occurred in particular circumstances. In light of such complications, however, both positions share the conclusion that a human being who is not known to be dead should be considered alive.

Second, neither position advocates loosening the standards for determining death on the basis of currently known clinical and pathophysiological facts. There is a well-developed third philosophical position that is often considered alongside the two that are the main focus of this chapter. This third position maintains that there can be two deaths – the death of the *person*, a being distinguished by the capacities for thought, reason, and feeling, and the death of the *body* or the *organism*. From the perspective of this third philosophical position, an individual who suffers a brain injury that leaves him incapacitated with regard to certain specifically human powers is rightly regarded as "dead as a person." The still living body that remains after this death is not a human being in the full sense. Philosopher John Lizza discusses the living organism left behind after the "person" has died in the following way:

> Advocates of a consciousness-related formulation of death do not consider such a being to be a living person. In their view, a person cannot persist through the loss of all brain function or even the loss of just those brain functions required for consciousness and other mental functions. . . [W]hat remains alive must be a different sort of being. . .a form of life created by medical technology. . .Whereas a person is normally transformed into a corpse at his or her death, technology has intervened in this natural process and has made it possible. . .for a person's remains to take the form of an artificially sustained, living organism devoid of the capacity for consciousness and any other mental function.[1]

Thus, advocates of this third position effectively maintain that in certain cases there can be two deaths rather than one. In such cases, they argue, a body that has ceased to be a person (having "died" the first death) can be treated as deceased – at least in certain ways. For example, according to some advocates of this position, it would be permissible to remove the organs of such individuals while their hearts continue to beat. The patients most often cited as potential

heart-beating organ donors, based on this concept of death, are PVS [persistent vegetative state] patients and anencephalic newborns (babies born with very little, if any, brain matter other than the brainstem). Organ retrieval in such cases might entail the administration of sedatives to the allegedly "person-less" patient because some signs of continued "biological life" (such as the open eyes and spontaneous breathing of the PVS patient) would be distracting and disturbing to the surgeons who procure the patient's organs.

Serious difficulties afflict the claim that something that can be called "death" has occurred even as the body remains alive. One such difficulty is that there is no way to know that the "specifically human powers" are irreversibly gone from a body that has suffered any injury shy of total brain failure. In [an earlier] chapter, we cited neurologist Steven Laureys's observation that it is impossible to ascertain scientifically the inward state of an individual – and features of this inward state (e.g., thinking and feeling) are always cited as marks of a distinctively *human* or *personal* life. It is very important here to recall the marked differences in appearance between the individual with total brain failure and the individual with another "consciousness-compromising" condition. The latter displays several ambiguous signs – moving, waking up, and groaning, among others – while the former remains still and closed off from the world in clinically ascertainable ways.[2]

A related problem with this "two deaths" position is that it expands the concept of death beyond the core meaning it has had throughout human history. Human beings are members of the larger family of living beings, and it is a fundamental truth about living beings that every individual – be it plant or animal – eventually dies. Recent advances in technology offer no warrant for jettisoning the age-old idea that it is not as persons that we die, but rather as members of the family of living beings and as animals in particular. The terminus of the transformation that occurs when a human being is deprived by injury of certain mental capacities, heartbreaking as it is, is not *death*. We should note, again, that some technological interventions administered to the living might be deemed *futile* – that is, ineffective at reversing or ameliorating the course of disease or injury – and that an ethically valid decision might be made to withdraw or withhold such interventions. There is no need, however, to call an individual *already dead* in order to justify refraining from such futile interventions.

In summary, the two positions that we present in this chapter share the conviction that death is a single phenomenon marking the end of the life of a biological organism. Death is the definitive end of life and is something more complete and final than the mere loss of "personhood."

I   Position One: There Is No Sound Biological Justification for Today's Neurological Standard

The neurological standard for death based on total brain failure relies fundamentally on the idea that the phenomenon of death can be *hidden*. The metaphor employed by the President's Commission [. . .] expresses this idea: When a ventilator supports the body's vital functions, this technological intervention obscures our view of the phenomenon. What seem to be signs of continued life in an injured body are, in fact, misleading artifacts of the technological intervention and obstacles to ascertaining the truth. To consult brain-based functions, then, is to look through a "second window" in order to see the actual condition of the body.

The critical thrust of Position One can be summarized in this way: There is no reliable "second window" on the phenomenon of death. If its presence is not made known by the signs that have always accompanied it – by breathing lungs and a beating heart – then there is no way to state with confidence that death has occurred. Only when all would agree that the body is ready for burial can that body, with confidence, be described as dead. If blood is still circulating and nutrients and oxygen are still serving to power the work of diverse cells, tissues, and organ systems,

then the body in which these processes are ongoing cannot be deemed a corpse.

Soon after the Harvard committee argued that patients who meet the criteria for "irreversible coma" are already dead, some philosophers and other observers of the committee's work advanced an opposing view. The counterarguments presented then by one such philosopher, Hans Jonas, are still useful in framing the objections raised today against the neurological standard. In his 1974 essay, "Against the Stream," Jonas dissented from the Harvard committee's equation of "irreversible coma" and death and counseled, instead, a conservative course of action:

> We do not know with certainty the borderline between life and death, and a definition cannot substitute for knowledge. Moreover, we have sufficient grounds for suspecting that the artificially supported condition of the comatose patient may still be one of life, however reduced – i.e., for doubting that, even with the brain function gone, he is completely dead. In this state of marginal ignorance and doubt the only course to take is to lean over backward toward the side of possible life.[3]

With these words, Jonas underscored a point that is pivotal to Position One: There can be uncertainty as to where the line between life and death falls even if we are certain that death is a biologically real event. In patients with total brain failure, the transition from living body to corpse is in some measure a mystery, one that may be beyond the powers of science and medicine to penetrate and determine with the finality that is possible when most human beings die.

Have advances in the scientific and clinical understanding of the spectrum of neurological injury shown that Jonas's stance of principled (and therefore cautious) uncertainty was incorrect? Today we have a more fine-grained set of categories of, as he put it, "artificially supported. . .comatose patients" – some of whom meet the criteria for total brain failure and others who have hope of recovering limited or full mental function. Only the first group is considered to be dead by today's "brain death" defenders. Even with respect to this group, however, there is still reason to wonder if our knowledge of their condition is adequate for labeling them as dead. If there are "sufficient grounds," as Jonas put it, for suspecting that their condition may still be one of life, then a stance of principled and hence cautious uncertainty is still the morally right one to take.

This line of inquiry brings us to Shewmon's criticisms [. . .] of the accepted pathophysiological and clinical picture of patients with "brain death" (total brain failure). Do Shewmon's criticisms constitute the "sufficient grounds" to which Jonas appeals? To answer this question, these criticisms and the evidence supporting them must first be considered in greater depth.

In 1998, the journal *Neurology* published an article by Shewmon entitled, "Chronic 'Brain Death': Meta-Analysis and Conceptual Consequences." In that article, Shewmon cites evidence for the claim that neither bodily disintegration nor cessation of heartbeat *necessarily* and *imminently* ensues after brain death.[4] Shewmon's evidence is drawn from more than one hundred documented cases that demonstrate survival past one week's time, with one case of survival for more than fourteen years.[i] Furthermore, he demonstrates that such factors as age, etiology, and underlying somatic integrity variably affect the survival probability of "brain dead" patients. Observing that asystole (the absence of cardiac contractions colloquially known as "flatline") does not necessarily follow from "brain death," Shewmon concludes that it is the overall integrity of the body (the "underlying somatic plasticity") *rather than the condition of the brain* that exerts the strongest influence on survival. These facts seem to contradict the dominant view that the loss of brain function, in and of itself, leads the body to "fall apart" and eventually to cease circulating blood.

Critics of this meta-analysis have challenged the data on which Shewmon based his conclusions, claiming that many of the patients in the cases that he compiles might not have been properly diagnosed with whole brain death (in our usage, total brain failure). They also point out the rarity with which such cases are encountered, compared with the frequency of rapid descent to asystole for patients accurately

diagnosed.[ii] To point out the rarity of prolonged survival, however, is to admit that the phenomenon does, in some cases, occur. Whether it might occur more often is difficult to judge because patients with total brain failure are rarely treated with aggressive, life-sustaining interventions for an extended time.

If it is possible – albeit rare – for a body without a functioning brain to "hold itself together" for an indefinite period of time, then how can the condition of total brain failure be equated with biological death? Or, to put the question in Jonas's terms, does this fact not give "sufficient grounds" for suspecting that such patients might still be alive, although severely injured? The case for uncertainty about the line between life and death is further strengthened by considering the somatic processes that clearly continue in the body of a patient with total brain failure.

In a paper published in the *Journal of Medicine and Philosophy* in 2001, Shewmon details the integrated functions that continue in a body in the condition of "brain death." Table 1 reproduces a list of somatically integrative functions that are, in Shewmon's words, "*not* mediated by the brain and possessed by at least some [brain dead] bodies."[5]

Readers not well-versed in human physiology might find this list hard to follow. Its significance, however, can be simply stated: It enumerates many clearly identifiable and observable physiological mechanisms. These mechanisms account for the continued health of vital organs in the bodies of patients diagnosed with total brain failure and go a long way toward explaining the lengthy survival of such patients in rare cases. In such cases, globally coordinated work continues to be performed by multiple systems, all directed toward the sustained functioning of the body as a whole. If being alive as a biological organism requires being a whole that is more than the mere sum of its parts, then it would be difficult to deny that the body of a patient with total brain failure can still be alive, at least in some cases.

None of this contradicts the claim that total brain failure is a unique and profound kind of *incapacitation* – and one that may very well warrant or even morally *require* the withdrawal of life-sustaining interventions.

Table 1   Physiological Evidence of "Somatic Integration"[6]

- Homeostasis of a countless variety of mutually interacting chemicals, macromolecules and physiological parameters, through the functions especially of liver, kidneys, cardiovascular and endocrine systems, but also of other organs and tissues (e.g., intestines, bone and skin in calcium metabolism; cardiac atrial natriuretic factor affecting the renal secretion of renin, which regulates blood pressure by acting on vascular smooth muscle; etc.);
- Elimination, detoxification and recycling of cellular wastes throughout the body;
- Energy balance, involving interactions among liver, endocrine systems, muscle and fat;
- Maintenance of body temperature (albeit at a lower than normal level and with the help of blankets);
- Wound healing, capacity for which is diffuse throughout the body and which involves organism-level, teleological interaction among blood cells, capillary endothelium, soft tissues, bone marrow, vasoactive peptides, clotting and clot lysing factors (maintained by the liver, vascular endothelium and circulating leucocytes in a delicate balance of synthesis and degradation), etc.;
- Fighting of infections and foreign bodies through interactions among the immune system, lymphatics, bone marrow, and microvasculature;
- Development of a febrile response to infection;
- Cardiovascular and hormonal stress responses to unanesthetized incision for organ retrieval;
- Successful gestation of a fetus in a [brain dead] pregnant woman;
- Sexual maturation of a [brain dead] child;
- Proportional growth of a [brain dead] child.

According to some defenders of the concept of medical futility, there is no obligation to begin or to continue treatment when that treatment cannot achieve any good or when it inflicts disproportionate burdens on the patient who receives it or on his or her family. Writing many years before the somatic state and the prognostic possibilities of total brain failure were well-characterized, Jonas emphasized the need to accept that sustaining life and prolonging dying is not always in the patient's interest:

> The question [of interventions to sustain the patient] cannot be answered by decreeing that death has already occurred and the body is therefore in the domain of things; rather it is by holding, e.g., that it is humanly

not justified – let alone demanded – to artificially prolong the life of a brainless body. . .the physician can, indeed should, turn off the respirator and let the "definition of death" take care of itself by what then inevitably happens.[7]

To summarize, Position One does *not* insist that medicine or science can know that all or even some patients with total brain failure are still living. Rather, Position One makes two assertions in light of what we now know about the clinical presentation and the pathophysiology of total brain failure. The first is that there are "sufficient grounds" for doubt as to whether the patient with this condition has died. The second is that in the face of such persistent uncertainty, the only ethically valid course is to consider and treat such a patient as a still living human being. Finally, such respectful consideration and treatment does not preclude the ethical withdrawal or withholding of life-sustaining interventions, based on the judgment that such interventions are futile.

II   Position Two: There *Is* a Sound Biological Justification for Today's Neurological Standard

Position One is the voice of "principled and hence cautious uncertainty." We should not claim to know facts about life and death that are beyond the limits of our powers to discern, especially when the consequence might be to place a human being beyond the essential and obligatory protections afforded to the living. The recent critical appraisals of total brain failure ("whole brain death") offered by Shewmon and others only underscore the limits to our ability to discern the line between life and death.

Position Two is also motivated by strong moral convictions about what is at stake in the debate: The bodies of deceased patients should not be ventilated and maintained as if they were still living human beings. The respect owed to the newly dead demands that such interventions be withdrawn. Their families should be spared unnecessary anguish over purported "options" for treatment. Maintaining the body for a short time to facilitate organ transplantation is a reasonable act of deference to the need for organs and to the opportunity for generosity on the part of the donor as well as the family. Notwithstanding this need and opportunity, the true moral challenge that faces us is to decide in each case whether the patient is living or has died. To help us meet that challenge, the clinical and pathophysiological facts that call the neurological standard into question should be re-examined and re-evaluated. On the basis of such a re-examination and re-evaluation, Position Two seeks to develop a better rationale for continuing to use the neurological standard to determine whether a human being has died.

A   The Work of the Organism as a Whole

Early defenders of the neurological standard of "whole brain death" relied on the plausible intuition that in order to be a living organism any animal, whether human or non-human, must be a *whole*. Ongoing biological activity in various cells or tissues is not in itself sufficient to mark the presence of a living organism. After all, some biological activity in cells and tissues remains for a time even in a body that all would agree is a corpse. Such activity signifies that disparate *parts* of the once-living organism remain, but not the organism *as a whole*. Therefore, if we try to specify the moment at which the "wholeness" of the body is lost, that moment must come before biological activity in all of its different cells or tissues has ceased. As Alexander Capron, former executive director of the President's Commission, has repeatedly emphasized, the fact that this moment is *chosen* does not mean that it is *arbitrary*; the choice is not arbitrary if it is made in accordance with the most reasonable interpretation of the biological facts that could be provided.[iii]

The neurological standard's early defenders were not wrong to seek such a principle of wholeness. They may have been mistaken, however, in focusing on the *loss of somatic integration* as the critical sign that the organism is no longer a whole. They interpreted – plausibly but perhaps incorrectly – "an organism as a whole" to mean "an organism whose parts are working together in an integrated way." But, as we have seen, even in a patient with total brain failure, some of the body's parts continue to work together in an integrated way for some time – for example, to fight infection, heal wounds, and maintain temperature. If these kinds of integration were sufficient to identify the presence of a living "organism as a whole," total brain failure could not serve as a criterion for organismic death, and the neurological standard enshrined in law would not be philosophically well-grounded.

There may be, however, a more compelling account of *wholeness* that would support the intuition that after total brain failure the body is no longer an organismic whole and hence no longer alive. That account, which we develop here with Position Two, offers a superior defense of "total brain failure" as the standard for declaring death. With that account, death remains a condition of the organism as a whole and does not, therefore, merely signal the irreversible loss of so-called higher mental functions. But reliance on the concept of "integration" is abandoned and with it the false assumption that the brain is the "integrator" of vital functions. Determining whether an organism remains a *whole* depends on recognizing the persistence or cessation of the fundamental vital *work* of a living organism – the work of self-preservation, achieved through the organism's need-driven commerce with the surrounding world. When there is good reason to believe that an injury has irreversibly destroyed an organism's ability to perform its fundamental vital work, then the conclusion that the organism as a whole has died is warranted. Advocates of Position Two argue that this is the case for patients with total brain failure. To understand this argument, we must explore at some length this idea of an organism's "fundamental work."

All organisms have a *needy* mode of being. Unlike inanimate objects, which continue to exist through inertia and without effort, every organism persists only thanks to its own exertions. To preserve themselves, organisms *must* – and *can* and *do* – engage in commerce with the surrounding world. Their constant need for oxygenated air and nutrients is matched by their ability to satisfy that need, by engaging in certain activities, reaching out into the surrounding environment to secure the required sustenance. This is the definitive work of the organism *as an organism*. It is what an organism "does" and what distinguishes every organism from non-living things.[iv] And it is what distinguishes a *living* organism from the dead body that it becomes when it dies.

The work of the organism, expressed in its commerce with the surrounding world, depends on three fundamental capacities:

1. Openness to the world, that is, receptivity to stimuli and signals from the surrounding environment.
2. The ability to act upon the world to obtain selectively what it needs.
3. The basic felt need that drives the organism to act as it must, to obtain what it needs and what its openness reveals to be available.

Appreciating these capacities as mutually supporting aspects of the organism's vital work will help us understand why an individual with total brain failure should be declared dead, even when ventilator-supported "breathing" masks the presence of death.

To preserve itself, an organism must be open to the world. Such openness is manifested in different ways and at many levels. In higher animals, including man, it is evident most obviously in consciousness or felt awareness, even in its very rudimentary forms. When a PVS patient tracks light with his or her eyes, recoils in response to pain, swallows liquid placed in the mouth, or goes to sleep and wakes up, such behaviors – although they may not indicate *self-consciousness* – testify to the organism's essential, vital openness to its surrounding world. An organism that behaves in such a way cannot be dead.

Self-preserving commerce with the world, however, involves more than just openness or receptivity. It also requires the ability to *act* on one's own behalf – to take in food and water and, even more basically, to breathe. Spontaneous breathing is an indispensable action of the higher animals that makes metabolism – and all other vital activity – possible. Experiencing a

felt inner need to acquire oxygen (and to expel carbon dioxide) and perceiving the presence of oxygen in its environment, a living body is moved to act on the world (by contracting its diaphragm so that air will move into its lungs). An organism that breathes spontaneously cannot be dead.

Just as spontaneous breathing in itself reveals an organism's openness to and ability to act upon the world, it also reveals a third capacity critical to the organism's fundamental, self-preserving work: What animates the motor act of spontaneous breathing, in open commerce with the surrounding air, is the inner experience of need, manifesting itself as the drive to breathe. This need does not have to be consciously felt in order to be efficacious in driving respiration. It is clearly not consciously felt in a comatose patient who might be tested for a remaining rudimentary drive (e.g., with the "apnea" test). But even when the drive to breathe occurs in the absence of any self-awareness, its presence gives evidence of the organism's continued impulse to live. This drive is the organism's own impulse, exercised on its own behalf, and indispensable to its continued existence.[v]

As a vital sign, the *spontaneous action of breathing* can and must be distinguished from the technologically supported, *passive condition of being ventilated* (i.e., of having one's "breathing" replaced by a mechanical ventilator). The natural work of breathing, even apart from consciousness or self-awareness, is itself a sure sign that the organism as a whole is doing the work that constitutes – and preserves – it as a whole. In contrast, artificial, non-spontaneous breathing produced by a machine is not such a sign. It does not signify an activity of the organism as a whole. It is not driven by *felt need*, and the exchange of gases that it effects is neither an achievement of the organism nor a sign of its genuine vitality. For this reason, it makes sense to say that the operation of the ventilator can obscure our view of the arrival of human death – that is, the death of the human organism as a working whole. A ventilator causes the patient's chest to heave and the lungs to fill and thereby *mimics* the authentic work of the organism. In fact, it mimics the work so well that it enables some systems of the body to keep functioning – but it does no more than that. The simulated "breathing" that the ventilator makes possible is not, therefore, a *vital sign:* It is not a sign that the organism is accomplishing its vital work and thus remains a living whole.[vi]

We have examined the phenomenon of breathing in order to understand and explain a living organism's "needful openness" to the world – a needful openness lacking in patients with total brain failure. Having done this, however, we must also emphasize that an animal cannot be considered dead simply because it has lost the ability to breathe spontaneously. Even if the animal has lost that capacity, other vital capacities might still be present. For example, patients with spinal cord injuries may be permanently apneic or unable to breathe without ventilatory support and yet retain full or partial possession of their conscious faculties. Just as much as striving to breathe, signs of consciousness are incontrovertible evidence that a living organism, a patient, is alive.

If there are no signs of consciousness *and* if spontaneous breathing is absent *and* if the best clinical judgment is that these neurophysiological facts cannot be reversed, Position Two would lead us to conclude that a once-living patient has now died. Thus, on this account, total brain failure can continue to serve as a criterion for declaring death – not because it necessarily indicates complete loss of integrated somatic functioning, but because it is a sign that this organism can no longer engage in the essential work that defines living things.

B   Comparison with the UK Standard

Although the terms may be different, the concepts presented here to defend the use of total brain failure as a reasonable standard for death are not wholly new. A similar approach to judging the vital status of a patient diagnosed as "brain dead," emphasizing the crucial importance of both spontaneous breathing and the capacity for consciousness, was advocated by the late British neurologist Christopher Pallis.[8] His conceptual justification for this argument was influential in gaining acceptance for a neurological standard in the United Kingdom.[vii]

Like this report's Position Two, Pallis attempted to strike a balance between the need to be "functionalist" and the need to remain rooted in the biological facts of total brain failure. He stated in very direct terms that the relevant functions that were irreversibly absent from the patient with a destroyed brainstem were *the ability to breathe* and *the capacity for consciousness.* When challenged as to why these two functions should be singled out, Pallis pointed to what he called "the sociological context" for basic concepts of life and death. In the West, he maintained, this context is the Judeo-Christian tradition in which "breath" and "consciousness" are two definitive features of the human soul:

> The single matrix in which my definition is embedded is a sociological one, namely Judeo-Christian culture. . . The "loss of the capacity for consciousness" is much the same as the "departure of the conscious soul from the body," just as "the loss of the capacity to breathe" is much the same as the "loss of the breath of life."[9]

Pallis also pointed to "the widespread identity, in various languages, of terms denoting *soul* and *breath.*"[10] A challenge to this approach can be framed with two questions: First, are consciousness and breathing the *only* or the *most important* culturally significant features of the soul? And second, does this argument about traditional beliefs, bound to a particular culture, provide a sufficient rationale for a standard applicable to the transcultural, universal phenomenon of human death?

Position Two agrees with Pallis's emphasis on certain functions in preference to others, but it avoids the limitations of his approach, that is, its dependence on a particular culture. Position Two does this by taking the loss of the impulse to breathe and the total loss of engagement with the world as the cessation of the most essential functions of the organism as a whole. In this way, it builds upon an insight into biological reality, an insight latent in culture-bound notions of "breath of life" and "departure of the conscious soul from the body." It does so by articulating a philosophical conception of the biological realities of organismic life. To repeat, an organism is the unique sort of being that it is because it *can* and *must* constantly act upon and be open to its environment. From this philosophical-biological perspective, it becomes clear that a human being with a destroyed brainstem has lost the functional capacities that define organismic life.

On at least one important point, however, our Position Two and the UK neurological standard part company. The UK standard follows Pallis in accepting "death of the brainstem," rather than total brain failure, as a sufficient criterion for declaring a patient dead. Such a reduction, in addition to being conceptually suspect, is clinically dangerous because it suggests that the confirmatory tests that go beyond the

bedside checks for apnea and brainstem reflexes are simply superfluous. As noted [earlier], it is important to seek clarity on where a patient is on the path to the endpoint of total brain infarction. Only if the destructive cycle of infarction and swelling has reached this endpoint can the irreversibility of the patient's condition be known with confidence. Ultimately, the decision to perform these confirmatory tests (beyond those targeted at brainstem functions, for example, angiography or EEG) belongs to the attending clinician. The counsel offered here is one of caution in reaching a diagnosis with such important consequences. Only in the presence of a certain diagnosis of total brain failure do the arguments that seek to interpret this clinical finding hold weight.

Notes

i This patient experienced a cardiac arrest in January 2004, more than twenty years after the diagnosis of "brain death." A report on the case, including the brain-only autopsy performed, appears in S. Repertinger, et al., "Long Survival Following Bacterial Meningitis-Associated Brain Destruction," *J Child Neurol* 21, no. 7 (2006): 591–5.

ii Wijdicks and Bernat, in a response to the Shewmon article, commented: "These cases are anecdotes yearning for a denominator." E. F. Wijdicks and J. L. Bernat, "Chronic 'Brain Death': Meta-Analysis and Conceptual Consequences," *Neurology* 53, no. 6 (1999): 1538–45.

iii Capron comments: "In part, any definition 'is admittedly arbitrary in the sense of representing a choice,' as the President's Commission stated in defending the view that the brain's function is more central to human life than are other necessary organs. . . But the societally determined view of what constitutes death is not 'arbitrary in the sense of lacking reasons.' . . . The 'cultural context' of the standards for determining death includes the generally held view that human death, like the death of any animal, is a natural event. Even in establishing their 'definition,' members of our society act on the basis that death is an event whose existence rests on certain criteria recognized rather than solely invented by human beings." A. M. Capron, "The Report of the President's

Commission on the Uniform Determination of Death Act," in *Death: Beyond Whole Brain Criteria*, ed. R. Zaner (The Netherlands: Kluwer Academic Publishers, 1988), 156–7. See, also, A. M. Capron, "The Purpose of Death: A Reply to Professor Dworkin," *Indiana Law J* 48, no. 4 (1973): 640–6.

iv The account here focuses on the details of organismic life that are manifested in the "higher animals" or, perhaps more precisely, the *mammals*. How these arguments might be modified and extended to other sorts of organisms (e.g., bacteria or plants) is beyond the scope of this discussion.

v The significance of this account of breathing may be more apparent if we contrast it with the more reductive account provided by Shewmon in his influential 2001 paper that criticized a "somatic integration rationale" for a whole brain standard for human death. Shewmon wrote:

If "breathing" is interpreted in the "bellows" sense – moving air in and out of the lungs – then it is indeed a brain-mediated function, grossly substituted in [brain dead] patients by a mechanical ventilator. But this is a function not only of the brain but also of the phrenic nerves, diaphragm and intercostal muscles; moreover, it is not a somatically integrative function or even a vitally necessary one... It is merely a condition for somatic integration itself. On the other hand, if "breathing" is understood in the sense of "respiration," which strictly speaking refers to the exchange of oxygen and carbon dioxide, then its locus is twofold: (1) across the alveolar lining of the lungs, and (2) at the biochemical level of the electron transport chain in the mitochondria of every cell in the body. (Shewmon, "Brain and Somatic Integration," 464.)

In his eagerness to debunk what he considers the myth of lost somatic integration, Shewmon fails to convey the essential character of breathing. We might summarize his account of breathing as follows:

Breathing = Inflation and deflation of a bellows + Diffusion at the alveoli + Cellular respiration

But Shewmon misses the critical element: the *drive* exhibited by the whole organism to bring in air, a drive that is fundamental to the constant, vital working of the whole organism. By ignoring the essentially *appetitive* nature of animal breathing, Shewmon's account misses the relevance of breathing as incontrovertible evidence that "the organism as a whole" continues to be *open to* and *at work upon* the world, achieving its own preservation. The breathing that keeps an organism alive is not merely the operation of a "bellows" for which a mechanical ventilator might substitute. Bringing air into the body is an integral part of an organism's mode

of being as a *needy* thing. More air will be brought in if metabolic need demands it and the body *feels* that need, as for example during exercise or in a state of panic or injury. The "respiration" taking place at the cellular level can be understood adequately only in the context of the work of the whole organism – the work of breathing.

vi If the view presented here is correct, that is, if the presence of spontaneous breathing truly reveals a persistent drive of the organism as a whole to live, we can better understand the force of a rhetorical question sometimes posed to those who view the loss of "higher" mental and psychological capacities as a sufficient criterion for declaring death. "Would you," they may be asked, "bury a patient who continues to breathe spontaneously?" Quite naturally, we recoil from such a thought, and we do so for reasons that the account given above makes clear. The striving of an animal to live, a striving that we can discern even in its least voluntary form (i.e., breathing), indicates that we still have among us a living being – and not a candidate for burial.

vii Other countries have adopted this conceptual framework as well. The Canadian Forum that issued its recommendations in 2006 followed the UK approach in adopting "irreversible loss of the capacity for consciousness combined with the irreversible loss of all brain stem functions, including the capacity to breathe" as the definition of neurologically determined death. Shemie, et al., "Neurological Determination of Death: Canadian Forum," S1–13.

References

1   J. P. Lizza, "The Conceptual Basis for Brain Death Revisited: Loss of Organic Integration or Loss of Consciousness?" *Adv Exp Med Biol* 550 (2004): 52.

2   S. Laureys, A. M. Owen, and N. D. Schiff, "Brain Function in Coma, Vegetative State, and Related Disorders," *Lancet Neurol* 3, no. 9 (2004): 537–46.

3   H. Jonas, "Against the Stream," in *Philosophical Essays: From Ancient Creed to Technological Man* (Englewood Cliffs, NJ: Prentice-Hall, 1974), 138.

4   D. A. Shewmon, "Chronic 'Brain Death': Meta-Analysis and Conceptual Consequences," *Neurology* 51, no. 6 (1998): 1538–45.

5   Shewmon, "Brain and Somatic Integration," 467. Author's emphasis.

6   Shewmon, "The Brain and Somatic Integration: Insights into the Standard Biological Rationale for Equating 'Brain Death' with Death," 457–78.

7   Jonas, "Against the Stream," 136.

8   C. Pallis and D. H. Harley. *ABC of Brainstem Death.* Second ed. London: BMJ Publishing Group, 1996; C. Pallis, "On the Brainstem Criterion of Death," in *The Definition of Death: Contemporary Controversies,* ed. S. J. Youngner, R. M. Arnold, and R. Schapiro (Baltimore: The Johns Hopkins University Press, 1999), 93–100.

9   Pallis, "On the Brainstem Criterion of Death," 96.

10 Ibid.

37

An Alternative to Brain Death

Jeff McMahan

Some Common but Mistaken Assumptions about Death

Most contributors to the debate about brain death share certain assumptions. They believe that the concept of death is univocal, that death is a biological phenomenon, that it is necessarily irreversible, that it is paradigmatically something that happens to *organisms*, that we are human organisms, and therefore that our deaths will be deaths of organisms. These claims are supposed to have moral significance. It is, for example, only when a person dies that it is permissible to extract her organs for transplantation.

It is also commonly held that our univocal notion of death is the permanent cessation of integrated functioning in an organism and that the criterion for determining when this has occurred in animals with brains is the death of the brain as a whole – that is, brain death. The reason most commonly given for this is that the brain is the irreplaceable master control of the organism's integration.

Before presenting my own view, let me say something about a couple of these assumptions and about the case for brain death. It is, perhaps, a measure of the heretical cast of my mind that I reject all of these widely shared assumptions.

I do not think the concept of death is univocal. When Jesus says that "whosoever liveth and believeth in me shall never die," he does not mean that some human organisms will remain functionally integrated forever. He means that believers will never cease to exist. (Admittedly, Jesus did not use the English word "die." But this seemed an intelligible use of the word to the translators.)

But "death" also has a biological meaning. It makes sense to say that when a unicellular organism, such as an ameba, undergoes binary fission, it ceases to exist; but in the biological sense it does not die. There is no cessation of functioning that turns this once-living organism into a corpse. So death as a biological phenomenon is different from the ceasing to exist of a living being and may or may not involve an entity's ceasing to exist. It is intelligible, for example, to say that when an animal organism dies, it does not cease to exist. Rather, it simply becomes a corpse. The living animal becomes a dead animal – but nothing ceases to exist until the animal organism disintegrates.

Original publication details: Jeff McMahan, "Alternative to Brain Death," pp. 47–48 from *Journal of Law, Medicine and Ethics* 34 (2006). Includes only the section "An Alternative Understanding of Brain Death," with some editing to remove references to the earlier section. Reproduced with permission of Sage Publications Ltd.

Bioethics: An Anthology, Fourth Edition. Edited by Udo Schüklenk and Peter Singer.
Editorial material and organization © 2022 John Wiley & Sons, Inc. Published 2022 by John Wiley & Sons, Inc.

I also do not think our concept of death makes it a necessary truth that death is irreversible. If that were true, the claim that Lazarus was raised from the dead, or that Jesus was resurrected, would be incoherent. I think these claims are false; but if it were a conceptual truth that death is irreversible, they would not be false, but nonsensical.

I do think, however, that there is something true and important in the idea that death as a biological phenomenon is irreversible. It may well be a conceptual truth that an organism can be revived from death only by a violation of the laws of nature – that is, only by a literal miracle of the sort that Jesus is thought by some to have performed. For in cases not involving miracles, if an organism that was thought to be dead is restored to integrated functioning, our tendency is to conclude that we were mistaken in assuming that it was dead. (Subsequent references to irreversibility should be understood as having the implicit qualification "except by miracle.")

Some people, of course, will say that the organism was dead but was non-miraculously restored to life. To make this claim acceptable, they will need to offer good reasons for thinking the organism was dead, given that it is now alive. For reasons that I will give later, I think that nothing of importance depends on this. It is just a question of how we use certain words. But for those who believe that we are organisms and that we always have special value or sanctity while we are alive, this is a very important issue indeed.

[. . .]

An Alternative Understanding of Death

I accept that it is largely correct to say that a human organism dies when it irreversibly loses the capacity for integrated functioning among its various major organs and subsystems. But the death of a human organism will necessarily be *my* death only if I am an organism. The view that we are organisms is the most important of the widely shared assumptions that

I noted at the outset. But, as I mentioned, I think it is mistaken.

The question whether we are organisms is not a biological question, or even a scientific question – just as it is not a scientific question whether a statue and the lump of bronze of which it is composed are one and the same thing or distinct substances. Whether we are organisms is also, and more obviously, not an ethical question. It is a metaphysical question.

There are two arguments that convince me that the answer to this question is "no." One appeals to the hypothetical case of brain transplantation – or, better yet, cerebrum transplantation. If my cerebrum were successfully grafted onto the brain stem of my identical twin brother (whose own cerebrum had been excised), I would then exist in association with what was once his organism. What was formerly my organism would have an intact brain stem and might, therefore, be idling nicely in a persistent vegetative state without even mechanical ventilation. Since I can thus in principle exist separately from the organism that is now mine, I cannot be identical with it.

The second argument appeals not to a science fiction scenario but to an actual phenomenon: dicephalus. Certain instances of dicephalic twinning, in which two heads sprout from a single torso, seem to be clear cases in which a single organism supports the existence of two distinct people. The transitivity of identity prevents us from saying that *both* these people *are* that organism; for that implies that the people are identical, that is, that there are not really two people but only one. And because each twin's relation to the organism is the same as the other's, it cannot be that one twin but not the other is the organism. The best thing to say, therefore, is that neither of them is identical to the organism. Since we are essentially the same kind of thing they are, we cannot be organisms either.

If I am right that we are not organisms, what are we? The most widely held alternative view is that each of us is essentially a cartesian soul – that is, a nonmaterial conscious entity that in life is linked with a particular brain and body but at death continues to exist and indeed remains conscious and is psychologically continuous with the person prior to death. Because the soul, so conceived, is nonphysical, it can be individuated only by reference to a single field of consciousness. Thus, any conscious state that is not accessible in my field of consciousness must belong to a different person, or soul. This conception of the soul is, however, undermined by what we know about the results of hemispheric commissurotomy – a procedure in which the tissues connecting a patient's cerebral hemispheres are surgically severed. This procedure gives rise, at least in certain experimental settings, to two separate centers of consciousness in a single human organism. If persons were cartesian souls, we would have to conclude that the procedure creates two persons where formerly there was only one. Since this is clearly not what happens, we cannot be cartesian souls.[1]

How should we think about the problem of determining what kind of thing we essentially are? Here is a quick thought-experiment. Imagine that you were facing the prospect of progressive dementia. At what point would you cease to exist? To most of us it seems clear that you would persist at least as long as the brain in your body retained the capacity for consciousness. For there would be somebody there, and who might it be, if not you? But would you still survive if your brain irreversibly lost the capacity for consciousness? It seems that the only thing there that might qualify as you would be a living human organism. But if I am right that you are not a human organism and there would be nothing else there for you to be, it seems that you must have ceased to exist when your brain lost the capacity for consciousness. I infer from this that you are in fact a mind, a mind that is necessarily embodied.

Recall now my earlier claim that the concept of death is not univocal. The term "death" can refer to our ceasing to exist (as in the earlier quotation from Jesus) or it can refer to a biological event in the history of an organism. This makes things easy; for we already have the two concepts of death that we require if I am right that we are not organisms.

An organism dies in the biological sense when it loses the capacity for integrated functioning. The best criterion for when this happens is probably a circulatory-respiratory criterion. There is bound to be considerable indeterminacy about how much functional integration is required for life in an organism. But if we are not organisms, this is of little consequence.

What it is important to be able to determine is when we die in the nonbiological sense – that is, when we cease to exist. If we are embodied minds, we die or cease to exist when we irreversibly lose the capacity for consciousness – or, to be more precise, when there is irreversible loss of function in those areas of the brain in which consciousness is realized. The best criterion for when this happens is a higher-brain criterion – for example, what is called "cerebral death." But I do not pretend to any expertise here.

Note that when I say the right criterion of our death is a higher-brain criterion, I am not claiming that a human organism in a persistent vegetative state is dead. If persistent vegetative state involves the loss of the capacity for consciousness, then neither you nor I could ever exist in a persistent vegetative state. But you could be survived by your organism, which could remain biologically alive in a persistent vegetative state even though you were dead (that is, had ceased to exist). My view thus avoids the embarrassing implication of most proposals for a higher-brain criterion of death that an organism with spontaneous respiration and heartbeat might be dead.

From an ethical point of view, what matters is not whether an organism remains alive, but whether one of us continues to exist. Of course, we cannot survive unless our organisms remain alive (though this might change if brain transplantation were to become possible). Indeed, although brain death is not sufficient for the biological death of a human organism, it is sufficient for the death or ceasing to exist of a person.

The problematic cases are those in which a person has ceased to exist but her organism remains alive. Might it be permissible to remove the organs from such an organism for transplantation? I believe that it would be, provided that this would not be against the expressed will of the person whose organism it was. But if the person had consented in advance, there would be no moral objection to killing the unoccupied organism in order to use its organs to save the lives of others.

The organism itself cannot be harmed in the relevant sense, it has no rights, and it is not an appropriate object of respect in the Kantian sense. I believe that the treatment of a living but unoccupied human organism is governed morally by principles similar to those that govern the treatment of a corpse. The latter also cannot be harmed or possess rights. But respect for the person who once animated a corpse dictates that there are certain things that must not be done to it. Taking its organs for transplantation with the person's prior consent is not one of these.

Reference

1   For further argument, see J. McMahan, *The Ethics of Killing: Problems at the Margins of Life* (New York: Oxford University Press: 2002): 7–24.

Advance Directives

38

Life Past Reason

Ronald Dworkin

We turn finally to what might be the saddest of the tragedies we have been reviewing. We must consider the autonomy and best interests of people who suffer from serious and permanent dementia, and what the proper respect for the intrinsic value of *their* lives requires. The most important cause of dementia is Alzheimer's disease, a progressive disease of the brain named after a German psychiatrist and neuropathologist, Alois Alzheimer, who first identified and described it in 1906. Patients in the late stages of this disease have lost substantially all memory of their earlier lives and cannot, except periodically and in only a fragmented way, recognize or respond to other people, even those to whom they were formerly close. They may be incapable of saying more than a word or two. They are often incontinent, fall frequently, or are unable to walk at all. They are incapable of sustaining plans or projects or desires of even a very simple structure. They express wishes and desires, but these change rapidly and often show very little continuity even over periods of days or hours.

Alzheimer's is a disease of physiological deterioration. Nerve terminals of the brain degenerate into a matted plaque of fibrous material. Though researchers have expressed some hope that treatment can be developed to slow that degeneration,[1] no such treatment has yet been established, and there is apparently little prospect of dramatically reversing very advanced brain deterioration. A specialist describes the degeneration as occurring "gradually and inexorably, usually leading to death in a severely debilitated, immobile state between four and twelve years after onset."[2] But according to the US Office of Technology Assessment, death may be delayed for as long as twenty-five years.[3]

Our discussion will focus only on the disease's late stages. I shall not consider, except in passing, the present structure of legal rights and other provisions for demented or mentally incapacitated people, or the present practices of doctors and other custodians or officials who are charged with their care. Nor shall I attempt any report of the recent research into genetic and other features of such diseases, or into their diagnosis, prognosis, or treatment. All these are the subjects of a full literature.[4] I will concentrate on the question of what moral rights people in the late stages of dementia have or retain, and of what is best for them. Is

Original publication details: Ronald Dworkin, "Life Past Reason," pp. 218–229 from *Life's Dominion: An Argument about Abortion, Euthanasia, and Individual Freedom* (New York: Knopf, 1993). © 1993 by Ronald Dworkin. Reproduced with permission of Alfred A. Knopf, an imprint of the Knopf Doubleday Publishing Group, a division of Random House LLC. All rights reserved.

Bioethics: An Anthology, Fourth Edition. Edited by Udo Schüklenk and Peter Singer.
Editorial material and organization © 2022 John Wiley & Sons, Inc. Published 2022 by John Wiley & Sons, Inc.

some minimum level of mental competence essential to having any rights at all? Do mentally incapacitated people have the same rights as normally competent people, or are their rights altered or diminished or extended in some way in virtue of their disease? Do they, for example, have the same rights to autonomy, to the care of their custodians, to dignity, and to a minimum level of resources as sick people of normal mental competence?

These are questions of great and growing importance. In 1990, the Alzheimer's Association estimated that four million Americans had the disease, and as Alzheimer's is a disease of the elderly, the number is expected to increase as the population continues to age. In 1989, a Harvard Medical School study estimated that 11.3 percent of the American population sixty-five or over probably had Alzheimer's. The estimated prevalence increased sharply with age: 16.4 percent of people between seventy-five and eighty-four were estimated to have Alzheimer's, and a stunning 47.55 percent of those over eighty-five.[5] (Other studies, using a narrower definition of the disease, suggest a significantly lesser but still alarming prevalence.[6]) The incidence of the disease is comparable in other countries. According to the Alzheimer's Disease Society in Britain, for example, 20 percent of people over eighty are afflicted, more than half a million people have the disease, and that figure will rise to three-quarters of a million in thirty years.[7] Alzheimer's cost is staggering, both for the community and for individuals. Dennis Selkoe, a leading expert on the disease, said in 1991, "The cost to American society for diagnosing and managing Alzheimer's disease, primarily for custodial care, is currently estimated at more than $80 billion annually."[8] In 1992, the annual cost of nursing home care in the United States for one individual with Alzheimer's ranged from $35,000 to $52,000.[9]

Each of the millions of Alzheimer's cases is horrible, for the victims and for those who love and care for them. A recent book dedicated "to everyone who gives a '36-hour day' to the care of a person with a dementing illness" describes the lives of some of these patients in chilling detail, not just in the final, immobile last stages, but along the way.

Often, Mary was afraid, a nameless shapeless fear. . . .People came, memories came, and then they slipped away. She could not tell what was reality and what was memory of things past. . . .The tub was a mystery. From day to day she could not remember how to manage the water: sometimes it all ran away, sometimes it kept rising and rising so that she could not stop it.. . .Mary was glad when her family came to visit. Sometimes she remembered their names, more often she did not.. . .She liked it best when they just held her and loved her.

Even though Miss Ramirez had told her sister over and over that today was the day to visit the doctor, her sister would not get into the car until she was dragged in, screaming, by two neighbors. All the way to the doctor's office she shouted for help and when she got there she tried to run away.

Mr. Lewis suddenly burst into tears as he tried to tie his shoelaces. He threw the shoes in the wastebasket and locked himself, sobbing, in the bathroom.[10]

When Andrew Firlik was a medical student, he met a fifty-four-year-old Alzheimer's victim whom he called Margo, and he began to visit her daily in her apartment, where she was cared for by an attendant. The apartment had many locks to keep Margo from slipping out at night and wandering in the park in a nightgown, which she had done before. Margo said she knew who Firlik was each time he arrived, but she never used his name, and he suspected that this was just politeness. She said she was reading mysteries, but Firlik "noticed that her place in the book jumps randomly from day to day; dozens of pages are dogeared at any given moment.. . .Maybe she feels good just sitting and humming to herself, rocking back and forth slowly, nodding off liberally, occasionally turning to a fresh page." Margo attended an art class for Alzheimer's victims – they all, including her, painted pretty much the same picture every time, except near the end, just before death, when the pictures became more primitive. Firlik was confused, he said, by the fact that "despite her illness, or maybe somehow because of it, Margo is undeniably one of the happiest people I have ever known." He reports, particularly, her pleasure at eating peanut-butter-and-jelly sandwiches. But, he asks, "When a person can no longer accumulate new memories as the old rapidly fade, what remains? Who is Margo?"[11]

I must now repeat an observation that I have made before: we are considering the rights and interests not of someone who has always been demented, but of someone who was competent in the past. We may therefore think of that person, in considering his rights and interests, in two different ways: as a *demented* person, emphasizing his present situation and capacities, or as a person who has *become* demented, having an eye to the course of his whole life. Does a competent person's right to autonomy include, for example, the power to dictate that life-prolonging treatment be denied him later, or that funds not be spent on maintaining him in great comfort, even if he, when demented, pleads for it? Should what is done for him then be in his contemporary best interests, to make the rest of his life as pleasant and comfortable as possible, or in the best interests of the person he has been? Suppose a demented patient insists on remaining at home, rather than living in an institution, though this would impose very great burdens on his family, and that we all agree that people lead critically better lives when they are not a serious burden to others. Is it really in his best interests, overall, to allow him to become such a burden?

A person's dignity is normally connected to his capacity for self-respect. Should we care about the dignity of a dementia patient if he himself has no sense of it? That seems to depend on whether his past dignity, as a competent person, is in some way still implicated. If it is, then we may take his former capacity for self-respect as requiring that he be treated with dignity now; we may say that dignity now is necessary to show respect for his life as a whole. Many prominent issues about the rights of the demented, then, depend on how their interests now relate to those of their past, competent selves.[12]

Autonomy

It is generally agreed that adult citizens of normal competence have a right to autonomy, that is, a right to make important decisions defining their own lives for themselves. Competent adults are free to make poor investments, provided others do not deceive or withhold information from them, and smokers are allowed to smoke in private, though cigarette advertising must warn them of the dangers of doing so. This autonomy is often at stake in medical contexts.[13] A Jehovah's Witness, for example, may refuse blood transfusions necessary to save his life because transfusions offend his religious convictions. A patient whose life can be saved only if his legs are amputated but who prefers to die soon than to live a life without legs is allowed to refuse the operation. American law generally recognizes a patient's right to autonomy in circumstances like those.[14] But when is that right lost? How far, for example, do mentally incapacitated people have a right to make decisions for themselves that others would deem not in their best interests?[15] Should Mary, the woman who couldn't recognize relatives or manage a tub, be allowed to spend or give away her money as she wishes, or to choose her own doctors, or to refuse prescribed medical treatment, or to decide which relative is appointed as her guardian? Should she be allowed to insist that she be cared for at home, in spite of her family's opinion that she would get better care in an institution?

There may, of course, be some other reason, beyond autonomy, for allowing Mary and other demented people to do as they please. For example, if they are prevented from doing as they wish, they may become so agitated that we do them more harm than good by opposing them, even though the decision they make is not itself in their interests. But do we have reason to respect their decision even when this is not so, even when we think it would be in their best interests, all things considered, to take some decision out of their hands?

We cannot answer that question without reflecting on the point of autonomy, that is, on the question of why we should ever respect the decisions people make when we believe that these are not in their interests. One popular answer might be called the *evidentiary* view: it holds that we should respect the decisions people make for themselves, even when we regard these decisions as imprudent, because each person generally knows what is in his own best interests better than anyone else.[16] Though we often think that someone has made a mistake in judging what is in his own interests, experience teaches us that in most cases we are wrong to think this. So we do better, in the long run, to recognize a general right to autonomy, which we always respect, than by reserving the right to interfere with other people's lives whenever we think they have made a mistake.

If we accepted this evidentiary account of autonomy, we would not extend the right of autonomy to decisions made by the seriously demented, who, having altogether lost the power to appreciate and engage in reasoning and argument, cannot possibly know what is in their own best interests as well as trained specialists, like doctors, can. In some cases, any presumption that demented people know their own interests best would be incoherent: when, for example, as is often the case, their wishes and decisions change radically from one bout of lucidity to another.

But in fact the evidentiary view of autonomy is very far from compelling. For autonomy requires us to allow someone to run his own life even when he behaves in a way that he himself would accept as not at all in his interests.[17] This is sometimes a matter of what philosophers call "weakness of the will." Many people who smoke know that smoking, all things considered, is not in their best interests, but they smoke anyway. If we believe, as we do, that respecting their autonomy means allowing them to act in this way, we cannot accept that the point of autonomy is to protect an agent's welfare. And there are more admirable reasons for acting against what one believes to be in one's own best interests. Some people refuse needed medical treatment because they believe that other people, who would then have to go without it, need it more. Such people act out of convictions we admire, even if we do not act the same way, and autonomy requires us to respect their decisions. Once again, the supposed explanation of the right to autonomy – that it promotes the welfare of people making apparently imprudent decisions – fails to account for our convictions about when people have that right.

All this suggests that the point of autonomy must be, at least to some degree, independent of the claim that a person generally knows his own best interests better than anyone else. And then it would not follow, just because a demented person may well be mistaken about his own best interests, that others are entitled to decide for him. Perhaps the demented have a right to autonomy after all.

But we must try to find another, more plausible account of the point of autonomy, and ask whether the demented would have a right to autonomy according to it. The most plausible alternative emphasizes the integrity rather than the welfare of the choosing agent; the value of autonomy, on this view, derives from the capacity it protects: the capacity to express one's own character – values, commitments, convictions, and critical as well as experiential interests – in the life one leads. Recognizing an individual right of autonomy makes self-creation possible. It allows each of us to be responsible for shaping our lives according to our own coherent or incoherent – but, in any case, distinctive – personality. It allows us to lead our own lives rather than be led along them, so that each of us can be, to the extent a scheme of rights can make this possible, what we have made of ourselves. We allow someone to choose death over radical amputation or a blood transfusion, if that is his informed wish, because we acknowledge his right to a life structured by his own values.

The integrity view of autonomy does not assume that competent people have consistent values or always make consistent choices, or that they always lead structured, reflective lives. It recognizes that people often make choices that reflect weakness, indecision, caprice, or plain irrationality – that some people otherwise fanatical about their health continue to smoke, for example. Any plausible integrity-based theory of autonomy must distinguish between the general point or value of autonomy and its consequences for a particular person on a particular occasion. Autonomy encourages and protects people's general capacity to lead their lives out of a distinctive sense of their own character, a sense of what is important to and for them. Perhaps one principal value of that capacity is realized only when a life does in fact display a general, overall integrity and authenticity. But the right to autonomy protects and encourages the capacity in any event, by allowing people who have it to choose how far and in what form they will seek to realize that aim.

If we accept this integrity-based view of the importance of autonomy, our judgement about whether incapacitated patients have a right to autonomy will turn on the degree of their general capacity to lead a life in that sense. When a mildly demented person's choices are reasonably stable, reasonably continuous with the general character of his prior life, and inconsistent and self-defeating only to the rough degree that the choices of fully competent people are, he can be seen as still in charge of his life, and he has a right to autonomy for that reason. But if his choices and demands, no matter how firmly expressed, systematically or randomly contradict one another, reflecting no coherent sense of self and no discernible even short-term aims, then he has presumably lost the capacity that it is the point of autonomy to protect. Recognizing a continuing right to autonomy for him would be pointless. He has no right that his choices about a guardian (or the use of his property, or his medical treatment, or whether he remains at home) be respected for reasons of autonomy. He still has the right to beneficence, the right that decisions on these matters be made in his best interests; and his preferences may, for different reasons, be important in deciding what his best interests are. But he no longer has the right, as competent people do, himself to decide contrary to those interests.

"Competence" is sometimes used in a task-specific sense, to refer to the ability to grasp and manipulate information bearing on a given problem. Competence in that sense varies, sometimes greatly, even among ordinary, nondemented people; I may be more competent than you at making some decisions and less competent at others. The medical literature concerning surrogate decision making for the demented points out, properly, that competence in this task-specific sense is relative to the character and complexity of the decision in question.[18] A patient who is not competent to administer his complex business affairs

may nevertheless be able to grasp and appreciate information bearing on whether he should remain at home or enter an institution, for example.

But competence in the sense in which it is presupposed by the right to autonomy is a very different matter. It means the more diffuse and general ability I described: the ability to act out of genuine preference or character or conviction or a sense of self. There will, of course, be hard cases in which we cannot know with any confidence whether a particular dementia patient is competent in that sense. But we must make that overall judgement, not some combination of judgements about specific task capability, in order to decide whether some mentally incapacitated patient has a right to autonomy.[19] Patients like Mary have no right that *any* decision be respected just out of concern for their autonomy. That may sound harsh, but it is no kindness to allow a person to take decisions against his own interests in order to protect a capacity he does not and cannot have.

So neither the evidentiary view of autonomy nor the more plausible integrity view recommends any right to autonomy for the seriously demented. But what about a patient's *precedent* autonomy? Suppose a patient is incompetent in the general, overall sense but that years ago, when perfectly competent, he executed a living will providing for what he plainly does not want now. Suppose, for example, that years ago, when fully competent, Margo had executed a formal document directing that if she should develop Alzheimer's disease, all her property should be given to a designated charity so that none of it could be spent on her own care. Or that in that event she should not receive treatment for any other serious, life-threatening disease she might contract. Or even that in that event she should be killed as soon and as painlessly as possible? If Margo had expressed any of those wishes when she was competent, would autonomy then require that they be respected now by those in charge of her care, even though she seems perfectly happy with her dog-eared mysteries, the single painting she repaints, and her peanut-butter-and-jelly sandwiches?

If we had accepted the evidentiary view of autonomy, we would find the case for respecting Margo's past directions very weak. People are not the best judges of what their own best interests would be under circumstances they have never encountered and in which their preferences and desires may drastically have changed. But if we accept the integrity view, we will be drawn to the view that Margo's past wishes must be respected. A competent person making a living will providing for his treatment if he becomes demented is making exactly the kind of judgement that autonomy, on the integrity view, most respects: a judgement about the overall shape of the kind of life he wants to have led.

This conclusion is troubling, however, even shocking, and someone might want to resist it by insisting that the right to autonomy is *necessarily* contemporary: that a person's right to autonomy is only a right that his present decisions, not past ones that he has since disowned, be respected. Certainly that is the normal force of recognizing autonomy. Suppose that a Jehovah's Witness has signed a formal document stipulating that he is not to receive blood transfusions even if out of weakness of will he requests one when he would otherwise die. He wants, like Ulysses, to be tied to the mast of his faith. But when the moment comes, and he needs a transfusion, he pleads for it. We would not think ourselves required, out of respect for his autonomy, to disregard his contemporary plea.

We can interpret that example in different ways, though, and the difference is crucial for our present problem. We might say, first, that the Witness's later plea countermanded his original decision because it expressed a more contemporary desire. That presumes that it is only right to defer to past decisions when we have reason to believe that the agent still wishes what he wanted then. On that view, precedent autonomy is an illusion: we treat a person's past decision as important only because it is normally evidence of his present wishes, and we disregard it entirely when we know that it is not. On the other hand, we might say that the Witness's later plea countermanded his original decision because it was a fresh exercise of his autonomy, and that disregarding it would be treating him as no longer in charge of his own life. The difference between these two views about the force

of precedent autonomy is crucial when someone changes his mind *after* he has become incompetent – that is, when the conditions of autonomy no longer hold. Suppose that the same accident that made a transfusion medically necessary for the Witness also deranged him, and that while still plainly deranged he demands the transfusion. On the first view, we would not violate his autonomy by administering it, but on the second, we would.

Which of the two views about the force of past decisions is more persuasive? Suppose we were confident that the deranged Witness, were he to receive the transfusion and live, would become competent again and be appalled at having had a treatment he believed worse for him than dying. In those circumstances, I believe, we would violate his autonomy by giving him the transfusion. That argues for the second view about the force of past decisions, the view that endorses precedent autonomy as genuine. We refuse to give the deranged Witness a transfusion not because we think he really continues to want what he wanted before – this is not like a case in which someone who objects to a given treatment is unconscious when he needs it – but because he lacks the necessary capacity for a fresh exercise of autonomy. His former decision remains in force because no new decision by a person capable of autonomy has annulled it.

Someone might say that we are justified in withholding the transfusion only because we know that the Witness would regret the transfusion if he recovered. But that prediction would make no difference if he was fully competent when he asked for the transfusion and desperate to live at that moment, though very likely to change his mind again and be appalled tomorrow at what he has done. Surely we should accede to his request in those circumstances. What makes the difference, when we are deciding whether to honor someone's plea even though it contradicts his past deep convictions, is whether he is now competent to make a decision of that character, not whether he will regret making it later.

Our argument for the integrity view, then, supports a genuine doctrine of precedent autonomy. A competent person's right to autonomy requires that his past decisions about how he is to be treated if he becomes demented be respected even if they contradict the desires he has at that later point. If we refuse to respect Margo's precedent autonomy – if we refuse to respect her past decisions, though made when she was competent, because they do not match her present, incompetent wishes – then we are violating her autonomy on the integrity view. This conclusion has great practical importance. Competent people who are concerned about the end of their lives will naturally worry about how they might be treated if they become demented. Someone anxious to ensure that his life is not then prolonged by medical treatment is worried precisely because he thinks that the character of his whole life would be compromised if it were. He is in the same position as people who sign living wills asking not to be kept alive in a hopeless medical condition or when permanently vegetative. If we respect *their* past requests, as the Supreme Court has

decided American states must do, then we have the same reasons for respecting the wishes not to be kept alive of someone who dreads not unconsciousness but dementia.

The argument has very troubling consequences, however. The medical student who observed Margo said that her life was the happiest he knew. Should we really deny a person like that the routine medical care needed to keep her alive? Could we ever conceivably *kill* her? We might consider it morally unforgivable not to try to save the life of someone who plainly enjoys her life, no matter how demented she is, and we might think it beyond imagining that we should actually kill her. We might hate living in a community whose officials might make or license either of those decisions. We might have other good reasons for treating Margo as she now wishes, rather than as, in my imaginary case, she once asked. But still, that violates rather than respects her autonomy.

Notes

1 Doctors are now investigating treatments that include reducing the presence in the brain of toxic substances that may play a role in neurodegeneration, enhancing the supply of trophic factors (which facilitate neuronal repair and growth) and neurotransmitters that are missing or deficient in Alzheimer's patients, and controlling diet-related factors such as blood glucose levels that appear to affect mental functioning in the elderly. See Dennis J. Selkoe, "Aging Brain, Aging Mind," *Scientific American*, 135 (September 1992); Robert J. Joynt, "Neurology," *Journal of the American Medical Association*, 268 (1992), 380; and Andrew A. Skolnick, "Brain Researchers Bullish on Prospects for Preserving Mental Functioning in the Elderly," *Journal of the American Medical Association*, 267 (1992), 2154.

2 Selkoe, "Amyloid Protein and Alzheimer's Disease," *Scientific American* (November 1991), 68.

3 OTA document, "Losing a Million Minds," OTA-BA-323 (1987), 14.

4 Legal provision and practices of custodial care are discussed in several of the papers contained in the OTA document, "Losing a Million Minds." For discussions of clinical diagnosis and histopathology, see, for example,

Guy McKhann et al., "Clinical Diagnosis of Alzheimer's Disease: Report of the NINCDS-ADRDA Work Group Under the Auspices of Department of Health and Human Services Task Force on Alzheimer's Disease," *Neurology*, 34 (1984), 939; Christine M. Hulette et al., "Evaluation of Cerebral Biopsies for the Diagnosis of Dementia," *Archives of Neurology*, 49 (1992), 28; Selkoe, "Amyloid Protein and Alzheimer's Disease"; and M. Farlow et al., "Low Cerebrospinal-fluid Concentrations of Soluble Amyloid β-protein Precursor in Hereditary Alzheimer's Disease," *The Lancet*, 340 (1992), 453.

5 Evans et al., "Estimated Prevalence of Alzheimer's Disease in the United States," *Milbank Quarterly*, 68 (1990), 267.

6 In 1992, the continuing Framingham Study determined the prevalence of dementia in its study cohort as 23.8 percent from ages eighty-five to ninety-three. See Bachman et al., "Prevalence of Dementia and Probable Senile Dementia of the Alzheimer Type in the Framingham Study," *Neurology*, 42 (January 1992), 42. For a discussion of the differences between the studies cited in this and the preceding note, see Selkoe, "Aging Brain, Aging Mind."

7   See "UK: Dementia Condition Alzheimer's Disease Will Hit 750,000 in 30 Years," *The Guardian*, July 6, 1992.

8   Selkoe, "Amyloid Protein and Alzheimer's Disease," 68.

9   See Abstract, *Journal of the American Medical Association*, 267 (May 27, 1992), 2809 (summarizing Welch et al., "The Cost of Institutional Care in Alzheimer's Disease," *Journal of the American Geriatric Society*, 40 [1992], 221).

10 Nancy L. Mace and Peter V. Rabins, *The 36-Hour Day: A Family Guide to Caring for Persons with Alzheimer's Disease, Related Dementing Illnesses, and Memory Loss in Later Life* (Baltimore: Johns Hopkins University Press, 1981, 1991).

11 See Andrew D. Firlik, "Margo's Logo," *Journal of the American Medical Association*, 265 (1991), 201.

12 I should mention another great practical problem about the relationship between a demented person and the competent person he once was. Should the resources available to a demented patient depend on what he actually put aside when he was competent, by way of insurance for his own care in that event? Insurance schemes, both private schemes and mandated public schemes, play an important part in the way we provide resources for catastrophes of different sorts. But is the insurance approach the proper model to use in thinking about provision for the demented? That must depend on whether we believe that a competent person has the appropriate prudential concern for the incompetent person he might become, and that in turn depends on knotty philosophical problems about the concept of personal identity. I cannot discuss, in this book, either that philosophical problem or any of the other serious problems about the justice of financing the extraordinarily expensive care of demented patients in different ways. I have discussed both at some length, however, in a report, "Philosophical Problems of Senile Dementia," written for the United States Congress Office of Technology Assessment in Washington, DC, and available from that office.

13 See discussion in Allen E. Buchanan et al., "Surrogate Decision-Making for Elderly Individuals Who Are Incompetent or of Questionable Competence,"

November 1985, a report prepared for the Office of Technology Assessment.

14 See George J. Annas and Leonard H. Glantz, "Withholding and Withdrawing of Life-Sustaining Treatment for Elderly Incompetent Patients: A Review of Appellate Court Decisions," September 16, 1985, a report prepared for the Office of Technology Assessment.

15 I am assuming, in this discussion, that it can be in a person's overall best interests, at least sometimes, to force him to act otherwise than as he wants – that it can be in a person's overall best interests, for example, to be made not to smoke, even if we acknowledge that his autonomy is to some degree compromised, considered in itself, as against his interests.

16 Buchanan et al., "Surrogate Decision-Making."

17 There is an important debate in the economic literature on the question whether it can be rational to act against one's own best interests. The better view is that it can. See, for example, Amartya Sen, "Rational Fools: A Critique of the Behavioural Foundations of Economic Theory," *Philosophy and Public Affairs*, 6, no. 4 (Summer 1977).

18 See Buchanan et al., "Surrogate Decision-Making." Questions of task-sensitive competence are plainly relevant to the issues considered in the Buchanan report. But when the argument against surrogate decision making relies on the autonomy of the demented person affected by these decisions, the overall, non-task-sensitive sense of competence is also relevant.

19 Problems are presented for this judgement of overall integrity capacity when a patient appears only periodically capable of organizing his life around a system of desires and wishes. He seems able to take command of his life sometimes, and then lapses into a more serious stage of dementia, becoming lucid again only after a substantial intervening period, at which time the desires and interests he expresses are very different, or even contradictory. It would be a mistake to say that such a patient has the capacity for autonomy "periodically." The capacity autonomy presupposes is of necessity a temporally extended capacity: it is the capacity to have and act out of a personality.

39

Dworkin on Dementia
Elegant Theory, Questionable Policy

Rebecca Dresser

In his most recent book, *Life's Dominion: An Argument about Abortion, Euthanasia, and Individual Freedom*,[1] Ronald Dworkin offers a new way of interpreting disagreements over abortion and euthanasia. In doing so, he enriches and refines our understanding of three fundamental bioethical concepts: autonomy, beneficence, and sanctity of life. It is exciting that this eminent legal philosopher has turned his attention to bioethical issues. *Life's Dominion* is beautifully and persuasively written; its clear language and well-constructed arguments are especially welcome in this age of inaccessible, jargon-laden academic writing. *Life's Dominion* also is full of rich and provocative ideas; in this article, I address only Dworkin's remarks on euthanasia, although I will refer to his views on abortion when they are relevant to my analysis.

Professor Dworkin considers decisions to hasten death with respect to three groups: (1) competent and seriously ill people; (2) permanently unconscious people; and (3) conscious, but incompetent people, specifically, those with progressive and incurable dementia. My remarks focus on the third group, which I have addressed in previous work,[2] and which

in my view poses the most difficult challenge for policymakers.

I present Dworkin's and my views as a debate over how we should think about Margo. Margo is described by Andrew Firlik, a medical student, in a *Journal of the American Medical Association* column called "A Piece of My Mind."[3] Firlik met Margo, who has Alzheimer disease, when he was enrolled in a gerontology elective. He began visiting her each day, and came to know something about her life with dementia.

Upon arriving at Margo's apartment (she lived at home with the help of an attendant), Firlik often found Margo reading; she told him she especially enjoyed mysteries, but he noticed that "her place in the book jump[ed] randomly from day to day." "For Margo," Firlik wonders, "is reading always a mystery?" Margo never called her new friend by name, though she claimed she knew who he was and always seemed pleased to see him. She liked listening to music and was happy listening to the same song repeatedly, apparently relishing it as if hearing it for the first time. Whenever she heard a certain song, however, she smiled and told Firlik that it reminded her of her

Original publication details: Rebecca Dresser, "Dworkin on Dementia: Elegant Theory, Questionable Policy," pp. 32–38 from *Hastings Center Report* 25: 6 (November/December 1995). Reproduced with permission of John Wiley & Sons.

deceased husband. She painted, too, but like the other Alzheimer patients in her art therapy class, she created the same image day after day: "a drawing of four circles, in soft rosy colors, one inside the other."

The drawing enabled Firlik to understand something that previously had mystified him:

> Despite her illness, or maybe somehow because of it, Margo is undeniably one of the happiest people I have known. There is something graceful about the degeneration her mind is undergoing, leaving her carefree, always cheerful. Do her problems, whatever she may perceive them to be, simply fail to make it to the worry centers of her brain? How does Margo maintain her sense of self? When a person can no longer accumulate new memories as the old rapidly fade, what remains? Who is Margo?

Firlik surmises that the drawing represented Margo's expression of her mind, her identity, and that by repeating the drawing, she was reminding herself and others of that identity. The painting was Margo, "plain and contained, smiling in her peaceful, demented state."

In *Life's Dominion*, Dworkin considers Margo as a potential subject of his approach. In one variation, he asks us to suppose that

> years ago, when fully competent, Margo had executed a formal document directing that if she should develop Alzheimer's disease. . .she should not receive treatment for any other serious, life-threatening disease she might contract. Or even that in that event she should be killed as soon and as painlessly as possible. (p. 226)

He presents an elegant and philosophically sophisticated argument for giving effect to her prior wishes, despite the value she appears to obtain from her life as an individual with dementia.

Dworkin's position emerges from his inquiry into the values of autonomy, beneficence, and sanctity of life. To understand their relevance to a case such as Margo's, he writes, we must first think about why we care about how we die. And to understand that phenomenon, we must understand why we care

about how we live. Dworkin believes our lives are guided by the desire to advance two kinds of interests. *Experiential* interests are those we share to some degree with all sentient creatures. In Dworkin's words:

> We all do things because we like the experience of doing them: playing softball, perhaps, or cooking and eating well, or watching football, or seeing *Casablanca* for the twelfth time, or walking in the woods in October, or listening to *The Marriage of Figaro*, or sailing fast just off the wind, or just working hard at something. Pleasures like these are essential to a good life – a life with nothing that is marvelous only because of how it feels would be not pure but preposterous. (p. 201)

But Dworkin deems these interests less important than the second sort of interests we possess. Dworkin argues that we also seek to satisfy our *critical* interests, which are the hopes and aims that lend genuine meaning and coherence to our lives. We pursue projects such as establishing close friendships, achieving competence in our work, and raising children, not simply because we want the positive experiences they offer, but also because we believe we should want them, because our lives as a whole will be better if we take up these endeavors.

Dworkin admits that not everyone has a conscious sense of the interests they deem critical to their lives, but he thinks that "even people whose lives feel unplanned are nevertheless often guided by a sense of the general style of life they think appropriate, of what choices strike them as not only good at the moment but in character for them" (p. 202). In this tendency, Dworkin sees us aiming for the ideal of integrity, seeking to create a coherent narrative structure for the lives we lead.

Our critical interests explain why many of us care about how the final chapter of our lives turns out. Although some of this concern originates in the desire to avoid experiential burdens, as well as burdens on our families, much of it reflects the desire to escape dying under circumstances that are out of character with the prior stages of our lives. For most people, Dworkin writes, death has a "special, symbolic importance: they want their deaths, if possible, to express and in that way vividly to confirm the values they believe most important to their lives" (p. 211). And because critical interests are so personal and widely varied among individuals, each person must have the right to control the manner in which life reaches its conclusion. Accordingly, the state should refrain from imposing a "uniform, general view [of appropriate end-of-life-care] by way of sovereign law" (p. 213).

Dworkin builds on this hierarchy of human interests to defend his ideas about how autonomy and beneficence should apply to someone like Margo. First, he examines the generally accepted principle that we should in most circumstances honor the competent person's autonomous choice. One way to justify this principle is to claim that people generally know better than anyone else what best serves their interests; thus, their own choices are the best evidence we have of the decision that would most protect their welfare. Dworkin labels this the *evidentiary* view of autonomy. But Dworkin believes the better explanation for the respect we accord to individual choice lies in what he calls the *integrity* view of autonomy. In many instances, he contends, we grant freedom to people to act in ways that clearly conflict with their own best interests. We do this, he argues, because we want to let people "lead their lives out of a distinctive sense of their own character, a sense of what is important to them" (p. 224). The model once again assigns the greatest moral significance to the individual's critical interests, as opposed to the less important experiential interests that also contribute to a person's having a good life.

The integrity view of autonomy partially accounts for Dworkin's claim that we should honor Margo's prior choice to end her life if she developed Alzheimer disease. In making this choice, she was exercising, in Dworkin's phrase, her "precedent autonomy" (p. 226). The evidentiary view of autonomy fails to supply support for deferring to the earlier decision, Dworkin observes, because "[p]eople are not the best judges of what their own best interests would be under circumstances they have never encountered and in which their preferences and desires may drastically have

changed" (p. 226). He readily admits that Andrew Firlik and others evaluating Margo's life with dementia would perceive a conflict between her prior instructions and her current welfare. But the integrity view of autonomy furnishes compelling support for honoring Margo's advance directives. Margo's interest in living her life in character includes an interest in controlling the circumstances in which others should permit her life as an Alzheimer patient to continue. Limiting that control would in Dworkin's view be "an unacceptable form of moral paternalism" (p. 231).

Dworkin finds additional support for assigning priority to Margo's former instructions in the moral principle of beneficence. People who are incompetent to exercise autonomy have a right to beneficence from those entrusted to decide on their behalf. The best interests standard typically has been understood to require the decision that would best protect the incompetent individual's current welfare.[4] On this view, the standard would support some (though not necessarily all) life-extending decisions that depart from Margo's prior directives. But Dworkin invokes his concept of critical interests to construct a different best interests standard. Dworkin argues that Margo's critical interests persist, despite her current inability to appreciate them. Because critical interests have greater moral significance than the experiential interests Margo remains able to appreciate, and because "we must judge Margo's critical interests as she did when competent to do so" (p. 231), beneficence requires us to honor Margo's prior preferences for death. In Dworkin's view, far from providing a reason to override Margo's directives, compassion counsels us to follow them, for it is compassion "toward the whole person" that underlies the duty of beneficence (p. 232).

To honor the narrative that is Margo's life, then, we must honor her earlier choices. A decision to disregard them would constitute unjustified paternalism and would lack mercy as well. Dworkin concedes that such a decision might be made for other reasons – because we "find ourselves unable to deny medical help to anyone who is conscious and does not reject it" (p. 232), or deem it "morally unforgiveable not to try to save the life of someone who plainly enjoys her life" (p. 228), or find it "beyond imagining that we should actually kill her" (p. 228), or "hate living in a community whose officials might make or license either of [Margo's] decisions" (pp. 228–9). Dworkin does not explicitly address whether these or other aspects of the state's interest in protecting life should influence legal policy governing how people like Margo are treated.

Dworkin pays much briefer attention to Margo's fate in the event that she did not explicitly register her preferences about future treatment. Most incompetent patients are currently in this category, for relatively few people complete formal advance treatment directives.[5] In this scenario, the competent Margo failed to declare her explicit wishes, and her family is asked to determine her fate. Dworkin suggests that her relatives may give voice to Margo's autonomy by judging what her choice would have been if she had thought about it, based on her character and personality. Moreover, similar evidence enables them to determine her best interests, for it is her critical interests that matter most in reaching this determination. If Margo's dementia set in before she explicitly indicated her preferences about future care, "the law should so far as possible leave decisions in the hands of [her] relatives or other people close to [her] whose sense of [her] best interests. . .is likely to be much sounder than some universal, theoretical, abstract judgement" produced through the political process (p. 213).

Life's Dominion helps to explain why the "death with dignity" movement has attracted such strong support in the United States. I have no doubt that many people share Dworkin's conviction that they ought to have the power to choose death over life in Margo's state. But I am far from convinced of the wisdom or morality of these proposals for dementia patients.

Advance Directives and Precedent Autonomy

First, an observation. Dworkin makes an impressive case that the power to control one's future as an incompetent patient is a precious freedom that our society should go to great lengths to protect. But how strongly do people actually value this freedom? Surveys show that a relatively small percentage of the US population engages in end-of-life planning, and that many in that group simply designate a trusted relative or friend to make future treatment decisions, choosing not to issue specific instructions on future care.[6] Though this widespread failure to take advantage of the freedom to exercise precedent autonomy may be attributed to a lack of publicity or inadequate policy support for advance planning, it could also indicate that issuing explicit instructions to govern the final chapter of one's life is not a major priority for most people. If it is not, then we may question whether precedent autonomy and the critical interests it protects should be the dominant model for our policies on euthanasia for incompetent people.

Dworkin constructs a moral argument for giving effect to Margo's directives, but does not indicate how his position could be translated into policy. Consider how we might approach this task. We would want to devise procedures to ensure that people issuing such directives were competent, their actions voluntary, and their decisions informed. In other medical settings, we believe that a person's adequate understanding of the information relevant to treatment decision-making is a prerequisite to the exercise of true self-determination. We should take the same view of Margo's advance planning.

What would we want the competent Margo to understand before she chose death over life in the event of dementia? At a minimum, we would want her to understand that the experience of dementia differs among individuals, that for some it appears to be a persistently frightening and unhappy existence, but that most people with dementia do not exhibit the distress and misery we competent people tend to associate with the condition. I make no claims to expertise in this area, but my reading and discussions with clinicians, caregivers, and patients themselves suggest that the subjective experience of dementia is more positive than most of us would expect. Some caregivers and other commentators also note that patients' quality of life is substantially dependent on their social and physical environments, as opposed to the neurological condition itself.[7] Thus, the "tragedy" and "horror" of dementia is partially attributable to the ways in which others respond to people with this condition.

We also would want Margo to understand that Alzheimer disease is a progressive condition, and that options for forgoing life-sustaining interventions will arise at different points in the process. Dworkin writes that his ideas apply only to the late stages of Alzheimer disease, but he makes implementation of Margo's former wishes contingent on the mere development of the condition (pp. 219, 226). If we were designing policy, we would want to ensure that competent individuals making directives knew something about the general course of the illness and the points at which various capacities are lost. We would want them to be precise about the behavioral indications that should trigger the directive's implementation. We would want them to think about what their lives could be like at different stages of the disease, and about how invasive and effective various possible interventions might be. We would want to give them the opportunity to talk with physicians, caregivers, and individuals diagnosed with Alzheimer disease, and perhaps, to discuss their potential choices with a counselor.

The concern for education is one that applies to advance treatment directives generally, but one that is not widely recognized or addressed at the policy level. People complete advance directives in private, perhaps after discussion with relatives, physicians, or attorneys, but often with little understanding of the meaning or implications of their decisions. In one study of dialysis patients who had issued instructions on treatment in the event of advanced Alzheimer disease, a subsequent inquiry revealed that almost two-thirds of them wanted families and physicians to have some freedom to override the directives to protect their subsequent best interests.[8] The patients' failure to include this statement in their directives indicates that the instructions they recorded did not reflect their actual preferences. A survey of twenty-nine people participating in an advance care planning workshop found ten agreeing with both of the following

inconsistent statements: "I would never want to be on a respirator in an intensive care unit"; and "If a short period of extremely intensive medical care could return me to near-normal condition, I would want it."[9] Meanwhile, some promoters of advance care planning have claimed that subjects can complete directives during interviews lasting fifteen minutes.[10]

We do not advance people's autonomy by giving effect to choices that originate in insufficient or mistaken information. Indeed, interference in such choices is often considered a form of justified paternalism. Moreover, advance planning for future dementia treatment is more complex than planning for other conditions, such as permanent unconsciousness. Before implementing directives to hasten death in the event of dementia, we should require people to exhibit a reasonable understanding of the choices they are making.[11]

Some shortcomings of advance planning are insurmountable, however. People exercising advance planning are denied knowledge of treatments and other relevant information that may emerge during the time between making a directive and giving it effect. Opportunities for clarifying misunderstandings are truncated, and decision-makers are not asked to explain or defend their choices to the clinicians, relatives, and friends whose care and concern may lead depressed or imprudent individuals to alter their wishes.[12] Moreover, the rigid adherence to advance planning Dworkin endorses leaves no room for the changes of heart that can lead us to deviate from our earlier choices. All of us are familiar with decisions we have later come to recognize as ill-suited to our subsequent situations. As Dworkin acknowledges, people may be mistaken about their future experiential interests as incompetent individuals. A policy of absolute adherence to advance directives means that we deny people like Margo the freedom we enjoy as competent people to change our decisions that conflict with our subsequent experiential interests.[13]

Personal identity theory, which addresses criteria for the persistence of a particular person over time, provides another basis for questioning precedent autonomy's proper moral and legal authority. In *Life's*

Dominion, Dworkin assumes that Margo the dementia patient is the same person who issued the earlier requests to die, despite the drastic psychological alteration that has occurred. Indeed, the legitimacy of the precedent autonomy model absolutely depends on this view of personal identity. Another approach to personal identity would challenge this judgement, however. On this view, substantial memory loss and other psychological changes may produce a new person, whose connection to the earlier one could be less strong, indeed, could be no stronger than that between you and me.[14] Subscribers to this view of personal identity can argue that Margo's earlier choices lack moral authority to control what happens to Margo the dementia patient.

These shortcomings of the advance decision-making process are reasons to assign less moral authority to precedent autonomy than to contemporaneous autonomy. I note that Dworkin himself may believe in at least one limit on precedent autonomy in medical decision-making. He writes that people "who are repelled by the idea of living demented, totally dependent lives, speaking gibberish," ought to be permitted to issue advance directives "stipulating that if they become permanently and seriously demented, and then develop a serious illness, they should not be given medical treatment except to avoid pain" (p. 231). Would he oppose honoring a request to avoid all medical treatment, including pain-relieving measures, that was motivated by religious or philosophical concerns? The above remark suggests that he might give priority to Margo's existing experiential interests in avoiding pain over her prior exercise of precedent autonomy. In my view, this would be a justified limit on precedent autonomy, but I would add others as well.

Critical and Experiential Interests: Problems with the Model

What if Margo, like most other people, failed to exercise her precedent autonomy through making an advance directive? In this situation, her surrogate decision-makers are to apply Dworkin's version of the best interests standard. Should they consider, first and foremost, the critical interests she had as a competent person? I believe not, for several reasons. First, Dworkin's approach to the best interests standard rests partially on the claim that people want their lives to have narrative coherence. Dworkin omits empirical support for this claim, and my own observations lead me to wonder about its accuracy. The people of the United States are a diverse group, holding many different world views. Do most people actually think as Dworkin says they do? If I were to play psychologist, my guess would be that many people take life one day at a time. The goal of establishing a coherent narrative may be a less common life theme than the simple effort to accept and adjust to the changing natural and social circumstances that characterize a person's life. It also seems possible that people generally fail to draw a sharp line between experiential and critical interests, often choosing the critical projects Dworkin describes substantially because of the rewarding experiences they provide.

Suppose Margo left no indication of her prior wishes, but that people close to her believe it would be in her critical interests to die rather than live on in her current condition. Dworkin notes, but fails to address, the argument that "in the circumstances of dementia, critical interests become less important and experiential interests more so, so that fiduciaries may rightly ignore the former and concentrate on the latter" (p. 232). Happy and contented Margo will experience clear harm from the decision that purports to advance the critical interests she no longer cares about. This seems to me justification for a policy against active killing or withholding effective, non-burdensome treatments, such as antibiotics, from dementia patients whose lives offer them the sorts of pleasures and satisfactions Margo enjoys. Moreover, if clear evidence is lacking on Margo's own view of her critical interests, a decision to hasten her death might actually conflict with the life narrative she envisioned for herself. Many empirical studies have shown that families often do not have a very good sense of their relatives' treatment preferences.[15] How will Margo's life narrative be improved by her family's decision to hasten death, if there is no clear indication that she herself once took that view?

I also wonder about how to apply a best interests standard that assigns priority to the individual's critical interests. Dworkin writes that family members and other intimates applying this standard should decide based on their knowledge of "the shape and character of [the patient's] life and his own sense of integrity and critical interests" (p. 213). What sorts of life narratives would support a decision to end Margo's life? What picture of her critical interests might her family cite as justification for ending her life now? Perhaps Margo had been a famous legal philosopher whose intellectual pursuits were of utmost importance to her. This fact might tilt toward a decision to spare her from an existence in which she can only pretend to read. But what if she were also the mother of an [intellectually disabled] child, whom she had cared for at home? What if she had enjoyed and valued this child's simple, experiential life, doing everything she could to protect and enhance it? How would this information affect the interpretation of her critical interests as they bear on her own life with dementia?

I am not sure whether Dworkin means to suggest that Margo's relatives should have complete discretion in evaluating considerations such as these. Would he permit anyone to challenge the legitimacy of a narrative outcome chosen by her family? What if her closest friends believed that a different conclusion would be more consistent with the way she had constructed her life? And is there any room in Dworkin's scheme for surprise endings? Some of our greatest fictional characters evolve into figures having little resemblance to the persons we met in the novels' opening chapters. Are real-life characters such as the fiercely independent intellectual permitted to become people who appreciate simple experiential pleasures and accept their dependence on others?

Finally, is the goal of respecting individual differences actually met by Dworkin's best interests standard? Although Dworkin recognizes that some people believe their critical interests would be served by a decision to extend their lives as long as is medically possible (based on their pro-life values), at times he

implies that such individuals are mistaken about their genuine critical interests, that in actuality no one's critical interests could be served by such a decision. For example, he writes that after the onset of dementia, nothing of value can be added to a person's life, because the person is no longer capable of engaging in the activities necessary to advance her critical interests (p. 230). A similar judgement is also evident in his discussion of an actual case of a brain-damaged patient who "did not seem to be in pain or unhappy," and "recognized familiar faces with apparent pleasure" (p. 233). A court-appointed guardian sought to have the patient's life-prolonging medication withheld, but the family was strongly opposed to this outcome, and a judge denied the guardian's request. In a remark that seems to conflict with his earlier support for family decision-making, Dworkin questions whether the family's choice was in the patient's best interests (p. 233). These comments lead me to wonder whether Dworkin's real aim is to defend an objective nontreatment standard that should be applied to all individuals with significant mental impairment, not just those whose advance directives or relatives support a decision to hasten death. If so, then he needs to provide additional argument for this more controversial position.

The State's Interest in Margo's Life

My final thoughts concern Dworkin's argument that the state has no legitimate reason to interfere with Margo's directives or her family's best interests judgement to end her life. A great deal of *Life's Dominion* addresses the intrinsic value of human life and the nature of the state's interest in protecting that value. Early in the book, Dworkin defends the familiar view that only conscious individuals can possess interests in not being destroyed or otherwise harmed. On this view, until the advent of sentience and other capacities, human fetuses lack interests of their own that would support a state policy restricting abortion. A policy that restricted abortion prior to this point would rest on what Dworkin calls a *detached* state interest in protecting human life. Conversely, a policy that restricts abortion after fetal sentience (which coincides roughly with viability) is supported by the state's *derivative* interest in valuing life, so called because it derives from the fetus's own interests (pp. 10–24, 168–70). Dworkin believes that detached state interests in ensuring respect for the value of life justify state prohibitions on abortion only after pregnant women are given a reasonable opportunity to terminate an unwanted pregnancy. Prior to this point, the law should permit women to make decisions about pregnancy according to their own views on how best to respect the value of life. After viability, however, when fetal neurological development is sufficiently advanced to make sentience possible, the state may severely limit access to abortion, based on its legitimate role in protecting creatures capable of having interests of their own (pp. 168–70).

Dworkin's analysis of abortion provides support, in my view, for a policy in which the state acts to protect the interests of conscious dementia patients like Margo. Although substantially impaired, Margo retains capacities for pleasure, enjoyment, interaction, relationships, and so forth. I believe her continued ability to participate in the life she is living furnishes a defensible basis for state limitations on the scope of her precedent autonomy, as well as on the choices her intimates make on her behalf. Contrary to Dworkin, I believe that such moral paternalism is justified when dementia patients have a quality of life comparable to Margo's. I am not arguing that all directives regarding dementia care should be overridden, nor that family choices should always be disregarded. I think directives and family choices should control in the vast majority of cases, for such decisions rarely are in clear conflict with the patient's contemporaneous interests. But I believe that state restriction is justified when a systematic evaluation by clinicians and others involved in patient care produces agreement that a minimally intrusive life-sustaining intervention is likely to preserve the life of someone as contented and active as Margo.

Many dementia patients do not fit Margo's profile. Some are barely conscious, others appear frightened,

miserable, and unresponsive to efforts to mitigate their pain. Sometimes a proposed life-sustaining treatment will be invasive and immobilizing, inflicting extreme terror on patients unable to understand the reasons for their burdens. In such cases, it is entirely appropriate to question the justification for treatment, and often to withhold it, as long as the patient can be kept comfortable in its absence. This approach assumes that observers can accurately assess the experiential benefits and burdens of patients with neurological impairments and decreased ability to communicate. I believe that such assessments are often possible, and that there is room for a great deal of improvement in meeting this challenge.

I also believe that the special problems inherent in making an advance decision about active euthanasia justify a policy of refusing to implement such decisions, at the very least until we achieve legalization for competent patients without unacceptable rates of error and abuse.[16] I note as well the likely scarcity of health care professionals who would be willing to participate in decisions to withhold simple and effective treatments from someone in Margo's condition, much less to give her a lethal injection, even if this were permitted by law. Would Dworkin support a system that required physicians and nurses to compromise their own values and integrity so that Margo's precedent autonomy and critical interests could be advanced? I seriously doubt that many health professionals would agree to implement his proposals regarding dementia patients whose lives are as happy as Margo's.

We need community reflection on how we should think about people with dementia, including our possible future selves. Dworkin's model reflects a common response to the condition: tragic, horrible, degrading, humiliating, to be avoided at all costs. But how much do social factors account for this tragedy? Two British scholars argue that though we regard dementia patients as "the problem," the patients

> are rather less of a problem than *we*. *They* are generally more authentic about what they are feeling and doing; many of the polite veneers of earlier life have been stripped away. *They* are clearly dependent on others, and

usually come to accept that dependence; whereas many "normal" people, living under an ideology of extreme individualism, strenuously deny their dependency needs. *They* live largely in the present, because certain parts of their memory function have failed. *We* often find it very difficult to live in the present, suffering constant distraction; the sense of the present is often contaminated by regrets about the past and fears about the future.[17]

If we were to adopt an alternative to the common vision of dementia, we might ask ourselves what we could do, how we could alter our own responses so that people with dementia may find that life among us need not be so terrifying and frustrating. We might ask ourselves what sorts of environments, interactions, and relationships would enhance their lives.

Such a "disability perspective" on dementia offers a more compassionate, less rejecting approach to people with the condition than a model insisting that we

should be permitted to order ourselves killed if this "saddest of the tragedies" (p. 218) should befall us. It supports as well a care and treatment policy centered on the conscious incompetent patient's subjective reality; one that permits death when the experiential burdens of continued life are too heavy or the benefits too minimal, but seeks to delay death when the patient's subjective existence is as positive as Margo's appears to be. Their loss of higher-level intellectual capacities ought not to exclude people like Margo from the moral community nor from the law's protective reach, even when the threats to their well-being emanate from their own former preferences. Margo's connections to us remain sufficiently strong that we owe her our concern and respect in the present. Eventually, the decision to allow her to die will be morally defensible. It is too soon, however, to exclude her from our midst.

Notes

1 Ronald Dworkin, *Life's Dominion: An Argument about Abortion, Euthanasia, and Individual Freedom* (New York: Knopf, 1993; Vintage, 1994).

2 See, for example, Rebecca Dresser, "Missing Persons: Legal Perceptions of Incompetent Patients," *Rutgers Law Review*, 609 (1994): 636–47; Rebecca Dresser and Peter J. Whitehouse, "The Incompetent Patient on the Slippery Slope," *Hastings Center Report*, 24, no. 4 (1994): 6–12; Rebecca Dresser, "Autonomy Revisited: The Limits of Anticipatory Choices," in *Dementia and Aging: Ethics, Values, and Policy Choices*, ed. Robert H. Binstock, Stephen G. Post, and Peter J. Whitehouse (Baltimore, MD: Johns Hopkins University Press, 1992), pp. 71–85.

3 Andrew D. Firlik, "Margo's Logo," *JAMA*, 265 (1991): 201.

4 See generally Dresser, "Missing Persons."

5 For a recent survey of the state of advance treatment decision-making in the US, see "Advance Care Planning: Priorities for Ethical and Empirical Research," Special Supplement, *Hastings Center Report* 24, no. 6 (1994).

6 See generally "Advance Care Planning." The failure of most persons to engage in formal end-of-life planning does not in itself contradict Dworkin's point that

most people care about how they die. It does suggest, however, that people do not find the formal exercise of precedent autonomy to be a helpful or practical means of expressing their concerns about future life-sustaining treatment.

7 See generally Dresser, "Missing Persons," 681–91; Tom Kitwood and Kathleen Bredin, "Towards a Theory of Dementia Care: Personhood and Well Being," *Ageing and Society*, 12 (1992): 269–87.

8 Ashwini Sehgal et al., "How Strictly Do Dialysis Patients Want Their Advance Directives Followed?" *JAMA*, 267 (1992): 59–63.

9 Lachlan Forrow, Edward Gogel, and Elizabeth Thomas, "Advance Directives for Medical Care" (letter), *New England Journal of Medicine*, 325 (1991): 1255.

10 Linda L. Emanuel et al., "Advance Directives for Medical Care – A Case for Greater Use," *New England Journal of Medicine*, 324 (1991): 889–95.

11 See Eric Rakowski, "The Sanctity of Human Life," *Yale Law Journal*, 103 (1994): 2049, 2110–11.

12 See Allen Buchanan and Dan Brock, "Deciding for Others," in *The Ethics of Surrogate Decisionmaking* (Cambridge: Cambridge University Press, 1989), at

101–7 for discussion of these and other shortcomings of advance treatment decision-making.

13 See generally Rebecca Dresser and John A. Robertson, "Quality-of-Life and Non-Treatment Decisions for Incompetent Patients: A Critique of the Orthodox Approach," *Law, Medicine & Health Care*, 17 (1989): 234–44.

14 See Derek Parfit, *Reasons and Persons* (New York: Oxford University Press, 1985), pp. 199–379.

15 See, e.g., Allison B. Seckler et al., "Substituted Judgment: How Accurate Are Proxy Predictions?" *Annals of Internal Medicine*, 115 (1992): 92–8.

16 See generally Leslie P. Francis, "Advance Directives for Voluntary Euthanasia: A Volatile Combination?" *Journal of Medicine & Philosophy*, 18 (1993): 297–322.

17 Kitwood and Bredin, "Towards a Theory of Dementia Care," 273–4.

Voluntary Euthanasia and Medically Assisted Suicide

40

The Note

Chris Hill

An open letter to anyone who wants to understand why I've checked out. It's very personal, pretty horrible and perhaps a bit shocking. I hope that those of you who knew me well enough find it unnecessary to read this.

Well, this is it – perhaps the hardest thing you've ever had to read, easily the most difficult thing I've ever attempted to write. To understand my over-whelming sense of loss and why I chose to take my own life, you need to know a bit about my life before and after my accident. Let's take a closer look.

I was born at one of the best times in one of the world's best countries – Australia. I had more than the proverbial happy childhood. Great parents, world travel, a good education and fabulous experiences like Disneyland, swimming with a wild dolphin in the turquoise waters of the Bahamas, riding across the desert sands around the Egyptian pyramids and much more.

Later, after the travel bug had bitten good and hard, I set out on my own adventures. I can remember only a fraction of them, but many rich images come flooding back. I stood on the lip of a live volcano in Vanuatu and stared down into the vision of hell in its throat; I watched the morning sun ignite Himalayan peaks

in a blaze of incandescent glory; smoked hashish with a leper in an ancient Hindu temple; danced naked under the stars with the woman I love on a tropical beach that left a trail of phosphorescent blue footsteps behind us; skied waist-deep powder snow in untracked Coloradon glades; soared thermals to 8,000 feet in a hang-glider and have literally flown with the eagles. In Maryland, on midsummer nights redolent with the smell of freshly ploughed earth, I rode past fields lit by the twinkling light of a billion fireflies. I've ridden a motorcycle at 265 km/h on a Japanese racetrack and up to the 5,000 metre snowline on an Ecuadorian volcano. And speaking of riding, what haven't I seen from behind the bars of a motorcycle? More than 200,000 kilometres in over a dozen countries embracing everything from some of the world's most spectacular wilderness areas to its greatest cities and vast slums containing millions of impoverished souls.

Along the way I picked up a decent education, including two university degrees, and learnt another language. All this and so much more – more than most people would experience in several lifetimes.

Perhaps most importantly of all, everywhere I've been I enjoyed the support of a caring family, the

Original publication details: Chris Hill, "The Note," pp. 9–17 from Helga Kuhse (ed.), *Willing to Listen, Wanting to Die* (Ringwood, Australia: Penguin Books, 1994).

Bioethics: An Anthology, Fourth Edition. Edited by Udo Schüklenk and Peter Singer.

company of good friends and, more than once, the rewards of being involved in a caring relationship. They – you, if you're reading – are ultimately what made my life as rich as it was, and I thank you.

I was lucky enough to know love, and I indulged in lust. I enjoyed exotic erotica with perhaps more than a hundred women of many different nationalities in places that ranged from the bedroom to a crowded ship's deck on the Aegean Sea, fields, rivers, trees, beaches, cars and motorcycles. There's been a *ménage à trois* in various combinations and even a few outright orgies. How wonderful to have been sexually active in the pre-AIDS era. I record this not as an exercise in testosterone-fuelled chest-beating, but to point out that sex was an important part of my life, and so that you can better understand my sense of loss.

In short, I once lived life to the max, always grateful that I had the opportunity to do just that, and always mindful to live for today because there may be no tomorrow.

Just as well, it seems. After my hang-gliding accident – how ironic that something I loved so much could destroy me so cruelly – tomorrows were nothing but a grey void of bleak despair. I was paralysed from the chest down, more than three-quarters dead. A talking head mounted on a bloody wheelchair. No more of the simple pleasures I once took for granted. No walking, running, swimming, riding motorcycles, the wonderful feel of grass, sand or mud underfoot, nothing. The simplest of everyday tasks – getting up, having a shower, getting dressed – became an enormous hassle and the source of endless frustration. That in itself was completely shattering physically and emotionally, but I lost so much more than mobility. I lost my dignity and self-respect. I would forever be a burden on those around me and I didn't want that no matter how willingly and unthinkingly family and friends assumed that burden. Every time I had to ask someone to do something for me, every time I was dragged up a damn step, was like thrusting a hot blade into the place where my pride used to be.

All that was bad enough, but there was so much more. No balance. My every action was as graceless as a toy dog nodding in the back of some beat-up car. No ability to regulate my body temperature properly – in a sense I was cold-blooded, more like a lizard than a human being. And without abdominal muscles I couldn't cough, sneeze, shout, blow out a candle or even fart.

Worse still, I couldn't shit or piss. Those body functions had to be performed manually, which meant sticking a 30-centimetre-long silicon tube up my willie four times a day so I could drain myself into a plastic bag, and sticking a finger up my arse every second day to dig out the shit. Sometimes both procedures drew blood. They always made me shudder with revulsion, but I had a powerful incentive to persevere. Autonomic dysreflexia it's called, the potentially fatal rise in blood pressure and excruciating headache that occurs if body waste isn't properly removed and backs up. I had a taste of it in hospital once, and that was enough.

Despite this regimen, there was no guarantee I wouldn't shit or piss my pants in public or wake up wallowing in it. Can you imagine living with that uncertainty? Can you imagine the shame and humiliation when it actually happened? Unbearable abominations that made me feel less than human. For me, it was no way to live.

There's more. I wept every morning when I saw myself in the mirror. I'd become a hunchback with a bloated pot belly above withered legs with muscles as soft and useless as marshmallow. It was an unbearable sight for someone who was once so grateful for being blessed with such an athletic and healthy body. Paraplegia meant that I also had to live with the constant possibility of pressure sores, ugly ulcers that can require months of hospitalization to cure. They're common. So are urinary tract infections and haemorrhoids. I suffer from both, and they also usually lead back to hospital sooner or later. I would rather die than return to hospital.

Then there was the pain in my shoulder. A damaged nerve meant that two muscles in my left shoulder didn't work and they wasted away, leaving the others to compensate and me with a pain that frequently made simple actions difficult. Then there were swollen ankles, which once meant sleeping with pillows under my feet so they could drain overnight. My chest became hypersensitive, which may sound like fun but meant that I felt like I was wearing an unbearably scratchy woollen jumper over bare skin. And after sitting in the chair for a few hours my bum, which shouldn't have had any sensation, felt like it was on fire. There were also tinea, crutch rot, headaches. . .The list of horrors was endless, and I haven't even mentioned some of the worst ones.

While at Moorong [Spinal Unit] I began to wake with pins and needles – loss of sensation – in my hands and arms. Sometimes it took hours to pass, and I began to fear losing what little I had left. That was unbearable. Tethering, nerves pinched by the scar tissue formed around the broken bones in my neck, I was told. The doctors talked about tests and surgery on my neck, wrists. Forget it. There was no way I'd return to hospital, let alone for such delicate, radical and debilitating surgery.

All my many pleasures had been stripped from me and replaced by a hellish living nightmare. The mere sight of someone standing up, a child skipping, a bicyclist's flexing leg muscles, were enough to reduce me to tears. Everything I saw and did was a stinging reminder of my condition and I cried constantly, even behind the jokes and smiles. I was so tired of crying. I never imagined that anyone could hurt so bad and cry so much. I guarantee that anybody who thinks it can't have been too bad would change their mind if they lived in my body for a day.

People kill animals to put them out of their misery if they're suffering even a tiny part of what I had to put up with, but I was never given the choice of a dignified death and I was very bitter about that. I could accept that accidents happen and rarely asked 'why me?', but I felt that the legislature's and the medical profession's attitude of life at any cost was an inhumane presumption that amounted to arrogance. And what of the dollar cost? My enforced recovery and rehabilitation cost taxpayers at least $150,000 by my rough count, money that wouldn't have been wasted had anybody bothered to ask me how I felt about the whole thing and what I'd like to do.

I had one good reason for living, of course, and her name is Lee-Ann, the best thing that ever happened to me. Wonderful Lee-Ann, without whom I would have gone insane long before now. But I wept whenever I thought of us together. What future could we have? No matter how hard I worked and how much I achieved, she would inevitably be a nursemaid in a million different ways, and I hated that, no matter that she so willingly and lovingly assumed the burden.

Nor would I condemn her to spend her nights sleeping with a sexless wooden lump twitching with spasm. That's right, sexless – impotent. Stripped of my sexuality, I felt that I'd lost part of my essence, the very core of my masculinity. I was even denied the sensual pleasure of embrace, because from the chest down I couldn't feel warmth, didn't even know if someone was touching me. I love Lee-Ann, but she deserves better than the pointless life I could offer, and I believe that I'm giving her another chance at happiness no matter how much pain I cause in the short term. Someone so desirable – open, honest, natural, loyal, with a great sense of humour and a figure the desire of men and envy of women – has a better chance than most of finding the happiness she deserves, and I hope with all my heart she finds it.

I had other reasons for living, of course – my family and friends. I remember, many years ago, lying on the verandah roof of a colonial mansion in the mountains of northern Burma. A shooting star streaked through the clear night sky and I made a wish. I wished for health, wealth and happiness for all those I loved and cared about. I repeated that wish several times in the following years and was enormously gratified to gradually see it come to pass for most of my family and friends. I'm not suggesting that my wishes had anything to do with their various successes – that was largely the result of their own efforts and the occasional dash of good fortune. But after my accident, even the joy I derived from seeing the happiness of those I cared about went sour for me. Seeing others get on with their lives, doing what I no longer could, was terribly distressing for me. I couldn't live my life vicariously through other people's satisfactions and achievements.

I was a self-centred person and I'd always done what I wanted, had my own reasons for living.

Mum and Dad, you often said that you didn't care what I did as long as I was happy. I expect that many of my friends felt the same way. Well, I was terminally, unbearably unhappy with no way out – except death. I know others have come to terms with paraplegia, or even quadriplegia, and managed to lead successful, apparently normal and happy lives. I've met and been encouraged by some of them. I tips me hat to them, for they have done what I cannot. Then again, perhaps I have done what they could not. Four attempts taught me that it takes an enormous amount of courage to commit suicide. Unfortunately, I didn't find the examples of others in my position motivating or inspirational. For me, life as a para was so far from the minimum I considered acceptable that it just didn't matter. It's quality of life, not quantity, that's important.

It's a challenge, many of you said. Bullshit. My life was just a miserable existence, an awful parody of normalcy. What's a challenge without some reward to make it worthwhile?

Despite that, I gave it a go. I worked hard – harder than I ever have at anything – to try and rebuild my life. I tried picking up the threads and doing whatever I was still capable of. I went out to shops, theatres and restaurants, even a concert. I learnt to drive again, and worked. I hated every second of it with a passion I'd never felt before. What good is a picnic when you can't play with the kids and dogs and throw a frisbee? What's the point of going to a gig if you can't dance when the music grips you? I used to be a player, not a spectator, and my new existence (life seems too strong a word) was painful, frustrating and completely unsatisfying.

At least you can still work, some said. Great. I liked my job, the caring, talented and generous people I worked with and especially where we worked. But it was still just a job, and as you all know, I worked to live, not lived to work. Work was never a reason for living for me. And what of the future? Where would I go, what would I do? There's no future for a wheelchair-bound journalist, not one with my interests anyway. I'd never be able to do any of the things, like travel and adventure, that drew me to journalism in the first place and ultimately made the long office hours worth-while.

I accepted death – embraced it eagerly, in fact, after so many months of the nightmare – without fear or regret. I had a full, rewarding and successful life by any measure, and in my last weeks I couldn't think of a single thing I'd always wanted to do but hadn't yet done. Well, actually, I guess I can think of a few things, but they don't amount to much. I'd always wanted to ride a Harley or drive a convertible Porsche, and I would have loved to have been 'stoked in the green room' – ridden a tube. Surfing would definitely have been the next sport I would have taken up. I've got a pretty good idea of the buzz it offers, and I think I would have liked it. Anyway, death is the last great adventure, and I was ready for it. I wasn't religious – how could anyone believe in a just, compassionate and almighty God after seeing and experiencing what I have? – but I felt quietly confident that whatever lay beyond had to be something more, something better, if anything.

I had one enormous regret, of course. I didn't want to hurt anyone the way I know I have.

I wish it didn't have to be this way. I didn't want to make those I love suffer, and the knowledge that I would bring awful grief to those I least wanted to hurt in the world compounded my own misery unbelievably. I'm so sorry. I hope you can find it in your hearts to forgive me. I wish you could see death as I did, as a release, something to celebrate, and be happy for me. I would rather have thrown a raging party and simply have disappeared at dawn with your blessings and understanding. Of course, it could never have happened that way. At any rate, I thank you all for making my last months as happy as they were, for your optimism and support, for the rays of light with which you pierced my gloom. My condition was permanent; I can only hope your grief fades quickly with the healing passage of time.

Chris Hill
10 February 1993

Statement

I have decided to take my own life for reasons detailed in the accompanying note. It is a fully considered decision made in a normal, rational state of mind and I have not been influenced or assisted by anyone else. Suicide is not a crime and I have the right not to be handled or treated against my will, *so I absolutely forbid anyone to resuscitate or interfere with me while I continue to live, unless it is to end my suffering. Anyone who disregards this notice will be committing a civil and criminal offence against me.*

In the event that I do not die, I wish to be placed under the care of Dr George Quittner at Mosman Hospital.

Chris Hill

41

When Self-Determination Runs Amok

Daniel Callahan

The euthanasia debate is not just another moral debate, one in a long list of arguments in our pluralistic society. It is profoundly emblematic of three important turning points in Western thought. The first is that of the legitimate conditions under which one person can kill another. The acceptance of voluntary active euthanasia would morally sanction what can only be called "consenting adult killing." By that term I mean the killing of one person by another in the name of their mutual right to be killer and killed if they freely agree to play those roles. This turn flies in the face of a long-standing effort to limit the circumstances under which one person can take the life of another, from efforts to control the free flow of guns and arms, to abolish capital punishment, and to more tightly control warfare. Euthanasia would add a whole new category of killing to a society that already has too many excuses to indulge itself in that way.

The second turning point lies in the meaning and limits of self-determination. The acceptance of euthanasia would sanction a view of autonomy holding that individuals may, in the name of their own private, idiosyncratic view of the good life, call upon others, including such institutions as medicine, to help them pursue that life, even at the risk of harm to the common good. This works against the idea that the meaning and scope of our own right to lead our own lives must be conditioned by, and be compatible with, the good of the community, which is more than an aggregate of self-directing individuals.

The third turning point is to be found in the claim being made upon medicine: it should be prepared to make its skills available to individuals to help them achieve their private vision of the good life. This puts medicine in the business of promoting the individualistic pursuit of general human happiness and wellbeing. It would overturn the traditional belief that medicine should limit its domain to promoting and preserving human health, redirecting it instead to the relief of that suffering which stems from life itself, not merely from a sick body.

I believe that, at each of these three turning points, proponents of euthanasia push us in the wrong direction. Arguments in favor of euthanasia fall into four general categories, which I will take up in turn: (1) the moral claim of individual self-determination and

Original publication details: Daniel Callahan, "When Self-Determination Runs Amok," pp. 52–55 from *Hastings Center Report* 22: 2 (March/April 1992). Reproduced with permission of John Wiley & Sons.

Bioethics: An Anthology, Fourth Edition. Edited by Udo Schüklenk and Peter Singer.

well-being; (2) the moral irrelevance of the difference between killing and allowing to die; (3) the supposed paucity of evidence to show likely harmful consequences of legalized euthanasia; and (4) the compatibility of euthanasia and medical practice.

Self-Determination

Central to most arguments for euthanasia is the principle of self-determination. People are presumed to have an interest in deciding for themselves, according to their own beliefs about what makes life good, how they will conduct their lives. That is an important value, but the question in the euthanasia context is, What does it mean and how far should it extend? If it were a question of suicide, where a person takes her own life without assistance from another, that principle might be pertinent, at least for debate. But euthanasia is not that limited a matter. The self-determination in that case can only be effected by the moral and physical assistance of another. Euthanasia is thus no longer a matter only of self-determination, but of a mutual, social decision between two people, the one to be killed and the other to do the killing.

How are we to make the moral move from my right of self-determination to some doctor's right to kill me – from *my* right to *his* right? Where does the doctor's moral warrant to kill come from? Ought doctors to be able to kill anyone they want as long as permission is given by competent persons? Is our right to life just like a piece of property, to be given away or alienated if the price (happiness, relief of suffering) is right? And then to be destroyed with our permission once alienated?

In answer to all those questions, I will say this: I have yet to hear a plausible argument why it should be permissible for us to put this kind of power in the hands of another, whether a doctor or anyone else. The idea that we can waive our right to life, and then give to another the power to take that life, requires a justification yet to be provided by anyone.

Slavery was long ago outlawed on the ground that one person should not have the right to own another,

even with the other's permission. Why? Because it is a fundamental moral wrong for one person to give over his life and fate to another, whatever the good consequences, and no less a wrong for another person to have that kind of total, final power. Like slavery, dueling was long ago banned on similar grounds: even free, competent individuals should not have the power to kill each other, whatever their motives, whatever the circumstances. Consenting adult killing, like consenting adult slavery or degradation, is a strange route to human dignity.

There is another problem as well. If doctors, once sanctioned to carry out euthanasia, are to be themselves responsible moral agents – not simply hired hands with lethal injections at the ready – then they must have their own *independent* moral grounds to kill those who request such services. What do I mean? As those who favor euthanasia are quick to point out, some people want it because their life has become so burdensome it no longer seems worth living.

The doctor will have a difficulty at this point. The degree and intensity to which people suffer from their diseases and their dying, and whether they find life more of a burden than a benefit, has very little directly to do with the nature or extent of their actual physical condition. Three people can have the same condition, but only one will find the suffering unbearable. People suffer, but suffering is as much a function of the values of individuals as it is of the physical causes of that suffering. Inevitably in those circumstances, the doctor will in effect be treating the patient's values. To be responsible, the doctor would have to share those values. The doctor would have to decide, on her own, whether the patient's life was "no longer worth living."

But how could a doctor possibly know that or make such a judgement? Just because the patient said so? I raise this question because, while in Holland at a euthanasia conference, the doctors present agreed that there is no objective way of measuring or judging the claims of patients that their suffering is unbearable. And if it is difficult to measure suffering, how much more difficult to determine the value of a patient's statement that her life is not worth living?

However one might want to answer such questions, the very need to ask them, to inquire into the physician's responsibility and grounds for medical and moral judgement, points out the social nature of the decision. Euthanasia is not a private matter of self-determination. It is an act that requires two people to make it possible, and a complicit society to make it acceptable.

Killing and Allowing to Die

Against common opinion, the argument is sometimes made that there is no moral difference between stopping life-sustaining treatment and more active forms of killing, such as lethal injection. Instead I would contend that the notion that there is no morally significant difference between omission and commission is just wrong. Consider in its broad implications what the eradication of the distinction implies: that death from disease has been banished, leaving only the actions of physicians in terminating treatment as the cause of death. Biology, which used to bring about death, has apparently been displaced by human agency. Doctors have finally, I suppose, thus genuinely become gods, now doing what nature and the deities once did.

What is the mistake here? It lies in confusing causality and culpability, and in failing to note the way in which human societies have overlaid natural causes with moral rules and interpretations. Causality (by which I mean the direct physical causes of death) and culpability (by which I mean our attribution of moral responsibility to human actions) are confused under three circumstances.

They are confused, first, when the action of a physician in stopping treatment of a patient with an underlying lethal disease is construed as *causing* death. On the contrary, the physician's omission can only bring about death on the condition that the patient's disease will kill him in the absence of treatment. We may hold the physician morally responsible for the death, if we have morally judged such actions wrongful omissions. But it confuses reality and moral judgement to see an omitted action as having the same causal status as one that directly kills. A lethal injection will kill both a healthy person and a sick person. A physician's omitted treatment will have no effect on a healthy person. Turn off the machine on me, a healthy person, and nothing will happen. It will only, in contrast, bring the life of a sick person to an end because of an underlying fatal disease.

Causality and culpability are confused, second, when we fail to note that judgements of moral responsibility and culpability are human constructs. By that I mean that we human beings, after moral reflection, have decided to call some actions right or wrong, and to devise moral rules to deal with them. When physicians could do nothing to stop death, they were not held responsible for it. When, with medical progress, they began to have some power over death – but only its timing and circumstances, not its ultimate inevitability – moral rules were devised to set forth their obligations. Natural causes of death were not thereby banished. They were, instead, overlaid with a medical ethics designed to determine moral culpability in deploying medical power.

To confuse the judgements of this ethics with the physical causes of death – which is the connotation of the word *kill* – is to confuse nature and human action. People will, one way or another, die of some disease; death will have dominion over all of us. To say that a doctor "kills" a patient by allowing this to happen should only be understood as a moral judgement about the licitness of his omission, nothing more. We can, as a fashion of speech only, talk about a doctor *killing* a patient by omitting treatment he should have provided. It is a fashion of speech precisely because it is the underlying disease that brings death when treatment is omitted; that is its cause, not the physician's omission. It is a misuse of the word *killing* to use it when a doctor stops a treatment he believes will no longer benefit the patient – when, that is, he steps aside to allow an eventually inevitable death to occur now rather than later. The only deaths that human beings invented are those that come from direct killing – when, with a lethal injection, we both cause death and are morally responsible for it. In the case of omissions, we do not cause death even if we may be judged morally responsible for it.

This difference between causality and culpability also helps us see why a doctor who has omitted a treatment he should have provided has "killed" that patient while another doctor – performing precisely the same act of omission on another patient in different circumstances – does not kill her, but only allows her to die. The difference is that we have come, by moral convention and conviction, to classify unauthorized or illegitimate omissions as acts of "killing." We call them "killing" in the expanded sense of the term: a culpable action that permits the real cause of death, the underlying disease, to proceed to its lethal conclusion. By contrast, the doctor who, at the patient's request, omits or terminates unwanted treatment does not kill at all. Her underlying disease, not his action, is the physical cause of death; and we have agreed to consider actions of that kind to be morally licit. He thus can truly be said to have "allowed" her to die.

If we fail to maintain the distinction between killing and allowing to die, moreover, there are some disturbing possibilities. The first would be to confirm many physicians in their already too-powerful belief that, when patients die or when physicians stop treatment because of the futility of continuing it, they are somehow both morally and physically responsible for the deaths that follow. That notion needs to be abolished, not strengthened. It needlessly and wrongly burdens the physician, to whom should not be attributed the powers of the gods. The second possibility would be that, in every case where a doctor judges medical treatment no longer effective in prolonging life, a quick and direct killing of the patient would be seen as the next, most reasonable step, on grounds of both humaneness and economics. I do not see how that logic could easily be rejected.

Calculating the Consequences

When concerns about the adverse social consequences of permitting euthanasia are raised, its advocates tend to dismiss them as unfounded and overly speculative. On the contrary, recent data about the Dutch experience suggests that such concerns are right on target. From my own discussions in Holland, and from articles on that subject, I believe we can now fully see most of the *likely* consequences of legal euthanasia.

Three consequences seem almost certain, in this or any other country: the inevitability of some abuse of the law; the difficulty of precisely writing, and then enforcing, the law; and the inherent slipperiness of the moral reasons for legalizing euthanasia in the first place.

Why is abuse inevitable? One reason is that almost all laws on delicate, controversial matters are to some extent abused. This happens because not everyone will agree with the law as written and will bend it, or ignore it, if they can get away with it. From explicit admissions to me by Dutch proponents of euthanasia, and from the corroborating information provided by the Remmelink Report and the outside studies of Carlos Gomez and John Keown, I am convinced that in the Netherlands there are a substantial number of cases of nonvoluntary euthanasia, that is, euthanasia undertaken without the explicit permission of the person being killed. The other reason abuse is inevitable is that the law is likely to have a low enforcement priority in the criminal justice system. Like other laws of similar status, unless there is an unrelenting and harsh willingness to pursue abuse, violations will ordinarily be tolerated. The worst thing to me about my experience in Holland was the casual, seemingly indifferent attitude toward abuse. I think that would happen everywhere.

Why would it be hard to precisely write, and then enforce, the law? The Dutch speak about the requirement of "unbearable" suffering, but admit that such a term is just about indefinable, a highly subjective matter admitting of no objective standards. A requirement for outside opinion is nice, but it is easy to find complaisant colleagues. A requirement that a medical condition be "terminal" will run aground on the notorious difficulties of knowing when an illness is actually terminal.

Apart from those technical problems there is a more profound worry. I see no way, even in principle, to write or enforce a meaningful law that can guarantee effective procedural safeguards. The reason is obvious yet almost always overlooked. The euthanasia transaction will ordinarily take place within the boundaries of the private and confidential doctor–patient relationship. No one can possibly know what takes place in that context unless the doctor chooses to reveal it. In Holland, less than 10 percent of the physicians report their acts of euthanasia and do so with almost complete legal impunity. There is no reason why the situation should be any better elsewhere. Doctors will have their own reasons for keeping euthanasia secret, and some patients will have no less a motive for wanting it concealed.

I would mention, finally, that the moral logic of the motives for euthanasia contain within them the ingredients of abuse. The two standard motives for euthanasia and assisted suicide are said to be our right of self-determination, and our claim upon the mercy of others, especially doctors, to relieve our suffering. These two motives are typically spliced together and presented as a single justification. Yet if they are considered independently – and there is no inherent reason why they must be linked – they reveal serious problems. It is said that a competent, adult person should have a right to euthanasia for the relief of suffering. But why must the person be suffering? Does not that stipulation already compromise the principle of self-determination? How can self-determination have any limits? Whatever the person's motives may be, why are they not sufficient?

Consider next the person who is suffering but not competent, who is perhaps demented or intellectually disabled. The standard argument would deny euthanasia to that person. But why? If a person is suffering but not competent, then it would seem grossly unfair to deny relief solely on the grounds of incompetence. Are the incompetent less entitled to relief from suffering than the competent? Will it only be affluent, middle-class people, mentally fit and savvy about working the medical system, who can qualify? Do the incompetent suffer less because of their incompetence?

Considered from these angles, there are no good moral reasons to limit euthanasia once the principle

of taking life for that purpose has been legitimated. If we really believe in self-determination, then any competent person should have a right to be killed by a doctor for any reason that suits him. If we believe in the relief of suffering, then it seems cruel and capricious to deny it to the incompetent. There is, in short, no reasonable or logical stopping point once the turn has been made down the road to euthanasia, which could soon turn into a convenient and commodious expressway.

Euthanasia and Medical Practice

A fourth kind of argument one often hears both in the Netherlands and in this country is that euthanasia and assisted suicide are perfectly compatible with the aims of medicine. I would note at the very outset that a physician who participates in another person's suicide already abuses medicine. Apart from depression (the main statistical cause of suicide), people commit suicide because they find life empty, oppressive, or meaningless. Their judgement is a judgement about the value of continued life, not only about health (even if they are sick). Are doctors now to be given the right to make judgements about the kinds of life worth living and to give their blessing to suicide for those they judge wanting? What conceivable competence, technical or moral, could doctors claim to play such a role? Are we to medicalize suicide, turning judgements about its worth and value into one more clinical issue? Yes, those are rhetorical questions.

Yet they bring us to the core of the problem of euthanasia and medicine. The great temptation of modern medicine, not always resisted, is to move beyond the promotion and preservation of health into the boundless realm of general human happiness and well-being. The root problem of illness and mortality is both medical and philosophical or religious. "Why must I die?" can be asked as a technical, biological question or as a question about the meaning of life. When medicine tries to respond to the latter, which it is always under pressure to do, it moves beyond its proper role.

It is not medicine's place to lift from us the burden of that suffering which turns on the meaning we assign to the decay of the body and its eventual death. It is not medicine's place to determine when lives are not worth living or when the burden of life is too great to be borne. Doctors have no conceivable way of evaluating such claims on the part of patients, and they should have no right to act in response to them. Medicine should try to relieve human suffering, but only that suffering which is brought on by illness and dying as biological phenomena, not that suffering which comes from anguish or despair at the human condition.

Doctors ought to relieve those forms of suffering that medically accompany serious illness and the threat of death. They should relieve pain, do what they can to allay anxiety and uncertainty, and be a comforting presence. As sensitive human beings, doctors should be prepared to respond to patients who ask why they must die, or die in pain. But here the doctor and the patient are at the same level. The doctor may have no better an answer to those old questions than anyone else; and certainly no special insight from his training as a physician. It would be terrible for physicians to forget this, and to think that in a swift, lethal injection, medicine has found its own answer to the riddle of life. It would be a false answer, given by the wrong people. It would be no less a false answer for patients. They should neither ask medicine to put its own vocation at risk to serve their private interests, nor think that the answer to suffering is to be killed by another. The problem is precisely that, too often in human history, killing has seemed the quick, efficient way to put aside that which burdens us. It rarely helps, and too often simply adds to one evil still another. That is what I believe euthanasia would accomplish. It is self-determination run amok.

42

When Abstract Moralizing Runs Amok

John Lachs

Moral reasoning is more objectionable when it is abstract than when it is merely wrong. For abstractness all but guarantees error by missing the human predicament that needs to be addressed, and worse, it is a sign that thought has failed to keep faith with its mission. The function of moral reflection is to shed light on the difficult problems we face; it cannot perform its job without a clear understanding of how and why certain of our practices come to seem no longer satisfactory.

It is just this grasp of the problem that is conspicuously lacking in Daniel Callahan's assault on euthanasia in "Self-Determination Run Amok"[1] [*sic*]. The rhetoric Callahan unleashes gives not even a hint of the grave contemporary moral problems that euthanasia and assisted suicide, a growing number of people now think, promise to resolve.

Instead, we are offered a set of abstract distinctions calculated to discredit euthanasia rather than to contribute to a sound assessment of it. Thus, Callahan informs us that suffering "brought on by illness and dying as biological phenomena"[2] is to be contrasted with suffering that comes from "anguish or despair at the human condition." The former constitutes the proper concern of medicine (so much for psychiatry!), the latter of religion and philosophy. Medication is the answer to physical pain; euthanasia can, therefore, be only a misconceived response to worries about the meaning of existence. Those who believe in it offer a "swift lethal injection" as the "answer to the riddle of life."

This way of putting the matter will come as a surprise to those who suffer from terrible diseases and who no longer find life worth living. It is grotesque to suppose that such individuals are looking for the meaning of existence and find it, absurdly, in a lethal injection. Their predicament is not intellectual but existential. They are not interested in the meaning of life but in acting on their belief that their own continued existence is, on balance, of no further benefit to them.

Those who advocate the legalization of euthanasia and the practice of assisted suicide propose them as answers to a serious and growing social problem. We now have the power to sustain the biological existence of large numbers of very sick people, and we use this

Original publication details: John Lachs, "When Abstract Moralizing Runs Amok," pp. 10–13 from *The Journal of Clinical Ethics* 5: 1 (Spring 1994). Reproduced with permission of The Journal of Clinical Ethics.

power freely. Accordingly, individuals suffering from painful terminal diseases, Alzheimer's patients, and those in a persistent vegetative state are routinely kept alive long past the point where they can function as human beings. They must bear the pain of existence without the ability to perform the activities that give life meaning. Some of these people feel intensely that they are a burden to others, as well as to themselves, and that their speedy and relatively dignified departure would be a relief to all concerned. Many observers of no more than average sensitivity agree that the plight of these patients is severe enough to justify such desires.

Some of these sufferers are physically not in a position to end their lives. Others could do so if they had the necessary instruments. In our culture, however, few have a taste for blowing out their brains or jumping from high places. That leaves drugs, which almost everyone is accustomed to taking, and which everyone knows can ease one peacefully to the other side.

The medical profession has, however, acquired monopoly power over drugs. And the danger of legal entanglement has made physicians wary of helping patients hasten their deaths in the discreet, humane way that has been customary for centuries. The result is that people who want to die and for whom death has long ceased to be an evil can find no way out of their misery. Current and growing pressures on the medical profession to help such sufferers are, therefore, due at least partly to medicine itself. People want physicians to aid in their suicides because, without such help, they cannot end their lives. This restriction of human autonomy is due to the social power of medicine; it is neither surprising nor morally wrong, therefore, to ask those responsible for this limitation to undo some of its most noxious effects. If the medical profession relinquished its hold on drugs, people could make effective choices about their future without the assistance of physicians. Even limited access to deadly drugs, restricted to single doses for those who desire them and who are certified to be of sound mind and near the end of life, would keep physicians away from dealing in death.

Unfortunately, however, there is little sensible public discussion of such policy alternatives. And these policy

alternatives may, in any case, not satisfy Callahan, who appears to believe that there is something radically wrong with anyone terminating a human life. Because he plays coy, his actual beliefs are difficult to make out. He says the notion that self-determination extends to suicide "might be pertinent, at least for debate."[3] But his argument against euthanasia sidesteps this issue: he maintains that even if there is a right to kill oneself, it is not one that can be transferred. The reason for this is that doing so would lead to "a fundamental moral wrong" – that of one person giving over "his life and fate to another."

One might wonder how we know that transferring power over oneself is "a fundamental moral wrong." Callahan appears to entertain the idea with intuitive certainty, which gives him the moral and the logical high ground and entitles him to demand a justification from whoever disagrees. But such intuitions are problematic themselves: is fervent embrace of them enough to guarantee their truth? Morality would be very distant from the concerns of life if it depended on such guideposts placed here and there in the desert of facts, unrelated to each other or to anything else. Their message, moreover, makes the guide posts suspect: it comes closer to being an echo of tradition or an expression of current views than a revelation of eternal moral truths.

Most important, the very idea of a right that intrinsically *cannot* be handed on is difficult to grasp. Under normal circumstances, to have a right is to be free or to be entitled to have or to do something. I have a right, for example, to clean my teeth. No one else has the right to do that without my consent. But I can authorize another, say my sweetheart or my dental hygienist, to do it for me. Similarly, I can assign my right to my house, to my left kidney, to raising my children, to deciding when I rise, when I go to sleep, and what I do in between (by joining the Army), and by a power of attorney even to pursuing my own interest.

To be sure, the transfer of rights is not without limits. My wife and I can, for example, give over our right to our children, though we cannot do so for money. I can contract to slave away for ten hours a day cooking hamburgers, but I cannot sell myself to be, once and for all, a slave. This does not mean, however, that some rights are intrinsically nontransferable. If my right to my left kidney were nontransferable, I could neither sell it nor give it away. But I can give it away, and the only reason I cannot sell it is because sales of this sort were declared, at some point, to be against public policy. We cannot sell ourselves into slavery for the same reason: human societies set limits to this transfer of rights on account of its unacceptable costs.

The case is no different with respect to authorizing another to end my life. If I have a right to one of my kidneys, I have a right to both. And if I can tell a needy person to take one of them, I can tell two needy people to take one each. There is nothing *intrinsically* immoral about this, even though when the second helps himself I die. Yet, by dying too soon, I may leave opportunities unexplored and obligations unmet. Unscrupulous operators may take advantage of my goodwill or naiveté. The very possibility of such acts invites abuse. For these or similar reasons, we may decide that giving the first kidney is morally acceptable, but giving the second is not. The difference between the two acts, however, is not that the first is generous while the second is "a fundamental moral wrong," but that the second occurs in a context and has consequences and costs that the first does not.

Only in terms of context and cost, therefore, can we sensibly consider the issue of the morality of euthanasia. Moving on the level of abstract maxims, Callahan misses this point altogether. He declares: "There are no good moral reasons to limit euthanasia once the principle of taking life. . .has been legitimated."[4] Serious moral reflection, though it takes principles into account, is little interested in legitimating *them*. Its focus is on determining the moral acceptability of certain sorts of actions performed in complex contexts of life. Consideration of the circumstances is always essential: it is fatuous, therefore, to argue that if euthanasia is ever permissible, then "any competent person should have a right to be killed by a doctor for any reason that suits him."[5]

We can achieve little progress in moral philosophy without the ability and readiness to make relevant distinctions. Why, then, does Callahan refuse to acknowledge that there are important differences between the situation of a terminally ill patient in grave pain who wants to die and that of a young father in the dental chair who wishes, for a moment, that he were dead? Callahan's reason is that he thinks all judgments about the unbearability of suffering and the worthlessness of one's existence are subjective and, as such, parts of a "private, idiosyncratic view of the good life."[6] The amount of our suffering "has very little directly to do" with our physical condition, and so the desire to end life is capricious and unreliable. If medicine honored such desires, it would "put its own vocation at risk" by serving "the private interests" of individuals.

I cannot imagine what the vocation of medicine might be if it is not to serve the private interests of individuals. It is, after all, my vision of the good life that accounts for my wish not to perish in a diabetic coma. And surgeons certainly pursue the private interests of their patients in removing cancerous growths and in providing face-lifts. Medicine does not surrender its vocation in serving the desires of individuals: since health and continued life are among our primary wishes, its career consists in just this service.

Nevertheless, Callahan is right that our judgments about the quality of our lives and about the level of our suffering have a subjective component. But so do the opinions of patients about their health and illness, yet physicians have little difficulty in placing these perceptions in a broader, objective context. Similarly, it is both possible and proper to take into account the objective circumstances that surround desires to terminate life. Physicians have developed considerable skill in relating subjective complaints to objective conditions; only by absurd exaggeration can we say that the doctor must accept either all or none of the patient's claims. The context of the young father in the dental chair makes it clear that only a madman would think of switching from novocaine to cyanide when he moans that he wants to be dead. Even people of ordinary sensitivity understand that the situation of an old person whose friends have all died and who now suffers the excruciating pain of terminal cancer is morally different.

The question of the justifiability of euthanasia, as all difficult moral questions, cannot be asked without specifying the details of context. Dire warnings of slippery slopes and of future large-scale, quietly conducted exterminations trade on overlooking differences of circumstance. They insult our sensitivity by the suggestion that a society of individuals of good will cannot recognize situations in which their fellows want and need help and cannot distinguish such situations from those in which the desire for death is rhetorical, misguided, temporary, or idiotic. It would indeed be tragic if medicine were to leap to the aid of lovelorn teenagers whenever they feel life is too much to bear. But it is just as lamentable to stand idly by and watch unwanted lives fill up with unproductive pain.

Callahan is correct in pointing out that, in euthanasia and in assisted suicide, the physician and the patient must have separate justifications for action. The patient's wish is defensible if it is the outcome of a sound reflective judgment. Such judgments take into account the current condition, pending projects, and long-term prospects of the individual and relate them to his or her permanent interests and established values. As all assessments, these can be in error. For this reason, persons soliciting help in dying must be ready to demonstrate that they are of sound mind and thus capable of making such choices, that their desire is enduring, and that both their subjective and their objective condition makes their wish sensible.

Physicians must first decide whether their personal values permit them to participate in such activities. If they do, they must diligently examine the justifiability of the patient's desire to die. Diagnosis and prognosis are often relatively easy to ascertain. But we are not without resources for a sound determination of the internal condition of individuals either: extensive questioning on multiple occasions, interviews with friends and loved ones, and exploration of the life history and values of people contribute mightily to understanding their state of mind. Physicians who are prepared to aid individuals with this last need of their lives are not, therefore, in a position where they have to believe everything they hear and act on every request. They must make independent judgments

instead of subordinating themselves as unthinking tools to the passing desires of those they wish to help. This does not attribute to doctors "the powers of the gods." It only requires that they be flexible in how they aid their patients and that they do so with due caution and on the basis of sound evaluation.

Callahan is once again right to be concerned that, if allowed, euthanasia will "take place within the boundaries of the private and confidential doctor–patient relationship."[7] This does, indeed, invite abuse and permit callous physicians to take a casual attitude to a momentous decision. Callahan is wrong, however, in supposing that this constitutes an argument against euthanasia. It is only a reason not to keep euthanasia secret, but to shed on it the wholesome light of publicity. Though the decision to terminate life is intensely private, no moral consideration demands that it be kept the confidential possession of two individuals. To the contrary, the only way we can minimize wrong decisions and abuse is to require scrutiny of the decision, prior to action on it, by a suitable social body. Such examination, including at least one personal interview with the patient, should go a long distance toward relieving Callahan's concern that any law governing euthanasia would have "a low enforcement priority in the criminal justice system."[8] With formal social controls in place, there should be very little need for the involvement of courts and prosecutors.

To suppose, as Callahan does, that the principle of autonomy calls for us to stand idly by, or even to assist, whenever and for whatever reason people want to end their lives is calculated to discredit both euthanasia and autonomy. No serious moralist has ever argued that self-determination must be absolute. It cannot hold unlimited sway, as Mill and other advocates of the principle readily admit, if humans are to live in a society. And morally, it would cut no ice if murderers and rapists argued for the legitimacy of their actions by claiming that they flow naturally and solely from who they are.

The function of the principle of autonomy is to affirm *a* value and to shift the burden of justifying infringements of individual liberty to established social and governmental powers. The value it affirms is that of individual agency expressed in the belief that, through action and suffering and death, the life of each person enjoys a sort of private integrity. This means that, in the end, our lives belong to no one but ourselves. The limits to such self-determination or self-possession are set by the demands of social life. They can be discovered or decided upon in the process of moral reflection. A sensible approach to euthanasia can disclose how much weight autonomy carries in that context and how it can be balanced against other, equally legitimate but competing values.

In the hands of its friends, the principle of self-determination does not run amok. What runs amok in Callahan's version of autonomy and euthanasia is the sort of abstract moralizing that forgets the problem it sets out to address and shuts its eye to need and suffering.

Notes

1   D. Callahan, "Self-Determination Run Amok," *Hastings Center Report* 22 (March–April 1992): 52–5. [See also Chapter 41 in this *Anthology*.]
2   Ibid., 55.
3   Ibid., 52.
4   Ibid., 54.
5   Ibid.
6   Ibid., 52.
7   Ibid., 54.
8   Ibid.

43

Physician-Assisted Death and Severe, Treatment-Resistant Depression

Bonnie Steinbock

Should people suffering from untreatable psychiatric conditions be eligible for physician-assisted death (PAD)? Although most jurisdictions that allow for PAD require physical, and typically terminal, illness as an eligibility condition, PAD for psychiatric conditions is permitted in four European countries (Belgium, Luxembourg, the Netherlands, and Switzerland) and possibly Canada.[1]

In Belgium and the Netherlands, the countries that have received the greatest attention on this issue, PAD is permitted, though rare, for psychiatric conditions, so long as the criteria of due care are met.[2] These criteria require that the physician be convinced that the request of the patient is voluntary and well considered, the patient is suffering unbearably without prospect of improvement, the patient is informed about his situation and prospects, and there are no reasonable alternatives to relieve suffering. Two further conditions are required: an independent physician must be consulted, and the method used must be performed with due medical care and attention.

The case for expanding the criteria is based on the idea that the request for PAD may be as justifiable in certain kinds of psychiatric illness as it is in the case of terminal illness. If we accept PAD in one case, on this line, we should be equally willing to accept it in the other. This, of course, assumes that PAD is justifiable in the case of terminal illness, an assumption I will be making in this chapter. The question I am addressing is not the justification for PAD in general, but only whether the eligibility criteria should be expanded to include psychiatric conditions.

Some maintain that it is obviously wrong to offer PAD to people with severe psychiatric conditions, while others think that it is obviously right. I reject both views. The issue is complicated, and there are multiple factors to consider. I acknowledge that there are, or could be, particular cases of psychiatric illness in which the request for PAD would be justified. However, I will argue that the fact that PAD for psychiatric illness might be justifiable in particular cases does not entail that it is a justifiable change in public policy. At this point, we do not have sufficiently robust answers to many of the relevant issues. For this reason, I argue that, at this point, allowing PAD for psychiatric conditions is not warranted.

Original publication details: Bonnie Steinbock, "Physician-Assisted Death and Severe, Treatment-Resistant Depression," pp. 30–42 from *Hastings Center Report* 47: 5 (2017), updated by the author for this edition (2021). Reproduced with permission of John Wiley & Sons.

Supporters of expansion argue that limiting PAD to those suffering from terminal illness is arbitrary and illogical. For example, Udo Schüklenk and Suzanne van de Vathorst argue that severely depressed patients with treatment-resistant disorder have as good a claim as those suffering from terminal illness, since their suffering can be just as unbearable.[3] Indeed, their claim may be better since, as another commentator notes, "for the suffering caused by depression, we do not have the kind of palliative care available which can, in most cases of physical suffering, eliminate the pain."[4] In addition, precisely because such patients are not terminally ill, their suffering may last for years, or even the rest of their lives. Finally, severe depression may not be treatable. Why shouldn't psychiatrists who have nothing else to offer their suffering patients be able to help them to die, if that is what they want?

Those who think that people with major depressive disorder should not have the option of assisted dying typically base their opposition on concerns about two factors: voluntariness and treatment-resistance. They doubt that such requests can ever be seen as truly voluntary, given that the disease can impair decision-making capacity. In addition, a common symptom of depression is "suicidal ideation." The request for assisted dying may simply be a manifestation of the disease and not a rational, considered decision. Moreover, it is alleged that the requirement that there are no reasonable alternatives to alleviate suffering, as in the due care criteria in Belgium and the Netherlands, cannot be met since it is always possible that a new treatment, a new therapist, or a change in environment might makes the patient's life worth living, even if a permanent cure is not possible.[5]

These are all compelling arguments deserving of in-depth examination. First, however, I need to review some terminological points.

Terminology

Physician-assisted death can take two forms: euthanasia and physician-assisted suicide. "Euthanasia" is the deliberate ending of life for reasons of compassion or the good of the one who is killed. It is also referred to as "mercy-killing." Euthanasia is often divided into sub-categories: voluntary, nonvoluntary, and involuntary. Nonvoluntary euthanasia refers to the killing of individuals who are incapable of giving consent, such as infants and the severely cognitively impaired. Whether and under what conditions nonvoluntary euthanasia is justified is beyond the scope of this paper. "Involuntary euthanasia" refers to euthanasia performed on individuals who do not want to die or who have not been given the chance to express their views on the matter. In my view, "involuntary euthanasia" is a misnomer. It clearly is not done out of compassion for unbearable suffering (as nonvoluntary euthanasia might be), since a patient who wants to go on living, despite suffering, does not regard that suffering as unbearable. What the Nazi doctors did was not euthanasia but murder. In this chapter, I use "euthanasia" to mean "voluntary euthanasia."

Euthanasia is usually accomplished by lethal injection on the part of a physician. By contrast, in physician-assisted suicide (PAS), the physician does not participate in the action that causes death, but rather, on the request of the patient, prescribes lethal medication, which the patient swallows. The difference between euthanasia and PAS turns solely on who administers the lethal dose. In the Netherlands, both euthanasia and assisted suicide are permitted. This is reflected in the Dutch term for physician-assisted death, EAS, the abbreviation for euthanasia and assisted suicide.

Does the difference between euthanasia and assisted suicide have legal significance? It does in the United States, where euthanasia is illegal everywhere, but physician-assisted suicide, or aid-in-dying, as it is now called, is legal in ten jurisdictions: California, Colorado, the District of Columbia, Hawaii, Montana, Maine, New Jersey, Oregon, Vermont, and Washington. The distinction lacks legal significance in Canada, Belgium, and the Netherlands, where both euthanasia and physician-assisted suicide are permitted. As a matter of practice, however, most Dutch physicians who are willing to help their patients die prefer administering euthanasia to PAS, as being safer and more reliable.

What is the reason for regarding euthanasia, but not aid-in-dying, as morally impermissible? Presumably, it is that in euthanasia, the physician administers the lethal injection, *killing* the patient, whereas in aid-in-dying, the patient has to swallow the pills in order to die. The patient, then, not the doctor, is the final cause of death. But why should it matter morally who completes the process? The physician who writes the lethal prescription for the patient who wants to die plays an essential causal role in her death and, for that reason, is as much an agent of the patient's death as the physician who, at the request of the patient, administers a lethal injection.

Perhaps there is a pragmatic reason for banning euthanasia, namely, as protection against a last-second change of mind. Requiring that the patient actually puts the pills in her mouth and swallows means that there will be clear evidence that she really does want to die. The data from Oregon reveal that many people who request a prescription do not actually use it. They simply want the peace of mind that comes from knowing they have the pills if things get too bad. Simply not taking the pills might be psychologically easier than telling the doctor you have summoned to kill you to go away.

However, if there are pragmatic reasons to prefer aid-in-dying to euthanasia, there are also pragmatic reasons to prefer euthanasia to aid-in-dying. Dutch doctors regard euthanasia as safer, that is, more certain to cause death rather than leaving the patient worse off. Moreover, aid-in-dying is not available to people who physically cannot put the pills in their mouth or have lost the ability to swallow. Such individuals are not "death-eligible" in the United States, regardless of their suffering or unwavering desire to die. This strikes the Dutch as absurd. Why should the inability to swallow be relevant to getting assistance in dying? They have a point. The claim of an intrinsic moral difference between euthanasia and aid-in-dying is difficult to defend.

There are many terms for assisted suicide, including physician-assisted suicide, physician-assisted death, aid-in-dying, and medical aid in dying, or MAID as it is called in Canadian law. These terms are pretty much interchangeable, although there can be reasons for preferring one term to another. For example, some Americans have adopted the term MAID, while others reject it because they see it as including euthanasia, which is illegal in the United States.

The terms "assisted suicide" and "physician-assisted suicide" have come into increasing disfavor in the United States. The preferred term is aid-in-dying. Indeed, supporters of aid-in-dying will often strenuously deny that it is suicide. They maintain that suicide is, by its nature, pathological, whereas opting for death in the face of incurable illness that imposes great suffering can be a rational choice. However, even if most suicides are in fact pathological, that is, the result of psychiatric disorders, it does not follow that all suicides are or that suicide cannot be a rational choice.

Another reason for rejecting the term PAS is how it plays with focus groups. Compassion & Choices, a leading organization for the right to die, has found that people are much more supportive of aid-in-dying, as compared with physician-assisted suicide. If the goal is to garner political support, the smart move is to choose a term that people respond to favorably.

Philosophically, however, the term "aid-in-*dying*" suggests that assistance should be given only to those who are *dying*, that is, terminally ill. However, whether such assistance should be limited to those who are dying, or whether it should be available to those who are not dying, but who meet the other eligibility criteria, is a substantive moral issue. If we want to take that question seriously, it might be preferable to use the term "suicide" in a morally neutral way that merely characterizes the act as one of self-killing. It would then be a further question whether a particular request for assisted suicide was rational and warranted, or an irrational product of the depressed state. However, the important point is not what we call the practice, but rather that we do not beg any questions regarding eligibility criteria. This means that if we are to limit the practice to dying patients, we must give good reasons for that restriction.

All of the states that allow aid-in-dying in the United States require that the physician ascertain that the patient is terminally ill, defined as likely to die within six months. Since most patients with major depressive disorder are not terminally ill, this requirement automatically excludes them. In other countries, such as the Netherlands and Belgium, terminal illness is not a requirement. Instead, the focus is on unbearable suffering without prospect of improvement. Should terminal illness be a prerequisite for aid-in-dying?

Terminal Illness

Those who accept the terminal illness requirement often give the following rationale. It is that such patients are already dying and beyond medical treatment that can cure them or significantly prolong their lives. When they request assistance in dying, they are asking their physicians for a "good death": a death without undue suffering and on their own terms.

Many in the hospice movement reject PAD, on the grounds that suffering in the terminally ill can be adequately addressed with palliative care. Sadly, this is not always the case. Brittany Maynard, the young woman with terminal brain cancer who became the "poster child" for aid-in-dying in California, decided that hospice and palliative care were not good enough. She knew she might develop morphine-resistant pain and suffer radical personality changes and severe cognitive and motor loss. In addition, because the rest of her body was young and healthy, she might continue to exist in hospice for weeks or months, and her family would have to watch that. She wanted to die on her own terms and in her own way, and so she and her family moved to Oregon where aid-in-dying was legally available.[6]

Some physicians support the terminal illness requirement on the grounds of role responsibility. Physicians are supposed to cure illness, prolong life, and reduce suffering. If a patient is dying and nothing can be done to reverse the dying process, then healing is no longer possible. At that point, the physician's job shifts from trying to cure to relieving physical suffering and also to providing the kind of death that fits with the patient's values.

Undoubtedly, the role of physicians in the care of dying patients differs from their role in the care of curable patients. However, not all patients who are incurable are terminally ill, especially if by "terminal illness," we mean, "probably will die within six months." What about those who have "incurable, but not imminently terminal, progressive illnesses,"[7] such as amyotrophic lateral sclerosis (ALS) and the most severe cases of multiple sclerosis or Parkinson's disease? Such diseases can impose suffering and impairments and deficits that are just as terrible as those inflicted by, for example, terminal cancer. It seems arbitrary to allow aid-in-dying for terminally ill patients but to deny it to such patients.

Some who reject the terminal-illness criterion would nevertheless restrict PAD to physical illness, excluding psychiatric conditions. What is the rationale for this restriction on eligibility?

Suffering. It may be said that the suffering imposed by psychiatric conditions is often regarded as less severe than that caused by physical illness. However, this is a misunderstanding of the suffering of people with major depressive disorder. Clinical depression is not akin to feeling a bit bad.[8] The psychiatrist Kay Redfield Jamison, herself a sufferer of bipolar disorder, writes, "Suicidal depression is a state of cold, agitated horror and relentless despair. The things that you most love in life leach away. Everything is an effort, all day and throughout the night. There is no hope, no point, no nothing."[9]

Another powerful account of the suffering caused by severe depression is depicted in a video entitled "24 and Ready to Die."[10] It tells the story of Emily, a twenty-four-year-old Belgian who requested assisted dying in 2015. Emily tells the interviewer that she feels dead inside. Everything is pointless; she cannot envisage a future for herself. She feels as if there is a monster inside her ribcage that is trying to get out. She would cut herself and bang her head against a wall. This provided some relief, but it was only temporary. The hardest thing for her to bear, she said, was the knowledge that, within a short period, her agony would begin again. She attempted suicide several times. Emily's depression lasted most of her life. She remembers not wanting to live as early as the age of three. By the age of twelve, she had entered psychiatric care. When she began her request for assisted dying at the age of twenty-two, she had undergone multiple therapies, none of which was successful. After a two-year process, her psychiatrists agreed that there was nothing more that could be offered to her, and that they would provide her with an assisted death if she really wanted it. They stressed that she could change her mind at any time, and they would support her decision, whatever it was.

When the day came for Emily to die, she did change her mind. The reason she gives in the video is that her life during the two weeks prior to the scheduled euthanasia did not seem so terrible to her, perhaps because she knew her torment would not continue indefinitely. It is also possible that having her request granted by psychiatrists who clearly cared for her made Emily feel that her suffering was being taken seriously. Perhaps that contributed to her not wanting to die. Providing access to euthanasia might actually prevent some patients from taking their own lives: some people might be willing to go on living, at least for a while, if they know that there is the option of an assisted death if life becomes intolerable. As mentioned earlier, we know that in Oregon only just over half of people who receive the prescriptions for lethal drugs actually ingest them.[11] The others just want the security of knowing they have an escape. Unfortunately, in Emily's case, the decision to go on living was not long-lasting. According to an email I received (with Emily's permission), from one of her psychiatrists, Lieve Thienpont, "Emily's life is still a survival from day to day. It is very difficult to find the adequate residential form of help because there is no energy left to follow therapy and she can't survive in an ambulant setting. She had a bit of hope after she has left the date of the planned euthanasia last year, but now she is suffering again very much and continuously. She wants to restart her eu-request." She did so, and died on August 25, 2018, peacefully, surrounded by those she loved. Dr. Thienpont, who was abroad, was not with her.[12]

The case for allowing people with major depressive disorder to receive PAD is based both on the severity of their suffering and the assessment that there is no treatment that can alleviate their suffering. Schüklenk and van de Vathorst say that people with treatment-resistant depression "experience no joy in life, and have not for a long time, and they *are right* to think that this will not change, based on everything that is known at the time of their decision-making."[13] However, some are skeptical about whether they are indeed right. I turn now to the questions of whether some cases of this disorder are genuinely resistant to therapy and whether these cases can be identified.

Defining and Identifying Treatment-Resistant Depression

On one estimate, roughly 20 to 33 percent of all people suffering from clinical depression suffer from a treatment-resistant variety.[14] However, there is no operational, validated, and systematic definition for treatment-resistant depression. There is no consensus over what constitutes adequate treatment in terms of drug dosage and duration of therapy or on the number of failures of adequate treatment that a patient must experience before being considered treatment resistant.[15] As Thomas Schlaepfer and colleagues explain,

> In Europe, the Committee for Medicinal Products for Human Use (CHMP) has stated that a patient is considered to be therapy resistant when consecutive treatment with two antidepressants of different classes (different mechanism of action), used for a sufficient length of time and at an adequate dose, fail to induce an acceptable effect.
>
> . . ..However, "sufficient" and "adequate" are not defined and consensus from the wider psychiatric community is still required. In addition, true pharmacological resistance needs to be distinguished from resistance due to ongoing somatic or psychosocial problems.[16]

Some people are skeptical of the efficacy of *any* drug treatments for major depressive disorder in light of a recent study of clinical trials that revealed only a modest difference between drugs and placebo.[17] The majority of psychiatrists think that antidepressants can be helpful for many patients. However, a sizeable minority does not respond, and others may experience only a partial response.[18] Currently, antidepressant clinical trials have an effect size of 0.30, which is considered modest and less than impressive. (This is not unique to antidepressants. As Arif Khan and Walter Brown note, "Clinical trials of medications for other common disorders, such as hypertension, asthma and diabetes, have produced similar effect sizes, although attracting much less attention and criticism."[19])

Other possible treatments include nonpharmacological interventions, such as brain stimulation. As Schlaepfer et al. observe, "The archetypal stimulation therapy is electroconvulsive therapy (ECT), which has consistently been shown to be highly effective for the treatment of depression."[20] However, patients and their families often resist ECT because of side effects, especially cognitive impairments. Several new brain stimulation methods have been developed, including vagus nerve stimulation, transcranial magnetic stimulation, and deep brain stimulation. Some of these methods are invasive or have potentially serious side effects, so the risks must be carefully considered. Others pose fewer risks but seem to be of limited efficacy.[21] So far, there is no magic bullet for treating severe depression. Despite advances in the field, there are still unacceptably high rates of treatment-resistant depression.[22]

However, the issue is not only whether treatment-resistant depression exists but also whether physicians can accurately identify it. Some psychiatrists claim that it is impossible to know this and, therefore, from a clinical perspective, PAD is never justifiable. "In the case of an individual patient," Brendan Kelly and Declan McLoughlin state,

> it remains extremely difficult to predict whether therapy will produce an early response, a delayed response or no response. It is impossible to predict which patients will undergo spontaneous remission and when this will happen. These uncertainties are far more pronounced in psychiatric practice than in medical practice, to the extent that it is essentially impossible to describe any psychiatric illness as incurable, with the exception of

advanced brain damage as occurs in progressive neurodegenerative disorders such as Alzheimer's disease and Huntington's disease.[23]

This may overstate the difference between medical and psychiatric practice. Cancer patients who have been given a terminal diagnosis also go into spontaneous remission, and it is impossible to predict if this will occur and to which patients. In other areas in medicine, it is also extremely difficult to predict outcomes in individual cases. We may know that the risk of death or extreme impairment is very high in infants born prior to twenty-three weeks' gestation, but some of those babies do survive, and a very few of those survive without any impairment.[24] Uncertainty pervades most areas of medicine.

But suppose we grant that the uncertainty in psychiatry is greater than in other branches of medicine. Would this justify excluding psychiatric patients from choosing assisted dying? Schüklenk and van de Vathorst argue that it would not. So long as patients with treatment-resistant major depressive disorder meet the due care criteria, which include the ability to make medical decisions they are, in Schüklenk and van de Vathorst's view, "perfectly entitled to evaluate the likelihood of successful treatment becoming available and making end-of-life choices based on their evaluation of the state of the medical evidence that exists at the time when they wish to make their choices. It seems unreasonable for us to deny them this choice based on a hunch that a successful treatment might come around soon, or that they might experience a spontaneous, unexplained remission of symptoms."[25] This is a persuasive argument. Even if psychiatrists are uncertain about whether a patient might benefit from more treatments or newer treatments, surely competent patients should be able to make their own decisions about the risks and benefits of medical treatment, including (where this is legal) PAD. However, even if we acknowledge this, there is the further question of whether severely depressed patients can be competent to understand their condition and evaluate the likelihood of remission or successful treatment in the future.

Udo Schüklenk dismisses this issue as not worthy of discussion. He writes, "Decisionally capable mentally ill patients, who suffer from an irremediable severe condition that renders their lives not worth living in their considered judgment, should qualify for medical assistance in dying (MAID). Why is there even an argument against this?"[26] Why? Because some argue that decision-making capacity is impaired by the very condition that prompts the request for PAD and that it is not possible to know that the patient's request for assisted dying is genuinely voluntary and authentic and not simply "the depression talking." This claim merits serious investigation, not a dismissal.

Can Patients with Severe Major Depressive Disorder Be Competent to Request Assisted Dying?

The right of competent adult patients to make their own medical decisions, based on their values, is a fundamental tenet of contemporary medical ethics. This includes the right to refuse treatment, including life-sustaining treatment, even when physicians believe that undergoing the treatment would be the right decision. Decisions to refuse life-sustaining treatment are not made solely on the basis of objective facts about diagnosis, prognosis, and options for treatment. They are inevitably value laden, dependent on patients' views about the quality of their lives and what makes life worth living. The values of patients may not necessarily accord with the values of their physicians. Physicians can certainly reason with their patients and attempt to persuade them to accept life-sustaining treatment, but at the end of the day, the choice is the patient's.[27]

This right of self-determination belongs only to patients who are competent – that is, have decision-making capacity.[28] Those who lack decision-making capacity, such as children or those who are severely cognitively impaired, must have decisions made for them. But if they are competent, then they get to make their own decisions, according to their values,

even if others disagree. In the case of competent patients, autonomy trumps well-being.

It is important to remember that the emphasis on respect for autonomy in the case of competent patients is a fairly recent development in medicine. Until about the middle of the twentieth century, medical paternalism held sway. Physicians regarded themselves as primary decision-makers for their patients both because of their medical expertise and because illness itself could render patients vulnerable, dependent, and anxious, thereby reducing their ability to make the best medical decisions. Physicians saw their role as promoting patients' well-being, not their autonomy.[29]

Although the doctrine of informed consent and the right of patients to refuse treatment began to be part of U.S. case law beginning in the early twentieth century,[30] it wasn't until the 1970s that courts began recognizing a robust right of competent, adult patients to refuse medical treatment, including life-sustaining treatment, even against the advice of their doctors. At first, most doctors regarded informed consent as little more than a legal barrier, not a part of good medical practice.[31] While paternalism has never disappeared completely from medicine, and indeed, has seen some new defenses in the last fifteen years,[32] respect for autonomy, informed consent, and a right to refuse treatment are regarded as foundational in bioethics, in theory if not always in practice.

The situation in psychiatry, however, has been different. "Refusal of lifesaving psychiatric treatment is regarded as a symptom of an illness that psychiatrists treat," Mark Sullivan and Stuart Younger state, "rather than the rational choice of an autonomous patient that should be respected."[33] Moreover, unlike in medicine, where the burden of proof to show that an adult patient is incompetent falls on the physician, in psychiatry, when refusal of life-sustaining treatment occurs, the burden of proof of competence is on the patient who wishes to die. This has often meant that the decisions to refuse such treatment by patients with major depressive disorder who are also terminally ill have been ignored or overridden.

Sullivan and Younger think that this is a mistake. While they acknowledge that depression – especially when severe – can have a significant effect on a person's capacity to decide about medical treatment, they caution against assuming that depression, at least in its mild to moderate forms, necessarily distorts patients' judgments about lifesaving treatment. "Discriminating those cases in which depression impairs the capacity to make medical decisions from those cases in which it does not is best accomplished," Sullivan and Youngner argue, "through a systematic approach to assessment of competence."[34]

Assessing competence. Competence has two important features. First, in most cases, competence is *decision relative*.[35] For example, someone can be incompetent to manage his or her financial affairs but competent to make decisions about medical treatment. To be a competent decision-maker about medical treatment – to be able to give or withhold informed consent – one needs the ability to understand the information one is given about one's condition and the possible treatments, to reason about the information in order to weigh options, and to appreciate the significance of this information for one's own situation.[36] Second, competence is a *threshold concept*.[37] That is, either people are competent to make medical decisions, or they are not. This may sound strange, since the abilities required for making decisions, such as understanding, reasoning, and appreciation, can obviously vary a great deal between individuals. For this reason, it may seem that some individuals are highly competent, others adequately competent, and some barely competent. Why, then, treat competence as having a blanket yes-or-no answer? The reason is that a determination of incompetence removes from the individual the right to make important decisions about what happens to him and gives that right to someone else. Because it has this serious consequence, the question of competence must have a yes-or-no answer.

Allen Buchanan and Daniel Brock suggest a sliding scale approach for assessing competence, in which the standards for competence are more stringent when the stakes are higher. Since, in the case of refusing life-sustaining treatment, the likely outcome is the death of the patient, more stringent standards of competence are justifiable. Sullivan and Youngner note

that such flexibility appears to be a reasonable way to protect both patients' liberty and their well-being. At the same time, they warn against imposing standards of competence that allow physicians to regard patients as incompetent simply on the grounds that they are rejecting medical advice. "We want to make sure that patients have their facts right about a life and death decision, but we must allow them to hold different values concerning life and death," they explain.[38]

Major depressive disorder may not affect the abilities to understand and reason, but it may have a profound effect on attitude. In depression, things look bleak, and the prospect that things could change for the better seems remote or even impossible. Severely depressed individuals may not be able to appreciate the chances for recovery or remission. Anhedonia may make it impossible to imagine that life will offer any pleasures that will make it worth enduring the discomforts and indignities of medical treatment. Guilt and worthlessness may make individuals believe that suffering and death is deserved.[39] For example, one Dutch patient who received EAS for psychiatric reasons told researchers that "she had had a life without love and *therefore had no right to exist*" (emphasis added).[40] Such a statement is a red flag for distorted thinking, as opposed to a carefully considered, rational request to die.

Sullivan and Youngner emphasize that, before acceding to a wish to refuse lifesaving treatment, it is important to give optimal medical and psychiatric treatment. However, they also support the right of psychiatric patients to make such decisions:

> The doctrine of informed consent implies that medical decisions have inescapable personal as well as medical elements. In a pluralist secular society such as our own, it must be assumed – unless proven otherwise – that adults are competent to evaluate their own quality of life as tolerable or intolerable. Assessing one's quality of life as intolerable is distinct from being depressed. We must learn to identify those refusals of life-saving treatment that should be respected. The burden of proof concerning competence should be on the clinician who is seeking to override a refusal of treatment. The desire to die is by itself not adequate evidence of incompetence.[41]

Sullivan and Youngner discuss only the right to refuse life-sustaining treatment, not assisted dying. However, their arguments about decision-making capacity seem to apply equally to the request for PAD. Charles Baron explicitly makes this argument: "For decades, physicians and mental health professionals have been making decisions regarding the mental competence of patients who request cessation of life-prolonging treatment. There is no reason to think that the criteria or methodology for determining competence in those cases should be different from the criteria or methodology to be used in cases under the Oregon Act."[42] He asks, what reason is there to think that a person who can competently process the issues involved in requesting assistance in dying through having life-sustaining treatment removed cannot process those involved in requesting assistance in dying through ingesting a drug?

Some see an important difference between the right to refuse treatment and the right to assistance in dying. The right to refuse treatment is a right against bodily intrusion and is grounded in terms of bodily integrity. Franklin Miller writes, "It is deeply offensive to autonomy and dignity to fail to respect a competent patient's refusal of treatment following due consideration of the consequences and alternative options, forcing them to remain tethered to life support and without control over their body."[43] Physicians have an obligation not to impose treatment on a patient without the patient's informed consent. Indeed, without consent (except in emergency situations), an unwanted bodily intervention is technically a battery. Miller notes that there is no comparable right to receive lethal treatment by virtue of a request for assisted dying. Therefore, even if psychiatric patients have a right to refuse life-sustaining treatment, it does not follow that they have a right to assisted death.

I agree that the right to refuse treatment, including life-sustaining treatment, does not entail a right to assisted dying. Concerns about unwarranted expansion – slippery-slope worries – are greater in the case of assisted dying than in the case of respecting treatment refusals. For this reason, a society may accept the right to refuse treatment without being committed to taking the further step of legalizing assisted dying. Such a step would depend on an assessment of the risks and benefits of legalizing PAD and not simply follow from acceptance of the right to refuse treatment.

However, if a jurisdiction has legalized PAD, the distinction between the right to refuse life-sustaining treatment and the right to an assisted death is no longer pertinent, since patients are entitled to both if they meet the eligibility criteria. Moreover, it is unclear why this distinction should be relevant to the evaluation of competence in patients with major depressive disorder. Given that the stakes are the same in both cases (namely, the death of the patient), it seems that the criteria for determining competence should also be the same.

One more issue concerning the difference between the right to refuse life-sustaining treatment and the right to an assisted death needs addressing. The right to refuse treatment, including life-saving treatment, is not based on unbearable suffering, but on the right to bodily autonomy, in particular, the right not to have treatment imposed without giving informed consent. By contrast, suffering is part of the justification for PAD. It is either explicit or implicit in the law of the jurisdictions that allow PAD, except for Switzerland, which requires only the competence to decide. This gives rise to the following paradox.[44] The more severe the depression, the greater the suffering imposed and the more justifiable the offering of PAD. At the same time, the more severe the depressive disorder, the greater the likelihood that decision-making capacity is impaired and the less justifiable it is to provide PAD. Their intense suffering is crucial to the justification for giving them PAD, but that very suffering is likely to distort their thinking and cast doubt that their decision is voluntary and rational. Matthew Broome and Angharad de Cates note that "it is very unlikely that there is such a patient with TRD [treatment-resistant depression] who is both competent to make decisions about ending their own life, and that the same individual has no prospect for relief of their suffering."[45]

It should be noted that Broome and de Cates are not making the strong claim that it is impossible that there could be a patient who is both competent to make life-ending decisions and completely treatment resistant. Rather, they say that it is "very unlikely," and that seems consistent with the data provided by Sullivan and Youngner. Does it matter that there are likely to be very few, if any, severely depressed competent patients? If we view access to PAD as a matter of justice and the denial of PAD to competent patients with treatment-resistant major depressive disorder as discrimination, as Schüklenk and van de Vathorst do, then the fact that there will be few such patients is not relevant. Even if only one competent individual is denied the right to choose PAD, that is an injustice. However, from a policy perspective, the numbers do matter, a point to which I will return in the section on policy considerations.

Role Responsibility

One reason that has been given for why PAD should not be available to psychiatric patients is that this conflicts with the role of psychiatrists. "The concept of assisting – rather than preventing – suicide counters the core aims of psychiatric practice," Kelly and McLoughlin assert. "The shift of therapeutic role from alleviating psychic despair to facilitating suicide would be anathema to many psychiatrists."[46] This claim is supported by a recent official position from the Board of Trustees of the American Psychiatric Association: "The American Psychiatric Association, in concert with the American Medical Association's position on Medical Euthanasia, holds that a psychiatrist should not prescribe or administer any intervention to a non-terminally ill person for the purpose of causing death."[47]

Let us assume that many, or even most, psychiatrists oppose PAD for their non-terminally ill patients. What should we make of this? Does this opposition imply that providing PAD would be incompatible with the psychiatrists' role responsibility? The problem is that the same argument, based on role responsibility, has been made by opponents of *all* PAD. Physicians, it has been said, are healers, not killers. The challenge for those who accept PAD for

terminally ill patients but oppose it for those with severe, treatment-resistant depression on grounds of professional responsibility is to explain why the role-responsibility argument cannot also be made against all PAD.

Franklin Miller takes up this challenge.[48] His objection to PAD for treatment-resistant major depressive disorder does not stem from doubts about patient competence. He acknowledges that suicide may be rational from the perspective of some patients suffering from unremitting depression. His objection is rather that offering PAD to patients with treatment-resistant depression is incompatible with the goals of medicine. Those goals include promoting the health of patients. This is no longer possible for terminally ill and some incurably ill patients, at which point the goal of medicine shifts from restoring health to keeping patients comfortable until they die, that is, palliative care. PAD is consistent with professional integrity as a last resort when palliative care can no longer relieve their suffering.

The distinction between curative therapy and palliative care, important in the care of patients with physical illnesses, is not relevant in the case of major depressive disorder. There is no palliative care for this disorder; either the treatment works to relieve the symptoms of depression or it does not. If the patient does not respond to any of the available treatments for depression, there is no way to keep the patient comfortable. Therefore, one might reasonably ask, if there is nothing more a psychiatrist can do for the patient, and the patient is competent, and his desire to die is rational, why is it inconsistent with the professional integrity of the psychiatrist to help the patient to die? Miller's answer is to revert to the difficulty of identifying cases of genuinely treatment-resistant depression: "Despite the fact that a patient with depression has been resistant to a succession of standard treatments, it is doubtful that a clinician can know that the patient has no possibility of significant therapeutic help."[49]

However, this response has nothing to do with the goals of medicine, which underlie Miller's account of professional responsibility. Rather, Miller is expressing another sort of concern, namely, the ability of clinicians to know when a patient's depression really is resistant to treatment. That ability depends on the profession's ability to develop reliable guidelines for this type of depression. This is not a matter of role responsibility, since *if* reliable guidelines could be developed, presumably providing PAD to psychiatric patients would be compatible with professional responsibility. Nevertheless, it is an important policy concern to which I will return.

Slippery-Slope Concerns

Some commentators do not oppose, in principle, allowing competent patients with severe, treatment-resistant depression to choose PAD. Rather, they are afraid that if the eligibility criteria are expanded to allow this, then it will prove very difficult, if not impossible, to prevent providing PAD in cases that lie outside this rubric. They worry that expanding the criteria will lead to PAD for severely depressed patients who are not actually treatment-resistant but who would rather die than undergo treatment. They worry that PAD could be used on individuals who do not have mental illness of any sort but want to die because they suffer from what has been called "existential suffering," that is, they are tired of life.

Commentaries on Schüklenk and van de Vathorst's defense of assisted dying for treatment-resistant depression examine three cases in the Netherlands that raise concerns about a slippery slope. In one of these cases, no psychiatrist had been consulted to consider the competence of the patient and to review whether the patient's condition was really treatment resistant.[50] In another, the so-called Chabot case (named after the physician involved), a patient, Mrs. Boomsma, refused treatment for depression after the deaths of her sons. In the third, the patient, Mr. Brongersma, an eighty-six-year- old man, did not suffer from any diagnosed mental illness but wanted to die because he was tired

of life.[51] Do these cases indicate that expansion of eligibility criteria in the Netherlands has led to a slippery slope?

Schüklenk and van de Vathorst respond to the case where no psychiatrist was consulted by saying that they were careful to consider only treatment-resistant competent patients. They respond to the Brongersma case as being outside the scope of their paper, as they were advocating PAD only for individuals suffering from a diagnosed mental illness. They give the same response to the Chabot case, calling it outside the scope of their paper "because the patient had no wish to be cured from her depression because she felt depression to be an appropriate state to be in after the premature deaths of her two sons."[52] However, it is an insufficient response to a slippery-slope argument to say that an example falls outside the scope of cases with which one is concerned. Precisely the point of a slippery-slope argument is that, although the proposed policy begins with acceptable cases, it inevitably will lead to unacceptable cases, outside the scope originally envisaged.

How one should respond to a slippery-slope argument depends on the kind of slippery-slope argument that is made. These arguments are often divided into two types: empirical and logical. The empirical kind makes a factual prediction that a seemingly acceptable law or policy is likely to have unacceptable results. In the case of PAD, the concern is that it would not be limited to the most clearly justifiable cases – terminally ill patients who genuinely wish to die – but would inevitably expand to cases that are less clearly justifiable or not justifiable at all. Initial restrictions, such as terminal illness, unbearable suffering, and voluntariness, may well be jettisoned as social attitudes change. As one commentator expresses it, "Euthanasia and PAS, which originally would be regulated as a last-resort option in only very select situations, could, over time, become less of a last resort and be sought more quickly, even becoming a first choice in some cases."[53]

What makes many empirical slippery-slope arguments unacceptable is that they are often based on pure speculation. They claim to be making a prediction about what is likely to occur, but no empirical evidence is offered to support the claim that the dire predicted effects will actually occur. To the extent that an empirical slippery-slope argument is purely speculative, it has little or no weight and may even be regarded as a fallacy. In 2012, a group in the Netherlands that advocates for euthanasia opened the End of Life clinic, to consider requests from people who meet all the Dutch legal requirements for PAD but whose requests were turned down by their regular physicians. Many commentators believe that

this clinic indicates a troubling expansion of PAD. Barron Lerner and Arthur Caplan are particularly troubled by the provision of PAD to those who are "tired of living" and the fact that loneliness was often cited as the reason for wanting PAD: "Loneliness, even if accompanied by other symptoms, hardly seems a condition best addressed by offering death."[54] They allow that the efforts of physicians at the End of Life clinic may be ethically defensible if they are relieving unremitting suffering that cannot be relieved in any other way, but they wonder if the increase in rates of euthanasia represents "a type of reflexive, carte blanche acquiescence among physicians to the concept of patient self-determination. Or worse, is it simply easier for physicians to accede to these sad and ailing patients' wishes than to reembark on new efforts to relieve or cope with their suffering?"[55]

Part of their concern is that the numbers of people receiving PAD in the Netherlands are increasing. The number of patients who received euthanasia or assisted suicide for psychiatric reasons in the Netherlands went from twelve in 2012 to fifty-six in 2015.[56] Between 1,100 and 1,150 psychiatric patients are estimated to have requested euthanasia between 2015 and 2016; between sixty and seventy are estimated to have received it. The rest were turned down because the due care criteria were not met.[57] The numbers are indeed creeping up. Is this increase troubling evidence of a slippery slope or simply a reasonable response to the demand? How many cases of assisted death for psychiatric cases would be too many? I do not think there is any way to answer these questions. Moreover, surely what matters ultimately is not the number of cases but, rather, whether the granting of PAD was justified, that is, whether the request was truly voluntary and reasonable in the circumstances. The fact that roughly only six percent were granted the request suggests that it is not becoming routine to euthanize psychiatric patients in the Netherlands.

The need for empirical evidence is not present with logical slippery-slope arguments. Here the claim is not that allowing something that seems desirable, or at least benign, will lead to bad outcomes but, rather, that the acceptance of the original policy logically commits its supporters to other policies that they do not wish to support. A logical slippery-slope argument is thus a consistency argument.

An example of the logical version of a slippery-slope argument was evident in the debate about sodomy statutes in the United States nearly two decades ago. Those who supported such statutes argued that if the state were not allowed to criminalize homosexual behavior, then there could be no plausible grounds for mandating that marriage can only be between those of opposite sex.[58] Supporters of gay rights agreed, launching a movement to legalize same-sex marriage. Obviously, they did not regard the possibility of legalizing same-sex marriage as the bottom of a slippery slope but, rather, as a logical and proper extension of the right to marry the person you love, without regard to race, ethnicity, or gender.

In the case of PAD, the logical version can be used against safeguards typically built into death-with-dignity laws, such as terminal illness. If this right is based on the right to self-determination, then what justifies limiting it to those who have a terminal illness, or any illness at all? An American judge made the point this way: "The depressed twenty-one- year-old, the romantically-devastated twenty-eight-year-old, the alcoholic forty-year-old who choose suicide are also expressing their views of existence, meaning, the universe, and life; they are also asserting their personal liberty. If at the heart of the liberty protected by the Fourteenth Amendment is this uncurtailable ability to believe and to act on one's deepest beliefs about life, the right to suicide and the right to assistance in suicide are the prerogative of at least every sane adult.

The attempt to restrict such rights to the terminally ill is illusory."[59]

One way to respond to a logical slippery-slope argument is to accept the alleged logical commitment but to deny that it describes a bad outcome. This is what happened when Dutch law, originally interpreted as allowing PAD only for unbearable suffering caused by physical illness, was expanded to allow PAD for unbearable suffering caused by mental illness. PAD was further expanded in 2005, when the Royal Dutch Medical Association issued a report that supported euthanasia in some cases of existential suffering, although the report recommended that therapeutic and social solutions should be tried first.[60] It is not clear why Schüklenk and van de Vathorst reject the Dutch approach to the Brongersma case.

Perhaps in saying that the Brongersma case lies outside the scope of their paper, Schüklenk and van de Vathorst mean only that they have not thought about whether PAD should be given to those with existential suffering. If they had, then they might have agreed that including existential suffering is a logical extension of euthanasia policy. However, if their claim is that PAD should not be given to those suffering from existential suffering but only to those with diagnosed mental illness, specifically, severe treatment-resistant depression, then they owe us an explanation of why their arguments do not apply to existential suffering. Without such an explanation, they remain vulnerable to the logical form of a slippery-slope argument.

Public Policy Considerations

As I have argued, some of the arguments for an absolute exclusion of patients with severe, treatment-resistant depression from receiving PAD are weak. The rationale for a terminal-illness requirement, which would exclude those suffering only from mental illness, appears arbitrary and inconsistent with the two arguments underlying PAD, namely, autonomy and suffering. Indeed, the terminal-illness requirement forces those who have an incurable illness but who are not terminally ill to suffer much longer than those who are terminally ill. In addition, the suffering that patients with major depressive disorder endure is at least as severe as that experienced by patients with physical illness.

A stronger objection to PAD for severe, treatment-resistant depression stems from concerns about competence. However, if depressed patients who refuse life-sustaining treatment because they decide that death would be preferable can be determined to be competent, then why cannot depressed patients for whom there is no life-sustaining treatment to refuse also be determined to be competent to choose assisted death, using the same criteria?

Some psychiatrists argue that doctors cannot know that any patient is genuinely treatment resistant. Perhaps a different drug regimen or nonpharmaceutical approach might yield positive results. While this is always possible, it may not be realistic. An experimental approach that seems to yield results may not be available to the patient, depending on factors like geographical locale. Psychiatrists surely are sometimes warranted in the judgment that a particular patient with major depressive disorder is both competent and treatment resistant.

Consider Emily, the Belgian patient whose case was discussed above. Emily had undergone treatment for more than twelve years, but nothing helped. Several psychiatrists agreed, after two years of consultation and deliberation, that there was nothing more they could do for her. Their assessment of her as competent to make this decision seems well founded. Her request for euthanasia was not impulsive, as are most pathological suicides, but well considered. Nor did it stem from the belief that she was not worthy of living. She stated that she wished she could be cured but found living with severe depression that would never be alleviated unbearable.

I think we should concede that there probably are patients with major depressive disorder who are both competent and genuinely treatment resistant. They have as good a claim to PAD as patients with terminal illness. However, it is, in my view, a leap from acknowledging this to making the kind of claim that Schüklenk and van de Vathorst make: "Jurisdictions that are considering, or that have, decriminalised assisted dying are *discriminating unfairly* (emphasis added) against patients suffering from treatment-resistant depression if they exclude such patients from the class of citizens entitled to receive assistance in dying."[61]

The charge of unfair discrimination holds only if there is no good reason to exclude such patients. We have seen, however, that there are serious concerns about unjustified expansion. There is a significant gap between acknowledging that there are individual cases in which PAD would be ethically justified and creating a law or policy that reliably identifies such cases. Statutes and procedures are inherently general. They do not pick out specific instances in which something is justifiable or reasonable and allow these to be permitted. Rather, they must be drafted to cover many cases. Therefore, the issue is not whether a physician would be ethically justified in helping a particular individual to die. The issue is rather whether it is possible to draft a statute or policy that will cover the justifiable cases without putting vulnerable patients at undue risk. As a matter of policy, we need to be concerned about not only the competent patients with treatment-resistant depression who would be denied access to PAD but also those who are not competent or not really treatment resistant who might be swept up by a law that failed to distinguish them. This point is made by den Hartogh: "In the case of depressed patients, we have some reasons for extra caution: doubts about their decision-making capacities and about the stableness of their decisions. It is true that these doubts do not apply to all cases, but it is hard to think of institutional arrangements that will guarantee us to a sufficient extent that the exceptional cases are properly identified."[62]

One response might be that both the Dutch and the Belgians have created such institutional arrangements. In both countries, physicians are required to follow the due-care criteria and to report cases in which they have provided assisted dying. Regional review committees examine these cases, after the fact, to ensure that the due-care criteria have been followed, and physicians who do not abide by these criteria are liable to sanctions.

Appeal to the Dutch and Belgian models raises two questions. First, does it provide adequate safeguards against misuse? Some are skeptical. Kim and colleagues note, "The retrospective oversight system in the Netherlands generally defers to the judgments of the physicians who perform and report EAS [euthanasia and assisted suicide]. Whether the system provides sufficient regulatory oversight remains an open question that will require further study."[63] Second, would such a system be adaptable to the United States or Canada? In the classic article "Euthanasia: The Way We Do It, The Way They Do It: End-of-Life Practices in the Developed World,"[64] Margaret Battin points out that cultural differences among countries are relevant to the assessment of end-of-life practices. Dutch physicians tend to have a closer relationship with their patients than American physicians. They have typically known them and their families for years. They are probably in a better position than American doctors to know when a patient's request stems from a well-considered and reasonable assessment of her prospects and when it reflects a passing mood. Therefore, even if the Dutch system works well in the Netherlands, it does not follow that it could be transplanted to a country like the United States, where this kind of physician–patient relationship is often lacking.

Another question is whether the benefits of expanding the eligibility criteria for PAD outweigh the risks. Here, the numbers do matter. If Broome and de Cates are correct in thinking that the number of patients whose depression is both untreatable and severe enough to justify PAD but who are also competent to make the decision is very small, then it may be reasonable to judge that the risks outweigh the benefits.

The views of patients with major depressive disorder are also relevant here. It is well known that psychiatric patients are undertreated and discriminated against in access to treatment.[65] Do they regard not having access to PAD as unfair discrimination and an injustice? Or do they instead regard being considered eligible for PAD as a potentially threatening move in which helping them to die might replace trying to improve their lives? Research into the attitudes of people living with the disorder apparently has not been done, either in the United States or in the Netherlands.[66] My guess is that there are people on both sides of the issue, much as there is disagreement within the disability community regarding aid-in-dying in general.[67] Without more research, we simply do not know what the demand for aid-in-dying from competent, treatment-resistant patients would be. That information is essential to a realistic balance of the risks and benefits.

A final policy concern is political. It has been difficult enough in the United States to get aid-in-dying legislation passed. Only ten jurisdictions have aid-in-dying, and it is restricted everywhere to terminally ill patients. Given current attitudes, writing legislation that permits severely depressed patients to have access to PAD would make legalization much harder. It makes sense to start with the most persuasive cases, moving slowly to expand eligibility criteria when and if this seems warranted. At this point, I submit, we simply do not know.

Notes

1 Canada's position is alleged to be "ambiguous in law and currently under debate." R. M. Jones and A. I. F. Simpson, "Medical Assistance in Dying: Challenges for Psychiatry." *Frontiers in Psychiatry* 9 (2018): 678. Published online 2018 Dec 10. https://www.frontiersin.org/articles/10.3389/fpsyt.2018.00678/full. Accessed February 26, 2010.

2 L. Deliens and G. van der Wal, "The Euthanasia Law in Belgium and The Netherlands," *Lancet* 362 (2003): 1239–40.

3 U. Schüklenk and S. van de Vathorst, "Treatment-Resistant Major Depressive Disorder and Assisted Dying," *Journal of Medical Ethics* 41 (2015): 577–83.

4 A. Sagan, "Equal in the Presence of Death?" *Journal of Medical Ethics* 41, no. 8 (2015): 584.

5 F. G. Miller, "Treatment-Resistant Depression and Physician-Assisted Death," *Journal of Medical Ethics* 41, no. 11 (2015): 885–6, at 885.

6 B. Maynard, "My right to death with dignity at 29," http://www.cnn.com/2014/10/07/opinion/maynard-assisted-suicide-cancer-dignity/index.html. Accessed February 25, 2020

7 T. E. Quill, C. K. Cassel, D. E. Meier, "Care of the Hopelessly Ill: Proposed Clinical Criteria for Physician-Assisted Suicide," *New England Journal of Medicine*, 327, no. 19 (1992): 1380–3, at 1381.

8 Schülenk and van de Vathorst, at 578.

9 K. R. Jamison, "To Know Suicide," *New York Times*, August 16, 2014. Schüklenk and van de Vathorst quote this passage from Jamison. However, she may not be as pessimistic as they seem to be about the possibility of treatment. The subtitle of her editorial is, "Depression can be treated, but it takes competence."

10 "24 and Ready to Die." *The Economist*, November 10, 2015, https://www.youtube.com/watch?v=SWWkUzkfJ4M. Accessed Feb. 26, 2020.

11 Oregon Death with Dignity Act: 2015 Data Summary, p. 3.

12 Email communications from Dr. Lieve Thienpont, Feb. 28 and Mar. 1, 2020.

13 Schüklenk and van de Vathorst, "Treatment-Resistant Major Depressive Disorder and Assisted Dying," 581.

14 Ibid., 578, citing D. Souery et al, "Treatment-Resistant Depression," *Journal of Clinical Psychiatry* 67, s6 (2006): 16–22.

15 Souery et al, "Treatment-Resistant Depression."

16 T. E. Schlaepfer et al., "The Hidden Third: Improving Outcome in Treatment-Resistant Depression," *Journal of Psychopharmacology* 26, no. 5 (2012): 587–602, at 589.

17 A. Khan and W. A. Brown, "Antidepressants versus Placebo in Major Depression: An Overview," *World Psychiatry* 14, no. 3 (2015): 294–300.

18 Schlaepfer et al., "The Hidden Third," 588–9.

19 Khan and Brown, "Antidepressants versus Placebo in Major Depression," 299.

20 Schlaepfer et al., "The Hidden Third," 596.

21 Ibid., 597.

22 Ibid., 587.

23 B. D. Kelly and D. M. McLoughlin, "Euthanasia, Assisted Suicide and Psychiatry: A Pandora's Box," *British Journal of Psychiatry* 181 (2002): 278–9.

24 ScienceDaily, "Reasons Why Survival Rates of Extremely Premature Infants Differ by Hospital," May 6, 2015, https://www.sciencedaily.com/releases/2015/05/150506182707.htm. Accessed Feb. 27, 2020.

25 Schüklenk and van de Vathorst, "Treatment-Resistant Major Depressive Disorder and Assisted Dying," 581.

26 U. Schüklenk, "Why Mentally Ill People Should Of Course Be Eligible for Assisted Dying," The Globe and Mail, Feb. 18, 2020. https://www.theglobeandmail.com/opinion/article-why-mentally-ill-people-should-of-course-be-eligible-for-assisted/. Accessed Feb. 27, 2020

27 For an important discussion of *when* "the end of the day" is reached, see D. Cowart and R. Burt, "Confronting Death: Who Chooses, Who Controls?" *Hastings Center Report*, 1998, 28, no. 1 (1998): 14–24.

28 Technically, competence and capacity are different. Competence is a legal term, decided by a court. If someone is found to be incompetent, the court will assign a guardian to make decisions on the person's behalf. Capacity refers to an assessment of the person's psychological abilities to understand and appreciate information and form rational decisions. Capacity is determined by a physician, often a psychiatrist, not the judiciary. See R. J. Leo, "Competence and the Capacity to Make Treatment Decisions: A Primer for Primary Care Physicians," *The Primary Care Companion Journal of Clinical Psychiatry* 1, no. 5 (1999): 131–41.

29 See, for example, J. Katz, "Informed Consent — Must It Remain a Fairy Tale?" *Journal of Contemporary Health Law and Policy* 10 (1994): 69–91.

30 For example, in Schloendorff v. Society of New York Hospital, 105 N.E. 92, 93 (N.Y. 1914).

31 J. Katz, "Informed Consent — Must It Remain a Fairy Tale?" 79–80.

32 See, for example, E. H. Loewy, "In Defense of Paternalism," *Theoretical Medicine and Bioethics* 26, no. 6 (2005): 445–68.

33 M. D. Sullivan and S. J. Youngner, "Depression, Competence, and the Right to Refuse Lifesaving Medical Treatment," *American Journal of Psychiatry* 151, no. 7 (1994): 971–8.

34 Ibid., 974.

35 A. E. Buchanan and D. W. Brock, *Deciding for Others: The Ethics of Surrogate Decision Making* (Cambridge: Cambridge University Press, 1989), 18-20. Incompetence may be global in the case of very young children or the severely cognitively impaired, but in most cases, it is relative to a given decision.

36 T. Appelbaum and P. S. Grisso, "Assessing Patients' Capacity to Consent to Treatment," *New England Journal of Medicine* 319, no. 25 (1988): 1635–8.

37 Buchanan and Brock, *Deciding for Others*, 1989), 26–9.

38 Sullivan and Youngner, "Depression, Competence, and the Right to Refuse Lifesaving Medical Treatment," 975.

39 Ibid., 976.

40 S. Y. H. Kim et al., "Euthanasia and Assisted Suicide of Patients with Psychiatric Disorders in the Netherlands 2011 to 2014," *JAMA Psychiatry* 73, no. 4 (2016): 362–8, at 365.

41 Sullivan and Youngner, "Depression, Competence, and the Right to Refuse Lifesaving Medical Treatment," 976.

42 C. H. Baron, "Competency and Common Law: Why and How Decision- Making Capacity Criteria Should Be Drawn from the Capacity-Determination Process," *Psychology, Public Policy, and Law* 6, no. 2 (2000): 373–81, at 375.

43 Miller, "Treatment-Resistant Depression and Physician-Assisted Death," 886.

44 M. R. Broome and A. de Cates, "Choosing Death in Depression: A Commentary on 'Treatment-Resistant Major Depressive Disorder and Assisted Dying,'" *Journal of Medical Ethics* 41, no. 8 (2015): 586–7.

45 Ibid., p. 587.

46 Kelly and McLoughlin, "Euthanasia, Assisted Suicide and Psychiatry: A Pandora's Box," 278.

47 American Psychiatric Association, "Position Statement on Medical Euthanasia," 2016, cited in C. Lane, "At Last, American Psychiatrists Speak Out on Euthanasia," *Washington Post*, December 15, 2016.

48 Miller, "Treatment-Resistant Depression and Physician-Assisted Death."

49 Ibid., 885.

50 G. den Hartogh, "Why Extra Caution Is Needed in the Case of Depressed Patients," *Journal of Medical Ethics* 41 (2015): 588–9.

51 C. Cowley, "Treatment-Resistant Major Depressive Disorder and Assisted Dying," *Journal of Medical Ethics* 41 (2015): 585–6.

52 U. Schüklenk and S. van de Vathorst, "Treatment-Resistant Major Depressive Disorder and Assisted Dying: Response to Comments," *Journal of Medical Ethics* 42, no. 8 (2015): 589–91.

53 J. Pereira, "Legalizing Euthanasia or Assisted Suicide: The Illusion of Safeguards and Controls," *Current Oncology* 18, no. 2 (2011): e38–e42, at e40.

54 B. H. Lerner and A. L. Caplan, "Euthanasia in Belgium and the Netherlands: On a Slippery Slope?" *JAMA Internal Medicine* 175, no. 10 (2015): 1640–1, at 1640.

55 Ibid., 1642.

56 S. Boztas, "Netherlands Sees Sharp Increase in People Choosing Euthanasia Due to 'Mental Health Problems,'" *The Telegraph*, May 11, 2016.

57 K. Evenblij, H. R. W. Pasman, R. Pronk, & B. D. Onwuteaka-Philipsen, "Euthanasia and physician-assisted suicide in patients suffering from psychiatric disorders: a cross-sectional study exploring the experiences of Dutch psychiatrists," BMC Psychiatry 19, no. 74 (2019). https://bmcpsychiatry.biomedcentral.com/articles/10.1186/s12888-019-2053-3. Accessed Feb. 28, 2020.

58 See, for example, Justice A. Scalia's dissent in Lawrence v. Texas (02-102) 539 U.S. 558 (2003), 41 S. W. 3d 349.

59 Compassion in Dying v State of Washington 49 F3d 586 (1995), at 590–1.

60 The report has not been translated into English. It is described in T. Sheldon, "Dutch Euthanasia Law Should Apply to Patients 'Suffering through Living', Report Says," BMJ 330 (2005): 61.

61 Schüklenk and van de Vathorst, "Treatment-Resistant Major Depressive Disorder and Assisted Dying: Response to Comments," 577.

62 den Hartogh, "Why Extra Caution Is Needed in the Case of Depressed Patients," 588.

63 Kim et al., "Euthanasia and Assisted Suicide of Patients with Psychiatric Disorders in the Netherlands 2011 to 2014," 368.

64 M. Battin, "Euthanasia: The Way We Do It, The Way They Do It: End-of-Life Practices in the Developed World," *Journal of Pain and Symptom Management* 65, no. 5 (1991): 298-306; updated for and reprinted in B. Steinbock, A. J. London, and J. D. Arras, eds., *Ethical Issues in Modern Medicine: Contemporary Readings in Bioethics*, 8th ed. (New York: McGraw-Hill, 2013): 467–483, at 478–9.

65 See "The Neglect of Mental Illness Exacts a Huge Toll, Human and Economic," March 1, 2012, https://www.scientificamerican.com/article/a-neglect-of-mental-illness/. Accessed Feb. 29, 2020.

66 The National Alliance for the Mentally Ill has not released an official stance on physician-assisted death for those living with mental illness (personal communication from E. Brooks, HelpLine associate, National Alliance on Mental Illness.) The topic is not mentioned in the Public Policy Platform of NAMI, 12th edition (2016): https://www.nami.org/getattachment/Learn-More/Mental-Health-Public-Policy/Public-Policy-Platform-December-2016-(1).pdf. Accessed Feb. 29, 2020. In the Netherlands, the general public seems to be satisfied with the current guidelines, and patient groups contributed to their formulation. There are no surveys specifically of patients living with mental illness (personal communication from A. J. Tholen, medical director, University Center for Psychiatry, Groningen, the Netherlands.)

67 Not-Dead-Yet opposes legalization of assisted suicide and euthanasia as "deadly forms of discrimination" (Not Dead Yet, "Not Dead Yet Disability Activists Oppose Assisted Suicide as a Deadly Form of Discrimination," http://notdeadyet.org/assisted-suicide-talking-points. Accessed Feb. 29, 2020). By contrast, Compassion & Choices, an organization that supports physician aid-in-dying, cites polls in Connecticut, Massachusetts, and New Jersey that show that a strong majority of voters living with disabilities support aid-in-dying, at about the level of all voters. (See Compassion & Choices, "Medical Aid in Dying and People Living with Disabilities," at https://compassionandchoices.org/resource/medical-aid-dying-people-disabilities/. Accessed Feb. 29, 2020.)

44

Are Concerns about Irremediableness, Vulnerability, or Competence Sufficient to Justify Excluding All Psychiatric Patients from Medical Aid in Dying?

William Rooney, Udo Schüklenk, and Suzanne van de Vathorst

Introduction

A recent Canadian Supreme Court decision (*Carter v Canada*) found the country's ban on medical aid in dying (MAID) to be unconstitutional because it unduly infringed on the rights to life and to self-deliberation of consenting, competent adults with grievous and irremediable medical conditions (*Carter v Canada*, 2015. The court did not stipulate that MAID must occur only at the end of life (*Carter v Canada*, 2015). This leaves questions about some psychiatric patients' access to MAID unanswered.

Canada's government responded to the court's decision with new legislation. The recently-passed bill C-14 includes a restrictive access criterion – requiring a foreseeable natural death (no precise length of time is given) (Act, 2016). This requirement is quite vague, but clearly intends to restrict access to MAID to only terminal conditions. Such a requirement is not present in the *Carter* decision (*Carter v Canada*, 2015). This clause excludes some physical conditions, and all psychiatric conditions.

We build on positive arguments that individuals with certain psychiatric conditions should be eligible for MAID (Berghmans et al.; Schüklenk and van de Vathorst, 2015a). This paper demonstrates why regimes which provide MAID for physical conditions while restricting access for psychiatric patients are employing an arbitrary distinction. We respond to concerns about whether psychiatric patients can be determined to fulfill key criteria present in a number of contemporary MAID regimes (including Canada's). These include arguments that psychiatric patients cannot be reliably determined to have irremediable conditions, that they are too vulnerable to make a choice like MAID, and that they cannot reliably be determined to be competent. We will set aside questions about whether psychological and physical pain are analogous, which we will take as a given. Adulthood will also be assumed.

Original publication details: William Rooney, Udo Schüklenk, and Suzanne van de Vathorst, "Are Concerns about Irremediableness, Vulnerability, or Competence Sufficient to Exclude All Psychiatric Patients from Medical Aid in Dying?" pp. 326–343 from *Health Care Analysis* 26 (2018). Reproduced with permission of Springer Nature.

This piece, following previous arguments for granting some psychiatric patients' access to MAID, identifies treatment resistant depression (TRD) as a strong test case for an arguably irremediable psychiatric condition. We then investigate the concept of vulnerability, and what it requires of policy. Vulnerability is a poorly defined term, but even if we accept the label, it does not provide sufficient justification for restricting *all* TRD patients' access to MAID.

We argue that the central aspect of psychiatric patients' vulnerability is that it is difficult to determine whether they are competent. Still, while some psychiatric patients are incompetent, this does not prevent us from accurately identifying many competent ones. In our final section, we address some recent allegations concerning the Dutch MAID regime, pointing out that many of these observations are misleading or poorly substantiated. We conclude by discussing whether these problems, even if they were of the magnitude opponents of MAID believe them to be, could justify restrictive regimes like Canada's.

Critics of a MAID regime which includes psychiatric patients argue that it is difficult to determine if psychiatric patients exhibit an irremediable condition or if these individuals are competent. They then argue this uncertainty (in conjunction with patients' vulnerability) justifies barring all psychiatric patients from accessing MAID (Kim and Lemmens, 2016; Lemmens, 2016; Sheehan et al., 2017). Both of these criteria are present in a number of contemporary MAID regimes. Concerns that psychiatric patients cannot be determined to meet these criteria are then used to support the exclusion of every patient in this group. Our paper seeks to defend the claim that some psychiatric patients can be accurately determined to be competent and to have irremediable conditions. Given strong positive arguments for MAID, a blanket ban on psychiatric patients' access to this service (whenever it is enforced where patients with terminal illnesses are eligible for the same procedure) amounts to unjustifiable discrimination. Protecting psychiatric patients only requires that we ensure MAID is responsibly regulated. We support additional measures aimed at ensuring psychiatric patients have irremediable

conditions and are competent. We conclude, however, that concerns about irremediableness, vulnerability, and incompetence fall well short of the justificatory power needed to support an outright ban of such patients' access to MAID.

Irremediableness

What are treatment outcomes like for patients with treatment resistant depression?

TRD has justifiably been proposed as a good starting point for identifying an irremediable psychiatric condition; this is not to say all instances of TRD are irremediable, but that *some* cases ought to be considered as such (Schüklenk and van de Vathorst, 2015a). It has also been rightly noted that patients with TRD do not face uniformly poor treatment outcomes (Blikshavn et al., 2017; Kim and Lemmens, 2016). While a complete literature review on this subject is beyond the scope of this paper, we will sketch a picture of why TRD is an appropriate starting point for our argument. It is unquestionable that the needs of some patients with TRD are impossible to meet within a timeframe one can reasonably expect them to endure.

Discussion of treatment outcomes for any condition should begin by assessing the primary treatment options, and their effectiveness. Schüklenk and van de Vathorst (2015a) point out that there is significant skepticism about the efficacy of frontline treatments for major depressive disorder (antidepressants and cognitive therapy) in the literature. One recent meta-analysis of literature on selective serotonin reuptake inhibitors, a class of commonly used anti-depressant medications, provides further reason to be skeptical (Jakobsen et al., 2017).

Few studies define TRD or its outcomes in the same way (Fekadu, Wooderson, et al., 2009a). We describe the findings from two studies with well-defined conceptions of TRD that investigated the long-term outcomes for patients suffering from the condition. These will provide the foundation for our claim that at least some cases of this condition deserve to be understood as irremediable.

One multicenter study of 124 patients defined TRD as a depressive episode which withstands 2–6 different courses of treatment (Dunner et al., 2006) A systematic review of TRD studies observes that this constitutes a "well characterized" definition of TRD (Fekadu, Wooderson, et al., 2009a). The study found 1-year remission rates of 3.6% and 2-year remission rates of 7.8% (Dunner et al., 2006).

A more recent study of 118 patients with TRD (defined somewhat differently from the previous study) found very different rates of remission.[1] It promisingly observed a 48.3% rate of recovery (remission lasting at least 6 months) and a high rate of remission of 60.2% over a period ranging from 8–84 months (with a mean of approximately 20 months) (Fekadu, Rane, et al., 2012).

Comparing two studies with small sample sizes is likely to be unfruitful; here this is especially so, as the latter study considers longer time periods, uses different criteria for positive outcomes, does differ somewhat in its definition of TRD, and takes place in a specialized, tertiary care facility. Even though the second study finds better outcomes than the first, the picture of TRD it provides is still bleak. Over the course of the follow-up period, 54.7% of patients who could relapse, did relapse. Additionally, 60.7% of patients' experience during the follow-up period was spent in a symptomatic state (Fekadu, Rane, et al., 2012). Additionally, 39.8% failed to achieve remission throughout the entire follow-up period (a mean of approximately 20 months) (Fekadu, Rane, et al., 2012). The prospects many patients with TRD face are poor.

Even among these cases (treated in a specialist inpatient center), almost 40% of patients did not achieve remission despite long-term, high-quality psychiatric treatment (Fekadu, Rane, et al., 2012). This addresses one claim made by opponents of MAID for psychiatric patients that is meant to soften the reality of banning the practice. It is argued that a better resourced mental health service would make a significant difference to TRD patients' quality of life by allowing us to meet unmet needs (VPS, 2016). This is unlikely to be true for many patients. A ban on access to MAID will force a significant number of patients to live with intolerable suffering when specialist care fails.

Discerning between irremediable and remediable cases

Often presented alongside concerns about TRD and irremediableness is the claim (explicit or implicit) that it is hard to determine who will or will not achieve remission (Kim and Lemmens, 2016; Shaffer et al., 2016). That is, while one can point to particularly problematic cases of TRD, it would be difficult in practice to differentiate those patients from those with better outcomes. Inaccurate predictions could lead to avoidable deaths.

Studies of TRD show fairly consistently that patient prospects diminish with the number of prior unsuccessful treatments (Rush et al., 2006). Indeed, this makes up a central component of evidence-based metrics for staging TRD, like the Maudsley Staging Method (MSM; Fekadu, Wooderson, et al. 2009b). Scores like these can be effective tools to help single out irremediable cases. Recent work from the Netherlands has further refined this staging method to better identify cases of TRD specifically, with the DM-TRD (Peeters et al., 2016).

We recognize that tests like these are limited in their ability to determine a condition to be irremediable (indeed, not all cases of TRD are irremediable). These tools are useful, however, as objective measures of the type of judgments that we contend can be made about psychiatric illness. Physicians' predictions of an individual patient's treatment prospects can be well-informed by evidence-based assessments like these. In a conservative oversight regime, guidelines or cut-offs could be set which are partially based on these scores. We argue in favor of a system which relies on physician judgment – and conceivably produces a small number of false positives – to one which refuses MAID to all psychiatric patients.

Irremediableness cannot be understood as certainty that no treatment will succeed

Assessing irremediableness is to perform a cost-benefit analysis of given treatments on a case-by-case basis, making medical decisions based on the statistically likely outcome. Indeed, concern for patient welfare is one value organizations like the Dutch Psychiatric Association have in mind when they define irremediableness as they do; namely, that "there must be reasonable balance between the expected treatment results and the burden of treatment" as well as a "real prospect of improvement" within a "reasonable period of time" (Tholen et al., 2009).

This understanding of irremediableness can produce false positives, but that does not imply it is reckless. The calculus we support is crucial for limiting patient suffering. The alternative is to allow MAID only where we know for certain that patients could never possibly recover. This is epistemically impossible, and will likely exclude patients who will never actually recover (though this could not have been known). Such a standard ignores the reality of patient experiences. Its disrespect for patient choice results in continuing, foreseeable misery for individual patients.

This same argument is applicable in cases where individuals refuse certain treatments. Determining whether a disorder is irremediable depends on which treatments are being refused, and should reflect a balanced judgement about the potential costs and benefits for the patient. In instances where treatment that is highly likely to be beneficial is being refused (for instance, in the case of a recent diagnosis, or other similar circumstances) physicians would be right to refuse a request for MAID (Shaffer et al., 2016). If a physician deems there to be a well-justified refusal of a particular, likely ineffective treatment by a competent individual, however, it is understandable why such a refusal should not constitute a barrier to MAID.

Defending irremediableness that admits of false positives

A stronger challenge to our position observes that it is likely that some patients would die whose lives could have been made worth living, and worth preserving, as a result of proper treatment or future advances in treatment options Kim and Lemmens, 2016). Other arguments against MAID for psychiatric patients gesture towards documented cases of miraculous recoveries after lasting depressive episodes (Blikshavn et al., 2017). We accept that MAID for psychiatric patients could lead to a small number of avoidable deaths. Our proposition is neither risk free nor cost neutral (none are). Yet, given poor treatment prospects and better safeguards, we also observe that there will be very few cases like these. To refrain from offering this service in order to protect these individuals would force many more competent psychiatric patients who otherwise would have applied for MAID to face unbearable psychological suffering for the rest of their lives.

It is here where the fact that these conditions are not terminal makes banning MAID especially costly. While others argue that the cost of dying prematurely is magnified when the condition is not terminal, they fail to note that the cost of living on is also magnified (Kim and Lemmens, 2016; Lemmens, 2016). Individuals with these conditions face agony for the duration of their life, and – without assistance – the harms of failed suicide attempts. In the study of 118 patients mentioned previously, 60% of the sample had attempted suicide at least once (Fekadu, Rane, et al., 2012). The exact harms of failed attempts vary with the method, but the lethality required by all methods implies that failures can always lead to severe, lasting injuries.

In the event of a successful attempt, the costs of sudden suicides on family and friends are significant. Some estimate that there are 6 other individuals who experience a host of psychological harms (including elevated risk of depression, substance abuse, and even suicide) for every successful attempt (Pompili et al., 2013). Thienpont and others, in a study of 100 Belgian MAID applicants with psychiatric conditions, observe that that family members and friends of those who pursued MAID found the process more humane and anticipated a less difficult period of mourning than if patients had taken their lives on their own (Thienpont et al., 2015).

The cost of protecting a minute proportion of cases determined to be irremediable who can, in fact, achieve lasting remission is an excessively high one, which seems *prima facie* difficult to defend. Sound public policy is based on highly statistically likely outcomes; in this case, to focus on the exceptions would harm the majority of individuals who would have pursued MAID, and would require us to callously ignore needs which we will likely never be able to meet. As we will see later, this unreasonable focus on exceptions is at the heart of one Canadian campaign for a restrictive MAID regime.

Does the availability of MAID for non-terminal patients negatively impact care?

Another concern with MAID for irremediable psychiatric conditions is that patients could have their care negatively affected by its provision. Blikshavn and others worry that MAID introduces hopelessness into the doctor-patient relationship. This includes loss of hope in the patient, as well as in their physician (this is often referred to as transference and counter-transference). They suggest a number of harms which follow from doctors admitting hopelessness about their patients' prospects, including reinforcement of the patient's negative affective states, and diminished efficacy of treatments like cognitive behavioral therapy (CBT; (Blikshavn et al., 2017).

This issue exists in the doctor-patient relationship already. Insofar as the mechanism these authors describe relies on hopelessness in psychiatrists, it is unclear why any present determination that their patient is unlikely to recover would not have a similar if not identical effect. It seems difficult to argue that long-term psychiatric patients whose treatments have failed are unable to grasp their physicians' attitudes about their situation merely because MAID is unavailable. As for treatment efficacy, MAID is being considered because treatments have been tried and have failed; if those treatments become less effective, the patient's welfare is not meaningfully diminished. Others have made similar observations about hope in cases like these (Berghmans et al. 2013).

A separate concern is that MAID could negatively impact the services received by individuals with these conditions who choose to live out their lives. This is one reason why many palliative care organizations oppose MAID (Vulnerable Persons Standard [VPS], 2016). If MAID regimes lowered the quality of these services, this would represent a significant negative externality of MAID. The empirical reality, however, is that the exact opposite trend holds. For instance, Quebec and the Netherlands both tie MAID to palliative care, and investment in palliative care in the Netherlands has significantly increased since their assisted dying legislation was passed in 2002 (Bernheim et al., 2014). We would welcome an analogous policy for psychiatric care in other MAID regimes.

Irremediableness does not pose insurmountable obstacles for a responsible MAID regime. In the next section, we will address other concerns about vulnerability.

Vulnerability

Vulnerability, even in documents like the 'Vulnerable Persons Standard' (VPS) – a set of Canadian policy suggestions supported by anti-choice-, disability rights activists and academics – is a poorly defined term (VPS, 2016). Proponents of the VPS claim that autonomous choice is more limited than standard bioethical analyses claim, and, for many, constitutes an unachievable ideal. They argue that protocols and procedures need to accommodate for those who cannot choose. One central contention, which we reject, is that psychiatric patients' vulnerability justifies barring their access to MAID. Even if one concedes that these claims about vulnerability provide a true reflection of some people's life realities, a ban on the entire patient group is an indefensible response.

Why are psychiatric patients especially vulnerable?

The VPS identifies the causes of vulnerability as extraneous factors that influence a person's decision making

(VPS, 2016). There are a number of such causes that could affect any potential recipient of MAID (such as violence, abuse, fraud, poverty and unemployment) (VPS, 2016). These do little to explain why psychiatric patients are especially vulnerable, relative to terminal patients. Such a disparity must exist if differential treatment is to be justified. The VPS attempts to solve this problem by including hopelessness and depression themselves as factors which make an individual vulnerable by virtue of "distorted insight and judgment" (VPS, 2016).

The primary difference between the vulnerability of patients with terminal illnesses (who are allowed to access MAID in more restrictive regimes) and the vulnerability of psychiatric patients, then, appears to derive from concerns about competence. Competence has been the focus of recent academic papers on vulnerability as it relates to psychiatric conditions. It is employed as the primary reason offered for why psychiatric patients are particularly vulnerable, relative to patients with terminal illnesses (Kim and Lemmens, 2016; Lemmens, 2016). Many other proffered determinants of vulnerability (such as abuse, fraud, and poverty) do not seem to be more applicable to psychiatric patients than patients with terminal physical illnesses. Competence, of course, also has value independent of vulnerability; one must be competent in order to give informed consent for any medical procedure, and as such, this criterion is featured in all MAID policy that we have come across.

Is vulnerability a useful concept?

If competence is the concept underlying the special vulnerability of psychiatric patients, it is worth asking what purpose this extra terminology serves. The policy advanced by the VPS is a product of the unacceptable stereotyping of a diverse patient group. This is surprising, given that the stereotyping of groups of individuals is a well-documented problem in academic work on vulnerability (Levine et al. 2004). Speaking of 'vulnerable groups' is to formulate blanket statements which likely and unacceptably overlook a fair number of exceptions; it is not inconceivable that

only a small minority of members of such a group would qualify for the label 'vulnerable.' For instance, recognizing that certain groups have fewer competent individuals than would a sample of the general population is legitimate, but making conclusions about the competence of everyone in that group based on that observation is not. Supporters of the VPS do exactly this, coaxing out false conclusions about the interests and capabilities of all psychiatric patients by making general observations about this patient group.

Significant injustices result from a failure to discern between different individuals in a 'vulnerable group.' Historically, broad measures meant to protect vulnerable groups have justified the exclusion of competent individuals from participating in activities (such as clinical trials) even when those individuals consider their participation to be of net personal benefit (Rhodes, 2005). Such practices would appear unacceptable and discriminatory were it not for the cover provided by terminology like 'vulnerability.' This has led some to question the value of "dogmas" like 'protecting the vulnerable' (Rhodes, 2005).

'Vulnerable' is a particularly burdensome label for a population whose treatment prospects have been shown to be negatively impacted by social stigma (Corrigan, 2004). Combating stigma involves empowering mentally ill individuals, as empowerment can be understood as the opposite end of a continuum from stigma (Corrigan, 2002). Effective programs to combat stigma aim to educate others by providing a more nuanced, realistic view of mental illness (Corrigan, 2002). Yet those who insist that psychiatric patients as a group are vulnerable achieve the opposite of this goal. Labeling all psychiatric patients as vulnerable instead of recognizing individual cases enshrines in law a view of all individuals comprising that group as troubled and as unfit to control their own lives.

Even if one insists on classifying all psychiatric patients as 'vulnerable,' it is still not clear that banning MAID for all these patients is justifiable on the basis of that vulnerability. As much as we ought to protect vulnerable individuals from coercive, extraneous forces, we should also respect the ability of competent psychiatric patients to make choices, especially choices as significant as pursuing MAID. The importance of vulnerability, for those who believe it to be a useful concept, appears to be that vulnerable persons are often unable to make the same autonomous decisions as others. Restricting every member of a vulnerable group's ability to make a given decision, instead of working to determine who can and cannot make said decision, fails to recognize why we care about vulnerability in the first place (that is, to preserve self-determination and individual choice).

Does vulnerability shift the burden of proof?

While protecting vulnerable individuals is arguably important, the consequences of such protections must be weighed against competing rights and freedoms. In the regimes we are concerned with, excluding all psychiatric patients also represents differential treatment, which requires justification. As such, the burden of proof lies squarely on those individuals who are intending to restrict patient freedoms. The policy proposed must be minimally restrictive in its goal of protecting vulnerable individuals; it is up to those proposing this policy to prove this is the case. Calls to ban MAID for psychiatric patients which insist we 'play it safe' or 'err on the side of caution' are not appeals to the default state of affairs; they are insisting we make an exception to it.

Indeed, to see how we weigh vulnerability, consider how we treat concerns about competence in the *status quo*. The presumption of competence, for instance, is a principle which insists we respect individuals' autonomy, and substantiate claims of incompetence with proof. In addition, *Carter v Canada* observes that risks concerning patient competence are "already part and parcel of our medical system;" that is, they are assumed (and mitigated) in order to provide acceptable levels of care *Carter v Canada*, 2015). Our view is not that MAID for psychiatric patients would be risk free, but that it can be provided with a tolerable level of risk for a significant benefit – namely, to alleviate the needless suffering of competent patients with grievous and irremediable psychiatric conditions.

This observation from *Carter* helps us recognize the implications of the alternative: weighing vulnerability too heavily. If one accepts that vulnerability can justify barring psychiatric patients from making serious self-regarding decisions, the implications would reach far beyond MAID. For example, the same concerns about vulnerability can be brought against competent psychiatric patients' other rights. Insofar as these individuals are vulnerable, one could argue that government must not allow them to refuse treatment until psychiatric assessment can ensure with greater certainty that this is what they want. In Canada, this would be in tension with legal precedent – clashing with previous rulings that found competent psychiatric patients have the right to refuse treatment (*Starson v Swaze*, 2003).

Blanket bans on MAID for vulnerable groups of people, unlike restrictions, need to be justified by evidence that the practice cannot accommodate these individuals with an acceptable level of risk. Our next step is [to] cast doubt on the claim that no responsible MAID regime can ensure psychiatric patients are competent.

Assessing Competence

Physicians call the clinical assessment of one's ability to consent to treatment 'decision making capacity' (simply, capacity). It is correlated with competence, though the concepts are distinct (Kim, 2009). For the purposes of this discussion, we will treat capacity as the most relevant proxy for competence in medical decision making. We will use 'competence' or 'competent' as short-hand for the ability to make a well-considered request for MAID.

Can physicians effectively perform capacity assessments?

Recent challenges have raised concerns about capacity assessment, and ask if consultant psychiatrists can accurately determine whether patients can make a well-considered request for MAID (Kim and

Lemmens, 2016). A recent survey of consultant psychiatrists (primarily in the United States) found that most believed capacity assessment to be challenging, and training to be sub-optimal (Seyfried et al., 2013).

Generally, however, the survey's findings are acceptable. Only 11.2% of physicians surveyed found capacity assessments to be "much more challenging" than other tests, with the remainder finding these consultations to be "somewhat more challenging" (52.2%), on par (22.3%), or easier than other determinations (14.4%) (Seyfried et al., 2013).[2] This is not to say that these determinations are trivial or easy, but that they are clearly an established feature of medical practice, and 'challenging' should not be read as 'impossible'.

While training is a concern, it is one which can be easily addressed. Looking to other jurisdictions, there will likely be a very small number of requests for physician assisted suicide motivated primarily by psychiatric conditions. For instance, in the Netherlands (a country of 17 million people), there were 42, 41, and 56 cases of MAID for psychiatric conditions in 2013, 2014 and 2015 respectively. There were also 97, 81, and 109 cases of MAID for dementia in the same years (Uitspraken & Uitleg).[3] These were only cases that were approved by physicians (and therefore overseen by the Dutch retroactive review boards), and physicians likely rejected more. Even assuming there are ten requests for every one approved case, however, these numbers are manageable. Relatively few psychiatrists will be needed to serve this patient group, which allows for selection of professionals on the basis of high levels of experience and training. Even if such professionals would be scarcer than we assume, the solution to this problem would be as straightforward as the provision of training by government.

Arbitrarily high capacity test score cutoffs as an alternative to a ban

One way of performing capacity assessment, which has attempted to standardize the practice, is evidence-based testing. Many such tests exist, which vary in form (Kim and Lemmens, 2016). Given that literature critical of MAID often operates under the assumption that such methods are the most precise way of performing capacity assessments (and then claims that these are far from satisfactory for all patients), we will accept this for the sake of argument (Kim and Lemmens, 2016).

The most significant objection we have come across argues that capacity assessment as a practice is imprecise. Competence and capacity are not the same thing, and evidence-based tests for capacity do not perfectly track patient competence. Kim explains the concern in *Evaluation of Capacity to Consent to Treatment and Research* with reference to the Mini-Mental State Examination (MMSE), one test of capacity. Categorical determination of competence from test scores is most effective at extremes, but less so when abilities score in the middle of the range (Kim, 2009). This 'grey zone' casts doubt on the precision of evidence-based testing more generally; indeed, one can apply similar reasoning to (stronger, more universally accepted) tests such as the MacCAT variants. Without accurate capacity assessments, physicians may assist the deaths of individuals who, were they competent, might not have elected to pursue MAID.

The question remains whether this uncertainty justifies a ban, or if it instead motivates well-designed MAID policy which takes these difficulties into account. Kim observes that there is good evidence to suggest that the majority of severely depressed individuals without comorbidities can consent to treatments like electroconvulsive therapy (Kim, 2009). This entails that rational decisions concerning significant procedures are within the capabilities of many severely depressed individuals and that the well-defined section of the range could be larger than one might expect, despite the previously mentioned concerns about capacity assessments. The empirical facts about tests for capacity require us to grapple with the Sorites Paradox; we must discern between different 'sections' of a continuum when there is no easy demarcation between them. While there are obviously incompetent individuals and others who occupy a range of scores such that they may or may not be competent, others are clearly competent. It is this latter group we wish to highlight with this paper.

Kim (2009) continues his discussion of evidence-based testing by noting a number of studies which seek to determine effective cut-off scores for competence. Setting thresholds or guidelines, however, is consistent with our claim that *some* psychiatric patients are competent for the purposes of accessing MAID. A cautious MAID regime could include such minimum capacity scores. We do not seek to advocate for one test over others, and for the purposes of this paper, it suffices that such tests exist and can inform thresholds. Additionally, while we recognize clinical judgment is stressed over thresholds or cut-offs in the MacCAT variants, (Kim, 2009) certain high scores could be applied as guidelines in a regime that makes use of this particular tool. While evidence-based testing has weaknesses, high sections of the range provide greater confidence, and could be used to responsibly guide physicians' judgments in a permissive MAID regime.

This raises the question of where these guidelines ought to be set. There are a number of methods one can use to set a lower bound for evidence-based capacity assessments (Kim, 2009). It is important to keep in mind that a responsible MAID regime that includes psychiatric patients does not need to determine the lowest possible cut-off. An arbitrarily high threshold would reduce false-positives by using a more effective portion of the range, while also allowing some competent individuals to access MAID. Such a threshold would exclude the marginally competent, but even a measure as crude as this would be preferable to barring all psychiatric patients from accessing MAID. This serves as just one example of the multitude of options one must reject in order to support a ban.

The claim that capacity assessment for psychiatric patients poses an insurmountable challenge should be met with considerable skepticism. A successful case to ban MAID on account of concerns about competence must address all that we suggested, as well as other possibilities, such as prior review, multiple independent psychiatric consultations, different access for different psychiatric conditions, waiting periods, as well as other possible restrictions and safeguards. After considering all of these options, and any combination thereof, supporters of a ban would have to conclude that none can provide an acceptable level of confidence in the assessment of patient competence. This does not appear to be a defensible conclusion based on the arguments provided thus far, or on the empirical evidence provided by our opponents.

A last bastion of doubt about the possibility of a responsible MAID regime is based on reports from contemporary MAID regimes which include psychiatric patients. In the next section, we will address recent evidence from the Netherlands.

The Netherlands

Many of the concerns raised about MAID in the Netherlands simply do not have to be defended by supporters of a permissive assisted dying regime in Canada or elsewhere. For instance, even if it were the case that a psychiatric consultation was not required in another country, this would have no bearing on whether that would be the policy in other jurisdictions. We would support requiring such consultations, as has been recommended before (Schüklenk and van de Vathors, 2015b). Reviews of assisted dying in the Netherlands primarily highlight procedural issues like this, while insisting without further argument that those problems have no policy solutions a different system could provide. This conclusion does not follow.

There are also substantial differences in context which meaningfully affect policy outcomes. The Dutch MAID policy was introduced to codify existing practices (Nys, 2002). Policy was introduced into a country with a pre-existing practice and culture of physician assisted dying (Schüklenk et al., 2011). It would be a mistake to explain the results produced by a Dutch assisted dying regime simply in terms of formal institutions. The Dutch medico-legal context, both previously and at present, is not comparable to the current situation in Canada, or that of many jurisdictions which ban psychiatric patients from accessing MAID. Moreover, if the objective is to avoid abuses, then it is best to set up strong institutions collaboratively with doctors in order to shape the practice, rather than risk practice emerging without oversight.

The remainder of this paper will therefore investigate some specific problems raised about MAID in the Netherlands; however, a successful defense of these practices is not required to make a persuasive case for MAID for psychiatric patients elsewhere.

Opposition to the Dutch system

One broad concern questions the safeguards present in the Netherlands. The Dutch system of independent consultants and retroactive review is designed to oversee cases of MAID to ensure that 'due care' is provided; due care includes confirming that the physician assessed competence and irremediableness, among other criteria. In a recent article, Kim and Lemmens (2016) observe that, given the difficulties involved in assessing irremediableness and competence for psychiatric patients, there are a surprisingly low number of problem cases detected by the review boards. Their central observation is that, of the 110 cases of MAID for psychiatric conditions between 2011 and 2014 in the Netherlands, only one failed to meet due care criteria (Kim, Vries, and Peteet, 2016).

The argument that follows from this has two horns. First, opponents of MAID for competent psychiatric patients point to the very few cases found to breach due care criteria by the review boards present in the Netherlands. They argue that these seem unusually low given what they imagine failure rates should be. It is then suggested that these institutions may be failing to hold doctors to account. The second horn argues that, if the failure rates *are* as low as reported, then the criteria being used must be too vague and therefore admit of problematic practices.

The crux of this argument is the presumption that physician error is more common than the review boards detect. The remainder of this paper will critically examine the few studies that support this pivotal claim. Underlying objectors' concerns is the basic intuition that every individual makes mistakes, even medical professionals. Yet the Dutch regime for MAID involves consultations and second-opinions. It requires multiple individuals to all make the same

mistake. A permissive regime could incorporate further checks, if desired.

Physician disagreement

One source of controversy is an analysis of 66 out of 67 publicly available Dutch review board cases of MAID granted for psychiatric conditions from 2011 to mid-2014 (Kim, Vries, and Peteet, 2016). This represents approximately 61% of the 110 cases of MAID for psychiatric reasons during this time period. This time period was selected because review boards publicly disclosed all cases of MAID for patients with psychiatric conditions beginning in 2013 on the request of the minister of health. This was later stopped. All reviewed cases from 2013 are included in this number, but 2011, 2012 and 2014 have omissions for other reasons (Kim, Vries, and Peteet, 2016). Kim observes that confidentiality is one of these reasons. It is worth noting that the review boards' publication committee has a number of other goals, however; for instance, with the exception of cases subject to the health minister's request, the publication committee makes publication decisions based on the likelihood a given case represents new precedent (Doernberg et al., 2016). We can infer from this that more complex cases (that is, cases where judgments of a certain kind are being made for the first time) are more likely to be published than uncontroversial ones. Published cases are skewed towards a representation of the frontiers of the practice.

Kim and others highlight that physicians disagreed in 16 (24%) of cases. Specifically, physicians disagreed about capacity status in 8, irremediableness in 13, and unbearable suffering in 1 (cases could have multiple disagreements) (Kim, Vries, and Peteet, 2016). Two important questions should be asked in response to this: first, how (un)common is disagreement in medical practice; and second, what does disagreement signify? Not all disagreement is a sign of unreliable assessment, it may well be a reflection of the distinct individual experiences of different physicians. For instance, acquiescing to the judgment of the assisting physician is justifiable in cases where this individual had the most contact with the patient. Indeed, Kim recommends (speaking about treatment, not MAID) that the physician who oversaw prior medical decisions *should* be the individual responsible for evaluating capacity precisely for this reason (Kim, 2009). The premium placed on patient interaction provides justification for a degree of deference. Disagreement is acceptable in instances where there is a reason to favor one opinion over another.

Even if one finds disagreement unpalatable despite this analysis, these cases may be overrepresented in the sample. In keeping with the educational goals of the publication process, disagreement may have been the reason many of these cases were published in the first place.

Kim's most pointed concern is that, in most cases where disagreement occurred, the physician in charge of assisting death continued with the procedure without all disagreements having been resolved. This is a separate problem, and is a practice that we do not need to defend. Another regulatory regime could, for example, require that disagreement be well-documented and assessments explained in light of this disagreement, as well as mandate an arbitration procedure for when disagreement arises.

Specific concerns about capacity assessment in the Netherlands

Another study by Doernberg, Petteet, and Kim investigates capacity assessment in MAID cases in the Netherlands. Reassessing the same 66 cases of psychiatric MAID mentioned earlier, Kim and colleagues coded each file, documenting when specific medical terms were used, in order to determine how doctors assessed competence (Doernberg et al., 2016). The authors flagged specific decision making abilities (such as the ability to appreciate the consequences of a choice, 'appreciation').

They claim to find that physicians often made broad statements about competence without investigating specific decision making abilities (Doernberg et al., 2016). Rather than closely looking at individual cognitive abilities of their patients, doctors in the Netherlands assess a patient holistically as competent.

One thing to keep in mind is that the method used by Kim's study is quite limited. The published cases are brief summary documents written in plain language, and might lack technical details for that reason (as the authors acknowledge) (Doernberg et al., 2016).

Doernberg and colleagues insist that the educational goals of the panel imply that the review boards would have a vested interest in publishing as much information about capacity assessment as possible, were it available (Doernberg et al., 2016). For this reason, they argue that these case reports do accurately depict Dutch physicians' capacity assessments. This claim is highly optimistic for two reasons. First, the review boards merely seek to confirm that the attending physician was *convinced* of the patient's competence. Second, it is worth noting just how brief these reports actually are. Elsewhere, Kim observes that the mean length from 2011 through to 2014 was 1573, 1248, 1154, and 1117 words for each year, respectively (Kim, Vries, and Peteet, 2016). A recent blank template (with no patient information included) we received from the review board numbered 614 words.[4] These are indeed summary documents meant to encourage discussion, not grounds for accurate generalizations about medical practice.

Even if one accepts this criticism of capacity assessment in the Netherlands, the problem would only be that tools go unused, not that such tools do not exist. One can provide guidance which requires physicians to comment on specific decision making abilities. A more restrictive regime could require the use of evidence-based tests of each individual decision making ability, such as the MacArthur Competence Assessment Tool (specifically a variant designed for MAID). At best, Kim provides reasons for why it might be desirable to use a MacCAT variant to assess psychiatric patients' decision making abilities in a permissive MAID regime.

Trust in physicians

Assessments of competence and irremediableness require one to trust the judgment of doctors. Many of the objections addressed in this paper seem to find this idea unpalatable. As one might expect, half of our response is that oversight can improve this relationship, but the other half accepts that a not insignificant degree of trust in the judgments and professionalism of physicians is necessary, as it is in *all* medical practice. Simply because a policy requires us to put confidence in the judgments of physicians does not imply it is reckless. So long as these judgments are guided appropriately, and are overseen by authoritative review boards, trust in physicians' judgments is an acceptable risk.

Finally, there is more evidence that has fallen by the wayside in discussions about MAID. A recent report from the End of Life Clinic, a pro-MAID group in the Netherlands that provides the service, represents a rough lower bound for the rejection rate for individuals with psychiatric conditions applying for MAID. In their most recent report, of 419 requests from patients with psychiatric conditions, 383 (91%) were either rejected or withdrawn, with only 36 patients receiving MAID (Levenseinde Kliniek, 2015). Given that fewer than one in ten requests are approved, it appears that physicians are acting with significant discretion.

Even if there were reason to be concerned about Dutch practice, nothing would stop legislators in another jurisdiction from regulating MAID to ensure that similar problems could not occur. None of the concerns raised by proponents of a restrictive regime justify the blanket ban they are promoting.

Conclusion

We argued that some patients with TRD satisfy two key eligibility criteria for MAID, and that their alleged vulnerability should not be considered. We recommend that government focus on designing a MAID policy that includes and protects all competent individuals with irremediable conditions, rather than one which unjustifiably restricts the access of a significant patient group. Insofar as TRD patients are entitled to act in accordance with their rights, those who wish to restrict access to MAID bear the burden of proving that the measures they suggest are truly necessary for and proportionate to their goal. This requires government to argue that no system could provide MAID to eligible patients at an acceptable level of risk. There is a middle ground between a ban and unmanaged access to MAID; those who advocate for a ban must at least consider the various regulatory schemes which constitute this middle ground.

The contention that no responsible regime for MAID ought to include psychiatric patients is implausible. Neither concerns about the assessment of irremediableness nor about incompetence are sufficiently well supported to justify restricting access to MAID such that only terminally ill patients may access it. Specific problems reported in the Netherlands (even if one were to agree with critics' assessments) have not been shown to be necessary features of a permissive MAID regime.

Notes

1 It defined the condition similarly insofar as it used scores associated with treatment failure, but these scores also consider severity and length of the depressive episode.
2 Numbers sum to 100.1% due to rounding.

3 These data are separate because dementia is considered a neurological condition in the Netherlands.
4 Contact williamrichardrooney@gmail.com for a copy.

References

An act to amend the criminal code and to make related amendments to other Acts (medical assistance in dying). Bill C-14, Royal Assent, Jun. 17, 2016. (42nd Parliament, 1st session). Accessible at: https://www.parl.ca/DocumentViewer/en/42-1/bill/C-14/royal-assent

Berghmans, R., Widdershoven, G., & Widdershoven-Heerding, I. (2013). Physician-assisted suicide in psychiatry and loss of hope. *International Journal of Law and Psychiatry, 36*, 436–43. doi:10.1016/j.ijlp.2013.06.020.

Bernheim, J. L., Chambaere, K., Theuns, P., & Deliens, L. (2014). State of palliative care development in European Countries with and without legally regulated physician-assisted dying. *Health Care, 2*, 10–14. doi:10.12966/hc.02.02.2014.

Blikshavn, T., Husum, T. L., & Magelssen, M. (2017). Four reasons why assisted dying should not be offered for depression. *Journal of Bioethical Inquiry, 14*, 151–57. doi:10.1007/s11673-016-9759-4.

Carter v Canada (Attorney General), 2015 SCC 5. Accessible at: http://scc-csc.lexum.com/scc-csc/scc-csc/en/item/14637/index.do. Accessed 2 Dec 2016.

Corrigan, P. (2004). How stigma interferes with mental health care. *The American Psychologist, 59*, 614–25. doi:10.1037/0003-066X.59.7.614.

Corrigan, P. W. (2002). Empowerment and serious mental illness: Treatment partnerships and community opportunities. *Psychiatric Quarterly, 73*, 217–28. doi:10.1023/A:1016040805432.

Doernberg, S. N., Peteet, J. R., & Kim, S. Y. H. (2016). Capacity evaluations of psychiatric patients requesting assisted death in the Netherlands. *Psychosomatics, 57*, 556–65. doi:10.1016/j.psym.2016.06.005.

Dunner, D. L., Rush, A. J., Russell, J. M., Burke, M., Woodard, S., Wingard, P., et al. (2006). Prospective, long-term, multicenter study of the naturalistic outcomes of patients with treatment-resistant depression. *The Journal of Clinical Psychiatry, 67*, 688–95.

Fekadu, A., Rane, L. J., Wooderson, S. C., Markopoulou, K., Poon, L., & Cleare, A. J. (2012). Prediction of longer-term outcome of treatment-resistant depression in tertiary care. *The British Journal of Psychiatry: The Journal of Mental Science, 201*, 369–75. doi:10.1192/bjp.bp.111.102665.

Fekadu, A., Wooderson, S. C., Markopoulo, K., Donaldson, C., Papadopoulos, A., & Cleare, A. J. (2009a). What happens to patients with treatment-resistant depression? A systematic review of medium to long term outcome studies. *Journal of Affective Disorders, 116*, 4–11. doi:10.1016/j.jad.2008.10.014.

Fekadu, A., Wooderson, S. C., Markopoulou, K., & Cleare, A. J. (2009b). The Maudsley Staging Method for treatment-resistant depression: Prediction of longer-term outcome and persistence of symptoms. *The Journal of Clinical Psychiatry, 70*, 952–57. doi:10.4088/JCP.08m04728.

Jakobsen, J. C., Katakam, K. K., Schou, A., Hellmuth, S. G., Stallknecht, S. E., Leth-Møller, K., et al. (2017). Selective serotonin reuptake inhibitors versus placebo in patients with major depressive disorder. A systematic review with meta-analysis and Trial Sequential Analysis. *BMC Psychiatry, 17*, 58. doi:10.1186/s12888-016-1173-2.

Kim, S. Y. H. (2009). *Evaluation of capacity to consent to treatment and research (best practices for forensic mental health assessments)*. Oxford, New York: Oxford University Press.

Kim, S. Y. H., & Lemmens, T. (2016). Should assisted dying for psychiatric disorders be legalized in Canada? *Canadian Medical Association Journal*. doi:10.1503/cmaj.160365.

Kim, S. Y. H., Vries, R. G. D., & Peteet, J. R. (2016). Euthanasia and assisted suicide of patients with psychiatric disorders in the Netherlands 2011 to 2014. *JAMA Psychiatry, 73*, 362–68. doi:10.1001/jamapsychiatry.2015.2887.

Lemmens, T. (2016). The conflict between open-ended access to physician-assisted dying and the protection of the vulnerable: Lessons from Belgium's euthanasia regime in the post-Carter era. *Les grands conflits en droit de la santé (pp. 261–317)*. Yvon Blais: Montréal.

Levenseinde Kliniek – Jaarverslag. (2015). Accessible at: https://issuu.com/levenseindekliniek/docs/lk_jaarverslag_2015_def-lr/19?e=12736569/37030889. Accessed 7 Nov 2016 (in Dutch).

Levine, C., Faden, R., Grady, C., Hammerschmidt, D., Eckenwiler, L., Sugarman, J., et al. (2004). The limitations of "vulnerability" as a protection for human research participants. *The American Journal of Bioethics: AJOB, 4*, 44–9. doi:10.1080/15265160490497083.

Nys, H. (2002). A comparative analysis of the law regarding euthanasia in Belgium and the Netherlands. *Ethical Perspectives, 9*, 73–85.

Peeters, F. P. M. L., Ruhe, H. G., Wichers, M., Abidi, L., Kaub, K., van der Lande, H. J., et al. (2016). The Dutch Measure for quantification of Treatment Resistance in Depression (DM-TRD): An extension of the Maudsley Staging Method. *Journal of Affective Disorders, 205*, 365–71. doi:10.1016/j.jad.2016.08.019.

Pompili, M., Shrivastava, A., Serafini, G., Innamorati, M., Milelli, M., Erbuto, D., et al. (2013). Bereavement after the suicide of a significant other. *Indian Journal of Psychiatry, 55*, 256–63. doi:10.4103/0019-5545.117145.

Rhodes, R. (2005). Rethinking research ethics. *The American Journal of Bioethics, 5*, 7–28. doi:10.1080/15265160590900678.

Rush, A. J., Trivedi, M. H., Wisniewski, S. R., Nierenberg, A. A., Stewart, J. W., Warden, D., et al. (2006). Acute and longer-term outcomes in depressed outpatients requiring one or several treatment steps: A STAR*D report. *The*

American Journal of Psychiatry, 163, 1905–17. doi:10.1176/ajp.2006.163.11.1905.

Schüklenk, U., & van de Vathorst, S. (2015a). Treatment-resistant major depressive disorder and assisted dying. *Journal of Medical Ethics, 41*, 577–83. doi:10.1136/medethics-2014-102458.

Schüklenk, U., & van de Vathorst, S. (2015b). Treatment-resistant major depressive disorder and assisted dying: Response to comments. *Journal of Medical Ethics, 41*, 589–591. doi:10.1136/medethics-2015-102966.

Schüklenk, U., Van Delden, J. J. M., Downie, J., Mclean, S. A. M., Upshur, R., & Weinstock, D. (2011). End-of-life decision-making in Canada: The report by the royal society of Canada expert panel on end-of-life decision-making. *Bioethics, 25*, 1–4. doi:10.1111/j.1467-8519.2011.01939.x.

Seyfried, L., Ryan, K. A., & Kim, S. Y. H. (2013). Assessment of decision-making capacity: Views and experiences of consultation psychiatrists. *Psychosomatics, 54*, 115–23. doi:10.1016/j.psym.2012.08.001.

Shaffer, C. S., Cook, A. N., & Connolly, D. A. (2016). A conceptual framework for thinking about physician-assisted death for persons with a mental disorder. *Psychology, Public Policy, and Law, 22*, 141–57. doi:10.1037/law0000082.

Starson. v Swaze, 2003 SCC 32 Accessible at: http://scc-csc.lexum.com/scc-csc/scc-csc/en/item/2064/index.do. Accessed 2 Dec 2016.

Sheehan, K., Gaind, K. S., & Downar, J. (2017). Medical assistance in dying: Special issues for patients with mental illness. *Current Opinion in Psychiatry, 30*, 26–30. doi:10.1097/YCO.0000000000000298.

Tholen, A. J., Berghmans, R. L. P, Huisman, J., et al. (2009). Richtlijn omgaan met het verzoek om hulp bij zelfdoding door patiënten met een psychiatrische stoornis. Accessible at: http://steungroeppsychiaters.nl/wp-content/uploads/Richtlijn-hulp-bij-zelfdoding_NVvP-2009.pdf. Accessed 2 Dec 2016 (in Dutch).

Thienpont, L., Verhofstadt, M., Loon, T. V., Distelmans, W., Audenaert, K., & Deyn, P. P. D. (2015). Euthanasia requests, procedures and outcomes for 100 Belgian patients suffering from psychiatric disorders: A retrospective, descriptive study. *British Medical Journal Open, 5*, e007454. doi:10.1136/bmjopen-2014-007454.

Uitspraken & Uitleg | Regionale Toetsingscommissies Euthanasie. Accessible at: https://www.euthanasiecommissie.nl/uitspraken-en-uitleg. Accessed Dec 2016 (in Dutch).

Vulnerable Persons Standard. (2016) Accessible at: http://www.vps-npv.ca/. Accessed 8 Sept 2016.

Part V

Resource Allocation

Introduction

Needs, wants and desires have no limits, but resources are finite. This is true also of healthcare resources. As a consequence not all healthcare needs and wants can be satisfied. Even if a society greatly increased its healthcare budget to meet more healthcare needs, it would still be the case that even more healthcare needs could be met, and more lives saved, if only even more money and resources were available. But money spent on healthcare cannot be spent on other things we value and want – better schools and roads, clean water, national parks, public housing, and so on.

Given the finiteness of healthcare resources, we thus need to find some ethically defensible way of allocating these resources.

It is sometimes suggested that these decisions be left to the market, or the ability of consumers to pay. But most developed countries have adopted public policies – guided by social welfare and justice considerations – that provide some basic level of healthcare to the poor and other vulnerable groups, who would otherwise die because they cannot afford to pay for private healthcare insurance or care. This means that a market-oriented way of allocating healthcare resources is at best inadequate and that the problem of finding another ethically defensible way of allocating scarce healthcare resources still awaits an answer.

Allocation questions arise at different levels of decision-making and, depending on which level they arise, are commonly referred to as "macro" or "micro allocation" decisions:

1. How much of the national budget should be devoted to healthcare as opposed to, say, schools, roads, public housing, defence, and so on?
2. How much of the healthcare budget should be spent on different areas within healthcare – say, on maternal healthcare vis-à-vis neonatal intensive care, dialysis, heart transplants, and so on?
3. If not enough resources are available to treat or save everyone within particular areas of medicine, who should have access to the last intensive care bed, or be the recipient of a donor heart?

Questions 1 and 2 are generally regarded as macro-allocation issues, and the kinds of questions raised by 3 are regarded as micro-allocation issues. Contributions to this Part of the *Anthology* focus mainly on questions 2 and 3, and do not address most of the issues raised by question 1.

Resource allocation poses some of the most challenging and perplexing ethical questions in the field of bioethics. In this brief introduction to the field, we can do no more than raise a small number of issues.

Bioethics: An Anthology, Fourth Edition. Edited by Udo Schüklenk and Peter Singer.
Editorial material and organization © 2022 John Wiley & Sons, Inc. Published 2022 by John Wiley & Sons, Inc.

Decisions that affect directly who will or will not have access to a particular scarce healthcare resource are always being made, but usually in a manner that is not noticed. In 2020, as the novel coronavirus that scientists named SARS-CoV-2 spread around the world, millions of people became infected and became ill with the disease COVID-19. For those most seriously affected, being placed in an intensive care bed and attached to a ventilator was the only hope of survival. In some countries, including the United States and Italy, however, there were not enough ventilators to provide one for every patient likely to benefit from one. The need to make life and death decisions thus suddenly began making headlines. Some people think it is inappropriate for humans to make these "God-like" decisions. Rather than develop and defend particular selection criteria, they say that we should rely on a random strategy, most commonly "first come, first served," even if this will save fewer lives than, for example, giving priority to those with the best chances of benefiting from the scarce resource.

It was against that background that the first item in this section, a debate between Peter Singer and Lucy Winkett on whether to give priority to younger people, was published. Singer argues that we should seek to maximize not the number of lives we save, but the number of life-years, and to do this we should, other things being equal, give preference to younger people. Winkett does not want us to make judgments that, in her view, depart from the idea that every human being is of equal worth.

In "The Value of Life," an article written many years before the coronavirus pandemic, John Harris offered a different argument against allowing age to play a role in the allocation of scarce healthcare resources, but one that would still have allowed favoring young patients over elderly ones. Harris holds that age is – in all situations bar one – morally irrelevant as long as we don't know when we will die, and have a fervent wish to live. The only time when age might become relevant, Harris argues, is when one person has had a reasonable life-span or a "fair innings" (traditionally thought to consist of three score and ten years, although as life expectancy increases in most countries, many would now extend that to at least 80 years), and the other person has not. In this case, Harris holds, even though both might fervently wish to live, only the younger person could claim that she has been deprived of a fair innings (which the other person has had), over and above the loss of life itself.

Economists typically hold that public resources should be spent so as to maximize the satisfaction of human needs, wants, or preferences. Healthcare economists have developed the idea of the QALY (Quality Adjusted Life Year) as a unit of measure of the benefits gained by various ways of using healthcare resources. The idea behind the QALY is that years of good quality are better than years of poor quality, and as long as the quality is positive, more years of life are better than fewer. On this basis we can compare the benefits gained by spending our dollars on different forms of treatment or prevention of ill-health. One common objection to the use of the QALY is that it seems to imply that, other things beings being equal, it is better to prolong the lives of those who are healthy rather than of those who are disabled. This seems to put people with disabilities under a kind of double jeopardy – first they are disabled, and then for that reason when they need scarce healthcare resources in order to survive, they are less likely to get them. Nick Beckstead and Toby Ord confront this objection in "Bubbles Under the Wallpaper: Healthcare Rationing and Discrimination." They argue that, unpalatable as this implication of the use of QALYs may seem, it may well be better than any alternative method of allocating healthcare resources.

Another area of medicine in which we need to make life and death decisions because of scarce resources is organ transplantation. It is now possible to successfully transplant several different organs, including kidneys, livers, hearts, lungs, and pancreases. Organ transplants can save or prolong lives. But organs for transplant are scarce (see also Part VI Obtaining Organs), and many potential recipients will die while on waiting lists for a suitable organ.

In "Rescuing Lives: Can't We Count?" Paul T. Menzel focuses on multiple organ transplants – where a patient needs more than one organ – and argues against the use of the "first come, first served" strategy in this context. Instead, Menzel urges us to "count before we cut", that is, distribute organs in a way that will save more lives rather than fewer.

Menzel directs his argument only against the transplant of multiple organs on a first-come-first-served basis and does not say what allocation principle or principles should be employed over and above the principle that we should save more lives rather than fewer lives. He does not say, for example, whether considerations such as the length and/or quality of a life saved should count, and whether factors such as the patient's age or her "social worth" are morally relevant.

Is responsibility for one's own ill-health a morally relevant consideration? Alvin H. Moss and Mark Siegler raise this question regarding alcoholism when they ask "Should Alcoholics Compete Equally for Liver Transplantation?" Alcohol-related end-stage liver disease is the principal cause of liver failure and avoiding alcohol abuse prevents it. Alcoholics who do not change their consumption habits are therefore responsible for their liver failure in a way in which non-alcoholics are not. Given this, non-alcoholic patients who develop liver failure due to no fault of their own should, the authors conclude, have priority over alcoholics.

Is this view defensible, or is it undermined by the recognition that social and genetic factors predispose some people to certain life-styles and diseases? Public policies do not generally attempt to distinguish between those who are and those who are not responsible for their diseases; by-pass surgery, for example, is generally provided not only to lean joggers, but also to overweight hamburger-consuming "couch potatoes" – and perhaps for good reasons. After all, who would ultimately determine whether a patient is or is not (fully) responsible for her condition? A distant bureaucrat, a busy doctor, or a committee? Even though it is not, in some sense of the term, "fair" that those who are responsible for their disease should have the same access to a scarce resource, one might take the view that it would be undesirable to write this principle into transplant protocols, public policies or laws.

45

In a Pandemic, Should We Save Younger Lives?

Peter Singer and Lucy Winkett

YES – Peter Singer

If we are faced with a tragic choice, as doctors already have been in some countries because they do not have enough ventilators for all the Covid-19 patients who will die without one, then – other things being equal – it is more important to save younger lives, because younger people are likely to live longer.

The "other things being equal" clause is essential. I am not suggesting we should put a 40-year-old with incurable cancer on the last ventilator rather than a healthy 70-year-old. The illness eliminates the usual expectation that the younger person will live longer.

For most people, life is positive. They don't want to die. To be diagnosed with a disease that will bring about death in a short time is one of the worst things that can happen to them. Putting aside those suffering from severe depression, or in chronic pain, or with other major health problems, people want to continue to live. They do things like eating healthy food, exercising, and having regular medical checkups to avoid dying. That is why we try to save lives.

We all know, however, that we are going to die. No one thinks that healthy food, exercise or medical check-ups will enable us to live forever. So when we try to stay healthy, what we are trying to do is to live as long as we can, compatibly with having a positive quality of life for the years that remain to us.

This common sense attitude is entirely reasonable. If life is a good, then, other things being equal, it is better to have more of it rather than less. And the same judgment is reasonable when it comes to saving the lives of others. It is a greater tragedy to die at 40 than to die at 80, and if we cannot prevent both deaths, we should choose the less tragic one.

NO – Lucy Winkett

Of course on the surface of it, it looks reasonable enough to prioritise saving younger lives, a bit like women and children first onto the lifeboat (although I suspect that was always more chivalry than biology). But no. Because hidden in this seemingly reasonable choice in extremis is a set of assumptions that become more worrisome the more they are explored.

Two initial questions occur: for whom is it more important to save a young life than another life? Of course it will be more important for the individual concerned, just as clearly as it will be bad for the lives not chosen. But how is it more intrinsically good? For society? For the survival of the species?

Original publication details: Peter Singer and Lucy Winkett, "The Duel: Is It More Important to Save Younger Lives?, *Prospect*, May 4, 2020. Reproduced courtesy of the authors and *Prospect* magazine.

Bioethics: An Anthology, Fourth Edition. Edited by Udo Schüklenk and Peter Singer.

Certainly not for the planet. And how is it beneficial to society as a whole that a definition of a disembodied "good" be the guiding principle for the inevitably messy and contingent decisions made in an emergency room?

The second question is that of value. By answering "yes," are we not simply replacing quality of life with length? The apocryphal stories of the saving of a young Adolf Hitler – sometimes by a soldier during the First World War, sometimes by a priest when he nearly drowned – may not be "true" in close detail but express something of the paradoxical nature of this question.

And perhaps this is my greatest objection to the answer "yes" to this question. It's very good to debate these things publicly and openly, but in the end, the whole project is flawed: the project of making comprehensive (closed) ethical statements about decisions that should be as much based on the clinical experience of human beings in the room as on any imposed rules about length of life. With guidance, of course, and some regulation to prevent abuse, in the end, experience, wisdom, humanity and trust in judgment are just as important. And this, even if – although I have no idea how this can be determined either – "other things" are judged to be "equal."

YES

You ask: "for whom is it more important to save a young life than another life?" Adding: "Of course it will be more important for the individual concerned, just as clearly as it will be bad for the lives not chosen." Yes, but that raises a further question: "Would it be equally bad for each of the two individuals not to be chosen?" Suppose that both are female UK citizens, one 30 and the other 90. The younger one can expect to live an additional 50 years, while the older one can only expect 4.6 years. If longer life is generally good – and if not, why save anyone? – then saving the older-person can be expected to bring about less than a tenth as much of this good as saving the younger one.

You then ask: "But how is it more intrinsically good?" There are many different theories about what is intrinsically good, and I can't go into that debate here, so I will have to be dogmatic and say that continuing to enjoy life with a positive level of wellbeing is intrinsically good, and – yes – the more years of such life are enjoyed, the greater the intrinsic good.

Should we set aside such ethical principles in favour of relying on "experience, wisdom, humanity and trust in judgment," as you suggest? For those who think that this is likely to work well, even when healthcare professionals are under pressure in an overburdened hospital, I recommend reading Sheri Fink's account of what happened in a New Orleans hospital after Hurricane Katrina, *Five Days at Memorial: Life and Death in a Storm-Ravaged Hospital*. Without clear ethical guidance, people's biases come to the fore, and they are likely to favour those with whom they identify over those who are less like them.

NO

The last point you make is an excellent one; but I take it also to be a powerful illustration of some of the challenge I am trying to make to any notion that an overarching ethical rule can satisfactorily be applied in matters of life and death. Because ethics themselves are necessarily contingent, and change over time depending on contemporary attitudes towards ontological difference, along with differences of geography, ability, nationality and so on.

If you and I were having this debate in a different generation, we might be arguing about the relative value of saving people with different skin tones, or genders. In toxic corners of the internet, this is still debated. But thankfully ethical rules have changed fundamentally overtime, otherwise I wouldn't have been taught to read or write in order to join the debate at all.

Age is another thing people cannot change about themselves, yet is still used to set ethical rules. If we're going down this route, I would be equally free to argue the opposite – to settle the saving of lives by rewarding their achievement, rather than their potential. Under this alternative way of ruling, an older person might be valued more highly because of the wisdom gained through their life experience – wisdom that is much needed to navigate a society through a crisis. The younger life might have potential, but as yet unproven and unfulfilled. Therefore the fewer years of proven sagacity from the old should be valued more highly than the longer life of (potential) foolishness from the young.

I don't believe this by the way, but outline it as a way of illustrating that hard and fast rules give the illusion of clarity for the rest of us, while my experience is that this cool clarity dissolves amid the dust and fury of actually saving lives. An alternative way of equipping medical professionals is, rather than giving them a blanket rule about age, instilling in them a regularly scrutinised confidence in their own judgment, with ongoing robust debate in ethics and unconscious bias throughout their careers, rooted in real life cases. Then leave them to it. Of course, prosecute them when they abuse their power but by and large back them as the ones in the (emergency) room.

YES

The ethical judgments we make should take account of all the consequences of our actions, and these consequences are contingent, but ethics itself is not contingent. If some cultures think that it is right to give priority to people of one race or gender, all that shows is that some cultures get it wrong. You implicitly acknowledge this when you refer to those corners of the internet in which racism is defended not simply as different, but as toxic.

I am arguing that when we cannot save everyone, we should choose to save those who are likely to live longer, and this usually implies saving those who are younger. You are, of course, free to argue for different ethical priorities. But this is not simply a matter of expressing different tastes, nor of voicing the views that are dominant in our cultural backgrounds. We are seeking to persuade others that we are right, and to do

that we must give reasons for our views. If saving the old really did lead to greater wisdom and better ways of navigating through a crisis, then that would be a strong reason against the position I am defending. But I see no evidence of this, and you acknowledge that you don't believe it either.

You appear to believe that medical professionals prefer to be left to their own judgment. My experience is different. For many years, I taught intensive bioethics courses for healthcare professionals, and many senior people, including intensive care unit directors, spoke of the difficulty of making life and death decisions on the run, without guidance from rules or principles, and sometimes in the face of passionate opposition from the families of the patients. It would be much better, they suggested, to be able to appeal to general principles that they could use to justify and explain their decisions. "Give priority to the young" is such a principle.

NO

The beginning and end of life raise particularly acute and sometimes excruciating ethical questions, perhaps because the consequences of decisions taken at those points are not, unlike some outcomes provoked by racist or homophobic views for example, reversible or redeemable. I believe that all human life is of equal value, regardless of length, and am with the 18th-century poet Thomas Mordaunt whose pithy conclusion is sometimes found on the gravestones of those who die young: "one crowded hour of glorious life/ Is worth an age without a name."

Perhaps in the end it is that judgment of worth that might helpfully provide a place to rest, for my side of the argument at least. Of course I am persuaded by the argument that maximising the time a person has to live also maximises their capacity to live well and therefore seems a good choice. But it obviously maximises their capacity to do harm too. That's why, in my view, time by itself can't carry ethical worth. If ethics is about good and bad, value and waste, about our right and wrong action, our well- or ill-judged treatment of others, then having more time to do any of it must always be a double-edged sword.

I take the point about confusion in ICU and having some parameters to work with, which I have accepted from the beginning. But doctors' preference for rules also might betray a concern that in an increasingly litigious society, blame falls heavily and expensively on the individual without a clear demonstration that the rules have been followed, to the letter of the law.

In a more mature, emotionally literate and (I would say it, wouldn't I) spiritually attentive society, the ethics of birth and death would be narrated entirely differently – relying on excellent science, but also displaying a good deal more humility about the mystery of both. Death is very often a painful tragedy, most especially for the ones left behind. But it isn't always a failure. For the flourishing of human society, it's just as important for its members to learn how to die as to, say, organise a fair and functioning tax system. Saving the old is a sign that our values are rooted in the fundamental equality of all, and that's the only society I really want to live in.

46

The Value of Life

John Harris

Suppose that only one place is available on a renal dialysis programme or that only one bed is vacant in a vital transplantation unit or that resuscitation could be given in the time and with the resources available to only one patient. Suppose further that of the two patients requiring any of these resources, one is a 70-year-old widower, friendless and living alone, and the other a 40-year-old mother of three young children with a husband and a career.

Or suppose that following a major disaster medical resources were available to save the lives of only half those for whom medical care was vital for life. Or, less dramatically, suppose that in the next two years, only half of 200 patients waiting for surgery that will alleviate severe discomfort can be accommodated in the only available hospital. Suppose further and finally that all candidates stand an equal chance of maximum benefit from any of the available treatments. Whom should we treat and what justifies our decision?

Many will think that in the first case preference should be given to the young mother rather than the old friendless widower, that this is obviously the right choice. There might be a number of grounds

for such a decision. Two of these grounds have to do with age. One indicates a preference for the young on the grounds that they have a greater expectation of life if they are restored to health. The other favours the young simply because their life is likely to be fuller and hence more valuable than that of the older person. Another consideration to which many will want to give some weight is that of the number of people dependent on or even caring about a potential victim. It is sometimes also considered relevant to give weight to the patient's probable usefulness to the community or even their moral character before a final decision is made. And of course these considerations may be taken together in various combinations.

In the case of a major disaster related problems arise. If say a policy of triage[1] has identified the only group of victims to be treated, those for whom medical intervention will make the difference between life and death, but there are still not enough resources to help all such persons, then, again, many will hold that the right thing to do is help the young or those with dependants and so on first.

Original publication details: John Harris, "The Value of Life," pp. 87–102 from *The Value of Life* (London: Routledge, 1985). © 1985 Routledge. Reproduced with permission of Taylor & Francis Books UK.

Bioethics: An Anthology, Fourth Edition. Edited by Udo Schüklenk and Peter Singer.
Editorial material and organization © 2022 John Wiley & Sons, Inc. Published 2022 by John Wiley & Sons, Inc.

Those who believe that they ought to select the patient or patients to be saved on any of the above criteria will believe that they must show preference for some types or conditions of person over others. Another available strategy is of course to decline to choose between people in any way that involves preferring one patient, or one sort of person, to another. Perhaps the easiest way of declining to show such a preference is to toss a coin or draw lots to decide who shall be helped. I want to consider what might count as a good reason for preferring to help some patients rather than others where all cannot be helped and also whether our intuitive preference for saving the younger and more useful members of society can be sustained.

I   The Moral Significance of Age

Many, perhaps most, people feel that, in cases like the one with which we began, there is some moral reason to save the 40-year-old mother rather than the 70-year-old widower. A smaller, but perhaps growing, group of people would see this as a sort of 'ageist' prejudice which, in a number of important areas of resource allocation and care, involves giving the old a much worse deal than the younger members of society. This is an exceptionally difficult issue to resolve. A number of the ways of thinking about the issue of the moral relevance of age yield opposed conclusions or seem to tug in opposite directions.

I want first to look at an argument which denies that we should prefer the young mother in our opening example. It is an anti-ageist argument so that is what I will call it, but it is not perhaps the usual sort of argument used to defend the rights of the old.

The anti-ageist argument

All of us who wish to go on living have something that each of us values equally although for each it is different in character, for some a much richer prize than for others, and we none of us know its true extent. This thing is of course 'the rest of our lives'.

So long as we do not know the date of our deaths then for each of us the 'rest of our lives' is of indefinite duration. Whether we are 17 or 70, in perfect health or suffering from a terminal disease, we each have the rest of our lives to lead. So long as we each fervently wish to live out the rest of our lives, however long that turns out to be, then if we do not deserve to die, we each suffer the same injustice if our wishes are deliberately frustrated and we are cut off prematurely. Indeed there may well be a double injustice in deciding that those whose life expectation is short should not benefit from rescue or resuscitation. Suppose I am told today that I have terminal cancer with only approximately six months or so to live, but I want to live until I die, or at least until I decide that life is no longer worth living. Suppose I am then involved in an accident and, because my condition is known to my potential rescuers and there are not enough resources to treat all who could immediately be saved, I am marked among those who will not be helped. I am then the victim of a double tragedy and a double injustice. I am stricken first by cancer and the knowledge that I have only a short time to live and I'm then stricken again when I'm told that because of my first tragedy a second and more immediate one is to be visited upon me. Because I have once been unlucky I'm now no longer worth saving.

The point is a simple but powerful one. However short or long my life will be, so long as I want to go on living it then I suffer a terrible injustice when that life is prematurely cut short. Imagine a group of people all of an age, say a class of students all in their mid-twenties. If fire trapped all in the lecture theatre and only twenty could be rescued in time, should the rescuers shout 'youngest first!'? Suppose they had time to debate the question or had been debating it 'academically' before the fire? It would surely seem invidious to deny some what all value so dearly merely because of an accident of birth? It might be argued that age here provides no criterion precisely because although the lifespans of such a group might be expected to vary widely, there would be no way of knowing who was most likely to live longest. But suppose a reliable astrologer could make very realistic estimates or, what amounts to the same thing, suppose the age range of the students to be much greater, say 17 to 55. Does not the invidiousness of selecting by birth-date remain? Should a 17-year-old be saved before a 29-year-old or she before the 45-year-old and should the 55-year-old clearly be the last to be saved or the first to be sacrificed?

Our normal intuitions would share this sense of the invidiousness of choosing between our imaginary students by reason of their respective ages, but would start to want to make age relevant at some extremes, say if there were a 2-day-old baby and a 90-year-old grandmother. We will be returning to discuss a possible basis for this intuition in a moment. However, it is important to be clear that the anti-ageist argument denies the relevance of age or life expectancy as a criterion absolutely. It argues that even if I know for certain that I have only a little space to live, that space, however short, may be very precious to me. Precious, precisely because it is all the time I have left, and just as precious to me on that account as all the time you have left is precious to you, however much those two time spans differ in length. So that where we both want, equally strongly, to go on living, then we each suffer the same injustice[2] when our lives are cut short or are cut further short.[3]

It might seem that someone who would insist on living out the last few months of his life when by 'going quietly' someone else might have the chance to live for a much longer time would be a very selfish person. But this would be true only if the anti-ageist argument is false. It will be true only if it is not plausible to claim that living out the rest of one's life could be equally valuable to the individual whose life it is irrespective of the amount of unelapsed time that is left. And this is of course precisely the usual situation when individuals do not normally have anything but the haziest of ideas as to how long it is that they might have left.

I think the anti-ageist argument has much plausibility. It locates the wrongness of ending an individual's life in the evil of thwarting that person's desire to go on living and argues that it is profoundly unjust to frustrate that desire merely because some

of those who have exactly the same desire, held no more strongly, also have a longer life expectancy than the others. However, there are a number of arguments that pull in the opposite direction and these we must now consider.

The fair innings argument

One problem with the anti-ageist argument is our feeling that there is something unfair about a person who has lived a long and happy life hanging on grimly at the end, while someone who has not been so fortunate suffers a related double misfortune, of losing out in a lottery in which his life happened to be in the balance with that of the grim octogenarian. It might be argued that we could accept the part of the anti-ageist argument which focuses on the equal value of unelapsed time, if this could be tempered in some way. How can it be just that someone who has already had more than her fair share of life and its delights should be preferred or even given an equal chance of continued survival with the young person who has not been so favoured? One strategy that seems to take account of our feeling that there is something wrong with taking steps to prolong the lives of the very old at the expense of those much younger is the fair innings argument.

The fair innings argument takes the view that there is some span of years that we consider a reasonable life, a fair innings. Let's say that a fair share of life is the traditional three score and ten, seventy years. Anyone who does not reach 70 suffers, on this view, the injustice of being cut off in their prime. They have missed out on a reasonable share of life; they have been short-changed. Those, however, who do make 70 suffer no such injustice, they have not lost out but rather must consider any additional years a sort of bonus beyond that which could reasonably be hoped for. The fair innings argument requires that everyone be given an equal chance to have a fair innings, to reach the appropriate threshold but, having reached it, they have received their entitlement. The rest of their life is the sort of bonus which may be cancelled when this is necessary to help others reach the threshold.

The attraction of the fair innings argument is that it preserves and incorporates many of the features that made the anti-ageist argument plausible, but allows us to preserve our feeling that the old who have had a good run for their money should not be endlessly propped up at the expense of those who have not had the same chance. We can preserve the conclusion of the anti-ageist argument, that so long as life is equally valued by the person whose life it is, it should be given an equal chance of preservation, and we can go on taking this view until the people in question have reached a fair innings.

There is, however, an important difficulty with the fair innings argument. It is that the very arguments which support the setting of the threshold at an age which might plausibly be considered to be a reasonable lifespan equally support the setting of the threshold at any age at all, so long as an argument from fairness can be used to support so doing. Suppose that there is only one place available on the dialysis programme and two patients are in competition for it. One is 30 and the other 40 years of age. The fair innings argument requires that neither be preferred on the grounds of age since both are below the threshold and are entitled to an equal chance of reaching it. If there is no other reason to choose between them we should do something like toss a coin. However, the 30-year-old can argue that the considerations which support the fair innings argument require that she be given the place. After all, what's fair about the fair innings argument is precisely that each individual should have an equal chance of enjoying the benefits of a reasonable lifespan. The younger patient can argue that, from where she's standing, the age of 40 looks much more reasonable a span than that of 30, and that she should be given the chance to benefit from those ten extra years.

This argument generalized becomes a reason for always preferring to save younger rather than older people, whatever the age difference, and makes the original anti-ageist argument begin to look again the more attractive line to take. For the younger person can always argue that the older has had a fairer innings, and should now give way. It is difficult to stop whatever span is taken to be a fair innings collapsing

towards zero under pressure from those younger candidates who see their innings as less fair than that of those with a larger share.

But perhaps this objection to the fair innings argument is mistaken? If seventy years is a fair innings it does not follow that the nearer a span of life approaches seventy years, the fairer an innings it is. This may be revealed by considering a different sort of threshold. Suppose that most people can run a mile in seven minutes, and that two people are given the opportunity to show that they can run a mile in that time. They both expect to be given seven minutes. However, if one is in fact given only three minutes and the other only four, it's not true that the latter is given a fairer running time: for people with average abilities four minutes is no more realistic a time in which to run a mile than is three. Four minutes is neither a fair threshold in itself, nor a fairer one than three minutes would be.

Nor does the argument that establishes seven minutes as an appropriate threshold lend itself to variation downwards. For that argument just is that seven is the number of minutes that an average adult takes to run a mile. Why then is it different for lifespans? If three score and ten is the number of years available to most people for getting what life has to offer, and is also the number of years people can reasonably expect to have, then it is a misfortune to be allowed anything less however much less one is allowed, if nothing less than the full span normally suffices for getting what can be got out of life. It's true that the 40-year-old gets more time than the 30-year-old, but the frame of reference is not time only, but time normally required for a full life.[4]

This objection has some force, but its failure to be a good analogy reveals that two sorts of considerations go to make an innings fair. For while living a full or complete life, just in the sense of experiencing all the ages of man,[5] is one mark of a fair innings, there is also value in living through as many ages as possible. Just as completing the mile is one value, it is not the only one. Runners in the race of life also value ground covered, and generally judge success in terms of distance run.

What the fair innings argument needs to do is to capture and express in a workable form the truth that while it is always a *misfortune* to die when one wants to go on living, it is not a *tragedy* to die in old age; but it is, on the other hand, both a tragedy and a misfortune to be cut off prematurely. Of course ideas like 'old age' and 'premature death' are inescapably vague, and may vary from society to society, and over time as techniques for postponing death improve. We must also remember that, while it may be invidious to choose between a 30- and a 40-year-old on the grounds that one has had a fairer innings than the other, it may not be invidious to choose between the 30- and the 65-year-old on those grounds.

If we remember, too, that it will remain wrong to end the life of someone who wants to live or to fail to save them, and that the fair innings argument will only operate as a principle of selection where we are forced to choose between lives, then something workable might well be salvaged.

While 'old age' is irredeemably vague, we can tell the old from the young, and even the old from the middle-aged, so that, without attempting precise formulation, a reasonable form of the fair innings argument might hold; and might hold that people who had achieved old age or who were closely approaching it would not have their lives further prolonged when this could only be achieved at the cost of the lives of those who were not nearing old age. These categories could be left vague, the idea being that it would be morally defensible to prefer to save the lives of those who 'still had their lives before them' rather than those who had 'already lived full lives'. The criterion to be employed in each case would simply be what reasonable people would say about whether someone had had a fair innings. Where reasonable people would be in no doubt that a particular individual was nearing old age *and* that that person's life could only be further prolonged at the expense of the life of someone that no reasonable person would classify as nearing old age, then the fair innings argument would apply, and it would be justifiable to save the younger candidate.

In cases where reasonable people differed or it seemed likely that they would differ as to whether people fell into one category or the other, then the anti-ageist argument would apply and the inescapable choice would have to be made arbitrarily.

But again it must be emphasized that the fair innings argument would only operate as a counsel of despair, when it was clearly impossible to postpone the deaths of all those who wanted to go on living. In all other circumstances the anti-ageist argument would apply.

So far so good. There are, however, further problems in the path of the anti-ageist argument and some of them are also problems for the fair innings argument.

Numbers of lives and numbers of years

One immediate problem is that, although living as long as possible, however long that turns out to be, will normally be very important to each individual, it seems a bad basis for planning health care or justifying the distribution of resources.

Suppose a particular disease, cancer, kills 120,000 people a year. Suppose further that a drug is developed which would prolong the lives of all cancer victims by one month but no more. Would it be worth putting such a drug into production? What if, for the same cost, a different drug would give ten years' complete remission, but would only operate on a form of cancer that affects 1,000 people? If we cannot afford both, which should we invest in? Or what if there is only one place on a renal dialysis programme and two patients who could benefit, but one will die immediately without dialysis but in six months in any event. The other will also die immediately without dialysis but with such help will survive for ten years. Although each wants the extra span of life equally badly, many would think that we ought to save the one with the longer life expectancy, that she is the 'better bet'.

All of these cases are an embarrassment for the anti-ageist argument, for our reaction to them implies that we do value extra years more. But how much more?

Extra life-time versus extra lives

If we choose to save one person for a predicted span of sixty years, rather than saving five people each for a predicted span of ten years, we have gained ten extra life years at the cost of overriding the desires of four extra people.[6]

So far we have looked at the issue of whether we should count length of life or desire to live as the most important factor when deciding which of two people should be saved. If all things are equal, there can be no reason to prefer one to the other and so we should choose in a way that does not display preference, by lot, for example. The question that seems so difficult is what, if any, difference should length of life make to such choices?

The anti-ageist argument says that it should make no difference, but the cases we have just been examining seem to pull the other way. And if we are persuaded by such cases this seems to imply that we do think length of life or life expectancy gives additional value to lives and so constitutes a factor which must be given some weight. One consequence of this is that we should think it more important to save one 10-year-old rather than five 60-year-olds (if we take 70 as an arbitrary maximum).[7] Equally, it would be better to save one 20-year-old rather than two 50-year-old people, for we would again save ten life years by so doing. Or one 15-year-old rather than two 45-year-olds (a saving of five life years) and so on.

It is just at this point that the anti-ageist argument seems to require resuscitation, for there is surely something invidious about sacrificing two 45-year-olds to one 15-year-old. To take the 'life years' view seems to discount entirely the desires and hopes and life plans of people in middle age, whenever an importunate youngster can place herself in the balance against them. But we do not normally think it better to save a 15-year-old rather than a 45-year-old when we cannot save both, so why should we think it better to save a 15-year-old rather than *two* 45-year olds?

For those who do favour saving one 15-year-old rather than two 45-year-olds, there is another difficulty. The life-time view seems to commit us to favouring total life-time saved rather than total number of people saved, with bizarre consequences. Suppose I could prolong the lives of 121,000 people for one month? This would yield a saving of 121,000 life months. Alternatively I could develop a drug which would give ten more years of life to 1,000 people. This would yield a saving of 120,000 life months. Thus,

on the time-span view, we should choose to extend the lives of 121,000 people by one month rather than 1,000 people by ten years each. So, what started out by looking as though it constituted an objection to the anti-ageist argument actually supports it in some circumstances. For, while we should favour length of life, where numbers of lives balanced against one another are equal, we should favour numbers of lives where, summed together, they yield a greater contribution to the total amount of life-time saved.

Unfortunately the force of the comparison between extending the lives of 120,000 people for one month or 1,000 for ten years was to encourage us to think that life-time saved was more important than numbers of lives saved. Its support for this conclusion now seems less decisive. What it seems to indicate is a very complicated calculus in which allocation of resources would be dependent on the amount of life-time such allocation could save. It would also lead to some bizarre orderings of priority, and not necessarily to those envisaged by enthusiasts of such a scheme.

One such enthusiast, Dr Donald Gould, produced the following scenario:

> Calculations are based on the assumption that all who survive their first perilous year ought then to live on to the age of 70. . .In Denmark for example, there are 50,000 deaths a year, but only 20,000 among citizens in the 1–70 bracket. These are the ones that count. The annual number of life years lost in this group totals 264,000. Of these 80,000 are lost because of accidents and suicides, 40,000 because of coronary heart disease, and 20,000 are due to lung disease. On the basis of these figures, a large proportion of the 'health' budget ought to be spent on preventing accidents and suicides and a lesser. . .amount on attempting to prevent and cure heart and lung disease. Much less would be spent on cancer which is predominantly a disease of the latter half of life, and which therefore contributes relatively little to the total sum of life years lost. . .No money at all would be available for trying to prolong the life of a sick old man of 82.[8]

The first thing to note about Gould's scenario is, that while deaths before the age of 70 may be the only life years *considered to have been lost*,[9] it does not follow that there is no reason to attempt to *gain* life years by prolonging the lives of the over-seventies if that seems feasible. For example, if a reasonable prognosis is that the life of the 70-year-old could be prolonged for five years by some intervention, then that is still a gain of five life years. This can have important consequences, for it means that it would be quite wrong to write off all care for the over-seventies. Suppose a simple procedure would add one year to the lives of all septuagenarians. This would yield a huge gain in life years spread over a whole population. Suppose, as is perhaps likely, the number of septuagenarians in Denmark was over 260,000, then the number of life years saved by adding a further year to their lives would exceed the total to be gained by all the measures to prevent accidents, suicides, heart disease and so on. This would then become the chief priority for health care spending.

Gould starts his calculations after 'the first perilous year' but this cut-off point would require justification. We might well conclude, persuaded by his general line of argument, that neonatal and postnatal care would have the first priority for resources.

The life-time position then can support a wide variety of practices and may lead to a policy of achieving small gains in lifespan for large numbers of people rather than to the sorts of substantial gains for those individuals with most to lose that its supporters seem to have principally in mind.

Threshold of discrimination It is tempting to think that we might be able to get over some of the problems of the life-time position by arguing that we can discount small gains in time as below the level of discrimination, in the sense that the benefit to the individual which accrued from living for a comparatively short period of extra time was nugatory. This might solve a few of the problems for the life-time position which arise from the necessity it imposes of favouring one group of people over another, wherever and whenever they are sufficiently numerous that the total life-time saved by rescuing them, even for a negligibly short period, exceeds that which might be saved by rescuing another smaller group who would live longer

individually, but shorter collectively. However, the problem will remain wherever the amount of life-time to be saved is just enough to be worth having (or is thought so to be by those whose time it is) but seems a poor return on the investment required to procure it or in terms of other savings, including savings of longer individual life-time, that might be made instead.

People versus policies We are strongly inclined to believe that where, for example, we can prolong the lives of 120,000 people by one month or 1,000 people by ten years that we should do the latter and that it is better to use a scarce resource to save the life of someone who is likely to live on for at least ten years rather than that of someone who will die in six months in any event. This inclination makes it look as though what we must in fact value is length of life-time rather than simply saving lives. But valuing life-time can be as dangerous to our moral intuitions as is the anti-ageist argument. Again, it might be tempting to believe that a policy of devoting resources to saving individual lives for as long as possible was better than simply maximizing life-time saved. There might be a number of different grounds for such a belief. One such ground would be the expectation that procedures which could prolong individual lives by a substantial period would lead to a greater saving of life-time in the long term than would procedures which merely postponed death for a month or so. But in the absence of any strong evidence for such a conclusion this expectation would be at best an act of faith and at worse a pious hope. Is there any way out?

The fallacy of life-time views

Suppose various medical research teams to be in competition for all research funds available and that one team could demonstrate that it was capable of producing an elixir of life that would make anyone taking it immortal. Suppose further that the entire world medical research budget, if applied to this end, would produce just enough elixir for one dose, and that nothing less than a full dose would have any effect at all. The life-time view suggests that all the money should go to making one person immortal rather than, say, to an alternative project by which another team could make everyone on earth live to a flourishing 80![10]

But there is an obvious fallacy in this argument which reveals a defect in the whole life-time approach. Making one person immortal will produce a saving of no more life years than would the alternative of making everyone on earth live to a flourishing 80. So long as the world itself and its population lasts as long as the immortal (and how – and where – could he last longer?) there would be no net increase in life years lived. Indeed, so long as there is either a stable or an increasing world population, from the life years point of view, it matters not at all who lives and who dies, nor does it matter how many years anyone survives. For, so long as those who die are replaced on a one-for-one or better than a one-for-one basis, there will be no loss of life years. Nor will there be any gain in life years when particular individuals live for longer. For if the overall world population is stable then prolonging the life of particular individuals does not increase the total number of life years the world contains. And if the world population is increasing then it is highly unlikely that prolonging the lives of particular people will fuel that increase. Indeed the reverse is more likely to be the case with the survival of people beyond child-bearing age having a retarding effect on the rate of increase.

In the context of a stable or of an increasing world population, any idea that any policy which did not have the effect of increasing the population in fact made any contribution to the amount of life-time saved would be an illusion.

We do not then have always to calculate the probable net saving in life-time of any particular policy or therapy, before knowing what to do, and can revert to the more customary consideration of the numbers of lives that might be saved or lost. This, however, highlights once again the problems of whether lives that can only be saved for relatively short periods of time (that can only be prolonged by a few months say) are as worth saving as those for whom the prognosis in terms of life expectancy is much longer. A manoeuvre that seems to capture our intuitions here involves modifying the life-time view into a worthwhile life-time view.

Worthwhile life-time

While to many just staying alive may be the most important consideration, and while they may even wish to continue to live even at appalling cost in terms of pain, disability and so on even, as we have seen,[11] where their lives are hardly worth living, they of course prefer to live worthwhile lives. So that, while any life might be better than no life, people generally expect medical care to concern itself not simply with preventing death but with restoring worthwhile existence.

Many sorts of thing will go to diminish the worth of life just as many and various considerations go to make life valuable and these will differ from individual to individual. For the moment we are just concerned with the question of how life expectancy operates as one of these.

If someone were sentenced to death and told that the execution would take place at dawn the next day, they would not, I imagine, be excessively overjoyed if they were then informed that the execution had been postponed for one month. Similarly if the prognosis for a particular disease were very accurate indeed, to be told that one had only seven months to live would not be dramatically less terrible than to be told one had six months to live. There are two related reasons for this. The first is simply that the prospect of imminent death colours, or rather discolours, existence and leaves it joyless. The second is that an almost necessary condition for valuing life is its open-endedness. The fact that we do not normally know how long we have to live liberates the present and leaves us apparently free to plan the future without having to be constantly aware of the futility of so doing.[12] If life had a short and finite (rather than indefinite) future, most things would not seem to be worth doing and the whole sense of the worth of life as an enterprise would evaporate.[13]

In the light of these considerations many people would not much value such short periods of remission, and support for policies which could at best produce such small gains might well be slight. However, some might well value highly the chance of even a small share of extra time. So far from emptying their life of meaning, it might enable them to 'round it off' or complete some important task or settle or better arrange their affairs. It might, so far from being of no value, be just what they needed to sort their life out and make some sort of final sense of it.

We have frequently noted the extreme difficulty involved in discounting the value of someone's life where we and they disagree about whether or not it is worth living, and we have also noted the injustice of preferring our assessment to theirs when so much is at stake for them. In view of all this it would be hard to prefer our judgement to theirs here.

Perhaps the problem would in reality be a small one. These dilemmas only arise where we cannot both help some people to live for relatively short periods *and* at the same time help others to live for much longer ones. Where there is no such conflict there is no question that we should go on helping people to stay alive for just so long as they want us to. However, the fact that hard cases are rare does not mean that we can turn our backs on them.

Fair innings or no ageism?

We have then two principles which can in hard cases pull in opposite directions. What should we do in the sorts of hard cases we have been considering? First, we should be clear that while the very old and those with terminal conditions are alike, in that they both have a short life expectancy, they may well differ with respect to whether or not they have had a fair innings. I do not believe that this issue is at all clear-cut but I am inclined to believe that where two individuals both equally wish to go on living for as long as possible our duty to respect this wish is paramount. It is, as I have suggested, the most important part of what is involved in valuing the lives

of others. Each person's desire to stay alive should be regarded as of the same importance and as deserving the same respect as that of anyone else, irrespective of the quality of their life or its expected duration.

This would hold good in all cases in which we have to choose between lives, except one. And that is where one individual has had a fair innings and the other not. In this case, while both equally wish to have their lives further prolonged one, but not the other, has had a fair innings. In this case, although there is nothing to choose between the two candidates from the point of view of their respective will to live and both would suffer the injustice of having their life cut short when it might continue, only one would suffer the further injustice of being deprived of a fair innings – a benefit that the other has received.

It is sometimes said that it is a misfortune to grow old, but it is not nearly so great a misfortune as not to grow old. Growing old when you don't want to is not half the misfortune that is not growing old when you do want to. It is this truth that the fair innings argument captures. So that while it remains true, as the anti-ageist argument asserts, that the value of the unelapsed possible lifespan of each person who wants to go on living is equally valuable however long that span may be, the question of which person's premature death involves the greater injustice can be important. The fair innings argument points to the fact that the injustice done to someone who has not had a fair innings when they lose out to someone who has is significantly greater than in the reverse circumstances. It is for this reason that in the hopefully rare cases where we have to choose between candidates who differ only in this respect that we should choose to give as many people as possible the chance of a fair innings.

Notes

1 Triage is a policy for coping with disasters where resources are insufficient to provide the normal standard of care for all. It involves dividing survivors into three groups: those who will die in any event, those who will live in any event, and those for whom care will make the difference

between life and death. Care is then given only to this last group. The argument is that this is the most economical use of resources where resources are insufficient to help all.

2 This may be a rash assumption because of the voluntary nature of many risks.

3 Of course if I don't value it because it is so short as to be scarcely worth having then the point does not apply in such a case.

4 I owe this objection to Tom Sorrel and am greatly in his debt here and elsewhere in this chapter for his generous and penetrating criticisms and comments.

5 No non-sexist form is available here, nor is one desirable since a different formulation would lose the resonance of the phrase.

6 Jonathan Glover, *Causing Death and Saving Lives* (Harmondsworth: Penguin, 1977), p. 221.

7 I'm assuming 70 as the full measure of life expectancy of healthy people and that all candidates are healthy in the sense that there is no reason to regard their life expectancy as less than average.

8 Quoted by Jonathan Glover (see note 6), p. 221. I am indebted here and elsewhere to Glover's stimulating discussion of these matters.

9 Because any figure of life expectancy will be arbitrary and one has to be taken.

10 The elixir of life example which prompted this argument about the fallacy of life-time views in stable or increasing populations I owe to Tom Sorrel, whose formulation of it I largely use.

11 See chapter 2 in *The Value of Life* (1985), from which this extract is taken.

12 Many people have argued of course that it is always futile to plan for the future because the inevitability of our world's ultimate destruction makes everything futile.

13 For the record we should note that small gains in life-time will only seem to be worthless to those who gain them if it is known that they will be short. If the potential beneficiaries are kept in ignorance of the fact that they can be granted only a short remission then the extra time will not be clouded by the futility deriving from its short duration and the gain, though small, will be as worthwhile as any other segment of their lives of comparable duration. Of course the deception may not be justified.

47

Bubbles under the Wallpaper
Healthcare Rationing and Discrimination

Nick Beckstead and Toby Ord

The ethics of priority setting in public health is both difficult and crucial. It involves hard questions about life and death on a scale that ranges from choices for individual patients to health strategies for the entire world's population. The problems arise because we simply do not have enough resources to provide everyone with all the medical care they need. We must therefore make seemingly impossible choices.

Over the last forty years, a standard has emerged for facing such choices: the QALY approach. A Quality Adjusted Life Year (QALY) is a unit for measuring the gains from medical interventions and is designed to be equivalent to the health gained by saving a year of life at full health. To determine how many QALYs are gained by a medical intervention, one looks at the length and (health-related) quality of a person's remaining lifespan, both with and without the intervention. The length is measured in years, and the quality at a given time is assigned a weight between 0 and 1, where 1 is full health and 0 is a quality of life equivalent to death. The length of life is multiplied by the weight, so that (for example) ten years of life

at full health is worth 10 QALYs, as is 20 years of life with a condition that has a quality of life weighting of 0.5 (a weighting commonly assigned to blindness). Once a QALY value is assigned to the person's future with the intervention and to their future without it, the difference between these is the gain due to the intervention. This method can thus measure benefits gained through the extension of life, as well as through the improvement of one's quality of life, or combinations of the two.

The QALY approach to priority setting is, roughly speaking, to rank all possible health interventions in terms of the ratio of QALYs gained to dollars spent and then to fund these interventions in order of their cost-effectiveness. This approach has a clear and important rationale: given a fixed health budget, it leads to the largest possible health gains. As such, it has been very successful in terms of promoting aggregate health.[1]

However, some ethicists and policy makers are concerned that the QALY approach achieves these gains in health at the expense of justice. For while it is uncontroversial that one gains in health by extending

Original publication details: Nick Beckstead and Toby Ord, "Bubbles under the Wallpaper: Healthcare Rationing and Discrimination," a paper presented to the conference "Valuing Lives" New York University, March 5, 2011, © Nick Beckstead and Toby Ord, reproduced with permission of the authors. The chapter draws on Nick Beckstead and Toby Ord, "Rationing and Rationality: The Cost of Avoiding Discrimination," pp. 232–239 from N. Eyal et al. (eds.), *Inequalities in Health: Concepts, Measures, and Ethics* (Oxford: Oxford University Press, 2013). Reproduced with permission of Oxford University Press.

one's life, or by raising the health-related quality of a given period of one's life, the QALY approach also produces a seemingly unsatisfactory conclusion: since a healthy person gains more QALYs from having their life extended than does a person with a disability, other things being equal, we should save the life of a healthy person over that of a disabled person. This objection has been forcibly made by John Harris (who described it as 'double jeopardy' for the disabled),[2] and it rose to national prominence in the United States after attempts to use the QALY approach in the state of Oregon were overturned on anti-discrimination grounds.[3]

The status of this objection is thus of key importance with respect to priority setting in healthcare. Is the current approach unjust? If so, should we make large sacrifices in terms of aggregate health in order to remedy it? Or does the objection rest on a mistake, in which case these large sacrifices would be in vain?

Bubbles under the Wallpaper

Attempts to resolve this problem have not met with great success. A solution favoured by Erik Nord and others involves ignoring quality-weights when deciding to whom we should give a life-saving treatment, provided the people to be saved regard their lives as worth living.[4] As Magnus Johannesson has pointed out,[5] Nord's proposal would sometimes conflict with individual preferences: it would sometimes rank one treatment higher than another, though this would be worse for someone and better for no one. Johannesson offers his own proposal, which also faces devastating objections.[6] In looking at such proposals, one gets the feeling that the task may be like trying to get a bubble out from behind the wallpaper; pushing down in one place simply moves the bubble elsewhere.

In this paper, we confirm this intuition by showing that *any* attempt to set priorities in health will face a highly counter-intuitive conclusion, often one of the counter-intuitive conclusions that people have tried to avoid in the above cases.[7] To see how this works, consider the following simplified case:[8]

Example

Alice and Beth were both perfectly healthy 20-year-olds, but have recently contracted an unusual disease. This disease will kill them very soon unless treated, and even then they will suffer from serious complications, such as blindness and/or a reduced lifespan. To make matters worse, there are not enough resources to treat them both. There are, however three possible treatment options outlined in the table:

	Option X	Option Y	Option Z
Alice	45 years (blind)	–	–
Beth	–	60 years (blind)	35 years (full health)

In X, Alice is treated and will live for 45 years but will lose her sight. Because Beth was infected by a slightly weaker strain, there are two treatment options available to her: in Y, she will live for 60 years but will lose her sight, in Z she will live for only 35 years, but will retain her sight. Beth has been asked which of options Y and Z she prefers, and (after considerable research and reflection) she arrived at a strong preference for 35 years of life with full health over 60 years of life with blindness (this is in line with most people's preferences and with the commonly used QALY ratings).

Which of these options should we choose? Let us first consider them pair-wise: in other words, which would we choose if it were a choice between only X and Y, only Y and Z, or only X and Z. We will then see that there are three problems that we would like to avoid:

1. *Preference for smaller benefits* X produces a smaller benefit for Alice than Y does for Beth. Since there is nothing else to distinguish between the two people, choosing X over Y demonstrates a morally perverse preference for producing smaller benefits rather than larger ones.

2. *Pointless violation of autonomy* Y is worse than Z for Beth and they are equally bad for Alice. Choosing Y over Z thus involves violating Beth's autonomy

for no gain at all (in fact, to produce what she and experts both regard as a worse outcome).

3. *Disability discrimination* Z provides fewer years of life for Beth than X provides for Alice. The only thing Z has in its favour is that Beth would be at full health, whereas X would leave Alice with a disability. Thus, choosing Z over X involves discriminating on the grounds of disability.

We are thus left with a cycle of preferences: we must choose Y over X in order to avoid *Preference for smaller benefits*, we must choose Z over Y to avoid *Pointless violation of autonomy*, and we must choose X over Z to avoid *Disability discrimination*.[9] However, this puts us in a very precarious position. Having cyclic preferences opens one up to so-called 'money pump' arguments. For example, consider the following. If you think it is important to choose Y over X given a choice between the two, then presumably you would be prepared to sacrifice something – at least a single penny – to choose Y in such a case. Similarly if you think the same thing between Y and Z, and between Z and X then you would be prepared to pay a penny to transfer in each of these cases. But this would leave you back where you began: with option X and slightly less money. Moreover, you would still be prepared to trade a penny to move from X to Y and could be made to go around this cycle until you had very little money remaining. Of course it is not just money that can be 'pumped' but anything of value.[10]

We could thus add a fourth problem:

4. *Cyclic preferences* Choosing Y over X, Z over Y, and X over Z, is an example of cyclic preferences, which violate the conditions of rational choice theory and leave one open to irrational behaviour such as money pumping.

It can be easily seen that any way of ranking health outcomes will therefore satisfy one of these four undesirable conditions. Given this conclusion, we must give up on producing a system of priority setting that avoids these problems and learn to live with the least of the evils, whichever it may be.

A Rights-Based Approach?

When confronted with this problem, it may seem natural to reach for a certain kind of rights-based approach. On this approach, when we have equally expensive treatments but can save only one person's life, the person who stands to gain the most life-years (ignoring any quality adjustments) is awarded the right to treatment. The person may then select the treatment that she most prefers to receive, under the advisement of her doctor.

Thus, if the choices are X and Z, Alice would be awarded the right to treatment and we would choose option X. Whereas if option Y were also available, Beth would receive the right to treatment, and since she prefers option Z to option Y, we would choose option Z.

In this section, we show that this approach faces considerable difficulties. These difficulties arise because the approach suffers from *Cyclic preferences*. Objections of this kind can be extended to other theories that suffer from *Cyclic preferences*, so the section can also be viewed as a way of illustrating the problems associated with embracing *Cyclic preferences*.

To see that this approach suffers from *Cyclic preferences* but avoids 1–3, note that in pairwise cases, it chooses Y over X, Z over Y, and X over Z. The rights-based approach therefore cannot be applied across all individual cases without leaving the decision maker open to being money pumped. This is unlikely to arise in practice, but casts doubt upon the rationality of the approach.

Cyclic preferences also lead to another strange problem for the rights-based approach. Note that the rights-based approach chooses X out of the options X and Z, but when Y is added to the set of options, it switches its choice to Z. In decision theory, this is known as violating the *Independence of irrelevant alternatives*.[11] This violation may not seem like a deep defect: after all, it emerges naturally from a seemingly reasonable system of rights, and partially as a result of the autonomous choice of individuals. However, if we extend the example, we can see cases where this violation of the *Independence of irrelevant alternatives* seems particularly unreasonable.

First, let us add a few details to the Alice and Beth case. Suppose that for each treatment (*X*, *Y*, or *Z*) that could be delivered, there is a corresponding vial of medicine which must be administered. After this, the patient must receive a very uncommon medicine, of which the clinic has only a single dose. Following the rights-based approach, the doctor decides on option *Z*, so he walks over to the table and selects vial *Z*, then fills a syringe with it. Just as he is about to inject Beth with this medicine, he hears a small crash: vial *Y* has just fallen off the table and shattered, making treatment *Y* unavailable. The doctor then realises that it would now be wrong to give treatment *Z*, as it has become a choice between only *X* and *Z*, so he goes back to the table and fills a syringe from vial *X* to give to Alice instead.

There is something very odd about this behaviour. This example brings the dependence on irrelevant alternatives to the fore and casts doubt upon whether the rights-based approach is a reasonable protocol.

Alternatively, consider a case in which the doctor knows that they have treatment *X* and *Z* available, but can't remember whether they have any of treatment *Y*. In this case, the doctor is uncertain of which is the right treatment to deliver. If *Y* is available, he must administer treatment *Z* to Beth (to avoid a *Pointless violation of autonomy*), but if it is not, then he must administer *X* to Alice (to avoid *Disability discrimination*). Since these are both weighty problems that adherents to the rights-based approach want to avoid, it is thus imperative for the doctor to spend some time searching the clinic to see if *Y* is available, or perhaps telephoning suppliers, even though he will not actually use it. More extreme examples could be constructed if the doctor would need to run moderately expensive tests in order to see if option *Y* was available or not.

Finally, consider a case in which we can help either Charles or Dan. They are both healthy 20-year-olds who were struck by a similar disease to Alice and Beth. To begin with, suppose that there are two options, *P* and *Q*, where *P* involves giving Charles 10 more years to live at full health and *Q* involves giving Dan 12 more years to live, but he would lose his sight. In this case, the rights-based approach would suggest treating Dan.

	Option P	Option Q	Option R	Option S	...
Charles	10 years (full health)	–	14 years (blind)	–	...
Dan	–	12 years (blind)		16 years (blind & deaf)	...

But now suppose that there was a third option, *R*, in which Charles could live for 14 years at the expense of being blind. Like most people, Charles does not prefer this to 10 years at full health, but if option *R* is available, then the rights-based approach recommends treating Charles. Now suppose there is a fourth option, *S*, where Dan could live for 16 years but would be both blind and deaf. Dan does not prefer this to 12 years with blindness and hearing, but now the rights-based approach would recommend treating Dan. Notice that we are now deciding between *P* and *Q* (which are the only options that will conceivably be chosen) on the basis of *R* and *S*. One could imagine a long sequence of increasingly irrelevant alternatives, the existence of which keeps swinging the balance between *P* and *Q*. Moreover, as it is very important on this view whether such options exist, we would often be required to spend some time and money investigating whether such options exist before making our decisions.

We thus find that the rights-based approach looks increasingly unreasonable. As noted above, these examples can be extended to other theories that possess *Cyclic preferences*, thereby demonstrating how important it is for a theory to avoid this problem.

Randomness to the Rescue?

Many philosophers are convinced on independent grounds that fairness requires us to leave some of our most important decisions up to chance, so it is natural to wonder whether a move to lotteries could resolve the present problem. The purpose of a lottery system is to give each person a fair chance of being treated – where this may be an equal chance or a chance weighted by how much the person involved stands to gain.[12]

Although lotteries may seem like a sensible solution in a case where we must allocate treatments to a small number of individuals in the same hospital, they seem less sensible as a general approach to priority setting. Given the numbers of people affected, we are most concerned with getting global priorities right. On that note, it is hard to believe that the government should draw numbers in order to decide which kinds of medical research to fund, which kinds of doctors to hire, or which kinds of treatments are worth funding. We won't pretend to have established that lotteries are unreasonable in this setting, but we note that randomness does not look promising as a solution to our problem, at least on the most important level.

However, even in its most plausible application, a lottery approach affords no traction on our problem. To defend this claim, we can give an argument that is highly analogous to the one given earlier. The first step is simply to use analogues of 1–3 that apply to gambles. In this case, we'd like to avoid policies that have any of the following three undesirable properties:

1★ *Preference for smaller benefits★* When the potential treatments are X and Y, the policy allows Alice at least as great a chance as Beth even though Alice and Beth are equally healthy and Beth would live for an additional 15 years.[13]

2★ *Pointless violation of autonomy★* When the potential treatments include Y and Z, the policy allocates a non-zero probability to Y, even though Beth prefers treatment Z and Beth's favoured treatment would come at no one else's expense.

3★ *Disability discrimination★* When the potential treatments are X and Z, the policy demands a lottery over X and Z that gives Beth at least a great a chance as Alice, even though (i) Beth stands to gain fewer years of life and (ii) we would favour Alice if she were not disabled.[14]

In the previous section, avoiding 1–3 required having cyclic preferences over X, Y, and Z. Here, we replace that cyclic ranking with another. In this case the relation 'A merits more probability than B, when the choices are A and B' turns out to be cyclic. To avoid *Preference for smaller benefits★*, we must give Y more probability than X. To avoid *Pointless violation of autonomy★*, we must give Z more probability than Y. To avoid *Disability discrimination★*, we must give X more probability than Z. That this relation could be cyclic is strange in itself. More importantly, it seems that we are dealing with the same problem all over again. Intuitively, treatment A should get more probability than treatment B only if we should prefer that treatment A be given rather than that treatment B be given. And, for the reasons noted above, we should not have cyclic preferences.

In case it seems that the problem just noted can somehow be avoided, note that it is impossible to satisfy 1★–3★ if we want to avoid a policy with the following undesirable (disjunctive) property:

4★ *Dependence on irrelevant treatments★*

a. The policy allows that adding a potential treatment for one person could decrease her odds of being treated. Intuitively, it would be unfair (and bizarre) to decrease a person's odds of being treated on the grounds that additional possible ways of curing that person (and no one else) were discovered, or

b. The policy allows that adding a potential treatment for one person could decrease another person's chances of being treated, even though the first person prefers an alternative treatment that is already available. Intuitively, the person whose chances decrease could complain that she was being given a lesser chance for irrelevant reasons.

We relegate the proof that it is impossible to avoid all of 1★–4★ to a note, since the argument is slightly more technical than the previous one.[15] The basic problem is that any lottery system that avoids *Preference for smaller benefits★*, *Pointless violation of autonomy★*, and *Dependence on irrelevant treatments★* will give more probability to Z than X when the choices are X, Y, and Z. On the other hand, any lottery system that avoids *Disability discrimination*★ and *Dependence on irrelevant treatments*★ will give at least as much probability to X as it does to Z. It is not possible to have both.

This result about lotteries can be viewed as a generalization of our original argument. Whatever the merits of randomization elsewhere, a move to lotteries cannot solve the present problem.

Conclusion

We have shown that it is impossible for a moral theory to provide guidance in multi-person trade-offs between length of life and quality of life without facing one of four very challenging conclusions. Of these, we think that the ones most likely to be accepted are *Disability discrimination* and *Cyclic preferences*. Thus, while we have not explicitly argued in favour of the QALY approach and its controversial applications in situations with respect to life-saving treatment for the disabled, we have shown it to be substantially

more plausible in light of the challenges faced by all of its competitors. This makes it a lot less clear that we should change the QALY system and thereby throw away the great health gains it has achieved.

We should also note, in passing, that the specific issues addressed here are part of a wider problem in the discourse on ethical theories. Some systems, such as the QALY approach, make their consequences clearly known in advance, making them easy targets for attack by intuitive counterexample. A single, confidently held, pre-theoretic judgment is often regarded as enough to reject such a position. Incomplete competitors frequently avoid this challenge because it is usually hard to see what problems an incomplete alternative will face. In the present case we were able to produce an argument that applies to *all* competitors to the QALY approach, getting around the issue of underspecification, but unfortunately this is not always possible. Proponents of highly incomplete ethical positions must be careful when challenging more systematic competitors; the next impossibility argument may be around the corner, even if no one has been clever enough to discover it yet.

Notes

1 Here we are setting aside some important issues. For example, the QALY system will only maximize health gains if the weights are appropriately chosen. In practice, this can be difficult. But this is orthogonal to the issues that we discuss here. For the sake of argument, we assume that we are dealing with a system with reasonably chosen weights.

2 Harris (1987). See Singer et al. (1995) for a response to Harris.

3 For more on the Oregon cost-setting exercise, see Hadorn (1991).

4 Nord et al. (1999).

5 Johannesson (2001).

6 Nord et al. (2003).

7 In an economist's vocabulary, we do this by establishing an *impossibility theorem*. We show that certain intuitively inevitable constraints on a fair system for prioritizing health are impossible to meet.

8 Note that in this case there is no pre-existing disability. In such cases, prioritarian and egalitarian adjustments to the QALY framework make no significant difference to which option is chosen. Some might argue that, in this kind of case, there is nothing wrong with favouring the healthy over the blind. To address this point, we could change the case so that Alice became blind five years ago. Our analysis of the revised case would remain the same.

9 Note that we are using the term 'cyclic preferences' in a broad sense, referring both to cycles of preferences within a given set of options, and cycles of preferences across sets of options (such as the present case).

10 The status of money pump arguments is somewhat controversial. Sometimes they are used to argue that rational people do not have cyclic preferences. In that context, it is assumed that rational people always choose A over B when they prefer A to B. But someone who

believes in the rationality of cyclic preferences may deny this, pointing to cases of strategic reasoning that appear to be counterexamples to this generalization. We need not settle this issue here. What's true is that if policy-makers want to set healthcare priorities using a ranking system that they can follow in general, the ranking system will be susceptible to a money pump if the ranking is cyclic.

11 This strange feature arises directly from the *Cyclic preferences*: one cannot stabilise a cyclic system of preferences in the case where all three options are presented at once without violating the *Independence of irrelevant alternatives*.

12 Broome (1984).

13 Some people may be tempted to think that it isn't so bad to satisfy *Preference for smaller benefits*⋆ on the grounds that a fair coin toss is the appropriate response to this case. We think that a difference of 15 years should be enough to make this implausible. We could adjust the case by choosing a more debilitating condition and allowing an even larger gap in years. For this solution to work in general, one must be willing to do fair coin tosses even when the difference in benefits could be very great. We find this idea absurd; it is anathema to the very idea of priority setting in health care.

14 To avoid *Disability discrimination*⋆ one must give Alice a greater chance of being treated when the choices are X and Z (equal chances would not be allowed). We can run a version of our argument using another version

of this requirement that allows giving each person an equal chance in this situation. To see this, note that we make use of a weak inequality rather than a strict one in line 6 of the proof in note 15.

15 We proceed by assuming the four conditions do not hold and deriving a contradiction. For some simplifying notation, let $\Pr(A{:}ABC)$ be the probability assigned by a lottery to A when the alternatives are A, B, and C. Likewise, $\Pr(B{:}BC)$ is the probability assigned to B when the alternatives are B and C. Then we can argue as follows:

1	$\Pr(Y{:}XY) > \Pr(X{:}XY)$	to avoid *Preference for smaller benefits*⋆
2	$\Pr(Y \text{ or } Z{:}XYZ) > \Pr(X{:}XYZ)$	to avoid *Dependence on irrelevant treatments*⋆ and satisfy 1
3	$\Pr(Y{:}XYZ) = 0$	to avoid *Pointless violation of autonomy*⋆
4	$\Pr(Z{:}XYZ) = \Pr(Y \text{ or } Z{:}XYZ)$	from 3 and probability theory
5	$\Pr(Z{:}XYZ) > \Pr(X{:}XYZ)$	from 2 and 4
6	$\Pr(X{:}XZ) \geq \Pr(Z{:}XZ)$	to avoid *Disability discrimination*⋆
7	$\Pr(X{:}XYZ) \geq \Pr(Z{:}XYZ)$	to avoid *Dependence on irrelevant treatments*⋆ and to satisfy 6
8	contradiction!	from 5 and 7

References

Broome, John. 1984. Selecting people randomly. *Ethics* 95: 38–55.

Hadorn, David C. 1991. The Oregon priority-setting exercise: quality of life and public policy. *Hastings Center Report* 21(3): 11–16.

Harris, John. 1987. QALYfying the value of life. *Journal of Medical Ethics* 13: 117–23.

Johannesson, Magnus. 2001. Should we aggregate relative or absolute changes in QALYs? *Health Economics* 10: 573–7.

Nord, Erik, et al. 1999. Incorporating societal concerns for fairness in numerical valuations of health programs. *Health Economics* 8: 25–39.

Nord, Erik, Paul Menzel and Jeff Richardson. 2003. The value of life: individual preferences and social choice. A comment to Magnus Johannesson. *Health Economics* 12: 873–7.

Singer, Peter, et al. 1995. Double jeopardy and the use of QALYs in health care allocation. *Journal of Medical Ethics* 21: 144–50.

48

Rescuing Lives
Can't We Count?

Paul T. Menzel

On 16 September 1993, five-year-old Laura Davies of Manchester, England, received small and large intestines, stomach, pancreas, liver, and two kidneys in a fifteen-hour transplant operation at Children's Hospital of Pittsburgh. The National Health Service paid for little of her care, but scores of private donors responded to newspaper publicity and her parents' appeals to provide the half-million pounds and more required for her various operations. In this case, where was medical technology taking us?

Laura died on 11 November. According to her Manchester physician at the time of the operation, however, Laura had a "better than 50–50 chance." After all, the three previous child recipients of multiple organs at Pittsburgh since the advent of a new antirejection drug in 1992 are still alive. It is thus difficult to dismiss the willingness of Laura's parents and physicians to proceed as using her for their own emotional or scientific purposes. Though surely "experimental," the surgery was the only chance Laura had.

And if anyone, either then or now in light of her death, claims that the 50–50 odds were inflated, a straightforward reply is available: maybe you're right, but let us employ this procedure, now and at other times, to see. Plucky Laura herself seemed to put the "guinea pig" charge to rest. "I'm not worried," she told reporters at a press conference. Then she ended the session with a song.

A standard objection to high expense-per-benefit care also does not apply: funded privately by response to special appeal, Laura's care does not come at the expense of anyone else whom limited funds might have saved. With a child like this and the money pouring in from donations, why should we dispute her parents' and physicians' decision? On a medical mission? Sure. Carried away? In the circumstances, seemingly not.

Still, something has been missed that is very problematic about Laura's aggressive care: in the attempt to save her, a greater number of other lives were sacrificed. It's a straightforward function of the marked scarcity of organs. Nearly half the children now on organ transplant waiting lists die before they get them. We should all be able to see the big picture: if one person at the head of the queue gets four scarce organs instead of one, four others somewhere down the queue, not one, never get any.

Original publication details: Paul T. Menzel, "Rescuing Lives: Can't We Count?" pp. 22–23 from *Hastings Center Report* 24: 1 (1994). Reproduced with permission of John Wiley & Sons.

Both the British and the US publics seem reluctant to recognize this. Take Pennsylvania's Governor Casey last spring. At first his waiting only a few days before receiving a heart–liver transplant met with skepticism: had he been allowed to jump the queue because of his political status? The Pittsburgh transplant center quickly replied: absolutely not, he was treated as any other multiple organ failure patient would have been. Because of the multiple failure, his need was more urgent. With the political queue-jumping charge rebuffed, the critics backed off.

But if organs are scarce, and those used in multiple scarce organ transplants could virtually always have saved more lives if used on others, what can possibly justify any multiple organ transplant candidate's elevation to the top of the queue? Except in the event of an extremely rare match, only two readily understandable explanations seem available, and neither justifies what was done.

One is pushing outward the medical frontier: carry out Casey's and Davies's more challenging operations despite the current sacrifice of a greater number of others' lives, and we will eventually develop new, effective forms of lifesaving. But this sort of argument represents the most extreme kind of medical adventurism. With the scarcity of organs virtually certain to continue – especially for children and infants, where we are already getting close to maximum contribution – what is the likelihood that multiple organ transplants will *ever* cease to use up on one person what could have saved several? A totally Pollyannaish view of future organ supply drives the "experimental development" argument. We should experiment with multiple scarce organ transplants only if we have good reason to believe that sometime in the future we will have ample supply. But there is every reason to think we will *never* have that!

The other readily understandable explanation is an odd view of "urgency." The Pittsburgh surgeons appear to regard the failure of both a heart and a liver as constituting more urgent need. This too falls apart upon examination. Certainly I am as close to death's door if "just" my heart fails as I am if my heart and liver both fail. Where, in "only heart failure," is there any lack of real urgency?

To say that Governor Casey or Laura Davies have greater medical need because they require two or seven organs instead of one betrays, I suppose, a kind of "Dunkirk Syndrome": thinking that the more *difficult* the rescue was, the greater was the need at the time. Admittedly, nations and doctors understandably feel in such circumstances that they have pulled off something more *miraculous* – in fact they have! But where in that pride in greater effort or thankfulness for greater luck is hidden any more urgent *need*?

So advancement of medical technology and urgent medical need utterly fail to justify multiple scarce-organ transplants. Their defense would have to invoke either of two much more difficult explanations. One is a direct, jolting challenge to the moral relevance of numbers at all in these kinds of acute care situations: there simply is no obligation to save the greater number. Such a position gets a foothold in our thinking through the claim that each and every individual deserves an equal chance of being saved; we should therefore flip coins to determine whether we will save the one or the four, not save the four right off because they are the greater number. Regardless of the merits of this view in academic philosophical terms,[1] however, it hardly fits the transplant setting. We continually strive to expand the organ pool. Why? To save more lives, obviously. If with that expanded supply we end up saving no more people than before because we use up enough of our organ bank on multiple organ recipients, what has been the point of our supply expansion efforts?

A second difficult explanation is at least anchored in some actual social reactions. Little objection to the occasional practice of using up multiple scarce organs on one recipient comes from competing single-organ patients, patients' families, or their representatives. The reason, I suspect, is that the context of waiting together on a queue is already transparently and pervasively infused with luck – the luck of the right organ and a good match arriving at the right time for one candidate, but not for another. Living continually with such grave unknowns may lead people to celebrate unselfishly when anyone gets saved. No patient begrudges another's sheer luck; all understand that there is no rhyme, reason, or desert in the outcome anyhow. Once in that laudable mindset, people may not even attend to the numbers. The many cast no challenging glance into the eyes of the few. Challenge, defense, claim – here, all are out of court. It's as if the many even consent to their own lack of rescue as long as someone is saved.

I am intrigued by this possibility of consent,[2] but I suspect that our surmisals here about the empathetic consent of organ failure patients who wait unsuccessfully on the queue are romantic and quite distort their actual feelings. Most of the real competitor potential recipients out there somewhere on the queue do not sit together in a transplant center's waiting room, directly sharing one another's fortune. In any case, why should those in the society who manage the process of organ procural and disbursement not empathize sequentially with *all* who might be saved, thereby letting the numbers of real, equally invaluable rescuable persons build up to turn their decision? Again, in terms of persuasive justifications, multiple scarce-organ transplants strike out.

Surgeons, the press, and the public need to face up to these considerations in cases like Laura Davies.

How can transplant centers justify ultimately letting two or more persons somewhere down the queue likely die because they have drawn so much out of the organ bank to save one? And why should the press play along with this lifesaving delusion and publicize appeals to unknowing financial donors without telling them the morally relevant facts? If donors knew, why should they feel good about having contributed to a net *non*-lifesaving project? In the whole situation, only Laura Davies's parents, in their attachment to their child, come out clean.

Worse yet, the essential problem in the multiple scarce organ cases portends bigger trouble. It has ominous implications for the distribution of other scarce health care resources. If in multiple organ transplants we are blind to the real lives of competing potential beneficiaries, where they, too, are acutely ill, how much more blind will we be in typical contexts of distributing scarce monies where the competing beneficiaries are more distant, and certainly not on any queue of named individuals?

Let's count before we cut.

Notes

1 Frances M. Kamm, *Morality, Mortality: Death and Whom to Save From It*, vol. 1 (New York: Oxford University Press, 1993), pp. 75–122. See also J. Taurek, "Should the Numbers Count?" *Philosophy and Public Affairs*, 6, no. 4 (1977): 293–316; and Derek Parfit, "Innumerate Ethics," *Philosophy and Public Affairs*, 7, no. 4 (1978): 285–301.

2 The attempt to discern the implications of consent to risk drove most of this author's reasoning in *Strong Medicine: The Ethical Rationing of Health Care* (New York: Oxford University Press, 1990).

49

Should Alcoholics Compete Equally for Liver Transplantation?

Alvin H. Moss and Mark Siegler

Until recently, liver transplantation for patients with alcohol-related end-stage liver disease (ARESLD) was not considered a treatment option. Most physicians in the transplant community did not recommend it because of initial poor results in this population[1] and because of a predicted high recidivism rate that would preclude long-term survival.[2] In 1988, however, Starzl and colleagues[3] reported 1-year survival rates for patients with ARESLD comparable to results in patients with other causes of end-stage liver disease (ESLD). Although the patients in the Pittsburgh series may represent a carefully selected population,[3,4] the question is no longer Can we perform transplants in patients with alcoholic liver disease and obtain acceptable results? but Should we? This question is particularly timely since the Health Care Financing Administration (HCFA) has recommended that Medicare coverage for liver transplantation be offered to patients with alcoholic cirrhosis who are abstinent. The HCFA proposes that the same eligibility criteria be used for patients with ARESLD as are used for patients with other causes of ESLD, such as primary biliary cirrhosis and sclerosing cholangitis.[5]

Should Patients with ARESLD Receive Transplants?

At first glance, this question seems simple to answer. Generally, in medicine, a therapy is used if it works and saves lives. But the circumstances of liver transplantation differ from those of most other lifesaving therapies, including long-term mechanical ventilation and dialysis, in three important respects:

Nonrenewable resource

First, although most lifesaving therapies are expensive, liver transplantation uses a nonrenewable, absolutely scarce resource – a donor liver. In contrast to patients with end-stage renal disease, who may receive either a transplant or dialysis therapy, every patient with ESLD who does not receive a liver transplant will die. This dire, absolute scarcity of donor livers would be greatly exacerbated by including patients with ARESLD as potential candidates for liver transplantation. In 1985, 63,737 deaths due to hepatic disease occurred in the

Original publication details: Alvin H. Moss and Mark Siegler, "Should Alcoholics Compete Equally for Liver Transplantation?" pp. 1295–1298 from *Journal of the American Medical Association* 265: 10 (1991). © 1991 American Medical Association. All rights reserved.

United States, at least 36,000 of which were related to alcoholism, but fewer than 1,000 liver transplants were performed.[6] Although patients with ARESLD represent more than 50% of the patients with ESLD, patients with ARESLD account for less than 10% of those receiving transplants (*New York Times.* April 3, 1990:B6[col 1]). If patients with ARESLD were accepted for liver transplantation on an equal basis, as suggested by the HCFA, there would potentially be more than 30,000 additional candidates each year. (No data exist to indicate how many patients in the late stages of ARESLD would meet transplantation eligibility criteria.) In 1987, only 1,182 liver transplants were performed; in 1989, fewer than 2,000 were done.[6] Even if all donor livers available were given to patients with ARESLD, it would not be feasible to provide transplants for even a small fraction of them. Thus, the dire, absolute nature of donor liver scarcity mandates that distribution be based on unusually rigorous standards – standards not required for the allocation of most other resources such as dialysis machines and ventilators, both of which are only *relatively* scarce.

Comparison with cardiac transplantation

Second, although a similar dire, absolute scarcity of donor hearts exists for cardiac transplantation, the allocational decisions for cardiac transplantation differ from those for liver transplantation. In liver transplantation, ARESLD causes more than 50% of the cases of ESLD; in cardiac transplantation, however, no one predominant disease or contributory factor is responsible. Even for patients with end-stage ischemic heart disease who smoked or who failed to adhere to dietary regimens, it is rarely clear that one particular behavior caused the disease. Also, unlike our proposed consideration for liver transplantation, a history of alcohol abuse is considered a contraindication and is a common reason for a patient with heart disease to be denied cardiac transplantation.[7,8] Thus, the allocational decisions for heart transplantation differ from those for liver transplantation in two ways: determining a cause for end-stage heart disease is less certain,

and patients with a history of alcoholism are usually rejected from heart transplant programs.

Expensive technology

Third, a unique aspect of liver transplantation is that it is an expensive technology that has become a target of cost containment in health care.[9] It is, therefore, essential to maintain the approbation and support of the public so that organs continue to be donated under appropriate clinical circumstances – even in spite of the high cost of transplantation.

General guideline proposed

In view of the distinctive circumstances surrounding liver transplantation, we propose as a general guideline that patients with ARESLD should not compete equally with other candidates for liver transplantation. We are *not* suggesting that patients with ARESLD should *never* receive liver transplants. Rather, we propose that a priority ranking be established for the use of this dire, absolutely scarce societal resource and that patients with ARESLD be lower on the list than others with ESLD.

Objections to Proposal

We realize that our proposal may meet with two immediate objections: (1) Some may argue that since alcoholism is a disease, patients with ARESLD should be considered equally for liver transplantation.[10] (2) Some will question why patients with ARESLD should be singled out for discrimination, when the medical profession treats many patients who engage in behavior that causes their diseases.[11] We will discuss these objections in turn.

Alcoholism: How is it similar to and different from other diseases?

We do not dispute the reclassification of alcoholism as a disease.[12] Both hereditary and environmental factors contribute to alcoholism, and physiological, biochemical, and genetic markers have been associated with increased susceptibility.[13] Identifying alcoholism as a disease enables physicians to approach it as they do other medical problems and to differentiate it from bad habits, crimes, or moral weaknesses. More important, identifying alcoholism as a disease also legitimizes medical interventions to treat it.[14]

Alcoholism is a chronic disease,[12,15] for which treatment is available and effective. More than 1.43 million patients were treated in 5,586 alcohol treatment units in the 12-month period ending October 30, 1987.[16] One comprehensive review concluded that more than two thirds of patients who accept therapy improve.[17] Another cited four studies in which at least 54% of patients were abstinent a minimum of 1 year after treatment.[18] A recent study of alcohol-impaired physicians reported a 100% abstinence rate an average of 33.4 months after therapy was initiated. In this study, physician–patients rated Alcoholics Anonymous, the largest organization of recovering alcoholics in the world, as the most important component of their therapy.[19]

Like other chronic diseases – such as type I diabetes mellitus, which requires the patient to administer insulin over a lifetime – alcoholism requires the patient to assume responsibility for participating in continuous treatment. Two key elements are required to successfully treat alcoholism: the patient must accept his or her diagnosis and must assume responsibility for treatment.[20,21] The high success rates of some alcoholism treatment programs indicate that many patients can accept responsibility for their treatment. ARESLD, one of the sequelae of alcoholism, results from 10 to 20 years of heavy alcohol consumption. The risk of ARESLD increases with the amount of alcohol consumed and with the duration of heavy consumption.[22] In view of the quantity of alcohol consumed, the years, even decades, required to develop ARESLD, and the availability of effective alcohol treatment, attributing personal responsibility for ARESLD to the patient seems all the more justified. We believe, therefore, that even though alcoholism is a chronic disease, alcoholics should be held responsible for seeking and obtaining treatment that could prevent the development of late-stage complications such as ARESLD. Our view is consistent with that of Alcoholics Anonymous: alcoholics are responsible for undertaking a program for recovery that will keep their disease of alcoholism in remission.[23]

Are we discriminating against alcoholics?

Why should patients with ARESLD be singled out when a large number of patients have health problems that can be attributed to so-called voluntary health-risk behavior? Such patients include smokers with chronic lung disease; obese people who develop type II diabetes; some individuals who test positive for the human immunodeficiency virus; individuals with multiple behavioral risk factors (inattention to blood pressure, cholesterol, diet, and exercise) who develop coronary artery disease; and people such as skiers, motor-cyclists, and football players who sustain activity-related injuries. We believe that the health care system should respond based on the actual medical needs of patients rather than on the factors (eg, genetic, infectious, or behavioral) that cause the problem. We also believe that individuals should bear some responsibility – such as increased insurance premiums – for medical problems associated with voluntary choices. The critical distinguishing factor for treatment of ARESLD is the scarcity of the resource needed to treat it. The resources needed to treat most of these other conditions are only moderately or relatively scarce, and patients with these diseases or injuries can receive a share of the resources (ie, money, personnel, and medication) roughly equivalent to their need. In contrast, there are insufficient donor livers to sustain the lives of all with ESLD who are in need.[24] This difference permits us to make some discriminating choices – or to establish priorities – in selecting candidates for liver transplantation based on notions of fairness. In addition, this reasoning enables us to offer patients with alcohol-related medical and surgical problems their fair share of relatively scarce resources, such as blood products, surgical care, and intensive care beds, while still maintaining that their claim on donor livers is less compelling than the claims of others.

Reasons Patients with ARESLD Should Have a Lower Priority on Transplant Waiting Lists

Two arguments support our proposal. The first argument is a moral one based on considerations of fairness. The second one is based on policy considerations and examines whether public support of liver transplantation can be maintained if, as a result of a first-come, first-served approach, patients with ARESLD receive more than half the available donor livers. Finally, we will consider further research necessary to determine which patients with ARESLD should be candidates for transplantation, albeit with a lower priority.

Fairness

Given a tragic shortage of donor livers, what is the fair or just way to allocate them? We suggest that patients who develop ESLD through no fault of their own (eg, those with congenital biliary atresia or primary biliary cirrhosis) should have a higher priority in receiving a liver transplant than those whose liver disease results from failure to obtain treatment for alcoholism. In view of the dire, absolute scarcity of donor livers, we believe it is fair to hold people responsible for their choices, including decisions to refuse alcoholism treatment, and to allocate organs on this basis.

It is unfortunate but not unfair [to] make this distinction.[25] When not enough donor livers are available for all who need one, choices have to be made, and they should be founded on one or more proposed principles of fairness for distributing scarce resources.[26,27] We shall consider four that are particularly relevant:

- To each, an equal share of treatment.
- To each, similar treatment for similar cases.
- To each, treatment according to personal effort.
- To each, treatment according to ability to pay.

It is not possible to give each patient with ESLD an *equal share*, or, in this case, a functioning liver. The problem created by the absolute scarcity of donor livers is that of inequality; some receive livers while others do not. But what is fair need not be equal. Although a first-come, first-served approach has been suggested to provide each patient with an equal chance, we believe it is fairer to give a child dying of biliary atresia an opportunity for a *first* normal liver than it is to give a patient with ARESLD who was born with a normal liver a *second* one.

Because the goal of providing each person with an equal share of health care sometimes collides with the realities of finite medical resources, the principle of *similar treatment for similar cases* has been found to be helpful. Outka[26] stated it this way: "If we accept the case for equal access, but if we simply cannot, physically cannot, treat all who are in need, it seems more just to discriminate by virtue of categories of illness, rather than between rich ill and poor ill." This principle is derived from the principle of formal justice, which, roughly stated, says that people who are equal in relevant respects should be treated equally and that people who are unequal in relevant respects should be treated differently.[27] We believe that patients with ARESLD are unequal in a relevant respect to others with ESLD, since their liver failure was preventable; therefore, it is acceptable to treat them differently.

Our view also relies on the principle of *To each, treatment according to personal effort*. Although alcoholics cannot be held responsible for their disease, once their condition has been diagnosed they can be held responsible for seeking treatment and for preventing the complication of ARESLD. The standard of personal effort and responsibility we propose for alcoholics is the same as that held by Alcoholics Anonymous. We are not suggesting that some lives and behaviors have greater value than others – an approach used and appropriately repudiated when dialysis machines were in short supply.[26–30] But we are holding people responsible for their personal effort.

Health policymakers have predicted that this principle will assume greater importance in the future. In the context of scarce health care resources, Blank[31] foresees a reevaluation of our health care priorities, with a shift toward individual responsibility and a renewed emphasis on the individual's obligation to society to maximize one's health. Similarly, more than a decade ago, Knowles[32] observed that prevention of disease requires effort. He envisioned that the next major advances in the health of the American people would be determined by what individuals are willing to do for themselves.

To each, treatment according to ability to pay has also been used as a principle of distributive justice. Since alcoholism is prevalent in all socioeconomic strata, it is not discrimination against the poor to deny liver transplantation to patients with alcoholic liver disease.[33] In fact, we believe that poor patients with ARESLD have a stronger claim for a donor liver than rich patients, precisely because many alcohol treatment programs are not available to patients lacking in substantial private resources or health insurance. Ironically, it is precisely this group of poor and uninsured patients who are most likely not to be eligible to receive a liver transplant because of their inability to pay. We agree with Outka's view of fairness that would discriminate according to categories of illness rather than according to wealth.

Policy considerations regarding public support for liver transplantation

Today, the main health policy concerns involve issues of financing, distributive justice, and rationing medical care.[34–37] Because of the many deficiencies in the US health care system – in maternal and child health, in the unmet needs of the elderly, and in the millions of Americans without health insurance – an increasing number of commentators and drawing attention to the trade-offs between basic health care for the many and expensive, albeit lifesaving care for the few.[9,25,38,39]

Because of its high unit cost, liver transplantation is often at the center of these discussions, as it has been in Oregon, where the legislature voted to eliminate Medicaid reimbursement for all transplants except kidneys and corneas.[9] In this era of health care cost containment, a sense of limits is emerging and allocational choices are being made. Oregon has already

shown that elected officials and the public are prepared to face these issues.

In our democracy, it is appropriate that community mores and values be regarded seriously when deciding the most appropriate use of a scarce and nonrenewable organ symbolized as a "Gift of Life." As if to underscore this point, the report of the Task Force on Organ Transplantation recommended that each donated organ be considered a national resource for the public good and that the public must participate in decisions on how to use this resource to best serve the public's interests.[40]

Much of the initial success in securing public and political approval for liver transplantation was achieved by focusing media and political attention not on adults but on children dying of ESLD. The public may not support transplantation for patients with ARESLD in the same way that they have endorsed this procedure for babies born with biliary atresia. This assertion is bolstered not only by the events in Oregon but also by the results of a Louis Harris and Associates[41] national survey, which showed that lifesaving therapy for premature infants or for patients with cancer was given the highest health care priority by the public and that lifesaving therapy for patients with alcoholic liver disease was given the lowest. In this poll, the public's view of health care priorities was shared by leadership groups also polled: physicians, nurses, employers, and politicians.

Just because a majority of the public holds these views does not mean that they are right, but the moral intuition of the public, which is also shared by its leaders, reflects community values that must be seriously considered. Also indicative of community values are organizations such as Mothers Against Drunk Driving, Students Against Drunk Driving, corporate employee assistance programs, and school student assistance programs. Their existence signals that many believe that a person's behavior can be modified so that the consequences of behavior such as alcoholism can be prevented.[42] Thus, giving donor livers to patients with ARESLD on an equal basis with other patients who have ESLD might lead to a decline in public support for liver transplantation.

Should Any Alcoholics Be Considered for Transplantation? Need for Further Research

Our proposal for giving lower priority for liver transplantation to patients with ARESLD does not completely rule out transplantation for this group. Patients with ARESLD who had not previously been offered therapy and who are now abstinent could be acceptable candidates. In addition, patients lower on the waiting list, such as patients with ARESLD who have been treated and are now abstinent, might be eligible for a donor liver in some regions because of the increased availability of donor organs there. Even if only because of these possible conditions for transplantation, further research is needed to determine which patients with ARESLD would have the best outcomes after liver transplantation.

Transplant programs have been reluctant to provide transplants to alcoholics because of concern about one unfavorable outcome: a high recidivism rate. Although the overall recidivism rate for the Pittsburgh patients was only 11.5%, in the patients who had been abstinent less than 6 months it was 43%.[2] Also, compared with the entire group in which 1-year survival was 74%, the survival rate in this subgroup was lower, at 64%.[2]

In the recently proposed Medicare criteria for coverage of liver transplantation, the HCFA acknowledged that the decision to insure patients with alcoholic cirrhosis "may be considered controversial by some."[5] As if to counter possible objections, the HCFA listed requirements for patients with alcoholic cirrhosis: patients must meet the transplant center's requirement for abstinence prior to liver transplantation and have documented evidence of sufficient social support to ensure both recovery from alcoholism and compliance with the regimen of immunosuppressive medication.

Further research should answer lingering questions about liver transplantation for ARESLD patients: Which characteristics of a patient with ARESLD can predict a successful outcome? How long is abstinence necessary to qualify for transplantation? What type of a social support system must a patient have to ensure good results? These questions are being addressed.[43] Until the answers are known, we propose that further transplantation for patients with ARESLD be limited to abstinent patients who had not previously been offered alcoholism treatment and to abstinent treated patients in regions of increased donor liver availability and that it be carried out as part of prospective research protocols at a few centers skilled in transplantation and alcohol research.

Comment

Should patients with ARESLD compete equally for liver transplants? In a setting in which there is a dire, absolute scarcity of donor livers, we believe the answer is no. Considerations of fairness suggest that a first-come, first-served approach for liver transplantation is not the most just approach. Although this decision is difficult, it is only fair that patients who have not assumed equal responsibility for maintaining their health or for accepting treatment for a chronic disease should be treated differently. Considerations of public values and mores suggest that the public may not support liver transplantation if patients with ARESLD routinely receive more than half of the available donor livers. We conclude that since not all can live, priorities must be established and that patients with ARESLD should be given a lower priority for liver transplantation than others with ESLD.

References

1   Scharschmidt B.F. Human liver transplantation: analysis of data on 540 patients from four centers. *Hepatology.* 1984; 4:95S–101S.

2   Kumar S., Stauber R.E., Gavaler J.S., et al. Orthotopic liver transplantation for alcoholic liver disease. *Hepatology.* 1990; 11:159–64.

3   Starzl T.E., Van Thiel D., Tzakis A.G., et al. Orthotopic liver transplantation for alcoholic cirrhosis. *JAMA.* 1988; 260:2542–4.

4   Olbrisch M.E. and Levenson J.L. Liver transplantation for alcoholic cirrhosis. *JAMA.* 1989; 261:2958.

5   Health Care Financing Administration. Medicare program: criteria for Medicare coverage of adult liver transplants. *Federal Register.* 1990; 55:3545–53.

6   Office of Health Technology Assessment, Agency for Health Care Policy Research. *Assessment of Liver Transplantation.* Rockville, MD: US Dept of Health and Human Services; 1990: 3, 25.

7   Schroeder J.S. and Hunt S. Cardiac transplantation update 1987. *JAMA.* 1987; 258:3142–5.

8   Surman O.S. Psychiatric aspects of organ transplantation. *Am J Psychiatry.* 1989; 146:972–82.

9   Welch H.G. and Larson E.B. Dealing with limited resources: the Oregon decision to curtail funding for organ transplantation. *N Engl J Med.* 1988; 319:171–3.

10 Flavin D.K., Niven R.G., and Kelsey J.E. Alcoholism and orthotopic liver transplantation. *JAMA.* 1988; 259:1546–7.

11 Atterbury C.E. The alcoholic in the lifeboat: should drinkers be candidates for liver transplantation? *J Clin Gastroenterol.* 1986; 8:1–4.

12 Mendelson J.H. and Mello N.K. *The Diagnosis and Treatment of Alcoholism.* 2nd ed. New York, NY: McGraw-Hill International Book Co; 1985:1–20.

13 Blum K., Noble E.P., Sheridan P.J., et al. Allelic association of human dopamine D_2 receptor gene in alcoholism. *JAMA.* 1990; 263:2055–60.

14 Aronson M.D. Definition of alcoholism. In: Barnes H.N., Aronson M.D., and Delbanco T.L., eds. *Alcoholism: A Guide for the Primary Care Physician.* New York, NY: Springer-Verlag NY Inc; 1987; 9–15.

15 Klerman G.L. Treatment of alcoholism. *N Engl J Med.* 1989; 320:394–5.

16 *Seventh Special Report to the US Congress on Alcohol and Health.* Washington, DC: US Dept. Health and Human Services; 1990. Publication 90–1656.

17 Saxe L. *The Effectiveness and Costs of Alcoholism Treatment: Health Technology Case Study No. 22.* Washington, DC: Congress of the United States, Office of Technology Assessment; 1983; 3–6.

18 Nace E.P. *The Treatment of Alcoholism.* New York, NY: Brunner/Mazel Publishers; 1987; 43–6.

19 Galanter M., Talbott D., Gallegos K., Ruberstone E. Combined Alcoholics Anonymous and professional care for addicted physicians. *Am J Psychiatry.* 1990; 147:64–8.

20 Johnson B. and Clark W. Alcoholism: a challenging physician–patient encounter. *J Gen Intern Med.* 1989; 4:445–52.

21 Bigby J.A. Negotiating treatment and monitoring recovery. In: Barnes H.N., Aronson M.D., and Delbanco T.L., eds. *Alcoholism: A Guide for the Primary Care Physician.* New York, NY: Springer Verlag NY Inc; 1987; 66–72.

22 Grant B.F., Dufour M.C., and Harford T.C. Epidemiology of alcoholic liver disease. *Sem Liver Dis.* 1988; 8:12–25.

23 Thoreson R.W. and Budd F.C. Self-help groups and other group procedures for treating alcohol problems. In: Cox W.M., ed. *Treatment and Prevention of Alcohol Problems: A Resource Manual.* Orlando, FL: Academic Press Inc; 1987; 157–81.

24 Winslow G.R. *Triage and Justice.* Berkeley: University of California Press; 1982:39–44, 133–150.

25 Engelhardt H.T. Jr. Shattuck Lecture: allocating scarce medical resources and the availability of organ transplantation. *N Engl J Med.* 1984; 311:66–71.

26 Outka G. Social justice and equal access to health care. *J Religious Ethics.* 1974; 2:11–32.

27 Beauchamp T.L. and Childress J.F. *Principles of Biomedical Ethics.* 3rd ed. New York, NY: Oxford University Press; 1989:; 256–306.

28 Ramsey P. *The Patient as Person.* New Haven, Conn: Yale University Press; 1970; 242–52.

29 Fox R.C. and Swazey J.P. *The Courage to Fail.* 2nd ed. Chicago, Ill: University of Chicago Press, 1978; 226–65.

30 Annas G.J. The prostitute, the playboy, and the poet: rationing schemes for organ transplantation. *Am J Public Health.* 1985; 75:187–9.

31 Blank R.H. *Rationing Medicine.* New York, NY: Columbia University Press; 1988; 1–37, 189–252.

32 Knowles J.H. Responsibility for health. *Science.* 1977; 198:1103.

33 Moore R.D, Bone L.R., Geller G., Marmon J.A., Stokes E.J., and Levine D.M. Prevalence, detection, and treatment of alcoholism in hospitalized patients. *JAMA.* 1989; 261:403–7.

34 Fuchs V.R. The 'rationing' of medical care. *N Engl J Med.* 1984; 311:1572–3.

35 Daniels N. Why saying no to patients in the United States is so hard: cost containment, justice, and provider autonomy. *N Engl J Med.* 1986; 314:1380–3.

36 Callahan D. Allocating health resources. *Hastings Cent Rep.* 1988; 18:14–20.

37 Evans R.W. Health care technology and the inevitability of resource allocation and rationing decisions. *JAMA.* 1983; 249:2047–53, 2208–19.

38 Thurow L.C. Learning to say no. *N Engl J Med.* 1984; 311:1569–72.

39 Caper P. Solving the medical care dilemma. *N Engl J Med.* 1988; 318:1535–6.

40 Task Force on Organ Transplantation. *Organ Transplantation: Issues and Recommendations.* Washington, DC: US Dept of Health and Human Services; 1986; 9.

41 Louis Harris and Associates. *Making Difficult Health Care Decisions.* Boston, Mass: The LORAN Commission; 1987; 73–89.

42 Fishman R. *Alcohol and Alcoholism.* New York, NY: Chelsea House Publishers; 1986; 27–34.

43 Beresford T.P., Turcotte J.G., Merion R., et al. A rational approach to liver transplantation for the alcoholic patient. *Psychosomatics.* 1990; 31:241–54.

Part VI

Obtaining Organs

Introduction

In organ transplantation solid organs and tissues – as distinct from blood or cells – are removed from the body of one individual (the organ donor) and placed into the body of another. Organs can be taken from living or from dead donors. Solid organs available for transplantation are scarce, and some of the difficult ethical issues raised by the problem of scarcity are discussed in Part V Resources Allocation. When distributing scarce resources, the primary focus is on the criteria that determine who should have access to the resource – given that the resource cannot be made available to everyone. The essays in the present Part of the *Anthology*, on the other hand, focus primarily on those from whom the organs are obtained, and on some of the important ethical issues raised by different approaches to the procurement of organs, and attempts to increase their supply.

In "Organ Donation and Retrieval: Whose Body is it, Anyway?", Eike-Henner W. Kluge starts by presenting the widely shared view that a paid organ procurement system would do little for the poor. Unable to afford the organs, they would, Kluge writes, "become the walking organ banks of the well-to-do." Kluge then proceeds to address the question of how organ shortages might be alleviated.

While most countries have rejected commercial systems – opting instead for an approach that limits the freedom of individuals to decide what will happen to their bodies during their lifetime and after death – there are great variations between the different approaches taken by different countries and states. Countries like Australia for example, have "opting in" systems of organ donation. Under an "opting in" system people can volunteer to donate organs after their death. Some European countries, including Belgium, Spain, and France, have adopted "opting out" systems. Here the assumption is that all citizens are potential organ donors, unless they opt out of the system, that is, withdraw their presumed consent.

Kluge supports various steps, including the adoption of presumed-consent legislation, to alleviate the shortage of organs for transplantation. In the absence of such laws, he also advocates making use of another source of organs that can become available without a change in the law, but merely a change in the way in which transplant societies work. At present, the protocols of transplant societies in countries with "opting in" legislation typically require the consent of the next of kin, even when the prior wishes of the deceased person are clear. Organ retrieval will not proceed without the next of kin's consent. The fact that the wishes of relatives can thus trump the wishes of deceased family members, runs counter, Kluge argues, to contemporary consent laws, which state

Bioethics: An Anthology, Fourth Edition. Edited by Udo Schüklenk and Peter Singer.
Editorial material and organization © 2022 John Wiley & Sons, Inc. Published 2022 by John Wiley & Sons, Inc.

that a competent person's consent to organ donation is "full" and "binding".

Violation of consent is, however, not – Kluge continues his argument – the only or most important consequence of transplant societies insisting on next-of-kin consent: this insistence also entails that the organ shortage is greater than it needs to be and people are dying while waiting for an organ. As Kluge concludes, "not only does that violate the autonomous decision of the donor, it also costs lives."

It is common ground between Kluge and Janet Radcliffe-Richards and her colleagues ("The Case for Allowing Kidney Sales") that the shortage of organs for transplantation causes suffering and death and that this tragic toll could be reduced if more organs were available. Unfortunately, in that respect there has been little change since these articles were published, in 1998–9. As Debra Satz reports in "Ethical Issues in the Supply and Demand of Human Kidneys," several new techniques have been employed in attempts to increase the supply of kidneys (including some that Kluge suggests) but it remains true that many people are suffering and dying because of the shortage of kidneys for transplantation. Satz indicates that in the United States alone, several thousand patients on the waiting list for a kidney die every year, some of whom would not have died if a kidney had been available.

For most commodities, a shortage leads to an increase in price which in turn provides a greater incentive to potential sellers, thus increasing the supply and overcoming, or at least reducing, the shortage. At present (2020) the sale of organs is illegal everywhere except in Iran, and international bodies like the United Nations and the World Health Organization support an international ban on organ sales. This has not put a stop to the international illegal market in kidneys.

The suggestion that it should be possible to buy and sell organs usually receives an extremely hostile reception both in the popular media and among members of professional organizations involved with organ transplantation. Radcliffe-Richards et al. urge professionals to reconsider the issue with a more open mind. The usual arguments against the sale of kidneys are, they contend, surprisingly weak, and the best explanation of their acceptance is that they are a way to justify our almost automatic feeling of repugnance at the idea of buying and selling human body parts. But the burden of justifying a prohibition that causes a great deal of avoidable death and suffering is heavy, and feelings of disgust are not sufficient to discharge it.

Debra Satz's discussion of the ethical issues in the supply and demand of human kidneys – a chapter from her book *Why Some Things Should Not Be for Sale: The Moral Limits of Markets* – responds to the voices that have recently been raised in support of re-examining the ban on kidney sales. Drawing on recent research, she casts doubt on the claim that offering payment for kidneys would increase the supply, noting that it might cause altruistic donations to decline. Still, she acknowledges that at some price, the offer of payment will no doubt increase the net supply of kidneys. Would selling kidneys be wrong even if it did increase the supply, and thus save lives? Would it, for instance, be wrong because people in desperate poverty are not in a position to give their free consent to the sale of their bodily organs? Do we want a world in which the poor survive by selling their organs to the rich? Satz carefully considers these and other objections to a market for organs, and asks whether various forms of regulation could help to overcome them. Whatever else one might think about her reasoning, she has certainly moved the discussion well beyond rationalizations for a feeling of repugnance.

In the last essay in this Part, John Harris puts forward an ingenious proposal to increase the supply of organs, and to give each of us as long and healthy a life as is possible. On the face of it, his proposed "survival lottery" appears to be an eminently sensible scheme that has the potential to save large numbers of lives, and increase everybody's chances of reaching a ripe old age. But is Harris making a serious proposal, or is he instead provoking us to re-examine our assumptions about the extent to which it would be desirable to pool our risks in order to preserve lives?

50

Organ Donation and Retrieval

Whose Body is it Anyway?

Eike-Henner W. Kluge

One of the most important advances in acute care medicine over the last thirty years has been the development of organ transplantation. In many instances, such as end-stage liver and heart disease, organ transplantation saves lives. In others, such as kidney disease, organ transplantation frees patients from dependence on expensive medical technology and allows them to resume an almost normal mode of existence. From a humane perspective, this makes organ transplantation very attractive.

The benefits of organ transplantation are not confined to patients. Kidney transplantation is economically more cost-effective than continued renal dialysis of patients; and as transplantation techniques become more sophisticated for other organs, similar cost savings will be realized in other areas as well. Therefore, as health-care resources are increasingly being diminished, transplantation emerges as an appealing health-care modality.

However, organ transplantation depends on the availability of organs. All countries are experiencing an acute shortage of human organs for transplantation. At any given time and in any jurisdiction, there are hundreds of people waiting for transplants.[1] Quite literally, they are waiting for a new lease on life. That is why transplant societies in all countries are doing their best to raise organ donor awareness so that more people will donate their organs; and why medical establishments and surgical teams are working to improve their techniques of organ recovery and transplantation. When the lack of a suitable organ may mean death, every organ counts and no organ may be wasted.

The responses to this organ shortage have been varied. Some countries treat human organs and bodies as commodities that belong to the individual person and that may be sold by these individuals for a valuable consideration. This lets economics decide who will have access to transplantable organs and entails that market forces determine how organ shortages are dealt with. If the shortage is severe – so goes the theory – prices for organs will go up, sellers will appear in the market-place and the shortage will thus be alleviated.

Most countries have rejected this position for several reasons. *First*, they believe that people have such

Original publication details: Eike-Henner W. Kluge, "Organ Donation and Retrieval: Whose Body Is It Anyway?" © 1999 Eike-Henner W. Kluge.

a close association with their bodies that to consider bodies and organs as property is tantamount to considering the people themselves as chattels. Hence they maintain that neither bodies nor body parts may be bought or sold. *Second*, they believe that if the ownership (and hence sale) of bodies or body parts were to be allowed, this would lead to a state of affairs where the rich would take advantage of the poor by offering such high prices for human organs that the poor would be unable to resist the enticement. The poor would therefore become the walking organ banks of the well-to-do. While this might alleviate the organ shortage in the case of affluent persons in need of organs, it would do nothing about the transplantation needs and the availability of organs for the poor.

In contrast, therefore, most countries have adopted the position that, while there is no ownership in human bodies, everyone has a right to decide what shall happen with her or his own body and that this right extends even beyond death. Beyond this, however, there is no general agreement. Some countries have instituted presumed consent legislation. That is to say, they have passed laws which mandate that, unless people have explicitly stipulated that they do not wish to be organ donors, their organs will be retrieved once they are dead. Other countries view organ donation as a supererogatory act that cannot reasonably be expected of all persons. Consequently they have passed laws which state that specific agreement to donation is a *sine qua non* for organ retrieval, and that this agreement must come either from the potential donor during her or his life time or, in the case of persons who have not made a decision in this matter, from those who are legally in possession of the body after the person is dead. These usually are the next of kin.

Unquestionably, the voluntary approach to organ donation can easily exacerbate the shortage of transplantable organs simply because potential donors (or their relatives) may be reluctant to agree to donation. This reluctance may be grounded in religious precepts which construe the removal of an organ as the sacrilegious mutilation of the body and hence consider it anathema. Alternatively, the refusal may be grounded

in a psychological perspective that finds organ retrieval personally offensive on aesthetic grounds. Finally, the refusal to donate may be based on a mere misunderstanding about the process of retrieval itself and the nature of death. Specifically, it may be based on the assumption that death occurs only when there is a complete and irremediable cardiovascular collapse of the body which cannot be alleviated even by mechanical ventilation. This leads to the refusal to allow organ retrieval until after all such attempts have proved unsuccessful – which effectively guarantees that the relevant organs have also deteriorated beyond the point of usefulness for transplantation.

A further contribution to the shortage of organs lies in the fact that many potential donors are simply unaware of the option of donation. Hence organs that otherwise might well be donated are never retrieved.

There is little that can be done about a refusal to donate which finds its basis in religious conviction, short of changing the tenets of the relevant religion or prohibiting adherence to the religion itself. Neither of these is morally acceptable. With due alteration of details, similar considerations apply to refusals to donate that are based on personal aesthetics.

On the other hand, organ shortages that are grounded in misinformation or in ignorance of the option of donation can be alleviated by properly focused and conducted educational campaigns. Physicians can be encouraged to raise the subject of donation with their patients, to educate them about the benefits of donation and to explain to them the nature of death. Further, transplant societies can maximize the chance of retrieving donated organs by establishing organ donor registers which list everyone who has agreed to being a donor. On the death of such a person, it would be known immediately whether that person had agreed to donation.

Furthermore, it has been suggested that all jurisdictions adopt presumed consent legislation. In this way, it is hoped, the supply of organs will be increased because refusal to donate would have to be explicitly expressed.

However, there is a readily available supply of organs which does not require the establishment of registers or changes in the current laws. Access to this supply does not require a change in anything – except in the way in which the various transplant societies work.

More precisely, in many countries that have consent legislation, the law states that the consent of a competent person is "full" and "binding" authority for the removal of that person's organs after death for the purposes of transplantation. In legal terms, the word "full" means that if someone has given consent, then this consent is sufficient and no one else needs to be asked for permission, while the term "binding" means that others may not overrule the consent of the donor and substitute their own wishes. Such consent is usually signified by an organ donor card or an organ donor sticker on the person's driver's licence.

Almost without exception, the organ retrieval protocols of most transplant societies are out of step with these provisions. Almost invariably, they state that the consent of the next of kin is required for organ retrieval *even when there is a donor card or sticker*. They further state that if the next of kin refuse the donation, the organs will not be retrieved.

In countries which have consent legislation that recognizes the individual's right to donate, these protocols clearly violate the law. In the great scheme of things, that may not be too important. However, what *is* important is that, because of these protocols, many organs that could be retrieved and used to save lives are never recovered. In other words, because of these protocols, the current organ shortage is greater than it needs to be, people are on waiting lists when they do not have to be, and people are dying while waiting for a suitable organ.

These are preventable deaths. They are therefore tragic. They are all the more tragic because they have ramifications far beyond the immediate sphere of the donor and the prospective recipient: they have implications for the availability of health care in general. Every organ that is not retrieved represents increased health-care costs for society. Health-care resources are finite: What is given to the one is taken away from the other. Therefore the impact of this non-retrieval affects not only the person who could have received the organ but everyone in the health-care system as a whole.

These protocols also have serious ethical implications for the ethics of informed consent. What the transplant societies are in effect saying with their guidelines is that the informed donor consent will not be considered binding if the donor is no longer capable of enforcing her or his wishes. Such an attitude sends the message that organ donation really doesn't mean anything: that the wishes of others really carry the day. If that practice were to be adopted in other areas of health care, informed consent would become meaningless. In fact, it would become a farce. It is surprising that, under the circumstances, anyone bothers to donate organs at all!

The transplant societies have argued that to retrieve organs against the wishes of the next of kin runs the danger of being perceived as ghouls, and that the negative publicity that would surround such actions might well result in a drop in organ donation. That is why they have proposed the establishment of a donor register, and that the law be changed in all jurisdictions in favour of presumed consent.

Unquestionably, the establishment of organ donor registers would be useful. So would the proposed change in legislation. Unfortunately, however, neither of these comes to grips with the real issue; and more important, neither of them would change the situation.

A register is useful only if the donors who are registered actually have their organs retrieved upon death. There is nothing inherent in a register to ensure that this would take place.

As to the proposed consent legislation, it would still leave the possibility that the next of kin might say *no* to organ retrieval even though the donor him- or herself had not said *no*. Therefore unless, under presumed consent legislation, the next of kin were *not asked for their consent*, the number of organ retrievals would not go up. The same number of next of kin who now refuse consent would also refuse their consent under the new legislation. The only way to avoid this would be not to ask the next of kin (or to ignore what they might say) and simply go on the assumption that, if the person had not wanted her or his organs retrieved, he or she would have said so. Therefore these proposed laws would work *only if the transplant societies acted the way they are supposed to act even under the current laws*. There is considerable justification for doubting that this would be the case.

The crux of the matter is really this: do people have the right to decide what shall be done with their body after they are dead? In particular, do they have the right to donate their organs in order to save lives? The answer may vary from society to society. However, once such a right is recognized, the ethics of informed consent entails that the donor's decision should not be overruled – or ignored – simply because others are uncomfortable with that decision. Not only does that violate the autonomous decision of the donor, it also costs lives. If others – e.g., the next of kin – are uncomfortable with the donor's decision, what is called for is not a refusal to follow the donor's last bequest but appropriate education and counselling in the ethics of donation and informed consent.

Always following the wishes of organ donors would not do away with the current shortage of organs. However, this shortage would not be so great if the donated organs were in fact retrieved, if the wishes of donors were followed – and if the ethics of informed consent were taken seriously. When every organ is a life, can one be less than ethical?

Note

1   Personal communication with various transplant organizations in Canada, US and Europe.

51

The Case for Allowing Kidney Sales

Janet Radcliffe-Richards, A. S. Daar, R. D. Guttmann,
R. Hoffenberg, I. Kennedy, M. Lock, R. A. Sells and N. Tilney
and for the International Forum Transplant Ethics

When the practice of buying kidneys from live vendors first came to light some years ago, it aroused such horror that all professional associations denounced it[1, 2] and nearly all countries have now made it illegal.[3, 4] Such political and professional unanimity may seem to leave no room for further debate, but we nevertheless think it important to reopen the discussion.

The well-known shortage of kidneys for transplantation causes much suffering and death. Dialysis is a wretched experience for most patients, and is anyway rationed in most places and simply unavailable to the majority of patients in most developing countries.[5] Since most potential kidney vendors will never become unpaid donors, either during life or posthumously, the prohibition of sales must be presumed to exclude kidneys that would otherwise be available. It is therefore essential to make sure that there is adequate justification for the resulting harm.

Most people will recognise in themselves the feelings of outrage and disgust that led to an outright ban on kidney sales, and such feelings typically have a force that seems to their possessors to need no further justification. Nevertheless, if we are to deny treatment to the suffering and dying we need better reasons than our own feelings of disgust.

In this paper we outline our reasons for thinking that the arguments commonly offered for prohibiting organ sales do not work, and therefore that the debate should be reopened.[6, 7] Here we consider only the selling of kidneys by living vendors, but our arguments have wider implications.

The commonest objection to kidney selling is expressed on behalf of the vendors: the exploited poor, who need to be protected against the greedy rich. However, the vendors are themselves anxious to sell,[8] and see this practice as the best option open to them. The worse we think the selling of a kidney, therefore, the worse should seem the position of the vendors when that option is removed. Unless this appearance is illusory, the prohibition of sales does even more harm than first seemed, in harming vendors as well as recipients. To this argument it is replied that the vendors' apparent choice is not genuine. It is said that they are likely to be too uneducated to understand the risks, and that this precludes informed consent. It is also claimed that, since they are coerced

Original publication details: Janet Radcliffe-Richards et al., "The Case for Allowing Kidney Sales," pp. 1950–1952 from *The Lancet* 351: 9120 (June 27, 1998). Reproduced with permission of Elsevier.

Bioethics: An Anthology, Fourth Edition. Edited by Udo Schüklenk and Peter Singer.

by their economic circumstances, their consent cannot count as genuine.[9]

Although both these arguments appeal to the importance of autonomous choice, they are quite different. The first claim is that the vendors are not competent to make a genuine choice within a given range of options. The second, by contrast, is that poverty has so restricted the range of options that organ selling has become the best, and therefore, in effect, that the range is too small. Once this distinction is drawn, it can be seen that neither argument works as a justification of prohibition.[7]

If our ground for concern is that the range of choices is too small, we cannot improve matters by removing the best option that poverty has left, and making the range smaller still. To do so is to make subsequent choices, by this criterion, even less autonomous. The only way to improve matters is to lessen the poverty until organ selling no longer seems the best option; and if that could be achieved, prohibition would be irrelevant because nobody would want to sell.

The other line of argument may seem more promising, since ignorance does preclude informed consent. However, the likely ignorance of the subjects is not a reason for banning altogether a procedure for which consent is required. In other contexts, the value we place on autonomy leads us to insist on information and counselling, and that is what it should suggest in the case of organ selling as well. It may be said that this approach is impracticable, because the educational level of potential vendors is too limited to make explanation feasible, or because no system could reliably counteract the misinformation of nefarious middlemen and profiteering clinics. But, even if we accepted that no possible vendor could be competent to consent, that would justify only putting the decision in the hands of competent guardians. To justify total prohibition it would also be necessary to show that organ selling must always be against the interests of potential vendors, and it is most unlikely that this would be done.

The risk involved in nephrectomy is not in itself high, and most people regard it as acceptable for living related donors.[10] Since the procedure is, in principle, the same for vendors as for unpaid donors, any systematic difference between the worthwhileness of the risk for vendors and donors presumably lies on the other side of the calculation, in the expected benefit. Nevertheless the exchange of money cannot in itself turn an acceptable risk into an unacceptable one from the vendor's point of view. It depends entirely on what the money is wanted for.

In general, furthermore, the poorer a potential vendor, the more likely it is that the sale of a kidney will be worth whatever risk there is. If the rich are free to engage in dangerous sports for pleasure, or dangerous jobs for high pay, it is difficult to see why the poor who take the lesser risk of kidney selling for greater rewards – perhaps saving relatives' lives,[11] or extricating themselves from poverty and debt – should be thought so misguided as to need saving from themselves.

It will be said that this does not take account of the reality of the vendors' circumstances: that risks are likely to be greater than for unpaid donors because poverty is detrimental to health, and vendors are often not given proper care. They may also be underpaid or cheated, or may waste their money through inexperience. However, once again, these arguments apply far more strongly to many other activities by which the poor try to earn money, and which we do not forbid. The best way to address such problems would be by regulation and perhaps a central purchasing system, to provide screening, counselling, reliable payment, insurance, and financial advice.[12]

To this it will be replied that no system of screening and control could be complete, and that both vendors and recipients would always be at risk of exploitation and poor treatment. But all the evidence we have shows that there is much more scope for exploitation and abuse when a supply of desperately wanted goods is made illegal. It is, furthermore, not clear why it should be thought harder to police a legal trade than the present complete ban.

Furthermore, even if vendors and recipients would always be at risk of exploitation, that does not alter the fact that, if they choose this option, all alternatives must seem worse to them. Trying to end exploitation by prohibition is rather like ending slum dwelling by bulldozing slums: it ends the evil in that form, but only by making things worse for the victims. If we want to protect the exploited, we can do it only by removing the poverty that makes them vulnerable, or, failing that, by controlling the trade.

Another familiar objection is that it is unfair for the rich to have privileges not available to the poor. This argument, however, is irrelevant to the issue of organ selling as such. If organ selling is wrong for this reason, so are all benefits available to the rich, including all private medicine, and, for that matter, all public provision of medicine in rich countries (including transplantation of donated organs) that is unavailable in poor ones. Furthermore, all purchasing could be done by a central organisation responsible for fair distribution.[12]

It is frequently asserted that organ donation must be altruistic to be acceptable,[13] and that this rules out payment. However, there are two problems with this claim. First, altruism does not distinguish donors from vendors. If a father who saves his daughter's life by giving her a kidney is altruistic, it is difficult to see why his selling a kidney to pay for some other operation to save her life should be thought less so. Second, nobody believes in general that unless some useful action is altruistic it is better to forbid it altogether.

It is said that the practice would undermine confidence in the medical profession, because of the association of doctors with money-making practices. That, however, would be a reason for objecting to all private practice; and in this case the objection could easily be met by the separation of purchasing and treatment. There could, for instance, be independent trusts[12] to fix charges and handle accounts, as well as to ensure fair play and high standards. It is alleged that allowing the trade would lessen the supply of donated cadaveric kidneys.[14] But, although some possible donors might decide to sell instead, their organs would be available, so there would be no loss in the total. And

in the meantime, many people will agree to sell who would not otherwise donate.

It is said that in parts of the world where women and children are essentially chattels there would be a danger of their being coerced into becoming vendors. This argument, however, would work as strongly against unpaid living kidney donation, and even more strongly against many far more harmful practices which do not attract calls for their prohibition. Again, regulation would provide the most reliable means of protection.

It is said that selling kidneys would set us on a slippery slope to selling vital organs such as hearts. But that argument would apply equally to the case of the unpaid kidney donation, and nobody is afraid that that will result in the donation of hearts. It is entirely feasible to have laws and professional practices that allow the giving or selling only of non-vital organs. Another objection is that allowing organ sales is impossible because it would outrage public opinion. But this claim is about western public opinion: in many potential vendor communities, organ selling is more acceptable than cadaveric donation, and this argument amounts to a claim that other people should follow western cultural preferences rather than their own. There is, anyway, evidence that the western public is far less opposed to the idea than are medical and political professionals.[15]

It must be stressed that we are not arguing for the positive conclusion that organ sales must always be acceptable, let alone that there should be an unfettered market. Our claim is only that none of the familiar arguments against organ selling works, and this allows for the possibility that better arguments may yet be found.

Nevertheless, we claim that the burden of proof remains against the defenders of prohibition, and that, until good arguments appear, the presumption must be that the trade should be regulated rather than banned altogether. Furthermore, even when there are good objections at particular times or in particular places, that should be regarded as a reason for trying to remove the objections, rather than as an excuse for permanent prohibition.

The weakness of the familiar arguments suggests that they are attempts to justify the deep feelings of repugnance which are the real driving force of prohibition, and feelings of repugnance among the rich and healthy, no matter how strongly felt, cannot justify removing the only hope of the destitute and dying. This is why we conclude that the issue should be considered again, and with scrupulous impartiality.

References

1   British Transplantation Society Working Party, Guidelines on living organ donation. *BMJ* 293 (1986), pp. 257–8.
2   The Council of the Transplantation Society, Organ sales. *Lancet* 2 (1985), pp. 715–16.
3   World Health Organization. A report on developments under the auspices of WHO (1987–1991). Geneva: WHO, 1992: 12–28.
4   P.J. Hauptman and K.J. O'Connor, Procurement and allocation of solid organs for transplantation. *N Engl J Med* 336 (1997), pp. 422–31.
5   R.S. Barsoum. Ethical problems in dialysis and transplantation: Africa. In: C.M. Kjellstrand and J.B. Dossetor, eds. *Ethical problems in dialysis and transplantation*: Netherlands: Kluwer Academic Publishers, 1992: 169–82.
6   J. Radcliffe-Richards, Nephrarious goings on: kidney sales and moral arguments. *J Med Philosoph. Netherlands: Kluwer Academic Publishers*, 21 (1996), pp. 375–416.
7   J. Radcliffe-Richards, From him that hath not. In: C.M. Kjellstrand and J.B. Dossetor, eds. *Ethical problems in dialysis and transplantation*. Netherlands: Kluwer Academic Publishers, 1992: 53–60.

8   M.K. Mani. The argument against the unrelated live donor, ibid. 164.
9   R.A. Sells, The case against buying organs and a futures market in transplants. *Trans Proc* 24 (1992), pp. 2198–2202.
10 A.D. Daar, W. Land, T.M. Yahya, K. Schneewind, T. Gutmann, and A. Jakobsen, Living-donor renal transplantation: evidence-based justification for an ethical option. *Trans Reviews* 11 (1997), pp. 95–109.
11 J.B. Dossetor and V. Manickavel, Commercialisation: the buying and selling of kidneys. In: C.M. Kjellstrand and J.B. Dossetor, eds. *Ethical problems in dialysis and transplantation*. Netherlands: Kluwer Academic Publishers, 1992: 61–71.
12 R.A. Sells, Some ethical issues in organ retrieval 1982–1992. *Trans Proc* 24 (1992), pp. 2401–3.
13 R. Sheil, Policy statement from the ethics committee of the Transplantation Society. *Trans Soc Bull* 3 (1995), p. 3.
14 J.S. Altshuler and M.J. Evanisko. *JAMA* 267 (1992), p. 2037.
15 R.D. Guttmann and A. Guttmann, Organ transplantation: duty reconsidered. *Trans Proc* 24 (1992), pp. 2179–80.

52

Ethical Issues in the Supply and Demand of Kidneys

Debra Satz

Societies sometimes ban the sale of goods whose supply they actually wish to support or encourage.[1] Examples include bans on markets in votes, children, and human organs. In the United States sales of organs such as kidneys are currently illegal, and those needing transplants must rely on altruistic donation. From an economic perspective, an organ ban appears inefficient, as it seems likely that payments to donors would elicit greater supply, thereby reducing chronic shortages. From a libertarian perspective, a ban on organ sales is an illegitimate infringement on personal liberty; allowing people to sell their own body parts is merely a way of recognizing their legitimate sphere of control.[2] Nonlibertarian proponents of a market in human organs also argue that a ban on sales is morally dubious because lives would be saved by the increased supply.

The idea of establishing a kidney market is now attracting unprecedented support among those involved in transplantation, as well as among economists and medical ethicists. This chapter examines the values at stake. But I also raise a distinct consideration that is relevant to these markets: the link between markets and motives. Unlike the cases of child labor, bonded labor, sex, and surrogacy, we have an interest in motivating people to act in ways that increase the supply of transplant organs.

Brief Background: The Status Quo Systems of Kidney Procurement

Despite the prima facie case for organ markets just noted, kidney selling is currently illegal in every developed society in the world.[3] The United Nations and the European Union have instructed their member countries to prohibit the sale of body parts. The World Health Organization has interpreted the Universal Declaration of Human Rights as prohibiting the sale of organs. Indeed most of the globe's countries have enacted legal bans of such sales, although states differ dramatically in their enforcement capacity, and a black market thrives in many countries.

In the United States people can donate their kidneys after death or while they are alive only out of altruism. The Uniform Anatomical Gift Act,

Original publication details: Debra Satz, "Ethical Issues in the Supply and Demand of Human Kidneys," pp. 189–206 from *Why Some Things Should Not Be for Sale: The Moral Limits of Markets* (New York: Oxford University Press, 2010). based on an article from *Proceedings of the Aristotelian Society 2* (2010). Reproduced with permission of Oxford University Press and the Aristotelian Society.

drafted in 1984 (the same year the National Organ Transplantation Act was enacted), made it illegal for anyone to receive any payment, or "valuable consideration," for providing an organ. Instead those who need kidneys must rely largely on individual or social exhortation to induce people to donate. The result is that most live donations come from close relatives or intimates, with parents entrusted to make decisions about whether a child can serve as a donor for a sibling or relative. Individuals have a right to donate their kidneys to loved ones, but not a right to sell them.

Cadaver organs in the United States come from two main groups: those who explicitly consented to have their organs used after their death, whether through a living will or indicating a wish to be a donor on a driver's license, and those who are *presumed* to have consented. More than fifteen states rely on presumed consent laws, whereby someone who undergoes a mandatory autopsy (often in the context of a homicide) is presumed to have consented to the use of some of his organs unless he explicitly objected to such donations prior to his death.[4] (In the United States presumed consent laws are limited to bodies under the authority of the coroner or medical examiner.)

Individuals also have the right *not* to donate their organs; *no* society makes kidney donation mandatory. Current US law protects living persons from having their organs taken from them without their consent, even in cases in which another person's life is at stake.[5] If exhortation fails to secure an organ, the person needing the donation has no (legal) recourse but instead must wait his turn on the transplant list.[6] Currently there are long queues for obtaining a kidney. In the United States alone there were more than fifty thousand Americans on the waiting list for a kidney in 2003. That same year there were twelve thousand donors.[7] This means that thirty-eight thousand people were carried over onto the 2004 waiting list, along with the year's new additions to that list. Many people wait years before an organ becomes available. Several thousand people die each year in the United States alone while waiting for an organ transplant.[8] Some of these people would not have died had an organ been available for them at the time they needed it most.[9]

A number of European societies rely on an opt-out system of organ procurement rather than the opt-in system used in the United States. In many nations – including Austria, Belgium, Denmark, Finland, France, Italy, Luxemburg, Norway, Singapore, and Spain – all individuals are presumed to consent to allow their organs to be used after their death for the benefit of others. In an opt-out system the default position is that every individual's organs are available on her demise, although each individual is permitted to rebut the presumption (to opt out), usually signaled by an explicit notation on a driver's license.[10]

Moving toward an opt-out baseline allocation system could be a justified social policy if it saved lives, but it does not appear to solve the shortage of organs needed for transplant. Shortages remain in many European countries, including in those that rely on opt-out allocation systems.[11] In fact some studies suggest that the choice of opt-out systems over opt-in systems often makes little difference to the ultimate numbers of organs procured.[12] This result might seem counterintuitive, but there are three reasons why changing the default starting point might not increase the yield of organs. First, many countries with opt-out systems give relatives a right of refusal with respect to cadaveric donations, even when the deceased indicated support for such donations. And relatives frequently choose to forgo donation for religious or personal reasons. Second, many procured organs are simply not suitable for transplantation; the deceased may have been very old or very sick or not found in time for his organs to be useful after death.[13] And the ability to effectively procure an organ, to safely and quickly remove it and deliver it for transplantation, seems to depend crucially on institutional factors.[14] Third, given burgeoning rates of obesity and diabetes and longer life spans, the numbers of people needing kidney transplants continues to grow at a faster rate than do increases in the supply.

Anti-Market Considerations

As we have seen, the free market has considerable appeal: freedom of contract is taken to promote liberty;

competitive markets are supposed to pay each input what it deserves (its marginal product); and markets tend to be extremely efficient mechanisms for the production and distribution of goods. Given the shortages in available kidneys and the strong interests at stake, it is not surprising that when a kidney was offered for sale on eBay the bidding reached $5.8 million before being shut down by the administrators of the site because the sale would violate US law.[15]

Despite such considerations, I think there are reasons to be wary of jumping on the growing bandwagon for a market in human kidneys. Some of these reasons turn on nonideal features in a nonideal world and can be addressed through regulation; some of these reasons would hold in any realistic world.

Does a Market Ban Necessarily Decrease the Supply of Available Organs?

In his famous study *The Gift Relationship*, Richard Titmuss argued that a purely altruistic system for procuring blood is superior to a system that relies on a combination of altruistic donation plus a market.[16] Comparing the American and British systems of procuring blood, he demonstrated that a system of donated blood (the British system) is superior in quality to a system that also uses purchased blood (the American system), in part because blood sellers have a reason to conceal their illnesses, whereas altruistic blood donors do not. Furthermore Titmuss claimed that offering financial incentives for blood leads those in need of money to supply too frequently, endangering their own health. According to Titmuss, an altruistic system is not only more ethical, but it also produces a blood supply of higher quality.

Titmuss also argued, to the surprise of many economists, that a system that relied only on altruistic donation might be more *efficient* than a market system for blood. He claimed that, with respect to blood, the introduction of markets "represses the expression of altruism [and] erodes the sense of community."[17] If blood is treated as a commodity with an associated price tag, some people who would have donated

when doing so bestowed the "gift of life" now decline to donate. Therefore blood supply would not necessarily be increased by the addition of a market; indeed Titmuss hypothesized that the net result of introducing a market for blood in England would be *less* blood of inferior quality.

This might seem surprising. Insofar as we are simply adding a new choice (i.e., selling blood) to a set of existing options, why should any of the existing options (i.e., donating blood), or their attractiveness to altruistic individuals, change?[18] Why should policies that appeal to self-interest also lead people to act in a less public-spirited way?

Consider the following real-life experiment, which illustrates the market effect that Titmuss conjectured on motivation. Faced with parents who habitually arrived late to pick up their children at the end of the day, six Haifa day care centers imposed a fine for such parental lateness. They hoped that the fines would give these parents a self-interested reason to arrive on time. The parents responded to the fine by *doubling* the amount of time they were late.[19] Even when the fine was revoked three months later the enhanced lateness continued. One plausible interpretation of this result is that the fine undermined the parents' sense that they were morally obligated not to take advantage of the day care workers; instead they now saw their lateness as a commodity that could be purchased.

This result has been replicated using carefully designed experiments. The experimental economist Bruno Frey and others have examined circumstances where *intrinsic motivation* is partially destroyed when price incentives are introduced.[20] An action is intrinsically motivated when it is performed simply because of the satisfaction the agent derives from performing the action. Whereas conventional economic analysis assumes that offers for monetary compensation will increase the willingness to accept otherwise unwanted projects, Frey found that support for building a noxious nuclear waste facility in a neighborhood actually *decreased* when monetary compensation to host it was offered. His study suggests that in cases where individuals are civically minded, using price incentives will not increase but can actually decrease levels of support for civic actions. For an intrinsically motivated agent, performing an act for money is simply not the same act when it is performed for free.[21] The presence of monetary incentives can crowd out a person's intrinsic reasons for performing the given action, changing the attractiveness of the options he faces. For example, in the nuclear waste example, citizens may feel bribed by the offer of money. In the case of timely day care pickup, altruistic concern for the teachers may be replaced by self-interested calculation about the worth of avoiding the fine.

This kind of crowding-out altruism result is not inevitable; the market can also be harnessed in a socially beneficial and more *altruistic* direction. A study of the introduction of a market wherein people purchased access to express carpool lanes in San Diego found that the program's initiation correlated with increased overall traffic in the express lanes, decreased traffic in the main lanes, and a significant *increase* in carpooling levels. (Carpoolers have access to the express lanes but do not have to pay for this access.) The author hypothesizes that the most likely explanation for the increase in carpoolers is that new drivers were attracted to carpooling by a *relative* monetary benefit: they felt better about getting for free what others pay for.[22]

If these case studies are illustrative, markets can change social norms. And if introducing a market does affect intrinsic motivations, we cannot a priori predict in which direction the net change of behavior will go. In the nuclear waste example we get less prosocial behavior, but the reverse is true in the carpooling example. Of course, kidney markets and blood markets are different from markets in access to faster commuting. Donations of organs and blood often involve questions of life and death, not simply convenience, and so it may well be that different motivations are invoked in those performing altruistic actions, motivations that are more likely to be vulnerable to crowding out.

Would the introduction of a kidney market actually serve to reduce supply by crowding out those with altruistic motivations? Even if kidney markets drove out altruists, it is still possible that the net supply of kidneys would be increased. Maybe there are more potential extrinsically motivated donors than

donors who are only, or primarily, intrinsically motivated. Furthermore if the amount of organs procured through a market remained inadequate, increasing the price of organs would likely lead to more nonaltruistic donors. In Friedrich Dürrenmatt's splendid tragedy, *The Visit of the Old Lady*, an incredibly rich woman who had been wronged in her youth by her lover now offers the residents of her hometown $1 million to kill him. At first the offer is angrily rejected by the citizens as deeply immoral, but the woman induces them to raise their consumption and take on debts. Finally as they accommodate themselves to their new level of comfort, they decide to kill the lover who refused to accept paternity for her child so many years ago. Perhaps in the cases Frey and others examined the monetary rewards were simply insufficient to motivate people or offered before people had a chance to get used to the idea.[23]

It is also important to consider whether, if there are crowding-out effects on people with altruistic motivations, it is the case that *all* extrinsic rewards for giving up a kidney – including rewards to one's heirs after one's death, lifetime medical benefits, and payment of funeral costs – would have the same crowding-out effects as cash.[24]

Perhaps legalizing kidney sales decreases altruistic donation and at the same time increases the net supply of organs, at least if the price is right.[25] Whether or not it does so is an especially relevant consideration if a person's support for or opposition to organ markets rests solely on the effects of such markets on supply. Because the positive case for organ markets does largely rest on such grounds, it is clearly relevant to whether that case is a good one; moral motivations may be more fragile than we often assume. But whether the introduction of markets increases or decreases supply may not be decisive for some opponents of kidney markets; some people believe that kidney selling is wrong even if it increases supply.

Vulnerability

For some a kidney sale is objectionable because it is a paradigmatic *desperate exchange*, an exchange no one would ever make unless faced with no reasonable alternative. A kidney is, in the words of one organ market critic, the "organ of last resort."[26] Many people object to organ markets precisely because they believe that these markets would allow others to exploit the desperation of the poor. This objection to desperate exchanges is often associated with a paternalistic concern that sellers would actually be harmed by the sale of their organs, but that given their desperation they would sell their organs if it were legal.

A defender of organ markets might argue that the worries about exploitation could be addressed through regulation: by eliminating organ brokers who capture much of the price of the organ; by allowing open competition that is precluded by the black market; and by enforcing the terms of contracts. To address this concern, it might also be argued that organ donation should be legal only in contexts in which people are not likely to be desperately poor.[27]

Weak Agency

Whereas ideal markets involve fully informed participants, [. . .] many markets do not, and in fact cannot, function on that basis. This is sometimes because market transactions involve consequences that can be known only in the future. Kidney transplants involve surgical operations and, like all surgical operations, entail risks. In a careful study of India's kidney sellers, 86 percent of the participants in the study reported a marked deterioration in their health following their nephrectomy.[28] Although one kidney is capable of cleansing the blood if it is functioning well, the removal of a kidney leaves the seller vulnerable to future problems if the remaining kidney becomes damaged or if its filtering capability declines. (In fact the decrease in filtering capacity is a normal byproduct of aging.) Needless to say, the poor in the developing world who sell their kidneys have no health insurance and no claim on an additional kidney if their remaining one fails to function properly. Moreover, although most studies of kidney transplants have reported few adverse effects for the donors, these studies have been

overwhelmingly conducted in wealthy countries; we simply do not know whether people in poor countries do as well with only one kidney as those in rich countries. Health risks are likely to be greater in places where people have little access to clean water or adequate nutrition and often are engaged in difficult manual labor.

Two other findings in the study of Indian kidney sellers relate to concerns with weak agency. First, an overwhelming majority of those interviewed (79 percent) said that they regretted their decision and would not recommend that others sell a kidney. Second, a majority of sellers interviewed (71 percent) were married women. Given the weak position of women in Indian society, the voluntary nature of the sales is questionable. The most common explanation offered by wives as to why they and not their husbands sold their organs were that the husbands were the family's income source (30 percent) or were ill (28 percent). Of course, as the authors of the study point out, most of the interviews of women were conducted in the presence of their husbands or other family members, so they may have been reluctant to admit to being pressured to donate.

Weak agency is a serious problem for those who wish to base their defense of the market in organs on the right of a person to make her own decisions with respect to her body parts, and this is especially true when the weak agency is connected to significant harm. The fact that most organ sellers would not recommend the practice suggests that potential sellers would be unlikely to sell a kidney if they were better informed about the outcomes of their sale.[29] Perhaps it is difficult to imagine what it means to lose a kidney before one actually experiences the loss. When we couple the information problems with the lack of benefit, the case for allowing a kidney market is thereby weakened.[30]

A defender of organ markets might reply that the appropriate response to the diminished agency of sellers is simply to make sure they are better informed about the likely consequences of their transactions. For example, organ sellers could be required to take classes dealing with the risks of live organ donation and to demonstrate that they understand the likely consequences of giving up a kidney. However, given the horrific poverty that many sellers face, and perhaps their lack of education, it is unclear to what extent they will refrain from undertaking the transaction simply because of the risks. Additionally, in poorer countries regulatory institutions are weak and underfunded.

Note, however, that the argument from weak agency – lack of information about how a seller will feel in the future about her kidney sale – might lead us to discourage altruistic organ donations as well as paid donations. That is, weak agency doesn't really single out what is problematic about the kidney *market*.[31] If the potential health risks for donors are substantial, then perhaps all such transfers from living donors should be banned. (And it is doubtful whether altruistic donation is really made from the vantage point of full information and in the context of a range of choices. Family members are often under enormous pressure to donate and, as we have seen, parents are free to donate the organs of their own children.)

It is also important to consider just how substantial the potential harms are to organ donors and sellers. Currently we allow people to engage in risky occupations (e.g., work in nuclear reactor plants); we do not prohibit markets enabling people to engage in risky behaviors such as cigarette smoking and skydiving; and we rely on financial incentives in military recruitment, which also exposes individuals to grave risks. So, to the extent that the argument from weak agency is compelling because it is predictive of harm, it is important to consider whether or not the potential harms are worse than from other sales that we currently permit.[32]

Equal Status Considerations

Current black markets in kidneys certainly reflect the different market situations of buyer and seller. Most sellers are extremely poor; most buyers are at least comparatively wealthy. It has been keenly noted that international organ markets transfer organs from poor to rich, third world to first world, female to male, and nonwhite to white. Indeed the fact that there is increasing pressure to allow kidneys to be bought and sold itself arguably reflects the fact that those who seek to purchase them tend to have the cash to be able to do so.[33] Contrast this with the situation of poor people whose health needs currently go unmet. Despite the fact that urgent health needs are shared by millions (billions?) of desperately poor people, poor people have little cash. Therefore their health needs tend to get far less attention than the health needs of the comparatively wealthy.

A system that relied on a kidney market of individual buyers and sellers for procurement and distribution would have the consequence that poor people would disproportionately be the organ sellers of the world and rich people the likely recipients.[34] By contrast, a procurement system that relies on donation is much more likely to have suppliers that come from all classes of people. Indeed Titmuss found just such a contrast between the American and British systems of blood donation.[35]

In his haunting novel *Never Let Me Go*, Kazuo Ishiguro imagines a world in which human clones are created to serve as organ donors for others.[36] Before these created humans are middle-aged, they start to donate their vital organs. At the end of the novel these purposely created humans "complete," that is, give up the last vital organs they have for transplantation into others, and then die. Along these lines critics of proposed organ markets have charged that such markets will effectively turn desperately poor people into "spare parts" for the rich. In her response to the argument that such organ markets nevertheless transfer money to the poor, Organs Watch founder Nancy Scheper-Hughes caustically quips, "Perhaps we should look for better ways of helping the destitute than dismantling them."[37]

There is surely something disturbing about the picture of poor people supplying the rich with vital organs, just as the world Ishiguro portrays, where some are created to supply others with needed organs, is unsettling. Still, it is important to realize that there are many services that the poor of this world already provide for the rich that are not reciprocally provided by the rich for the poor. Few, if any, wealthy people take hazardous jobs in mines or work in nuclear power plants or are employed cleaning other people's latrines. Societies justify such tasks by pointing out that they are socially necessary and that what is important is that those who perform these tasks are justly compensated under conditions that meet health and safety standards. Given that, the inequality between suppliers doesn't pick out what is especially objectionable about a kidney market.

At the same time I think the critics raise the legitimate concern that kidney markets might actually *worsen* existing inequalities based on class. Such markets could expand inequality's scope by including body parts in the scope of things that money gives a person access to. There are people who have little or no money currently waiting on kidney transplant lists. To a large extent the selection of the person who receives a kidney for transplant is independent of his ability to pay. By contrast, a kidney market might mean that kidneys go to the highest bidders. But shouldn't kidneys be allocated on the basis of need, length of time waiting, and medical suitability and not on the basis of ability to pay?

Theoretically, of course, a legalized organ market could be regulated to ensure that rich and poor have access to kidneys, with the government providing funding for the organ purchases of poor buyers. Through subsidy and insurance the government *could* seek to make the demand for kidneys independent of the wealth of the buyer. Additionally the government might devote itself to finding donors for poorer patients.[38] From an egalitarian viewpoint, these regulations are desirable. Indeed the government might create a monopsony in which it was the *only* legal buyer of organs. And it could buy these organs using a future market, in which people are paid for their organs only after their death as a way of staving off coercive ploys. However, even if a government took such measures, it remains difficult for any government with limited resources and other priorities to make

kidney allocation via a market completely independent of the wealth of the donor. Establishing a maximum price for kidneys under a monopsony might recreate the shortages that the kidney market was designed to overcome, especially if the availability of subsidized kidneys created a moral hazard problem.[39]

The Integrity of the Body

Three of the concerns that I have detailed thus far – weak agency, vulnerability, and the possibility that poor people will become suppliers of organ parts for the rich – can be dealt with through regulating the kidney market rather than blocking it. The concern about whether or not markets will increase supply is different: markets may decrease altruistic donation of organs under any realistic background social conditions, even in the context of regulation.

There is an additional consideration about kidney markets, [. . .]: the way that adding a choice to a choice set changes the other choices that are available to the agent. I want to consider the ways that the existence of kidney markets might make some poor people worse off than they would otherwise be. Although this consideration isn't decisive – the banning of kidney markets makes others in desperate need of a kidney worse off than they would otherwise be – I think it has been missing from the current enthusiasm for organ markets and needs to be addressed. This consideration prompts us to think about the ways that a person's internal resources can differ from their external resources, a point that will resonate with specific egalitarian approaches.

The idea I want to explore here is that even if restrictions on kidney sales are beneficial from the point of view of an individual seller, they may be harmful to others. This is because allowing such markets as a widespread practice, as a pattern of repeated and regular exchanges backed up by laws, has effects on the nature of the choices that are available to people. While proponents of kidney markets usually focus on individual transactions within given environments, the introduction of markets can change environments (including, as we have seen, by possibly altering motivations). Consider that where the practice of kidney selling is widespread, kidneys are viewed as potential collateral and moneylenders acquire incentives to seek out additional borrowers as well as to change the terms of loans. The anthropologist Lawrence Cohen found that in areas of India where kidney selling was relatively common, creditors placed additional pressures on those who owed them money.[40] Cohen notes, "In the Tamil countryside with its kidney belts, debt is primary. . . . Operable *women are vehicles for debt collateral.*"[41]

Cohen's finding suggests that if kidney selling became widespread, a poor person who did *not* want to sell her kidney might find it harder to obtain loans.[42] Ceteris paribus, the credit market allocates loans to people who can provide better collateral. If a kidney market exists, the total amount of collateral rises, which means that those without spare kidneys or those that refuse to sell them, will get fewer loans than before, assuming that the supply of loanable funds is more or less fixed. In other words, these people are made worse off by the kidney market. If this is so, then although allowing a market in kidneys expands a single individual's set of choices, if adopted in the aggregate it may reduce or change the available choices open to others, and those others will be worse off. They will have less effective choices insofar as they will no longer be able to find reasonable loan rates without mortgaging their organs. Once we see the effects of a kidney market on those who are not party to the transactions, we can no longer say that such markets have no harmful consequences.

Of course this argument is true of other linked markets; many markets generate pecuniary externalities. Recall that a pecuniary externality is an effect of production or transactions on outside parties through prices and not through direct resource allocations. For example, the introduction of a market in second homes in a rural community may price some first-time buyers out of the housing market in that community. But people who find kidney markets troubling do not necessarily find markets in second homes troubling. So my point about the effect of a kidney market on other

people's choice sets does not settle the issue of whether that market should be blocked. Instead it leads us to ask, Should people have to pay a cost for their unwillingness to sell their organs? And if not, why not?

If we view kidneys as resources analogous to other resources we have, whether money or apples, it is unclear why we should not have to part with that resource if we wish to secure credit. But many people resist this analogy. They seem to tacitly believe, following Ronald Dworkin, that we have good reason to draw a "prophylactic line" around the body, a line "that comes close to making [it] inviolate, that is, making body parts not part of social resources at all."[43] I concur that there is something to this line of thought, and indeed that a horror at the thought of the conscription of our bodies by others may lie behind the repugnance people feel toward kidney markets, but my endorsement of it as a reason to block kidney markets is a bit tentative because it does not take into account the person who may be dying for lack of a kidney. Nevertheless it is worth stressing that whether or not this line of argument is ultimately successful, it offers a different perspective on kidney markets from one that focuses on the fact that a trade entered into out of desperation is also a trade that is likely to be exploitive, overreaching, or otherwise extremely unfair.[44] That is, this objection holds even if we think that the terms of trade are fair and that the choice made by the seller is not one of desperation.

Policy

I've analyzed the discomfort people feel with kidney markets in terms of vulnerability, weak agency, harmful outcomes, inequality, and motivations, looking at the case for curtailing such markets based on these considerations under both existing and more ideal circumstances. Many problems with kidney markets arise precisely because such markets are not likely to be ideal markets, but rather markets in which there are widespread market failures: weak agency, significant pockets of monopoly power, and human desperation leading to exploitation and inadequate pricing. Much of the repugnance that people feel toward kidney markets arises from the potential for harm stemming from the circumstances in which sellers are found: poverty, lack of clean water and basic health care, and grueling labor. Market regulation may go some way to mitigating the problems along the dimensions of weak agency, although it is unlikely to make the problem of desperate world poverty go away. It is also possible that any potential harms from giving up a kidney can be addressed by mandating appropriate follow-up care, ensuring access to a replacement organ if needed, and perhaps banning the international trade of kidneys. But again, in parts of the world this may be difficult to enforce. One way of mitigating the possibility of harmful outcomes for sellers would be to have purchased organs taken only after the seller's death – a kind of futures market in organs.

Even with the ban on kidney markets and even with little follow-up or no care, people who are desperate are likely to resort to the black market. If the state is too weak to enforce the ban or not particularly inclined to do so, a black market in organs will thrive, as it does in parts of India, Pakistan, and Brazil. According to many observers, the sale of organs on the black market has reached alarming proportions in the third world, especially as advanced medical technology spreads. Regulating a legalized kidney market rather than relying on a black market would arguably go some way in redressing the worries about exploitation and one-sided terms of sale. If properly regulated, an organ market might be structured to discourage sales from extremely poor donors.

But this is where the argument from pecuniary externalities becomes relevant. Allowing the desperately poor to sell their organs as a social practice will have an effect on the choices that are open to those who do not want to participate in such a market. Some may think that it is inappropriate to make people pay a cost for exercising their choice not to sell their kidney. This issue also needs to be considered in policy design.

The problem of inequality, of turning poor people into "spare parts" for the rich, can also be addressed, at least in part, by regulation. Instead of relying on a competitive market we might create a monopsony, with the state the only legal buyer, and distribute on the basis of medical need. We might provide for the state to purchase organs for poor recipients. Nonetheless if there is a market there is likely to be greater stratification by wealth in organ donors and recipients than is currently the case. This may be significant for many reasons, not least of which is that it might "repress the expression of altruism and erode the sense of community."

Reflecting on the values at stake in different kinds of markets helps us to see why kidney markets are different from apple markets. Some of the values that I have discussed are internal to the functioning of markets: perfect information is assumed by the efficiency theorems of welfare economics; if the introduction of a market actually serves to decrease supply, then there is no social cost to banning it. Some of these values are external to the functioning of markets – in matters of life and death urgent needs should trump ability to pay – but widely shared. Some of these external values are more controversial: the list of goods that no one should have to pay a price for refusing to sell.

I want to conclude by briefly considering how a number of recent proposals for kidney markets, some of which are now being debated among policymakers, fare along the dimensions I have set out: vulnerability, weak agency, harmful individual outcomes, and harmful social inequality. The proposals I consider are (1) competitive markets governing supply and demand, in other words, treating kidneys like apples; (2) competitive markets governing supply only and distributing either on the basis of need or supplementing market distribution with subsidized distribution to the poor; (3) competitive futures markets with organs given up only after death; and (4) matching-in kind exchanges, where a patient with a willing donor who has an incompatible blood type can trade with another such incompatible patient-donor pair.[45]

A *yes* in table 1 indicates a problem along a dimension; a *no* indicates a relatively low (but not necessarily unproblematic) score.[46] As can be seen from this schematic, a pure competitive market in kidneys appears to be the most problematic, scoring fairly high on all parameters. By contrast, a market in apples would not normally score high along all these dimensions. Given

Table 1   Evaluating alternative methods of organ allocation

Market/Allocation	Weak agency	Vulnerability	Individual harm	Harmful social inequality
Competitive market in supply and demand	Yes, although could be mitigated by informed consent	Yes	Yes: harm to very poor seller; externalities to other poor	Yes
Competitive market in supply only; government monopsony	Yes: see above	Yes	Yes: see above	No
Futures markets	No	No, unless this gives people an incentive to hasten the death of future donors	No	No
Matching-in kind exchanges	Possible: see above	No	No	No
Altruistic donation	Possible: see above	No	No	No

the imperfect information, the potential for harmful outcomes, and the inequality in access to urgently needed goods (kidneys), I think we should view this market as morally unacceptable.

On my view, the greater the extent to which the concerns raised along the various dimensions can be addressed, the more acceptable is the market. Even for those who worry about the pecuniary effects of such markets – changing the terms of trade for those who do not want to participate in such markets – the question is whether mechanisms can be found that would prevent kidney sales from entering into other kinds of contracts, for example, as loan collateral or as a means of eligibility for social services.

And if these considerations cannot be adequately addressed, whether through information dissemination, regulation, income transfer, or some other means, other possibilities need to be considered, including increased exhortation to donate. I do not want to lose sight of the fact that in addition to the potential for harm to the seller from a kidney market, there is also the potential to extend the life of a person who would otherwise die. Much more could be done to encourage the altruistic donation of organs. Meanwhile, given the desperation on both the buyer and seller sides of the equation, the search for solutions to the shortage of transplantable organs is likely to be with us for a long time to come.[47]

Notes

1   Thanks to Caleb Perl and Jose Campos for research assistance. Thanks also to Joe Shapiro, whose undergraduate honors thesis at Stanford, "The Ethics and Efficacy of Banning Human Kidney Sales," prompted me to think harder about this topic. I was the co-advisor of his thesis with Ken Arrow. Thanks to Ben Hippen for comments on a longer version of this chapter. Thanks also to the audience at the Aristotelian Society, the editor of the Society's proceedings, David Harris, and to Annabelle Lever, Eric Maskin, and Josh Cohen for written comments.

2   This libertarian view confronts serious questions about the scope of control a person has over her body. For example, does a person have the right to sell all of her organs, even if it means her death? Does my right to use my body as I wish mean that I can walk naked into my office? More to the point, do rights to bodily autonomy and integrity entail rights to *sell* one's body or body parts? Cécile Fabre has recently argued that, under many circumstances, justice requires conferring on the sick a right to confiscate the superfluous body parts of healthy individuals. See Fabre, *Whose Body Is It*

Anyway: Justice and the Integrity of the Person (Oxford: Oxford University Press, 2006). Her argument depends on a close analogy between body parts and external resources and perhaps an overly optimistic view about the state's ability to fairly enforce the organ distribution policy.

3   Among undeveloped nations only Iran presently has a legalized kidney market.

4   Michelle Goodwin, *Black Markets: The Supply and Demand of Body Parts* (Cambridge: Cambridge University Press, 2006), 119–22.

5   In *McFall v. Shimp*, 10 Pa. D&C.3d 90 (Ch. Ct. 1978) a man (McFall) who would surely die without a bone marrow transplant, sought an injunction to require his cousin (Shimp) to donate bone marrow, a procedure that would have posed little risk but considerable pain. The court refused to grant the injunction, and the man subsequently died. In *Curran v. Bosze*, 566 N.E.2d 1319 (Ill. 1990) the Illinois Supreme Court refused to grant a noncustodial parent's request that his own twin three-year-old children be compelled to undergo blood testing and possible bone marrow harvesting to save the life of their twelve-year-old half-brother. (The half-brother died while the case was still being decided.)

6   Or perhaps I should say *lists*, since in the United States there is a national list as well as lists at regional transplant centers.

7   Goodwin, *Black Markets*, 40. Goodwin also importantly notes that there are racial disparities in how long people have to wait for a kidney, as well as racial differences in rates of organ donation. African Americans, for example, wait longer on lists and also donate organs less frequently than whites.

8   This figure also includes those who die while waiting for a heart to become available for transplant.

9   See Living Legacy Registry, Donation Statistics, at http://livinglegacy.org.

10   Some object that opt-out systems do not really allow for individual consent because many people do not have adequate information about their society's default position on cadaver organs. According to critics, opt-out systems are really systems of organ conscription. Those who would not have wished to donate their organs after their death, if they had properly reflected on this while they were alive, are forcibly drafted into donation: their actual consent is sidestepped. But *even if this were true*, that is, even if most people comply

with such systems only out of ignorance, the critics' argument is insufficient to rebut those who favor such systems, since an analogous charge could be brought against opt-in systems. In opt-in systems there are likely to be people who have never thought about whether or not their organs should be available for others upon their death, yet would have ex ante preferred that they were. In opt-in donation systems, such people are simply presumed to have consented to nondonation and thus are forcibly drafted into nondonation; their consent to nondonation, in other words, is also sidestepped. Different attitudes about the respective degrees of coerciveness of opt-out and opt-in systems undoubtedly reflect different views about the extent to which an individual has strong ownership claims over her body parts, even after her death. The different default starting positions reflect, at least in part, different attitudes and preferences about social claims on cadaver organs. But these attitudes and preferences are themselves reciprocally influenced by framing effects and starting points. That is, *whichever* default position we choose for organ donation, opt in or opt out, may change the likelihood of certain choices over others. Initial allocations, expectations, and laws about a person's organs form a starting point that affects her individual preferences and judgments. Because every society must have some donation or nondonation starting point, every society faces the question of deciding how this starting point should be determined.

11   See the data collected by Spain's Organización Nacional de Trasplantes, at http://ont.es. See also Newsletter *Transplant: International Figures on Organ Donation and Transplantation*, vol. 10, no 1. Madrid: Fundación Renal, 2005.

12   Remco Coppen et al., "Opting-out Systems: No Guarantee for Higher Donation Rates," *Transplant International*, 18 (2005): 1275–9.

13   Those who receive their kidneys from live donors tend to fare better than those who receive their kidneys from cadavers. See Editorial, "Renal Transplantation from Living Donors," *British Medical Journal* 318 (1999): 409–10; P. I. Terasaki, J. M. Cecka, D. W. Gjertson, and S. Takemoto, "High Survival Rates of Kidney Transplants from Spousal and Living Unrelated Donors," *New England Journal of Medicine*, 333 (1995): 333–6.

14   See Kieran Healy, *Last Best Gifts: Altruism and the Market for Human Blood and Organs* (Chicago: University of Chicago Press, 2006).

15 Cited in Paul Seabright, *The Company of Strangers: A Natural History of Economic Life* (Princeton: Princeton University Press, 2004), 151–2.

16 Richard Titmuss, *The Gift Relationship: From Human Blood to Social Policy* (New York: Random House, 1971).

17 Titmuss, *Gift Relationship*, 314.

18 Arrow, "Gifts and Exchanges," *Philosophy and Public Affairs*, 1 (1972): 343–62.

19 See Uri Gneezy and Aldo Rustichini, "A Fine Is a Price," *Journal of Legal Studies*, 29 (1) (Jan. 2000): 1–18.

20 Bruno Frey and Felix Oberholzer-Gee, "The Cost of Price Incentives: An Empirical Analysis of Motivation Crowding Out," *American Economic Review*, 87 (4) (Sept. 1997): 746–55.

21 See Elizabeth Anderson, *Value in Ethics and Economics* (Cambridge, MA: Harvard University Press, 1993).

22 Lior Jacob Strahilevitz, "How Changes in Property Regimes Influence Social Norms: Commodifying California's Carpool Lanes," *Indiana Law Journal*, 75 (2000): 1231–96.

23 Uri Gneezy and Aldo Rustichini, "Pay Enough or Don't Pay at All," *Quarterly Journal of Economics*, 115 (3) (2000): 791–810. Frey discusses the Dürrenmatt play in Bruno S. Frey, Felix Oberholzer-Gee, and Reiner Eichenberger, "The Old Lady Visits Your Backyard: A Tale of Morals and Markets," *Journal of Political Economy*, 104 (6) (1996): 1297–1313.

24 Thanks to Ben Hippen for the point that not all extrinsic rewards need have the same consequences for altruistic donation.

25 A. J. Ghods, S. Savaj, and P. Khosravani, "Adverse Effects of a Controlled Living Unrelated Donor Renal Transplant Program on Living Related and Cadaveric Kidney Transplantation," *Transplantation Proceedings*, 32 (2000): 541.

26 Nancy Scheper-Hughes, "Keeping an Eye on the Global Traffic in Human Organs," *The Lancet*, 361 (2003): 1645–8, at 1645.

27 If we are concerned about desperation, banning kidney markets itself does nothing to rectify the desperate conditions that prompt such sales. If our concern with kidney markets is the desperation that is prompting the sale, it does no good to close off the sale but leave the circumstances that yielded the desperation in place. In fact, given the desperation, sellers and buyers may still resort to a black market, with a host of attendant abuses even more exploitive, overreaching, or unfair than a legalized market would be.

28 Madhav Goyal et al., "Economic and Health Consequences of Selling a Kidney in India," *Journal of the American Medical Association*, 288 (2002): 1589–93.

29 Indebtedness is a fact of life in many of the areas where kidney selling is widespread. The Goyal study found that 96 percent of sellers interviewed sold a kidney to pay off a debt; 74 percent were still in debt at the time of the survey, six years later. In fact, this study of 305 kidney sellers in Chennai, India, found that after selling a kidney family income actually declined. Many sellers experienced pain and were unable to work. Participants were also paid little for their organs, and often substantially less than they were promised. So even when they were able to stave off the moneylenders for a few years, they were soon in debt again.

30 Goyal et al., "Economic and Health Consequences," report that although people sell their kidneys to get out of debt, sellers are frequently in debt again within several years of the sale.

31 In the case of altruistic donation, our concerns about sellers' agency is presumably mitigated by the fact that the suppliers of kidneys are likely to come from many economic groups and not simply from the desperately poor, who also tend to be uneducated.

32 Recent studies have found that donating a kidney does not damage donors' health or reduce their life span, and they are less likely to develop kidney failure than the general population. See H. N. Ibrahim et al., "Long-Term Consequences of Kidney Donation," *New England Journal of Medicine*, 360 (5) (2009): 459–69. Of course, as I have stressed, the results of kidney donation in the developed world may not tell us very much about kidney donation in the undeveloped world. For one thing, donors in the United States, where this study was undertaken, are very carefully screened for health risks.

33 Joe Shapiro makes this observation as a framing background for his discussion of the morality of kidney markets. See "The Ethics and Efficacy of Banning Human Kidney Sales," Undergraduate thesis, Stanford University.

34 Christian Williams, "Note. Combating the Problems of Human Rights Abuses and Inadequate Organ Supply through Presumed Donative Consent," *Case Western Reserve Journal of International Law* 26 (1994): 315.

35 Titmuss, *Gift Relationship*. Goodwin, *Black Markets*, draws attention to racial disparities in who gives and who gets an organ.

36 Kazuo Ishiguro, *Never Let Me Go* (London: Faber & Faber, 2005). Recently, an article in the *New York Times* by Andrew Pollack raised concerns about the sale of plasma by poor Mexicans to centers run by pharmaceutical companies at the US and Mexico border. See "Is Money Tainting the Plasma Supply?" Dec. 6, 2010, Sunday Business section, p. 1.

37 Nancy Scheper-Hughes, quoted in Michael Finkel, "Complications," *New York Times Magazine*, May 27, 2001, 32. The term *transplant tourism* refers to wealthy individuals or their brokers from the developed world flying halfway around the world to less developed countries searching for organ sellers.

38 See Shapiro, "Ethics and Efficacy," 120.

39 To what extent would the availability of kidneys through a market indemnify individuals against the effects of bad health choices? Thanks to Annabelle Lever for pressing this point.

40 Lawrence Cohen, "Where It Hurts: Indian Material for an Ethics of Organ Transplantation," *Zyogon*, 38 (3) (2003): 663–88.

41 Cohen, "Where It Hurts, 673.

42 I have made an analogous argument about child labor: the availability of child labor decreases the price of unskilled adult labor and thereby makes it harder for families to refrain from putting their children to work.

43 Ronald Dworkin, "Comment on Narveson: In Defense of Equality," *Social Philosophy and Policy*, 1 (1983): 24–40, at 39.

44 Michael Walzer, *Spheres of Justice* (New York: Basic Books, 1983), 102.

45 Alvin E. Roth, Tayfun Sonmez, and M. Utka Unver, "Pairwise Kidney Exchange," *Journal of Economic Theory*, 125 (2) (2005): 151–88.

46 The idea for this chart comes from Ravi Kanbur, "On Obnoxious Markets," in Steve Cullenberg and Prasanta Pattanaik (eds.), *Globalization, Culture and the Limits of the Market* (New Delhi: Oxford University Press, 2004).

47 An earlier version of this chapter appeared as Debra Satz, "The Moral Limits of Markets: The Case of Human Kidneys," *Proceedings of the Aristotelian Society*, 108, part 3 (2008).

53

The Survival Lottery

John Harris

Let us suppose that organ transplant procedures have been perfected; in such circumstances if two dying patients could be saved by organ transplants then, if surgeons have the requisite organs in stock and no other needy patients, but nevertheless allow their patients to die, we would be inclined to say, and be justified in saying, that the patients died because the doctors refused to save them. But if there are no spare organs in stock and none otherwise available, the doctors have no choice, they cannot save their patients and so must let them die. In this case we would be disinclined to say that the doctors are in any sense the cause of their patients' deaths. But let us further suppose that the two dying patients, Y and Z, are not happy about being left to die. They might argue that it is not strictly true that there are no organs which could be used to save them. Y needs a new heart and Z new lungs. They point out that if just one healthy person were to be killed his organs could be removed and both of them be saved. We and the doctors would probably be alike in thinking that such a step, while technically possible, would be out of the question. We would not say that the doctors were killing their patients if they refused to prey upon the healthy to save the sick. And because this sort of surgical Robin Hoodery is out of the question we can tell Y and Z that they cannot be saved, and that when they die they will have died of natural causes and not of the neglect of their doctors. Y and Z do not however agree, they insist that if the doctors fail to kill a healthy man and use his organs to save them, then the doctors will be responsible for their deaths.

Many philosophers have for various reasons believed that we must not kill even if by doing so we could save life. They believe that there is a moral difference between killing and letting die. On this view, to kill A so that Y and Z might live is ruled out because we have a strict obligation not to kill but a duty of some lesser kind to save life. A. H. Clough's dictum 'Thou shalt not kill but need'st not strive officiously to keep alive' expresses bluntly this point of view. The dying Y and Z may be excused for not being much impressed by Clough's dictum. They agree that it is wrong to kill the innocent and are prepared to agree to an absolute prohibition against so doing. They do not agree, however, that A is more innocent than they are. Y and Z

Original publication details: John Harris, "The Survival Lottery," pp. 81–87 from *Philosophy* 50 (1975). © 1975 Royal Institute of Philosophy. Reproduced with permission of Cambridge University Press.

Bioethics: An Anthology, Fourth Edition. Edited by Udo Schüklenk and Peter Singer.
Editorial material and organization © 2022 John Wiley & Sons, Inc. Published 2022 by John Wiley & Sons, Inc.

might go on to point out that the currently acknowledged right of the innocent not to be killed, even where their deaths might give life to others, is just a decision to prefer the lives of the fortunate to those of the unfortunate. A is innocent in the sense that he has done nothing to deserve death, but Y and Z are also innocent in this sense. Why should they be the ones to die simply because they are so unlucky as to have diseased organs. Why, they might argue, should their living or dying be left to chance when in so many other areas of human life we believe that we have an obligation to ensure the survival of the maximum number of lives possible.

Y and Z argue that if a doctor refuses to treat a patient, with the result that the patient dies, he has killed that patient as sure as shooting, and that in exactly the same way, if the doctors refuse Y and Z the transplants that they need, then their refusal will kill Y and Z, again as sure as shooting. The doctors, and indeed the society which supports their inaction, cannot defend themselves by arguing that they are neither expected, nor required by law or convention, to kill so that lives may be saved (indeed, quite the reverse) since this is just an appeal to custom or authority. A man who does his own moral thinking must decide whether, in these circumstances, he ought to save two lives at the cost of one, or one life at the cost of two. The fact that so called 'third parties' have never before been brought into such calculations, have never before been thought of as being involved, is not an argument against their now becoming so. There are, of course, good arguments against allowing doctors simply to haul passers-by off the street whenever they have a couple of patients in need of new organs. And the harmful side-effects of such a practice in terms of terror and distress to the victims, the witnesses and society generally, would give us further reason for dismissing the idea. Y and Z realize this and have a proposal, which they will shortly produce, which would largely meet objections to placing such power in the hands of doctors and eliminate at least some of the harmful side-effects.

In the unlikely event of their feeling obliged to reply to the reproaches of Y and Z, the doctors might offer the following argument: they might maintain that a man is only responsible for the death of someone whose life he might have saved, if, in all the circumstances of the case, he ought to have saved the man by the means available. This is why a doctor might be a murderer if he simply refused or neglected to treat a patient who would die without treatment, but not if he could only save the patient by doing something he ought in no circumstances to do – kill the innocent. Y and Z readily agree that a man ought not to do what he ought not to do, but they point out that if the doctors, and for that matter society at large, ought on balance to kill one man if two can thereby be saved, then failure to do so will involve responsibility for the consequent deaths. The fact that Y's and Z's proposal involves killing the innocent cannot be a reason for refusing to consider their proposal, for this would just be a refusal to face the question at issue and so avoid having to make a decision as to what ought to be done in circumstances like these. It is Y's and Z's claim that failure to adopt their plan will also involve killing the innocent, rather more of the innocent than the proposed alternative.

To back up this last point, to remove the arbitrariness of permitting doctors to select their donors from among the chance passers-by outside hospitals, and the tremendous power this would place in doctors' hands, to mitigate worries about side-effects and lastly to appease those who wonder why poor old A should be singled out for sacrifice, Y and Z put forward the following scheme: they propose that everyone be given a sort of lottery number. Whenever doctors have two or more dying patients who could be saved by transplants, and no suitable organs have come to hand through 'natural' deaths, they can ask a central computer to supply a suitable donor. The computer will then pick the number of a suitable donor at random and he will be killed so that the lives of two or more others may be saved. No doubt if the scheme were ever to be implemented a suitable euphemism for 'killed' would be employed. Perhaps we would begin to talk about citizens being called upon to 'give life' to others. With the refinement of transplant procedures such a scheme could offer the chance of saving large numbers of lives that are now lost. Indeed, even taking into account the loss of the lives of donors, the numbers of untimely deaths each year might be dramatically reduced, so much so that everyone's chance of living to a ripe old age might be increased. If this were to be the consequence of the adoption of such a scheme, and it might well be, it could not be dismissed lightly. It might of course be objected that it is likely that more old people will need transplants to prolong their lives than will the young, and so the scheme would inevitably lead to a society dominated by the old. But if such a society is thought objectionable, there is no reason to suppose that a programme could not be designed for the computer that would ensure the maintenance of whatever is considered to be an optimum age distribution throughout the population.

Suppose that inter-planetary travel revealed a world of people like ourselves, but who organized their society according to this scheme. No one was considered to have an absolute right to life or freedom from interference, but everything was always done to ensure that as many people as possible would enjoy long and happy lives. In such a world a man who attempted to escape when his number was up or who resisted on the grounds that no one had a right to take his life might well be regarded as a murderer. We might or might not prefer to live in such a world, but the morality of its inhabitants would surely be one that we could respect. It would not be obviously more barbaric or cruel or immoral than our own.

Y and Z are willing to concede one exception to the universal application of their scheme. They realize that it would be unfair to allow people who have brought their misfortune on themselves to benefit from the lottery. There would clearly be something unjust about killing the abstemious B so that W (whose heavy smoking has given him lung cancer) and X (whose drinking has destroyed his liver) should be preserved to over-indulge again.

What objections could be made to the lottery scheme? A first straw to clutch at would be the desire for security. Under such a scheme we would never know when we would hear *them* knocking at the door. Every post might bring a sentence of death, every sound in the night might be the sound of boots on the stairs. But, as we have seen, the chances of actually being called upon to make the ultimate sacrifice might be slimmer than is the present risk of being killed on the roads, and most of us do not lie trembling a-bed, appalled at the prospect of being dispatched on the morrow. The truth is that lives might well be more secure under such a scheme.

If we respect individuality and see every human being as unique in his own way, we might want to reject a society in which it appeared that individuals were seen merely as interchangeable units in a structure, the value of which lies in its having as many healthy units as possible. But of course Y and Z would want to know why A's individuality was more worthy of respect than theirs.

Another plausible objection is the natural reluctance to play God with men's lives, the feeling that it is wrong to make any attempt to re-allot the life opportunities that fate has determined, that the deaths of Y and Z would be 'natural', whereas the death of anyone killed to save them would have been perpetrated by men. But if we are able to change things, then to elect not to do so is also to determine what will happen in the world.

Neither does the alleged moral difference between killing and letting die afford a respectable way of rejecting the claims of Y and Z. For if we really want to counter proponents of the lottery, if we really want to answer Y and Z and not just put them off, we cannot do so by saying that the lottery involves killing and object to it for that reason, because to do so would, as we have seen, just beg the question as to whether the failure to save as many people as possible might not also amount to killing.

To opt for the society which Y and Z propose would be then to adopt a society in which saintliness would be mandatory. Each of us would have to recognize a binding obligation to give up his own life for others when called upon to do so. In such a society anyone who reneged upon this duty would be a murderer. The most promising objection to such a society, and indeed to any principle which required us to kill A in order to save Y and Z, is, I suspect, that we are committed to the right of self-defence. If I can kill A to save Y and Z then he can kill me to save P and Q, and it is only if I am prepared to agree to this that I will opt for the lottery or be prepared to agree to a man's being killed if doing so would save the lives of more than one other man. Of course there is something paradoxical about basing objections to the lottery scheme on the right of self-defence since, *ex hypothesi*, each person would have a better chance of living to a ripe old age if the lottery scheme were to be implemented. None the less, the feeling that no man should be required to lay down his life for others makes many people shy away from such a scheme, even though it might be rational to accept it on prudential grounds, and perhaps even manda-tory on utilitarian grounds. Again, Y and Z would reply that the right of self-defence must extend to them as much as to anyone else; and while it is true that they can only live if another man is killed, they would claim that it is also true that if they are left to die, then someone who lives on does so over their dead bodies.

It might be argued that the institution of the sur-vival lottery has not gone far to mitigate the harmful side-effects in terms of terror and distress to victims, witnesses and society generally, that would be occa-sioned by doctors simply snatching passers-by off the streets and disorganizing them for the benefit of the unfortunate. Donors would after all still have to be procured, and this process, however it was carried out, would still be likely to prove distressing to all concerned. The lottery scheme would eliminate the arbitrariness of leaving the life and death decisions to the doctors, and remove the possibility of such terrible power falling into the hands of any individ-uals, but the terror and distress would remain. The effect of having to apprehend presumably unwill-ing victims would give us pause. Perhaps only a long period of education or propaganda could remove our

abhorrence. What this abhorrence reveals about the rights and wrongs of the situation is, however, more difficult to assess. We might be inclined to say that only monsters could ignore the promptings of con-science so far as to operate the lottery scheme. But the promptings of conscience are not necessarily the most reliable guide. In the present case Y and Z would argue that such promptings are mere squeamishness, an over-nice self-indulgence that costs lives. Death, Y and Z would remind us, is a distressing experience whenever and to whomever it occurs, so the less it occurs the better. Fewer victims and witnesses will be distressed as part of the side-effects of the lottery scheme than would suffer as part of the side-effects of not instituting it.

Lastly, a more limited objection might be made, not to the idea of killing to save lives, but to the involvement of 'third parties'. Why, so the objection goes, should we not give X's heart to Y or Y's lungs to X, the same number of lives being thereby preserved and no one else's life set at risk? Y's and Z's reply to this objection differs from their previous line of argu-ment. To amend their plan so that the involvement of so called 'third parties' is ruled out would, Y and Z claim, violate their right to equal concern and respect with the rest of society. They argue that such a pro-posal would amount to treating the unfortunate who need new organs as a class within society whose lives are considered to be of less value than those of its more fortunate members. What possible justification could there be for singling out one group of peo-ple whom we would be justified in using as donors but not another? The idea in the mind of those who would propose such a step must be something like the following: since Y and Z cannot survive, since they are going to die in any event, there is no harm in putting their names into the lottery, for the chances of their dying cannot thereby be increased and will in fact almost certainly be reduced. But this is just to ignore everything that Y and Z have been saying. For if their lottery scheme is adopted they are not going to die anyway – their chances of dying are no greater and no less than those of any other participant in the lottery whose number may come up. This ground for confining selection of donors to the unfortunate therefore disappears. Any other ground must discriminate against Y and Z as members of a class whose lives are less worthy of respect than those of the rest of society.

It might more plausibly be argued that the dying who cannot themselves be saved by transplants, or by any other means at all, should be the priority selection group for the computer programme. But how far off must death be for a man to be classified as 'dying'? Those so classified might argue that their last few days or weeks of life are as valuable to them (if not more valuable) than the possibly longer span remaining to others. The problem of narrowing down the class of possible donors without discriminating unfairly against some sub-class of society is, I suspect, insoluble.

Such is the case for the survival lottery. Utilitarians ought to be in favour of it, and absolutists cannot object to it on the ground that it involves killing the innocent, for it is Y's and Z's case that any alternative must also involve killing the innocent. If the absolutist wishes to maintain his objection he must point to some morally relevant difference between positive and negative killing. This challenge opens the door to a large topic with a whole library of literature, but Y and Z are dying and do not have time to explore it exhaustively. In their own case the most likely candidate for some feature which might make this moral difference is the malevolent intent of Y and Z themselves. An absolutist might well argue that while no one intends the deaths of Y and Z, no one necessarily wishes them dead, or aims at their demise for any reason, they do mean to kill A (or have him killed). But Y and Z can reply that the death of A is no part of their plan, they merely wish to use a couple of his organs, and if he cannot live without them. . .*tant pis*! None would be more delighted than Y and Z if artificial organs would do as well, and so render the lottery scheme otiose.

One form of absolutist argument perhaps remains. This involves taking an Orwellian stand on some

principle of common decency. The argument would then be that even to enter into the sort of 'macabre' calculations that Y and Z propose displays a blunted sensibility, a corrupted and vitiated mind. Forms of this argument have recently been advanced by Noam Chomsky (*American Power and the New Mandarins*) and Stuart Hampshire (*Morality and Pessimism*). The indefatigable Y and Z would of course deny that their calculations are in any sense 'macabre', and would present them as the most humane course available in the circumstances. Moreover they would claim that the Orwellian stand on decency is the product of a closed mind, and not susceptible to rational argument. Any reasoned defence of such a principle must appeal to notions like respect for human life. Hampshire's argument in fact does, and these Y and Z could make conformable to their own position.

Can Y and Z be answered? Perhaps only by relying on moral intuition, on the insistence that we do feel there is something wrong with the survival lottery and our confidence that this feeling is prompted by some morally relevant difference between our bringing about the death of A and our bringing about the deaths of Y and Z. Whether we could retain this confidence in our intuitions if we were to be confronted by a society in which the survival lottery operated, was accepted by all, and was seen to save many lives that would otherwise have been lost, it would be interesting to know.

There would, of course, be great practical difficulties in the way of implementing the lottery. In so many cases it would be agonizingly difficult to decide whether or not a person had brought his misfortune on himself. There are numerous ways in which a person may contribute to his predicament, and the task of deciding how far, or how decisively, a person is himself responsible for his fate would be formidable. And in those cases where we can be confident that a person is innocent of responsibility for his predicament, can we acquire this confidence in time to save him? The lottery scheme would be a powerful weapon in the hands of someone willing and able to misuse it. Could we ever feel certain that the lottery was safe from unscrupulous computer programmers? Perhaps we should be thankful that such practical difficulties make the survival lottery an unlikely consequence of the perfection of transplants. Or perhaps we should be appalled.

It may be that we would want to tell Y and Z that the difficulties and dangers of their scheme would be too great a price to pay for its benefits. It is as well to be clear, however, that there is also a high, perhaps an even higher, price to be paid for the rejection of the scheme. That price is the lives of Y and Z and many like them, and we delude ourselves if we suppose that the reason why we reject their plan is that we accept the sixth commandment.[1]

Note

1   Thanks are due to Ronald Dworkin, Jonathan Glover, M. J. Inwood and Anne Seller for helpful comments.

Part VII

Ethical Issues in Research

Introduction

Research ethics has grown rapidly since the advent of the 1947 Nuremberg Code, a guidance document written in response to the coming-to-light of atrocities committed by Nazi biomedical researchers on prisoners in the Nazi concentration camps. The Code spelled out the most basic requirements research involving human participants would have to meet in order to be considered ethical. Since then ethicists were among those drafting national and international guidance documents concerning appropriate conduct in biomedical research.

This Part of the *Anthology* consists of three broad areas, the first section comprises articles looking at various aspects of research involving humans, the second section looks at research involving non-human animals, and the last section investigates questions of academic freedom.

Experimentation with Humans

Medical research involving human participants differs substantially from medical treatment. While medical treatment focuses on the healthcare needs of individual patients, medical research is a scientific enterprise. It seeks to gain a better understanding of biological processes in humans and aims to develop new drugs and other treatments, for future therapeutic use. Another way of putting this is to say that medical therapy is directed at the welfare of particular, identifiable patients, whereas medical research on humans seeks to improve the health and well-being of patients as a whole.

One of the central ethical issues in experimentation on humans is that human individuals may be subjected to invasive and even risky procedures, for the sake of others. This has led some people to suggest that research should be conducted not on humans, but on nonhuman animals, human cells and by way of computer modeling. Scientists argue that at least some experimentation on human beings is necessary; the knowledge gained by experimenting on nonhuman animals, cells and so on, does not always tell us how complex human organisms will respond to biomedical interventions.

Today, it is widely agreed that at least some research on autonomous human beings is morally permissible, provided the research participants have given their voluntary informed consent. This leaves unanswered the question of whether, and if so when, experimentation may be performed on those who cannot consent – for example, human infants, the mentally disabled, and human embryos.

The assumption that consent is crucial to the moral permissibility of research on autonomous human

Bioethics: An Anthology, Fourth Edition. Edited by Udo Schüklenk and Peter Singer.

research subjects has not always prevailed. We mentioned already that at the end of World War II the world became aware of monstrous examples of medical research conducted in the name of medical science by German and Japanese doctors, on non-consenting prisoners, in utter disregard of their interests or rights. Unsurprisingly, perhaps, the earlier mentioned Nuremberg Code was set up, the first principle of which states that "The voluntary consent of the human subject is absolutely essential. . ." Although this was well-intentioned, it quickly became clear that a number of vitally important research projects could not be undertaken, for instance research involving diseases that render patients incapable of giving consent. Subsequent international guidance documents, such as the World Medical Association's Declaration of Helsinki, address this problem.

However, it is important to note that it was not only in dictatorships like Nazi Germany that unethical research took place. Healthcare professionals in many other nations – including the United States – have engaged in practices that ignored the rights or interests of their research participants. Some 20 years after the end of World War II, Henry K. Beecher published an article entitled "Ethics and Clinical Research" in a leading medical journal. He provided evidence there that hundreds of patients in the United States had been unaware of the risks of the research they participated in, and that hundreds more did not even know they were participating in research.[1]

Since the publication of Beecher's article in the mid-1960s, various international, national, and professional statements and regulations on human experimentation have been issued, and many countries have set up research ethics committees, in attempts to regulate and oversee research. Among the most influential of these was the so-called "Belmont Report," a document produced over a 5-year period by a national Commission, comprising the nation's leading experts, that was established by the United States Congress in 1973. Its responsibility was the drafting of regulations recommended to federal government agencies to protect research participants. The commission produced the "Belmont Report: Ethical Principles and

Guidelines for the Protection of Human Subjects of Research," excerpts of which we include here as the first reading. It established the ethical principles that would be guiding research funded by the United States government, going forward. The foundational principles included respect for persons, beneficence, and justice. The Belmont Report helpfully spelled out what the meaning of these principles was for informed consent, the sound balancing of risks and benefits, and the just selection of research participants.

Let's assume a researcher has succeeded in designing an ethically sound clinical trial protocol. She would then depend on recruiting participants willing to volunteer their time and bodies, otherwise her trial could not proceed. Sometimes these participants are patients, but that does not have to be the case. Some research designs pose significant risks to research participants, for instance in phase 1 clinical trials that are designed to establish whether or not a particular drug is safe to take, and at what dosage levels. The next set of articles discuss the question of whether or not we have a moral obligation to participate in research, and, if there is such an obligation, what kind of obligation that is.

John Harris answers this question in the affirmative. He thinks that our traditional approach to the issue got it all wrong. Research participation is not a supererogatory individual act but actually is morally incumbent on us. In "Scientific Research is a Moral Duty" he makes his case for our moral obligation to participate in clinical research. Harris argues that the moral obligation to participate in clinical research is based on our obligation to assist others in need, as well as on fairness-related consideration. He thinks it is unfair to be a free rider on other research participants' risk-taking. Given that we all benefit to some extent from clinical research, and so from others' risk-taking, it is incumbent on us to volunteer for participation in clinical research, too.

Sandra Shapshay and Kenneth D. Pimple concede in their article "Participation in Research is an Imperfect Moral Duty: A Response to John Harris" that we have a general moral obligation to benefit others, including by means of participation in research. However, they argue that this obligation is merely an imperfect obligation, that is, an obligation not requiring us to participate in particular research projects. Kantian imperfect duties permit duty bearers sometimes to ignore what is owed. On other occasions they permit us to act in benevolent ways toward others while still choosing not to participate in clinical research.

Over the last two decades a global debate has ensued over the question of how to avoid exploitation of trial participants in research undertaken in low-income countries by researchers from high-income countries. In the next set of readings this is discussed from different perspectives, using a controversial real-world clinical trial as an example.

Particularly pressing and difficult ethical issues are raised by internationally sponsored trials in developing countries, where very different social and economic circumstances separate researchers from research subjects. The debate over a clinical trial involving the administration of an anti-viral to pregnant HIV-infected women and their infants after birth is a good example of this. While today the state of medical science has moved on, and these kinds of drugs are much more widely available, as well as affordable, in low-income countries than they were when this trial occurred, it is worth considering the issues, because they continue to occur involving other drugs and other illnesses.

Millions of women in some developing countries are HIV positive and may pass the virus on to their children during pregnancy and birth. Administration of an antiretroviral drug during pregnancy, at birth, and to the infants after birth in a regime known as ACTG 076 can substantially reduce HIV infections in infants. Soon after the regime's effectiveness had been established, it became the standard treatment for HIV-positive pregnant women in high-income countries, but its potential remained largely unrealized in low-income countries because of the drug's exorbitant cost. This led to a decision to conduct a number of trials of less expensive treatment regimes, involving a lower dosage of the drug, in a number of developing countries. Here the experimental regime was tested not against the proven ACTG 076 treatment, but

against a placebo control. In a placebo trial, one group of research participants receives a substance known to be ineffective, in order to give a basis of comparison with the other group, who are receiving the drug to be tested. The researchers wanted to know whether the experimental regime was better than doing nothing, which was the local standard of care at the time. The availability of an effective treatment regime in high-income countries meant that it would be unethical to undertake such a trial there. Does the absence of an effective treatment in developing countries mean that it is ethical to do trials there that would not be ethical in developed countries? Is it ethical to subject trial participants in low-income countries knowingly to a standard of care – in this case, a placebo – lower than the global gold standard that would be required in high-income countries?

In "Unethical Trials of Interventions to Reduce Perinatal Transmission of the Human Immunodeficiency Virus in Developing Countries" Peter Lurie and Sidney M. Wolfe argue that a trial design involving lower standards of clinical care than would be acceptable in high-income countries is morally wrong and involves a gross violation of human rights. While attempts have been made to defend research protocols using placebo groups in developing countries by arguing that the research participants were volunteers, and nobody was worse off than they would have been (given that no effective treatment was available to them in these countries), Lurie and Wolfe charge that the adoption of such a standard would create an incentive to use those who have the least access to healthcare as subjects in research.

Ugandan healthcare workers Danstan Bagenda and Philippa Musoke-Mudido disagree. They argue, in "We're Trying to Help our Sickest People, Not Exploit Them," that it is somewhat presumptuous for critics from developed countries to think that they can lay down ethical research standards for others when these critics are unfamiliar with local conditions.

If the principles governing the ethics of medical research must take account of differences between cultures and regions, arguably these principles should also be sensitive to changed circumstances within a single region. As indicated in our Introduction to Part V, the 2020 coronavirus pandemic forced some countries to reconsider traditional ethical positions about allocating scarce resources. The pandemic also meant that some sections of society – for example, healthcare workers – were exposed to a high risk of becoming infected with the virus. Exposing them to this risk was seen as justified by the number of lives that would be saved by their work. In "Pandemic Ethics: The Case for Risky Research," Peter Singer and Richard Yetter Chappell argue that if it is permissible to expose some members of society to a high risk in order to minimize the overall harm the virus causes, then it is also permissible to expose fully informed volunteers to a comparable level of risk. In order to shorten the process for obtaining a vaccine against a virus that is causing thousands of deaths every day, therefore, we would be justified in using informed volunteers in a human challenge trial, in which they are deliberately exposed to the virus to test the efficacy of a potential vaccine.

Experimentation with Animals

The seventeenth-century French philosopher René Descartes thought that nonhuman animals, including mammals and vertebrates, were insensitive automata, lacking consciousness. Today, physiological studies and behavioral observations leave little doubt that mammals and birds have conscious experiences. It seems probable that all vertebrates, and some invertebrates, such as octopuses, do as well. They can experience pain, suffering and discomfort, and their lives can go better or worse for them. If this were not the case, animal experimentation would raise few ethical issues. The ethical debate over whether, and if so when, nonhuman animals – mice, rabbits, cats, dogs, rhesus monkeys and chimpanzees, for example – can justifiably be used in medical and biomedical research is premised on the belief that animals can experience distressing mental states.

Some people object to all experimentation on nonhuman animals. Many others – often persuaded by the view that experimentation can bring great benefits to humans (and sometimes to animals) – hold

that nonhuman animals may at least sometimes justifiably be used in research. The readings in this section focus on the second position, and on the kinds of argument that might be advanced for and against it. This position is typically held in conjunction with the view that painful or dangerous research is more easily justified when conducted on animals than when conducted on humans.

The view that non-human animals deserve lesser consideration than humans is sometimes defended by appeal to religious teachings – for example, that the God of Judaism and Christianity has given humans dominion over animals, and that only humans but not "brutes" have immortal souls, or are made in the image of God. Religious appeals, however, address only a limited audience. They will be unpersuasive to those who subscribe to a different religion or to no religion at all.

Other defenses of a moral divide between humans and nonhuman animals rely on non-religious premises. The philosophy of the eighteenth-century German philosopher Immanuel Kant ("Duties towards Animals"), for example, centers on rationality and the capacity for autonomous action, which he regarded as the most ethically significant characteristics of humans. Rational beings, capable of autonomous action are, according to Kant, ends in themselves; non-rational animals, on the other hand, "are there merely as means to an end". This does not entail that rational agents may inflict needless cruelty on animals. Being cruel to animals, Kant thought, will be bad for our relations with other humans, "for he who is cruel to animals becomes hard also in his dealings with men." In other words, we should refrain from inflicting needless suffering on an animal, not because it is bad for the animal, but rather because it is bad for humans. It is worth noting that Christine Korsgaard, arguably the leading contemporary moral philosopher working within a Kantian moral framework, strongly disagrees with Kant's view of animals. She thinks that Kant made the mistake of confusing what it takes to be moral *agent,* that is, someone capable of acting morally, with what it takes to be a moral *patient*, that is, a being with moral rights, or to whom we have moral duties. Without rationality or autonomy, one cannot be a moral agent, but one can, she asserts, be a moral patient.[2]

In a footnote to *An Introduction to the Principles of Morals and Legislation,* the late eighteenth and early nineteenth century British philosopher and reformer Jeremy Bentham urged – as one would expect from the founding father of English utilitarianism – that humans and animals have an important morally relevant characteristic in common: the capacity for pain and pleasure. In contrast to Kant, Bentham wrote: "The question is not, Can they *reason?* Nor, Can they *talk?* but, Can they *suffer?*" According to Bentham, sentience or the capacity to experience pleasure and pain entitles a being to moral consideration. Animals matter morally because they are sentient. Bentham thought it wrong to inflict unnecessary pain and suffering on animals, not because our doing so harms humans, but because it harms the animals themselves.

The articles in this section by Nathan Nobis and Dario L. Ringach form a symposium, originally published in the *American Journal of the Medical Sciences,* debating the ethics of using animals as research subjects. Nobis's article is a careful attempt to construct a valid argument from widely accepted premises. At the outset, as he is writing for readers not trained in philosophy or ethics, he sets out the methods of argument he will use. And as he is also writing for an audience that is likely to include many who carry out experiments on animals, and others who draw on the results of such research, he seeks to make his conclusion difficult to escape. Readers who disagree with his conclusion must either reject his premises, or show that the conclusion does not follow from them.

For his premise, Nobis draws on two examples of research – the Tuskegee Syphilis Study and the Willowbrook Case – that are today universally condemned as unethical. In both these cases, researchers infected human participants with diseases – syphilis in the former, and hepatits in the latter – in order to learn more about the diseases. If we share the standard view that this was wrong, Nobis asks, how can we defend doing similar things to nonhuman animals? After examining various attempts to explain why it

might be wrong to do such things to humans, but right to do them to nonhuman animals, he concludes that none of these attempts succeed, and therefore we should accept that harmful nontherapeutic experimentation on animals cannot be justified.

Ringach is a scientist who experiments on animals. To his credit, and unlike many in his position, he does not hide from the public gaze, but is willing to defend his practice openly, so that there can be an open and informed debate on the use of animals in research.

Ringach begins by presenting evidence against some frequently voiced factual claims, but then turns his attention to ethical arguments. After arguing against those who take the absolutist view that no harmful research on animals can ever be justified, he considers a utilitarian critique that accepts the possibility of justifiable uses of animals in research, but insists that we should give equal consideration to the interests of both humans and nonhuman animals, where these interests are similar. Addressing this view, Ringach asserts that "The relevant question for the utilitarian is, has animal research so far, as a field, produced sufficiently important benefits as to be justified?"

Utilitarians might challenge this claim, for utilitarianism looks forward, rather than backward, and deals with the justification of each act, rather than of an entire field of research. Moreover, utilitarians will weigh benefits against costs, both to the animal subjects of the research, and the opportunity costs of using resources on research on animals rather than in other ways.

In the final chapter on animal experimentation Carolyn P. Neuhaus draws our attention to the implications of genome editing techniques, like CRISPR, for research on brain disorders. While in the past animal models typically relied on small animals like mice, CRISPR would permit researchers to overcome some of the difficulties in modeling these illnesses more accurately in larger animals and nonhuman primates. Neuhaus asks whether such research is ethically defensible. Her answer is that it is not ethically defensible. Precisely what makes it possible to model human brain disorders closely in nonhuman primates is also what should give us reason not to use such animals, namely their developmental closeness to us. Neuhaus advocates instead in favor of using human participants, human biospecimens and organoids. She flags the obvious epistemological advantages of using human brains and human tissues for such research. These advantages should also increase the benefits humans can derive from such research. Neuhaus notes that even with human participants 90% of compounds tested in clinical trials fail. Given that they typically rely on animal models not many benefits are derived from the suffering these animals are subjected to. This is especially disconcerting if nonhuman primates who are developmentally particularly close to us are used for such research.

Academic Freedom and Research

The fact that we think it necessary to add this new section to the fourth edition of our *Anthology* says something about the way in which assumptions about the freedom of researchers to conduct research and publish their views have been called into question by an increasing number of incidents during recent years. Politically motivated protests against research have led to researchers being intimidated and threatened with violence, to offers of academic positions being withdrawn from researchers, and to attempts to prevent researchers from speaking at universities and other venues. Some of the protests have come from conservatives, objecting, for example, to the article on "After-Birth Abortion" by Giubilini and Minerva that can be found in Part IV, Chapter 31, of this volume, but the recent increase in the number of attempts to restrict freedom in research has come largely from progressives targeting research about differences between different demographic groups, or between men and women, and about transgender issues.

In this atmosphere, John Stuart Mill's classic statement of the case for freedom of thought and expression, here extracted from his *On Liberty*, is as relevant as ever. Mill warns us that we should not assume that we are infallible. The opinion we are trying to suppress may be true, as many suppressed opinions have been. Perhaps more significant today, however, is Mill's further argument that even if the opinion we wish to suppress is false, the truth that we are trying to protect by suppressing alternative views will become "a dead dogma, not a living truth," unless it is "fully, frequently, and fearlessly discussed". Those who teach philosophy and bioethics know that this is right. In order to educate others to think for themselves, and not merely to parrot the views the teacher takes to be true, a view needs to be challenged. As Mill said, "if opponents of all important truths do not exist, it is indispensable to imagine them and supply them with the strongest arguments which the most skillful devil's advocate can conjure up."

The two other articles in this section discuss whether freedom to conduct research extends to research into cognitive differences between races, or between men and women. Janet A. Kourany asks "Should Some Knowledge Be Forbidden?" She acknowledges that normally we should support a right to freedom of speech, but she also notes some exceptions that are commonly accepted as justified, for example to prevent the spread of knowledge about how to modify a virus so as to produce a pandemic. From this she draws the conclusion that research that causes serious harm may legitimately be restricted. She refers to evidence that researching cognitive differences between blacks and whites, or men and women, can harm blacks and women. The right to freedom of speech thus comes into conflict with the right to equality, and she thinks that here too, freedom should give way to the need to prevent harm to less privileged members of our society.

With this conclusion, James R. Flynn forcefully disagrees. Flynn is best known for his discovery of the "Flynn effect," a demonstration that there has been a sustained increase in intelligence, as measured by non-standardized IQ tests, over the twentieth century. These gains must be due to environmental factors rather than genetic factors. Flynn himself pointed out the relevance of the substantial, environmentally based, IQ gain over time to the debate about whether cognitive differences between blacks and whites have a genetic or environmental basis when he wrote, in an influential article published in 1999:

> . . . an environmental explanation of the racial IQ gap need only posit this: that the average environment for Blacks in 1995 matches the quality of the average environment for Whites in 1945. I do not find that implausible.[3]

Despite spending much of his working life arguing against those who have said that group differences in intelligence are largely genetic, Flynn is adamant in his support of freedom to do scientific research in this area. Whereas Kourany believes that investigating cognitive differences between blacks and whites will be harmful to blacks, Flynn says "Ignorance of reality always extracts its price." In his 1999 article, he asked "Would anyone who holds humane ideals prefer to pursue them in a fantasy world rather than the real world?" We are more likely to be able to bring about social equality, he believes, if we know where to look for the causes of the present inequality.

Notes

1 Henry K. Beecher, "Ethics and Clinical Research", *New England Journal of Medicine* 1966; 274: 1354–60.

2 Christine Korsgaard, *Fellow Creatures: Our Obligations to the Other Animals,* Oxford University Press, Oxford, 2018.

3 Flynn, J. R. (1999). Searching for justice: The discovery of IQ gains over time. *American Psychologist, 54*(1), 5–20. doi: 10.1037/0003-066X.54.1.5

Experimentation with Humans

Belmont Report
Ethical Principles and Guidelines for the Protection of Human Subjects of Research

National Commission for the Protection of Human Subjects of Biomedical and Behavioral Research

Scientific research has produced substantial social benefits. It has also posed some troubling ethical questions. Public attention was drawn to these questions by reported abuses of human subjects in biomedical experiments, especially during the Second World War. During the Nuremberg War Crimes Trials, the Nuremberg Code was drafted as a set of standards for judging physicians and scientists who had conducted biomedical experiments on concentration camp prisoners. This code became the prototype of many later codes[1] intended to assure that research involving human subjects would be carried out in an ethical manner.

The codes consist of rules, some general, others specific, that guide the investigators or the reviewers of research in their work. Such rules often are inadequate to cover complex situations; at times they come into conflict, and they are frequently difficult to interpret or apply. Broader ethical principles will provide a basis on which specific rules may be formulated, criticized and interpreted.

Three principles, or general prescriptive judgments, that are relevant to research involving human subjects

are identified in this statement. Other principles may also be relevant. These three are comprehensive, however, and are stated at a level of generalization that should assist scientists, subjects, reviewers and interested citizens to understand the ethical issues inherent in research involving human subjects. These principles cannot always be applied so as to resolve beyond dispute particular ethical problems. The objective is to provide an analytical framework that will guide the resolution of ethical problems arising from research involving human subjects.

This statement consists of a distinction between research and practice, a discussion of the three basic ethical principles, and remarks about the application of these principles.

A   Boundaries between Practice and Research

It is important to distinguish between biomedical and behavioral research, on the one hand, and the practice

Original publication details: National Commission for the Protection of Human Subjects of Biomedical and Behavioral Research, U.S. Department of Health, Education and Welfare, "The Belmont Report: Ethical Principles and Guidelines for the Protection of Human Subjects of Research," 1978, pp. 1–20. Public domain.

of accepted therapy on the other, in order to know what activities ought to undergo review for the protection of human subjects of research. The distinction between research and practice is blurred partly because both often occur together (as in research designed to evaluate a therapy) and partly because notable departures from standard practice are often called "experimental" when the terms "experimental" and "research" are not carefully defined.

For the most part, the term "practice" refers to interventions that are designed solely to enhance the well-being of an individual patient or client and that have a reasonable expectation of success. The purpose of medical or behavioral practice is to provide diagnosis, preventive treatment or therapy to particular individuals.[2] By contrast, the term "research" designates an activity designed to test a hypothesis, permit conclusions to be drawn, and thereby to develop or contribute to generalizable knowledge (expressed, for example, in theories, principles, and statements of relationships). Research is usually described in a formal protocol that sets forth an objective and a set of procedures designed to reach that objective.

When a clinician departs in a significant way from standard or accepted practice, the innovation does not, in and of itself, constitute research. The fact that a procedure is "experimental," in the sense of new, untested or different, does not automatically place it in the category of research. Radically new procedures of this description should, however, be made the object of formal research at an early stage in order to determine whether they are safe and effective. Thus, it is the responsibility of medical practice committees, for example, to insist that a major innovation be incorporated into a formal research project. [3]

Research and practice may be carried on together when research is designed to evaluate the safety and efficacy of a therapy. This need not cause any confusion regarding whether or not the activity requires review; the general rule is that if there is any element of research in an activity, that activity should undergo review for the protection of human subjects.

B   Basic Ethical Principles

The expression "basic ethical principles" refers to those general judgments that serve as a basic justification for the many particular ethical prescriptions and evaluations of human actions. Three basic principles, among those generally accepted in our cultural tradition, are particularly relevant to the ethics of research involving human subjects: the principles of respect for persons, beneficence and justice.

1   Respect for persons

Respect for persons incorporates at least two basic ethical convictions: first, that individuals should be treated as autonomous agents, and second, that persons with diminished autonomy are entitled to protection. The principle of respect for persons thus divides into two separate moral requirements: the requirement to acknowledge autonomy and the requirement to protect those with diminished autonomy.

An autonomous person is an individual capable of deliberation about personal goals and of acting under the direction of such deliberation. To respect autonomy is to give weight to autonomous persons' considered opinions and choices while refraining from obstructing their actions unless they are clearly detrimental to others. To show a lack of respect for an autonomous agent is to repudiate that person's considered judgments, to deny an individual the freedom to act on those considered judgments, or to withhold information necessary to make a considered judgment, when there are no compelling reasons to do so.

However, not every human being is capable of self-determination. The capacity for self-determination matures during an individual's life, and some individuals lose this capacity wholly or in part because of illness, mental disability, or circumstances that severely restrict liberty. Respect for the immature and the incapacitated may require protecting them as they mature or while they are incapacitated.

Some persons are in need of extensive protection, even to the point of excluding them from activities which may harm them; other persons require little protection beyond making sure they undertake activities freely and with awareness of possible adverse consequences. The extent of protection afforded should depend upon the risk of harm and the likelihood of benefit. The judgment that any individual lacks autonomy should be periodically reevaluated and will vary in different situations.

In most cases of research involving human subjects, respect for persons demands that subjects enter into the research voluntarily and with adequate information. In some situations, however, application of the principle is not obvious. The involvement of prisoners as subjects of research provides an instructive example. On the one hand, it would seem that the principle of respect for persons requires that prisoners not be deprived of the opportunity to volunteer for research. On the other hand, under prison conditions they may be subtly coerced or unduly influenced to engage in research activities for which they would not otherwise volunteer. Respect for persons would then dictate that prisoners be protected. Whether to allow prisoners to "volunteer" or to "protect" them presents a dilemma. Respecting persons, in most hard cases, is often a matter of balancing competing claims urged by the principle of respect itself.

2 Beneficence

Persons are treated in an ethical manner not only by respecting their decisions and protecting them from harm, but also by making efforts to secure their well-being. Such treatment falls under the principle of beneficence. The term "beneficence" is often understood to cover acts of kindness or charity that go beyond strict obligation. In this document, beneficence is understood in a stronger sense, as an obligation. Two general rules have been formulated as complementary expressions of beneficent actions in this sense: (1) do not harm and (2) maximize possible benefits and minimize possible harms.

The Hippocratic maxim "do no harm" has long been a fundamental principle of medical ethics. Claude Bernard extended it to the realm of research, saying that one should not injure one person regardless of the benefits that might come to others. However, even avoiding harm requires learning what is harmful; and, in the process of obtaining this information, persons may be exposed to risk of harm. Further, the Hippocratic Oath requires physicians to benefit their patients "according to their best judgment." Learning what will in fact benefit may require exposing persons to risk. The problem posed by these imperatives is to decide when it is justifiable to seek certain benefits despite the risks involved, and when the benefits should be foregone because of the risks.

The obligations of beneficence affect both individual investigators and society at large, because they extend both to particular research projects and to the entire enterprise of research. In the case of particular projects, investigators and members of their institutions are obliged to give forethought to the maximization of benefits and the reduction of risk that might occur from the research investigation. In the case of scientific research in general, members of the larger society are obliged to recognize the longer term benefits and risks that may result from the improvement of knowledge and from the development of novel medical, psychotherapeutic, and social procedures.

The principle of beneficence often occupies a well-defined justifying role in many areas of research involving human subjects. An example is found in research involving children. Effective ways of treating childhood diseases and fostering healthy development are benefits that serve to justify research involving children – even when individual research subjects are not the direct beneficiaries. Research also makes it possible to avoid the harm that may result from the application of previously accepted routine practices that on closer investigation turn out to be dangerous. But the role of the principle of beneficence is not always so unambiguous. A difficult ethical problem remains, for example, about research that presents more than minimal risk without immediate prospect of direct benefit to the children involved. Some have argued that such research is inadmissible, while others have pointed out that this limit would rule out much research promising great benefit to children in the future. Here again, as with all hard cases, the different claims covered by the principle of beneficence may come into conflict and force difficult choices.

3 Justice

Who ought to receive the benefits of research and bear its burdens? This is a question of justice, in the sense of "fairness in distribution" or "what is deserved." An injustice occurs when some benefit to which a person is entitled is denied without good reason or when some burden is imposed unduly. Another way of conceiving the principle of justice is that equals ought to be treated equally. However, this statement requires explication. Who is equal and who unequal? What considerations justify departure from equal distribution? Almost all commentators allow that distinctions based on experience, age, deprivation, competence, merit and position do sometimes constitute criteria justifying differential treatment for certain purposes. It is necessary, then, to explain in what respects people should be treated equally. There are several widely accepted formulations of just ways to distribute burdens and benefits. Each formulation mentions some relevant property on the basis of which burdens and benefits should be distributed. These formulations are (1) to each person an equal share, (2) to each person according to individual need, (3) to each person according to individual effort, (4) to each person according to societal contribution, and (5) to each person according to merit.

Questions of justice have long been associated with social practices such as punishment, taxation and political representation. Until recently these questions have not generally been associated with scientific research. However, they are foreshadowed even in the earliest reflections on the ethics of research involving human subjects. For example, during the 19th and early 20th centuries the burdens of serving as research subjects fell largely upon poor ward patients, while the benefits of improved medical care flowed primarily to private patients. Subsequently, the exploitation of unwilling prisoners as research subjects in Nazi concentration camps was condem[n]ed as a particularly flagrant injustice. In this country, in the 1940s, the Tuskegee syphilis study used disadvantaged, rural black men to study the untreated course of a disease that is by no means confined to that population. These subjects were deprived of demonstrably effective treatment in order not to interrupt the project, long after such treatment became generally available.

Against this historical background, it can be seen how conceptions of justice are relevant to research involving human subjects. For example, the selection of research subjects needs to be scrutinized in order to determine whether some classes (*e.g.,* welfare patients, particular racial and ethnic minorities, or persons confined to institutions) are being systematically selected simply because of their easy availability, their compromised position, or their manipulability, rather than for reasons directly related to the problem being studied. Finally, whenever research supported by public funds leads to the development of therapeutic devices and procedures, justice demands both that these not provide advantages only to those who can afford them and that such research should not unduly involve persons from groups unlikely to be among the beneficiaries of subsequent applications of the research.

C   Applications

Application of the general principles to the conduct of research leads to consideration of the following requirements: informed consent, risk/benefit assessment, and the selection of subjects of research.

1   Informed consent

Respect for persons requires that subjects, to the degree that they are capable, be given the opportunity to choose what shall or shall not happen to them. This opportunity is provided when adequate standards for informed consent are satisfied.

While the importance of informed consent is unquestioned, controversy prevails over the nature and possibility of an informed consent. Nonetheless, there is widespread agreement that the consent process can be analyzed as containing three elements: information, comprehension and voluntariness.

Information. Most codes of research establish specific items for disclosure intended to assure that subjects are given sufficient information. These items generally include: the research procedure, their purposes, risks and anticipated benefits, alternative procedures (where therapy is involved), and a statement offering the subject the opportunity to ask questions and to withdraw at any time from the research. Additional items have been proposed, including how subjects are selected, the person responsible for the research, etc.

However, a simple listing of items does not answer the question of what the standard should be for judging how much and what sort of information should be provided. One standard frequently invoked in medical practice, namely the information commonly provided by practitioners in the field or in the locale, is inadequate since research takes place precisely when a common understanding does not exist. Another standard, currently popular in malpractice law, requires the practitioner to reveal the information that reasonable persons would wish to know in order to make a decision regarding their care. This, too, seems insufficient since the research subject, being in essence a volunteer, may wish to know considerably more about risks gratuitously undertaken than do patients who deliver themselves into the hands of a clinician for needed care. It may be that a standard of "the reasonable volunteer" should be proposed: the extent and nature of information should be such that persons, knowing that the procedure is neither necessary for their care nor perhaps fully understood, can decide whether they wish to participate in the furthering of knowledge. Even when some direct benefit to them is anticipated, the subjects should understand clearly the range of risk and the voluntary nature of participation.

A special problem of consent arises where informing subjects of some pertinent aspect of the research is likely to impair the validity of the research. In many cases, it is sufficient to indicate to subjects that they are being invited to participate in research of which some features will not be revealed until the research is concluded. In all cases of research involving incomplete disclosure, such research is justified only if it is clear that (1) incomplete disclosure is truly necessary to accomplish the goals of the research, (2) there are no undisclosed risks to subjects that are more than minimal, and (3) there is an adequate plan for debriefing subjects, when appropriate, and for dissemination of research results to them. Information about risks should never be withheld for the purpose of eliciting the cooperation of subjects, and truthful answers should always be given to direct questions about the research. Care should be taken to distinguish cases in which disclosure would destroy or invalidate the research from cases in which disclosure would simply inconvenience the investigator.

Comprehension. The manner and context in which information is conveyed is as important as the information itself. For example, presenting information in a disorganized and rapid fashion, allowing too little time for consideration or curtailing opportunities for questioning, all may adversely affect a subject's ability to make an informed choice.

Because the subject's ability to understand is a function of intelligence, rationality, maturity and language, it is necessary to adapt the presentation of the information to the subject's capacities. Investigators are responsible for ascertaining that the subject has comprehended the information. While there is always an obligation to ascertain that the information about risk to subjects is complete and adequately comprehended, when the risks are more serious, that obligation increases. On occasion, it may be suitable to give some oral or written test of comprehension.

Special provision may need to be made when comprehension is severely limited – for example, by conditions of immaturity or mental disability. Each class of subjects that one might consider as incompetent (*e.g.,* infants and young children, mentally disabled patients, the terminally ill and the comatose) should be considered on its own terms. Even for these persons, however, respect requires giving them the opportunity to choose to the extent they are able, whether or not to participate in research. The objections of these subjects to involvement should be honored, unless the research entails providing them a therapy unavailable elsewhere. Respect for persons also requires seeking the permission of other parties in order to protect the subjects from harm. Such persons are thus respected both by acknowledging their own wishes and by the use of third parties to protect them from harm.

The third parties chosen should be those who are most likely to understand the incompetent subject's situation and to act in that person's best interest. The person authorized to act on behalf of the subject should be given an opportunity to observe the research as it proceeds in order to able to withdraw the subject from the research, if such action appears in the subject's best interest.

Voluntariness. An agreement to participate in research constitutes a valid consent only if voluntarily given. This element of informed consent requires conditions free of coercion and undue influence. Coercion occurs when an overt threat of harm is intentionally presented by one person to another in order to obtain compliance. Undue influence, by contrast, occurs through an offer of an excessive, unwarranted, inappropriate or improper reward or other overture in order to obtain compliance. Also, inducements that would ordinarily be acceptable may become undue influences if the subject is especially vulnerable.

Unjustifiable pressures usually occur when persons in positions of authority or commanding influence – especially where possible sanctions are involved – urge a course of action for a subject. A continuum of such influencing factors exists, however, and it is impossible to state precisely where justifiable persuasion ends and undue influence begins. But undue influence would include actions such as manipulating a person's choice through the controlling influence of a close relative and threatening to withdraw health services to which an individual would otherwise be entitled.

2   Assessment of risks and benefits

The assessment of risks and benefits requires a careful arrayal of relevant data, including, in some cases, alternative ways of obtaining the benefits sought in the research. Thus, the assessment presents both an opportunity and a responsibility to gather systematic and comprehensive information about proposed research. For the investigator, it is a means to examine whether the proposed research is properly designed. For a review committee, it is a method for determining whether the risks that will be presented to subjects are justified. For prospective subjects, the assessment will assist the determination whether or not to participate.

The Nature and Scope of Risks and Benefits. The requirement that research be justified on the basis of a favorable risk/benefit assessment bears a close relation to the principle of beneficence, just as the moral requirement that informed consent be obtained is derived primarily from the principle of respect for persons. The term "risk" refers to a possibility that harm may occur. However, when expressions such as "small risk" or "high risk" are used, they usually refer (often ambiguously) both to the chance (probability) of experiencing a harm and the severity (magnitude) of the envisioned harm.

The term "benefit" is used in the research context to refer to something of positive value related to health or welfare. Unlike "risk," "benefit" is not a term that expresses probabilities. Risk is properly contrasted to probability of benefits, and benefits are properly contrasted with harms rather than risks of harm. Accordingly, so-called risk/ benefit assessments are concerned with the probabilities and magnitudes of possible harms and anticipated benefits. Many kinds of possible harms and benefits need be taken into account. There are, for example, risks of psychological harm, physical harm, legal harm, social harm and economic harm and the corresponding benefits. While the most likely types of harms to research subjects are those of psychological or physical pain or injury, other possible kinds should not be overlooked.

Risks and benefits of research may affect the individual subjects, the families of the individual subjects, and society at large (or special groups of subjects in society). Previous codes and federal regulations have required that risks to subjects be outweighed by the sum of both the anticipated benefit to the subject, if any, and the anticipated benefit to society in the form of the knowledge to be gained from the research. In balancing these different elements, the risks and benefits affecting the immediate research subject will normally carry special weight. On the other hand, interests other than those of the subject may on some occasions be sufficient by themselves to justify the risks involved in the research, so long the subjects' rights have been protected. Beneficence thus requires that we protect against risk of harm to subjects and also that we be concerned about the loss of the substantial benefits that might be gained from research.

The Systematic Assessment of Risks and Benefits. It is commonly said that benefits and risks must be "balanced" and shown to be "in a favorable ratio." The metaphorical character of these terms draws attention to the difficulty of making precise judgments. Only on rare occasions will quantitative techniques be available for the scrutiny of research protocols. However, the idea of systematic, nonarbitrary analysis of risks and benefits should be emulated insofar as possible. This ideal requires those making decisions about the justifiability of research to be thorough in the accumulation and assessment of information about all aspects of the research, and to consider alternatives systematically. This procedure renders the assessment of research more rigorous and precise, while making communication between review board members and investigators less subject to misinterpretation, misinformation and conflicting judgments. Thus, there should first be a determination of the validity of the presuppositions of the research; then the nature, probability and magnitude of risk should be distinguished with as much clarity as possible. The method of ascertaining risks should be explicit, especially where there is no alternative to the use of such vague categories as small or slight risk. It should also be determined whether an investigator's estimates of the probability of harm or benefits are reasonable, as judged by known facts or other available studies.

Finally, assessment of the justifiability of research should reflect at least the following considerations: (i) Brutal or inhumane treatment of human subjects is never morally justified. (ii) Risks should be reduced to those necessary to achieve the research objective. It should be determined whether it is in fact necessary to use human subjects at all. Risk can perhaps never be entirely eliminated, but it can often be reduced by careful attention to alternative procedures. (iii) When research involves significant risk of serious impairment, review committees should be extraordinarily insistent on the justification of the risk (looking usually to the likelihood of benefit to the subject – or, in some rare cases, to the manifest voluntariness of the participation). (iv) When vulnerable populations are involved in research, the appropriateness of involving them should itself be demonstrated. A number of variables go into such judgments, including the nature and degree of risk, the condition of the particular population involved, and the nature and level of the anticipated benefits. (v) Relevant risks and benefits must be thoroughly arrayed in documents and procedures used in the informed consent process.

3   Selection of subjects

Just as the principle of respect for persons finds expression in the requirements for consent, and the principle of beneficence in risk/benefit assessment, the principle of justice gives rise to moral requirements that there be fair procedures and outcomes in the selection of research subjects.

Justice is relevant to the selection of subjects of research at two levels: the social and the individual. Individual justice in the selection of subjects would require that researchers exhibit fairness: thus, they should not offer potentially beneficial research on to some patients who are in their favor or select only "undesirable" persons for risky research. Social justice requires that a distinction be drawn between classes of subjects that ought, and ought not, to participate in any particular kind of research, based on the ability of members of that class to bear burdens and on the appropriateness of placing further burdens on already burdened persons. Thus, it can be considered a matter of social justice that there is an order of preference in the selection of classes of subjects (*e.g.,* adults before children) and that some classes of potential subjects (*e.g.,* the institutionalized mentally infirm or prisoners) may be involved as research subjects, if at all, only on certain conditions.

Injustice may appear in the selection of subjects, even if individual subjects are selected fairly by investigators and treated fairly in the course of the research. This injustice arises from social, racial, sexual and cultural biases institutionalized in society. Thus, even if individual researchers are treating their research subjects fairly, and even if IRBs [Institutional Review Boards] are taking care to assure that subjects are selected fairly within a particular institution, unjust social patterns may nevertheless appear in the overall distribution of the burdens and benefits of research. Although individual institutions or investigators may not be able to resolve a problem that is pervasive in their social setting, they can consider distributive justice in selecting research subjects.

Some populations, especially institutionalized ones, are already burdened in many ways by their infirmities and environments. When research is proposed that involves risks and does not include a therapeutic component, other less burdened classes of persons should be called upon first to accept these risks of research, except where the research is directly related to the specific conditions of the class involved. Also, even though public funds for research may often flow in the same directions as public funds for health care, it seems unfair that populations dependent on public health care constitute a pool of preferred research subjects if more advantaged populations are likely to be the recipients of the benefits.

One special instance of injustice results from the involvement of vulnerable subjects. Certain groups, such as racial minorities, the economically disadvantaged, the very sick, and the institutionalized may continually be sought as research subjects, owing to their ready availability in settings where research is conducted. Given their dependent status and their frequently compromised capacity for free consent, they should be protected against the danger of being involved in research solely for administrative convenience, or because they are easy to manipulate as a result of their illness or socioeconomic condition.

Notes

1   Since 1945, various codes for the proper and responsible conduct of human experimentation in medical research have been adopted by different organizations. The best known of these codes are the Nuremberg Code of 1947, the Helsinki Declaration of 1964 (revised in 1975), and the 1971 Guidelines (codified into Federal Regulations in 1974) issued by the US Department of Health, Education, and Welfare. Codes for the conduct of social and behavioral research have also been adopted, the best known being that of the American Psychological Association, published in 1973.

2   Although practice usually involves interventions designed solely to enhance the well-being of a particular individual, interventions are sometimes applied to one individual for the enhancement of the well-being of another (e.g., blood donation, skin grafts, organ transplants) or an intervention may have the dual purpose of enhancing the well-being of a particular individual, and, at the same time, providing some benefit to others (e.g., vaccination, which protects both the person who is vaccinated and society generally). The fact that some forms of practice have elements other than immediate benefit to the individual receiving an intervention, however, should not confuse the general distinction between research and practice. Even when a procedure applied in practice may benefit some other person, it remains an intervention designed to enhance the well-being of a particular individual or groups of individuals; thus, it is practice and need not be reviewed as research.

3   Because the problems related to social experimentation may differ substantially from those of biomedical and behavioral research, the Commission specifically declines to make any policy determination regarding such research at this time. Rather, the Commission believes that the problem ought to be addressed by one of its successor bodies.

55

Scientific Research is a Moral Duty

John Harris

Science is under attack. In Europe, America, and Australasia in particular, scientists are objects of suspicion and are on the defensive.[i]

"Frankenstein science"[5] is a phrase never far from the lips of those who take exception to some aspect of science or indeed some supposed abuse by scientists. We should not, however, forget the powerful obligation there is to undertake, support, and participate in scientific research, particularly biomedical research, and the powerful moral imperative that underpins these obligations. Now it is more imperative than ever to articulate and explain these obligations and to do so is the subject and the object of this paper.

Let me present the question in its starkest form: is there a moral obligation to undertake, support and even to participate in serious scientific research? If there is, does that obligation require not only that beneficial research be undertaken but also that "we", as individuals and "we" as societies be willing to support and even participate in research where necessary?

Thus far the overwhelming answer given to this question has been "no", and research has almost universally been treated with suspicion and even hostility by the vast majority of all those concerned with the ethics and regulation of research. The so called "precautionary approach"[6] sums up this attitude, requiring dangers to be considered more likely and more serious than benefits, and assuming that no sane person would or should participate in research unless they had a pressing personal reason for so doing, or unless they were motivated by a totally impersonal altruism. International agreements and protocols – for example, the *Declaration of Helsinki*[7] and the *CIOMS Guidelines*[8] – have been directed principally at protecting individuals from the dangers of participation in research and ensuring that, where they participate, their full informed consent is assured. The overwhelming presumption has been and remains that participation in research is a supererogatory, and probably a reckless, act not an obligation.

Suspicion of doctors and of medical research is well founded. In the modern era it stems from the aftermath of the Nazi atrocities and from the original Helsinki declaration prompted, although rather belatedly, by the Nazi doctors' trial at Nuremberg.[9,10] More recently it has been fuelled by further examples

Original publication details: John Harris, "Scientific Research Is a Moral Duty," pp. 242–248 from *Journal of Medical Ethics* 31: 4 (2005). Reproduced with permission of BMJ Publishing Group Ltd.

of extreme medical arrogance and paternalism. The Tuskegee Study of Untreated Syphilis,[11] for example, in which 412 poor African-American men were deliberately left untreated from 1932–1972 so that the natural history of syphilis could be determined.[12] Even when it became known that penicillin was effective against syphilis they were left untreated. More recently in the UK a major scandal caught the public imagination and reflected serious medical malpractice; it involved the unauthorised and deceitful post-mortem removal and retention of organs and tissue from children.[13] (For a commentary on some of the major issues concerning this case see my paper "Law and regulation of retained organs: the ethical issues".[14])

These and many other cases seem to provide ample justification for the presumption of suspicion of, and even hostility to, medical research. Vigilance against wrongdoing is, however, one thing; the inability to identify wrongdoing with the result that the good is frustrated and harm caused is quite another.

This paper challenges and seeks to reverse the presumption against medical research.

When we ask whether there is a moral obligation to support and even to participate in serious scientific research we need first to be clear that we are talking of research directed toward preventing serious harm or providing significant benefits to humankind. In all cases the degree of harm or benefit must justify the degree of burden on research subjects, individuals, or society. This balance will be explored below. Of course the research must also be serious in the sense that the project is well designed and with reasonable prospect of leading to important knowledge that will benefit persons in the future.[ii]

Two separate but complementary lines of argument underpin a powerful obligation to pursue, support, and participate in scientific research.

Do No Harm

The first is one of the most powerful obligations that we have, the obligation not to harm others. Where our actions will, or may probably prevent serious harm then if we can reasonably (given the balance of risk and burden to ourselves and benefit to others) we clearly should act because to fail to do so is to accept responsibility for the harm that then occurs. (I set out arguments for and the basis of this duty in *Violence and Responsibility*.[15]) This is the strong side of a somewhat weaker, but still powerful duty of beneficence, our basic moral obligation to help other people in need. This is sometimes called "the rule of rescue".[16] Most, if not all diseases create needs, in those who are affected, and in their relatives, friends, and carers and indeed in society. Because medical research is a necessary component of relieving that need in many circumstances, furthering medical research becomes a moral obligation. This obligation is not limited to actual physical participation in research projects, but also involves supporting research in other ways, for instance economically, at the personal, corporate, and societal levels and indeed politically.

Fairness

Second, the obligation also flows from an appeal to basic fairness. This is sometimes expressed as an appeal to the unfairness of being a "free rider". We all benefit from the existence of the social practice of medical research. Many of us would not be here if infant mortality had not been brought under control, or antibiotics had not been invented. Most of us will continue to benefit from these and other medical advances (and indeed other advances such as clean drinking water and sanitation). Since we accept these benefits, we have an obligation in justice to contribute to the social practice which produces them. We may argue that since we could not opt out of advances that were made prior to our becoming capable of autonomous decision making we are not obliged to contribute. It may, however, still be unfair to accept their benefits and implies also that we will forgo the fruits of any future advances.[17] Few, however, are willing to do so, and even fewer are really willing to forgo benefits that have been created through the sacrifices of others when their own hour of need arises!

It should be clear how what I am claiming relates to the principle which is sometimes called the "principle of fairness" developed by Herbert Hart and later used by John Rawls.[18,19] That principle may be interpreted as saying "those who have submitted to . . . restrictions have a right to similar acquiescence on the part of those who have benefited from their submission".[20] Here I am not suggesting an *enforceable* obligation to participate based on fairness although such an enforceable obligation would, as we shall see, certainly in some circumstances be justified by the argument of this paper. Nor am I proposing any *right* possessed by those who participate, to similar acquiescence on the part of those who benefit. Being a free rider *is*, however, unfair and people always have a moral reason not to act unfairly. This moral reason is probably enough to justify an enforceable obligation but we do not have to use compulsion as a strategy of first resort. It is surely powerful enough, however, to rebut some of the presumptions against an obligation to support and participate in research.

There may be specific facts about me and my circumstances that absolve me from the obligation to be a research subject in a given situation. This could be the case if I have just participated in other burdensome experiments and there are other potential research subjects who have not done so, or if participation would create excessive burdens for me that it would not create for other potential participants. This does not show that the general obligation we have identified does not exist, just that it, like most other or perhaps all moral obligations, can be overridden by other moral considerations in specific circumstances.[iii]

The Moral Imperative for Research

We all benefit from living in a society, and, indeed, in a world in which serious scientific research is carried out and which utilises the benefits of past research. It is both of benefit to patients and research subjects and in their interests to be in a society which pursues and actively accepts the benefits of research and where research and its fruits are given a high priority. We

all also benefit from the knowledge that research is ongoing into diseases or conditions from which we do not currently suffer but to which we may succumb. It makes us feel more secure and gives us hope for the future, for ourselves and our descendants, and for others for whom we care. If this is right, then I have a strong general interest that there be research, and in all well founded research; not excluding but not exclusively, research on me and on my condition or on conditions which are likely to affect me and mine. All such research is also of clear benefit to me. A narrow interpretation of the requirement that research be of benefit to the subject of the research is therefore perverse.[21]

Moreover, almost everyone now living, certainly everyone born in high income industrialised societies, has benefited from the fruits of past research. We all benefit – for example, either from having been vaccinated against diseases such as polio, smallpox, and others or because others have been vaccinated we benefit from the so called "herd" immunity; or we benefit (as in the case of smallpox) from the fact that the disease has actually been eradicated. To take another obvious example, almost at random, we all benefit from the knowledge of connections between diet, exercise, and heart disease. This knowledge enables us to adopt preventive strategies and gives us ways of calculating our level of personal risk.

In view of these considerations there is a clear moral obligation to participate in medical research in certain specific circumstances. This moral obligation is, as we have seen, straightforwardly derivable from either of two of the most basic moral obligations we have as persons.

This entails that there are circumstances where an adult, competent person ought to participate in research, even if participating is not in his or her best interests narrowly defined. If I am asked to give a blood sample for a worthwhile research project, or if I am asked if tissue removed during an operation may be retained for research or therapeutic use, I may have to think in the following way: in the case of giving the blood sample I may say to myself: "I hate needles and the sight of my own blood!" Equally with retained tissue or organs I may feel that since I understand little of the future uses for my tissue it would be safer to say "no".

In each case we will suppose that the disease being investigated is not one that I or anyone I know is likely ever to get, so giving this blood sample or allowing the use of excised tissue is not in my best interests narrowly conceived. In this situation doing what is best, all things considered, therefore seems to entail not doing what is best for myself, not pursuing my own best interests. However, this is not really so. Some of my main interests have not been identified and taken into account in this hypothetical train of thought. One of these is my interest in taking myself seriously as a reflective moral agent, and my interest in being taken seriously by others. Identifying my moral obligations, and acting on them is not contrary to my interests, but is an integral part of what makes me a moral agent.[iv]

More importantly, however, as we have seen, I do have a powerful interest in living in a society and indeed in a world in which scientific research is vigorously pursued and is given a high priority.

Do Universal Moral Principles Deny This Claim?

A number of the most influential international protocols on science research seem to contradict the claims so far made and we must now examine these more closely.[22] One of the most widely cited principles is contained in a crucial paragraph of the World Medical Association's *Declaration of Helsinki*, adopted by the 52nd General Assembly, in Edinburgh, Scotland, in October 2000.

> In medical research on human subjects, considerations related to the wellbeing of the human subject should take precedence over the interests of science and society. (WMA,[7] para 5)

This paragraph is widely cited in support of restrictions on scientific research and is interpreted as requiring that all human subject research is in the narrowly conceived interests of the research subjects themselves. This article of faith has become almost unchallengeable.

We need first to examine more closely the idea of what is or is not in someone's interests. (Here the argument echoes that of my paper, "Ethical genetic research".[3]) In this paper I shall neither follow nor consider what other commentators have made of this idea but attempt a rigorous analysis of the meaning of the concepts involved. We should note at the outset that what is or is not in a particular individual's interests is an objective matter. While subjects have a special role to play in determining this, we know that human beings are apt to act against their own interests. Indeed the idea of respect for persons which underpins this guideline has two clear and sometimes incompatible elements, namely, concern for welfare and respect for autonomy. Because people often have self harming preferences (smoking, drug abuse, selfless altruism, etc) they are sometimes bad judges of their interests.

The interests of the subject *cannot* be paramount nor can they automatically take precedence over other interests of comparable moral significance. Such a claim involves a straightforward mistake: being or becoming a research subject is not the sort of thing that could conceivably augment either someone's moral claims or, for that matter, her rights. *All* people are morally important and, with respect to one another, each has a claim to equal consideration. No one has a claim to overriding consideration. To say that the interests of the subject must take precedence over those of others, if it means anything, must be understood as a way of reasserting that a researcher's narrowly conceived professional interests must not have primacy over the human rights of research subjects. (The researcher may also have specific contractual duties to them.) As a general remark about the obligations of the research community, the health care system, society or indeed of the world community, it is not, however, sustainable.

This is not of course to say that human rights are vulnerable to the interests of society whenever these can be demonstrated to be greater. On the contrary, it is to say that the rights and interests of research subjects are just the rights and interests of persons and must be balanced against comparable rights and interests of other persons. In the case of medical research the contrast is not between vulnerable individuals on the one hand and an abstract entity such as "society" on the other, but rather between two different groups of vulnerable individuals. The rights and interests of research subjects are surely not served by privileging them at the expense of the rights and interests of those who will benefit from research. Both these groups are potentially vulnerable, neither is obviously prima facie more vulnerable or deserving of special protection.

It is important to emphasise that the point here is not that there is some general incoherence in the idea of sometimes privileging the rights and interests of particularly vulnerable groups in order to guarantee to them the equal protection that they need and to which they are entitled. Rather I am suggesting two things. The first is that all people have equal rights and entitlement to equal consideration of interests. The second is that any derogation from a principle as fundamental as that of equality must be justified by especially powerful considerations.

Finally, although what is or is not in someone's interests is an objective matter about which the subject her (or him) self may be mistaken, it is usually the best policy to let people define and determine "their own interests". While it is if course possible that people will misunderstand their own interests and even act against them, it is surely more likely that people will understand their own interests best. It is also more respectful of research subjects for us to assume that this is the case unless there are powerful reasons for not so doing – for example, in cases of research on young children, mental patients, and others whom it is reasonable to assume may not be adequately competent.

Is There an Enforceable Obligation to Participate in Research?

It is widely recognised that there is clearly sometimes an obligation to make sacrifices for the community or an entitlement of the community to go so far as to deny autonomy and even violate bodily integrity in the public interest and this obligation is recognised in a number of ways.[23]

There are a perhaps surprisingly large number of cases where we accept substantial degrees of compulsion or coercion in the interests of those coerced and in the public interest. Numerous examples can be given: limiting access to dangerous or addictive drugs or substances; control of road traffic, including compulsory wearing of car seat belts; vaccination as a requirement – for example, for school attendance or travel; screening or diagnostic tests for pregnant mothers or for newborns; genetic profiling for those suspected of crimes; quarantine for some serious communicable diseases; compulsory military service; detention under mental health acts; safety guidelines for certain professional activities of HIV positive people, and compulsory attendance for jury service at criminal trials. Some societies make voting compulsory, taxation is omnipresent, universal education for children, requiring as it does compulsory attendance in school, is another obvious example. All these involve some denial of autonomy, some imposition of public standards even where compliance is not based on the competent consent of individuals. These are, however, clearly exceptional cases where overriding moral considerations take precedence over autonomy. Might medical research be another such case?

Mandatory Contribution to Public Goods

The examples cited above demonstrate a wide range of what we might term "mandatory contribution to public goods".[v] I will take one of these as a model for how we might think about participation in science research. (For use of this principle in a different context see my paper, "Organ procurement – dead interests, living needs".[24] Taxation is of course the clearest and commonest example.)

All British citizens between 18 and 70[vi] are liable for jury service.

They may be called, and unless excused by the court, must serve. This may involve a minimum of 10 days but sometimes months of daily confinement in a jury box or room, whether they consent or not. However, although all are liable for service only some are actually called. If someone is called and fails to appear they may be fined. Most people will never be called but some must be if the system of justice is not to break down. Participation in, or facilitation of, this public good is mandatory. There are many senses in which participation in vaccine or drug trials involve features relevantly analogous to jury service. Both involve inconvenience and the giving up of certain amounts of time. Both are important public goods. It is this latter feature that is particularly important. Although jury service (or compulsory attendance as a witness) is an integral part of "due process", helping to safeguard the liberty and rights of citizens, the same is also true of science research. Disease and infirmity have profound effects on liberty and while putting life threatening criminals out of circulation or protecting the innocent from wrongful imprisonment is a minor (numerically speaking) product of due process, life saving is a major product of science research. If compulsion is justifiable in the case of due process the same or indeed more powerful arguments would surely justify it in the case of science research.

Of course "compulsion" covers a wide range of possible measures. Compulsion may simply mean that something is legally required, without there being any legal penalties for non-compliance. Such legal requirement may of course also be supported by various penalties or incentives, from public disapproval and criticism, fines or loss of tax breaks on the one hand, to imprisonment or forcible attendance or participation further along the spectrum. To say that it would be legitimate to make science research compulsory is not to say that any particular methods of compulsion are necessarily justified or justifiable. While it seems clear that mandatory participation in important public goods is not only justifiable but also widely accepted as justifiable in most societies, as the examples above demonstrate, my own view is that voluntary means are always best and that any form

of compulsion should be a last resort to be used only when consensual means had failed or where the need for a particular research activity was urgent and of overwhelming importance. If the arguments of this paper are persuasive, compulsion should not be necessary and we may expect a climate more receptive to both the needs and the benefits of science. However, to point out that compulsion may be justifiable in some circumstances in the case of science research establishes that a fortiori less stringent means are justifiable in those circumstances.

I hope it is clear that I am not here advocating mandatory participation in research, merely arguing that it is in principle justifiable, and may in certain circumstances become justified in fact. There is a difference between ethics and public policy. To say that something is ethical and therefore justifiable is not the same as either saying it is justified in any particular set of circumstances, nor is it to recommend it nor yet to propose it as a policy for either immediate nor yet for eventual implementation. I believe that consensual participation is always preferable and that persuasion by a combination of evidence and rational argument is always the most appropriate way of achieving social and moral goals. This paper is an attempt to do precisely this. I believe, for example, that conscription into the armed forces is justifiable, but I am not recommending, still less advocating its reintroduction into the UK at this time. The distinction between ethical argument and policy proposal is crucial but is almost always ignored, particularly by the press and news media that report on these matters. In this paper I am intending to do ethics; this is not a policy proposal although it contains one policy proposal, which we will come to in due course.

If I am right in thinking that medical research is a public good, that may *in extremis* justify compulsory participation, then a number of things may be said to follow:

- It should not simply be assumed that people would not wish to act in the public interest, at least where the costs and risks involved are minimal. In the absence of specific evidence to the contrary, if any assumptions are made, they should be that people are public spirited and would wish to participate. (I talk here of minimal risk in the sloppy fashion usual in such contexts. "Risk" is, however, ambiguous between "degree of danger" and "probability of occurrence of danger". Risk may of course be minimal in either or both of these senses.)

- It may be reasonable to presume that people would not consent (unless misinformed or coerced) to do things contrary to their own and to the public interest. The reverse is true when (as with vaccine trials) participation is in both personal and public interest.

- If it is right to claim that there is a general obligation to act in the public interest, then there is less reason to challenge consent and little reason to regard participation as actually or potentially exploitative. We do not usually say: "are you quite sure you want to" when people fulfil their moral and civic obligations. We do not usually insist on informed consent in such cases, we are usually content that they *merely* consent or simply acquiesce. When, for example, I am called for jury service no one says: "only attend if you fully understand the role of trial by jury, due process, etc in our constitution and the civil liberties that fair trials guarantee".

If these suggestions are broadly acceptable and an obligation to participate in research is established, this may well become one of the ways in which research comes to be funded in the future.

We must weigh carefully and compassionately what it is reasonable to put to potential participants in a trial for their free and unfettered consideration. Provided, however, potential research subjects are given full information, and are free to participate or not as they choose, then the only remaining question is whether it is reasonable to permit people freely to choose to participate, given the risks and the sorts of likely gains. Is it reasonable to ask people to run whatever degree of risk is involved, to put up with the inconvenience and intrusion of the study, and so on in all the circumstances of the case? These circumstances

will include both the benefits to them personally of participating in the study and the benefits that will flow from the study to other persons, persons who are of course equally entitled to our concern, respect, and protection. (If they are.) Putting the question in this way makes it clear that the standards of care and levels of protection to be accorded to research subjects who have full information must be, to a certain extent, study relative.

It is crucial that the powerful moral reasons for conducting science research are not drowned by the powerful reasons we have for protecting research subjects. There is a balance to be struck here, but it is not a balance that must always and inevitably be loaded in favour of the protection of research subjects. They are entitled to our concern, respect, and protection to be sure, but they are no more entitled to it than are, say, the people whom, for example, HIV/AIDS or other major diseases are threatening and killing on a daily basis.[vii]

It is surely unethical to stand by and watch three million people die this year of AIDS alone and avoid taking steps to prevent this level of loss, steps, which will not put lives at risk and which are taken only with the fully informed consent of those who participate.

Fully informed consent is the best guarantor of the interests of research subjects. While not foolproof, residual dangers must be balanced against the dangers of not conducting the trial or the research, which include the massive loss of life that possibly preventable diseases cause. These residual dangers include the difficulties of constructing suitable consent protocols and supervising their administration in rural and isolated communities and in populations which may have low levels of formal education.

An interesting limiting case is that in which the risks to research subjects are significant and the burdens onerous but where the benefits to other people are equally significant and large. In such a case the research is both urgent and moral but conscription would almost certainly not be appropriate because of the unfairness of conscripting any particular individual to bear such burdens in the public interest. That is not of course to say that individuals should not be willing to bear such burdens nor is it to say that it is not their moral duty so to do. In fact the history of science research is full of examples of people willing to bear significant risks in such circumstances, very often these have been the researchers themselves. (For one prominent example, that of Barry Marshall's work, in which he swallowed Heliobacter pylori bacteria, thereby poisoning himself, to test a bacterial explanation for peptic ulcers.[25])

Benefit Sharing

I have so far said nothing about the public/private divide in research funding and about the fact that much of the research we have referred to has been carried out in the private sector for profit. This has inevitably led both to a concentration on what the comedian Tom Lehrer memorably called "diseases of the rich" and on diseases and conditions where, for whatever reason, a maximum return on investment is to be expected. In this paper there is room simply to note that the duty to participate in research is not a duty to enable industry to profit from moral commitment or basic decency, and that fairness and benefit sharing as well as the widest and fairest possible availability of the products of research is, as we have seen, an essential part of the moral force of the arguments for the obligation to pursue research. Benefit sharing must therefore be part of any mechanisms for implementing the arguments of this paper.

A New Principle of Research Ethics

A new principle of research ethics suggests itself as an appropriate addition to the *Declaration of Helsinki*:

> Biomedical research involving human subjects cannot legitimately be neglected, and is therefore both permissible and mandatory, where the importance of the objective is great and the risks to and the possibility of exploitation of fully informed and consenting subjects is small.

For an earlier version of this principle applied in the context of genetics see my paper, "Ethical genetic research on human subjects".[3]

Thus while fully informed consent and the continuing provision to research subjects of relevant information does not eliminate all possibility of exploitation, it does reduce it to the point at which it could no longer be ethical to neglect the claims and the interests of those who may benefit from the research. It should be noted that it is fully informed consent, and the concern and respect for the individual that it signals, which severs all connection with the Nazi experiments and the concerns of Nuremberg, and which rebuts spurious comparisons with the Tuskegee study. It is this recognition of the obligation to show equal concern and respect for all persons, which is the defining characteristic of justice.[26] The recognition that the obligation to do justice applies not only to research subjects but also to those who will benefit from the research must constitute an advance in thinking about international standards of research ethics.

On Whom Does the Obligation to Participate in Research Fall?

The Declaration of Helsinki (paragraph 19) states:

> Medical research is only justified if there is a reasonable likelihood that the populations in which the research is carried out stand to benefit from the results of the research. (WMA,[7] para 19)

Me and My Kind

It is sometimes claimed that where consent is problematic or, as perhaps with genetic research on archival material, where the sources of the material are either dead or cannot be traced, that research may be legitimate if it is for the benefit of the health needs of the subjects or of people with similar or related disorders. See, for example, the CIOMS guidelines (CIOMS,[8] guideline 6: p 22). The suggestion that research which is not directly beneficial to the patient be confined to research that will benefit the category of patients to which the subject belongs seems not only untenable but also offensive. What arguments sustain the idea that the most appropriate reference group is that of fellow sufferers from a particular disease, Alzheimer's, for example? Surely any moral obligation I have to accept risk or harm for the benefit of others is not plausibly confined to those others who are narrowly like me. This is surely close to claiming that research should be confined to others who are "black like me" or "English like me" or "God fearing like me"? The most appropriate category is surely "a person like me". (I make a distinction between humans and persons which is not particularly pertinent in this context but which explains my choice of terminology.[27, 28])

Children and the Incompetent

What, however, about children?[1] Do they have an obligation to participate in research and if they have, is a parent justified in taking it into account in making decisions for the child?

If children are moral agents, and most of them, except very young infants are, then they have both obligations and rights; and it will be difficult to find any obligations that are more basic than the obligation to help others in need. There is therefore little doubt that children share the obligation argued for in this paper, to participate in medical research. A parent or guardian is accordingly obliged to take this obligation into account when deciding on behalf of her child and is justified in assuming that the person they are making decisions for is or would wish to be, a moral person who wants to or is in any event obliged to discharge his or her moral duties. If anything is presumed about what children would have wished to do in such circumstances the presumption should surely be that they would have wished to behave decently and would not have wished to be free riders. If we simply consult their best interests (absent the possibility of a valid consent) then again, as this paper has

shown, participation in research is, other things being equal, in their best interests. Because of the primacy of autonomy in the structure of this argument we should, however, be cautious about enrolling those who cannot consent in research and should never force resisting incompetent individuals to participate. It also follows from principles of justice and fairness that those who are not competent to consent should not be exploited as prime candidates for research. We should always therefore prefer autonomous candidates and only use those who cannot consent when such individuals are essential for the particular research contemplated and where competent individuals cannot, because of the nature of the research, be used – for example, because the research is into an illness which only affects children or those with a particular condition which affects competence. In those extreme cases in which we might contemplate mandatory participation the same will hold. The incompetent should only be used where competent individuals cannot be research subjects because of the nature of the research itself.

Inducements to Participate in Research

Before concluding, a word needs to be said about inducements to research. Most research ethics protocols and guidelines are antipathetic to inducements. The CIOMS guidelines – for example, state that if inducements to subjects are offered "[t]he payments should not be so large, however, or the medical services so extensive as to induce prospective subjects to consent to participate in the research against their better judgment (undue inducement)" (CIOMS,[8] guideline 7).

However, the gloss the CIOMS document offers on this guideline is perhaps confused. It states: "Someone without access to medical care may or may not be unduly influenced to participate in research simply to receive such care" (CIOMS,[8] pp 28ff). The nub of the problem is the question what is it that makes inducement *undue*? If inducement is undue when it undermines "better judgment", then it cannot simply be the level of the inducement nor the fact that it is the inducement that makes the difference between participation and non-participation that undermines better judgment. If this were so, all jobs with attractive remuneration packages would constitute "undue" interference with the liberties of subjects and anyone who used their better judgment to decide whether a total remuneration package plus job was attractive would have been unduly influenced.[viii]

Surely, it is only if things are very different that influence becomes undue. If, for example, it were true that no sane person would participate in the study and only incentives would induce them to disregard "better judgment" or "rationality", or if the study were somehow immoral, or participation was grossly undignified and so on, would there be a legitimate presumption of undue influence.

Grant a number of assumptions: that research is well founded scientifically; that it has important objectives which will advance knowledge; that the subjects are at minimal risk, and that the inconvenience and so on, of participation is not onerous. Then surely it is not only in everyone's best interests that *some* people participate but also in the interests of those who do. *Better judgment* surely will not indicate that any particular person should not participate. Of course someone consulting personal interest and convenience might not participate: "it's too much trouble, not worth the effort, rather inconvenient" and so on. However, removing the force of *these sorts of objections* with incentives is not undermining *better judgment* any more than is making employment attractive.[29–31]

Of course inducements may be undue in a different sense. If, for example, a research subject were a drug addict and she were to be offered the drug of her choice to participate, or subjects were blackmailed into participating in research, then in such cases we might regard the inducements as undue. It is important, however, to note that here the influence or inducement is undue, not because it is improper to offer incentives to participate, nor because participation is

against the best interests of the subject, nor because the inducements are coercive in the sense that they are irresistible, but rather because the *type of incentive* offered is illegitimate or against the public interest or immoral in itself.

If I offer you a million dollars to do something involving minimal risk and inconvenience, something that is good in itself, is in your interests, and will benefit mankind, my offer may be irresistible but it will not be coercive. If, however, I threaten you with torture unless you do the same thing, my act will be coercive even if you were going to do it whether or not I threatened you. I should be punished for my threat or blackmail or criminal offer of illegal substances, but surely you should none the less do the deed and your freedom to do it should not be curtailed because of my wrongdoing in attempting to force your hand in a particular way. The wrong is not that I attempted to force your hand but resides rather in the wrongness of the methods that I chose. This is the distinction between undue inducement and inducements which are undue. "Undue inducement" is the improper offering of inducements, improper because no inducements should be offered. It is this that it referred to in the various international protocols we have been examining and which is almost always wrongly understood and applied. "Inducements which are undue", refer to the nature of the inducement, not to the fact of it being offered at all. This is an important but much neglected distinction. Here it is the nature of the inducement that is undue rather than the fact of inducements of some sorts (even irresistible sorts) being offered.

We can see that offering incentives, perhaps in the form of direct payment or tax concessions to people to participate in research, or, for example, to make archive samples available for research would not be unethical. We tend to forget that law and morality are methods of encouraging and indeed enforcing morality. Approval and inducements are others. All are acceptable if the conduct they promote is ethical and worthwhile. Where science research is both of these, encouragement and, as we have seen, enforcement are justifiable.

Conclusion

There is then a moral obligation to participate in medical research in certain contexts.[ix]

This will obviously include minimally invasive and minimally risky procedures such as participation in biobanks, provided safeguards against wrongful use are in place. The argument concerning the obligation to participate in research should be compelling for anyone who believes there is a moral obligation to help others, and/or a moral obligation to be just and do one's share. Little can be said to those whose morality is so impoverished that they do not accept either of these two obligations.

Furthermore we are justified in assuming that a person would want to discharge his or her moral obligations in cases where we have no knowledge about their actual preferences. This is a way of recognising them as moral agents. To do otherwise would be to impute moral turpitude as a default. Parents making decisions for their children are therefore fully justified in assuming that their child will wish to do that which is right, and not do that which is wrong.

Notes

i In this paper I use arguments developed for a paper I wrote with my colleague Søren Holm. See our paper "Should we presume moral turpitude in our children?";[1] my chapter "Research on human subjects, exploitation and global principles of ethics";[2] and my paper "Ethical genetic research".[3] Recently these themes have been taken up by Martyn Evans. See his paper "Should patients be allowed to veto their participation in clinical research,"[4]

ii Here the argument is restricted to research projects that are not merely aimed at producing knowledge. Unless an increase in knowledge is a good in itself (a question I will not discuss here) some realistic hope of concrete benefits to persons in the future is necessary for the validity of our arguments.

iii It is perhaps also worth pointing out that there is a separate question about whether this moral obligation should be enforced on those who do not discharge it voluntarily. This is not a question I will discuss here.

iv I owe this formulation of the interest I have in being a moral agent to Søren Holm.

v I use this term in a non-technical sense.

vi Those over 65 may be excused if they wish.

vii Of course the historical explanation of the *Declaration of Helsinki* and its concerns lies in the Nuremberg trials and the legacy of Nazi atrocities. We are, however, I believe, in real danger of allowing fear of repeating one set of atrocities to lead us into committing other new atrocities.

viii The CIOMS gloss on their own guidelines creates a kind of Catch 22 which is surely unreasonable and unwarranted. Wherever the best proven diagnostic and therapeutic methods are guaranteed by a study in a context or for a population who would not normally expect to receive them, this guideline would be broken. The CIOMS guideline four therefore surely contradicts and violates not only the *Declaration of Helsinki* but also its own later guideline 14.

ix This obligation has been partly endorsed by the Hugo Ethics Committee in its *Statement on Human Genomic databases*.[32] However, like so many statements by august ethics committees the Hugo statement contains not a single argument to sustain its proposals or conclusions. This paper and those referred to in references 1, 2, 3, and 4 provide the missing arguments. For a critique of the operation of national and international ethics committees see the introduction to my book, *Bioethics*.[33]

References

1 Harris J. and Holm S. Should we presume moral turpitude in our children? Small children and consent to medical research. *Theor Med* 2003; 24:121–9.

2 Harris J. Research on human subjects, exploitation and global principles of ethics. In: Lewis A.D.E. and Freeman M., eds. *Current legal issue 3: law and*

medicine. Oxford: Oxford University Press, 2000: 379–99.

3 Harris J. Ethical genetic research. *Jurimetrics* 1999; 40:77–93.

4 Evans H.M. Should patients be allowed to veto their participation in clinical research? *J Med Ethics* 2004; 30:198–203.

5 Williams C., Kitzinger J., and Henderson L. Envisaging the embryo in stem cell research: rhetorical strategies and media reporting of the ethical debates. *Sociol Health Illn* 2003; 5:783–814.

6 Harris J. and Holm S. Extended lifespan and the paradox of precaution. *J Med Philos* 2002; 27:355–68.

7 World Medical Association. *Declaration of Helsinki*. Adopted by the 52nd General Assembly, Edinburgh, Scotland Oct 2000: note of clarification of para 29 added by the WMA General Assembly, Washington, 2002.

8 Council for International Organisations of Medical Sciences (CIOMS). *Guidelines*. Geneva: CIOMS, 2002.

9 Caplan A.L., ed. *When medicine went mad*. Totowa: Humana Press, 1992.

10 Glover J. *Humanity: a moral history of the twentieth century*. London: Jonathan Cape, 1999, part 6.

11 Angell M. The ethics of clinical research in the Third World. *N Engl J Med* 1997; 337:847.

12 Anon. Twenty years after: the legacy of the Tuskegee syphilis study. *Hastings Cent Rep* 1992; 22:29–40.

13 *The Royal Liverpool Children's Inquiry Report*. London: The Stationery Office, London, 2001.

14 Harris J. Law and regulation of retained organs: the ethical issues. *Legal Studies* 2002; 22:527–49.

15 Harris J. *Violence and responsibility*. London: Routledge & Kegan Paul, 1980.

16 Barry B. *Justice as impartiality*. Oxford: Clarendon Press, 1995: 228.

17 Jonas H. Philosophical reflections on experimenting with human subjects. In: Freund P.A., ed. *Experimentation with human subjects*. London: Allen and Unwin, 1972.

18 Hart H.L.A. Are there any natural rights? *Oxford Review* No 4, 1967; Feb.

19 Rawls J. *A theory of justice*. Cambridge: Harvard University Press, 1972.

20 Nozick R. *Anarchy, state and Utopia*. Oxford: Basil Blackwell, 1974: 90.

21 Harris J. The ethics of clinical research with cognitively impaired subjects. *Ital J Neurol Sci* 1997; 18:9–15.

22 Harris J. and Holm S. Why should doctors take risks? Professional responsibility and the assumption of risk. *J R Soc Med* 1997; 90:625–9.

23 Harris J. Ethical issues in geriatric medicine. In: Tallis R.C. and Fillett H.M., eds. *Textbook of geriatric medicine and gerontology* [6th ed]. London: Churchill Livingstone, 2002.

24 Harris J. Organ procurement – dead interests, living needs. *J Med Ethics* 2003; 29:130–5.

25 Marshall B. [See now https://www.nobelprize.org/prizes/medicine/2005/marshall/biographical/

26 Dworkin R. *Taking rights seriously*. London: Duckworth, 1977.

27 Harris J. *The value of life*. London: Routledge and Kegan Paul, 1985, ch 1.

28 Harris J. The concept of the person and the value of life. *Kennedy Inst Ethics J* 1999; 9:293–308.

29 Wilkinson M. and Moore A. Inducements Revisited. *Bioethics* 1997; 11:114–30.

30 McNeill P. Paying people to participate in research: why not? *Bioethics* 1997; 11:390–7.

31 Harris J. *Wonderwoman and Superman: the ethics of human biotechnology*. Oxford: Oxford University Press, 1992, ch 6.

32 Hugo Ethics Committee. *Statement on human genomic databases*, http://www.hugo-international.org/Resources/Documents/CELS_Statement-HumanGenomicDatabase_2002.pdf

33 Harris J, ed. *Bioethics: Oxford readings in philosophy series*. Oxford: Oxford University Press, 2001: 1–25.

56

Participation in Biomedical Research is an Imperfect Moral Duty

A Response to John Harris

Sandra Shapshay and Kenneth D. Pimple

In his paper "Scientific research is a moral duty" [chapter 55 in this *Anthology*], John Harris[1] intends to encourage individuals to volunteer as subjects in biomedical research by arguing that supporting biomedical research is a moral obligation, both for individuals and society. Although we agree that biomedical research is an important social good, we find Harris's arguments for the thesis that individuals have a moral duty to participate in serious scientific research to be unconvincing.

Most of Harris's arguments concern the moral duty of individuals, on which we will focus our attention. In our view, the moral duty of a society to support biomedical research is better approached separately.

The bulk of this paper will concern Harris's substantive arguments in making his case that those of us who have benefited from modern medical science – virtually all of us living in industrialised nations – have a moral obligation to volunteer as research subjects, but first we wish to touch briefly on his rhetorical strategy.

In our judgement, Harris makes a serious rhetorical mistake by engaging in hyperbole. For example,

Harris cites paragraph A.5 of the World Medical Association's *Ethical principles for medical research involving human subjects*,[2] commonly referred to as the Declaration of Helsinki.

> In medical research on human subjects, considerations related to the well-being of the human subject should take precedence over the interests of science and society.

According to Harris, "this paragraph is widely cited in support of restrictions on scientific research and is interpreted as requiring that all human subject research is in the narrowly conceived interests of the research subjects themselves. This article of faith has become almost unchallengeable" (p 243).

Unfortunately, Harris does not offer a single citation to support this claim. We know of no instance in which this paragraph has been so narrowly construed, and we suggest that such a construal conflates research with therapy, which is obviously contrary to the purpose of the Declaration. Indeed, Harris's later interpretation of this paragraph accords closely with

Original publication details: Sandra Shapshay and Kenneth D. Pimple, "Participation in Research Is an Imperfect Moral Duty: A Response to John Harris," pp. 414–417 from *Journal of Medical Ethics* 33 (2007). Reproduced with permission of BMJ Publishing Group Ltd.

Bioethics: An Anthology, Fourth Edition. Edited by Udo Schüklenk and Peter Singer.

our own, and, in our belief, with the majority opinion: "To say that the interests of the subject must take precedence over those of others … must be understood as a way of reasserting that a researcher's narrowly conceived professional interest must not have primacy over the human rights of research subjects" (p 244).

Harris also hyperbolises in his first sentence, stating: "Science is under attack", and admonishes us to remember "the powerful moral obligation there is to undertake, support, and participate in scientific research, particularly biomedical research, and the powerful moral imperative that underpins these obligations" (p 242). But by the end of his article, he qualifies the moral duty to participate in biomedical research nearly out of existence.

Here, our aim is to show that Harris's arguments succeed only in showing that such participation and support is one moral good among many, but that there is no moral duty to support and/or participate in biomedical research per se, except, perhaps, in rare emergency situations. We will show this by focusing on the two major ethical principles that Harris employs: the principles of beneficence and fairness. We will detail why each ethical principle yields only a weaker discretionary obligation to help others in need and to reciprocate for sacrifices that others have made for the public good.

The Principle of Beneficence

Harris claims polemically that "the overwhelming presumption has been and remains that participation in research is a supererogatory, and probably a reckless, act, not an obligation" (p 242). This presumption should be abandoned, he argues, based on the "rule of rescue":

> Where our actions will, or may probably prevent serious harm then if we can reasonably (given the balance of risk and burden to ourselves and benefit to others) we clearly should act because to fail to do so is to accept responsibility for the harm that then occurs. (p 242)

He calls this rule "the stronger side" of the principle of beneficence, the duty to help others in need.[i]

On this basis of the rule of rescue, Harris argues that if our actions can prevent some harm, and we can reasonably perform those actions, then we ought so to act. This understanding of the principle is reminiscent of Singer's[3] famous statement: "If it is in our power to prevent something bad from happening, without thereby sacrificing anything of comparable moral importance, we ought, morally, to do it." Singer supports this obligation through the pond case: Imagine you are the only adult in view when you see a toddler drowning in a shallow pond. Clearly, you should rescue the child even if your clothes will be drenched.

However, the rule of rescue in the case of biomedical research would have to be derived from a rather different case: 50 agents surround the pond and 20 toddlers are in distress: one child is drowning, another is lost, a third is being attacked by a dog, etc, and neither you nor any of the other agents is uniquely situated to help any particular child. In this more analogous case, it would be strange to argue that every agent is obliged to save the drowning child, especially at the cost of the other 19 children. Clearly, each agent may justifiably choose which child to help.[ii]

Harris's application of the rule of rescue can be schematised as follows:

1. If our actions can prevent serious harm, and we can reasonably perform those actions, then we ought to act so.
2. Many diseases cause serious harm.
3. Medical research is a necessary component of preventing or relieving those harms.
4. Therefore, if we can take reasonable steps to further medical research (by volunteering as a research participant), we have an obligation to do so.

We accept premises 2 and 3 as true statements. However, premise 1 requires further specification: we should determine whether our moral duty to prevent serious harm when we reasonably can means that we have a duty

a. to prevent any and all serious harm whenever we reasonably can; or

b. to prevent only the most serious harm when we reasonably can; or

c. to prevent some subset of serious harm of our own choice when we reasonably can.

It seems that in order for Harris's argument to be valid, he must call on (a), the most general and stringent formulation. If our duty were only to prevent (b) the most serious harm, or if our duty were to prevent (c) some subset of serious harm of our own choice, it is not clear why the serious harms caused by disease in particular should necessarily entail a claim on us for our help. With the less general formulations of the rule of rescue, one might justifiably decide to prevent other forms of serious harm, say, political persecution, or illiteracy. It is only if we are duty-bound to prevent any and all serious harms when we reasonably can that we are obliged to prevent disease in particular. Without the most general formulation, we would be quite justified in working to prevent harm to at-risk youth instead of participating in biomedical research, even if we were reasonably capable of so participating.

But the most general formulation of the rule of rescue, "that we ought to prevent any and all serious harm, when we reasonably can", is implausible largely because it is over-demanding. Otherwise put, this form of the rule of rescue amounts to the act utilitarian injunction, always to act so as to minimise harm or bad states of affairs (the negative construal of the principle of utility). Bernard Williams[4] has forcefully criticised act utilitarianism on the grounds that it "makes integrity as a value more or less unintelligible" because it enjoins the agent to factor his or her own deepest commitments and projects in life equally alongside all the other factors in the utility calculus. As there are, as a matter of fact, so many opportunities to minimise harm, one is duty-bound to devote most of one's time and resources to preventing poverty, hunger, war and any number of other serious harms, rather than to other less useful projects.

A person who consistently acts on this formulation of the rule of rescue would become nothing more than "a channel between the input of everyone's projects, including his own, and an output of optimific decision". This principle thus reduces him to a harm-minimising conduit and destroys his personal integrity – the union of his actions with his own deepest convictions and projects in life. With Williams,[4] we argue, the most general formulation of the rule of rescue is profoundly alienating.

It might be argued that the qualifier "when we reasonably can" salvages individual integrity; it can hardly be considered "reasonable" to expect everyone to abandon all of their personal goals to minimise all serious harm. If this is what Harris intends, however, he is in fact endorsing a weaker formulation of the principle of beneficence, (c) above: where we reasonably can, we ought to prevent some subset of serious harm, of our own choice. If we do adopt this weaker formulation, we are left without a duty to participate in biomedical research per se. Rather, we are left with an imperfect duty to choose from all possible harms those which we will strive to prevent.

A Kantian imperfect duty is a duty to adopt certain ends – one's own perfection and the happiness of others. Accordingly, one may not totally neglect the happiness of others or the perfection of oneself, but one has a good deal of latitude in what one does to achieve these ends. According to Kant scholar Thomas Hill,

> imperfect duties allow us to do what we please on some occasions … [f]or example, though we have an imperfect duty of beneficence we may sometimes pass over an opportunity to make others happy simply because we would rather do something else.[5]

Despite some controversy concerning just how much latitude Kantian imperfect duties allow,[6] on reading (c) of Harris's principle, one may surely discharge one's imperfect obligation to prevent harm to others by volunteering at an animal shelter, or by donating money to Oxfam, or by participating in medical research – but one cannot be said to have a duty to do the latter, in particular.

Perhaps Harris's argument could be saved by use of version (b) of the rule of rescue – namely, "we have an obligation to prevent the most serious harm, when we reasonably can." By this formulation, one would be obliged to address only the most serious harms one reasonably could. Surely, the most significant harms facing people in the world today are not those which must be addressed through biomedical research. Citing statistics from the United Nations Development Report of 2002, Thomas Pogge[7] writes,

> poverty is far and away the most important factor in explaining health deficits. Because they are poor, 815 million persons are malnourished, 1.1 billion lack access to safe water, 2.4 billion lack access to basic sanitation, more than 880 million lack access to health services, and approximately 1 billion have no adequate shelter.

This staggering amount of suffering is due to preventable poverty, not due to disease.

Furthermore, Pogge argues that much poverty is due to global institutions (lending and trade practices) that exploit poor nations. Citizens of democratic, industrialised nations are thus materially implicated in the poverty-related harms caused in part by global institutions. It stands to reason that we have much more of an obligation to rectify the injustice that our own democratically elected governments have caused than to try to alleviate disease-related suffering in which we are not materially implicated. If we accept formulation (b) of the rule of rescue, we ought rather to work to change unjust institutions that foster poverty rather than participate in biomedical research.

We have analysed the rule of rescue following Harris's lead, but a similar analysis could be done along any of a number of dimensions:

- Are we obliged to rescue only persons in our own household, or those in our physical presence, or those we know to exist, or any potential persons (those untold billions not yet born)?
- Are we obliged to prevent only obvious and imminent harms, or likely harms, or potential but unlikely harms?
- Are we required to take action only if it will assure the prevention of harm, or if it is likely to prevent harm, or if it might possibly prevent harm?

We believe that the conclusion would be the same no matter which of these dimensions were pursued: the more extreme and stringent a formulation, the less reasonable it is to construe it as a perfect moral obligation.

Essentially, the main problem with Harris's overall argument so far is that he sets up a false dilemma: either participation in research is supererogatory or it is a positive and perfect moral obligation. However, there is a third possibility: The rule of rescue may constitute an "imperfect obligation", meaning that we must make others' happiness our end, and act in good faith to help some others some of the time, but we may justifiably use our own discretion as to whom, how and how much to help.[iii] Thus, we can say that participation in research per se is not morally obligatory, but neither is it supererogatory; it is one way in which people may choose to discharge their imperfect obligation to help others.

The Principle of Fairness

The second principle which Harris invokes to show that we have a positive moral obligation to support/participate in biomedical research, is the principle of fairness developed by H L A Hart[8] and John Rawls[9]. As Harris puts it, as all of us (at least all members of industrialised countries[iv]) benefit from the existence of medical research, and we all accept these benefits (eg, through vaccines, public sanitation, personal medical services, etc), "we have an obligation in justice to contribute to the social practice which produces them."[1] In other words, if one accepts the benefits of biomedical research, then one ought to support the endeavour which makes those benefits possible in the first place; otherwise one would be acting unfairly as a "free rider".

Although this line of argument is far more promising than the previous one, it does not stand up to close scrutiny. Let us begin with a literal free-rider scenario. For the sake of argument, assume that the Berlin S-Bahn system runs more efficiently when all riders pay for and stamp their own tickets, with minimal enforcement. On the basis of this added effi-ciency, every resident of Berlin enjoys more generous public services. Hans, who is wealthy, decides that he will derive maximal personal benefit if he does not pay to ride – he enjoys all of the advantages of oth-ers' cooperation, but does not pay the price. Clearly Hans's action is unfair, and he has a perfect duty not to act unfairly in this way.

Harris implicitly draws a parallel between the classic free rider and the individual who benefits from but who does not personally participate in biomedical research. But there are two significant differences between these situations. The first difference concerns one's freedom to choose to use the benefit. In the case of Hans, he is certainly free not to ride the S-Bahn if he does not want to pay. He could walk or bike instead. But the benefi-ciary of biomedical research is not similarly free not to enjoy the fruits of the research. In our modern indus-trialised societies, as a child one does not choose to be immunised or brought up with modern sanitation. An adult could certainly decline further enjoyment of such benefits, but, as the benefits of biomedical research are ubiquitous in modern society, this would require one to move to the wilderness or what's left of it.

This disanalogy is morally significant because, if one does not truly choose to accept the benefits of such research, it is hard to see how one is thereby respon-sible for supporting the institutions that bestow those benefits, whereas Hans, our free rider, must explicitly choose to ride the S-Bahn and is thus responsible for playing fair by paying the fare.

Furthermore, the people who are harmed by Hans's free riding are the same people who would benefit from his cooperation. This is not likely to be the case with participation in medical research, where, due to the lag between trials and interventions, one generally benefits from past participation and is likely to benefit those in the future, not present partici-pants in research.[v] Even if I owe a duty of reciprocity to those living people who participated in medical research, or to the descendants of those who partici-pated in the past, if I have benefited from vaccinations, am I obliged to participate in vaccination research? What about mental health research? The list can be extended indefinitely. As in the case of beneficence, the more comprehensively a moral duty is construed, the less credible it is.

To the extent that we are obliged to discharge our debts for benefits "in kind", we can find ourselves with directly conflicting moral obligations. If not for the service of Allied military men and women, we would be living under a Nazi dictatorship; therefore, we have a moral obligation to enlist in the military. But if not for the sacrifices of conscientious objectors and war protesters, governments would be less con-strained in choosing when to go to war; therefore, we should resist military operations.

There are many ways in which we ought to refrain from "free riding", but we cannot reasonably be expected to do them all. Harris might reply that those who have many other obligations imposed on them by the principle of fairness can only reasonably be expected to reciprocate – namely, biomedical research when it is easy for them to do so. He cites two exam-ples of obligatory participation in biomedical research when doing so seems not to be in one's best interest, narrowly construed:

> If I am asked to give a blood sample for a worthwhile research project, or if I am asked if tissue removed during an operation may be retained for research or therapeutic use [I should accede].[1]

This is what the duty to participate in biomedical research boils down to for Harris: when participation requires nothing more than a minor inconvenience, you should. We find it difficult to disagree with this extraordinarily modest conclusion, which is akin to asserting that telling the truth is a moral duty as long as it is convenient to do so.

But at this point, Harris implicitly concedes that the obligation to participate in biomedical research is only part of a discretionary duty to help others. In the cases Harris mentions, the demands are quite trivial. Insofar as the demand of participating is greater, in terms of time, hardship or risk, a person is justified in spending his or her time, money and effort in dis-charging her imperfect obligations in another way.

Conclusions

We have argued, contra Harris, that any duty to participate in biomedical research must be understood as part of a more general imperfect duty to promote the welfare of others. Any candid attempt to persuade people to volunteer as research participants should acknowledge this, emphasising that such participation helps to sustain a moral good.

While Harris does not succeed in proving the point he set out to prove, his line of reasoning supports what we believe is an important conclusion: we have a general obligation to support just institutions insofar as we benefit from them. The principle of fairness better supports a societal obligation to promote research in a way that protects subjects and distributes the fruits of research fairly. But, as individuals faced with multiple worthy collective enterprises, and finite lives, we must each decide how to discharge our duty to do our fair share, rather than being browbeaten into choosing one tactic over another.

Notes

i   This section of Harris's article is confused. It is headed "Do no harm" and cites "the duty not to harm others", which we would call "non-maleficence". We agree that the obligation of non-maleficence is stronger than the obligation of beneficence, but the rule of rescue falls more happily under beneficence (which involves taking positive actions to do good) than non-maleficence (which involves avoiding or refraining from actions that cause harm).

ii   We are indebted to an anonymous reviewer for bringing this significant disanalogy to our attention.

iii   We are arguing that the rule of rescue may be seen as an imperfect duty when an agent is not uniquely situated to do the rescuing.

iv   Except, of course, in the US, where approximately 46 million people do not have reliable access to healthcare. By Harris's account, the principle of fairness would compel Britons more strongly than Americans to support biomedical research because in the US such research is not a truly public good.

v   We gained an appreciation of this salient point from an anonymous reviewer.

References

1   Harris J. Scientific research is a moral duty. *J Med Ethics* 2005; 31:242–8.

2   World Medical Association. *Declaration of Helsinki: ethical principles for medical research involving human subjects,* 2004.

3   Singer P. Famine, affluence, and morality. *Philos Public Aff* 1972; 1:229–43.

4   Williams B. A critique of utilitarianism. In: Smart J.J.C and Williams B., eds. *Utilitarianism, for and against.* Cambridge: Cambridge University Press, 1990: 82–117.

5   Hill T.E. *Dignity and practical reason in Kant's moral theory.* Ithaca: Cornell University Press, 1992.

6   Baron M. *Kantian ethics almost without apology.* Ithaca: Cornell University Press, 1995.

7   Pogge T. Responsibilities for poverty-related ill health. *Ethics Int Aff* 2002; 16:71–9.

8   Hart H.L.A. Are there any natural rights? *Oxford Review* No. 4 1967.

9   Rawls J. *A theory of justice.* Cambridge: Harvard University Press, 1971.

57

Unethical Trials of Interventions to Reduce Perinatal Transmission of the Human Immunodeficiency Virus in Developing Countries

Peter Lurie and Sidney M. Wolfe

It has been almost three years since the Journal [the *New England Journal of Medicine*][1] published the results of AIDS Clinical Trials Group (ACTG) Study 076, the first randomized, controlled trial in which an intervention was proved to reduce the incidence of human immunodeficiency virus (HIV) infection. The antiretroviral drug zidovudine, administered orally to HIV-positive pregnant women in the United States and France, administered intravenously during labor, and subsequently administered to the newborn infants, reduced the incidence of HIV infection by two thirds.[2] The regimen can save the life of one of every seven infants born to HIV-infected women.

Because of these findings, the study was terminated at the first interim analysis and, within two months after the results had been announced, the Public Health Service had convened a meeting and concluded that the ACTG 076 regimen should be recommended for all HIV-positive pregnant women without substantial prior exposure to zidovudine and should be considered for other HIV-positive pregnant women on a case-by-case basis.[3] The standard of care for HIV-positive pregnant women thus became the ACTG 076 regimen.

In the United States, three recent studies of clinical practice report that the use of the ACTG 076 regimen is associated with decreases of 50 percent or more in perinatal HIV transmission.[4-6] But in developing countries, especially in Asia and sub-Saharan Africa, where it is projected that by the year 2000, 6 million pregnant women will be infected with HIV,[7] the potential of the ACTG 076 regimen remains unrealized primarily because of the drug's exorbitant cost in most countries.

Clearly, a regimen that is less expensive than ACTG 076 but as effective is desirable, in both developing and industrialized countries. But there has been uncertainty about what research design to use in the search for a less expensive regimen. In June 1994, the World Health Organization (WHO) convened a group in Geneva to assess the agenda for research on perinatal HIV transmission in the wake of ACTG 076.

Original publication details: Peter Lurie and Sidney M. Wolfe, "Unethical Trials of Interventions to Reduce Perinatal Transmission of the Human Immunodeficiency Virus in Developing Countries," pp. 853–856 from *New England Journal of Medicine* 337: 12 (September 1997). © 1997 Massachusetts Medical Society. Reproduced with permission of Massachusetts Medical Society.

The group, which included no ethicists, concluded, "Placebo-controlled trials offer the best option for a rapid and scientifically valid assessment of alternative antiretroviral drug regimens to prevent [perinatal] transmission of HIV."[8] This unpublished document has been widely cited as justification for subsequent trials in developing countries. In our view, most of these trials are unethical and will lead to hundreds of preventable HIV infections in infants.

Primarily on the basis of documents obtained from the Centers for Disease Control and Prevention (CDC), we have identified 18 randomized, controlled trials of interventions to prevent perinatal HIV transmission that either began to enroll patients after the ACTG 076 study was completed or have not yet begun to enroll patients. The studies are designed to evaluate a variety of interventions: antiretroviral drugs such as zidovudine (usually in regimens that are less expensive or complex than the ACTG 076 regimen), vitamin A and its derivatives, intrapartum vaginal washing, and HIV immune globulin, a form of immunotherapy. These trials involve a total of more than 17,000 women.

In the two studies being performed in the United States, the patients in all the study groups have unrestricted access to zidovudine or other antiretroviral drugs. In 15 of the 16 trials in developing countries, however, some or all of the patients are not provided with antiretroviral drugs. Nine of the 15 studies being conducted outside the United States are funded by the US government through the CDC or the National Institutes of Health (NIH), 5 are funded by other governments, and 1 is funded by the United Nations AIDS Program. The studies are being conducted in Côte d'Ivoire, Uganda, Tanzania, South Africa, Malawi, Thailand, Ethiopia, Burkina Faso, Zimbabwe, Kenya, and the Dominican Republic. These 15 studies clearly violate recent guidelines designed specifically to address ethical issues pertaining to studies in developing countries. According to these guidelines, "The ethical standards applied should be no less exacting than they would be in the case of research carried out in [the sponsoring] country."[9] In addition, US regulations governing studies performed with federal funds domestically or abroad specify that research procedures must "not unnecessarily expose subjects to risk."[10]

The 16th study is noteworthy both as a model of an ethically conducted study attempting to identify less expensive antiretroviral regimens and as an indication of how strong the placebo-controlled trial orthodoxy is. In 1994, Marc Lallemant, a researcher at the Harvard School of Public Health, applied for NIH funding for an equivalency study in Thailand in which three shorter zidovudine regimens were to be compared with a regimen similar to that used in the ACTG 076 study. An equivalency study is typically conducted when a particular regimen has already been proved effective and one is interested in determining whether a second regimen is about as effective but less toxic or expensive.[11] The NIH study section repeatedly put pressure on Lallemant and the Harvard School of Public Health to conduct a placebo-controlled trial instead, prompting the director of Harvard's human subjects committee to reply, "The conduct of a placebo-controlled trial for [zidovudine] in pregnant women in Thailand would be unethical and unacceptable, since an active-controlled trial is feasible."[12] The NIH eventually relented, and the study is now under way. Since the nine studies of antiretroviral drugs have attracted the most attention, we focus on them in this article.

Asking the Wrong Research Question

There are numerous areas of agreement between those conducting or defending these placebo-controlled studies in developing countries and those opposing such trials. The two sides agree that perinatal HIV transmission is a grave problem meriting concerted international attention; that the ACTG 076 trial was a major breakthrough in perinatal HIV prevention; that there is a role for research on this topic in developing countries; that identifying less expensive, similarly effective interventions would be of enormous benefit, given the limited resources for medical care in most developing countries; and that randomized studies can help identify such interventions.

The sole point of disagreement is the best comparison group to use in assessing the effectiveness of less-expensive interventions once an effective intervention has been identified. The researchers conducting the placebo-controlled trials assert that such trials represent the only appropriate research design, implying that they answer the question, "Is the shorter regimen better than nothing?" We take the more optimistic view that, given the findings of ACTG 076 and other clinical information, researchers are quite capable of designing a shorter antiretroviral regimen that is approximately as effective as the ACTG 076 regimen. The proposal for the Harvard study in Thailand states the research question clearly: "Can we reduce the duration of prophylactic [zidovudine] treatment without increasing the risk of perinatal transmission of HIV, that is, without compromising the demonstrated efficacy of the standard ACTG 076 [zidovudine] regimen?"[13] We believe that such equivalency studies of alternative antiretroviral regimens will provide even more useful results than placebo-controlled trials, without the deaths of hundreds of newborns that are inevitable if placebo groups are used.

At a recent congressional hearing on research ethics, NIH director Harold Varmus was asked how the Department of Health and Human Services could be funding both a placebo-controlled trial (through the CDC) and a non-placebo-controlled equivalency study (through the NIH) in Thailand. Dr Varmus conceded that placebo-controlled studies are "not the only way to achieve results."[14] If the research can be satisfactorily conducted in more than one way, why not select the approach that minimizes loss of life?

Inadequate Analysis of Data from ACTG 076 and Other Sources

The NIH, CDC, WHO, and the researchers conducting the studies we consider unethical argue that

differences in the duration and route of administration of antiretroviral agents in the shorter regimens, as compared with the ACTG 076 regimen, justify the use of a placebo group.[15–18] Given that ACTG 076 was a well-conducted, randomized, controlled trial, it is disturbing that the rich data available from the study were not adequately used by the group assembled by WHO in June 1994, which recommended placebo-controlled trials after ACTG 076, or by the investigators of the 15 studies we consider unethical.

In fact, the ACTG 076 investigators conducted a subgroup analysis to identify an appropriate period for prepartum administration of zidovudine. The approximate median duration of prepartum treatment was 12 weeks. In a comparison of treatment for 12 weeks or less (average, 7) with treatment for more than 12 weeks (average, 17), there was no univariate association between the duration of treatment and its effect in reducing perinatal HIV transmission ($P = 0.99$) (Gelber R: personal communication). This analysis is somewhat limited by the number of infected infants and its post hoc nature. However, when combined with information such as the fact that in non-breast-feeding populations an estimated 65 percent of cases of perinatal HIV infection are transmitted during delivery and 95 percent of the remaining cases are transmitted within two months of delivery,[19] the analysis suggests that the shorter regimens may be equally effective. This finding should have been explored in later studies by randomly assigning women to longer or shorter treatment regimens.

What about the argument that the use of the oral route for intrapartum administration of zidovudine in the present trials (as opposed to the intravenous route in ACTG 076) justifies the use of a placebo? In its protocols for its two studies in Thailand and Côte d'Ivoire, the CDC acknowledged that previous "pharmacokinetic modelling data suggest that [zidovudine] serum levels obtained with this [oral] dose will be similar to levels obtained with an intravenous infusion."[20]

Thus, on the basis of the ACTG 076 data, knowledge about the timing of perinatal transmission, and pharmacokinetic data, the researchers should have had every reason to believe that well-designed shorter regimens would be more effective than placebo. These findings seriously disturb the equipoise (uncertainty over the likely study result) necessary to justify a placebo-controlled trial on ethical grounds.[21]

Defining Placebo as the Standard of Care in Developing Countries

Some officials and researchers have defended the use of placebo-controlled studies in developing countries by arguing that the subjects are treated at least according to the standard of care in these countries, which consists of unproven regimens or no treatment at all. This assertion reveals a fundamental misunderstanding of the concept of the standard of care. In developing countries, the standard of care (in this case, not providing zidovudine to HIV-positive pregnant women) is not based on a consideration of alternative treatments or previous clinical data, but is instead an economically determined policy of governments that cannot afford the prices set by drug companies. We agree with the Council for International Organizations of Medical Sciences that researchers working in developing countries have an ethical responsibility to provide treatment that conforms to the standard of care in the sponsoring country, when possible.[9] An exception would be a standard of care that required an exorbitant expenditure, such as the cost of building a coronary care unit. Since zidovudine is usually made available free of charge by the manufacturer for use in clinical trials, excessive cost is not a factor in this case. Acceptance of a standard of care that does not conform to the standard in the sponsoring country results in a double standard in research. Such a double standard, which permits research designs that are unacceptable in the sponsoring country, creates an incentive to use as research subjects those with the least access to health care.

What are the potential implications of accepting such a double standard? Researchers might inject live malaria parasites into HIV-positive subjects in China in order to study the effect on the progression of HIV infection, even though the study protocol had been rejected in the United States and Mexico. Or researchers might randomly assign malnourished San (Bushmen) to receive vitamin-fortified or standard bread. One might also justify trials of HIV vaccines in which the subjects were not provided with condoms or state-of-the-art counseling about safe sex by arguing that they are not customarily provided in the developing countries in question. These are not simply hypothetical worst-case scenarios; the first two studies have already been performed,[22,23] and the third has been proposed and criticized.[24]

Annas and Grodin recently commented on the characterization and justification of placebos as a standard of care: "'Nothing' is a description of what happens; 'standard of care' is a normative standard of effective medical treatment, whether or not it is provided to a particular community."[25]

Justifying Placebo-Controlled Trials by Claiming They Are More Rapid

Researchers have also sought to justify placebo-controlled trials by arguing that they require fewer subjects than equivalency studies and can therefore be completed more rapidly. Because equivalency studies are simply concerned with excluding alternative interventions that fall below some preestablished level of efficacy (as opposed to establishing which intervention is superior), it is customary to use one-sided statistical testing in such studies.[11] The numbers of women needed for a placebo-controlled trial and an equivalency study are similar.[26] In a placebo-controlled trial of a short course of zidovudine, with rates of perinatal HIV transmission of 25 percent in the placebo group and 15 percent in the zidovudine group, an alpha level of 0.05 (two-sided), and a beta level of 0.2, 500 subjects would be needed. An equivalency study with a transmission rate of 10 percent in the group receiving the ACTG 076 regimen, a difference in efficacy of 6 percent (above the 10 percent), an alpha level of 0.05 (one-sided), and a beta level of 0.2 would require 620 subjects (McCarthy W: personal communication).

Toward a Single International Standard of Ethical Research

Researchers assume greater ethical responsibilities when they enroll subjects in clinical studies, a precept acknowledged by Varmus recently when he insisted that all subjects in an NIH-sponsored needle-exchange trial be offered hepatitis B vaccine.[27] Residents of impoverished, postcolonial countries, the majority of whom are people of color, must be protected from potential exploitation in research. Otherwise, the abominable state of health care in these countries can be used to justify studies that could never pass ethical muster in the sponsoring country.

With the increasing globalization of trade, government research dollars becoming scarce, and more attention being paid to the hazards posed by "emerging infections" to the residents of industrialized countries, it is likely that studies in developing countries will increase. It is time to develop standards of research that preclude the kinds of double standards evident in these trials. In an editorial published nine years ago in the Journal, Marcia Angell stated, "Human subjects in any part of the world should be protected by an irreducible set of ethical standards."[28] Tragically, for the hundreds of infants who have needlessly contracted HIV infection in the perinatal-transmission studies that have already been completed, any such protection will have come too late.

References

1 Connor E.M., Sperling R.S., Gelber R., et al. Reduction of maternal–infant transmission of human immunodeficiency virus type 1 with zidovudine treatment. *N Engl J Med* 1994; 331:1173–80.

2 Sperling R.S., Shapiro D.E., Coombs R.W., et al. Maternal viral load, zidovudine treatment, and the risk of transmission of human immunodeficiency virus type 1 from mother to infant. *N Engl J Med* 1996; 335:1621–9.

3 Recommendations of the US Public Health Service Task Force on the use of zidovudine to reduce perinatal transmission of human immunodeficiency virus. MMWR Morb Mortal Wkly Rep 1994; 43(RR-11): 1–20.

4 Fiscus S.A., Adimora A.A., Schoenbach V.J., et al. Perinatal HIV infection and the effect of zidovudine therapy on transmission in rural and urban counties. *JAMA* 1996; 275:1483–8.

5 Cooper E., Diaz C., Pitt J., et al. Impact of ACTG 076: use of zidovudine during pregnancy and changes in the rate of HIV vertical transmission. In: Program and abstracts of the Third Conference on Retroviruses and Opportunistic Infections, Washington, DC, January 28–February 1, 1996. Washington, DC: Infectious Diseases Society of America, 1996: 57.

6 Simonds R.J., Nesheim S., Matheson P., et al. Declining mother to child HIV transmission following perinatal ZDV recommendations. Presented at the 11th International Conference on AIDS, Vancouver, Canada, July 7–12, 1996, abstract.

7 Scarlatti G. Paediatric HIV infection. Lancet 1996; 348: 863–8.

8 Recommendations from the meeting on mother-to-infant transmission of HIV by use of antiretrovirals, Geneva, World Health Organization, June 23–25, 1994.

9 World Health Organization. International ethical guidelines for biomedical research involving human subjects. Geneva: Council for International Organizations of Medical Sciences, 1993.

10 45 CFR 46.111(a)(1).

11 Testing equivalence of two binomial proportions. In: Machin D, Campbell MJ. Statistical tables for the design of clinical trials. Oxford, England: Blackwell Scientific, 1987: 35–53.

12 Brennan T.A. Letter to Gilbert Meier, NIH Division of Research Ethics, December 28, 1994.

13 Lallemant M. and Vithayasai V. A short ZDV course to prevent perinatal HIV in Thailand. Boston: Harvard School of Public Health, April 28, 1995.

14 Varmus H. Testimony before the Subcommittee on Human Resources, Committee on Government Reform and Oversight, US House of Representatives, May 8, 1997.

15 Draft talking points: responding to Public Citizen press conference. Press release of the National Institutes of Health, April 22, 1997.

16 Questions and answers: CDC studies of AZT to prevent mother-to-child HIV transmission in developing countries. Press release of the Centers for Disease Control and Prevention, Atlanta. (Undated document.)

17 Questions and answers on the UNAIDS sponsored trials for the prevention of mother-to-child transmission:
background brief to assist in responding to issues raised
by the public and the media. Press release of the United
Nations AIDS Program. (Undated document.)

18 Halsey N.A., Meinert C.L., Ruff A.J., et al. Letter to
Harold Varmus, Director of National Institutes of Health.
Baltimore: Johns Hopkins University, May 6, 1997.

19 Wiktor S.Z. and Ehounou E. A randomized placebo-
controlled intervention study to evaluate the safety
and effectiveness of oral zidovudine administered in
late pregnancy to reduce the incidence of mother-to-
child transmission of HIV-1 in Abidjan, Côte d'Ivoire.
Atlanta: Centers for Disease Control and Prevention.
(Undated document.)

20 Rouzioux C., Costagliola D., Burgard M., et al. Timing
of mother-to-child HIV-1 transmission depends on
maternal status. AIDS 1993; 7:Suppl 2:S49–S52.

21 Freedman B. Equipoise and the ethics of clinical
research. N Engl J Med 1987; 317:141–5.

22 Heimlich H.J., Chen X.P., Xiao B.Q., et al. CD4
response in HIV-positive patients treated with malaria
therapy. Presented at the 11th International Conference
on AIDS, Vancouver, BC, July 7–12, 1996, abstract.

23 Bishop W.B., Laubscher I., Labadarios D., Rehder
P., Louw M.E., Fellingham S.A. Effect of vitamin-
enriched bread on the vitamin status of an isolated
rural community – a controlled clinical trial. S Afr Med
J 1996; 86:Suppl:458–62.

24 Lurie P., Bishaw M., Chesney M.A., et al. Ethical,
behavioral, and social aspects of HIV vaccine
trials in developing countries. JAMA 1994;
271:295–301.

25 Annas G. and Grodin M. An apology is not enough.
Boston Globe. May 18, 1997: C1–C2.

26 Freedman B., Weijer C., and Glass K.C. Placebo orthodoxy in clinical research. I. Empirical and methodological
myths. J Law Med Ethics 1996; 24:243–51.

27 Varmus H. Comments at the meeting of the Advisory
Committee to the Director of the National Institutes
of Health, December 12, 1996.

28 Angell M. Ethical imperialism? Ethics in international
collaborative clinical research. N Engl J Med 1988;
319:1081–3.

58

We're Trying to Help Our Sickest People, Not Exploit Them

Danstan Bagenda and Philippa Musoke-Mudido

Every day, like the beat of a drum heard throughout Africa, 1,000 more infants here are infected with HIV, the virus that causes AIDS. At Old Mulago Hospital, we are trying to educate people about AIDS, as well as study new therapies to prevent the disease's rampant spread. Recently, some of these studies have been attacked, with comparisons made to the notorious Tuskegee experiment in which black men in the United States were denied treatment for syphilis. Tuskegee? Is this really what is happening here in our mother–child clinic?

Our country lies in the heart of Africa, along the Great Rift Valley and Lake Victoria. It is one of those hardest hit by the AIDS epidemic. A few years ago, visitors here in the capital were greeted by the macabre sight of empty coffins for sale – piled in pyramids from adult to baby size – along the main road. These grim reminders have since been removed by city authorities, but the AIDS epidemic is omnipresent. In this city of 1 million, about one out of every six adults is infected with HIV. Hospitals and clinics like ours, which provide free medical care and therefore serve the poorest communities, are stretched beyond their resources.

At the Mulago Hospital, where more than 20,000 women deliver each year, we are trying to find effective therapies to stop transmission of HIV from pregnant women to their babies. About one in five babies becomes infected with HIV during pregnancy and delivery. If the mother breast-feeds her baby, there is an additional 15- to 25-percent chance that the baby will later become infected. There is no available treatment for the disease in Uganda. After careful consideration among researchers from developing and developed countries, the World Health Organization (WHO) recommended in 1994 that the best way to find safe and effective treatment for sufferers in countries in the developing world is to conduct studies in which new treatments, better tailored to the local population, are compared with placebos (inactive pills).

Women who enroll in our studies undergo intensive education and individual counseling. They are given a comprehensive consent form, written in the local language, which they are encouraged to take home and discuss with their families. It describes the potential risks of participating in the study and their chances of receiving a placebo. Only when they and their counselors are satisfied that all questions have been answered are they asked to sign the form. Our careful attention to these measures has consistently met the standards of national and international ethical review committees.

Results from a clinical trial in the United States and France, known as the ACTG 076 protocol, showed as long ago as 1994 that, if a mother takes zidovudine (AZT) daily from the middle of her pregnancy until delivery, receives intravenous AZT during delivery, gives her infant oral AZT for the first six weeks of life and does not breast-feed, the transmission of HIV from mother to child can be reduced by two-thirds. The ACTG 076 protocol immediately became the recommended therapy in the United States. But it is not possible to simply transplant this protocol to Uganda for three main reasons: At a cost of between $800 and $1,000 per person, it is far too expensive; it requires treatment to begin in the middle of a pregnancy; and it means mothers must abstain from breast-feeding.

Some critics in the United States have asserted that we should compare new therapies with the ACTG 076 protocol rather than with a placebo. But, in Uganda, the government health expenditure is $3 per person per year, and the average citizen makes less than $1 per day. We think it is unethical to impose expensive treatment protocols that could never be used here. The situations are not parallel. In America, for instance, antibiotics are often over-prescribed; but here in Uganda we have difficulty even obtaining many needed antibiotics – to treat common complaints like ear infections. It is also naive to assume that what works for Americans will work for the rest of the world. Differences in nutrition, economics, societal norms and culture, and the frequency of tropical diseases make such extrapolations dangerously ethnocentric and wrong.

Many pregnant women here never show up for prenatal care and, of those who do, 70 percent make their first visit after the 30th week of pregnancy – too late for the US treatment protocol. Should we make a study available only to the minority of women who come early for care and tell the others, sorry, you came too late? We need to find treatments that will reach the most women possible – ones that can be given late in pregnancy or during labor.

There is also a huge gap between the United States and Uganda in breast-feeding practices. Should we apply the ACTG 076 protocol and tell women in the clinic not to breast-feed and instead give their babies infant formula? Access to clean water is a formidable challenge here, and we still remember the shocking epidemics of infant diarrhea and mortality in the early 1970s, when multinational companies shamelessly marketed formula in Africa. Despite the known risks of transmitting HIV through breast milk, the Ugandan Ministry of Health, UNICEF and WHO still encourage African women to breast-feed, as the nutritional benefits outweigh the risks of HIV transmission.

There are other factors we need to take into account. Every day, we treat both mothers and infants for malaria and iron deficiency. Both diseases contribute to anemia, which is also a major side effect of AZT. We are worried that AZT will exacerbate anemia in women and infants here. If we are to find out whether the new treatments are safe, the best way is to compare them with a placebo. How could we evaluate the safety of a new treatment if we compared it with the treatment used in America – one that has its own side effects? Could we really tell Ugandans that we had evaluated a new therapy for side effects using the best possible methods?

The AIDS epidemic has touched all our lives. Each of the 90 staff members in the mother–child health clinic has lost a family member, a loved one or a close friend. There is no dividing line between patients with HIV and those of us who care for them. A few years ago, we all chipped in money when a staff member needed to pay for the burial of a loved one, but recently we realized that we were all giving and receiving the same.

The ethical issues in our studies are complicated, but they have been given careful thought by the local community, ethicists, physicians and activists. Those who can speak with credibility for AIDS patients in

Africa are those who live among and know the people here or have some basic cross-cultural sensitivity. We are suspicious of those who claim to speak for our people, yet have never worked with them. Callous accusations may help sell newspapers and journals, but they demean the people here and the horrible tragedy that we live daily.

In the next several months, we expect to see results from our study and others like it in Ivory Coast, South Africa, Tanzania and Thailand. We hope they will help bring appropriate and safe therapies to the people of the developing world. That hope is the driving force that brings us back to our work in the clinic after each of the all-too-frequent burials.

59

Pandemic Ethics

The Case for Risky Research[1]

Peter Singer and Richard Yetter Chappell

The COVID-19 pandemic has upset ordinary moral assumptions. Restrictions on freedom of movement and association, to an extent previously unthinkable in liberal democracies, are now widely accepted as necessary. This is a significant revision to the ethics that guides our everyday lives. Few, in contrast, have shown such willingness to rethink the moral assumptions that guide our research into possible solutions to the pandemic. When so much is at stake, complacency and moral inertia cost lives.

In this paper, we will defend a principle of *risk parity*: if it is permissible to expose some members of society (e.g. health workers, or the economically vulnerable) to a certain level of *ex ante* risk in order to minimize overall harm from the virus, then it is permissible to expose fully informed volunteers to a comparable level of risk in the context of promising research into the virus. We then apply this principle to three examples of risky research: skipping animal trials for promising treatments, human challenge trials to speed up vaccine development, and low-dose controlled infection or "variolation".

The Principle of Risk Parity

Research ethics normally prohibits exposing human research participants to significant risks. The overriding aim is to prevent exploitation by researchers whose interests may not coincide with the interests of individual patients or volunteers. Art. 8 of the Declaration of Helsinki (WMA 2013) reads:

> While the primary purpose of medical research is to generate new knowledge, this goal can never take precedence over the rights and interests of individual research subjects.

We agree that participants' rights must not be violated, but suggest that participants' "interests" must be understood broadly to include any altruistic interest they may have in helping society to fight the pandemic.

In a pandemic, we all face heightened risks. As a result, restrictions on promising research (beyond the basic requirement of informed consent, confirmed via ethics committee approval) could easily prove

Original publication details: Richard Yetter Chappell and Peter Singer, "Pandemic Ethics: The Case for Risky Research," pp. 1–8 from *Research Ethics* 16: 3–4 (2020). Reproduced with permission of Sage Publications Ltd.

counterproductive. The overriding aim must be to avoid a potentially catastrophic toll.

When grave risks are widespread, care is required to ensure that in protecting individuals against the risk of exploitation by researchers, we do not implicitly condemn everyone – including those we are protecting – to the far greater risks that would result from the pandemic continuing to spread, unchecked by the knowledge we could have gained from research using informed volunteers.

We are not suggesting any weakening of the basic requirement that medical researchers must scrupulously obtain the informed consent of their research participants. Requiring informed consent goes a long way to prevent or mitigate the greatest risks of unethical, exploitative research. Requiring informed consent would have sufficed to prevent the great atrocities of twentieth-century medical research, including those performed by Nazi and Japanese researchers on prisoners, in the United States the Tuskegee syphilis study, and in New Zealand the "Unfortunate Experiment" (Paul and Brookes 2015). The scrutiny of a research ethics committee may provide additional oversight. But such committees should bear in mind the immense risk to innocent people of blocking promising pandemic research, in contrast to the swiftly-diminishing moral returns to further risk-mitigating requirements beyond that of informed consent. In a pandemic, only the weightiest of moral reasons can justify preventing or delaying research that promises to help society to mitigate the catastrophic toll.

Many altruistic and public-spirited individuals want to play their part in overcoming the pandemic or at least reducing the huge toll it is taking on our society. This also became apparent during the Ebola crisis. Within minutes of an announcement from a Canadian Health Centre, "the phones started ringing and e-mails began arriving from people who wanted to . . . .. be injected with an experimental vaccine that might cause aches and fever – but could protect against the Ebola virus" (Tangwa, Browne, and Schroeder 2018). Altruism and public spirit were particularly apparent as there was no risk of contracting the virus in Canada.

To do their part in the fight against COVID-19, some serve as health workers, or other essential workers, with a high risk of exposure to the virus as a result. Others stay at home, suffering social and economic costs in order to slow the pandemic's spread. When considering these various risks and costs, it is also important to note that they are not all freely chosen. Many people paying these costs do so unwillingly, coerced by their employer or by the state, in a way that compounds the total moral cost of the situation.

Compare this to the situation in which fully informed volunteers help to fight the pandemic by participating in promising (but risky) research. Often such research is blocked on the grounds that it "raises ethical questions." It does, of course, raise ethical questions. But so does slowing promising research, which extends the expected moral costs of the pandemic to everyone. The longer it takes to find an effective means of preventing the virus from killing people or making them seriously ill, the more deaths there will be, the more people there will be who are forced into dire poverty, and the more coerced individuals will suffer costs to which *they* never consented. Should we instead allow research participants to *voluntarily* undertake a comparable level of *ex ante*[2] risk in order to help relieve vast numbers of others of their burdens? Even non-Utilitarians ought to answer this question in the affirmative.

The (theory-neutral) principle of *risk parity* tells us that risks incurred in the course of medical research are not intrinsically more morally problematic than risks arising in other contexts. There is no rational basis for allowing health workers and others to be exposed to high risk, and then refusing to allow research participants to voluntarily take on comparable levels of risk (for comparable or greater benefit). The cogency of defending research risks by comparing them to non-research activities is also suggested by Miller and Joffe (2009) as well as London (2006).

Given the immense and ongoing global harm caused by the pandemic, speeding promising research has immense expected value. And since the costs borne by informed volunteers are consensual, in contrast to many of the costs imposed on others in society, important non-utilitarian values such as *respect for autonomy* (Macklin 2003) are also better served by permitting (indeed, encouraging) such research.

Much of the public discourse surrounding pandemic research ethics reveals an implicit failure to appreciate this principle of risk parity. For example, Paul Duprex, Director of the Center for Vaccine Research at the University of Pittsburgh, has cautioned against risky research in the present context, insisting that we must "be absolutely certain that we don't do something for the greater good which is highly detrimental for that individual [volunteer research participant]" (Morning Ireland 2020 at 32:15). The comment was made in an interview for Irish National Radio. Regrettably, the interviewer did not press him on why we shouldn't be similarly concerned about other individuals, for whom delayed research in the context of the pandemic would prove even more detrimental.

When thousands of individuals are dying every day and millions more are suffering ongoing social and economic harms, any delay to promising research is clearly disastrous. We hope that defenders of conventional research ethics will rise to address this challenge. To reiterate, this is not about premeditatedly sacrificing some individuals for the greater good of the many. It is not a crude utilitarian tradeoff that neglects or violates anyone's rights. This is about allowing competent adults to choose to act altruistically within the context of medical research to address the pandemic, just as we allow (or worse: require) others to act altruistically in non-research contexts while the pandemic is ongoing.

One interesting argument that Duprex (Morning Ireland 2020 at 31:47) does offer involves a kind of skepticism regarding whether informed consent is even possible given how little we know about COVID-19: "Are [research participants] fully informed, whenever we really only have a small amount of the information?" The implicit assumption seems to be that you cannot give informed consent to taking a risk without knowing exactly what the risk is (ideally, perhaps, knowing the *objective chances* of each possible outcome). But this assumption is far-fetched. What more plausibly matters for informed consent is that

participants understand and accept whatever known *and unknown* risks apply *in light of our current epistemic situation*.[3] When the researchers themselves are highly uncertain about the outcome of a procedure, and what hidden vulnerabilities might result in a seemingly healthy participant suffering unexpected harms, they need to clearly communicate this uncertainty. Most candidates, facing such uncertain risks, would reasonably choose to refrain from participating in the trial, and that decision must certainly be respected. But others may reasonably choose to go ahead, accepting the risks (both known and unknown), in order to help fight the pandemic. This choice, too, should be respected.

Applying the Principle of Risk Parity to COVID-19 Research – Three Examples

While it is ultimately up to medical researchers to identify the most promising lines of research, we can here indicate three broad avenues within which greater tolerance for risky research (in line with the principle of risk parity) could plausibly save lives during the pandemic.

(1) Conventional standards require that new drugs be tested on animals before clinical trials with humans are permitted. For COVID-19, we suggest that sufficiently promising treatments (and vaccine candidates) should jump to human clinical trials as soon as is reasonably possible, bypassing the usual lengthy period of animal testing. This measure has already been taken in a vaccine trial in Seattle, which attracted considerable criticism from research ethicists:

> A clinical trial for an experimental coronavirus vaccine has begun recruiting participants in Seattle, but researchers did not first show that the vaccine triggered an immune response in animals, as is normally required (Lanese 2020).

There is a precedent for such a move. In 1986, when AZT first showed promising results in the treatment of AIDS, patients demanded that the drug be made available without going through animal testing (Park 2017). The Food and Drug Administration licensed it, saving many lives. AIDS had a much higher fatality rate than COVID-19, but even so, if we fully inform COVID-19 patients about the risks of taking part in an experimental treatment trial, they may reasonably choose to take that risk. When we consider the broader humanitarian benefits of confirming a treatment's (or vaccine's) effectiveness much sooner than would otherwise be possible, not to mention the reduced animal suffering involved, there is a strong moral case for allowing volunteers to make that choice.

(2) Similar arguments support allowing human challenge trials to speed development of a vaccine (Eyal et al 2020). According to the World Health Organization (WHO 2016):

Human challenge trials are trials in which participants are intentionally challenged (whether or not they have been vaccinated) with an infectious disease organism. This challenge organism may be close to wild-type and pathogenic, adapted and/or attenuated from wild-type with less or no pathogenicity, or genetically modified in some manner.

Ordinarily, testing a candidate vaccine means waiting months to see whether injected research participants are less prone to infection. Deliberately exposing vaccinated volunteers to the virus could produce results much more quickly. Strikingly, there is no shortage of volunteers willing to undergo such a trial. More than 14,000 volunteers from more than 100 countries have already signed up to do so (Ramgopal 2020).

(3) Finally, consider research into low-dose controlled voluntary infection, or "variolation," widely used to inoculate against smallpox before the discovery of vaccination (Boylston 2012). Princeton University researchers Joshua Rabinowitz and Caroline Bartman (2020) have emphasized the importance of viral dose: people who receive a low dose of a virus are more likely to recover than those who receive a high dose, and this holds for coronaviruses too. Robin Hanson

(2020) notes that, historically, variolation has reduced infection mortality by factors ranging from 3 to 30. This all seems to suggest a strong *prima facie* case for exploratory research into SARS-CoV-2 variolation as a possible vaccine-substitute.

Some may object that it would be unethical to deliberately expose volunteers to a potentially lethal virus. But does this assumption really make sense in our current context? The seriousness of the coronavirus pandemic cuts both ways: more risk from the initial low dose infection, but greater benefits if it does protect the volunteers. For instance, if we can gain solid evidence that receiving a low dose of the virus (variolation) leads to a mild case of COVID-19, and that such mild cases then bring immunity to further exposure to the virus, we would have found a means of saving a considerable number of lives – and millions of livelihoods – in the absence of a vaccine. Even the most optimistic scientists assume that COVID-19 vaccine development will last at least 12 months (Deutsch 2020), and there is no guarantee that such optimism will be vindicated. It therefore seems both prudent and ethical to investigate alternatives by inviting healthy young adults to volunteer to receive a low dose of the virus, followed by quarantine and medical observation.

In fact, some individuals have already sought deliberately to infect themselves via uncontrolled "coronavirus parties," despite medical experts urging them not to do so (Bauer 2020). It would be better for everyone were such individuals instead to have the opportunity to volunteer to receive a low dose of the virus as part of a carefully monitored trial. That would be safer for the participants than an uncontrolled infection, and the knowledge that we would gain from such a trial could guide us towards an earlier end to the pandemic.

There is too much that we do not know about COVID-19. The longer we take to find it out, the more lives will be lost. If volunteers, fully informed about the risks, are willing to help fight the pandemic by aiding promising research, there are strong moral reasons to gratefully accept their help. To refuse it would implicitly subject others to still graver risks.

Notes

1 Some passages of this essay appeared previously in Peter Singer and Richard Yetter Chappell, "Pandemic ethics: the case for experiments on human volunteers," *Washington Post,* April 27, 2020, https://www.washingtonpost.com/opinions/2020/04/27/pandemic-ethics-case-experiments-human-volunteers

2 Based on forecasts rather than actual results.

3 It is also worth noting that case fatality rates for COVID-19 vary roughly between "0.2% in Germany to 7.7% in Italy" (Roser et al 2020). Hence, one might argue that the risks taken by volunteers infected with the virus are at least *broadly* specifiable.

References

Bauer, G. (2020). Please, Don't Intentionally Infect Yourself. Signed, an Epidemiologist. *New York Times*. https://www.nytimes.com/2020/04/08/opinion/coronavirus-parties-herd-immunity.html. Accessed 11 May 2020.

Boylston, A. (2012). The Origins of Inoculation. *Journal of the Royal Society of Medicine, 105*(7), 309–13. doi:10.1258/jrsm.2012.12k044

Deutsch, J. (2020) How long will it take to develop a coronavirus vaccine? *Politico*. https://www.politico.eu/article/coronavirus-vaccine-how-long-will-it-take-to-develop/. Accessed 11 May 2020.

Eyal, N., Lipsitch, M., and Smith, P. (2020). Human Challenge Studies to Accelerate Coronavirus Vaccine Licensure. *The Journal of Infectious Diseases*. doi:10.1093/infdis/jiaa152

Hanson, R. (2020). Variolation (+ Isolation) May Cut Covid19 Deaths 3-30X. Overcoming Bias. http://www.overcomingbias.com/2020/03/variolation-may-cut-covid19-deaths-3-30x.html. Accessed 11 May 2020.

Lanese N (2020) Researchers fast-track coronavirus vaccine by skipping key animal testing first, *LiveScience*. https://www.livescience.com/coronavirus-vaccine-trial-no-animal-testing.html. Accessed 11 May 2020.

London, A. J. (2006). Reasonable risks in clinical research: A critique and a proposal for the Integrative Approach. *Statist Med, 25*: 2869–85. doi:10.1002/sim.2634

Macklin, R. (2003). Dignity is a useless concept. *BMJ 327*(7429), 1419–20. doi:10.1136/bmj.327.7429.1419

Miller, F. and Joffe, S. (2009). Limits to Research Risks. *Journal of Medical Ethics, 35*(7), 445–49. doi:10.1136/jme.2008.026062

Morning Ireland. (2020). The Race for a Vaccine, Podcast Interview, https://soundcloud.com/morning-ireland/the-race-for-a-vaccine. Accessed 11 May 2020.

Park, A. (2017). The Story Behind the First AIDS Drug. *TIME*. https://time.com/4705809/first-aids-drug-azt/. Accessed 11 May 2020.

Paul, C., and Brookes B. (2015). The rationalization of unethical research: Revisionist accounts of the Tuskegee syphilis study and the New Zealand "Unfortunate Experiment". *Am J Public Health*: *105*(10):e12–e19. doi:10.2105/AJPH.2015.302720

Rabinowitz, J. D. and Bartman C. R. (2020). These coronavirus exposures might be the most dangerous. *New York Times*. https://www.nytimes.com/2020/04/01/opinion/coronavirus-viral-dose.html. Accessed 11 May 2020.

Ramgopal, K. (2020). Why have 14,000 people volunteered to be infected with coronavirus? *NBC News*. https://www.nbcnews.com/health/health-news/why-have-14-000-people-volunteered-be-infected-coronavirus-n1203931/. Accessed 11 May 2020.

Roser, M, Ritchie, H., Ortiz-Ospina, E., and Hasell, J. (2020). Mortality risk of COVID-19. *Our World in Data*. https://ourworldindata.org/mortality-risk-covid#the-current-case-fatality-rate-of-covid-19. Accessed 11 May 2020.

Tangwa, G. B., Browne, K., and Schroeder, D. (2018). Ebola vaccine trials. In D. Schroeder, J. Cook, F, Hirsch, S. Fenet, and V. Muthuswamy (eds.), *Ethics Dumping*. Springer Briefs in Research and Innovation Governance. Springer, Cham.

World Health Organization (WHO) (2016) Human Challenge Trials for Vaccine Development: Regulatory considerations. https://www.who.int/biologicals/expert_committee/Human_challenge_Trials_IK_final.pdf. Accessed 11 May 2020.

World Medical Association (WMA) (2013) Declaration of Helsinki. Ethical principles for medical research involving human subjects. https://www.wma.net/policies-post/wma-declaration-of-helsinki-ethical-principles-for-medical-research-involving-human-subjects/. Accessed 11 May 2020.

Experimentation with Animals

60

Duties towards Animals

Immanuel Kant

Baumgarten speaks of duties towards beings which are beneath us and beings which are above us. But so far as animals are concerned, we have no direct duties. Animals are not self-conscious and are there merely as a means to an end. That end is man. We can ask, 'Why do animals exist?' But to ask, 'Why does man exist?' is a meaningless question. Our duties towards animals are merely indirect duties towards humanity. Animal nature has analogies to human nature, and by doing our duties to animals in respect of manifestations which correspond to manifestations of human nature, we indirectly do our duty towards humanity. Thus, if a dog has served his master long and faithfully, his service, on the analogy of human service, deserves reward, and when the dog has grown too old to serve, his master ought to keep him until he dies. Such action helps to support us in our duties towards human beings, where they are bounden duties. If then any acts of animals are analogous to human acts and spring from the same principles, we have duties towards the animals because thus we cultivate the corresponding duties towards human beings. If a man shoots his dog because the animal is no longer capable of service, he does not fail in his duty to the dog, for the dog cannot judge, but his act is inhuman and damages in himself that humanity which it is his duty to show towards mankind. If he is not to stifle his human feelings, he must practise kindness towards animals, for he who is cruel to animals becomes hard also in his dealings with men. We can judge the heart of a man by his treatment of animals. Hogarth depicts this in his engravings ('The Stages of Cruelty', 1757). He shows how cruelty grows and develops. He shows the child's cruelty to animals, pinching the tail of a dog or a cat; he then depicts the grown man in his cart running over a child; and lastly, the culmination of cruelty in murder. He thus brings home to us in a terrible fashion the rewards of cruelty, and this should be an impressive lesson to children. The more we come in contact with animals and observe their behaviour, the more we love them, for we see how great is their care for their young. It is then difficult for us to be cruel in thought even to a wolf. Leibniz used a tiny worm for purposes of observation, and then carefully replaced it with its leaf on the tree so that it should not come to harm through any act of his. He would have been sorry – a

Original publication details: Immanuel Kant, "Duties towards Animals," pp. 239–241 from *Lectures on Ethics,* trans. Louis Infield (London: Methuen, 1930).

natural feeling for a humane man – to destroy such a creature for no reason. Tender feelings towards dumb animals develop humane feelings towards mankind. In England butchers and doctors do not sit on a jury because they are accustomed to the sight of death and hardened. Vivisectionists, who use living animals for their experiments, certainly act cruelly, although their aim is praiseworthy, and they can justify their cruelty, since animals must be regarded as man's instruments; but any such cruelty for sport cannot be justified. A master who turns out his ass or his dog because the animal can no longer earn its keep manifests a small mind. The Greeks' ideas in this respect were high-minded, as can be seen from the fable of the ass and the bell of ingratitude. Our duties towards animals, then, are indirect duties towards mankind.

61

A Utilitarian View

Jeremy Bentham

What other agents then are there, which, at the same time that they are under the influence of man's direction, are susceptible of happiness? They are of two sorts: 1. Other human beings who are styled persons. 2. Other animals, which, on account of their interests having been neglected by the insensibility of the ancient jurists, stand degraded into the class of *things*.[1]

Note

1 Under the Gentoo and Mahometan religions, the interests of the rest of the animal creation seem to have met with some attention. Why have they not, universally, with as much as those of human creatures, allowance made for the difference in point of sensibility? Because the laws that are have been the work of mutual fear; a sentiment which the less rational animals have not had the same means as man has of turning to account. Why *ought* they not? No reason can be given. If the being eaten were all, there is very good reason why we should be suffered to eat such of them as we like to eat: we are the better for it, and they are never the worse. They have none of those long-protracted anticipations of future misery which we have. The death they suffer in our hands commonly is, and always may be, a speedier, and by that means a less painful one, than that which would await them in the inevitable course of nature. If the being killed were all, there is very good reason why we should be suffered to kill such as molest us: we should be the worse for their living, and they are never the worse for being dead. But is there any reason why we should be suffered to torment them? Not any that I can see. Are there any why we should *not* be suffered to torment them? Yes, several. The day has been, I grieve to say in many places it is not yet past, in which the greater part of the species, under the denomination of slaves, have been treated by the law exactly upon the same footing as, in England for example, the inferior races of animals are still. The day *may* come, when the rest of the animal creation may acquire those rights which never could have been withholden from them but by the hand of tyranny. The French have already discovered that the blackness of the skin is no reason why a human being should be abandoned without redress to the

Original publication details: Jeremy Bentham, "A Utilitarian View," section XVIII, IV from *An Introduction to the Principles of Morals and Legislation*, First published c. 1820. Public domain.

caprice of a tormentor. It may come one day to be recognized, that the number of the legs, the villosity of the skin, or the termination of the *os sacrum*, are reasons equally insufficient for abandoning a sensitive being to the same fate. What else is it that should trace the insuperable line? Is it the faculty of reason, or, perhaps, the faculty of discourse? But a full-grown horse or dog is beyond comparison a more rational, as well as a more conversable animal, than an infant of a day, or a week, or even a month, old. But suppose the case were otherwise, what would it avail? The question is not, Can they *reason?* nor, Can they *talk?* but, Can they *suffer?*

62

The Harmful, Nontherapeutic Use of Animals in Research is Morally Wrong

Nathan Nobis

I will present and defend some reasons to believe that a certain kind of medical and scientific research involving animals is morally wrong. The research that I argue is morally impermissible is that which is (a) harmful to animals, ie, it makes them worse off than they were, physically and/or psychologically, and is (b) nontherapeutic, ie, it is not intended to, or reasonably expected to, benefit the individual animals who are experimented on. Thus, I do not argue that (a) non-harmful research (eg, perhaps observational studies in the wild) is morally wrong or that (b) therapeutic research (ie, research reasonably expected to benefit an individual when there is no existing sufficiently effective treatment for some noninduced disease or injury) is wrong, even if the treatment turns out, unexpectedly and against the odds, to harm the animal. As analogous research concerning human beings is permissible, these forms of animal research are permissible as well.

A principle I appeal to in defending my thesis is this:

To better understand more controversial moral issues, we should try to use insights gained from thinking about less controversial moral issues that can be applied back to the more controversial issues.

To employ this principle, I begin by very briefly describing 4 less controversial cases concerning human experimentation. Two are historical cases that most readers will be familiar with; and 2 are generic, hypothetical cases:

Case 1. The Tuskegee Syphilis Study (This case is discussed in, among many other sources, Refs. 1 and 2.) (1932–72).
Brief summary: Poor African American men in Alabama with syphilis were falsely diagnosed (as having "bad blood"), given false treatment and then were not given effective treatment for syphilis when it was found (1957).
Case 2. The Willowbrook Children Case (This case is discussed in, among many other sources, Refs. 3 and 4) (1963–66).
Brief summary: Severely mentally challenged, institutionalized children were given hepatitis, without their parents' consent.
Case 3. Human Cadaver Research

Original publication details: Nathan Nobis, "Harmful, Nontherapeutic Use of Animals in Research is Morally Wrong," pp. 297–304 from *American Journal of the Medical Sciences* 342: 4 (October 2011). Reproduced with permission of Elsevier.

Brief summary: A cardiologist gets permission to study her patients' hearts after they die of natural causes, and she does so.

Case 4. Skin Tissue Research

Brief summary: A scientist acquires skin cells from consenting donors to study, and she does so.

For each of these cases, we can make, or have made, judgments about whether what was done was, or would be, morally permissible or morally wrong. In addition, we can explain why this is so, ie, we can give reasons for our moral judgments and we can defend our reasons from objections.

In light of readers' judgments about and justifications for them concerning these cases, the main reasoning I will present and defend in favor of my thesis concerning animals is the following:

Premise 1.   Harmful, nontherapeutic experimentation on (conscious, sentient) human beings – imposing disease, injury, addiction, pain, suffering, fear, distress, confinement and early death and so on – is morally wrong.

Premise 2.   This fact can be explained or justified: we can identify what it is about these human beings that makes such experimentation wrong.

Premise 3.   The best explanations for why these human experiments are morally wrong support belief that similarly harmful nontherapeutic experimentation on (conscious, sentient) animals is morally wrong also because these humans and animals share morally relevant properties.

Conclusion.   Therefore, harmful, nontherapeutic animal experimentation is morally wrong.

Premises 1 and 2 are uncontroversial. Some of the human research cases above, eg, 1 and 2, provide opportunities to confirm premise 1 and explain, by appealing to a variety of moral considerations, why certain kinds of research involving human beings are morally wrong. Other cases of morally permissible research above, eg, 3 and 4, allow for contrasts that can help illuminate those cases in which we judge that the research was morally wrong.

Premise 3 is thus where controversy lies. To support this premise, I appeal again to the principle of appealing to less controversial issues to address controversial ones and to reflective answers to these questions:

Why would it be wrong to experiment on you (the reader), or any other conscious, sentient human being, *in ways animals are experimented on*? What is it *about* you, or any such humans, that *makes* such experimentation morally wrong? *What do better answers to these questions imply for (any) animals?*

Thus, I argue that if we identify what it is about human beings that would make (and has made) "vivisecting" them wrong, ie, what properties or features such human beings have that best explain why such harmful experimentation is wrong, we see that many nonhuman beings have these same properties. As, I argue, there are no morally relevant differences between the human and animal vivisection cases, it follows that comparably harmful experiments on animals are morally wrong as well.

The structure of my article is as follows:

1. I explain my methods, which will involve presenting some basic logic and moral argument analysis skills. Philosophers are often not explicit about their methods: this is unfortunate because it can result in needless misunderstanding, especially for why certain common objections to arguments in defense of animals are weak, and generally less fruitful engagement with the issues.

2. I briefly mention some issues that many people want to discuss when ethical questions of animal use arise, but I am not going to discuss in detail. This is because these issues are irrelevant to questions concerning the morality of animal use. Using the argument analysis skills presented earlier, we see that these concerns are logically

irrelevant and/or needlessly complicate the issues and so can be avoided without loss.

3. I respond to some common arguments for the denial of my conclusion, ie, arguments in favor of the common response, "No, animal experimentation is morally permissible *because* . . ." Using the moral argument analysis skills developed earlier, I respond to some common objections to arguments similar to mine. My "respond to objections first" strategy is intended to defuse potentially defensive reactions and allow for a better reception of my positive case for my conclusion.

4. Finally, I return to my argument and offer support for premise (This case is discussed in, among many other sources, Refs. 3 and 4) that the best explanations for why these human experiments are wrong support belief that experimentation on many animals is wrong also. I explain why many animals are similar to many human beings in morally relevant ways, why various differences are morally irrelevant and thus protections due to many human beings are also due to many animals.

For better or worse, I will not discuss the arguments of specific animal research advocates. I have done this in many other (readily accessible) articles and reviews, and I invite readers to apply my general discussion to any particular arguments given in moral defense of animal research and to investigate for themselves whether my observations about how people tend to argue about these issues are accurate.

Also, it seems that more is written in moral opposition to animal experimentation than in its support. Many animal experimentation advocates realize this. For examples, Smith[5,6] observes in his 2010 book subtitled *The Human Cost of the Animal Rights Movement* that:

> Hundreds of books have been published on the issue of animal rights. Most of these . . . are decidedly on the pro side, with very few books written in explicit opposition.

Morrison[7] in his 2010 book subtitled *A Veterinarian's Reflections on the Animal Rights & Welfare Debate* reports that:

> [o]nly a few [scientists, in their speaking and writing] have directly confronted the 'philosophical underpinnings' of perspectives critical of animal experimentation.

A 2001 collection of essays, *Why Animal Experimentation Matters: The Use of Animals in Medical Research*, describes itself as a "much needed corrective to [a] cause that has up until now been too rarely challenged" (book flap).[8,9] My hope is that this article, with its methodological focus, will contribute to an increase of the quantity and quality of discussion of these issues.

Methods

First, I will present and explain some standard methods of analytic moral philosophers. They involve analyzing moral arguments using a set of logical tools. Most simply, such analysis involves asking "What do you mean?" and "Why think that?" of moral claims people make. Using these methods involves understanding a number of concepts.

First, there is the concept of an argument, which is a set of premises given in support of a conclusion. There are different conclusions about animal research ("it is morally permissible" and "it is morally wrong") and different premises can be, and are, given in support of various conclusions. Following the "Why think that?" question, the conclusion of an argument is the "that" and the premise(s) are the "why" one might accept that conclusion.

Conclusions and premises must be precise and clear. This relates to the "What do you mean?" question. Conclusions and premises are imprecise when the quantity or number of "things" in the claim is not stated, and so, we cannot tell exactly what is being said. Precision is important for animal ethics as many claims made in discussion of the topic are imprecise, eg, "Human beings are self-aware," "Animals are sentient," "Animal research saves lives," "Animal experimentation does not lead to cures," and so forth. These claims are all imprecise: eg, concerning the first claim, we do not know whether it is being said that *all* human beings are "self-aware" or just *some* of them (and, if so, *which* ones?). The others are also imprecise, more so when they contain more than 1 noun phrase or subject, eg, *all* or *some* "animal research" leads to *all* or *some* "cures"? Precision enables us to know what exact claim is being made, so we might try to determine whether it is true or false.

Premises and conclusions must also be made clear as the meanings of many words used in discussions of moral issues are not clear or are ambiguous: again, "What do you mean?" So, we often need to ask what people mean when they use a particular word, and new, distinct premises are derived from each possible meaning. The clarification of meanings is especially valuable in discussions of animals and ethics issues as the meanings of many terms used are not clear, eg, "rights," "persons," "equal," "important," "animals," "humans," "human beings," "human," and more.

A second important concept is that of an argument in logically valid form in which the premises lead, as a matter of logic, to the conclusion. This often involves adding premises essential to the form of the reasoning, so. To illustrate, consider this common example:

Premise.   Socrates is a man.
Conclusion.   Therefore, Socrates is mortal.

To get from the premise to the conclusion, we must add an additional premise:

Premise.   All men are mortal, or
                If someone is a man, then that someone
                is mortal.

In adding such a premise, the argument is put in logically valid form. Although this seems simple and obvious with this example, such premises are often not added to real world moral arguments, and so, the reasoning is not explicit. This is unfortunate because often such unstated premises are false, as we shall see concerning various arguments about animal research.

Some common patterns of logically valid arguments include these:

"Universal Generalization," the form of the Socrates argument above:

- "All A's are B's; X is an A; therefore X is a B," or
- "If X is an A, then X is a B. X is an A, so X is a B."

Modus Tollens:

- "If claim A is true, then claim B is true; but claim B is *not* true; therefore claim A is *not* true."

Modus Ponens:

- "If claim A is true, then claim B is true; claim A is true; therefore claim B is true."

In all cases, the mathematical structure of the entire pattern of reasoning must be displayed.

Third, there is the concept of a sound argument, which is an argument in (a) logically valid form with (b) true [or justified, reasonable] premises. Such premises might be moral claims, often moral principles that state that if an action has some features, then it has some deontic status (ie, morally permissible, obligatory or wrong), eg, "If an action is like *this*, then it is permissible" and "All actions with *these* features are wrong" or they might be empirical claims, evaluated by science or observation.

A fourth concept is that of a counterexample. Many common moral arguments, when put in logically valid form, have moral principles that can be shown false by counterexample, ie, an exception to the proposed principle. To give a nonmoral example, a counterexample to "All men are good dancers" is a man who is not a good dancer. A counterexample to "If someone does not have blue eyes, then that someone lacks a right to life," would, of course, be someone with blue eyes who has such a right. To develop a counterexample to a moral principle, we identify a principle's logical implications or consequences, ie, what would follow from it, as a matter of logic. If the principle implies something false, then the principle is false: if we reasonably believe it implies something false, then we have reason to believe the principle is false.

A fifth concept is that of "begging the question," which is to assume – ie, to accept without giving reasons in defense of – one's conclusion in a premise. This sometimes occurs by stating the conclusion in different words as a premise or by offering a premise that would not be accepted by someone unless she already accepted the argument's conclusion. Insofar as arguments are supposed to give reason to accept a conclusion, question-begging arguments fail to do this.

In addition to skills in using these concepts to identify and evaluate moral arguments, these intellectual and moral virtues are desirable: patience (as complex moral issues take time to understand and think through); understanding (especially the details of positions different from our own); openness to the possibility of error and the need for change (as we have been mistaken in our moral and scientific views before, so this might be the case here concerning animals) and self-awareness of potential conflicts of interest (as self-interest, real or perceived, can preclude unbiased moral inquiry and, at least, many people enjoy eating animals and their employment depends on animal use: these factors might influence the quality of one's thinking about these topics).

These argument analysis skills and virtues are best practiced and their value confirmed, in the context of other moral issues. Because of some unique aspects of ethical issues concerning animals, they are typically better addressed after careful discussions of other moral issues that are, in some important ways, arguably less controversial in certain ways.

Thus, discussion is usually more fruitful when we have already discussed the treatment of disabled newborns, abortion, euthanasia, absolute poverty and even sexual ethics, to name a few issues. Such discussion provides insight into concepts and distinctions that often arise in animal ethics, eg, personhood, being human or a "human being," possible moral differences between "doing" and "allowing," quality of life issues, the relevance of appeals to what "natural" and evolution and many other common moral concepts and distinctions. In addition, ethical theories – ie, general hypotheses about what makes actions morally permissible, obligatory or wrong – are often introduced and evaluated in discussions of practical moral issues. Readers are encouraged to, if they have not done so, review these topics to have stronger background understanding and practice in using argument analysis skills that they can apply to ethics and animals issues.[10–12]

Some Distracting Issues not Discussed in Detail

When the topic of the ethics of animal use arises, many people often want to talk about some other issues that have no logical connection to the topic and/or needlessly complicate the issues. As these issues distract from the core topic, I will explain why I will not discuss them.

Activists' behavior

First, some people want to complain about animal advocates, arguing that they engage in offensive, uncivil, illegal and/or counter productive activities: they wish to paint these activists as an unsavory lot.[13–15] They then seem to think that this shows that animal experimentation is morally permissible.

Although these observations might apply to some activists at most (and it also likely applies to some animal research activists), it is logically irrelevant to the ethics of animal use. This is because no activists' activity is ever relevant to the morality of any action. To see this clearly, consider a less controversial case: imagine someone reasoning either of these ways:

- "Some abortion critics behave badly; *therefore*, abortion is morally permissible."
- "Some 'pro-choice' advocates are really nice people; *therefore*, abortion is morally permissible."

Both arguments are unsound because, irrespective of the truth or falsity of the stated premise, when made logically valid, they rely on the following general principles that can be shown false by counterexamples:

- If some activists regarding action X behave badly, then doing action X is morally permissible.
- If some activists regarding action X behave well, then doing action X is morally wrong.

Although many people often want to discuss and evaluate some animal activists' activities, if these judgments are intended to show something about the ethics of animal use, they simply do not: they are an irrelevant distraction to that issue. These judgments might also reveal a question-begging view that animal experimentation must be morally permissible, so activists must be mistaken, but the reasons for and against that view about animal research are what should be focused on, not the behavior of any activists.

"Rights"

Second, people often want to frame ethics and animals issues in terms of "animal rights." They assert that animals do not have "rights," and so animal experimentation is not wrong. This argument, however, is unsound for a number of reasons, in part, because rights claims can be distracting and are needless.

First, about rights claims, we can rightly ask, "What do you mean?" There are legal rights, which are "man-made" and vary from time and place. Usually this is not the issue, as most animals who are be used in research have very few legal rights: few experiments on them are illegal, at least in the United States. However, whether a being has legal rights does not determine whether it has rights in any other sense, such as moral rights, which are typically considered universal and "natural," ie, not "man made." In addition, there are a variety of possible moral rights: eg, the right to life, the right to be treated with respect and not used as a mere means toward others ends, the right to not be harmed for others' benefits, the right to not be caused to suffer and so on.

A common difficulty with moral rights talk is that, often, the exact right in question – what exactly the right is to or from – is not specified, which creates confusion and misunderstanding. So, it is common for people to argue that animals do not have *some* specific moral right and then conclude that animals do not have *any* moral rights, which does not follow. In addition, the basis of the right – what is it about someone that would make them, such that they have that right – is not argued, which can give rights claims and denials a question-begging quality. Any claim or denial that someone has rights must specify the exact right in question and the reason(s) why someone has or lacks that right: often this is not done.

Another common misunderstanding that arises in using the term "rights" is due to accepting this false principle:

- If animals have no moral rights, then animal experimentation is morally permissible.

Although some people seem to think that the question of the ethics of animal use depends on whether animals have moral rights, this is not so. The nature and existence of moral rights for anyone, including human beings, is controversial: many moral theories deny them outright. These theories, however, do support thinking that certain kinds of human experimentation are morally wrong, but they just do not explain this using concepts of rights. Similarly, some people argue that animal experimentation is morally wrong, even if animals do not have moral rights: it's wrong for other reasons than rights-based reasons.

Given all this, the question of whether animals have rights, in any sense, can be seen as the distraction that it sometimes is.

"Equality," "importance," "status" and "standing"

Similar distractions arise in use of the terms "equal" and "important." It is often argued that "animals are not 'equal' to humans" or "animals are not 'as important' as humans" and then concluded that animal research is morally permissible. Sometimes it is also said that animals' "moral status" or "standing" is less than humans', or at a lower level, and so research is permissible.

However, what it means for beings (even human beings!) to be "equal" is not easy to explain, and what makes beings "important" (to who? for what?) is also unclear. Notions of "moral status" and "standing" are also unclear. Thus, we often do not know what people mean when they make these claims, and so, we cannot assess whether they are true or false ("why think that?"): again, these claims can have a question-begging quality to them, as assertions without explanation of meaning or defense.

However, as with rights claims, probably the most common misunderstanding that arises in using these terms is due to accepting these false principles:

- If animals are not "equal" to (any) humans, then animal experimentation is morally permissible.
- If animals are not "as important" to (any) humans, then animal experimentation is morally permissible.

Although these concepts of "importance" and "equality" need to be clarified ("what do you mean?"), and judgments involving them justified ("why think that?"), they seem to be false or, at least, in need of defense. Concerning the second, to say that A is not as important as B, does not imply that A is not important at all or that A is of so little importance that it can be harmed for B. Concerning the first, as quality is often explained in terms of equal consideration of interests, not equal consideration of interests does not imply no consideration of interests whatsoever.

Thus, some have argued that even if no animals' interests are deserving of equal consideration to any humans' interests, or no animals are as important or valuable as any humans, animals' interests are deserving of *some* level of consideration, such that experimentation on them is wrong or that animals are important or valuable enough that experimentation on them is wrong.[16,17] These more subtle positions need to be engaged more deeply.

In this section, I have discussed a number of issues and concepts that can distract from core ethics and animal experimentation issues. These are whether some specific, or kinds of, animal experiments are morally permissible, morally impermissible (ie, wrong) or morally obligatory (ie, impermissible or wrong to not do) and, most importantly, the reasons and arguments that can be given in favor of these conclusions.

Some Objections: "Animal Experimentation is Morally Permissible Because . . ."

I now turn to some common objections to my conclusion, ie, some arguments that [it] is false because animal research is morally permissible, and so, any arguments that it is wrong are unsound. I discuss these first to try to defuse potential defensiveness to my positive case and to show readers that it is be harder to morally justify animal research than they might have suspected. These arguments are evaluated as sound or unsound using the argument analysis concepts presented earlier: meaning-clarification, precision-clarification, adding unstated premises to make arguments logically valid and counterexamples to general moral principles.

These 3 common sets of arguments are the following.

"Scientific" arguments

"Humans benefit from animal research; there are no alternatives; it is necessary. *Therefore*, animal research is morally permissible."

"Necessary condition" arguments

"Animals are not rational, not moral agents, not contributors to culture, without a sense of the future, are not self-aware, and so forth. *Therefore*, animal research is morally permissible."

"Group-based" arguments

"Animals are not members of a *species*, *kind* or *group* that is rational, has moral agency, contributes to culture, is self-aware, and so forth. *Therefore*, animal research is morally permissible."

The first set of arguments all involve appeals to (imprecise) scientific claims which may or may not be true or evidence based. Some people seem to think that science settles moral question[s] of animal research, but it does not. This is because science never, in itself, answers any moral questions: formulating arguments in logically valid form helps make this clear.

It is worthwhile, however, to observe that there is a growing body of scientific literature that assesses the scientific evidence for common claims, typically asserted without any kind of evidence that would be required to try to support them, such as that there are significant human benefits from animal research, animal research is necessary for medical progress and so forth. Some of these recent articles include:

"Where is the evidence that animal research benefits humans?" *British Medical Journal*. Pound P, Ebrahim S, Sandercock P, Bracken M, Roberts I. 2004; 328:514–17.

> Reviewed six systematic reviews examining the extent to which animal experiments had informed human clinical research, and found that, although animal studies are intended to be conducted prior to human clinical trials to test for potential toxicity in two cases clinical trials were conducted concurrently with the animal studies, in three cases clinical trials were conducted despite evidence of harm from prior animal studies, in the remaining case the outcome of the animal study contradicted the findings of previous investigators, who appeared to have cited only studies that supported their prior views.

"Comparison of treatment effects between animal experiments and clinical trials: systematic review." *British Medical Journal*. Perel P, Roberts I, Sena E, Wheble P, Briscoe C, Sandercock P, Macleod M, Mignini LE, Jayaram P, Khan KS. 2007; 334:197.

> Compared treatment effects from systematic reviews of clinical trials with those of our own systematic review of the corresponding animal experiments. Discordance

between animal and human studies may be due to bias or to the failure of animal models to mimic clinical disease adequately.

"Medical progress depends on animal models – doesn't it?" *Journal of the Royal Society of Medicine*. Matthews RA. 2008: 101:95–8.

> Critical assessment of the oft-repeated claim that 'Virtually every medical achievement of the last century has depended directly or indirectly on research with animals.' Includes a quantitative analysis of the predictivity for human outcomes of animal models.

Additional research is summarized in Ray Greek and Niall Shank's *FAQS About the Use of Animals in Science* (University Press of America, 2009), their *Animal Models in Light of Evolution* (BrownWalker Press, 2009) and in Ray and Jean Greek's *Sacred Cows and Golden Geese: The Human Cost of Experiments on Animals* (Continuum, 2000) and *Species Science: Why Experiments on Animals Harm Humans* (Continuum, 2003).

Thus, there is evidence that common scientific assumptions about the human utility of animal experimentations are not evidence based and that they are likely false. If these scientific assumptions are false, then many of the empirical premises of the arguments below are false, and so these arguments are unsound.

"Benefits" arguments

The argument above is actually a number of distinct arguments. Here is one:

1. Humans benefit from animal experimentation.
C. Therefvore, animal experimentation is morally permissible.

To state this argument in logically valid form, however, ie, to display the complete reasoning, we must add this premise as well:

2. If humans benefit from action X, then action X is morally permissible.

There are many reasons to think that this argument should not be judged to be sound. First, premise 1 is imprecise: is the claim that all humans benefit from animal experimentation? Some humans? If so, which humans? Is the claim that all animal research is beneficial to (some?) humans? Some research benefits some humans? To evaluate this premise, this needs to be clarified: rarely is it.

Also, we also do not know what the conclusion is here: *all* animal research is permissible? *Some* of it? *Which?* These are all very different claims, and they often are not specified to evaluate the argument we need to know what is being said, as some understandings of premise 1 are false ("*all* humans benefit from *all* animal research") and some might be true ("*some* humans benefit from *some* animal research").

The deeper problems with this argument concern premise 2. First, it ignores harms to animals. If these are irrelevant, it is not explained why. If it is assumed that some benefits to some humans "outweigh" some harms to animals, no explanation is given for how this accounting is done or why we should think that the accounting favors humans ("why think that?"). Second, and most importantly, it is not said why it is permissible to harm animals to benefit humans. It is often wrong to harm humans to benefit other humans (especially when the harms are great, the harmed humans do not, or would not consent, and they themselves do not benefit from being harmed). If harms to animals should be treated differently, reasons why need to be given: often they are not. Third, premise 2 also ignores any harms to humans that result from animal research, direct harms or indirect harms, in terms of opportunity costs that result from it, if net benefits for humans from alternative courses of action not involving animal research would be greater.

Thus, to develop and defend a "benefits" argument, much more needs to be said: usually, however, few, if any, of these details are provided. Some of what is often said in defense of the argument will be discussed later in this article though and shown inadequate.

"Necessity" arguments

A second variant on this kind of argument, stated in logically valid form, is this:

1. Animal experimentation is "necessary."
2. If action X is "necessary," then action X is morally permissible.
3. Therefore, animal experimentation is morally permissible.

There are many reasons to think that this argument should not be judged to be sound also.

First, premise 1 is unclear: "What do you mean, necessary?" Claims that something is "necessary" are always incomplete as nothing is just plan[e] "necessary": something is necessary only relative to achieving a specific end or goal. Thus, to evaluate premise 1 that end, or those ends, must be specified. For various ends, it may be true or false that any, or even some, animal experimentation is indeed (causally, scientifically) "necessary" to achieve those ends: eg, if the goal is "medical progress," broadly understood, then it is surely false that animal experimentation is necessary for that, if the implication is that no other means of research or practice promotes medical progress (eg, clinical research, technology-based research, public health, distributing existing medical knowledge and access, education, prevention, etc.). Other claims of "necessity" are false as well, eg, that it is "necessary" to dissect or vivisect animals for medical training: this is demonstrably false insofar as there are highly competent physicians and medical personnel who did not train using animals.

If, however, the claim is that some specified animal research is (causally, scientifically) "necessary" to achieve some more specific, constrained end, then that claim might be true: there may be no other way to achieve that specific goal. Many people seem to think that this truth would show that animal experimentation is morally permissible, but it does not. This is because this revised premise, needed for a logically valid argument, is either false or question begging:

- If action X is "necessary" to achieve a goal, then action X is morally permissible.

That an action is "necessary" to achieve a goal, even a very worthy goal, does not in itself imply that it is morally permissible. There are moral constraints on achieving goals. We recognize this in the case of human research, eg, that it would be wrong to intentionally seriously harm some innocent, unconsenting human being (say, by vital organ theft) even if that were "necessary" to benefit some other human being, ie, if there truthfully was no other way to save that human. Insofar as this premise denies this for animals, it seems question begging insofar as it does not explain why it would be permissible to harm animals in cases of alleged "necessity" but not human beings.

Again, more explanation and defense of this argument is necessary to try to make a thorough attempt to show that it is sound.

"No alternatives" arguments

Third, there is this argument, stated in logically valid form:

1. There are "no alternatives" to animal experimentation.
2. If there are no alternatives to doing action X, then doing action X is morally permissible.
3. Therefore, animal experimentation is morally permissible.

Much of the discussion of this argument repeats what has already been said. First, premise 1 is unclear: there are "no alternatives" to animal research to try to achieve what end(s)? For some stated ends, this premise will be false, as there are other ways to achieve that end (or possibly better ends) and for others that will be true: eg, if one wants to experiment on animals for some reason, there is no alternative but to experiment on animals.

The second premise, however, is more troubling. Even if there is "no alternative" to doing some action that does not imply that the action is morally permissible. To think otherwise about animals seems to beg the question, ie, to merely assume that harming animals for research is permissible. The typical advocate

of this argument thinks that it would be wrong to seriously harm human beings in medical research even if there were "no alternatives" to doing so (ie, cases strongly analogous to animal research). However, if she thinks that the lack of "alternatives" makes animal research permissible, an explanation why this is so is needed. Some explanations for what justifies this difference will be evaluated soon.

Finally, it is worthwhile to observe that premise 1 is simply false: one "alternative" to doing animal research is just to not do it: people who engage in animal research are not compelled to do it. They surely could apply their talents elsewhere, if they chose to do so. Perhaps more human beings would benefit from that too.

"Necessary condition" arguments

I have argued that the arguments above appear question begging insofar as they apply one moral standard to human beings but a different standard to animals: they grant protections from harm for humans but permit harm to animals [but] do not explain why this difference in treatment is justified. Many respond by arguing that this difference in treatment and consideration can be justified by morally relevant differences between animals and human beings. Thus, we have arguments similar to these:

1. Animals are not "rational," do not understand moral concepts, are not "moral agents," are not "self-aware," do not "contribute to culture," are "not responsible for their actions," are not "no obligated to help others," do not create artworks, lack a religious sense and/or so on.
C. Therefore, animal research is morally permissible.

Premise 1 is intended to summarize many premises that attempt to identify differences between humans and animals: this premise could be broken up into separate premises and arguments. For some of these premises, we can rightly ask what they mean, eg, what it means to be "rational." However, some of these premises are true; others might be false.

What's important, however, is that the argument be put in logically valid form. To do this, we must add general premises such as these:

- If a being is not "rational," then it is morally permissible to experiment on that being.
- If a being is not "self-aware," then it is morally permissible to experiment on that being.
- If a being does not contribute to culture, then it is morally permissible to experiment on that being.

And so on. Premises such as these, however, can easily be shown false by *counterexamples*: there are many human beings (eg, the very young, very old, the mentally and emotionally challenged) who do not meet [these] arguments' *necessary condition(s)* for being wrong to experiment on. Insofar as these human beings are wrong to experiment on, even though they are not rational, self-aware, artistically gifted, etc. this shows that the italicized premises such as these above are false. Arguments such as these are unsound, and almost all advocates of animal research reject them.

Group-based arguments

In response to the refutation of the arguments above by way of glaring and obvious counterexamples to their major premises, some advocate this strategy: we should not focus on individual human beings – as some do not meet the proposed necessary conditions suggested above – but rather we should focus on the group(s), "kinds" or species that individual human beings are members of.[18,19] This kind of reasoning might involve premises such as the following:

- "Human beings, *as a group*, have done magnificent things, like create beautiful artworks, skyscrapers, and so forth. Animals have not."
- "Human beings, normally, in adult form, have sophisticated minds. Animals do not."
- "Human beings are the 'kind' of beings who are moral agents and are morally responsible. Animals are not."

These arguments concede that not all human beings have sophisticated minds. However, they hold that moral protections somehow result from sophisticated mental capacities: after all, this is why, according to these arguments, animal research is permissible, due to animals' lacking mental sophistication.

The problem is explaining how these properties of the group "transfer" to each individual, some of whom lack these properties, in a plausible, non ad hoc manner. Even if human beings "as a group" have done magnificent things (and perhaps that makes no sense), that does not seem to imply anything for human beings who did not participate in this. Also, perhaps we have also done some horrendously evil things as well "as a group": why the "good credit" would "transfer" to all human beings and not the bad credit, and perhaps deserved punishment, is hard to understand. Also although "normal" humans have various characteristics, "nonnormal" humans often lack some of them, and this can make a difference to how they should be treated: eg, if a very mentally challenged individual was treated similar to a "normal" adult in all ways, this would be very morally wrong. (Some might argue that a fetus or embryo will normally have sophisticated mental capacities or is the kind of being that does: would advocates of animal research who accept this argument [. . .] also think abortion is wrong?) Finally, each individual is many different "kinds" of beings: humans and animals are of some of the same "kinds," some different "kinds" and differing humans are of different "kinds" as well. The challenge is to explain which kinds are relevant in a plausible, explanatory manner.

In sum, it is not at all clear why we should believe that each individual human has all the moral characteristics that normal, mentally sophisticated human beings have. To put this another way, it is not at all clear what premises one would have to add to the (true!) premises above to construct an argument in logically valid form, and it is not clear why they would be true: insofar as individuals should be treated on their own merits, not on the merits of different groups they belong in, this argumentative strategy is unsuccessful. Thus, there are no good reasons to think premises such as these (essential for making these arguments logically valid) are true, and counterexamples can be developed to show them false:

- If human beings, as a group, have done magnificent things, then each individual human being is entitled to some "credit" for these accomplishments, even in cases they had nothing to do with them.
- If human beings, normally, in adult form, have sophisticated minds, and some other characteristics P depend on having sophisticated minds, then each individual human being has characteristics P, even when they lack sophisticated minds (or minds at all).
- If human beings are the "kind" of beings who are moral agents and are morally responsible, then all human beings have the moral properties of moral agents, even when they are not moral agents.

These are just a few common arguments given for the moral permissibility of animal research. I have argued that they are unsound or should not be evaluated as sound. Other arguments, and there are many, can be addressed using [. . .] these same analysis concepts and skills.

A Positive, Cumulative Case in Defense of Animals

In conclusion, I briefly turn to my positive case against much animal research. As mentioned, I advocate appealing to less controversial cases to better understand controversial ones. So we should ask what are the best, most fundamental explanations why would it be morally wrong to experiment on you, the reader and vulnerable humans, in ways that animals are experimented on? That is, if injuries were inflicted, diseases induced, harmful conditions and states created, drug addictions induced, painful procedures done, all (typically) ending in the loss of some human being's life, why would that be wrong? To go

back to my initial cases, why was what was done at Tuskegee and Willowbrook wrong?

This is not because we, or the victims in these cases, are (or were) biologically human. First, we can reasonably ask why is it wrong to harm biologically humans, suggesting that this is not a very deep explanation. Second, we can observe that many things that are biologically human are clearly permissible to kill or destroy: eg, various cells and tissues, at least, such as those in [the] Skin Cell and Human Cadaver Research cases above. Third, although somewhat controversially, we can observe that some entities that are biologically human are arguably permissible to kill or let die: eg, individuals whose quality of life has dropped significantly, perhaps so much, so that death is no longer harmful for them, perhaps due to the irreversible loss of consciousness. Thus, our biological humanity has little, in itself, to do with what we are owed, morally.

It is also not because we are "persons." Again, we can ask why it is wrong to harm persons. If the answer is that persons are rational, self-conscious beings and so killing them harms them, then "harm-ability" seems to be the fundamental explanation, not personhood. In addition, this explanation has to say something about harm-able human beings who do not meet its criteria for personhood, such as the Willowbrook children. If the answer is that we are "harm-able" and biologically human organisms, we can rightly wonder what biological humanity morally explains, as it does not seem to do anything on its own and the "harm-ability" can do the explanatory work on its own to explain why harming us for the sought benefit of others is wrong.

Thus, I argue that the fundamental moral explanation why certain kinds of human experiments are wrong appeal to harms to the victim: they are made worse off, physically and/or psychologically than they were. Conversely, research tends to be permissible when no one is harmed, as the Skin Cell and Cadaver cases help confirm. Thus, if any animals can be harmed, then there is a presumption of its wrongness. This presumption would be defeated if morally relevant differences between all humans being who are wrong to harm and all animals can be found; I critiqued some of these attempts above, found them wanting and set forth a set of methods that can be used to evaluate other attempts. My conjecture is that other arguments could be shown unsound using these methods.

So can any animals be harmed? Contemporary common sense and science supports thinking that many animals, at least mammals and birds, perhaps all vertebrates, can be harmed: they are conscious, have mental lives, are aware, can feel negative and positive feelings and sensations, can process information, have memory, can anticipate, have negative and positive emotions, have social lives, among other psychological capacities. Those attentive to scientific studies of animals regularly hear of new discoveries that their mental and emotional lives are richer than we ever expected: rarely do we hear of new studies providing evidence that any animals are less aware, less emotional, less cognizant than anyone expected.

For animals' minds that are as rich as the minds of humans who would be morally wrong to "vivisect," consistently requires thinking that these animals are also wrong to engage in harmful research on. The best explanations why it would be wrong to engage in harmful, nontherapeutic experiments on human beings have analogous implications for many animals, as they too are harmed without consent.

This kind of reasoning has been developed in a number of ways, by many moral philosophers. Regan[20–22] argues that all beings who are "subjects of lives," ie, have a certain level of a mental life, such

that they can be harmed, have inherent value and a moral right to not be used as a "mere means" for others; Rowlands[23] appeals to a John Rawls-inspired "Veil of Ignorance" unbiased decision making procedure, similar to a Golden Rule, to evaluate animal research: if we consider the issue from a unbiased perspective where our own identity is concealed from us, ie, we do not know our sex, race, age, intelligence and species, it would be irrational to accept animal research, as it could turn out, once the Veil is lifted, that we are its victim; and Peter Singer[24–26] appeals to the Principle of Equal Consideration of Interests and argues that it applies to all beings who have interests, human and nonhuman.

Many other philosophers, scientists and "popular" thinkers have developed complementary cases in defense of animals. Most have used the general strategy I have suggested: consider less controversial cases, understand them better and use [. . .] those insights [to] address the more controversial issues of animal use. In reviewing these cases, DeGrazia[27] observes that, "The leading book length works in this field exhibit a *near consensus* that the status quo of animal usage is ethically indefensible and that at least significant reductions in animal research are justified." If this consensus is mistaken, my hope is that this article, with its methodological focus, will help others more clearly and carefully explain what has gone wrong with all these moral arguments against animal research. My stronger hope is that this article, with its methodological focus, will help more people better understand why these arguments are likely sound.

References

1   Regan T, Animal rights, human wrongs: an introduction to moral philosophy. Lanham (MD): Rowman and Littlefield; 2003. p. 68–9.

2   Regan T. Empty cages: facing the challenge of animal rights. Lanham (MD): Rowman and Littlefield; 2004. p. 9–20, 38.

3   Regan T. Animal rights, human wrongs: an introduction to moral philosophy. Lanham (MD): Rowman and Littlefield; 2003; p. 78–9.

4   Regan T. Empty cages: animal rights and vivisection. In: Andrew I. Cohen and Christopher Heath Wellman, editors. Contemporary debates in applied ethics. Malden (MA): Blackwell; 2005. p. 77–90.

5   Smith W. A rat is a pig is a dog is a boy: the human cost of the animal rights movement. New York (NY): Encounter Books; 2010. p. 251.

6   Taylor A. Review of Wesley J. Smith's A rat is a pig is a dog is a boy: the human cost of the animal rights

movement. *Between Species Online J Study Philosophy Animals* 2010;13. Available at: http://digitalcommons.calpoly.edu/bts/vol13/iss10/14/. Accessed July 26, 2011.

7   Morrison A. An odyssey with animals: a veterinarian's reflections on the animal rights & welfare debate. New York (NY): Oxford University Press; 2009. p. 197–8.

8   Paul E.F. and Paul J., editors. Why animal experimentation matters: the use of animals in medical research, 1st ed. Piscataway (NJ): Transaction Publishers; 2001.

9   Nobis N. So why does animal experimentation matter? *AJOB* 2003; 3:1a.

10 Rachels J. The elements of moral philosophy, 6th ed. New York (NY): McGraw Hill; 2009.

11 Rachels J. The right thing to do: basic readings in moral philosophy, 5th ed. New York (NY): McGraw Hill; 2009.

12 Feldman R. Reason and argument, 2nd ed. Upper Saddle River (NJ): Prentice Hall; 1998.

13 Conn M. and Parker J. The animal research war. New York (NY): Palgrave Macmillan; 2008.

14 Smith W. A rat is a pig is a dog is a boy: the human cost of the animal rights movement. New York (NY): Encounter Books; 2010. p. 115–66.

15 Regan T. Empty cages: facing the challenge of animal rights. Lanham (MD): Rowman and Littlefield; 2004, p. 9–20.

16 Engel M. The mere considerability of animals. *Acta Analytica* 2001; 16:89–108.

17 DeGrazia D. Animal rights: a very short introduction. New York (NY): Oxford; 2002.

18 Nobis N. Carl Cohen's 'kind' argument for animal rights and against human rights. *J Appl Philosophy* 2004; 21:43–59.

19 Nobis N. and Graham D. Review of Tibor Machan's putting humans first: why we are nature's favorite. *J Ayn Rand Studies* 2006; 8:85–104.

20 Regan T. Animal rights, human wrongs: an introduction to moral philosophy. Lanham (MD): Rowman and Littlefield; 2003.

21 Regan T. Empty cages: facing the challenge of animal rights. Lanham (MD): Rowman and Littlefield; 2004. p. 37–76.

22 Regan T. The case for animal rights. Berkeley (CA): Berkeley; 1983.

23 Rowlands M. Animals like us. Brooklyn (NY): Verso; 2002.

24 Singer P. Animal liberation: the definitive classic of the animal movement, Reissue ed. New York (NY): Harper Perennial Modern Classics; 2009.

25 Singer P. Animal liberation, 1st ed. New York (NY): Harper; 1975.

26 Singer P. Practical ethics. New York (NY): Cambridge; 1999.

27 DeGrazia D. The ethics of animal research: what are the prospects for agreement? *Camb Q Healthc Ethics* 1999; 8:23–34.

63

The Use of Nonhuman Animals in Biomedical Research

Dario L. Ringach

Scientists have a duty to talk to the public.[1] Why? Because social policies need to be decided on the basis of rational grounds and facts. These include important issues ranging from climate change, to the goals of the space program, to the protection of endangered species, to the use of embryonic stem cells or animals in biomedical research. Both the public and policy makers need to understand not only the scientific justification for our work but also, in some cases, why we deem our studies to be morally justifiable.

The time is ripe for a more open, public and honest debate about the role of scientific experimentation in animals. What follows are some of my thoughts on this topic. I hope this perspective encourages other scientists to join the discussion and prompts opponents of animal research to create an atmosphere where civil discourse can take place, free of the threats, harassment and intimidation that are increasingly directed at biomedical scientists and their families.[2,3]

Criticism to the use of animals in biomedical research rests on varied scientific and ethical arguments. The discussion below is necessarily incomplete but represents an initial effort to answer some key objections. We start by addressing the opposition's claims regarding the validity of the scientific work to human health and then turn our attention to ethical issues.

Arguments Against the Use of Animals in Scientific Research

Let us first consider some common criticisms directed at the scientific basis for animal research.

Claim: Humans do not benefit from animal research

One extreme view holds that information gathered from animal research cannot, even in principle, be used to improve human health. It is often accompanied by catchy slogans such as "If society funds mouse models of cancer, we will find more cures for cancer in mice."[4] It is argued that the physiology of animals and humans are too different to allow results from animal research to be extrapolated to humans.[5]

Original publication details: Dario L. Ringach, "Use of Nonhuman Animals in Biomedical Research," pp. 305–313 from *American Journal of the Medical Sciences* 342: 4 (October 2011). Reproduced with permission of Elsevier.

Such a blanket statement is falsified by numerous cases where experimentation on animals has demonstrably contributed to medical breakthroughs. The experiments on cardiovascular and pulmonary function in animals that began with Harvey and continued with the Oxford physiologists[6] established the understanding of what the heart and lungs do and how they do it, on which the modern practice of internal medicine rests. Modern medical practice is inconceivable in the absence of the insights gained from these experiments. Anti-coagulants were first isolated in dogs; insulin was discovered in dogs and purified in rabbits; lung surfactants were first extracted and studied in dogs; rabbits were used in the development of *in vitro;* fertilization; mice in the development of efficient breast cancer drugs and so on.

For the sake of completeness, it must be noted that the other extreme – the notion that all medical advances are a result of animal research – is false as well. Important medical advances, such as sanitation and the discovery of aspirin, were conducted without the use of animals.

Claim: Animal research has a very low success rate

Here the claim is not that animal research has never produced benefits, but it has done so with a very low success rate, which in the minds of our opponents is enough to deem the work unacceptable.[5,7] But what does very low mean exactly? Is the term meant to be interpreted in absolute or relative terms? If the comparison is relative, then very low relative to what?

Absolute interpretation

If one is to interpret the success rate as an absolute figure, then the assertion does little more than restate what is an inherent property of the scientific method.[8] Scientific research involves a continuous cycle of 3 phases: postulating a theory that can account for the existing data, generating novel predictions from the theory and testing them experimentally. While searching for answers to difficult problems (such as developing a cure for cancer), it is expected for many

paths to lead to dead ends. This is a feature of science, not a bug. The scientific method allows us to rule out hypotheses proven wrong by data and systematically narrow down the list of possible explanations until we converge on an answer. History has shown, time and again, that such a strategy works, producing advances in everything from mathematics and physics, to life sciences and medicine. Incorrect hypotheses and negative findings are integral, fundamental and inseparable components of the scientific method.

Grasping the principles of the scientific method is not difficult. Accepting its consequences in the field of animal is hard. The implication is one we would naturally resist: animals, if used in scientific studies, will sometimes be used in experiments that do not yield immediate, tangible benefits.

We must understand and accept the fact that science does not provide recipes. There is no recipe that can ensure a particular type of work that will lead to a unified theory of physics. There is no line of research guaranteed to yield a proof or a rejection of a mathematical conjecture. There is no recipe that can ensure a particular type of work, whether using humans or animals, will lead to cures for cancer, paralysis or autism. Anyone claiming to know with certainty where the answers are to be found, or where they are not to be found, is simply not credible.

Relative interpretation

An alternative interpretation is that the success rate of animal research should be interpreted as relative to a baseline. The critics are vague about what this baseline is, but the implication seems to be the success rate one would achieve solely by human-based medical research.[7]

This claim can be verified because there is plenty of scientific research performed with human subjects alone, from cancer to Alzheimer's and Parkinson's disease. If there was an obvious advantage for such work in yielding new cures and therapies, we would certainly know by now. To the best of my knowledge, there are no data to support this view.

One may also interpret the baseline success rate as the one we all wish it could be. Patients and families that anxiously await new developments to treat their loved ones surely must feel the rate at which new therapies are generated is low. So does everyone else, including the physicians who care for the patients and the scientists who do their best to develop new cures and therapies as fast as they possibly can. We all wish that effective treatments could be developed faster. In the absence of a viable alternative, this lament is hardly an argument against the use of animals in medical research.

Finally, and perhaps most surprising, it has been stated that the success rate of animal research is comparable to that of astrology.[9] Our discoveries, we are told, are mere chance events that are not causally related to our investigations. The origin of the claim rests on anecdotes describing serendipitous discoveries in science. Yet, as Louis Pasteur commented, "Chance favors the prepared mind." What he meant, of course, is that an accidental observation will generate a finding only in the mind of someone who has been thinking about the problems for some time, and who is a keen observer.

Claim: Researchers must prove animals are necessary for their work

Faced with irrefutable causal links between animal studies and medical breakthroughs, opponents of animal research typically respond with a claim and a demand of their own.

The claim is that such research represents work performed decades ago.[5,7] On one hand, they accept that we have learned much about the respiratory, circulatory and digestive systems from animals that has been relevant for human health. On the other, they contend that the problems we face today are more complex and subtle. There is little or nothing left to be understood about basic biological function from animals that is relevant to human conditions. In other words, the entire field of animal research is declared to be exhausted of fundamental results.

Any scientist will be perplexed and baffled by such statements. Surely, the claims must come from those

with a poor appreciation of the time scales involved in bringing basic research results to the clinic. Indeed, it can take many years, even decades. For example, consider the development of electrocardiography, which relied on classic studies on bioelectricity in the 18th century by Galvani and Volta, with the first measurements of electrocardiograms in humans near the beginning of the 20th century.[10]

Second, only someone lacking in scientific humility can declare an entire field to be depleted of fundamental results. Can we imagine a similar claim made about mathematics or physics? After all, one may argue, these are areas of research that are more than 2,000 years old! What else could be left to discover? But our critics do not claim these fields to be depleted of results. Oddly enough, their claims are restricted just to those areas of scientific inquiry that involve the use of animals.

One can simply point to some recent examples to prove the claim false. Consider the development of Herceptin to fight breast cancer,[11–13] antivascular endothelial growth factor (VEGF) therapy for retinal vascular disorders[14–16] or RNAi drug delivery.[17–21] All these represent recent breakthroughs that were obtained by the scientific use of animals (including worms, mice and monkeys) in just the last 2 decades.

What about their demand? Our critics insist that if scientists are to claim that animals are necessary for their research, that a proof be provided showing there was no other way of obtaining the results that circumvented animal use.

What do scientists mean when they say animals are necessary in their work? In most cases, I submit the meaning is that animals are necessary in the sense that the data they seek requires the use of invasive methods, which we would not apply in humans because of the high risks involved and the resulting ethical concerns. Furthermore, it means that a reasonable effort was made to identify potential alternatives in which the data could have been collected without the use of animals. Thus, the necessity is partly an ethical one, not a scientific one. There is nothing in the science per se that would invalidate the use of invasive methods in human subjects. For example, cancerous tumors can certainly be grown in humans as they are in mice, but we do not consider the practice morally acceptable. In other cases, there are clear practical reasons for the selection of animal species. In many genetic studies, one needs to work with organisms that have short generational times, like fruit flies. In studying development, the ability to observe deep tissue *in vivo;*, such as in transparent zebrafish eggs, offers a tremendous practical advantage. Finally, animals allow scientists to control many external factors that might otherwise affect the outcome of experiments, such as diet, temperature, humidity and genetic composition, in ways that are not possible in humans.

In contrast, our critics often adopt a stricter interpretation of necessity, arguing that scientists are claiming that animal research is the only possible way to obtain the data they need, and they demand proof to this effect. In the words of Greek:[22]

> [. . .] the claimant must essentially prove a negative; that the discovery could not have been made any other way. Although difficult, this can be done and indeed must be done for the claimant to say the discovery was dependent on animal use.

This is an unreasonable demand based on a strawman argument. First, as noted above, this is not what scientists mean. Second, there are infinite possibilities that must be considered for one to prove that no other method could have generated the same result without the use of animals. Proving the positive, in contrast, should be simpler. Those with the absolute conviction that animals are unnecessary in biomedical research could prove their point by simply showing there is another way. Such a demonstration would be a tremendous contribution to society. Finally, as remarked by an anonymous reviewer, once a mountain has been reached, it is sometimes possible to look back down and find an alternate path that would have been easier or that might have avoided some segment. However, this does not mean one could have located that alternate path during the initial climb.

Claim: Animal models are not predictive of human responses

This claim is a centerpiece of many arguments. It effectively states that it is impossible to model human disease in animals because any treatments we develop in animals will not translate to humans. Prediction is no doubt a goal of scientific work and some, but not all, of animal research aims at modeling disease in human subjects.

Predictions are the fruits of theories that can be tested experimentally. If the prediction is false so is the theory, and a new one must be generated based on prior knowledge and the specific way in which the data falsified the theory. Interestingly, those that claim animal models are not predictive of human response take some literary license in restating the above along the following lines:[5,7]

> Predictions, generated from hypotheses, are not always correct. But if a modality or test or method is said to be predictive then it should get the right answer a very high percentage of the time [. . .]
>
> If a modality consistently fails to make accurate predictions then the modality cannot be said to be predictive simply because it occasionally forecasts a correct answer. The above separates the scientific use of the word predict from the layperson's use of the word, which more closely resembles the words forecast, guess, conjecture, project and so forth. [. . .]
>
> Many philosophers of science think a theory (and we add, a modality) could be confirmed or denied by testing the predictions it made.

This language delicately nudges the reader to equate different concepts, namely theory, hypothesis, modality and method. In this deceptively innocuous equation, resulting from either an honest misunderstanding or mischievous intent, lies the foundation to a seriously flawed argument.

For example, the statement:

> . . . if a modality or test or method is said to be predictive then it should get the right answer a very high percentage of the time

is not accurate. It is theories that generate predictions, not modalities or methods.

Consider the domain of physics. Here, physicists put forward mathematical theories of some natural phenomenon which, in turn, generate predictions. These predictions can be experimentally tested. If a prediction is falsified, so is the theory. When this occurs, scientists seek to understand how the data depart from the prediction and use prior knowledge and intuition to develop a new working hypothesis, which is embedded in a new theory. Mathematics is the language of physics – its methodology. Obviously, by using mathematical language, one can create many different theories. The overwhelming majority of them will be false. Science is difficult because most of the time our ideas turn out to be wrong.

The point is that one's ability to conjure up vast numbers of incorrect theories does not invalidate mathematics as a method in the physical sciences. Mathematics can in fact be used to arrive at accurate descriptions of how matter behaves. It makes no sense to describe this state of affairs by stating that mathematics (the modality) gets it right occasionally. Mathematics does not generate theories – people do.

A similar situation arises in the domain of biomedical research. Researchers create models of disease in animals by trying to replicate what they believe are the essential components at play. These animal models can then be used to generate predictions for therapeutic interventions, which can then be tested in human clinical trials. If a prediction is falsified, so is the animal model of disease. Let me repeat, it is the specific animal model that is falsified. When this happens, scientists seek to understand how the data depart from the prediction, what other factors were ignored that might play a role and use prior knowledge and intuition to develop a better, improved model. In the course of developing and refining such a model, scientists will go through many such cycles. A model is expected to be valid once it captures all the key ingredients of the human condition.

The fact that one can postulate inaccurate animal models of human disease does not invalidate the whole methodology of animal research, it merely shows the

work is difficult. But animal models can in fact be successful. It is a mistake to conclude that animal models get it right occasionally. The scientific question is not whether animals can be used to generate inaccurate models of human disease but whether they can be used to generate faithful ones. The answer is yes they can.

It is also worth noting that a theory can often capture partial patterns in the data. Thus, even though we might know a theory to be strictly incorrect, it can still be used to our benefit until refinements are developed. Consider the standard calculation of an object falling in a gravitational field based on Newton's laws of motion. The resulting model is only approximate and can be substantially improved by incorporating drag forces resulting from air resistance and how they depend on the shape of the object. And yet, for many purposes, the original model, although strictly incorrect, is sufficient to make reasonable predictions in many circumstances.

Similarly, some animal models may be strictly incorrect in that they do not capture all the behavior in the human condition, and improvements are clearly needed. However, they have predictive value, which make them utilizable until these refinements are worked out. One such example is the question of determining the first dose of potential new medicines to human subjects.[23]

The conditions for honest debate are eroded when critics cherry pick animal models that have poor predictive power, deliberately cite scientists who acknowledge these limitations out of context, completely ignore their explanations of what have they have learned from the results, disregard their ideas as to how the models can be improved and package such examples as proof that animal research is not predictive of human responses.[5] Such mischaracterization of scientific research must be forcefully rejected.

Claim: Basic research is knowledge for knowledge's sake

Animal models of disease are only 1 way in which animals are used in science. A substantial amount of research is aimed at understanding the basic biological processes of life and disease, so-called basic research. The function of cells, how they communicate, how they develop, how they age and how they die are all part of the foundations of biological science.

Some have characterized this research as "knowledge for knowledge's sake", the benefits of which, we are told, are so unlikely to materialize that one cannot possibly justify the use of animals in this type of work.[7] However, it is precisely such basic knowledge, from the abstract geometric theorems of ancient Greece, to the physical models of atoms and subatomic particles, to the inner workings of cells and organs that are responsible for our greatest scientific advancements. The mission of the National Institutes of Health (NIH) recognizes this fact in its opening statement,

> NIH's mission is to seek fundamental knowledge about the nature and behavior of living systems and the application of that knowledge to enhance health, lengthen life and reduce the burdens of illness and disability.

Implicit in this declaration is the acknowledgment that it is basic knowledge that drives advancements in our health and well being. Translational or applied research would not exist without basic knowledge as the raw material. Nevertheless, scientists engaged in basic research are continuously challenged to explain the value of their work. Approximately 35 years ago, the National Science Foundation was asked by the House Committee on Appropriations exactly this question:[24] "Why does the foundation persist in supporting research whose results have no apparent value to the American people?" The request prompted not only a response from National Science Foundation but also the compilation of an entire volume describing the multiple ways in which basic research has led to technological and medical advancement.[25] In its introduction, Isaac Asimov presented an eloquent defense of basic research and concluded:[25]

> [. . .] And now we stand in the closing decades of the twentieth century, with science advancing as never before in all sorts of odd, and sometimes apparently useless, ways. We've discovered quasars and pulsars in the distant heavens. Of what use are they to the average

man? Astronauts have brought back rocks from the moon at great expense. So what? Scientists discover new compounds, develop new theories, work out new mathematical complexities. What for? What's in it for you?
>
> No one knows what's in it for you right now, any more than Plato knew in his time, or Faraday knew, or Edison knew, or Einstein knew. But you will know if you live long enough; if not, your children or grandchildren will know. [. . .]
>
> In fact, unless we continue with science and gather knowledge, whether or not it seems useful on the spot, we will be buried under our problems and find no way out. Today's science is tomorrow's solution – and tomorrow's problems too – and, most of all, it is mankind's greatest adventure, now and forever.

Today's science is tomorrow's solution. Even though we might not be able to benefit directly from the basic research of today, we owe it to our children and our grandchildren to develop the knowledge that they will need to build a better future for their generation and those to come. Basic knowledge about life processes is part of this endeavor.

Claim: Alternatives to animal research already exist

To the scientist, this claim is perhaps the most infuriating of all, because it not only pertains to the scientific work, but it represents an attack on our ethical conduct. Scientists are effectively accused of engaging in animal research even though alternatives are supposedly available. The Humane Society of the United States web site states:[26]

> If animal experimentation was the hallmark of twentieth century biomedical research, sophisticated nonanimal methods are likely to characterize twenty-first century research. Many humane state-of-the-art alternatives to animal experiments have already been shown to be effective in advancing medical progress, cutting research costs and eliminating animal suffering.

We are told, for example, that today's computer simulations are advanced and detailed enough to be able to replace animals in many studies and that functional magnetic resonance imaging can be used to replace all our electrophysiologic studies of brain function in animals. This is utter nonsense. It is scientists who have developed these techniques, not the opponents of animal research. What reasons would we have to reject our own methods? Do the critics truly believe scientists engage in animal research despite the existence of viable alternatives? Apparently so. Greek[27] defends this notion by citing Upton Sinclair: "It is difficult to get a man to understand something when his salary depends upon his not understanding it." Other animal activists appear to believe in a vast conspiracy network that includes the NIH, the Center for Disease Control, the US Department of Agriculture and many scientific professional organizations, all of which work together to promote the practice of animal research for mere financial gain. Needless to say, such theories do not stand scrutiny.

Once again, these are shameful attacks that detract from honest debate. The methods suggested are already being used in conjunction with animal research but are incapable of replacing the studies that require access to cellular and molecular processes. Every single scientist I know will support and embrace the use of alternatives if and when they become available. None of them derives any pleasure in harming animals. It should also be noted that our funding agencies require each study submitted for consideration to justify the use of animals and species in each case and to clearly explain all the alternatives that have been considered and ruled out.

Ethics of Animal Research

Even if we grant that biomedical research using animals advances human/animal health and well being, one can still ask whether the work is ethically permissible. Moral philosophers bring important issues to the table that cannot be dismissed easily.[28–36] I believe that scientists ought to familiarize themselves with the arguments, understand that there are some complex

moral questions being raised and confront the ethical arguments directly.

It is useful to start by noting some points of agreement. I accept that history shows moral boundaries to be dynamic. One example suffices to make the point: at one time, society recognized slavery as morally acceptable, it is no longer so. Thus, animal research can neither be defended exclusively on the grounds that the work, today, is legal, well regulated, includes work aimed at replacing, refining and reducing the use of animals and is supervised by a multi-tiered oversight system, nor can it be justified exclusively based on public support. The justification of animal research requires an ethical argument as its core.

The Moral Status of Animals

Rights, properly defined, are claims (or potential claims) to be exercised against another within a community of moral agents.[37] Animals cannot have rights because they are not able to participate as autonomous rational agents in our moral community. You cannot bring a claim to a dog that attacked you. The dog cannot recognize your interests. This, however, does not preclude animals from having moral status.[38] A living being is said to have moral status if we are morally obliged to give weight to their interests independent of their utility to us. Both animals and humans may be considered to have interests in their well being, freedom and life and thus to have moral status.

What is the moral status of nonhuman animals? On one end of the spectrum, we find those that may think that animals have no moral status at all and that we can do with animals as we please. On the other end of the spectrum, we find those who think that the moral status of sentient animals is equal to that of humans.[33] My position lies in-between these extreme viewpoints. I believe moral status to be graded according to the cognitive capabilities of each living being. Unfortunately, the first hurdle faced by anyone sharing this view is that some theorists would reject moral status as possible accepting degrees.[36]

Elizabeth Harman is clear on this point:[39]

We have no reason to posit such degrees of moral status, so we can conclude that moral status is not a matter of degree but is rather on/off: a being has moral status or lacks it.

Francione agrees:[33]

We have two choices – and only two – when it comes to the moral status of animals.

And Regan[30] writes similarly in terms of the inherent value of animals:

Two options present themselves concerning the possession by moral agents of inherent value. First, moral agents might be viewed as having this value to varying degrees, so that some may have more of it than others. Second, moral agents might be viewed as having this value equally. The latter view is rationally preferable. [. . .] We must reject the view that moral agents have inherent value in varying degrees. All moral agents are equal in inherent value, if moral agents have inherent value.

Rejecting the Extremes of the Spectrum

The extreme views have the virtue that [they] are simple to understand and apply; the problem is that they are wrong. Most of us readily reject the Cartesian view that animals [are] mere things based on multiple scientific evidence, starting with the work of Darwin. I will therefore concentrate my effort into explaining my reasons for ruling out the other extreme – the animal rights view.

Animal rights theories posit that once a living being satisfies some basic characteristics (such as exhibiting a minimum level of sentience[33] or passing the subject-of-life criterion[30]), they attain the same moral status as that of a normal human. Such all-or-none theories of moral status admit a moral universe with 2 possible equivalence classes, one that includes rocks and a second one that includes normal humans.

Is this so? What would be the moral status of single-cell organisms, plankton, worms, coral reefs, mice, cats, monkeys and great apes? Do we accept that in each case we must equate their moral status to that of a rock or a human? My moral intuition rejects such conclusion and, along with it, the notion of all-or-none moral status.

I submit it would be morally permissible to save my child and not a mouse in a burning house scenario. Curiously, this intuition is shared by my opponents,[30,33] although they fail to recognize the implications. Francione[33] justifies his decision by explaining that, "I better understand what is at stake for the human than I do for the dog. But this is a matter of my own cognitive limitation and how it plays out in these extreme circumstances [. . .]."

It is important to recognize that his decision to consistently select a human over the animal in these circumstances cannot be derived from an application of animal rights theory. Instead, the theory directs us to flip a fair coin among 2 living beings with equal moral status to decide who should be saved. The justification offered, based on our cognitive limitation in understanding animal minds, ceases to be one at the same instant we recognize it as one. Clearly, we are free to overcome our limitations by doing what is right according to the theory: rendering a fair, random decision between 2 living beings of equal moral status. And yet, neither Francione nor Regan seems ready to act in such a way.

Further, Francione[33] clarifies that, "my decision to favor the human does not mean I am morally justified in using dogs in experiments or otherwise treating dogs exclusively as means to my ends." This is a straw man. The point is that his refusal to act according to the theory cannot be justified in any other way but one: the theory is wrong and must be rejected. In rejecting the animal rights theory, I am not subscribing to the notion that animals are things and we should be able to do with them as we please. I reject such attempt at robbing others of the possibility to argue for moral theories based on graded moral status of living beings.

The validity of all-or-none moral status has been questioned before, and indeed, the moral philosophy literature is much more complex than the animal right activist in the street seems to know or acknowledge.[38,40,41] In particular, the notion of a graded moral status (defined as the degree a being's interests are protected vis-a-vis other beings) has been defended as a reasonable, alternative possibility.[41] One such example is the sliding scale model, where the moral weight of someone's interests depends on the individual degree of cognitive, affective and social complexity.[41] In this model, scientific facts about animal cognition and how we interpret the minds of animals are key in deciding how we weigh their interests. And it is what we know about the minds of animals that must primarily guide our ethical judgments, which is not just how we feel about them.[42] Ethical boundaries may shift as we learn more about animal minds but, given our current knowledge, there is good reason to grant humans the highest moral status followed by great apes, dolphins, monkeys, higher mammals, rodents, insects and so on. The sliding scale model is fully compatible with the views of many scientists and certainly with the NIH guidelines, which requires the use of the simplest organism that can provide the scientific data without compromising the validity of the study.

It should be emphasized that once the 2 extreme positions on moral status are rejected, all the theoretical frameworks that remain standing can be reasonably characterized as animal welfarism of various degrees, and importantly, all of them would allow for animal experimentation to some extent.

Equal Consideration of Equal Interests

The principle of equal consideration calls for giving equal weight to relevantly similar interests. Utilitarian[35] and animal rights[30] theories are both based on the principle of equal consideration and constitute the central theories used to challenge scientific work with animals. Is equal consideration violated in biomedical research that use animals?

Clearly, in animal research, the ultimate cost to animals is the loss of life. Many philosophers agree,

however, that the interests of (normal) humans and animals in life are not relevantly similar.[41,43,44]

Human life is the execution of an aspiration – a life's plan. Human life is a process that cannot be reduced to mere living by satisfying our immediate biological needs.[43] Humans are not content with living, they need to live well and realize their ambitions. Among these ambitions is the need to transcend our biological lives in some shape or form, by contributing to science, arts and society, in ways that improve the well being of living beings in our planet. When these needs are denied, and despite having all their biological needs met, humans can willfully terminate their own life.

Interests in life are not relevantly similar among humans and animals – the same things are not at stake. In recognition of this fact, many philosophers who would agree that, when faced with a choice between the life of a mouse or a human in a burning house scenario, we might be well justified in choosing the human. The moral status of the mouse is not equal to that of the human. Below, I suggest scientists are making a similar choice when they decide to engage in animal research. Not in an abstract or hypothetical scenario, but a rather concrete one where lives are at stake.

Human Ability to Challenge Nature and Suffering is Unique

Humans can transcend their biological lives in ways that other animals cannot. Relevant to this discussion is the fact that humans are unique in their ability to study and understand nature, including the basic biological principles underlying life and disease processes. We have the unique ability to store and accumulate vast amounts of knowledge in perpetual form, securing benefits to all future generations, challenge nature by means of technological might and, in short, improve well being of all living creatures on the face of the planet.

Our abilities also carry a moral burden, as we often find ourselves having to make difficult decisions [. . .] that trade off human and animal life. As a concrete example, consider a patient with severe aortic stenosis, which has a mortality rate of approximately 75% 5 years after diagnosis. The patient's life can be saved by replacing the valve in his heart with one from a pig. Is it morally permissible to carry out such a procedure? In some respects, we are facing a burning house scenario: it is either a pig or a human. Those that consider the moral status of the pig equal to that of the patient must effectively condemn the patient to death for the same reasons we would not take the heart valve of another human as a replacement.

Another example comes from recent advances in neonatal care. The rate of premature birth has increased by 36% since the 1980s. Most babies born before 37 weeks of pregnancy are premature and are at risk of complications. In the United States alone, approximately 13% of babies are born prematurely and will spend the first few days of their life in the neonatal intensive care unit. Among babies born before the 34th week, 23,000 of them each year will suffer from respiratory distress syndrome. These babies lack a protein in their lungs (called surfactants) that keep the air sacs in the lungs from collapsing. If left untreated, these babies would die.

Surfactants were discovered, and their chemical composition was analyzed by experimentation in dogs.[45] The fruits of this research were translated into the treatments using surfactants in the 1990s, which reduced the death of babies from respiratory distress syndrome by approximately 50%. In other words, slightly more than 10,000 babies are saved every year, in the United States alone as a result of surfactant replacement therapy.[46] This amounts to more than 1 baby per hour. The use of the dogs in research produced these enormous benefits that are realized each hour when a proud mother goes back home carrying her newborn baby instead of doing so empty handed. Those that consider the moral status of dogs equal to that of human babies must have declared such research unethical.

When scientists are confronted with the incredible suffering caused by disease on one hand and faced with our proven ability to challenge such maladies on the other, we feel a moral imperative to act. True; under normal circumstances, nobody would want to inflict unnecessary harm to animals. But to the patients and their families, these are no normal circumstances; the scientist, in some cases, cannot see any other way to help them but to experiment in animals. Such is our plight, which was recognized in the words of Charles Darwin[47] when he wrote to the London Times:

> [. . .] I know that physiology cannot possibly progress except by means of experimenting on live animals, and I feel the deepest conviction that he who retards the progress of physiology commits a crime against mankind.

Utilitarian Considerations

What is the likelihood any 1 experiment will advance our knowledge and produce important benefits? Given our preceding discussion of the scientific method, it is clear there is a problem with deciding the moral worth of scientific work based on its consequence, because [. . .] the outcome is initially unknown.

Singer, for example, justified the use of monkeys in the development of a therapy for Parkinson's disease in a recent encounter with neuroscientist Tipu Aziz, who was explaining to Singer that:[48]

> To date 40,000 people have been made better with this [Parkinson's therapy], and worldwide at the time I would guess only 100 monkeys were used at a few laboratories.

To which, Singer replied:

> Well, I think if you put a case like that, clearly I would have to agree that was a justifiable experiment. I do not think you should reproach yourself for doing it, provided – I take it you are the expert in this, not me – that there was no other way of discovering this knowledge. I could see that as justifiable research.

The problem is that this is a *post hoc* justification. There was, of course, no way for anyone to know the experiments would yield such important benefits. One must ask how a utilitarian would respond had he/she been asked to approve the experiments before they were conducted.

Individual experiments cannot be justified based on utilitarian considerations unless we allow for some probabilistic calculus of cost/benefits. This is, as a matter of fact, the task performed by the Center for Scientific Review at the NIH, where a panel of experts evaluate and recommend scientific proposals so that our society can fund the most promising research as judged by our best scientific minds. This system is the one that has allowed the development of cutting-edge drugs and cures for conditions that would have surely killed our parents and grandparents.

The relevant question for the utilitarian is, has animal research so far, as a field, produced sufficiently important benefits as to be justified? I honestly believe that any person with basic knowledge of medical history must answer this question in the affirmative. Recall what medical science was merely a couple of generations ago: a visit to a physician might have resulted in a recommendation to induce vomiting, diarrhea or, more commonly, bleeding. Diphtheria, mumps, measles and polio were common and untreatable. Life expectancy in the United States was less than 50 years; it is now close to 80 years. Animal research was an integral part of these past achievements. Our generation benefits from treatments and medicines that our parents and grandparents only dreamt about. Moreover, our children, grandchildren and all future generations will benefit as well. Thus, any utilitarian calculation of the benefits will show that they are not merely astronomical, but infinite. Harms, of course, must also be counted, including the life of the animals used and any negative outcomes that might be attributed, in part, to the use of animals in research. When the costs and benefits are tallied, I believe we must agree animal research has been justified. It is doubtful this picture and our assessment of the work will change substantially in the near future.

What About Marginal Cases?

We are often challenged to spell out the criteria that makes some experiments justified in some animals but not in some humans that might have comparable interests. These criteria, we are explained, must be evaluated for each individual subject[30,35,37,49] (so-called moral individualism[50]). No matter what criteria are selected, it is likely we will find some humans (the senile, the severely mentally impaired or the minimally conscious patient) who would qualify for invasive research. We are then asked to be logically consistent and accept that we should also be experimenting in these human patients along with the animals.

First, I note that no matter what criteria are selected, the moral status of a rock, a dead cat, or human remains should all [be] equal to each other (they are all inanimate objects with no interests of their own). Although nobody will object to a child playfully kicking a rock, most will not feel comfortable with him kicking a dead cat for his or her amusement or using human remains in an art project for school. Clearly, there are relational properties that come into play about how to judge the moral status of deceased organisms or inanimate objects. We believe that we owe dignity to the deceased cat and human in ways that do not apply to the rock. Conversely, special relations call for some inanimate objects to have moral status because of their importance to humans, such as the Church of the Nativity, the Western Wall or the Black Stone in Mecca. Damaging such inanimate objects would certainly cause much human suffering, and consequently, these objects have higher moral status than others. As I discuss below, such relational properties might be integral to the definition of human kind as well.[51]

Second, if we insist on moral judgments being based on properties at the individual level alone, the resulting theory is not really practical. Moral individualism is a necessary condition to pose the marginal case scenario. But are we ready to evaluate every single individual we encounter in life to decide on his or her moral status? Are we to assess the child now crossing the street? And the dog walking along? And the squirrel that just rushed in front of our moving car? Consistency demands that we do, but applicability demands that we do not. A consistent moral theory that cannot be practiced has little value.

Instead, our daily behavior is aided by organizing the world into different categories (or kinds) of living beings and our assessment of their interests and moral status.[37] Our brain's ability to quickly recognize species membership makes such a kind a rather natural choice. This enables us to immediately recognize the interests of the squirrel running in front of our car and avoid running it over (there is really no need to assess the individual interests and moral status of this one particular squirrel). Thus, we must understand that interests of living beings can be assessed in most cases based on the normal life of its species.[51]

Human Relationships Are Unique: The Human Family

I happen to be writing this article as the world anxiously awaits the rescuing of 33 miners trapped in Chile. They have been entombed underground for 70 days, under 700 m of hard rock, in damp and hot conditions, in nearly complete darkness and physically and psychologically weakened. An estimated 1 billion people have been following the fate of a truly insignificant number of individuals. Thousands across many countries have mobilized to make the rescue possible. The economic cost of the operation is unknown, likely exorbitant, and appropriately irrelevant.

As miners start coming out of a small duct, the spectacle is surreal. Earth appears to be giving birth anew to those that a couple of months ago were presumed dead. Across the planet, people wipe tears of joy and celebrate the unique value of human life. We feel good because, for once, we acted according to what we think is the proper moral status of human life – the gold, machinery and financial cost is insignificant compared with the life of the miners. It is in these extreme circumstances that the human race is at once redeemed and when John Donne's words acquire extra meaning:

> No man is an Island, entire of itself; every man is a piece of the Continent, a part of the main; [. . .] any man's death diminishes me, because I am involved in Mankind; And therefore never send to know for whom the bell tolls; It tolls for thee.

It is here, then, that we realize that any moral theory that includes relational characteristics among human beings sets human (kind) apart in a unique way. And this argument has been articulated previously. It is accepted that we might be morally justified in giving one's immediate family higher moral status because of our special relations. Kittay[52] has argued that species membership can be considered an extension of such family and community membership concepts, agreeing with the notion that, "As humans, we are indeed a family."

Assuming Responsibility and Stewardship

Feelings of embarrassment and guilt are understandable responses to any emergent recognition of the unique moral status of human life. Embarrassment because innumerable animals, even entire species, have been wronged by our disregard for animal life and the environment. Guilt because we abhor discrimination, which makes us prone to misconstrue factual statements about evolutionary biology and interpret any implication of unequal moral status as an expression of human arrogance, bias and prejudice.

However, no amount of denial, guilt or embarrassment can erase or blur our differences. Declaring equality is not a remedy. To the contrary, a responsible and sensible sharing of the planet among all its inhabitants will result the sooner we acknowledge our differences. Accepting that evolution has put us in a place to be the stewards of our planet, its environment and all living creatures within it, carries a tremendous responsibility that we must accept and face.

Conclusion

The contributions of animal research to medical science and human health are undeniable. Scientific expertise, consensus and facts on the use of animal research must be weighed accordingly to have an honest, public discussion. When the majority of scientists see the work as scientifically justified, and so do the many professional medical and scientific organizations, the expert views cannot be simply dismissed based on wild claims of ulterior motives, self-interest and conspiracy theories.

Why is the use of animals in scientific experimentation morally permissible? In my view, it is because the moral status of animals is not equal to that of humans and because opting out of the research condemns our patients (both animal and human) to suffer and die of disease. Stopping the research would be, as Darwin correctly judged, a crime against humanity. I have come to appreciate the compassion animal activists have toward animals. Paradoxically, this compassion does not seem to extend to human patients. Hopefully, animal activists will come to accept that our work is driven similarly by an honest attempt at advancing knowledge and alleviating suffering and disease in the world.

I reject moral theories that posit all-or-none moral status for all living organisms. I identified the existence of moral theories that admit degrees of moral status, which are compatible with the practice and regulations of animal research (such as the sliding scale model). Thus, the responsible, regulated animal research with the goal of advancing medical knowledge and human health can be morally justified by a spectrum of existing theories.

The public must know that all those participating in animal research recognize our moral obligations to the welfare of the animals, to reduce the number used and the amount of suffering involved, and the need to develop alternative methods. Such recognition is embedded in our regulations (the Animal Welfare Act and NIH guidelines) and in specific federal programs that are designed to fund the search for alternatives to animal research. No doubt regulations and compliance systems can continuously be improved. Our society could also benefit by holding regular discussions about the science of animal cognition, and how such data could be used to promote animal welfare and provide guidelines as to the type of experimentation we deem permissible in different species.

Scientists have regularly spoken up in defense of animal research.[2,10,53,54] I now add my voice and encourage other scientists to share their opinions on this important topic. I trust that funding agencies and our public health officials will also find their participation in public dialog pertinent. The same applies to the many private medical foundations and patient groups that support the responsible use of animals in biomedical research. At stake is nothing short of the future health of the nation and our children.

References

1 Dean C. Am I making myself clear? A scientist's guide to talking to the public. Cambridge (MA): Harvard University Press; 2009.

2 Conn P.M. and Parker J.V. The animal research war. New York (NY): Palgrave Macmillan; 2008.

3 Smith W.J. A rat is a pig is a dog is a boy: the human cost of the animal rights movement. New York (NY): Encounter Books; 2009.

4 Greek C.R. The fruits of human-based research. Available at http://www.opposingviews.com/i/the-fruits-of-human-based-research. Accessed January 10, 2011.

5 Shanks N. and Greek C.R. Animal models in light of evolution. Boca Raton (FL): BrownWalker Press; 2009.

6 Frank R.G. Harvey and the Oxford physiologists: a study of scientific ideas. Berkeley & Los Angeles (CA): The University of California Press; 1980.

7 Greek R. and Greek J. Is the use of sentient animals in basic research justifiable? *Philos Ethics Humanit Med* 2010; 5:14.

8 Cohen M.R. and Nagel E. An introduction to logic and scientific method. New York (NY): Harcourt, Brace & Company; 1934.

9 Greek C.R. Strip mining for oil. Available at http://www.opposingviews.com/i/strip-mining-for-oil. Accessed January 10, 2011.

10 Comroe J.H. and Dripps R.D. Scientific basis for the support of biomedical science. *Science* 1976; 192:105–11.

11 Shepard H.M., Jin P., Slamon D.J., et al. Herceptin. *Handb Exp Pharmacol* 2008: 183–219.

12 Finn R.S. and Slamon D.J. Monoclonal antibody therapy for breast cancer: herceptin. *Cancer Chemother Biol Response Modif* 2003; 21:223–33.

13 Vogel C.L., Cobleigh M.A., Tripathy D., et al. First-line Herceptin monotherapy in metastatic breast cancer. *Oncology* 2001; 2:37–42.

14 van der Meel R., Symons M.H., Kudernatsch R., et al. The VEGF/Rho GTPase signalling pathway: a promising target for anti-angiogenic/anti-invasion therapy. *Drug Discov Today* 2011; 16:219–28.

15 Campa C. and Harding S.P. Anti-VEGF compounds in the treatment of neovascular age-related macular degeneration. *Curr Drug Targets* 2011; 12:173–81.

16 Waisbourd M., Goldstein M., and Loewenstein A. Treatment of diabetic retinopathy with anti-VEGF drugs. *Acta Ophthalmol* 2010; 89:203–7.

17 Gunther M., Lipka J., Malek A., et al. Polyethylenimines for RNAi-mediated gene targeting in vivo and siRNA delivery to the lung. *Eur J Pharm Biopharm* 2011; 77:438–49.

18 Mowa M.B., Crowther C., and Arbuthnot P. Therapeutic potential of adenoviral vectors for delivery of expressed RNAi activators. *Expert Opin Drug Deliv* 2010; 7:1373–85.

19 Dykxhoorn D.M. Advances in cell-type specific delivery of RNAi-based therapeutics. *IDrugs* 2010; 13:325–31.

20 Baigude H. and Rana T.M. Delivery of therapeutic RNAi by nanovehicles. *Chembiochem* 2009; 10: 2449–54.

21 Nguyen T., Menocal E.M., Harborth J., et al. RNAi therapeutics: an update on delivery. *Curr Opin Mol Ther* 2008; 10:158–67.

22 Greek C.R. Claims versus proof. Available at http://www.opposingviews.com/i/claims-versus-proof. Accessed January 10, 2011.

23 Greaves P., Williams A., and Eve M. First dose of potential new medicines to humans: how animals help. *Nat Rev Drug Discov* 2004; 3:226–36.

24 Wakeling P.R. A look behind research grant titles. *Appl Opt* 1976; 15: 576–91.

25 Kone E.H. and Jordan H.J. The greatest adventure: basic research that shapes our lives. New York (NY): Rockefeller University Press; 1974.

26 HSUS. Biomedical research; 2010.

27 Greek C.R. Rules of engagement. Available at http://www.opposingviews.com/i/rules-of-engagement. Accessed January 10, 2011.

28 Rollin B.E. Animal rights & human morality. Amherst (NY): Prometheus Books; 2006.

29 Taylor A. and Burbidge J.W. Animals & ethics: an overview of the philosophical debate. Peterborough (Ontario): Broadview Press; 2009.

30 Regan T. The case for animal rights. Berkeley (NY): University of California Press; 1983.

31 Regan T. Empty cages: facing the challenge of animal rights. Lanham (MD): Rowman & Littlefield; 2004.

32 DeGrazia D., Cohen C., and Regan T. The animal rights debate. *Ethics* 2003; 113:692–4.

33 Francione G.L. Introduction to animal rights: your child or the dog? Philadelphia (PA): Temple University Press; 2000.

34 Singer P. In defence of animals. New York (NY): Blackwell; 1985.

35 Singer P. Animal liberation. New York (NY): New York Review of Books; 1990.

36 DeGrazia, D. Moral status as a matter of degree? *Southern J Philos* 2008; 46:181–98.

37 Cohen C. The case for the use of animals in biomedical research. *New Engl J Med* 1986; 315:865–70.

38 Warren M.A. Moral status: obligations to persons and other living things (issues in biomedical ethics). New York (NY): Oxford University Press; 2000.

39 Harman E. The potentiality problem. *Philos Stud* 2003; 114:173–98.

40 McMahan J. The ethics of killing: problems at the margins of life. New York (NY): Oxford University Press; 2003.

41 Degrazia D. Equal consideration and unequal moral status. *South J Philos* 1993; 31:17–31.

42 Harris L.T. and Fiske S.T. The brooms in fantasia: neural correlates of anthropomorphizing objects. *Soc Cogn* 2008; 26:210–23.

43 Ortega y Gasset J. Man the technician. In: History as a system and other essays toward a philosophy of history. New York (NY): Norton & Company; 1962.

44 Frey R.G. Animal parts, human wholes: on the use of animals as a source of organs for human transplant. In: Humber J.M. and Almeder R.F., editors. Biomedical ethical reviews. Clifton (NJ): Humana; 1988. p. 89–101.

45 Wrobel S. and Clements J.A. Bubbles, babies and biology: the story of surfactant – second breath: a medical mystery solved. *FASEB J* 2004: 18.

46 Engle W.A. and Stark A.R. Surfactant replacement therapy for respiratory distress syndrome in the preterm and term neonate: congratulations and corrections. Reply. *Pediatrics* 2008; 121:1291–2.

47 Darwin C.R. Mr. Darwin on vivisection. *The Times of London* 1881; 10.

48 Walsh G. Father of animal activism backs monkey testing. Available at http://www.timesonline.co.uk/tol/news/uk/article650168.ece. Accessed January 10, 2011.

49 Nobis N. Interests and harms in primate research. *Am J Bioethics* 2009; 9:27–9.

50 Rachels J. Created from animals: the moral implications of Darwinism. Oxford: Oxford University Press; 1990.

51 Anderson E. Animal rights and the value of nonhuman live. In: Nussbaum M. and Sunstein C., editors. Rights for animals? Law and policy. Oxford: Oxford University Press; 2002.

52 Kittay E. At the margins of moral personhood. *Ethics* 2005;1 16: 100–31.

53 Gallistel C.R. Bell, Magendie, and the proposal to restrict the use of animals in neurobehavioral research. *Am Psychol* 1998; 36:357–60.

54 Morrison A.R. An odyssey with animals: a veterinarian's reflection on the animal rights & welfare debate. New York (NY): Oxford University Press; 2009.

64

Ethical Issues When Modelling Brain Disorders in Non-Human Primates

Carolyn P. Neuhaus

Introduction

Model organisms are created to study human diseases in non-human organisms. For example, mouse models of cancer allow researchers to describe biochemical mechanisms underlying tumour development and develop targeted therapies. The discovery of recombinant DNA in the 1970s made it possible to study genetic contributions to disease progression, too. Scientists since have improved methods for creating genetically modified model organisms.

The mouse is the most widely used model organism for various reasons. Humans and mice share about 90% of their DNA. Mice have short gestational periods, large litters and are inexpensive to house. Yet mouse models of disease are limited in scope. Knowledge gleaned from mouse models often does not translate into humans, especially for brain disorders.[1,2]

Known limitations of mouse models of disease prompted researchers to look to other non-human animals,[i] including non-human primates (NHPs), to generate disease models. Until recently, creating

large animal disease models was nearly impossible, but genome editors like CRISPR (Clustered Randomised Interspersed Palindromic Repeat) present a technological advance that brings genome engineering of larger animals within reach.[3] Some scientists have proposed creating models of brain disorders in NHPs.[5,6] Yet it is arguably the most ethically fraught use of genome editing in laboratory animals.

This paper starts with the assumption that creating model organisms is sometimes morally justified. Yet even granting that assumption, experiments involving NHPs ought to be held to a higher standard of justification than experiments involving other animals owing to differences in moral status between NHPs and other non-human animals. This paper is novel in asking: Insofar as NHPs are being considered for use as model organisms for brain disorders, can this be done ethically? The paper concludes that it cannot. Notwithstanding ongoing debate about NHPs' moral status, (1) animal welfare concerns, (2) the availability of alternative methods of studying brain disorders and (3) unmet expectations of benefit justify a stop on the creation of NHP model organisms to study

Original publication details: Carolyn P. Neuhaus, "Ethical Issues When Modelling Brain Disorders in Non-Human Primates," pp. 323–327 from *Journal of Medical Ethics* 44. Reproduced with permission of BMJ Publishing Group Ltd.

brain disorders. After clarifying some scientific and methodological starting points, these three areas are reviewed.

Trends in Disease Modelling Post-CRISPR

Genome editing works by inserting molecules into a cell that target and 'edit' a specified genomic sequence. CRISPR is not a breakthrough technology in the sense that it enables genome editing: Biologists have been using other methods to engineer genomes for decades. But CRISPR is more efficient, more precise and cheaper. Think of CRISPR as a much-improved 'find and replace' function in your word processor. CRISPR makes it possible for a standard molecular biology laboratory to edit almost any organism's genome.

Upon CRISPR's discovery in 2012, researchers quickly adopted the method to improve the process of creating rodent model organisms. Moving beyond rodents, researchers successfully edited an NHP embryo using CRISPR in 2014, providing proof of concept that CRISPR works in NHPs. A 2015 paper laid out an approach to generating NHP model organisms.[7] And in early 2016, a group of Chinese scientists reported creating macaques with a mutation in the MeCP2 gene, a mutation found in 90% of people with an autism-like disorder called Rett's syndrome. Macaques with the MeCP2 mutation exhibited self-mutilating and other 'autism-like' behaviours. Although the authors had not used CRISPR to achieve the desired genotype, they conclude: 'our findings pave the way for the efficient use of genetically engineered macaque monkeys for studying brain disorders'[8] (p101).

CRISPR, it is hoped, will allow researchers to study the significance of a gene or set of genes to the development of brain disorders such as autism, depression or Alzheimer's, and develop new therapeutics so desperately needed by humans with brain disorders. Researchers start with the hypothesis that particular genes or sets of genes *might* explain *part*

of the pathological processes underlying brain disorders. CRISPR could be used in NHP embryos to introduce point-specific edits thought to contribute to the development of brain disorders, and to introduce mutations at multiple points at the same time to observe in vivo; interactions among multiple genetic variants. Creating model organisms to study and compare results of different mutations – much less reproduce results – would require many animals. A potential moral advantage of new genome editors, from a utilitarian perspective, is that researchers might sacrifice fewer animals in the process of creating 'designed' model organisms.[7] Traditional approaches to breeding model organisms typically sacrifice many animals before achieving the desired genotype and phenotype.

Methodological Starting Point

Creation of NHP models of brain disorders is justified in part by the idea that NHPs are the *only* non-human animal that will yield knowledge about brain disorders. Other animals simply do not have enough in common with humans genetically, cognitively or emotionally to yield knowledge about human brains.

There is a moral problem with this justification, however. If NHPs have enough in common with humans to be useful model organisms, they likely occupy a level of moral status that would obligate us to protect them from being used in certain ways.[ii, 9–11] According to what's been called the 'commonsense' view of animals' moral status articulated best by DeGrazia, moral status varies with organisms' capacities, for example, sentience, consciousness, self-awareness, moral agency, participation in meaningful relationships, language and so on.[12] Different capacities generate morally weightier interests. Mice, by virtue of having the capacity to feel pain, have an interest in not being subjected to pain, but humans, by virtue of having the capacity for moral agency, also have an interest in preserving their agency. DeGrazia argues that human interests matter more, morally, than mouse interests; there is more at stake for humans. This view permits degrees of moral status ordered by the weightiness of interests. It is consistent with this view that we have some obligations to mice, for example, to avoid or at least reduce pain and suffering, but since human interests matter more, we are also justified in using mice, thereby thwarting their interests, to advance human interests.

Where do NHPs fall? Because of our inability to empirically verify whether NHPs have certain capacities, such as self-awareness or moral agency, where NHPs fall on the moral status hierarchy, and what we owe to them, remain contested.[iii] But to rearticulate a central problem in NHP use in research, if NHPs are enough like humans to yield knowledge about brain disorders, they likely also have a similar degree of moral status to humans, insofar as they likely have some common morally relevant capacities. Both the fact that NHPs are different from humans and the fact that NHPs are similar to humans are used to justify the conclusion that it is morally permissible to use NHPs to model human brain disorders.[13]

This unresolved question about NHPs' moral status has led many to stake the justification of NHP use on other facts about the research.[5,6,12,14] This paper adopts DeGrazia's 'commonsense' view of moral status and methodological approach to justifying animal use.[14] NHPs, insofar as they exhibit more capacities and have weightier interests than mice, have interests that merit serious moral consideration and require a strong justification for over-riding. Whether scientists are justified in using them in ways that thwart their interests depends on other aspects of the research. Three are considered: (1) to what extent NHPs' interests are thwarted when they are genetically modified to model brain disorders; (2) alternative ways to answer the scientific question at hand; and (3) the expectation of benefit from the research. Each of these issues, it will be argued, provides a reason to refrain from creating NHP model organisms.

Animal welfare

Animals used in research are likely to be used in ways that thwart their interests and diminish their quality of life. They will be subjected to pain as part of experiments. Additionally, captivity, restriction of movement and activity, and limited food choice all impact well-being. This section focuses on aspects of creating NHP model organisms that affect the organism's interests and quality of life – very generally, concerns related to animal welfare.

One concern is that the creation of model organisms may *introduce* capacities that render them of a higher moral status than their non-genetically edited peers. Some model organisms are created by introducing human stem cells into the animal embryo, creating a non-human/human chimaera. Chimaeras are non-human animals with human components, such as tissues, organs, genes or stem cells. Although not all model organisms are chimaeras, some are. One ethical concern asks whether mixing human and non-human species is morally permissible. A second concern is that the introduction of genetically human tissues, neurons or stem cells might enhance the moral status of chimaeric animals, for example, heightening self-awareness, but they will lack concomitant moral protections.[15]

This objection to the creation of chimaeric model organisms, however, exaggerates the extent to which most chimaeric model organisms are 'humanized'. Human neurons will function, at a very basic level, in mouse brains, but the structural and physical differences between mouse and human brains make it extremely unlikely that the chimaeric mouse has human-like cognitive or emotional capacities.[15] That being said, the risk of introducing morally relevant capacities into chimaeric model organisms may increase in NHPs owing to greater structural similarity between the NHP and human brain. This worry led Greely to recommend using genome editing rather than chimaeras to create model organisms to guard against introducing morally relevant capacities.[15]

Still, even if genome editing does not introduce morally relevant capacities, serious welfare concerns remain. Modelling human brain disorders in primates may substantially diminish organisms' welfare and quality of life. No matter what kinds of perceptual, cognitive or emotional capacities an organism possesses, it is uncontroversial to endorse RG Frey's assertion that every animal's life is:

> An unfolding series of experiences, that, depending on their quality, can make that creature's life go well or badly. Such a creature has a welfare that can be positively and negatively affected, depending on what we do to it, and with a welfare that can be enhanced and diminished.[16] (p184)

This characterisation of animals' lives does not assert that animals are aware of their experiences in some higher order or self-reflexive sense. It posits only that experiences can be made better or worse. It requires no argument or weighty claims about animals' mentation to say that a starved mouse has a worse quality of life than a sated mouse, or a monkey raised in isolation has a worse quality of life than a monkey in ethologically appropriate, social housing.

Introducing genetic variants that impede sociality, mobility or participation in relationships, or increase self-harm or mutilating behaviours, may be unethical because it substantially diminishes quality of life. Many objected on these grounds to Harlow's infamous social isolation experiments involving monkeys in the 1960s and 1970s.[17] Monkeys raised in isolation were reared to purposely cause psychological damage. As described by John Gluck, they had a seriously diminished quality of life compared with peers raised in social housing, evidenced by their self-mutilating behaviour, fear of other monkeys and difficulty adjusting to surroundings.[18] Genetically modified macaques in the aforementioned study of Rett's syndrome exhibited some of the same behaviours: increased stress response, repetitive behaviour and less social interaction.

Contrast social isolation with the temporary induction of cognitive, emotional or memory deficits. Deep brain stimulation (DBS), for example, allows researchers to temporarily 'turn on' or 'turn off' groups of neurons, and makes it possible to tease apart which parts of the brain are responsible for which functions and assess the extent of cognitive, emotional or memory function controlled by those areas. It is meant to induce *reversible* functional changes only for the duration of the experiment.

Mentioning DBS does not imply that its use always, or even ever, justified. Rather, its comparison to the creation of model organisms with social and cognitive deficits underscores methodological and moral differences between them. While DBS introduces temporary deficits, CRISPR-induced mutations would introduce permanent, *irreversible* changes to brain functioning, just as social isolation introduced irremediable social deficits and psychological sequelae.[18] By argument from analogy, researchers ought to refrain from introducing genetic variants that substantially, and permanently, diminish quality of life just as they ought to refrain from housing a monkey in ways that substantially, and permanently, diminish its quality of life.

Available alternatives

Notwithstanding animal welfare concerns, it may still be the case that only NHP models of brain disorders can provide knowledge about the genetic underpinnings of disease, owing to ethical challenges to engaging humans in research on brain disorders. This would seem to satisfy the moral condition that there are no alternative ways of identifying genetic underpinning of brain disorders or testing targeted gene therapies.[5,14] But is that criterion met? Rather than shift to NHP models of brain disorders to advance research on brain disorders, those who study brain disorders, and fund research on brain disorders, should consider first expanding research involving human subjects, as well as human biospecimens and organoids. Doing so may obviate the need – and so the moral justification – for creating NHP model organisms to study brain disorders. Expanding studies involving humans and human tissues also has epistemological advantages.

Research on certain brain disorders is tricky because people with brain disorders sometimes experience impairments to decision-making capacity (DMC) as a component or symptom of disease, as evidenced in some people with Alzheimer's disease, schizophrenia, autism and chronic depression.[19-23] Although there is wide variation in DMC among people diagnosed with brain disorders, this heightens concerns about ability to consent and properly weigh risks and benefits encountered in research. Well-intentioned protections of human research subjects with impaired DMC, however, serve to limit their participation in research, and, arguably, harm people more than help them.[24] Failing to do research on a disease category or population perpetuates disparities in health outcomes. Considered through the lens of justice, 'access to research, not just protection from its risks, is a constitutive part of the ethical mandates governing clinical research'[25] (p15).

One way to advance research on the genetic underpinnings of brain disorders would be to expand 'big data' projects that focus specifically on brain disorders to identify correlations between genetic variants and diagnoses. To this end, several projects are underway amassing biospecimens from people afflicted with brain disorders, including postmortem brain tissue. Contributing biospecimens to a biobank project poses less risk to participants than participation in a typical clinical trial, and ethical requirements for consent and oversight ought to reflect this.[26] Impairments to DMC associated with brain disorders, if they co-occur, do not necessarily pose a barrier to participation in genetic research that leverages big data. For studies where informed consent is required, several papers have proposed protections for people with impaired DMC: mandated use of a validated DMC assessment, relying on an 'auxiliary consenter', someone not affiliated with the study, to determine the patient's knowledge about the procedures, risks and the device, and seeking assent from research subjects on obtaining a proxy's consent.[27]

One problem with doing away with NHP modelling for brain disorders is that drug approval regulations typically require toxicology and pharmacokinetic testing of new drugs in animals prior to starting trials in humans, so expanding human persons' participation in research may not eliminate the use of animals in drug development. Still, animal models of the disease in question are not required; drugs need not be tested in a *specific* animal. Current US National Institutes of Health Director, Francis Collins, went as far to say, "the use of small and large animals to predict safety in humans is a long-standing but not always reliable practice in translational science" and "the use of animal models for therapeutic development and target validation is time consuming, costly, and may not accurately predict efficacy in humans".[28] Instead, he called for "more reliable efficacy models that are based on access to biobanks of human tissues, use of human embryonic stem cell and induced pluripotent stem cell models of disease, and improved validation of assays"[28] (at 3). The use of 'brains on a chip' derived from induced pluripotent stem cells is already underway in research on schizophrenia and autism. Expanding the toolbox to look at the genetic, enzymatic and biochemical processes underlying pathologies, as well as to assess toxicity and pharmacokinetics of new drugs, will impact the need – and so the moral justification – for model organisms of brain disorders. The assertion that NHP model organisms for brain disorders are the *only* way to access knowledge about the genetic underpinnings of disease or develop targeted therapies is, at the very least, questionable, given available alternatives.

It is worth noting that reducing reliance on animal models skirts epistemic problems associated with NHP models of brain disorders, too. The best model organism for a human disease is a human. Translational research requires a leap from model organisms to humans, which calls into question the model's relevance to understanding human brain disorders that involve cognitive, behavioural *and* psychological dysfunction. Benefits to humans are likely to be more substantial if human subjects with autism rather than autism-like macaques are used.[iv]

Expectation of benefit

It is commonly held that the use of animals in research is justified when experiments are expected to produce benefits to humanity.[5,6,14] Fully unpacking this moral requirement will have to wait, but one problem is that one cannot guarantee ahead of time that an experiment will produce the promised benefits. If anything, systematic reviews of the translational benefits of research involving animals suggest that research involving animals fails to directly benefit humans most of the time. More than 80% of potential therapeutics fail when tested in people.[1] Numbers within the field of behavioural neuroscience are even worse: 90% of compounds that enter human trials will fail.[2] A large contributing factor is that experiments are not performed at a level where conclusions drawn from studies involving animals can be validated or reproduced.[1] Additionally, experiments involving model organisms sometimes are not designed to produce generalisable knowledge.[2] Emphasising indeterminate benefits to humans in the justification of research involving animals may distract from determinate steps that ought to be taken to improve the quality and integrity of research, whether benefits to humans accrue.

Rather than focus on promised benefits, those reviewing proposed uses of animals should instead look for evidence that the experiment will produce generalisable knowledge that advances important human interests. Meeting this requirement does not require evidence that an experiment will produce direct, translational benefits to humans. Rather, it requires that experiments involving animals test a hypothesis that, whether proved or disproved, would advance important human interests. This means establishing (1) that the hypothesis is connected to advancing human interests, and (2) that the experiment is designed and will be performed in such a way as to prove one's hypothesis. When it comes to creating NHP model organisms of brain disorders, the first is established. Identifying genetic underpinnings of brain disorders and testing gene therapies undoubtedly advance human interests. The second needs further justification.

It is well beyond the scope of this paper to adjudicate among experimental designs. The point of raising this concern is to emphasise that, at a minimum, scientists should justify experimental design (beyond 'this is the way it's always been done') and show that their experiment is designed to prove or disprove a testable hypothesis. Although Jennings et al.[3] lay out plans for an ambitious international collaboration for creating and studying NHP model organisms in a systematic way, their paper does not cite Garner,[2] who is extremely critical of their experimental approach, attributing the failure to achieve translational benefits in the field of behavioural neuroscience to widely used methods of developing and validating model organisms.[2]

Ethicists must recognise that the quality of preclinical research is a scientific problem and a moral one. Poor quality undermines the basis for the entire research enterprise and puts human research subjects at great risk.[29] It is not yet established that creating NHP model organisms of brain disorders can be done in a way that can be validated, reproduced, blinded or otherwise meet the highest standards of research integrity at the preclinical stage. Until that is established, this means it should not be done at all.

Conclusion

The areas of concern reviewed in this paper support the conclusion that creating NHP models of brain disorders is not justified at this point, and may never be justified. Researchers must establish that there is something unique to learn from modelling brain disorders in NHPs that could not be learnt through expanding research involving humans with brain disorders. They should be expected to defend their experimental approach, and further they must show that introducing genetic variants associated with brain disorders does not substantially diminish NHP model organisms' quality of life. The lure of using new genetic technologies combined with the promise of novel therapeutics presents a formidable challenge to those who call for slow, careful and only necessary research involving NHPs. But researchers should not create macaques with social deficits or capuchin monkeys with memory deficits just because they can.

Notes

i Hereafter 'animals'.

ii Some theorists deny altogether that a possession of capacities is relevant to determining how we ought to treat organisms, in research or otherwise, and will disagree with this analysis of moral status.[9–11]

iii The same may be true of some humans who cannot self-report self-awareness or moral agency, which may seem to put NHPs and some humans in the same epistemic category with respect to moral status. It is precisely this issue that has led some to reject capacities-relative views of moral status.[10] Many thanks to an anonymous reviewer for pointing this out.

iv Many thanks to an anonymous reviewer for this point.

References

1 Perrin S. Preclinical research: make mouse studies work. *Nature* 2014; 507:423–5.

2 Garner J.P. The significance of meaning: why do over 90% of behavioral neuroscience results fail to translate to humans, and what can we do to fix it? *Ilar J* 2014; 55:438–56.

3 Jennings C.G., Landman R., Zhou Y., et al. Opportunities and challenges in modeling human brain disorders in transgenic primates. *Nat Neurosci* 2016; 19:1123–30.

4 Van Dam D. and De Deyn P.P. Non human primate models for Alzheimer's disease-related research and drug discovery. *Expert Opin Drug Discov* 2017; 12:187–200.

5 Weatherall D. The use of non-human primates in research: a working group report chaired by Sir David Weatherall FRS Fmedsci. 2006 https://mrc.ukri.org/documents/pdf/the-use-of-non-human-primates-in-research/ (accessed Feb 2017).

6 Barnhill A., Joffe S., and Miller F.G. The ethics of infection challenges in primates. *Hastings Cent Rep* 2016; 46:20–6.

7 Chen Y., Niu Y., and Ji W. Genome editing in non-human primates: approach to generating human disease models. *J Intern Med* 2016; 280:246–51.

8 Liu Z., Li X., Zhang J.T., et al. Autism-like behaviours and germline transmission in transgenic monkeys over-expressing MeCP2. *Nature* 2016;530: 98–102.

9 Liao S.M. The basis of human moral status. *J Moral Philos* 2010; 7:159–79.

10 Kittay E.F. At the margins of moral personhood. *Ethics* 2005; 116:100–31.

11 Rollins R. *A New Basis for Animal Ethics: telos and common sense*. Columbia, MO: University of Missouri Press, 2016.

12 DeGrazia D. Moral status as a matter of degree? *South J Philos* 2008;46:181–98.

13 This point is made often in animal ethics literature. For a recent and related discussion, see: Bovenkerk B. and Kaldewaij F. The use of animal models in behavioural neuroscience research. In: Lee G., Illes H., and Ohl F., eds. *Ethical issues in Behavioral Neuroscience*. Berlin, Germany: Springer-Verlag, 2015: 17–46.

14 DeGrazia D. and Sebo J. Necessary conditions for morally responsible animal research. *Camb Q Healthc Ethics* 2015; 24:420–30.

15 Greely H. Human/Nonhuman chimeras: Assessing the issues. In: Beauchamp T.L. and Frey R.G., eds. *The Oxford Handbook of Animal Ethics*. New York: Oxford University Press, 2011: 671–99.

16 Frey R.G. Utilitarianism and animals. In: Beauchamp T.L. and Frey R.G., eds. *The Oxford Handbook of Animal Ethics*. New York, NY: Oxford University Press, 2011: 172–97.

17 Singer P. *Animal Liberation*. New York: New York Review, 1975.

18 Gluck J. *Voracious Science, Vulnerable Animals*. Chicago: University of Chicago Press, 2016.

19 Kim S.Y., Caine E.D., Currier G.W., et al. Assessing the competence of persons with Alzheimer's disease in providing informed consent for participation in research. *Am J Psychiatry* 2001;158:712–7.

20 Carpenter W.T., Gold J.M., Lahti A.C., et al. Decisional capacity for informed consent in schizophrenia research. *Arch Gen Psychiatry* 2000; 57:533–8.

21 Luke L., Clare I.C., Ring H., et al. Decision-making difficulties experienced by adults with autism spectrum conditions. *Autism* 2012; 16:612–21.

22 Elliott C. Caring about risks. Are severely depressed patients competent to consent to research? *Arch Gen Psychiatry* 1997; 54:113–6.

23 Fisher C.E., Dunn L.B., Christopher P.P., et al. The ethics of research on deep brain stimulation for depression: decisional capacity and therapeutic misconception. *Ann N Y Acad Sci* 2012; 1265: 69–79.

24 Humphreys K., Blodgett J.C., and Roberts L.W. The exclusion of people with psychiatric disorders from medical research. *J Psychiatr Res* 2015; 70: 28–32.

25 Lyerly A.D., Little M.O., and Faden R. The second wave: toward responsible inclusion of pregnant women in research. *Int J Fem Approaches Bioeth* 2008; 1:5–22.

26 Rhodes R., Azzouni J., and Baumrin S.B., et al. *De Minimis* risk: a proposal for a new category of research risk. *Am J Bioeth* 2011; 11:1–7.

27 Alzheimer's Association. Research consent for cognitively impaired adults: recommendations for institutional review boards and investigators. *Alzheimer Dis Assoc Disord* 2004; 18:171–5.

28 Collins F.S. Reengineering translational science: the time is right. *Sci Transl Med* 2011; 3:90cm17.

29 Redman B.K. and Caplan A.L. Limited reproducibility of research findings: implications for the welfare of research participants and considerations for institutional review boards. *IRB: Ethics & Human Research* 2016; 38:8–10.

Academic Freedom and Research

65

On Liberty

John Stuart Mill

Chapter II: Of The Liberty of Thought and Discussion

[. . .] the peculiar evil of silencing the expression of an opinion is, that it is robbing the human race; posterity as well as the existing generation; those who dissent from the opinion, still more than those who hold it. If the opinion is right, they are deprived of the opportunity of exchanging error for truth: if wrong, they lose, what is almost as great a benefit, the clearer perception and livelier impression of truth, produced by its collision with error.

It is necessary to consider separately these two hypotheses, each of which has a distinct branch of the argument corresponding to it. We can never be sure that the opinion we are endeavouring to stifle is a false opinion; and if we were sure, stifling it would be an evil still.

First: the opinion which it is attempted to suppress by authority may possibly be true. Those who desire to suppress it, of course deny its truth; but they are not infallible. They have no authority to decide the question for all mankind, and exclude every other person from the means of judging. To refuse a hearing to an opinion, because they are sure that it is false, is to assume that their certainty is the same thing as absolute certainty. All silencing of discussion is an assumption of infallibility. Its condemnation may be allowed to rest on this common argument, not the worse for being common.

Unfortunately for the good sense of mankind, the fact of their fallibility is far from carrying the weight in their practical judgment, which is always allowed to it in theory; for while everyone well knows himself to be fallible, few think it necessary to take any precautions against their own fallibility, or admit the supposition that any opinion of which they feel very certain, may be one of the examples of the error to which they acknowledge themselves to be liable. Absolute princes, or others who are accustomed to unlimited deference, usually feel this complete confidence in their own opinions on nearly all subjects. People more happily situated, who sometimes hear their opinions disputed, and are not wholly unused to be set right when they are wrong, place the same unbounded reliance only on such of their opinions as are shared by

Original publication details: John Stuart Mill, "Of the Liberty of Thought and Discussion" (extract) from *On Liberty*, chapter II. First published 1859. Public domain.

Bioethics: An Anthology, Fourth Edition. Edited by Udo Schüklenk and Peter Singer.
Editorial material and organization © 2022 John Wiley & Sons, Inc. Published 2022 by John Wiley & Sons, Inc.

all who surround them, or to whom they habitually defer: for in proportion to a man's want of confidence in his own solitary judgment, does he usually repose, with implicit trust, on the infallibility of "the world" in general. And the world, to each individual, means the part of it with which he comes in contact; his party, his sect, his church, his class of society: the man may be called, by comparison, almost liberal and large-minded to whom it means anything so comprehensive as his own country or his own age. Nor is his faith in this collective authority at all shaken by his being aware that other ages, countries, sects, churches, classes, and parties have thought, and even now think, the exact reverse. He devolves upon his own world the responsibility of being in the right against the dissentient worlds of other people; and it never troubles him that mere accident has decided which of these numerous worlds is the object of his reliance, and that the same causes which make him a Churchman in London, would have made him a Buddhist or a Confucian in Peking. Yet it is as evident in itself as any amount of argument can make it, that ages are no more infallible than individuals; every age having held many opinions which subsequent ages have deemed not only false but absurd; and it is as certain that many opinions, now general, will be rejected by future ages, as it is that many, once general, are rejected by the present.

The objection likely to be made to this argument, would probably take some such form as the following. There is no greater assumption of infallibility in forbidding the propagation of error, than in any other thing which is done by public authority on its own judgment and responsibility. Judgment is given to men that they may use it. Because it may be used erroneously, are men to be told that they ought not to use it at all? To prohibit what they think pernicious, is not claiming exemption from error, but fulfilling the duty incumbent on them, although fallible, of acting on their conscientious conviction. If we were never to act on our opinions, because those opinions may be wrong, we should leave all our interests uncared for, and all our duties unperformed. An objection which applies to all conduct can be no valid objection to any conduct in particular.

It is the duty of governments, and of individuals, to form the truest opinions they can; to form them carefully, and never impose them upon others unless they are quite sure of being right. But when they are sure (such reasoners may say), it is not conscientiousness but cowardice to shrink from acting on their opinions, and allow doctrines which they honestly think dangerous to the welfare of mankind, either in this life or in another, to be scattered abroad without restraint, because other people, in less enlightened times, have persecuted opinions now believed to be true. Let us take care, it may be said, not to make the same mistake: but governments and nations have made mistakes in other things, which are not denied to be fit subjects for the exercise of authority: they have laid on bad taxes, made unjust wars. Ought we therefore to lay on no taxes, and, under whatever provocation, make no wars? Men, and governments, must act to the best of their ability. There is no such thing as absolute certainty, but there is assurance sufficient for the purposes of human life. We may, and must, assume our opinion to be true for the guidance of our own conduct: and it is assuming no more when we forbid bad men to pervert society by the propagation of opinions which we regard as false and pernicious.

I answer, that it is assuming very much more. There is the greatest difference between presuming an opinion to be true, because, with every opportunity for contesting it, it has not been refuted, and assuming its truth for the purpose of not permitting its refutation. Complete liberty of contradicting and disproving our opinion, is the very condition which justifies us in assuming its truth for purposes of action; and on no other terms can a being with human faculties have any rational assurance of being right.

When we consider either the history of opinion, or the ordinary conduct of human life, to what is it to be ascribed that the one and the other are no worse than they are? Not certainly to the inherent force of the human understanding; for, on any matter not self-evident, there are ninety-nine persons totally incapable of judging of it, for one who is capable; and the capacity of the hundredth person is only comparative; for the majority of the eminent men of every past generation held many opinions now known to be erroneous, and did or approved numerous things which no one will now justify. Why is it, then, that there is on the whole a preponderance among mankind of rational opinions and rational conduct? If there really is this preponderance – which there must be, unless human affairs are, and have always been, in an almost desperate state – it is owing to a quality of the human mind, the source of everything respectable in man, either as an intellectual or as a moral being, namely, that his errors are corrigible. He is capable of rectifying his mistakes by discussion and experience. Not by experience alone. There must be discussion, to show how experience is to be interpreted. Wrong opinions and practices gradually yield to fact and argument: but facts and arguments, to produce any effect on the mind, must be brought before it. Very few facts are able to tell their own story, without comments to bring out their meaning. The whole strength and value, then, of human judgment, depending on the one property, that it can be set right when it is wrong, reliance can be placed on it only when the means of setting it right are kept constantly at hand. In the case of any person whose judgment is really deserving of confidence, how has it become so? Because he has kept his mind open to criticism of his opinions and conduct. Because it has been his practice to listen to all that could be said against him; to profit by as much of it as was just, and expound to himself, and upon occasion to others, the fallacy of what was fallacious. Because he has felt, that the only way in which a human being can make some approach to the whole of a subject, is by hearing what can be said about it by persons of every variety of opinion, and studying all modes in which it can be looked at by every character of mind. No wise man ever acquired his wisdom in any mode but this; nor is it in the nature of human intellect to become wise in any other manner. The steady habit of correcting and completing his own opinion by collating it with those of others, so far from causing doubt and hesitation in carrying it into practice, is the only stable foundation for a just reliance on it: for, being cognizant of all that can, at least obviously, be said against him, and having taken up his position against all gainsayers knowing that he

has sought for objections and difficulties, instead of avoiding them, and has shut out no light which can be thrown upon the subject from any quarter – he has a right to think his judgment better than that of any person, or any multitude, who have not gone through a similar process.

It is not too much to require that what the wisest of mankind, those who are best entitled to trust their own judgment, find necessary to warrant their relying on it, should be submitted to by that miscellaneous collection of a few wise and many foolish individuals, called the public. The most intolerant of churches, the Roman Catholic Church, even at the canonization of a saint, admits, and listens patiently to, a "devil's advocate." The holiest of men, it appears, cannot be admitted to posthumous honors, until all that the devil could say against him is known and weighed. If even the Newtonian philosophy were not permitted to be questioned, mankind could not feel as complete assurance of its truth as they now do. The beliefs which we have most warrant for, have no safeguard to rest on, but a standing invitation to the whole world to prove them unfounded. If the challenge is not accepted, or is accepted and the attempt fails, we are far enough from certainty still; but we have done the best that the existing state of human reason admits of; we have neglected nothing that could give the truth a chance of reaching us: if the lists are kept open, we may hope that if there be a better truth, it will be found when the human mind is capable of receiving it; and in the meantime we may rely on having attained such approach to truth, as is possible in our own day. This is the amount of certainty attainable by a fallible being, and this the sole way of attaining it.

Strange it is, that men should admit the validity of the arguments for free discussion, but object to their being "pushed to an extreme;" not seeing that unless the reasons are good for an extreme case, they are not good for any case. Strange that they should imagine that they are not assuming infallibility when they acknowledge that there should be free discussion on all subjects which can possibly be doubtful, but think that some particular principle or doctrine should be forbidden to be questioned because it is so certain, that is, because they are certain that it is certain. To call any proposition certain, while there is anyone who would deny its certainty if permitted, but who is not permitted, is to assume that we ourselves, and those who agree with us, are the judges of certainty, and judges without hearing the other side.

[. . .]

Let us now pass to the second division of the argument, and dismissing the Supposition that any of the received opinions may be false, let us assume them to be true, and examine into the worth of the manner in which they are likely to be held, when their truth is not freely and openly canvassed. However unwillingly a person who has a strong opinion may admit the possibility that his opinion may be false, he ought to be moved by the consideration that however true it may be, if it is not fully, frequently, and fearlessly discussed, it will be held as a dead dogma, not a living truth.

[. . .]

If the cultivation of the understanding consists in one thing more than in another, it is surely in learning the grounds of one's own opinions. Whatever people believe, on subjects on which it is of the first importance to believe rightly, they ought to be able to defend against at least the common objections. But, someone may say, "Let them be taught the grounds of their opinions. It does not follow that opinions must be merely parroted because they are never heard controverted. Persons who learn geometry do not simply commit the theorems to memory, but understand and learn likewise the demonstrations; and it would be absurd to say that they remain ignorant of the grounds of geometrical truths, because they never hear any one deny, and attempt to disprove them." Undoubtedly: and such teaching suffices on a subject like mathematics, where there is nothing at all to be said on the wrong side of the question. The peculiarity of the evidence of mathematical truths is, that all the argument is on one side. There are no objections,

and no answers to objections. But on every subject on which difference of opinion is possible, the truth depends on a balance to be struck between two sets of conflicting reasons. Even in natural philosophy, there is always some other explanation possible of the same facts; some geocentric theory instead of heliocentric, some phlogiston instead of oxygen; and it has to be shown why that other theory cannot be the true one: and until this is shown and until we know how it is shown, we do not understand the grounds of our opinion. But when we turn to subjects infinitely more complicated, to morals, religion, politics, social relations, and the business of life, three-fourths of the arguments for every disputed opinion consist in dispelling the appearances which favor some opinion different from it. The greatest orator, save one, of antiquity, has left it on record that he always studied his adversary's case with as great, if not with still greater, intensity than even his own. What Cicero practised as the means of forensic success, requires to be imitated by all who study any subject in order to arrive at the truth. He who knows only his own side of the case, knows little of that. His reasons may be good, and no one may have been able to refute them. But if he is equally unable to refute the reasons on the opposite side; if he does not so much as know what they are, he has no ground for preferring either opinion. The rational position for him would be suspension of judgment, and unless he contents himself with that, he is either led by authority, or adopts, like the generality of the world, the side to which he feels most inclination. Nor is it enough that he should hear the arguments of adversaries from his own teachers, presented as they state them, and accompanied by what they offer as refutations. This is not the way to do justice to the arguments, or bring them into real contact with his own mind. He must be able to hear them from persons who actually believe them; who defend them in earnest, and do their very utmost for them. He must know them in their most plausible and persuasive form; he must feel the whole force of the difficulty which the true view of the subject has to encounter and dispose of, else he will never really possess himself of the portion of truth which meets and removes that difficulty. Ninety-nine in a hundred of what are called educated men are in this condition, even of those who can argue fluently for their opinions. Their conclusion may be true, but it might be false for anything they know: they have never thrown themselves into the mental position of those who think differently from them, and considered what such persons may have to say; and consequently they do not, in any proper sense of the word, know the doctrine which they themselves profess. They do not know those parts of it which explain and justify the remainder; the considerations which show that a fact which seemingly conflicts with another is reconcilable with it, or that, of two apparently strong reasons, one and not the other ought to be preferred. All that part of the truth which turns the scale, and decides the judgment of a completely informed mind, they are strangers to; nor is it ever really known, but to those who have attended equally and impartially to both sides, and endeavored to see the reasons of both in the strongest light. So essential is this discipline to a real understanding of moral and human subjects, that if opponents of all important truths do not exist, it is indispensable to imagine them and supply them with the strongest arguments which the most skillful devil's advocate can conjure up.

66

Should Some Knowledge Be Forbidden?
The Case of Cognitive Differences Research

Janet A. Kourany

For centuries scientists have claimed that women are intellectually inferior to men and blacks are inferior to whites. Although these claims have been contested and corrected for centuries, they still continue to be made. Meanwhile, scientists have documented the harm done to women and blacks by the publication of such claims. Can anything be done to improve this situation? Freedom of research is universally recognized to be of first-rate importance. Yet, constraints on that freedom are also universally recognized. I consider three of these constraints and argue for tighter restrictions on race- and gender-related cognitive differences research on their basis.

1 Introduction

Freedom of research is a fundamental right of scientists and an indispensable part of the scientific enterprise. This, at least, is what is said all over the world – in covenants of the United Nations, in charters and declarations of such bodies as the European Union and the World Congress for Freedom of Scientific Research, in the constitutions of nations, and in other places

as well. As a result, encroachments on scientific freedom are met with alarm: think not only of the recent heated debates concerning stem cell research but also of the widespread, sometimes passionate discussions surrounding the "politicization," "commercialization," and "militarization" of science. But how much freedom do scientists really need – or deserve?

The very question seems anathema. And yet, all the covenants and charters and declarations that recognize the right to freedom of research at the same time recognize, whether explicitly or implicitly, other important rights that can conflict with the right to freedom of research. Asking how much freedom scientists really need or deserve thus involves asking how the conflict between the right to freedom of research and these other rights is to be resolved. Only by resolving the conflict do we gain a clear understanding of the extent and depth of scientists' right to freedom of research. Of course, the answer in some areas is already largely settled. Take the right to human dignity and the integrity of the person and the right to environmental protection. These rights are already recognized to be constraints on scientists' right to freedom of research, constraints as politically

Original publication details: Janet A. Kourany, "Should Some Knowledge be Forbidden: The Case of Cognitive Differences Research," pp. 779–790 from *Philosophy of Science* 83 (December 2016). Reproduced with permission of University of Chicago Press.

legitimate as the national and international declarations that recognize the right to freedom of scientific research in the first place. Scientists are no more free in the way they conduct their research to compromise the safety or dignity of research participants than they are to endanger the environment. But what of other rights and their possible conflict with the right to freedom of research?

2 A Case Study: The Right to Equality versus the Right to Freedom of Research

Take the right to equality between men and women and between people of different racial and ethnic groups, a right as widely recognized as the right to freedom of research. Many have warned that the enforcement of this right to equality is threatened by certain kinds of scientific research – for example, by research investigating gender- and race-linked differences in cognitive abilities, particularly biologically based differences in cognitive abilities (see, e.g., Ceci and Williams 2009; Rose 2009). A glimpse at some of the claims emerging from this research helps us to understand what lies behind the warning.

Consider the research related to gender. For centuries scientists have claimed that women are intellectually inferior to men, and for centuries the basis for such inferiority has been located in biology. In the seventeenth century women's brains were claimed to be too "cold" and "soft" to sustain rigorous thought. In the late eighteenth century the female cranial cavity was claimed to be too small to hold a powerful brain. In the late nineteenth century the exercise of women's brains was claimed to be damaging to women's reproductive health – was claimed, in fact, to shrivel women's ovaries. In the twentieth century the lesser "lateralization" (hemispheric specialization) of women's brains compared to men's was claimed to make women inferior in visuospatial skills (including mathematical skills) (Schiebinger 1989; Fausto-Sterling 1992, 2000).

And now, in the beginning of the twenty-first century, the claims continue: that women's brains are smaller than men's brains, even correcting for differences of body mass; that women's brains have less white matter; that women's brains have less focused cortical activity (lower "neural efficiency"); that women's brains have lower cortical processing speed (lower conduction velocity in their white matter's axons); and so on. And once again these differences are being linked to differences in intellectual capacity: that people with smaller brains have lower IQ test scores; that less focused cortical activity is associated with lower intellectual performance; that lower cortical processing speed is associated with lower working memory performance, which is correlated with lower "fluid intelligence" scores; and so on (see Hamilton 2008 for more details). At the same time, much attention now focuses on the mappings of brain activity produced by brain imaging, particularly fMRIs (functional magnetic resonance imaging), and the differences in "emotional intelligence" these disclose. But once again the "male brain," the "systemizer" brain, comes out on top – is the more scientific brain, the more innovative brain, the more leadership-oriented brain, the more potentially "elite" brain, than the "female brain," the "empathizer" brain (Karafyllis and Ulshöfer 2008).

Of course, this is just a peek at the history of scientific claims regarding women's intellectual inferiority. The claims include not only these about the structure and functioning of women's brains but also ones about women's hormones, women's psychological propensities, women's genetic endowment, and women's evolutionary past – how all these are connected to intellectual inferiority; and the claims go back in history at least to Aristotle and his observation that women are literally misbegotten men, barely rational at all. And though these claims of intellectual inferiority continue to be contested and corrected, they also continue to be made, and the endless succession of claims and counterclaims both feeds on and helps to sustain the stereotype of intellectual inferiority associated with women.

Meanwhile, the effects are profound. For example, studies have documented the harm done to women and girls by the publication of scientific claims suggesting an innate female deficit in mathematics (see, e.g., Steele 1997; Spencer, Steele, and Quinn 1999; Dar-Nimrod and Heine 2006). Reports one of the researchers involved in these studies, social/personality psychologist Steven Heine of the University of British Columbia, "As our research demonstrates, just hearing about that sort of idea" – that female underachievement in mathematics is due to genetic factors rather than social factors – "is enough to negatively affect women's performance, and reproduce the stereotype that is out there" (quoted in Ceci and Williams 2010, 221). But that harm has been recognized for years. Virginia Woolf described it almost a century ago: "There was an enormous body of masculine opinion to the effect that nothing could be expected of women intellectually. Even if her father did not read out loud these opinions, any girl could read them for herself; and the reading, even in the nineteenth century, must have lowered her vitality, and told profoundly upon her work. There would always have been that assertion – you cannot do this, you are incapable of doing that – to protest against, to overcome" (Woolf 1929, quoted in Spencer et al. 1999, 5). Of course, much the same can be said of race-related cognitive differences research and the harm that it has caused.

Many have warned, then, that cognitive differences research threatens the enforcement of the right to equality and, hence, that scientists' freedom to pursue such research ought to be constrained by that right. But this response is far from universal (see, again, Ceci and Williams 2009; Rose 2009). Indeed, many others have warned that constraining scientists' freedom to pursue this research will cause us to lose valuable information, including all those discoveries that support rather than undermine the right to equality. And, in any case, they emphasize, constraining scientists' freedom to pursue this research is an unacceptable infringement of scientists' rights. The conflict between the right to equality and the right to freedom of research thus remains unresolved, and this despite years of debate on the subject. Under these conditions a plausible strategy might be to consider past precedents – cases in which the conflict between the right to freedom of research and other rights has been effectively resolved. Then we can try to model the resolution we seek on these other cases.

3   Past Precedents

Consider, then, three precedents that involved the right to freedom of research. The first two are relatively familiar, so discussion of them will be brief. Until the US National Institutes of Health Revitalization Act was passed in 1993, women and minority men tended to be neglected in US biomedical research – left out of clinical drug trials, left out of the definitions of diseases, left out of research agendas, their health needs largely ignored (see, e.g., Rosser 1994; Schiebinger 1999). What the Revitalization Act did was mandate the equal inclusion with white men of women and minority men in publicly funded US biomedical research and make funding contingent on that inclusion. This surely formed a constraint on scientists' freedom to design their own research programs, and it was justified by women's and minority men's right to equality – in this case their right to equality of access to health care.

Similarly, the earlier US National Research Act of 1974 mandated the formation of Institutional Review Boards to oversee all research that receives funding from what is now the Department of Health and Human Services. These review boards, themselves regulated by the Office for Human Research Protections of the Department of Health and Human Services, can reject, modify, or suspend any medical or behavioral research that fails to protect the rights and welfare (the right to life, the right to autonomy, the right to human dignity, etc.) of its human subjects (National Commission for the Protection of Human Subjects of Biomedical and Behavioral Research 1979). So here again, scientists' right to freedom of research has been constrained by other rights. Can a new constraint to protect human rights, this time in the area of cognitive differences research, be modeled on these two cases?

Certainly, there are important similarities among the cases. They all rule out as unacceptable harmful kinds of scientific enquiry, and thereby they all shape the kinds of knowledge scientific enquiry can deliver, but they do not shape that knowledge in any other way. So none can be said to censor particular kinds of knowledge. The National Research Act rules out as unacceptable harmful procedures for obtaining knowledge, not particular kinds of knowledge. If other ways are found to obtain the knowledge without harming research participants, that is perfectly acceptable, regardless of the content of the knowledge in question. The Revitalization Act rules out as unacceptable harmful − exclusionary and neglectful − kinds of research agendas, though it says nothing about the content of the knowledge that is gathered with those agendas. If it turns out that one or another group is, say, more prone to disease, that is also acceptable, though, of course, unfortunate. In a similar way, a constraint on cognitive differences research would rule out as unacceptable the kinds of harmful gender and racial group comparison questions that are included in that research and, thereby, the answers to those questions that continue to be circulated, though it would do this regardless of the content of the answers − that is, regardless of whether they bespeak equality or inequality of the groups in question.

Of course, ruling such questions out is controversial. Indeed, some maintain that science should rule no questions out. But if such questions are harmful to women and minority men, then surely they should be ruled out − in just the way in which the two other harmful kinds of scientific enquiry described above have been ruled out. And if so, a resolution of the conflict between the right to freedom of research and the right to equality in the area of cognitive differences research is at hand, one modeled on our first two precedents.

At this point, you will protest. There is nothing especially harmful, you will say, about seeking to determine who is better at something, or about seeking to determine whether some are as good at something as others, or else everything from spelling bees and team sports to college entrance examinations and

the Nobel Prize would be ruled out of bounds. What is problematic about cognitive differences research is not the questions asked or even the results sometimes obtained, but the prejudiced − the racist and sexist − context in which the research takes place. It is this context that makes the research disempowering. For example, whites do not typically feel demeaned or disempowered when it is reported that Asians have higher IQ scores than they. The result, in fact, seems of little consequence; IQ isn't everything. But when it is reported that whites have higher IQ scores than blacks, blacks do feel demeaned and disempowered. The difference, of course, is the racism that oppresses blacks and privileges whites. To be sure, finding out that blacks have lower IQ scores than whites, or that women are analytically weaker than men, could be the beginning of educational and training programs to work with the strengths and work on the weaknesses of every group to help make them the very best they can be, and even to use the special talents of each group to help the others. Finding these things out could be the beginning of innovative programs that support rather than undermine the right to equality. That this does not happen, or seldom happens, is a function of the sexism and racism of society, not the knowledge uncovered by cognitive differences research.

In short, there is nothing wrong with cognitive group differences research taken by itself. It is our society that is wrong, not the research. So why should we limit the freedom of scientists and the potentially interesting and important insights they might offer because of the shortcomings of the society in which they do their research? This is what I think you will say. And, although the argument falls short of compelling − cognitive differences research, after all, is far less benign than spelling bees, team sports, and the Nobel Prize, with their emphases on motivating hard work and rewarding achievement − still the societal context of such research is surely significant. Turn, then, to the third of my three precedents, a very new case involving the conflict between the right to freedom of research and the right to personal security (that is, the right not to be killed and not to be injured or abused – in the US Constitution, this is called the right to life). This time the case comes from synthetic genomics investigations within biomedical research.

4   The Third Precedent

In 2001, Australian researchers inadvertently produced a superstrain of mousepox, one that kills mice regardless of whether they have been vaccinated against mousepox or are naturally resistant to it. What the researchers had hoped to achieve, when they inserted the mouse IL-4 gene into the mousepox virus, was an altered virus that would provide a means of pest control by sterilizing mice. What the researchers did achieve was not only the superstrain of mousepox but very possibly also a technique for producing a superstrain of smallpox. In the wrong hands, this information could be deadly. Since there is no known treatment for smallpox – since vaccination is our only defense – having a vaccine-resistant strain of smallpox on the loose would produce havoc.

As if this weren't enough, in a second study in 2002, researchers at the State University of New York at Stony Brook stitched together strands of DNA that they had purchased via mail order, following the map of the polio virus RNA genome available on the Internet. Their technique resulted in the artificial synthesis of a "live" polio virus, one that paralyzes and kills mice. In this case, however, the researchers produced their deadly virus deliberately, "from scratch," using materials and information readily available to anyone, in order to demonstrate that terrorists might be able to make biological weapons without obtaining natural viruses.

In still further studies completed in 2005, researchers from the US Centers for Disease Control and Prevention, the Armed Forces Institute of Pathology, Mount Sinai School of Medicine, and the US Department of Agriculture pieced together viral fragments from hospital specimens and from the remains of a human victim dug up in Alaska to sequence the complete genome of the deadly Spanish flu virus, the virus that had killed an estimated 40–50 million

people worldwide in the winter of 1918–19. They then went ahead and re-created the virus, this virus that by then no longer existed anywhere on Earth. The re-created virus, the researchers found, was just as lethal as historical records had led them to expect: all the mice that were infected died within days, and Canadian, US, and Japanese researchers found the same outcome with monkeys in 2007.

Note that all these groundbreaking studies were carried out by top researchers, and all were published in top journals – the first in the *Journal of Virology* (Jackson et al. 2001) and the others in *Science* (Cello, Paul, and Wimmer 2002; Tumpey et al. 2005) and *Nature* (Taubenberger et al. 2005; Kobasa et al. 2007). And all these studies (as well as others that might have employed similar techniques to synthesize smallpox or Ebola) were said to promise unprecedented insights into some of the most virulent diseases ever known and the kinds of drugs and vaccines that might be developed to combat them. Nonetheless, many have argued that these studies should not have been done at all, or at least they should not have been published. Regarding the 1918 Spanish flu studies, for example, biosecurity experts have warned that (to use the wording given in a special report in *Nature* in 2005) "the risk that the recreated strain might escape is so high, it is almost a certainty" (von Bubnoff 2005, 794). Others charged that publishing the full genome of the 1918 influenza virus was worse than publishing the precise design for an atomic bomb, since creating and releasing the virus from the published genetic data would be easier than building and detonating an atomic bomb from only its design, given that rare materials such as plutonium and enriched uranium would not be needed, and releasing the virus would kill many more people than detonating an atomic bomb (Kurzweil and Joy 2005). And still others called the virus "perhaps the most effective bioweapons agent now known" (von Bubnoff 2005, 795). According to these experts, in short, the present "age of terrorism" in which the studies have been conducted, as well as the ever-present possibility of human error, have turned what the Centers for Disease Control called important health research into a very bad idea.

So, the context of research can shape the value of research – in biomedical research, given its context of terrorism, no less than in psychological research, given its context of sexism and racism. The controversial biomedical research described above, however, unlike the controversial psychological research described previously, has produced new policy constraints on the freedom of research. In 2003, for example, a joint "statement on scientific publication and security" appeared in *Science, Nature*, the *Proceedings of the National Academy of Sciences*, and the journals of the American Society for Microbiology. According to this statement, editors should screen and, if necessary, request modification of or even refuse to publish manuscripts if the editors "conclude that the potential harm of publication outweighs the potential societal benefits" (Journal Editors and Authors Group 2003). In 2004, the US National Research Council issued a comprehensive report, *Biotechnology Research in an Age of Terrorism*, commonly known as the Fink report (see National Research Council 2004). This report, as well as others appearing around the same time, emphasized the need for systematic reviews of potentially harmful life sciences research before the initiation of the research and at regular intervals thereafter, way before publication is at issue. The Fink report went on to identify the kinds of study that require this especially careful oversight, and it expanded the institutional framework already in place to carry out the oversight. It emphasized, as well, the need to develop a culture of responsibility within the life sciences to support and anticipate the oversight, to be accomplished by educational programs undertaken by all the professional societies in the life sciences, by group strategies coordinated by the major societies, and by the creation and promotion of codes of ethics detailing life scientists' social responsibilities. Finally, the Fink report recommended the establishment of a National Science Advisory Board for Biosecurity to provide the necessary advice, guidance, and resources for both the scientific community and the government regarding the system of review and oversight it proposed. This board was created in 2004, and it included both leading scientists and biosecurity experts.

Is there any reason new policy constraints like these for the life sciences should not be put into effect for the social sciences – new policy constraints that include research guidelines for weighing societal harms of research against societal benefits, that include educational programs and codes of ethics designed to foster a culture of responsibility among social scientists, and that include a new National Science Advisory Board for Social Research to provide advice, guidance, and resources for both the scientific community and the government? Such a board could count among its members both leading social scientists and representatives of the public at large, such as racial, ethnic, and gender group advocates. Is there any reason new policy constraints like these should not be put into effect for the social sciences? Reflecting, again, on the two cases described above, one from the social sciences (the case of cognitive differences research) and one from the life sciences (the case of recent synthetic genomics research), two reasons might be offered to say that the cases should not be treated similarly. The first reason is that the cognitive differences research in question does not pose harms to society anywhere near the harms posed by the recent synthetic genomics research. Hence, there is no need for similar constraints on scientific freedom in the two cases. The second reason is that such constraints might have very different effects in the two cases, limiting scientific progress in the one case but not in the other. What can be said in response to these considerations?

To begin with, it is clear that the kinds of synthetic genomics research described previously may cause great harm to certain people – to the people who work in the laboratories in which the research is carried out, to the people who live near those laboratories in whose midst the pathogens may escape, to the people who may end up targets of terrorists' use of the published results of the research, and so on. All these people, under the old system of standards for choosing, carrying out, and publishing research, might have gotten very sick or even died as a result of the research, though the degree of likelihood for these various effects is hotly debated (see, e.g., von

Bubnoff 2005 for some of the debate). As a result, special new constraints on scientific freedom were thought necessary to minimize the risks.

So, on the one hand, synthetic genomics research unconstrained may cause serious harm to various groups of people. On the other hand, cognitive differences research unconstrained, as previously stated, has already been shown to cause significant harm, though lesser harm than a serious illness, but for much longer periods than the length of an illness, to lots more people – to all the people whose self-esteem, self-efficacy, ambitions, and successes are lessened as a result of direct or indirect exposure to the research or aspects of the research (e.g., its results or even just its questions); to all the people whose self-esteem, self-efficacy, ambitions, and successes are lessened as a result of the treatment they receive from others who have been directly or indirectly exposed to the research or aspects of the research; and so on – in short, to all or most women and, in the United States at least, to most minority men and many men of color in other parts of the world. And these harms have gone on for centuries to this majority of society. Cognitive group differences research, then, arguably does pose harms to society near – perhaps even exceeding – the harms posed by the recent synthetic genomics research. If special constraints on scientific freedom are thought necessary in the one case, then why should they not be thought necessary in the other case as well?

But decisions of this kind must take into account their expected effects on science as well as society. And in the case of health research, it is claimed that the new constraints on scientific freedom will not limit scientific progress. Indeed, this was one of the desiderata built into the new policy. As the Fink report made clear, "any system of review and oversight must operate in ways that do not put the United States – and the world – at risk of losing the great potential benefits of biotechnology" (National Research Council 2004, 10). Some have gone further. They have claimed that even more stringent constraints than those now in place, constraints that would further restrict synthetic genomics research, will still not limit progress in health research, since, given the information already available, the controversial genomics research was not really needed (see, e.g., van Aken 2006, S12).

So, we have been assured that the new policy constraints on scientific freedom imposed on the life sciences will not limit scientific progress. But we can be equally assured that new policy constraints on scientific freedom in the social sciences will not limit scientific progress either. Indeed, we can write that into the policy, as the Fink report did. Moreover, as advocates for tighter restrictions in the life sciences have done, we can also question exactly how important to the overall goals of the social sciences race- and gender-related cognitive differences research really is, and we can also question the reasonableness of those goals that may make it important. For example, the synthetic genomics research described above has aroused great concern in the United States because of its national security implications. But surely cognitive differences research also has something akin to national security implications. After all, people of color from various national origins will soon be the majority in the United States, and women already are. As a result, the competence and productivity, indeed the flourishing, of minority populations and women are becoming central to our collective well-being. A kind of research that undermines this competence and productivity therefore also undermines our security, and goals that support such research thereby become suspect.

Of course, none of this precludes losses – to society as well as science – when scientists' freedom is constrained. New Zealand psychologist James Flynn's remarks in a recent debate in *Nature* on whether scientists should investigate cognitive group differences make this especially clear: "When you assert that a topic is not to be debated, you are foreclosing not some narrow statement of opinion on that topic, but the whole spiraling universe of discourse that it may inspire"; "I invite everyone to search the social-science literature of the past 34 years and ask whether or not they really wish that everything on the subject [of biologically based cognitive group differences], pro or con, was missing" (Flynn 2009, 146). But Flynn never considers the gains that might have occurred along with the losses had cognitive group differences research not been pursued during the past 34 years – the research that might have done far more to dismantle race- and gender-related injustice than the research to which Flynn and others contributed. Nor does Flynn consider the whole spiraling universe of discourse and benefits that might ensue if we now put a halt to cognitive group differences research. When we look at some of the newer work in child development in minority populations in the United States, how the old genetic deficit models and cultural deficit models of minority child development are being replaced by models that foreground and seek to build on minority competencies, strengths, and resourcefulness in the context of racism and poverty, or when we look at some of the work in feminist science studies over the past 30 years, how the old doubts whether women can make the same contributions to science as men have been replaced by studies showing the importantly different critical and constructive contributions to the sciences women have made, we get a hint of what this new discourse and these new benefits can be (for some of the newer models of minority child development, see, e.g., Garcia Coll et al. 1996; for some of the work in feminist science studies, see Kourany 2012).

5 Conclusion

The three precedents considered above – the US National Research Act of 1974, the US National Institutes of Health Revitalization Act of 1993, and the Fink report and related policy directives of 2003–4 – point to a resolution of the conflict between the right to freedom of research and the right to equality, a resolution that favors the right to equality. At least this seems to be the result in the context of cognitive group differences research. But the same result should follow in other contexts in which the right to freedom of research conflicts with the right to equality – such as in the context of public health and biomedical research, where the health needs of the more affluent are privileged over the health needs of the poor (see, e.g., Hotez 2008). In fact, taken together the three precedents considered above suggest a quite general conclusion: that scientists' right to freedom of research cannot be allowed to subvert other people's rights, whether those other people are research subjects inside the research context or recipients of the effects of the research outside it. The case of cognitive group differences research, if enacted into a fourth precedent, will simply add further strength and urgency to this conclusion. It will also move science closer to the forefront of social change rather than remain holding up the rear.

References

Ceci, Stephen and Wendy M. Williams. 2009. "Darwin 200: Should Scientists Study Race and IQ? YES: The Scientific Truth Must Be Pursued." *Nature* 457 (7231): 788–89. https://www.nature.com/articles/457788a.

——. 2010. *The Mathematics of Sex: How Biology and Society Conspire to Limit Talented Women and Girls.* New York: Oxford University Press.

Cello, Jeronimo, Aniko V. Paul, and Eckard Wimmer. 2002. "Chemical Synthesis of Poliovirus cDNA: Generation of Infectious Virus in the Absence of Natural Template." *Science* 297: 1016–18.

Dar-Nimrod, Ilan and Steven J. Heine. 2006. "Exposure to Scientific Theories Affects Women's Math Performance." *Science* 314 (5798): 435.

Fausto-Sterling, Anne. 1992. *Myths of Gender.* 2nd ed. New York: Basic.

——. 2000. *Sexing the Body: Gender Politics and the Construction of Sexuality.* New York: Basic.

Flynn, James. 2009. "Would You Wish the Research Undone?" *Nature* 458 (7235): 146.

Garcia Coll, Cynthia Gontran Lamberty, Renee Jenkins, Harriet Pipes McAdoo, Keith Crnic, Barbara Hanna Wasik, and Heidie Vázquez García. 1996. "An Integrative Model for the Study of Developmental Competencies in Minority Children." *Child Development* 67:1891–1914.

Hamilton, Colin. 2008. *Cognition and Sex Differences.* New York: Palgrave Macmillan.

Hotez, Peter J. 2008. "Neglected Infections of Poverty in the United States of America." *PLoS Neglected Tropical*

Diseases 2 (6): 1–11. https://journals.plos.org/plosntds/article?id=10.1371/journal.pntd.0000256.

Jackson, Ronald J., et al. 2001. "Expression of Mouse Interleukin-4 by a Recombinant Ectromelia Virus Suppresses Cytolytic Lymphocyte Responses and Overcomes Genetic Resistance to Mousepox." *Journal of Virology* 75:1205–10.

Journal Editors and Authors Group. 2003. "Uncensored Exchange of Scientific Results." *Proceedings of the National Academy of Sciences* 100 (4): 1464. http://www.pnas.org/content/100/4/1464.

Karafyllis, Nicole C., and Gotlind Ulshofer. 2008. *Sexualized Brains: Scientific Modeling of Emotional Intelligence from a Cultural Perspective.* Cambridge, MA: MIT Press.

Kobasa, Darwyn, et al. 2007. "Aberrant Innate Immune Response in Lethal Infection of Macaques with the 1918 Influenza Virus." *Nature 445*: 319–23.

Kourany, Janet. 2012. "Feminist Critiques: Harding and Longino." In *Philosophy of Science: The Key Thinkers*, ed. James Robert Brown. London: Continuum.

Kurzweil, Ray, and Bill Joy. 2005. "Recipe for Destruction." *New York Times*, October 17. http://www.nytimes.com/2005/10/17/opinion/17kurzweiljoy.html.

National Commission for the Protection of Human Subjects of Biomedical and Behavioral Research. 1979. "The Belmont Report: Ethical Principles and Guidelines for the Protection of Human Subjects of Research." Regulations and Ethical Guidelines, National Institutes of Health. http://www.hhs.gov/ohrp/regulations-and-policy/belmont-report/.

National Research Council. 2004. *Biotechnology Research in an Age of Terrorism.* Washington, DC: National Academies.

Rose, Steven. 2009. "Darwin 200: Should Scientists Study Race and IQ? NO: Science and Society Do Not Benefit." *Nature* 457 (7231): 786–88. https://www.nature.com/articles/457786a.

Rosser, Sue. 1994. *Women's Health – Missing from U.S. Medicine.* Bloomington: Indiana University Press.

Schiebinger, Londa. 1989. *The Mind Has No Sex?* Cambridge, MA: Harvard University Press.

———. 1999. *Has Feminism Changed Science?* Cambridge, MA: Harvard University Press.

Spencer, Steven J., Claude M. Steele, and Diane M. Quinn. 1999. "Stereotype Threat and Women's Math Performance." *Journal of Experimental Social Psychology* 35:4–28.

Steele, Claude M. 1997. "A Threat in the Air: How Stereotypes Shape Intellectual Identity and Performance." *American Psychologist* 52 (6): 613–29.

Taubenberger, Jeffery K., Ann H. Reid, Raina M. Lourens, Ruixue Wang, Guozhong Jin, and Thomas G. Fanning. 2005. "Characterization of the 1918 Influenza Virus Polymerase Genes." *Nature* 437 (7060): 889–93.

Tumpey, Terrence M., et al. 2005. "Characterization of the Reconstructed 1918 Spanish Influenza Pandemic Virus." *Science* 310:77–80.

van Aken, Jan. 2006. "When Risk Outweighs Benefit." *EMBO [European Molecular Biology Organization] Reports* 7 (Special Issue): S10–S13.

von Bubnoff, Andreas. 2005. "Special Report: The 1918 Flu Virus Is Resurrected." *Nature* 437 (October 6): 794–95.

Woolf, Virginia. 1929. *A Room of One's Own.* London: Hogarth.

67

Academic Freedom and Race
You Ought Not to Believe What You Think May Be True

James R. Flynn

There should be no academic sanctions against those who believe that were environments equalized, genetic differences between black and white Americans would mean that blacks have an IQ deficit. I will call this the genetic hypothesis as opposed to an environmental hypothesis. In passing, I wish to say that scholars who hold the genetic hypothesis are not thereby, guilty of racial bias. There is no doubt in my mind that Arthur Jensen was innocent of this (Flynn, 2013). Moreover, research into this question should not be forbidden. This is so, no matter what the outcome of the race and IQ debate, that is, no matter whether the evidence eventually dictates a genetically caused deficit of nil or 5 or 10 or 20 IQ points.

I will begin my case for this by discussing five propositions: (1) That the hypothesis is intelligible and subject to scientific investigation; (2) The advice that you ought not believe what you think may be true; (3) The advice that you ought not attempt to persuade those who may be in error; (4) The advice that you ought not to use the scientific method to enhance belief in the truth; (5) The use of sanctions to enforce the three pieces of moral advice just stated.

Note that 2, 3, and 4 are simply that, only 5 advocates sanctions to coerce the behavior of those who refuse to be advised.

1 An Intelligible Hypothesis

Four arguments are used to challenge the coherence of the hypothesis that "on average black Americans have inferior genes for IQ than white Americans." First, that it makes a racial distinction and that there are no such things as pure races, that is, there are no groups of humans that have interbred exclusively within one another during their evolutionary history. That is true but the hypothesis asserts only that there are two sociologically identifiable groups in question. Those who deny this would have to be against affirmative action: blacks must be sociologically identifiable for benefits to be conferred.

Second, that if groups are sociologically identified, when there is a trait difference, you cannot claim that there is a genetic difference. This is manifestly false. Watusi and pygmies are two sociologically identifiable

Original publication details: James R. Flynn, "Academic Freedom and Race: You Ought Not to Believe What You Think May Be True," pp. 127–131 from *Journal of Criminal Justice* 59 (2018). Reproduced with permission of Elsevier.

groups (they cannot be pure races because no such thing exists) and they differ on average for height. No scientist has ever doubted that genes are involved. Even prior to scientific investigation, they had sound empirical grounds: under conditions when food was plentiful within both groups, no one could find an adult pygmy that was as tall as an adult Watusi. A few years ago, Price et al. (2009) identified two genes involved in the iodide-dependent thyroid hormone pathway as likely causes.

A hypothetical example is instructive. Irish immigrants to America establish a town. Initially, they are randomly distributed in terms of residing north or south of the railway tracks. North becomes more desirable (better views, less fog, less flooding, etc.). Those who do better in school make more money, purchase homes north of the tracks, and tend to marry one another. Those who do worse make less money, tend to live south of the tracks, and wed one another. Within a few generations, there will be a mean IQ difference between these two sociologically defined groups with a genetic component. Anyone who denies this must assert that school does not affect income or that intelligence does not affect success at school or that intelligence is not influenced by whether those [who] have more children possess above or below average intelligence

Third, that unlike a tape measure, IQ tests are not culture free. This is true. I have advocated that societies at different stages of modernity should have IQ tests that prioritize cognitive abilities as each culture does (Flynn, 2016). In America, at the top of the list would be analytic abilities that predict success in the formal schooling that predicts occupational success. In Aboriginal society, top would be mapping abilities that predict how well you would do in finding water in a near-desert (mapping ability is also useful for London taxi drivers). It would be quite absurd to test Aborigines for logical analysis of abstractions that are missing when they cognize about how to make use of their concrete world.

But as Thomas Sowell has said, no one lives in a culture-free society. What you want in America are tests that are culturally significant in the society in which both blacks and whites live. Let us assume that blacks are genetically favored for skills that once fostered success among African tribal groups. That is little solace to blacks in Chicago who want their children to rise out of the ghetto and become food chemists. They would prefer that blacks are not genetically disadvantaged for cognitive skills that bring educational success. It is worth noting that IQs predict academic success at least as well for blacks as for whites. The fact that IQ tests are not culturally free is a double-edged sword: what you gain from better adaptation to a pre-industrial society is no compensation for what you lose if you stay in America.

We no longer hear much from those who once proposed a fourth argument: that all races share so many genes in common that it would be absurd to look for genetic differences (note: even this argument assumes the question is subject to investigation; they just think the answer is as obvious as height differences between Watusi and pygmies). We share 99% of our genes with bonobo chimpanzees. That 1% makes a huge difference in cognitive capacity: one hundredth of 1% might make a huge difference between socially identified groups.

2   Not Believing What You Think May Be True

This piece of moral advice is psychologically impossible. You cannot ask someone to deny to themselves what they think may be true. Coercing thought gets you into the realm of sanctions (the rack and the thumb-screw, or at least making job applicants for university posts take a loyalty oath about racial traits).

3   Not Discussing What Some Think To Be True

I am happy to discuss the race and IQ debate with colleagues who hold contrary views and do so at conferences and in the common room. I want to persuade and that is much more difficult if we both know that I have hidden behind my back an instrument of coercion. Telling someone that what they believe is morally remiss or telling them that if they persist in disagreeing, I will expose them is not my style. I got enough of this when defending democratic socialism during the McCarthy era. I take it as conceded that when we academics discuss this issue among ourselves, we will use evidence and persuasion as we do on all matters of substance.

4 Not Using Science to Investigate the Truth

To advise scholars that they should not systematically investigate race and IQ seems to me to raise the question of what we are afraid of: that we will discover that genes do play a significant role? A few years ago I addressed scholars at one of America's most distinguished universities who admitted that they had never approved a research grant that might clarify whether black and white had equivalent genes for IQ. I had some suggestions and said I knew that they might have reasons for ignoring them other than pessimism: they were just intimidated by the public furor that would ensue. That was not fair because they could not publicly admit that they curtailed scholarly research because of intimidation. They had to argue that the most trivial grant they had approved (something like whether chipmunks like Mozart) was more important than clarifying the causes of racial differences.

This may seem to prejudice the outcome of a systematic investigation. I do not intend this. The research should be done no matter what the outcome, as I will show. I am merely asking those who would forbid research to be honest (at least to themselves) about their own beliefs. I should add that, to my cost, I have discovered another motive that discourages research. Let us assume that it is not genes that cause the black IQ deficit. Then it must be environment and if it is environment, the most immediate environment, namely, black subculture, must be examined. If

causes exist there, we will hear rhetoric about blaming the victim. For example, a relevant cause might be black child-rearing practices. However, to avoid criticism, I am not going to disempower blacks by keeping them ignorant. Note the penalty for ignoring reality: no knowledge of causes, hard to alter effects. This is a theme to which we will return. Irish Americans were persecuted ("no Irish need apply, black man preferred"). The ultimate causes of their disadvantages were written in their history rather than their genes. But that history had engendered a subculture that had become an active cause in itself. Rather than merely dwelling on the sins of England, they really did have to change in order to reduce their alcoholism and domestic violence.

I know of no alternative to the scientific method to maximize accumulation of truth about the physical world and the causes of human behavior. If scholars are to debate this issue, do we not want the best evidence possible – and this can only come from science.

Assume that everyone who at present leans toward an environmental hypothesis eschewed scientific investigation. That would be equivalent to unilateral disarmament. The only science that would be done would be by those who at present lean toward a genetic hypothesis. Such a state of affairs carries its own price. Twice a year I get emails from young scholars who tell me how glad they are that they have read my work on race (Flynn, 1980, 2008 chapters 2–4; 2012 pp. 132–141). They say that up to then, they had assumed all the evidence was on the side of Jensen and Rushton and that the lack of any evidential rebuttal was a confession of bankruptcy. Research on race and IQ has competed with my chief interest of moral philosophy and earned me opprobrium. But I felt obliged to rectify the fact that the evidence on record in 1978 was not fair to the environmental hypothesis, and I was determined not to embrace unilateral disarmament. I did not, however, pre-judge the issue: I knew that the evidence can always go against you and results can be unwelcome.

Those who believe in the relative equality of the races may choose not to research race and IQ, but they have not thereby discovered something that turns all beliefs into ones of which they approve. There has never been a time since World War II during which all Americans had more "progressive" views on race than Arthur Jensen. He always emphasized overlap between the races for genes for IQ and stated that the brightest person in America might well be a black male (no sexism: there is some evidence that black women have a higher mean IQ than black males). I discovered this as a CORE (Congress of Racial Equality) chairman in the South in 1961, although I really knew it already from being raised in Washington DC. I know of no reputable scholar who has addressed this question whose conclusions were not at stark variance with those of the classical racist who abhors the notion that there is substantial overlap between the races for valued traits.

There will be bad science on both sides of the debate. The only antidote I know for that is to use the scientific method as scrupulously as possible.

5   From Advice to Sanctions

Everyone knows that universities apply sanctions to alter behavior among academics that refuse to accept the advice given thus far. A stated intention of doing race/gene research on a vita will mean no job; doing that research may mean no tenure, no promotion, no research grants, or even a campaign for dismissal. Some like Jensen, who are at a prestige university such as Berkeley, survive.

In the *Emile*, Rousseau included a long footnote in which he addresses the world of scholars. He knows that many of them are atheists but warns them against any attempt to spread atheism to the masses: the latter need the fear of hell as an incentive to compensate for or refrain from injustices. The notion that there is an elite who can discuss what may be true or false but who must present a united front to others on a point of dogma is recurrent in human history. Newton could not make known his doubts about the Trinity; Henry Sidgwick felt he ought to resign his fellowship at Cambridge because he could not accept the Anglican credo (he got the stipulation scrapped).

The use of sanctions against those who do not confine their views on race and IQ to the common room dictates limiting debate to the faculty, and turns an environmentalist position into a dogma in the sense that no wider discussion is allowed. That includes your students; and, of course, no sign of dissent can be allowed to reach the public (no frank interviews given, no research pursued, etc.). There are almost no courses on intelligence in psychology departments in America. When I ask staff why, they give the same answer: what if a student raised a hand and said, what do you think about the race and IQ debate? You either have a potted lying answer that makes the debate seem simpler than it is (every sophisticated environmentalist knows that Jensen has a case to answer), or you say, "well that goes beyond the scope of this course" (why?), or you admit heresy.

Universities should welcome a full discussion of any topic within their walls. In *On Liberty*, John Stuart Mill sets out why. Sanctions always assume that truth will be maximized by the winners of a prizefight (a test of political strength) rather than by free debate. Those who want to forbid discussion and scientific investigation ignore three things. There may be a truth hidden in an erroneous position that is not present elsewhere: we all owe Jensen a debt for exploding simplistic explanations of black under achievement, such as that it was merely a matter of class (matching black and white for SES [socioeconomic status] does not nearly eliminate the IQ gap). Having to defend your position means you can have knowledge rather than just right opinion. Let us assume that those of us who think the causes are environmental are correct. It is one thing for our students to believe correctly simply because they have been indoctrinated by a united front and another for them to be able to defend their position. Finally, truth gains vitality from being challenged rather than being an unquestioned inheritance. Converts to Christianity are often more pious than those who inherit their faith.

Mill closes by claiming that those who favor sanctions have presumptions to infallibility or absolute certainty. They are so sure of their position they are willing to use power to ensure that no case for another opinion is ever to be heard throughout the entire course of human history. This kind of ban is far more serious than it might seem. To kill an idea is to forfeit all rewards that may flow from reaction to that idea. If I had not read about Arthur Jensen and his research, with its emphasis on IQ and the general intelligence factor, I would never have documented massive IQ gain over time, or urged a revolution in the theory of intelligence, or connected cognitive gains and moral gains, or cooperated with Bill Dickens to formulate the Dickens/Flynn model, which unifies phenomena from the dynamics of cognitive development to the results of interventions. There are actually people who are still alive "because" of Jensen: those on death row who were proved to be mentally retarded thanks to application of the Flynn effect to their IQ test scores.

What kind of crystal ball do they have, those who wish the University of California at Berkeley had deleted Jensen from the history of ideas of our time? Was it not better to debate with him, and learn from that debate? Does academia really want to ally itself with those who reserve free discussion to Philosopher Kings, and create dogmas to deaden the minds of all others? However benevolent the intent, there is a flaw in imprinting beliefs in people's minds never to alter. The beliefs have become like instincts rather than reasoned conclusions. A creature with a frozen mind can qualify as an insect but it is not fully human.

6   The Dead Hand of Ignorance

By ignorance I mean unawareness of what science reveals about the real world. It always extracts a price. Let us assume the "worst" possible outcome of this debate: black American school children have a genetic deficit worth 20 IQ points. I cannot make this very plausible given that the present IQ gap is far less than that. We would have to assume either that blacks today are privileged environmentally or that some unlikely event had occurred: cosmic radiation has struck only black neighborhoods and caused harmful mutations. But if so, would we really want to be ignorant of that? Doubling the present IQ gap would mean that black

underperformance at school would be twice as evident as it is today. If we dogmatically assumed that only environmental factors were relevant, we would be embarking on a frantic scramble to identify them and one doomed to failure.

We need not be fanciful to assess the price of ignorance. Assume that the entire IQ gap between school children today (10 points) is genetic. Take the principal of a high school in an affluent neighborhood where both black and white students all come from professional homes. The principal may be doing everything he or she can think of to give the best education to all. However, if black students get worse grades than white students, there will inevitably be suspicion of institutional racism. Something has to be wrong if only the fact blacks find the environment less friendly. The principal may actually come to believe that she is remiss. The greatest tragedy is an innocent person suffering from guilt. In some pre-industrial societies people think dreams can kill. A person can be perfectly innocent of a murder but think they are guilty because of murderous dreams or thoughts. Again I say: ignorance of reality always extracts its price.

The following is not always true, but the constituency that wants to ban race/genes research includes many who have a "shoot the messenger mentality". They try to discredit IQ tests. I will not digress to show how mistaken they are but will only say that IQ tests provide priceless data about the cognitive development of parents and their children and the injustices the latter may suffer (Flynn, 2016). This does not mean IQ tests should be used for streaming. If that is to occur, it should be based on past academic performance, which is a better predictor of future academic performance than anything else.

7   The Appeal to Paradigms of Irrationality

Are there to be no limits on what the university will tolerate? Will academics offer courses on holocaust denial, or on the extraterrestrial sources of crop rings, or teach a course in Algebra using roman numerals? In passing, anyone who wanted to hire a room on the university campus to speak on such issues should be free to do so and treated with formal courtesy. If they are willing to have a critic nominated to debate their views, fine. If not, someone can hire the same room for a presentation immediately following. To ban them by force is to assume that university students, of all people, cannot make up their own minds about what to believe.

But allocating money to conduct such courses or finance research of this sort would test the resources of most universities (if there were many volunteers). To use such examples in order to ban research into a serious question is the rhetoric of an enemy of liberty. In my classes, I advocate giving the Nazi party the right to exist in America and publish its literature (if they plan violence or intimidation, there are plenty of laws that are relevant). Inevitably, a student will say, but what if we were living in Germany in 1930. The answer is that by 1930 free debate had given way to battles in the streets and only force could settle whether democracy survived. To pretend that such a situation existed in American in 1950 when the Communist Party was banned was the mark of an enemy of liberty. To appeal to extreme cases that show the university cannot make liberty absolute, in order to justify suppressing freedom of inquiry where it is perfectly possible, is the mark of an enemy of truth.

8   Compromises

Universities are the focus of irrational pressures that hope to compromise their purpose. I sympathize with an American university president who says something like the following.

You don't know how hard I struggle to maintain what freedoms we have. We are free to debate evolution versus intelligent design, atheism versus theism, socialism verses the welfare state versus the free market. Within limits, we can freely debate US foreign policy as long as we do not say too much about the Middle East. We do research without restriction into economics, philosophy, politics, and biology. We hire without prejudice in these areas (never entirely true: when I was a young academic during the height of the Cold War, the left had trouble; now the right have trouble). I simply *have* to trim my sails on race/genes research. I will try to defend you but must do so semi-dishonestly: publicly lament what you do but say we must not fire you because of academic freedom. And strictly in private, I suggest that you get research money from some source less inhibited.

This I can respect. What is far worse is the academic who marches with the legions that want to curtail academic freedom. They should be a pressure group on the side of freedom that helps the president fight in the trenches.

9   The Bright Light of Knowledge

I want to summarize some results that have come to light only because scientific investigation was not banned. They are not chosen to show that an evidential approach was worthwhile only because some of the evidence favors an environmental hypothesis. Rather they are chosen to show that knowledge is better than ignorance. The reader should assess whether or not we would be better off if the research had not been done.

Moore (1986) did a study [that] would have been forbidden by a prescription against race/gene research. She identified adoptees all of who were black and thereby, controlled for genetic differences between black and white. Of these, 23 were adopted by white middle-class couples and 23 adopted by black middle-class couples. The white and black adoptive mothers had the same number of years of schooling, that is, 16 years. As is characteristic of the black middle-class, the black fathers did not quite match the white fathers, with 15.6 years of schooling compared to 17.3 years. As a consequence, the income of the black homes was a bit lower, with a socio-economic index of 63.5 compared to 70.3, both quite respectable. When tested at age 8.5 (ages 7 to 10), the black-adopted black children had a mean IQ of 103.6 and the white-adopted black children a mean of 117.1, a difference of 13.5 IQ points. This easily matched the black-white IQ gap for that age at that time.

Her results were significant and their significance goes far beyond the fact that they count on the environmental side of the ledger. Moore observed (over two 20-minute periods) the mother's interaction with her child while the latter was trying to perform a difficult cognitive task. The mothers were told they could help their children. Although both sets of mothers had the same number of years of education, there was a sharp contrast. White mothers tended to smile, joke, give positive encouragement (that is an interesting idea), and applaud effort. Black mothers tended to frown, scowl, criticize (you know that doesn't look right), and express displeasure (you could do better than this if you really tried). Understandably, children were more likely to ask for help from white than black mothers when confronted with cognitive problems.

Remember the high school principal. Was she aware of these results, she would know that black underperformance at her school might well be a sign that black professional homes are on average less educationally efficient than white professional homes. Everyone accepts that the homes of East Asians are more efficient than those of whites. She might be able to gentle parents toward looking at their own behavior rather than looking for "institutional racism".

What would this mean? Asking the following questions: do black professionals sit down with their children and help with homework; are they too censorious when they do so; do non-professionals see their child's education as a chance to upgrade their own; is there a special effort made to repair deficiencies (or does the child hear "I was never any good at math either"); do older achieving children help younger non-achieving ones; is their praise for academic achievement more enthusiastic than for making a sports team (or when a child settles down to homework, does the father say, "let's go out behind the garage and shoot a few baskets"); can you get them to associate with at least some peers who are academic rather than the smart set (one can go too far

here: when Tom Sowell stopped at the library on the way home, his father beat him for hanging out on the street); do parents read good literature setting a model for their children; do parents perceive hanging out at shopping malls as the first symptom of mental illness.

Moore's numbers are too small for strong inference. However, if over the last 30 years, we had complied a complete register of all black children adopted and had the relevant parental data, we might have the numbers to put the issue beyond doubt. Forget the race and IQ debate. We could be certain that the black family environment is less cognitively challenging, and could try to alter real world behavior.

My research (Flynn, 2008) convinced me that there are other factors of black subculture worthy of investigation particularly youth culture: when half black and white school children (offspring of US occupation soldiers) were compared in Germany after World War II, their IQ profiles matched in terms of g loadings (loading on the general intelligence factor). Take my word for it that this is highly significant. The half- blacks being raised in Germany were simply dark-skinned Germans. What was missing was a black American youth subculture.

The Harvard sociologist Patterson (2006) has investigated black youth culture. The fact that he is black protects him from some, but only from some, opprobrium. He argues that young black males do not despise education and are aware of the benefits it brings, but that their youth culture offers rewards that they cannot resist. Dressing sharply, hanging out, sexual conquests, party drugs, and hip-hop music and its ambiance are powerfully attractive, and the admiration they get from both black and white peers bolsters self-esteem. White teenagers find imitating the postures of this culture attractive but they do not live it. Rather it is a hobby, something they set aside every time they think of the looming presence of the SAT (Scholastic Aptitude Test) that will determine their fate.

Perhaps survey data can be supplemented with something that helps us penetrate to the reality of black youth culture (cameras that record what actually goes on during the hours of homework reported?).

For now, I will add my own impressions for what they are worth. It seems to me that a subculture that legislates atypical speech and puts song and dance ahead of cognitively demanding leisure activity has to be a negative influence.

Finally, on the Nation's Report Card, between 1971 and 2008 (averaging scores for reading and mathematics), blacks gained 6.39 IQ points on whites and the final gap for all ages stood at 9.94 points. Using all Wechsler and Stanford-Binet standardization samples, Dickens and Flynn (2006) concluded that between 1972 and 2002, blacks gained 5.5 IQ points on whites and that the average gap had fallen to 10.0 points for ages 9 to 17. The two data sets offer remarkably similar results. The Dickens and Flynn data cover all ages between 4 and 24 and sadly, black IQ steadily loses ground on white IQ as children age. In 2002, the gap was only 4.6 points at age 4 rising to 16.6 points at age 24.

I believe the fact that the IQ gap increases suggests (but does not prove) that certain facets of black culture are an increasingly heavy burden with age. I offer a scenario in which child-rearing practices are eventually outweighed by teenage subculture, which in turn is outweighed by the high incidence of male blacks in prison during the "university years" and of young black women who become solo-parents (Flynn, 2012).

10   Armageddon

My most important point is this. The race and IQ debate has taken on the role of Armageddon, a war between the forces of righteousness (the environmentalists) and the armies of the night (those who posit genetic differences). This fixation has overshadowed the fact that there are real people out there. When they try to improve the prospects of their children, they will not be attempting to score one more point for the environmental side of the race and IQ debate. Enormously helpful things have come to light without regard as to which side of the debate was

being argued. Jensen's point that equating for SES does not close the black/white IQ or educational achievement gap was a step forward. Moore's point that factors more subtle than SES seemed to count was another step forward. Scholars should stop playing games and let science do its job. Those of us who have turned their research into a contest rather than a diagnosis should be ashamed. I am not exempt from this censure.

Anyone who ceases to research what environmental handicaps blacks have will have to acknowledge that what motivated them was not helping real people but the excitement of a contest.

I have no illusions, of course, that the debate about race and IQ will end. And I do not deny that it could have social and political consequences. Perhaps someday we will conclude that a portion of the present gap will prove to be genetic in origin. I do not want to sugar the pill but will only say I am not too alarmed. Unless you believe black and white environments are today equivalent, genes will count for less than 10 points among schoolchildren.

But even that would mean that the group socially-classified as black will on average have somewhat worse social statistics for unemployment, crime, and so forth. And the free market will always penalize black individuals to some degree by making it rational to classify them as members of their group rather than incur the cost of getting to know them as individuals. A landlady with a room to rent is confronted with a female Korean American and a black male youth. She will not hire a private detective to check them out. She is likely to play the statistical odds: an almost sure thing versus someone from a group one-third of whom are convicted felons.

I have tried to show how affirmative action can compensate individuals who are handicapped by their group membership (Flynn, 2008). This case has nothing to do with genes versus environment; it simply focuses on the fact that rational market actors must discriminate against blacks without regard for their personal traits. But I want to add that if genes are part of the gap, helping individuals will not mean equal outcomes for all social groups. As a group, blacks would tend to have worse social statistics than whites. Perhaps we can accept that. Assume that the lower job profile of Irish Americans compared to Chinese Americans is due in part to genes: I do not know one Irishman who cares (the English would be a different matter).

Then there is the struggle over racial quotas in the private job market and at universities. It is worth noting that such quotas do not exist in the United Kingdom. The case for quotas is fought out, at least at universities, on whether diversity outweighs lower SAT scores. Assume that those quotas disappear. Would it be a tragedy if blacks were matched with quality of university by educational competence? Blacks marginal at Harvard would be good students at Illinois, and blacks marginal at Illinois would be good students at Southern Illinois, and so on down the ladder. There is a price for the fiction that someone is competent to meet the pace of courses, and competence of competing students, when it is not so. Someone who would be encouraged to aspire to (and qualify for) a profession at Illinois may be daunted by the competition at Harvard.

Moreover, if blacks admitted with lower SAT scores really are competent to do well, that must be judged by the individual case. It has nothing to do with how genes and environment divide the IQ gap between blacks as a group and whites as a group. No doubt, real racists will seize upon a genetic component in the racial IQ gap as a defense of their position. But we know that in fact, it does not provide the classical racist with any defense at all. Better to confront them with the truth rather than a fiction, and whatever the rhetorical disadvantage, forfeiting

the benefits of knowledge over ignorance is too heavy a price to pay.

11 Some History and Rhetoric

Once Christians admitted that blacks had souls, slavery was doomed. As Thomas Sowell says, once you grant that black and white so overlap that the brightest person in America may be black, the real ball game is over. Whether all people as individuals, no matter whether black or white, get justice as fairness will be a test of our humanity. Nothing will be gained by systemic sanctions that protect ignorance.

Having made a rational case, it is allowable to use rhetoric to try to bring people's emotions into line with their heads. Assume that the data showed that black Americans had a mean IQ 5 points *above* white Americans. How many would still want to forbid academics from doing race/gene research? Would not casting aspersions on IQ tests be labeled as an outrageous attempt to hide from a truth that cried out for amelioration? Look into your hearts. Suppressing free inquiry is by its nature an expressive of contempt for truth by power. The truth can never be racist.

A final word to those who seek respectability by banning race/gene research: how much respectability would you get if your position were stated without equivocation? After all, those who refuse to investigate genetic equality between the races cannot label it true; yet if you openly say *it may not be true* would you not reap the whirlwind? Honesty dictates this assertion: "I do not know if genetic equality is true and do not want to know." Say that, and see if your views are deemed innocent rather than pernicious.

References

Dickens, W. T., and Flynn, J. R. (2006). Black Americans reduce the racial IQ gap: Evidence from standardization samples. *Psychological Science, 17,* 913–20.

Flynn, J. R. (1980). *Race, IQ, and Jensen.* London: Routledge.

Flynn, J. R. (2008). *Where Have All the Liberals Gone? Race, Class, and Ideals in America.* Cambridge University Press.

Flynn, J. R. (2012). *Are We Getting Smarter: Rising IQ in the Twenty-first Century.* Cambridge University Press.

Flynn, J. R. (2013). Arthur Robert Jensen. *Intelligence, 41,* 144–5.

Flynn, J. R. (2016). Does your family make you smarter? *Nature, Nurture, and Human Autonomy.* Cambridge University Press.

Moore, E. G. J. (1986). Family socialization and the IQ test performance of traditionally and transracially adopted black children. *Developmental Psychology, 22,* 317–26.

Patterson, O. (2006). *A poverty of the mind.* New York Times (Op-ed, Sunday, March 26, 2006).

Price, A. L., Tandon, A., Patterson, N., Barnes, K. C., Rafaels, N., Ruczinski, I., . . . Myers, S. (2009). Sensitive detection of chromosomal segments of distinct ancestry in admixed populations. *PLoS Genetics, 5,* 213–21.

Further Reading

Mill, J. S. (1859). *On Liberty.* London: John W. Parker & Son.

Rousseau, J.-J. (1979). *Emile, or On Education. Translation and notes by Allan Bloom.* New York: Basic Books.

Part VIII

Public Health Issues

Introduction

Public health ethics is concerned with ethical issues in public or community health. Simply put: problematic individual behavior has the potential to affect very large numbers of other people very quickly. Michael J. Selgelid reminds us of this in the introduction to his article "Ethics and Infectious Disease." The Black Death killed about 1/3 of Europe's population in the fourteenth century. At the heart of many problems in public health ethics is the vexing question of what limitations on individual freedoms are ethically defensible when the greater good of society is at stake. John Stuart Mill famously argued in his 1859 essay *On Liberty* (an extract from which appears in Part VII, Chapter 65, of this *Anthology*) that "the only purpose for which power can be rightfully exercised over any member of a civilized community, against his will is to prevent harm to others." Unfortunately, this does not help us a great deal, because the diseases we are concerned about in public health ethics will, if not contained, harm, and sometimes kill, many people. During the early stages of the 2020 crisis sparked by the spread of the novel coronavirus, known to scientists as SARS-CoV-2, disturbing videos circulated on social media showing Chinese officials in protective clothing forcibly dragging or carrying people out of buildings and putting them in vehicles to be quarantined. A Chinese government spokesperson defended the actions on the grounds that people who had the virus, or had been in close contact with others who had it, posed a threat to others, and if they resisted going into quarantine, they had to be compelled to do so.

Michael Selgelid's essay was written before the 2020 outbreak of COVID-19 put infectious disease into the headlines all over the world, but his contribution usefully lays out the territory of public health ethics. He explains the importance of looking at ethical issues in infectious diseases control, and provides a brief background discussion of the conflict between individual liberty and the greater good of society. He then proceeds to explain why some of the problems are also importantly problems of justice because they are inextricably linked to the living conditions of the world's poor and the world economic order that arguably gave rise to their plight.

Multiple drug resistant infectious diseases such as some strains of tuberculosis constitute significant public health threats. Jerome Amir Singh and colleagues, in their article "XDR-TB in South Africa: No Time for Denial or Complacency," look at (multiple)

Bioethics: An Anthology, Fourth Edition. Edited by Udo Schüklenk and Peter Singer.
Editorial material and organization © 2022 John Wiley & Sons, Inc. Published 2022 by John Wiley & Sons, Inc.

drug-resistant tuberculosis in South Africa. They consider it a serious threat to public health. Their article proposes that South Africa ought to consider temporary detainment of infected people to protect public health. They conclude, "forced isolation and confinement of individuals infected with XDR-TB and selected MDR-TB may be an appropriate and proportionate response in defined situations, given the extreme risk posed by both strains and the fact that less severe measures may be insufficient to safeguard public interest."

Although more than a decade has passed since this article was first published, XDR-TB remains a major health problem in South Africa, with Kwazulu-Natal province ranking among the worst-affected regions in the world for the disease.[1] The article's central argument could also be generalized to other diseases with a similar or greater ability to spread, and sufficiently serious implications for the population at risk.

Vijayaprasad Gopichandran, writing in the *Indian Journal of Medical Ethics*, focuses on the clinical ethics issues that arise in a global public health emergency such as the pandemic SARS-CoV-2. He notes the inherent conflict between public health responses that are population focused and clinical ethics that is patient focused. Patients suffer when 'infection control supersedes clinical care'. Gopichandran defends the use of experimental agents on compassionate grounds. Like Schüklenk in chapter 73 Gopichandran argues here that doctors' obligation to treat COVID-19 patients is contingent on reciprocity from the healthcare system in which they work. He urges policy makers to consider in their response to a threat like SARS-CoV-2 or Ebola virus the impact of their policies on all other patients.

Typically during flu season in many countries there is a heated public debate about whether we as individual citizens have a moral – and should possibly have a legal – obligation to get vaccinated. At issue is both the protection conferred on others by us being vaccinated, because our infection risk is significantly reduced, but also the eventual realization of herd immunity, which can be achieved when the number of vaccinated people is so large a proportion of the population that the disease does not have enough unvaccinated hosts to spread. Herd immunity thus provides protection even to the few who refuse to get vaccinated, either because in their health condition vaccination is contraindicated, or because of other objections that they may have. Alberto Giubilini, Thomas Douglas, and Julian Savulescu, in "The Moral Obligation to be Vaccinated: Utilitarianism, Contractualism and Collective Easy Rescue" contend that we have such an obligation. They argue first that utilitarianism, as well as two different types of deontological, or non-consequentialist, theories, support the view that there is an obligation to be vaccinated. They then acknowledge, however, that many people do not subscribe to any comprehensive ethical theory. Therefore they seek to justify the moral obligation to be vaccinated by appealing to a common intuition that they believe has a wide appeal: the rule of easy rescue, according to which if I can do something that, at relatively minor cost to me, would greatly benefit others, I have a moral obligation to do it. Giubilini and his colleagues then argue that this rule applies not only to individuals, but also to collectives. If a group of people can, at very low cost, provide the great good of herd immunity to others, it has a collective obligation to do so. Each individual member of the group then has an obligation to do his or her fair share of the burden of providing this good.

The last chapter in this Part, Neil Levy's "Taking Responsibility for Responsibility," shifts focus from infectious disease issues to non-communicable diseases like obesity. Levy is concerned about arguments that hold those suffering from so-called lifestyle diseases solely responsible for their predicament. He shows that there is a strong correlation between a person's socioeconomic status, and chronic disease, morbidity, and mortality. Low socioeconomic status is strongly correlated with higher likelihood of chronic disease. Levy argues that people of low socioeconomic status face many difficult-to-make choices in their daily lives, while at the same time struggling with a decreased capacity to make those choices. His analysis suggests that instead of focusing on ascertaining to what extent such people can be held responsible for their health-related predicaments, we ought to focus on the social determinants of health that are primarily responsible for these problems.

Reference

1   Thandi Kapwata et al., "Spatial distribution of extensively drug-resistant tuberculosis (XDR TB) patients in KwaZulu-Natal, South Africa," *PLOS One*, October 13, 2017. doi:10.1371/journal.pone.0181797

68

Ethics and Infectious Disease

Michael J. Selgelid

I Distribution of Research Resources

The '10/90 divide' is a phenomenon whereby 'less than 10 percent of [medical] research funds are spent on the diseases that account for 90% of the global burden of disease . . . [D]iseases affecting large proportions of humanity are given comparatively little attention.'[1] Because medical research so often aims at the promotion of profits rather than solutions to the world's most urgent medical problems, a majority of funds focus on the wants of a minority of the world's population – those who are relatively wealthy. As a result, health care is often unavailable to those who need it most.

A situation analogous to the 10/90 divide in medical research apparently holds true for research in bioethics. A quick flip through most bioethics texts and journals (or a visit to any number of websites) reveals attention on abortion, euthanasia, assisted reproduction, genetics, and doctor-patient relationships. To a large extent the issues examined one way or another involve advanced technologies or expensive interventions available primarily in wealthy developed nations. 'Distribution of resources' is a

common topic; but discussion here often (at least implicitly) concerns domestic allocation rather than issues of *international* justice. Greatly lacking, in comparison, is discussion of ethical issues involving infectious disease and the (related) health care situation in the developing world. Infectious diseases (such as AIDS, tuberculosis, and a variety of other emerging and reemerging pathogens) and the health care situation in developing countries pose some of the most serious problems of our times, but they have received relatively little attention from medical ethicists. In what follows I will (1) argue that the topic of infectious disease should be recognized as one of *the* most important topics for the discipline of bioethics, (2) briefly illustrate that it has received comparatively little attention from bioethicists,[2] and (3) attempt to explain why it has not received the attention it warrants.

II The Ethical Importance of Infectious Disease

The lack of bioethics discussion of infectious disease is both odd and unfortunate. Given that infectious

Original publication details: Michael J. Selgelid, "Ethics and Infectious Disease," pp. 272–289 from *Bioethics* 19: 3 (2005). Reproduced with permission of John Wiley & Sons.

Bioethics: An Anthology, Fourth Edition. Edited by Udo Schüklenk and Peter Singer.

disease was traditionally a – if not *the* – primary focus of medicine, for example, one would expect this to be obvious territory for a discipline concerned with 'medical ethics.'[3] More specific reasons why this should be recognized as one of the most relevant and important topics for bioethics are the following:

1. The historical and likely future consequences of infectious diseases are almost unrivalled,
2. Infectious diseases raise exceedingly difficult ethical questions of their own, and
3. The topic of infectious disease is closely connected to the topic of justice – which is a central concern of ethics.

1   Consequences

First, the paramount ethical importance of infectious diseases is illustrated by the fact that their consequences have been, and will likely continue to be, enormous. Epidemics have constituted some of the most catastrophic events in human history. The Black Death, for example, is famous for eliminating approximately one third of the European population between 1347 and 1350.[4] Another devastating epidemic occurred in 1918 when a nasty strain of influenza killed somewhere between 20 and 100 million people. According to the historian Alfred Crosby, the 1918 flu undoubtedly 'killed more humans than any other disease in a period of similar duration in the history of the world.'[5] Gina Kolata writes that the 1918 flu killed 'more Americans in a single year than died in battle in World War I, World War II, the Korean War, and the Vietnam War.'[6] (According to the *New York Times*, '[J]ust about everyone who has studied the disease says [that] a new pandemic is inevitable.')[7]

A third major killer, which has received high-profile attention in American newspapers recently, is smallpox. Smallpox allegedly killed more people in history than any other infectious disease. In the 20th Century alone it killed somewhere between 300 and 540 million people – or 'more than all the wars and epidemics [of that century] combined.'[8] Michael Oldstone claims that smallpox killed three times

more people during the 20th Century than were killed by all the wars of that period.[9] Although the disease was declared eradicated by the World Health Organization (WHO) in 1980, fears about smallpox have resurfaced. It has recently come to light that the Soviet Union, until its fall in the early 1990s, manufactured and froze tens of tons of smallpox for military purposes. Many are worried that stocks of the Soviet supply may have fallen into the hands of 'rogue nations' or terrorists. Experts claim that a smallpox bioterrorist attack could spark a catastrophic global epidemic now that the world population largely lacks immunity (because routine vaccination ended 20 or 30 years ago).[10] Modeling has shown that a smallpox attack could cause the devastation of (perhaps a series of) nuclear attack(s).

Smallpox aside, it is important to recognize that the enormous impact of infectious diseases is not just a matter of history. Infectious diseases are currently the world's largest 'killer[s] of children and young adults. They account for more than 13 million deaths a year – one in two deaths in developing countries.'[11] The rapidly growing HIV/AIDS epidemic perhaps provides the clearest illustration that infectious diseases continue to have the power of their past. AIDS is arguably 'the greatest health disaster in history.'[12] In 24 years, it has killed 20 million people (whereas the Black Death killed only 9 to 11 million people in Europe between 1346 and 1350).[13] HIV prevalence rates commonly exceed 30% (of adults) in sub-Saharan Africa, and similar scenarios may follow in parts of Asia and the former Soviet Union. As of 1999, anyway, only 5% of those infected could afford life-extending antiretroviral therapy.[14] In 2004, 3 million people died from AIDS, and 5 million people were newly infected with HIV. At the end of 2004, an estimated 39 million people were living with HIV.[15]

A related, but less well publicized, scenario involves the re-emergent spread of tuberculosis. Previously thought to be controlled, or at least considered controllable, TB was declared a global health emergency by the World Health Organization in 1993 and currently kills more people than ever before. 'Each year, 2 to 3 million people die from tuberculosis . . . despite the fact that the disease in its most common form is entirely preventable and treatable.'[16] One third of the world's population is infected with the latent form of the disease; and, a tenth of these are expected to develop active illness. 'It is estimated that between 2000 and 2020, nearly one billion people will be newly infected, 200 million people will get sick, and 35 million will die from TB – if control is not further strengthened.'[17] Of particular concern is the rise and spread of multi-drug resistant TB, resulting from the improper use of medication (in Russian prisons, for example).

The recent emergence and spread of SARS (Severe Acute Respiratory Syndrome) is, of course, the latest indicator that the impact of infectious diseases will continue to be severe. According to studies, the 'death rate from SARS may be . . . up to 55 percent in people 60 and older, and up to 13.2 percent in younger people . . . unless the numbers fall drastically, SARS would be among the infectious diseases with the highest death rates . . . By contrast, the influenza pandemic of 1918 . . . had an estimated mortality rate, overall, of 1 percent or less.'[18] In the meanwhile, there is no treatment, vaccine, or reliable diagnostic test for the SARS virus – which 'can survive on surfaces [such as doorknobs] for up to four days.'[19] Isolation, quarantine, travel advisories, travel restrictions, and related public health measures were put into effect; and the economic impact, alone, was staggering – '[j]ust a few weeks after SARS was identified, WHO [calculated] that the cost of the disease [was] already close to $30 billion.'[20]

It is now widely acknowledged that, in addition to posing global health and economic threats, AIDS and other infectious diseases threaten global security. Historical studies reveal that factors such as high infant mortality, low life expectancy, decreasing life expectancy, etc. – which are being severely affected in places like sub-Saharan Africa and the former Soviet Union – are among the most reliable indicators of major social upheaval. Given the serious historical and potential future consequences of infectious disease, it is no wonder that the CIA recently conducted (and published) a special investigation of *The Global Infectious Disease Threat and Its Implications for the United States.*[21] It is puzzling, on the other hand, that medical ethicists have not had more to say about infectious disease – compared to abortion, euthanasia, and genetics, for example, which have saturated the literature.

2   Difficult ethical questions

A second reason why infectious diseases warrant more of bioethics' attention is that they raise serious, difficult philosophical/ethical questions of their own. Obvious examples arise from the fact that infectious diseases can be contagious. Depending on the disease in question, infected individuals can threaten the health of other individuals or society as a whole. The public health measures required to protect other individuals and society from contagion (again, depending on the disease) might sometimes involve surveillance, mandatory testing, mandatory vaccination or treatment, notification of authorities or third parties, isolation (of individuals), quarantine (of entire regions), or travel restrictions. Because such public health care measures could infringe upon widely accepted basic human rights and liberties, we are here confronted with conflicting values.

An extremely difficult ethical question asks how, in situations of conflict, the utilitarian aim to promote the greater good in the way of public health should be balanced against libertarian aims to protect privacy and individual rights and liberties such as freedom of movement, and so on. Most philosophers, policy makers, and ordinary citizens would (upon reflection, I imagine) deny that *either* liberty or aggregate utility should *always* be given *absolute* priority over the other regardless of the degree (in terms of likelihood and severity) to which the other is threatened. So the challenge is to find a principled way of striking a balance between these presumably legitimate, but apparently conflicting, social aims in contexts involving diseases that are – to varying degrees[22] – contagious, deadly, or otherwise dangerous.[23] I will later say more about the difficulty of ethical issues raised by infectious disease.

3 Justice

Third, infectious disease should be recognized as a crucial topic for bioethics because the topic of infectious disease is closely connected to the topic of justice. Pathogens primarily prey upon the poor. Bad nutrition, dirty water, crowded living conditions, poor education, lack of access to basic medicines, disempowerment of women, and a complex host of other factors combine to make the populations of developing nations especially vulnerable to infectious diseases:

> Most deaths from infectious diseases occur in developing countries – the countries with the least money to spend on health care. In developing countries, about one third of the population – 1.3 billion people – live on incomes of less than $1 a day. Almost one in three children are malnourished. One in five are not immunized by their first birthday. And over one third of the world's population lack access to essential drugs.[24]

Today it is widely acknowledged that ailments called 'tropical diseases' are often not peculiar to tropical regions at all. To a large extent 'tropical diseases' are those that afflict poor developing countries, rather than necessarily tropical ones.[25] Sanitation, hygiene, vaccination, antibiotics, other drugs, and general improvements in living conditions have, in recent decades anyway, left privileged populations relatively sheltered from the scourges of the developing world.

Relationships between poverty and disease are well illustrated by the AIDS pandemic and the health care situation in Africa at the beginning of the 21st Century. Of the (roughly) 40 million people estimated to be living with HIV/AIDS in 2002, 28 million – or 70% – lived in sub-Saharan Africa.[26]

> [A]nd 95% [in 2001] live[d] in developing nations. Most of the infected people who live in these countries have no access to new or existing drugs for HIV/AIDS. But the problem of access to medications goes far beyond the HIV/AIDS pandemic: people in developing nations also cannot afford medications used to treat or prevent malaria, tuberculosis, cholera, dysentery, meningitis, and typhoid fever. The affordability problem also extends beyond a lack of access to new drugs designed to treat devastating, infectious diseases: 50% of people in developing nations do not have access to even basic medications, such as antibiotics, analgesics, broncho-dilators, decongestants, anti-inflammatory agents, anti-coagulants, or diuretics.[27]

The fact that those who are already worse-off in virtue of their poverty thus have their misfortunes compounded – as they are more likely to fall victim to disease – will strike most of us as an injustice in itself.[28] It seems especially unjust when the ailments that cause the already unfortunate to suffer and die are – sometimes easily and inexpensively – treatable or preventable with existing medications (that have often been developed at least partly through public funding). Egalitarians and utilitarians should agree on this point.

Poverty and (consequent) illness in many cases can also be attributed to what should be considered injustices even by staunch libertarians. As (one of) the wealthiest African nation(s), for example, South Africa should have been better able than its sub-Saharan neighbors to stave off AIDS. It has, however, famously failed to do so. This country has more HIV positive persons than any other country in the world; and, its (increasing) prevalence rate is estimated (from antenatal clinic data) to be almost 25% of adults.

> About 5 [million] South Africans are living with HIV and, at the current rate of infection, about half the country's teenagers under 15 can expect to contract it. By 2005 South Africa is likely to have about 1 [million] orphans.[29]

A recent Medical Research Council (MRC) report estimates that AIDS, which is already the leading cause of death in the country, will kill between four and seven million South Africans within a decade.[30]

This situation is not merely *unfortunate*. We here suffer social and political *injustice*. The facts that the current South African government (for mysterious reasons) consistently[31] but (apparently) illegitimately (1) challenged the causal link between HIV and

AIDS (and perhaps even the very existence of HIV and AIDS), (2) challenged the safety and efficacy of antiretroviral therapy, (3) suppressed scientific research which cast doubt on its HIV/AIDS stance,[32] (4) failed to provide inexpensive (or, in some cases, free) antiretroviral treatment to reduce the risk of mother-to-child transmission of HIV, (5) refused to comply with court orders requiring it to do so, (6) forbid provision of prophylactic antiretroviral therapy to rape victims (some of which were *gang-raped babies*, less than a year old),[33] and (7) over-spent on the military (in an apparently scandalous fashion) while under-spending on health care are only a part of what I have in mind.

The current state of AIDS in South Africa – and the government's failure to effectively deal with the situation – should also be attributed to wrongs with longer histories. The etiology of the AIDS epidemic is extremely complex; its present state is the result of a wide variety of social, political, economic, and historical factors. The new South African government's failure to ameliorate the situation is at least partly forgivable – or, in any case, explainable – by virtue of the fact that it had so many other enormous tasks to accomplish in the aftermath of apartheid. In addition to overhauling the political apparatus of the country, provision of decent education, housing, sanitation, and water to those who were victims of systematic racial oppression for decades – i.e. the vast majority of the population – posed monumental challenges for the new South African government. The shambles in which apartheid left this country is thus at least partly to blame for the health care *status quo*.[34] The fact that urbanization, overcrowded living conditions, migrant working conditions, poor education, fatalistic behavior, prostitution, and other ravishes of poverty (including poor nutrition, widespread infection with worms, and lack of treatment for other STDs[35]) each contribute to the AIDS epidemic – and are each (at least partly) the result of exploitative racist colonial oppressive practices – corroborates the point that the South African AIDS epidemic should largely be blamed on social injustice.

Similar things can be said about other developing nations where health care is compromised because of impoverishment resulting from colonialization, oppression, exploitation, protectionist trade policies, domestic corruption, failure of democracy, and so on. According to Solomon R. Benatar, for example, the poverty and consequent poor health of many in the developing world should be attributed to (militarization and) exploitative global economic activities involving irresponsible business practices of multinational corporations in particular. The result is a widening of the gap – in terms of both wealth and human rights protection – between the haves and have-nots.[36]

Pulitzer Prize-winning journalist Laurie Garrett provides an extreme example of the link between disease and injustice. In her recent book *Betrayal of Trust: The Collapse of Global Public Health*, she blames the famous 1995 Ebola (hemorrhagic fever) epidemic in Zaire (now the Democratic Republic of the Congo) on the corruption of the leader Mobutu who stole billions of dollars from public coffers, leaving public hospitals (which were primary *sources* of infection) in complete disarray and lacking the most basic supplies.

> Two things are clear: Ebola spread in Kikwit because the most basic, essential elements of public health were non-existent. And those exigencies were lacking in Kikwit – indeed, throughout Zaire – because Mobutu Sese Seko and his cronies had for three decades looted the national treasuries. Ebola haunted Zaire because of corruption and political repression . . . [Ebola's] emergence into human populations required the special assistance of humanity's greatest vices: greed, corruption, arrogance, tyranny, and callousness. What unfolded in Zaire in 1995 was not so much the rain forest terror widely depicted then in popular media worldwide as an inevitable outcome of disgraceful disconcern – even disdain – for the health of the Zairois public.[37]

Garrett implicates American meddling in the affair, insofar as the US government backed Mobutu and propped him into power. She insinuates CIA involvement with the murder of his predecessor Patrice Lumumba, unfavored because of supposedly socialist sympathies. In her earlier book *The Coming Plague: Newly Emerging Diseases in a World Out of Balance*,

Garrett suggests that the AIDS epidemic in Africa was at least partly fueled by the fact that underequipped hospitals in places like Congo sometimes had no choice but to use the same unsterilized syringes over and over and over again.

III   Why the Neglect?

Based on what I have said so far, one would expect that infectious disease would already be a typical topic of dedicated discussion in a discipline called 'medical ethics.' One would expect that there would be books on ethics and infectious disease and that articles and sections specifically devoted to ethical aspects of infectious diseases would be regular fare in bioethics journals and anthologies. In reality, however, 'infectious disease' is hardly found even in indexes of standard bioethics texts; and I have never seen a book on this general topic. An October 2002 Google (internet) search of the phrase 'ethics and infectious disease' yielded only 11 entries.[38] Six of these referred to a single project (of Margaret Battin), and some of the others were false positives. In March 2005 a similar search yielded 35 entries[39] – while a search of 'ethics and genetics' led to 5,100 entries.

1   High tech medicine

Why, then, has the topic been neglected by bioethics? It is likely that part of the explanation relates to the origins of the discipline of medical ethics itself. Although the roots of bioethics extend twenty-five hundred years back to the world of Hippocrates, bioethics' birth as an autonomous discipline is a relatively recent phenomenon. Medical ethics really came into its own during the last four or five decades, largely as a result of advancements in biological science and technology. With revolutionary developments in medical technology came unprecedented moral and policy dilemmas, and hence an academic discipline was born.[40] If this rough sketch of the birth of bioethics captures much truth, then there should be less surprise

that there has been a high-tech, wealthy-world slant to discussion within the discipline.

2   Optimism in medicine

A second probable reason why infectious disease has not received more attention of medical ethicists similarly relates to the timing of the birth of the discipline. The rise of bioethics coincided with a period of tremendous optimism in medicine. The development of antibiotics in the 1940's and the hugely successful Salk Polio vaccination program in the 1950's, and other developments such as the discovery of DDT, led the medical community to believe that infectious disease would soon be defeated through medical progress.[41] As early as

> 1948 U.S. Secretary of State George C. Marshall declared at the Washington, D.C., gathering of the Fourth International Congress on Tropical Medicine and Malaria that the conquest of all infectious diseases was imminent. Through a combination of enhanced crop yields to provide adequate food for humanity and scientific breakthroughs in microbe control, Marshall predicted, all the earth's microscopic scourges would be eliminated.[42]

In 1955 the World Health Organization decided to 'eliminate all malaria on the planet' via the eradication of mosquitoes with DDT. 'Few doubted that such a lofty goal was possible: nobody at the time could imagine a trend of worsening disease conditions; the arrow of history always pointed towards progress.'[43] 'By 1965, more than 25,000 different antibiotic products had been developed; physicians and scientists felt that bacterial diseases, and the microbes responsible, were no longer of great concern or of research interest.'[44] In 1967 U.S. Surgeon General William H. Stewart was so convinced of success that he told a White House gathering of health officers 'that it was time to close the book on infectious diseases and shift all national attention (and dollars) to what he termed "the New Dimensions" of health: chronic diseases.'[45] 'In 1972, the Nobel laureate Macfarlane Burnet concluded that "the most likely forecast about the future of infectious disease is that it will be very dull."[46] Fields such as bacteriology and parasitology appeared less important and subsequently fell out of vogue in the medical scientific community. The rise of medical ethics thus occurred at a time when it was popular – though perhaps hubristic – to think that infectious disease would no longer be a central concern of medicine. This presumably explains at least part of the neglect on the part of those concerned with medical ethics.

3 'The other'

AIDS, of course, has been on the scene for more than twenty years already – and thus overlaps with roughly half the lifespan of bioethics proper. And it has been clear for quite some time that malaria, TB, and other infectious diseases would not just disappear as planned. To the contrary, plenty of pathogens have developed more dangerous drug-resistant strains. And many morbid microbes – such as SARS and Ebola – have newly emerged during the last few decades.

A third reason why infectious diseases receive sparse discussion by academic ethicists is that they have likely been relegated as problems of 'the other.'[47] AIDS, for example, for a long time was, and perhaps still is, considered a problem for homosexuals, IV drug users, and poor black people in Africa. AIDS and other infectious diseases are, as has already been said, by far more prevalent in the developing world. Given that the vast majority of professional medical ethicists are straight, non-drug-injecting, relatively well-to-do whites who reside and work in wealthy developed nations, it should not be entirely unexpected that they have focused most on matters of more obvious central domestic concern, rather than problems of 'strangers' on the fringe of society and foreigners in faraway places. This third explanation involves both psychological and practical elements. Regarding the latter, (relatively conservative) university employers (and research funders) likely expect academic ethicists to focus most on pressing local issues rather than (radically) concentrating on international justice.[48] This has *explanatory* power, but I doubt it makes the

failure of medical ethicists to further discuss one of world's most consequential topics *excusable*. Ethics and morality essentially involve elements of impartiality; and, *tenured* professors, in any case, have substantial freedom to choose their topics.

4 Complexity

A fourth explanation of neglect by bioethicists relates to the complexity of the issues in question.[49] Traditional topics in medical ethics already require difficult interdisciplinary study. Expertise in both ethics and science are required to do bioethics well. Though many scholars have expertise in the discipline of ethics and many scholars expertise in scientific and technological aspects of biology and medicine, it is rare to find both kinds of expertise embodied in single individuals. One result is the relatively weak reputation of medical ethics within philosophical circles. Philosophers commonly complain about a 'low level' of discussion in medical ethics. This is attributed to the fact that (1) contributors with philosophical mastery in ethics often fail to get the science right and are thus unrealistic while (2) contributors with scientific backgrounds too often lack sufficient training in rigorous philosophical argumentation to get the ethics right, and (3) too few contributors are skilled enough in both areas to generate a consistently high level of discussion.

I have been discussing the challenging nature of the interdisciplinarity of medical ethics scholarship because I believe this difficulty is greatly exacerbated with discussion of infectious disease and the health care situation in the developing world. In addition to grounding in ethics and science/medicine (the latter of which is itself complicated by entry into the realm of epidemiology and drug-resistant pathogen emergence), we here need a greater grip on complex social, political, historic, and economic dynamics in order to *explain* – and thus comment upon the justice of – the current global healthcare situation.[50] A similarly broadened understanding is needed to realistically assess – and base moral/policy prescriptions upon – *predictions of impact*. Exploring the issues I have in mind requires more *empirical* work than most (medical) ethicists are likely to be trained for or accustomed to.[51] With regard to distribution of resource questions, confrontation with issues of international (rather than merely domestic) justice is an additional obvious way in which *theoretical* discussion is complicated.[52] The fact that infectious diseases do not respect international borders is just one of the ways in which the topic is inherently international. My fourth explanation, thus, is that questions concerning infectious disease and the healthcare situation in the developing world have been neglected by biomedical ethicists at least partly because of the *difficulty* of working on them.

5 Apparent ease

My fifth explanation, ironically, is that this area has been ignored because of a *misperception* that the questions raised are all-too-easy. The injustice of the situation, which has received substantial *media* attention at least, whereby AIDS medications are unavailable because they are unaffordable – at least partly because of prices set by profit-driven pharmaceutical companies – to populations in sub-Saharan Africa where they are by far needed most will strike many as a clear and blatant injustice. 'Of course this is wrong. Of course more should be done to make medication available to AIDS victims in Africa,' many might say, 'and you don't need to be a philosopher – or priest – to figure that out.' Questions about the justice of the health care situation in the developing world, where the innocent poor are sick and suffering, at first glance anyway, *appear* to lack the deep philosophical significance of questions upon which medical ethicists usually focus their attention.[53] Topics such as euthanasia and abortion, for example, raise what might look like deeper and more intellectually challenging issues: When is it morally permissible to kill another human being? What is a person? Upon what is the moral status of human beings based? What does quality of life consist in? Notice that emerging bioethical debates surrounding genetics and embryo/stem cell research often revolve around these same sorts of questions.

In comparison with these more theoretical (or perhaps *metaphysical*) questions, the injustice of a situation where tens of millions of (relatively innocent) people will soon suffer and die because they are too poor to buy medications might look like a no-brainer.

6 Religious hijacking

My final explanation of why infectious disease has not received more attention from bioethicists refers to the fact that bioethicists have been kept so occupied by discussion of *religious objections* to things like abortion, euthanasia, cloning, stem cell research, and so on. Contrary to Paul Farmer,[54] my own belief is that most bioethicists *are* (at heart, anyway) genuinely concerned about issues of justice. Liberal-minded bioethicists presumably would have focused much more attention on the topic of infectious disease and the injustice of the health care situation in the developing world if they hadn't been kept so busy battling the illiberal policy agenda (regarding abortion, euthanasia, cloning, stem cell research, etc.) advocated by the church.[55] Debate in bioethics has thus, to a large extent, been hijacked by religion.

Conclusion

I have offered six explanations of why ethical issues associated with infectious disease (and the related health care situation in the developing world) have not been more prominent in medical ethics literature. I have suggested that this is the case roughly because (1) bioethics was born (as an autonomous discipline) with advances in medical technology and thus has largely focused on these, (2) bioethics' birth and initial development (as an autonomous discipline) came at a time when it was believed that infectious disease would be conquered by medicine, (3) infectious diseases are often seen as problems of others, (4) bioethical research on infectious disease in the developing world is especially difficult because it is so empirical and interdisciplinary, (5) ethical questions about infectious disease (in the developing world) might not *appear* to pose the kinds of deep philosophical questions that academic ethicists are interested in, and (6) bioethics debate has been hijacked by the church. These are just suggestions; and this list is not meant to be exhaustive. Rather than choosing between these alternative explanations, I believe that they each likely capture *parts* of the story we are after. In any case, as argued above, it would be entirely wrong to explain the lack of discussion of infectious diseases by denying their central importance and/or relevance to the discipline of bioethics.

Notes

A version of this paper was presented at the VI World Congress of Bioethics, Brasilia, Brazil, October 2002.

1   K. Lee, and A. Mills. Strengthening Governance for Global Health Research. *British Medical Journal* 2000; 321: 775–6, at http://www.bmj.com/cgi/content/full/321/7264/775.

2   Although I shall not in this article discuss this point at great length, others who have worked in this area, such as Margaret Battin and Solomon Benatar, have agreed that it is quite correct. A similar point is made by (especially Chapter 8 of) P. Farmer. 2003. *Pathologies of Power: Health, Human Rights, and the New War on the Poor.* Los Angeles. University of California Press.

3   I shall use the expressions 'bioethics', 'biomedical ethics', and 'medical ethics', interchangeably.

4   P. Ziegler. 1969. *The Black Death.* London. Penguin.

5   A.W. Crosby. 1989. *America's Forgotten Epidemic: The Influenza of 1918.* Cambridge, UK. Cambridge University Press: 203.

6   G. Kolata. 1999. *Flu.* London. Pan Books: xii.

7   B. Gewen. 'The Great Influenza' and 'Microbial Threats to Health': Virus Alert. *The New York Times* March 14, 2004, available at: http://www.nytimes.com/2004/03/14/books/review/14GEWENT.html.

8   J. Miller, S. Engelberg & W. Broad. 2001. *Germs: The Ultimate Weapon.* London. Simon and Schuster: 58.

9   M.B.A. Oldstone. 1998. *Viruses, Plagues, and History.* New York. Oxford University Press: 3.

10 For more on smallpox, see M.J. Selgelid. Smallpox Revisited? *American Journal of Bioethics* 2003; 3, 1; and M.J. Selgelid. Bioterrorism and Smallpox Planning: Information and Voluntary Vaccination. *Journal of Medical Ethics* 2004; 30, 6: 558–560; available at http://jme.bmjjournals.com/cgi/reprint/30/6/558, accessed 1 March 2005.

11 World Health Organization. 1999. *Removing Obstacles to Healthy Development: Report on Infectious Diseases.* Geneva: WHO. At http://apps.who.int/iris/handle/10665/65847.

12 C. Gilbert. AIDS Draws New Attention. *Milwaukee Journal Sentinel*, 15 April, 2002.

13 L. Garrett. 2000. *Betrayal of Trust: The Collapse of Global Public Health.* New York. Hyperion: 474.

14 Ibid., p. 473.

15 UNAIDS: AIDS Epidemic Update, 2004. Available at www.unaids.org.

16 L.B. Reichman and J.H. Tanne. 2002. *Timebomb: The Global Epidemic of Multi-Drug-Resistant Tuberculosis.* New York. McGraw Hill: x–xi. See also P. Farmer. 1999. *Infections and Inequalities: The Modern Plagues.* Berkeley, CA. University of California Press.

17 World Health Organization. Tuberculosis, Fact Sheet No. 104, revised April 2000, p. 1.

18 L.K. Altman. Death Rate from SARS is Revised Upward. *International Herald Tribune* May 8, 2003.

19 Ibid.

20 Kickbusch. A Wake-Up Call for Global Health. *International Herald Tribune* April 29, 2003.

21 One conclusion of the report is that we should perhaps worry most about new infectious diseases – more dangerous than AIDS – likely to emerge in the future.

22 I highlight variation in severity to suggest that there is likely no simple, obvious answer to this question. I should here point out the practical importance, in addition to theoretical difficulty, of this kind of question. It is now widely acknowledged, for example, that quarantine policy is outdated and in need of revision. Biodefense planning and the emergence of SARS provide the most recent illustrations of the immediate importance of this issue.

23 This topic, of course, has not been altogether ignored. For discussion in the context of AIDS see U. Schüklenk. 1998. AIDS: Individual and 'Public' Interests, in *A Companion to Bioethics,* P. Singer & H. Kuhse. eds.

Oxford, UK. Blackwell: 343–54. For recent discussion of quarantine policy in light of the smallpox bioterrorist threat, see G.J. Annas. Bioterrorism, Public Health, and Civil Liberties. *The New England Journal of Medicine* 2002; 346: 1337–42.

24 World Health Organization, *Removing Obstacles to Health Department.*

25 N.L. Stepan. 2001. *Picturing Tropical Nature.* Ithaca, NY. Cornell University Press; L. Garrett. 1994. *The Coming Plague: Newly Emerging Diseases in a World Out of Balance.* New York. Penguin.

26 Gilbert, AIDS Draws New Attention.

27 D.B. Resnik. Developing Drugs for the Developing World: An Economic, Legal, Moral, and Political Dilemma. *Developing World Bioethics* 2001; 1: 11.

28 Others, to the contrary, might claim that this situation is 'unfortunate' but not necessarily 'unfair' or 'unjust'.

29 Fighting Back. *The Economist* May 11–17, 2002, 27.

30 R. Dorrington, D. Bourne, D. Bradshaw, R. Laubscher & I.M. Timaeus. The Impact of HIV/AIDS on Adult Mortality in South Africa. Burden of Disease Research Unit, Medical Research Council of South Africa.

31 At the time of this writing the South African Government appears to finally be changing its stance on HIV/AIDS.

32 This seemed to occur with regard to the above-mentioned MRC Report, for example.

33 Note that points (4)–(6), at least, appear to conflict with the South African constitution by failing to respect what are recognized as human rights here. The same thing may be said about the failure to provide antiretrovirals to HIV-positive South Africans more generally speaking.

34 See D. Webb. 1997. *HIV and AIDS in Africa.* London. Pluto Press; A. Whiteside & C. Sunter. 2000. *AIDS: The Challenge for South* Africa. Cape Town. Human & Rousseau; H. Marais. 2000. *To the Edge: AIDS Review 2000.* Pretoria, South Africa. University of Pretoria, Centre for the Study of AIDS.

35 Increased risk of HIV infection results, for example, in the presence of other untreated STDs or when immune systems are weakened from poor nutrition or infection with worms.

36 S.R. Benatar. Global Disparities in Health and Human Rights: A Critical Commentary. *American Journal of Public Health* 1998; 88: 295–300.

37 Garrett, *Betrayal of Trust,* p. 59.

38 Search conducted on October 30, 2002 at www.google.com.

39 Many of these referred to a more recent work of Ronald Bayer. There have of course been books and anthology sections on ethical issues associated with AIDS in particular. And Internet searches of 'Ethics and AIDS', as was pointed out by Peter Singer in discussion, will yield more results – i.e. 408 results on 1 March 2005. The fact remains, however, that discussion of infectious diseases in general (which would likely inform discussion of particular diseases such as AIDS) is lacking. In my opinion even AIDS – with the exception of doctor–patient relationship issues (especially the 'duty to treat') and AIDS-related international research ethics (especially the debate over 'standards of care') – has not received adequate attention in mainstream bioethics literature, given the magnitude of the problem. On 1 March 2005, in any case, a Google search of 'ethics and tuberculosis' yielded only 42 results (though tuberculosis kills two or three million persons per year) and 'ethics and malaria' yielded zero (though malaria kills one million per year). On the same date, 'ethics and stem cells' yielded 440 results – despite the newness of stem cell research (in comparison with AIDS).

40 The development of elaborate life-sustaining technologies made the question of euthanasia, for example, more urgent. I should note that – in addition to technological advance – the birth of bioethics was also importantly related to the civil rights movement of the 1960s. See H. Kuhse and P. Singer. 1998. What is Bioethics? A Historical Introduction, in *A Companion to Bioethics*, P. Singer and H. Kuhse eds. Oxford, UK. Blackwell: 3–11.

41 See Garrett, *The Coming Plague*, pp. 30–52, esp. pp. 30–1.

42 Ibid., pp. 30–1.

43 Ibid., p. 31. Not only did it fail, but this program was somewhat counter-productive. DDT-resistant mosquitoes returned in higher numbers than before; and misuse of medication promoted drug-resistant strains of malaria. By '1975 the worldwide incidence of malaria was about 2.5 times what it had been in 1961 . . . A new global iatrogenic form of malaria was emerging – "iatrogenic" meaning created as a result of medical treatment. In its well-meaning zeal to treat the world's malaria scourge, humanity had created a new epidemic' (p. 52).

44 Ibid., p. 36.

45 Ibid., p. 33.

46 Gewen, 'The Great Influenza'.

47 See H. Joffe. 1999. *Risk and the Other.* Cambridge, U.K. Cambridge University Press; & N.L. Stepan, *Picturing Tropical Nature,* for discussions of how AIDS and

tropical diseases, respectively, are regularly understood and portrayed as problems of others.

48 Udo Schüklenk suggested this point in conversation.

49 This was (independently) suggested by Mary Tjiattas. Peter Singer concurred in conversation.

50 I do not mean to imply that other issues in bioethics do not require appreciation of social, political, historical, and economic phenomena. My point is one of degree: assessment of the health care situation in the developing world *often* requires substantially *more* contact with these other disciplines. Others who have worked in this area will agree.

51 For further illustration of what I here have in mind see M.J. Selgelid. Ethics, Economics, and AIDS in Africa. *Developing World Bioethics* 2004; 4, 1: 96–105.

52 See D. Moellendorf. 2002. *Cosmopolitan Justice.* Boulder, Colorado. Westview Press.

53 This objection was (independently) raised by Julian Savulescu in discussion.

54 In discussion.

55 James William Ley, philosophy PhD student at the University of Sydney, encouraged explicit inclusion of this point.

69

XDR-TB in South Africa

No Time for Denial or Complacency

Jerome Amir Singh, Ross Upshur, and Nesri Padayatchi

On September 1, 2006, the World Health Organization (WHO) announced that a deadly new strain of extensively drug-resistant tuberculosis (XDR-TB) had been detected in Tugela Ferry (Figure 69.1), a rural town in the South African province of KwaZulu-Natal (KZN),[1] the epicentre of South Africa's HIV/AIDS epidemic. Of the 544 patients studied in the area in 2005, 221 had multi-drug-resistant tuberculosis (MDR-TB), that is, *Mycobacterium tuberculosis* that is resistant to at least rifampicin and isoniazid. Of these 221 cases, 53 were identified as XDR-TB (see Table 69.1 and [2]), i.e., MDR-TB plus resistance to at least three of the six classes of second-line agents.[3] This reportedly represents almost one-sixth of all known XDR-TB cases reported worldwide.[4] Of the 53, 44 were tested for HIV and all were HIV infected.

The median survival from the time of sputum specimen collection was 16 days for 52 of the 53 infected individuals, including six health workers and those reportedly taking antiretrovirals.[2] Such a fatality rate for XDR-TB, especially within such a relatively short period of time, is unprecedented anywhere in the world.

The Threat to Regional and Global Health

South Africa is one of the world's fastest growing tourist destinations,[5] home to millions of migrant labourers from neighbouring countries, and its ports and roads service several other African countries. Seroprevalence rates for HIV in South Africa, and in adjoining nations such as Lesotho and Swaziland, are very high. Cumulatively, these factors make for a potentially explosive international health crisis.

The threat to regional and global public health is thus clear,[6] and further underlined by reports that XDR-TB is now considered endemic to KZN,[7] as it has been reported in at least 39 hospitals throughout the province[8] and in other parts of the country.[9–11] At least 30 new cases of XDR-TB are reportedly detected each month in KZN alone.[12]

Original publication details: Jerome Amir Singh, Ross Upshur, and Nesri Padayatchi, "XDR-TB in South Africa: No Time for Denial or Complacency," PLoS Medicine 4: 1 (2007): e50. © 2007 Singh et al. Open access / CC BY 4.0.

Bioethics: An Anthology, Fourth Edition. Edited by Udo Schüklenk and Peter Singer.
Editorial material and organization © 2022 John Wiley & Sons, Inc. Published 2022 by John Wiley & Sons, Inc.

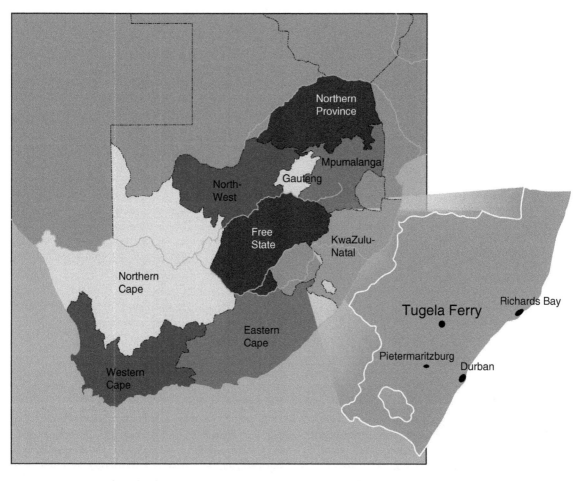

Figure 69.1   Map of South Africa showing Tugela Ferry in the province of KwaZulu-Natal, the epicentre of South Africa's HIV/AIDS epidemic

The True Extent of the Problem

Diagnosed cases of XDR-TB likely represent a small proportion of the true extent of the problem. The number of persons harbouring latent infections is unknown (and likely unknowable at present). Official statistics also likely underestimate the true prevalence of XDR-TB, as the current national TB guidelines prescribe the conditions under which *M. tuberculosis* susceptibility testing should be done.[13] These guidelines recommend susceptibility testing for those patients who have previously been treated for TB or fail to respond to treatment after two months of TB treatment, at which point there is a high treatment interruption rate. In addition, specialised laboratory facilities are required for such testing. Routine sputum culture and susceptibility testing of all patients suspected as having TB should form part of a multi-faceted approach to identifying and addressing TB drug resistance.

In recognition of the global threat posed by these factors, on September 9, 2006, WHO urged a response

Table 69.1 Characteristics of patients in South Africa with XDR-TB

Characteristic	No. (%)
Tuberculosis (TB) characteristics ($n = 53$):	
Pulmonary TB alone	40 (75%)
Pulmonary and extrapulmonary TB	13 (25%)
Sputum-smear positive	42 (79%)
Sputum-smear negative	11 (21%)
Previous TB treatment ($n = 47$):	
No previous treatment	26 (55%)
Previous treatment: cure or completed treatment	14 (30%)
Treatment default or failure	7 (15%)
Previous admission in past 2 y ($n = 42$)	
Admission for any cause	28 (67%)
No previous admission	14 (33%)

Data from Gandhi N.R., Moll A., Sturm A.W., Pawinski R., Govender T., et al. (2006) Extensively drug-resistant tuberculosis as a cause of death in patients co-infected with tuberculosis and HIV in a rural area of South Africa. *Lancet* 368: 1575–80. doi:10.1371/journal.pmed.0040050.t001

to the outbreak akin to recent global efforts to control severe acute respiratory syndrome (SARS) and bird flu.[14] The South African government's initial lethargic reaction to the crisis[15,16] and uncertainty amongst South African health professionals concerning the ethical, social, and human rights implications of effectively tackling this outbreak[17,18] highlight the urgent need to address these issues lest doubt and inaction spawn a full-blown XDR-TB epidemic in South Africa and beyond.

Factors Fuelling the Outbreak

Several well-documented factors, including high treatment interruption rates of drug-sensitive TB and consequent low cure rates, together with the HIV epidemic, have contributed to the emergence of MDR-TB and XDR-TB in South Africa and merit urgent remediation. For instance, the development of drug resistance may result from inappropriate treatment regimens (e.g., choice of drugs, dosage, duration of treatment), programme factors (e.g., irregular drug supply, incompetent health personnel), and patient

factors (e.g., poor adherence, mal-absorption). In fact, it could be said that the emergence of MDR-TB itself is evidence of the systematic failure of the global community to tackle a curable disease.

The factors that facilitate the spread of tuberculosis are well known and abundantly present in sub-Saharan Africa. Alongside inadequate healthcare system response, poverty and global inequity contribute to the worsening of the global TB situation.[19,20] According to South Africa's Medical Research Council, about half of adults in South Africa with active TB are cured each year, compared with 80% in countries with better resources. Moreover, nationally, about 15% of patients default on the first-line six-month treatment, while almost a third of patients default on second-line treatmen.[21] This highlights the urgent need for the health system (which includes health-care workers) to reinforce the DOTS (directly observed treatment, short-course) and DOTS-plus strategy, to revise current adherence counselling and public information strategies, and to actively promote avoidance of a "victim blaming approach". The emergence of MDR-TB and XDR-TB is an indicator of the poor implementation of South Africa's TB Control Programme.

A neglected but significant factor fuelling the MDR-TB and XDR-TB outbreaks in South Africa[22] is the lack of infection control in institutions, including the lack of simple administrative measures such as triaging of patients, as well as more sophisticated expensive environmental control measures, such as negative pressure rooms and personal respiratory protection (respirators). Infection control must be addressed in order to reduce the nosocomial transmission of these infections.

In the modern era, tuberculosis is recognised as a disease that preys upon social disadvantage.[23,24] Thus, the inadvertent deterrent impact that health and social welfare policies are having on the hospitalisation of such patients needs to be explored. Currently, 10 million South Africans – almost one in four citizens – are beneficiaries of some form of social welfare.[25] With unemployment in South Africa conservatively estimated at about 27% of the population,[26] social welfare grants often constitute the sole or primary income of many households. While South Africa does not have a formal universal health-care system, those who require but who cannot afford to pay for hospitalisation are often treated free of charge in the public sector.[27] However, current government policy stipulates that those who are hospitalised at state expense lose their social welfare benefits for the duration of their hospitalisation.

Faced with the prospect of being deprived of their gainful employment and/or having their welfare benefits suspended for the duration of hospitalisation – which in the case of MDR-TB or XDR-TB could last 18–24 months – many MDR-TB patients opt not to stay in hospitals, where their treatment adherence and resistance profile could be closely monitored by health personnel. Instead, understandably, these highly infectious individuals fail to receive appropriate therapy and are likely to default on adherence. They mix broadly in society among non-infected individuals, typically utilise public transport, and seek or continue their gainful employment. In so doing, they pose a significant public health risk to their families, co-workers, local community, and the wider public they encounter.

Given the cost of trying to manage a MDR-TB or XDR-TB epidemic,[28] the South African government ought to rethink its policy of suspending welfare benefits to patients with MDR-TB or XDR-TB for the duration of their hospitalisation. Moreover, it ought to consider extending welfare benefits to those infected patients who are gainfully employed as an incentive to draw such patients into the health system so that their adherence to anti-TB medication and resistance profile can be monitored. Although these measures will undoubtedly have cost implications for the government and may not adequately compensate patients for their lost income, they would at least serve as some form of incentive and encouragement for infected individuals to enter and remain in the health system, although admittedly, their confinement could conceivably be indefinite or until they die. It would also be a partial realisation of the reciprocity principle, which we explore below.

Factors That Could Undermine Efforts to Tackle the Outbreak

Several factors threaten to stymie efforts to control the XDR-TB outbreak in South Africa. Drug resistance can only be detected if a patient presents to the health system, a health-care worker suspects TB, an appropriate specimen is taken, facilities exist for smear and cultures, and if laboratories are equipped to do drug susceptibility testing. Moreover, because most hospital beds in South Africa are occupied by patients infected with opportunistic infections associated with HIV/AIDS, there is little or no spare capacity to accommodate patients with MDR-TB and XDR-TB. However, given the airborne transmission of TB and the grave threat that MDR-TB and XDR-TB pose immediately to such immunocompromised patients and, if the spread of XDR-TB is not abated, to global health, the government ought to reconsider its prioritisation of hospital resources. It seems that, at minimum, patients with XDR-TB requiring inpatient care should be housed in facilities independent both of patients with MDR-TB and patients who are immunocompromised. The containment of infectious patients with XDR-TB may arguably take precedence over any other patients not infected with highly infectious and deadly airborne diseases, including those with full-blown AIDS. This is an issue requiring urgent attention from the global community.

Is There a Role for Involuntary Detention?

The successful containment of TB, MDR-TB, and XDR-TB in South Africa and elsewhere carries human rights[29] and ethical implications. An important question that we must come to terms with is the extent to which judicially sanctioned restrictive measures should be employed to bring about control of what could develop into a lethal global pandemic.

As diagnosis of MDR-TB and XDR-TB can take several weeks, questions remain about what to do with patients suspected of being infected with MDR-TB or XDR-TB while awaiting susceptibility results. And once patients have been determined to be infected, there are questions about how long and how closely their clinical status should be monitored and under what conditions. Ideally, patients suspected of having TB should be isolated in an acute infectious diseases setting while awaiting anti-tuberculosis drug-susceptibility testing, and then triaged for further management based on these results. Current WHO guidelines recognise that this strategy is not feasible in resource-constrained environments. WHO recommends that persons with MDR-TB voluntarily refrain from mixing with the general public and from those susceptible to infection, while they are infectious and in ambulatory care.[30] The document is silent on what steps to take should such voluntary measures fail.

The emergence of XDR-TB indicates that the WHO strategy of allowing the patient to assume responsibility for mixing with the general public may be too permissive and more attention to strategies of infection control in the community is required. In general, from both an ethical and legal perspective, measures that rely on voluntary cooperation and are the least restrictive in terms of interfering with human rights are preferred. However, if such measures prove to be ineffective, then more restrictive measures may need to be contemplated. Such measures should be taken with due consideration for the possibility that they may increase disincentives to seek care. However, if due care is taken to provide for the rights and needs of those so detained and therapeutic goals are kept paramount, such measures could play an important role in containing XDR-TB before it spreads more generally in the population globally.

The use of involuntary detention may legitimately be countenanced as a means to assure isolation and prevent infected individuals possibly spreading infection to others. However, South African officials have raised human rights concerns in dealing with the country's XDR-TB and MDR-TB outbreaks,[18] although they have conceded that forcible treatment may be a viable option in tackling the outbreak.[31] Health workers and human rights advocates in South Africa and elsewhere

must be reminded that although a country's Bill of Rights may bestow a range of human rights on individuals, these rights can usually be restricted if doing so is reasonable and justifiable. They should be made aware of any national laws and municipal by-laws that permit the provision of involuntary treatment and isolation measures in the interests of public health.

Moreover, the judiciary often has the authority to issue orders compelling involuntary confinement/ hospitalisation and treatment, even against the wishes of an affected party, if doing so is in the public interest. This option should only be invoked if non-coercive measures have failed. Such an approach has been endorsed by the European Court on Human Rights (ECHR) in *Enhorn v. Sweden*.[32] The applicant in this case was an HIV-infected man who had infected another party and disobeyed the instructions of public health officials to desist from irresponsible and risky behaviour. The man complained to the ECHR that the compulsory isolation orders and his involuntary detention in a hospital had been in breach of Article 5(1) of the European Convention for the Protection of Human Rights and Fundamental Freedoms. This article states that "Everyone has the right to liberty and security of the person. No one shall be deprived of his liberty save in the following cases and in accordance with a procedure prescribed by law". Section 5(1)(e) provides for the situation at hand: "the lawful detention of persons for the prevention of the spreading of infectious diseases".

The applicant argued that the substantive provisions of Article 5 were not made out in his case, given that the detention did not constitute a proportionate response to the need to prevent the spread of infectious disease. The court held that any such detention must be in compliance with both the principle of proportionality and the requirement that there be an "absence of arbitrariness" such that other less severe measures have been considered and found to be insufficient to safeguard the individual and the public. This would entail that the deprivation of liberty was necessary in all circumstances.[33]

Moreover, for detention to comply with principles of proportionality and freedom from arbitrariness, it must be established that the detained person is suffering from an infectious disease, that the spread of disease is dangerous to public safety, and that the detention of the infected person is the last resort measure in order to prevent disease spread. The court ruled that the institution of detention for infectious disease must be appropriate to the nature of the disease. Where these conditions are satisfied, deprivation of liberty is justified, both on grounds of public policy and in order to provide medical treatment to the affected party. In ruling in favour of the applicant the court found that the compulsory isolation of the applicant by Swedish authorities ought to have been considered only as a last resort in order to prevent him from spreading HIV after less severe measures had been considered and found to be insufficient to safeguard the public interest. We believe that the forced isolation and confinement of individuals infected with XDR-TB and selected MDR-TB may be an appropriate and proportionate response in defined situations, given the extreme risk posed by both strains and the fact that less severe measures may be insufficient to safeguard public interest. Patients with XDR-TB should also be quarantined separately from those with MDR-TB, as the latter is potentially curable.

Although the justness and effectiveness of forcibly confining and treating patients with TB[34,35] has been called into question,[36] such an approach has met with some degree of success in the US,[37] where it helped bring down TB infection rates in states such as New York in the 1990s.[38] We would not argue for forcible treatment of patients with MDR-TB or XDR-TB, simply restriction of mobility rights of such individuals.

Emulation of New York's aforementioned successful approach in controlling its TB outbreak could empower health officials in South Africa and elsewhere to act decisively in tackling emerging XDR-TB and MDR-TB outbreaks. The consequences of not educating health workers of the state's powers in such instances were highlighted on September 12, 2006, in Johannesburg, Africa's commercial and air transport hub, when health workers allowed a patient diagnosed with XDR-TB, who refused to be hospitalised, to discharge herself. Although this patient was eventually traced and forcibly hospitalised five days after her self-discharge,[39] it remains unknown how many people she may have infected in the months between her sputum sample being taken and her eventual diagnosis in September 2006, and before she was traced after her self-discharge.

Questions also remain about how authorities should deal with patients with MDR-TB whom treatment has failed to cure as well as patients with XDR-TB in whom cure is unlikely as few active drugs remain. While isolating such patients until they die – which in the case of the slightly less deadly MDR-TB could be years – has been described as "ethically questionable and impractical,"[21] this option may, of necessity, need to be countenanced. It is not, *a priori*, unethical to restrict the movement of those whose infection poses risks to public health. It is a matter of what types of safeguards are put in place to assure the legitimacy of such acts.

There are many such justifications emerging in the field of public health ethics that recognise that prevention of harm and protection of public health are legitimate ethical norms.[40-42] Human rights doctrine also recognises the limitation of many rights in a public health emergency, provided the measures employed are legitimate, non-arbitrary, publicly rendered, and necessary. In this regard, section 25 of the Siracusa Principles on the Limitation and Derogation of Provisions in the International Covenant on Civil and Political Rights holds: "Public health may be invoked as a ground for limiting certain rights in order to allow a state to take measures dealing with a serious threat to the health of the population or individual members of the population. These measures must be specifically aimed at preventing disease or injury or providing care for the sick and injured."[43] It must be assured that detained individuals have appropriate legal council, and given the uncertainty of the duration of restrictions required, duly constituted independent tribunals could be established to oversee the process. At issue from a human rights perspective is whether such prolonged isolation represents the least restrictive means to achieve this goal and the extent of the belief in the severity of the threat. We do not intend to resolve this issue presently, but believe it is worth tabling for broader debate.

The use of legally sanctioned restrictive measures for the control of XDR-TB should not obscure the fact that being infected is not a crime. A strong reciprocal obligation is borne by authorities so wishing to invoke these measures. Those who are isolated require humane and decent living conditions. In fact the restriction of their liberties is more for a collective good than for their own. Thus every effort must be made to ensure conditions of living that preserve dignity. Harris and Holm have argued that all people with a communicable disease have a duty not to infect others. They stress, however, that "[i]t is . . . also a duty which we can expect people to discharge *only if they live in a community that does not leave them with all the burdens involved in discharging this duty*"[38] (italics ours). The task of global health is to help create these communities.

Conclusion

XDR-TB is a serious global health threat. It has the potential to derail the global efforts to contain HIV/AIDS, as broadly disseminated XDR-TB will prove to be a much more serious public health threat owing to its mode of transmission. The emergence of XDR-TB is also an uncomfortable reminder of the failure of health systems to control problems at a tractable scale. If, in the recent past, TB were to have been adequately managed when it was completely drug sensitive, we would not be in such a dire situation as is currently the case. This failure rests upon us all. We should begin to contemplate the response when we move to the predictable next phase: completely drug-resistant tuberculosis.

By December 1, 2006 – World AIDS Day – South Africa had reported more than 300 cases of XDR-TB[44] (based on the latest definition of XDR-TB, i.e., resistance to at least rifampicin and isoniazid, with resistance to one of the injectable drugs [kanamycin, amikacin, capreomycin] and one of the quinolones).

Given the South African government's poor track record in dealing with the country's HIV/AIDS epidemic and what is at stake if it adopts a similar lethargic and denialist response to the country's XDR-TB outbreak, the international community must be vigilant in monitoring the government's response to this emerging crisis. Although recent initiatives of the government[45,46] and the Medical Research Council of South Africa[28,47] are encouraging, these will hopefully not inspire complacency amongst officials.

While it is encouraging that the South African government invited the WHO to an October 2006 meeting on the emerging crisis,[48] it is worth noting that neither party raised the human rights and ethical dimensions of controlling the outbreak. Containing XDR-TB and selected MDR-TB will require an interdisciplinary approach[49] and the synergistic cooperation of all organs of the state, including, in particular, the judiciary, as well as various government departments. Moreover, the government should urgently consider devising strategies to control the disease amongst particularly high-risk groups such as prisoners and migrant labourers, which might necessitate the involvement of prisoner advocacy groups and neighbouring countries, respectively.

If WHO is sincere in calling for the XDR-TB outbreak in South Africa to be treated in the same light as SARS and bird flu, then global efforts to develop rapid diagnostic tests and novel treatment regimens must be stepped up. In addition to drug development, the appropriateness of using these technologies in countries with TB/HIV epidemics needs to be explored. The determination of XDR-TB requires specialised laboratories and quality assurance, particularly when testing for resistance to second-line antituberculosis agents. Moreover, while the diagnosis of MDR-TB may take weeks or months, new technologies, including liquid culture and PCR probes, can reduce this time. Efforts must be stepped up to sponsor and equip poor countries to address these challenges. Depending on how successfully the South African government controls the outbreak, as in the case of SARS, infection monitoring at hospitals, border posts, and airports may become necessary.

Given the ethical and legal implications of these measures, the experience of countries that were affected by SARS[50] could prove valuable in guiding South Africa to deal with its XDR-TB outbreak. Admittedly though, more is known of XDR-TB than was the case with SARS when it first emerged. In the meantime, South Africa must urgently reduce crowding in hospitals where patients with TB are being treated to reduce the risk of the infection spreading, drastically expand its surveillance of the disease, and rethink its current counselling, treatment, reporting, and tracing strategies. It must also devise measures to reduce contact between patients with TB and those suspected or confirmed with MDR-TB and XDR-TB in the weeks or months it takes to diagnose the latter two infections. It must also devise appropriate infection-prevention strategies for health workers treating such patients.

All reasonable attempts must be made to accommodate the interests of infected patients in a sensitive and humane manner, although, if necessary, the government must adopt a more robust approach towards uncooperative patients with MDR-TB and XDR-TB, which might necessitate favouring the interests of the wider public over that of the patient. Although such an approach might interfere with the patient's right to autonomy and will undoubtedly have human rights implications, such measures are reasonable and justifiable, and must be seen in a utilitarian perspective. Ultimately in such crises, the interests of public health must prevail over the rights of the individual.

References

1 South African Press Association (2006 September 1). New deadly TB strain detected in SA. Available: http://www.iol.co.za/news/south-africa/new-deadly-tb-strain-detected-in-sa-1.292028#.VYVW0PlVhBc.

2 Gandhi N., Moll A., Pawinski R., Zeller K., Lalloo U., et al. (2006) Favorable outcomes of integration of TB and HIV treatment in a rural South Africa: The Sizonqoba study [abstract]. 16th International AIDS Conference; 2006 13–18 August; Toronto, Canada. Abstract MOPE0181.

3 Centers for Disease Control and Prevention (2006). Emergence of Mycobacterium tuberculosis with extensive resistance to second-line drugs worldwide, 2000–2004. *MMWR Morb Mortal Wkly Rep* 55: 301–5. Available: http://www.medicalnewstoday.com/medicalnews.php?newsid=40511. Accessed 23 December 2006.

4 WHO (2006 September 5). Emergence of XDR-TB. WHO concern over extensive drug resistant TB strains that are virtually untreatable. Available: http://www.who.int/mediacentre/news/notes/2006/np23/en/index.html. Accessed 23 December 2006.

5 Pressly D. (2006 September 11). Foreign tourists boost SA coffers.

6 Editorial (2006). XDR-TB – a global threat. *Lancet* 368: 964.

7 Zulu X (2006 September 11). Super TB "now endemic in KZN". Available: http://www.iol.co.za/news/south-africa/super-tb-now-endemic-in-kzn-1.293133#.VYVSpflVhBc.

8 Staff reporter (2006 November 30). Report: Drug-resistant TB at 39 KZN hospitals. *Mail and Guardian*.

9 Smith C. and Clarke L. (2006 September 10). Prospect of TB epidemic sets medics trembling. Available: http://www.iol.co.za/news/south-africa/prospect-of-tb-epidemic-sets-medics-trembling-1.293002#.VYVYYPlVhBc.

10 McGregor S. (2006 September 11). New TB strain could fuel South Africa AIDS toll. Available: http://www.iol.co.za/news/south-africa/new-tb-strain-could-fuel-aids-toll-1.293202#.VYVd1flVhBc.

11 South African Press Association (2006 October 17). Extreme TB spreading across the nation – MRC. Available: http://www.iol.co.za/news/south-africa/extreme-tb-spreading-across-the-nation-mrc-1.297989#.VYVgd_lVhBc.

12 McGregor S. (2006 November 27). Hospital struggles with deadly SA TB. *Mail and Guardian*.

13 Department of Health, Republic of South Africa (2000). *The South African Tuberculosis Control Programme Practical Guidelines* Available: https://www.westerncape.gov.za/text/2003/tb_guidelines2000.pdf.

14 Reuters (2006 September 7). WHO urges South Africa to curb TB killer super-bug.

15 McGregor S. (2006 September 17). State slammed for "delayed reaction" to TB. Available: http://www.iol.co.za/news/south-africa/state-slammed-for-delayed-reaction-to-tb-1.293975#.VYVjj_lVhBc.

16 Clark L. and Smith C. (2006 September 10). Extreme TB outbreak just "tip of the iceberg". Available: http://www.iol.co.za/news/south-africa/extreme-tb-outbreak-just-tip-of-the-iceberg-1.293026#.VYVkIPlVhBc.

17 South African Associated Press, South African Broadcasting Corporation (2006 September 8). Drug-resistant TB: Whose rights should prevail?

18 Agence France-Presse (2006 October 24). South Africa's anti-TB fight hamstrung by Constitution.

19 Verma G., Upshur R.E., Rea E., and Benatar S.R. (2004). Critical reflections on evidence, ethics and effectiveness in the management of tuberculosis: Public health and global perspectives. *BMC Med Ethics* 12: E2.

20 Yong Kim J., Shakow A., Mate K., Vanderwarker C., Gupta R., et al. (2005). Limited good and limited vision: Multidrug-resistant tuberculosis and global health policy. *Soc Sci Med* 61: 847–59.

21 Beresford B (2006 September 8). Call to isolate TB victims. *Mail and Guardian*.

22 Sacks L.V., Pendle S., Orlovic D., Blumberg L., and Constantinou C. (1999). A comparison of outbreak- and nonoutbreak-related multidrug-resistant tuberculosis among human immunodeficiency virus-infected patients in a South African hospital. *Clin Infect Dis* 29: 96–101.

23 Benatar S. (2005). Why tuberculosis persists as a global problem. *Int J Tuberc Lung Dis* 9: 235.

24 Benatar S.R. (2006). Extensively drug resistant tuberculosis: Problem will get worse in South Africa unless poverty is alleviated. *BMJ* 333: 705.

25 SouthAfrica.info (2005 September 12). Spreading the social security net.

26 Statistics South Africa (September 2005). P0210 – Labour Force Survey (LFS). Available: www.statssa.gov.za/publications/P0210/P0210September2005.pdf.

27 Singh J.A., Govender M., and Reddy N. (2005). South Africa a decade after apartheid: Realising health through human rights. *Georgetown Journal of Poverty Law and Policy* 7: 355–88.

28 Medical Research Council of South Africa (2006). Managing multidrug-resistant TB: Legal implications. Available: http://www.mrc.ac.za/policybriefs/managingTB.pdf. Accessed 23 December 2006.

29 WHO (2001). *A human rights approach to TB: Stop TB guidelines for social mobilization.* Available: http://whqlibdoc.who.int/hq/2001/WHO_CDS_STB_2001.9.pdf. Accessed 23 December 2006.

30 WHO (2006). *Guidelines for the Programmatic Management of Drug-Resistant Tuberculosis.* Available: http://whqlibdoc.who.int/publications/2006/9241546956_eng.pdf. Accessed 23 December 2006.

31 De Lange D. (2006 October 25). Patients "could be quarantined".

32 European Court of Human Rights (2005). *Enhorn v. Sweden. ECHR 56529/00.*

33 Martin R. (2006). The exercise of public health powers in cases of infectious disease: Human rights implications. *Enhorn v. Sweden. Med Law Rev* 14: 132–43.

34 Connecticut Department of Public Health (2006). Tuberculosis quarantine laws.

35 Public Health Institute (2003). TB control and the law. Frequently asked questions on civil commitment.

36 Coker R. (2001). Just coercion? Detention of non-adherent tuberculosis patients. *Ann N Y Acad Sci* 953: 216–23.

37 William J., Burman W.J., Cohn D.L., Rietmeijer C.A., Judson F.N., et al. (1997). Short-term incarceration for the management of noncompliance with tuberculosis treatment. *Chest* 112: 57–62.

38 Harris J. and Holm S. (1995). Is there a moral obligation not to infect others? *BMJ* 311: 1215–17.

39 News24 (2006 September 13). Woman with killer TB found.

40 Kass N. (2001). An ethics framework for public health. *Am J Public Health* 91: 1776.

41 Childress J.F., Faden R., Gaare R.D., Gostin L.O., Kahn J., et al. (2002). Public health ethics: Mapping the terrain. *J Law Med Ethics* 30: 170–8.

42 Uphsur R. (2002). Principles for the justification of public health intervention. *Can J Public Health* 93: 101–3.

43 United Nations, Economic and Social Council, U.N. Sub-Commission on Prevention of Discrimination and Protection of Minorities (1984). Siracusa principles on the limitation and derogation of provisions in the International Covenant on Civil and Political Rights, Annex.

44 News24 (2006 November 23). 300+ cases of killer TB in SA.

45 Department of Health, Republic of South Africa (2006). TB crisis management plan.

46 Dlamini N. (2006 September 5). Department addresses extremely drug resistant TB in KZN. Available:

http://allafrica.com/stories/200609051470.html. Accessed 23 December 2006.

47 Dlamini N. and Dube S. (2006 September 7). Action plan developed to combat drug resistant TB.

48 South Africa Press Association/Agence France-Presse (2006 October 12). South Africa invites WHO experts for killer TB talks. Available: http://www.iol.co.za/news/south-africa/sa-invites-who-experts-for-killer-tb-talks-1.297401#.VYVsSflVhBc.

49 Lienhardt C. and Rustomjee R. (2006). Improving tuberculosis control: An interdisciplinary approach. *Lancet* 367: 949–50.

50 Working group of the University of Toronto Joint Centre for Bioethics (2003). *Ethics and SARS: Learning lessons from the Toronto experience.* Available: http://www.yorku.ca/igreene/sars.html. Accessed 18 September, 2006.

70

Clinical Ethics During the Covid-19 Pandemic

Missing the Trees for the Forest

Vijayaprasad Gopichandran

Introduction

The novel coronavirus, SARS-CoV2, has taken the world by storm (1). On the day this paper was written the virus had infected 2.2 million people worldwide and led to more than 1.53 lakh deaths (2). Many countries, including India, are seeing a surge in infections.

In the past few months, the world has been jolted into understanding the importance of public health measures as never before in the recent past. Physical distancing, quarantine of international travellers and their contacts, isolation of people with infection, hand hygiene measures, cough etiquette and wearing of face masks have all been promoted aggressively (3). One of the most forceful and harsh methods of physical distancing adopted by several countries is the lockdown of all travel, work, social, educational and economic activities for protracted periods of time (4). On the one hand there is an argument that states must intervene with such stringent public health measures to save lives and protect their people. But on the other, the huge losses and suffering, especially of the poor and marginalised, due to the lockdown are overwhelming (5). The balance of individual liberties and rights versus the public good is very difficult to achieve in such situations.

Multiple clinical ethics issues have also emerged during this pandemic response. This is the phenomenon of "missing the trees for the forest". In other words, so much attention is given to the macro-issues such as lockdown, physical distancing, isolation, quarantine, travel bans and other public health measures that their impact on the individual is neglected. This paper will focus on clinical ethics as it applies to two groups of people – people infected with the Covid-19 virus and people with "non-Covid-19" illnesses. It will attempt to draw out important ethical concerns and discuss the substantial moral distress that is faced by healthcare providers while handling these ethical conflicts. It will also argue that governments must set up and operate ethics consultations to help healthcare providers address the moral distress they will face.

Original publication details: Excerpted from Vijayaprasad Gopichandran, "Clinical Ethics During the Covid-19 Pandemic: Missing the Trees for the Forest," pp. 1–5 from *Indian Journal of Medical Ethics* 5: 3 (2020).

Clinical Ethics Challenges Arising in the Care of Covid-19 Patients

A number of ethical issues arise during the treatment of patients with Covid-19 (Table 70.1).

Treatment of Covid-19 patients as a means to an end

There is a fundamental difference of approach between clinical medicine and public health. While in clinical medicine the focus is on the individual patient, in public health it is on populations. Clinical medicine cares for individuals after the onset of illness and therefore lays emphasis on the alleviation of suffering, pain, psychological and emotional distress. On the other hand, public health works with healthy populations to prevent illness or the spread of infection. In pandemics like Covid-19 there is a very fluid distinction between these two approaches. Public health and population protection take priority and all interventions by the state are directed towards containment of infection and reduction of morbidity and mortality. Most decisions are driven by statistics and mathematical modelling based on numbers of those

susceptible, exposed, infected, or cured. Testing, detection, isolation, and treatment of individuals become a means to the greater end of keeping the numbers of infected persons low. The foundational tenets of clinical ethics including respect for the individual patient's rights, values, preferences, care for individual needs, avoiding unnecessary harm to and discrimination against infected persons, all take a back seat during such emergency situations (6). Clinicians whose primary training is in caring for individual patients, are forced to adopt public health strategies during pandemics and this leads to moral distress.

Based on the experience of the author and other clinicians providing care for patients with Covid-19, it is observed that patients in isolation wards are often alone without any social or psychological support. In order to reduce the risk of infection to healthcare providers, they do not visit these patients frequently. Even when they go on rounds or to check on patients, they are all in full personal protective equipment, looking like faceless robots, with no warm smile to reassure them. In fact, many health facilities have actually deployed robots to dispense food and medicines for patients in isolation wards, thus removing even minimal human contact (7). Touch, which is one of the most valuable modes of communication in a healthcare

Table 70.1   Ethical issues in the clinical care of patients with Covid-19

Type of Covid-19 illness	Treatment	Ethical considerations
Asymptomatic and minor illness	Isolation of asymptomatic individuals and those with minor illness in Covid Care Centres (CCC)	Cleanliness and maintenance of hotels, lodges, hostels which are converted to CCCs. Biomedical waste management in these centres Separation from family and relatives, loneliness Harm to mental health of the patients due to isolation
	Use of unproven treatments such as Hydroxychloroquine and Azithromycin	Adverse effects of drugs – torsade de pointes and other arrhythmias with HCQ Emergence of drug resistance especially for Azithromycin
Moderate to severe illness	Isolation of patients in Dedicated Covid Health Centres (DCHC)	Conversion of district level hospitals into DCHC – compromise in routine care
	Weak evidence of all available treatments	Doubtful efficacy and precarious benefit-risk balance
	Healthcare providers refusing to give care without adequate protection	Duty to care versus protection of health care providers Reciprocity in the form of adequate protection by PPE
Critical illness (ARDS, sepsis, septic shock)	Scarce resources	Deprivation of adequate care to those in need Triage of who should get priority over scarce resources Lack of dignity in death

provider-patient relationship is minimised to reduce transmission of infection. With curbing infection being the priority, many individuals are neglected and left to suffer alone and in silence. Hippocrates said, "Cure sometimes, treat often, comfort always." Covid-19 has made comforting the patient the least of the three priorities. Communication is one of the fundamental aspects of a good patient- provider relationship and in clinical medicine, it is not just verbal communication but associated cues like touch, physical presence, body language, facial expression, which help patients feel reassured and comforted. This aspect of the patient-provider relationship suffers during admission in isolation wards. Unfortunately, infection control supersedes clinical care.

Working with uncertain evidence and unproven therapies

When a pandemic occurs due to a new infective agent, without any definitive treatment or drug, all clinicians clutch at straws to somehow save lives. This is the case with the SARS-CoV2 virus too. Hydroxychloroquine, in combination with Azithromycin, features in the treatment protocol for moderate to severe illness in India (8). Some state treatment protocols also include Oseltamivir, originally a drug against influenza virus, in the treatment of mild to moderate illness (9). Other anti-viral drugs such as Lopinavir/Ritonavir, originally an oral combination therapy against HIV, is also being studied in many contexts. Umifenovir is a repurposed anti-viral agent of interest as a therapeutic agent. Nitazoxanine, an antihelminthic agent, has also been proposed as a treatment. Remdesivir, a broad spectrum anti-viral agent with potent in vitro; activity against SARS-CoV2 is said to be showing promising results (10). All these agents are still under clinical trial and none has so far been proven effective at the time of writing. Immunomodulatory agents such as Tocilizumab and Sarilumab are also under trial as agents to manage the "cytokine storm" that is associated with the Covid-19 illness. Treatment with convalescent plasma or hyperimmune immunoglobulin is being tried and reported to be successful (11).

Such immunoglobulin therapy is going to be tried in India as well.

At present, other than supportive treatments and management of typical syndromes like acute respiratory distress syndrome (ARDS), septicaemia, multiorgan dysfunction syndrome (MODS), and cytokine storm, there is no established treatment. As some of these treatments feature in state recommended protocols, there is a risk that patients and the community may mistake these for definitive treatments. Besides, some of these drugs have serious adverse effects and may result in greater harm than good. One such example is the use of hydroxychloroquine among patients with severe illness. Often, such patients are of advanced age and have multiple comorbidities. This puts them at greater risk of cardiac arrhythmias, a known side effect of hydroxychloroquine (12). Working with such uncertain evidence can also lead to moral distress among the providers. In such pandemics, clinicians are left with no choice but to try experimental therapies on compassionate grounds. However, the level of uncertainty and the distress that it causes must be acknowledged and clinicians must be supported to overcome this distress. A trustworthy and transparent line of communication about the level of evidence and status of new therapies must be established.

Duty to care versus right to protection

One of the most contentious issues globally during this pandemic has been the scarcity of personal protective equipment (PPE) for healthcare personnel working with Covid-19 patients (13). They are directly exposed to high viral loads and therefore susceptible to more severe illness. Deaths of healthcare providers due to Covid-19 illness have been reported in large numbers in Italy, China, the United States and many other countries (14). There is a debate on whether healthcare providers have the duty to care when the health system does not protect their health and safety through adequate provision of PPE. In the UK, doctors and nurses appeared in a video, pleading with the government to improve the supply of

PPE for their safety. This video was projected on to the walls of the Palace of Westminster (15). Doctors and nurses in Zimbabwe staged protests, and several resigned their jobs over lack of PPE (16). These examples highlight the global nature of the debate on duty to care versus right to protection.

Healthcare providers have multiple duties during such pandemic times, including the duty to care for their patients, the duty to protect themselves from getting infected so that they remain productive and in action throughout the period of the pandemic, the duty to protect their families and neighbourhoods, and to their colleagues, many of whom may become sick and have to go on leave, whose jobs they may have to cover, and finally a duty to society at large (17).

Nobody else can provide the unique and specialised services that healthcare providers can. They have spent years in learning these skills, and they must be put to maximum use during pandemics. There is a moral obligation based on a social contract between the healthcare provider and society that the provider will deliver healthcare services in time of need. While they have these duties to care, they also have the right to be protected from harm to themselves, because only then can they actually continue to serve society.

The General Medical Council (GMC) of the United Kingdom recommends that doctors must not refuse to treat patients because exposure will endanger their lives. Furthermore, the GMC recommends that striking the balance between serving during the time of need and protecting the health and welfare of healthcare providers must be ensured at the local level by providing adequate PPE to protect their health to the maximum extent possible (18). The American Medical Association adds that "physicians should balance the immediate benefit to the patients with their long-term ability to serve many patients" (19). The Code of Medical Ethics Regulations of the Medical Council of India, 2002, amended up to 2016, states that no physician can refuse to treat a patient during an emergency (20). There is no specific mention of the conundrum of duty to care versus protection of the self in the MCI code of medical ethics.

The emerging consensus across different international ethical guidance seems to be that duty to care during pandemics and emergency situations must be voluntary and must be associated with reciprocity from the health system, the government and society to protect providers. This can be in the form of provision of PPE, duty hours that offer adequate time for rest and recuperation, comfortable rooms to stay in while separated from family and loved ones, and adequate incentives in the form of monetary or non-monetary compensations. However, the fear, anxiety and guilt of transmitting the illness from patients to their loved ones is likely to cause substantial distress among healthcare providers and impact the care that they provide.

Rationing of scarce resources in pandemic situations

Though rationing of scarce resources is a public health concern, it has important implications for clinical care provision and clinical ethics. Many countries, including Italy and the United States, are facing a major resource crunch during the Covid-19 pandemic (13). Hospital beds, ventilators, medications, personal protective equipment for healthcare providers, are all becoming scarce resources. Clinicians are pushed into making morally contentious decisions on allocation of beds, ventilators and medicines. Making such decisions takes a heavy toll on the psyche of healthcare providers. Scarce resources are allocated based on ability to save most lives, ability to save most life years, priority to those who are likely to make significant contributions eg, healthcare providers, etc. These decision algorithms select a few patients in preference to others based on criteria such as age, presence of comorbidities, contribution to society etc, and having to make these decisions causes the clinician severe moral distress (21). Since these decisions have a significant impact on the community, active community engagement in order to understand community perspectives, values and priorities is important. Local guidelines must be developed to support healthcare providers in making rationing decisions that are relevant and acceptable to the community (22).

Dignity in death

Families of patients who die due to Covid-19 face serious emotional stress. Firstly, the patients die alone in the hospital isolation ward or the critical care unit. Their family and loved ones do not get a chance to say goodbye. The formalities of disposal of the body without contamination of the environment further place severe restrictions on certain important traditions and rituals that are performed as part of funeral rites. In a recent incident in Chennai, the cremation of the body of a doctor who died of Covid-19 infection was not allowed by the local community, for fear of contamination (23). This completely dehumanises the dead and strips the last shreds of their dignity. In some cases, patients die even before the test result for SARS-CoV2 come out, and this leads to delays in disposal of the body. All of these are also major causes of ethical distress for providers.

Clinical Ethics Considerations in the Care of "Non-Covid-19" Patients

Clinical ethics challenges arise during a pandemic in relation to "non-Covid-19" patients, such as denial of clinical care for non-emergency conditions, and lack of clinical support for mental illness. In the rush to prepare hospitals and health facilities to receive the deluge of patients with Covid-19, many hospitals at the district and medical college levels have been converted into dedicated Covid hospitals. Here, basic clinical services which are considered "non-emergency" have been suspended by a government advisory (24). This is done for two main reasons, ie hospitals are hot-beds of transmission of SARS-CoV2 and overcrowding in hospitals will make social distancing difficult to practise. In the current situation, most government health facilities have closed their non-emergency services and many private clinics and nursing homes have also been shut down in containment zones. Small, congested single-doctor clinics in many cities have also shut down because of the fear of community transmission of the

disease (25). Reproductive and child health services, including antenatal care, delivery services, post-natal care and care of the new born child including immunisation is likely to suffer due to closure of several hospitals as well as redirection of grassroots health workers to Covid-19 containment activities. The worst hit during this situation are patients who have chronic noncommunicable diseases such as diabetes, hypertension, cardiac diseases and chronic lung diseases. Many of these patients may not have an acute emergency. However, they will require long term medication, and have to face the effects of interruptions in their supply. Similarly, patients on long term drug treatment for tuberculosis and HIV are likely to suffer from shortages because of difficulties in reaching a health facility as well as supply chain problems. Patients on dialysis for chronic kidney disease, and those receiving treatment for cancer, also suffer due to access barriers and shut down of treatment facilities.

Prior experience from the Ebola pandemic of 2014–15 showed that deaths due to neglect of measles, malaria, HIV and tuberculosis were far more in number than Ebola deaths (26). The World Health Organisation released a document that outlined the key principles of maintaining essential health services during an outbreak situation (27). The Ministry of Health and Family Welfare, Government of India, followed by releasing a guidance on April 14 regarding maintaining essential health services through utilisation of non-Covid hospitals, empanelled private hospitals under the Pradhan Mantri Jan Arogya Yojna (PMJAY) – National Health Protection Scheme, telemedicine, home visits by frontline health workers and triaging patients in hospitals (28,29). The operational feasibility of these guidelines and the way they are implemented on the ground needs to be observed closely.

There are also reports of people suffering from mental health problems due to the prolonged lockdown as well as isolation and social distancing (29). These individuals do not have access to care for their mental health problems. Another group of individuals badly hit by this pandemic are those dependent on alcohol. Several instances of people dying due to alcohol withdrawal have been reported, as all alcohol

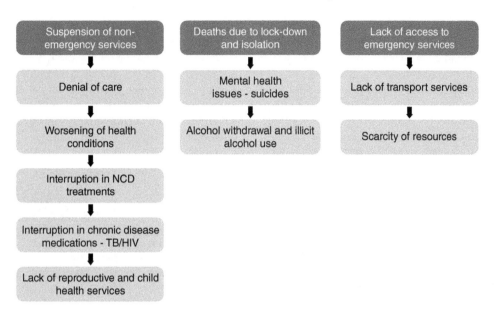

Figure 70.1 Ethical issues in clinical care of "non-Covid-19" patients

outlets were closed due to the lock down (30). There have also been instances of individuals consuming toxic substitutes for alcohol such as paint varnish and shaving lotion which led to their deaths. These patients suffered due to lack of clinical alcohol deaddiction, detoxification support. Though emergency medical services are open and functional in many hospitals, patients find access to the emergency services difficult due to the lockdown. Further, interruptions in the supply chain lead to many hospitals facing drug shortages, so that even the quality of the limited services available in hospitals is poor. The various ethical issues in the care of "non-Covid-19" patients are described in Figure 70.1.

Moral Distress of Healthcare Providers

The Covid-19 pandemic has laid bare the gross under-preparedness of most health systems in the world in the face of a major, catastrophic health event. The healthcare providers, namely doctors, nurses,

technicians and others are not in a situation to address these major ethical issues as described above. Some of these emerge from the conflict between their responsibility to the individual patient versus responsibility to the public during a public health crisis. Such ethical issues are a cause for severe moral distress among healthcare providers. In addition, healthcare providers face a serious dilemma as to whether they should turn whistle-blowers about the lack of PPE, lack of reasonable duty timings and suffering of vulnerable populations due to non-availability of non-Covid 19 services. They face probable punitive action that may extend to termination of service in some instances. The moral distress that healthcare providers are likely to face must be addressed (31). In addition to the numerous webinars on training healthcare providers to manage critical care of patients with Covid-19, infection prevention and control practices within the hospital and isolation ward settings, support must be offered through counselling to address moral distress arising while treating patients during pandemics. There are examples of a nurse in Italy and the finance minister of a German state who took their own lives probably because of the stress and irreconcilable moral distress arising from the pandemic (32,33). Support to healthcare providers to address moral conflicts can be offered as an ethics helpline within the hospital setting. The government must also focus on setting up Clinical Ethics Consultations, either on the telephone or through video conferencing for any healthcare provider or team faced with a moral conflict.

The most serious problems in clinical ethics during pandemic situations arise because of neglect of the trees while focusing on the forest. While prioritising prevention of the spread of infection, individual patients, their preferences, values and wellbeing are often neglected. This must be carefully weighed and considered while planning care during pandemic situations.

References

1   Lai C.-C., Shih T.-P., Ko W.-C., Tang H.-J., Hsueh P.-R. Severe acute respiratory syndrome coronavirus 2 (SARS-CoV-2) and corona virus disease-2019 (COVID-19): the epidemic and the challenges. *Int J Antimicrob Agents.* 2020 Mar; 55(3):105924.

2   World Health Organization. *Coronavirus disease 2019 (COVID-19) Situation Report – 84.* Geneva: WHO; 2020 [cited 2020 Apr 24]. Available from: https://www.who.int/docs/default-source/coronaviruse/situation-reports/20200413-sitrep-84-covid-19.pdf?sfvrsn=44f511ab_2

3   Wilder-Smith A., and Freedman D.O. Isolation, quarantine, social distancing and community containment: pivotal role for old-style public health measures in the novel coronavirus (2019-nCoV) outbreak. *J Travel Med.* 2020 Mar 13; 27(2):taaa020.

4   Lau H., Khosrawipour V., Kocbach P., Mikolajczyk A., Schubert J., Bania J., et al. The positive impact of lockdown in Wuhan on containing the COVID-19 outbreak in China. *J Travel Med.* 2020.

5   Wang Z. and Tang K. Combating COVID-19: health equity matters. *Nat Med.* 2020; 1.

6   Berlinger N., Wynia M.K., Powell T., Hester M., Milliken A., Fabi R., et al. Ethical framework for health care institutions responding to novel coronavirus SARS-CoV-2 (COVID-19) Guidelines for institutional ethics services responding to COVID-19 Managing uncertainty, safeguarding communities, guiding practice [Internet]. New York; 2020 Mar 16[cited 2020 Apr 25]. Available from: https://www.thehastingscenter.org/wp-content/uploads/HastingsCenterCovidFramework2020.pdf

7   Yang G.-Z., Nelson B.J., Murphy R.R., Choset H., Christensen H., Collins S.H., et al. Combating COVID-19 – The role of robotics in managing public health and infectious diseases. *Science Robotics.* 2020 Mar 25; 5(40):eabb5589 Available from: https://robotics.sciencemag.Org/content/5/40/eabb5589

8   Directorate General of Health Services. Revised guidelines on clinical management of COVID – 19. New Delhi; DGHS; 2020 Mar 31 [cited 2020 Apr 25]. Available from: https://www.mohfw.gov.in/pdf/RevisedNationalClinicalManagementGuidelineforCOVID1931032020.pdf

9   Department of Health and Family Welfare. Clinical Management Guidelines for Covid19. Chennai; DGFW; 2020 Apr 4[cited 2020 Apr 25].

10 Sanders J.M., Monogue M.L., Jodlowski T.Z., Cutrell and J.B. Pharmacologic treatments for coronavirus disease 2019 (COVID-19): A review. *JAMA.* 2020 Apr 13; Available from: https://doi.org/10.1001/jama.2020.6019

11 Shen C., Wang Z., Zhao F., Yang Y., Li J., Yuan J., et al. Treatment of 5 critically ill patients with COVID-19 with convalescent plasma. JAMA. 2020 Mar 27 [cited 2020 Apr 25], Available from: https://jamanetwork.com/journals/jama/fullarticle/2763983

12 Hasan S.S., Kow C.S., and Merchant H. Is it worth the wait? Should Chloroquine or Hydroxychloroquine be allowed for immediate use in CoViD-19? *Br J Pharm.* 2020 Mar 31 [cited 2020 Apr 25];5(1):745. Available from: https://pure.hud.ac.uk/en/publications/is-it-worth-the-wait-should-chloroquine-or-hydroxychloroquine-be-

13 Ranney M.L., Griffeth V., and Jha A.K. Critical supply shortages – the need for ventilators and personal protective equipment during the Covid-19 pandemic. *N Engl J Med.*2020 Mar25[cited 2020 Apr 26], Available from: https://www.nejm.org/doi/full/10.1056/NEJMp2006141

14 Adams J.G. and Walls R.M. Supporting the health care workforce during the COVID-19 global epidemic. *JAMA.* 2020 Mar 12[cited 2020 Apr 26],

Available from: https://jamanetwork.com/journals/jama/fullarticle/2763136

15 UK News. NHS staff make plea for PPE in video projected onto Palace of Westminster. Express and Star. 2020 Apr 17 [cited 2020 Apr 26]. Available from: https://www.expressandstar.com/news/uk-news/2020/04/17/nhs-staff-make-plea-for-ppe-in-video-projected-onto-palace-of-westminster/

16 Chingono N. Zimbabwe doctors and nurses down tools over lack of protective coronavirus gear. *CNN*. 2020 Mar 25[cited 2020 Apr 26]. Available from: https://edition.cnn.com/2020/03/25/africa/zimbabwe-doctors-nurses-ppe-strike/index.html

17 Simonds A.K. and Sokol D.K. Lives on the line? Ethics and practicalities of duty of care in pandemics and disasters. *EurRespir J.* 2009 Aug; 34(2):303–9.

18 General Medical Council. Good Medical Practice. Pandemic Influenza: Responsibilities of Doctors in a National Pandemic. London; 2009[withdrawn 2012 Nov], Available from: https://www.gmc-uk.org/-/media/documents/pandemic-influenza-2009---2012-55677705.pdf?la=en

19 Morin K., Higginson D., and Goldrich M. Physician obligation in disaster preparedness and response. *Camb Q Healthc Ethics*. 2006 Fall; 15(4):417–31.

20 Medical Council of India. Code of Medical Ethics Regulations. New Delhi: MCI;2002, amended up to 2016 Oct 8 [cited 2020 Apr 26] Available from: https://www.mciindia.org/CMS/rules-regulations/code-of-medical-ethics-regulations-2002

21 Emanuel E.J., Persad G., Upshur R., Thome B., Parker M., Glickman A., et al. Fair allocation of scarce medical resources in the time of Covid-19. *N Engl J Med*. 2020 Mar 23 [cited 2020 Apr 26], Available from: https://doi.org/10.1056/NEJMsb2005114

22 Biddison E.L.D., Faden R.R., Gwon H.S., Mareiniss D.P., Regenberg A.C., Schoch-Spana M., et al. Too many patients. A framework to guide statewide allocation of scarce mechanical ventilation during disasters. *Chest*. 2019; 155(4):848–54

23 Express News Service. Nellore doctor's cremation blocked by locals in Chennai. *New Indian Express*. 2020 Apr 14[cited 2020 Apr 26], Available from: www.newindianexpress.com/states/andhra-pradesh/2020/apr/14/nellore-doctors-cremation-blocked-by-locals-in-chennai-2129895.amp

24 Ministry of Health and Family Welfare. Advisory for hospitals and medical education institutions. New Delhi: MoHFW; 2020 [cited 2020 Apr 26].

25 Chitharanjan S. Small clinics shut down in Kozhikode due to Covid19 scare. The Times of India [Internet]. 2020 Apr 13[cited 2020 Apr 26]. Available from: https://timesofindia.indiatimes.com/city/kozhikode/small-clinics-shutdown-in-kozhikode-due-to-covid-19-scare/artideshow/75119896.cms

26 Elston J.W.T., Cartwright C., Ndumbi P., and Wright J. The health impact of the 2014–15 Ebola outbreak. *Public Health*. 2017 Feb; 143:60–70.

27 World Health Organization. COVID-19: Operational guidance for maintaining essential health services during an outbreak. Geneva: WHO; 2020 Mar 25[cited 2020 Apr 26], Available from: https://www.who.int/publications-detail/covid-19-operational-guidance-for-maintaining-essential-health-services-during-an-outbreak

28 Ministry of Health and Family Welfare. Enabling Delivery of Essential Health Services during the COVID 19 Outbreak: Guidance note. New Delhi: MoHFW; 2020 [cited 2020 Apr 26]. Available from: https://apps.who.int/iris/bitstream/handle/10665/331561/WHO-2019-nCoV-essential_health_services-2020.1-eng.pdf

29 Goyal K., Chauhan P., Chhikara K., Gupta P., and Singh M.P. Fear of COVID 2019: First suicidal case in India! *Asian J Psychiatr*. 2020 Feb27; 49:101989.

30 Nidheesh M. In God's own country, 1 died of Covid-19 but 7 commit suicide after alcohol ban. *Livemint*. 2020 Mar 29[cited 2020 Apr 26]. Available from: https://www.livemint.com/news/india/in-god-s-own-country-1-died-of-covid-19-but-7-commit-suicide-after-alcohol- ban-11585483376504.html

31 Mazanec P. Covid 19 Resource: Ethical dilemmas facing nurses during the Coronavirus crisis: Addressing moral distress. Sigma CNE Course, Sigma repository; 2020 Mar 26[cited 2020 Apr 26] Available from: https://sigma.nursingrepository.Org/handle/10755/20413

32 Steinbuch Y. Italian nurse with coronavirus kills herself over fear of infecting others. New York Post 2020 Mar 25[cited 2020 Apr 26]. Available from: https://nypost.com/2020/03/25/italian-nurse-with-coronavirus-kills-herself-amid-fears-of-infecting-others/

33 Rahn W. German state finance minister Thomas Schäfer found dead. *DW.com*. 2020 Mar 29[cited 2020 Apr 26], Available from: https://www.dw.com/en/german-state-finance-minister-thomas-schafer-found-dead/a-52948976

71

The Moral Obligation to be Vaccinated

Utilitarianism, Contractualism, and Collective Easy Rescue

Alberto Giubilini, Thomas Douglas, and Julian Savulescu

Introduction

Despite the success of vaccines in preventing and sometimes eradicating infectious diseases, and despite their demonstrated safety (Navin 2015, p. 6; CDC 2015a; Andre et al. 2008), many people today refuse vaccination for themselves or their children. In the US there has been a significant increase in cases of measles over the last few years due to increasingly widespread non-vaccination: in 2014, for example, there were 667 reported cases, the highest number since measles elimination was documented in the US in 2000 (CDC 2016a). Similarly, in different parts of Europe there were measles outbreaks in 2016 and 2017, due to a significant decrease in measles vaccination rates; for example, in Italy there were more than 3,300 cases of measles in the first half of 2017, 88% of which were not vaccinated and 7% of which received just one dose of vaccine (ECDC 2017). Before the introduction of the measles vaccination program in 1963, 3–4 million people in the US were infected by measles every year, and 4–500 of them died (CDC 2015b).

Some reasons for vaccine refusal derive from scepticism about the efficacy or safety of vaccines (Smith et al. 2011; Harmsen et al. 2013), while in other cases objections are based on philosophical or religious views about how humans should deal with diseases; for instance, the largest local outbreak of measles in the US in recent years (383 cases) occurred in 2014 in unvaccinated Amish communities in Ohio (CDC 2016a).

A high rate of vaccine refusal can compromise herd immunity, which is achieved when a sufficient proportion of the population is immune (Andre et al. 2008), and therefore the incidence of infection declines, which makes disease more unlikely to spread (Fine et al. 2011; Dawson 2007). The coverage rate required to realise herd immunity depends on the specific disease considered, but it typically ranges between 90 and 95%.

Herd immunity is a *collective good*, in the sense that it can be produced only through the cooperation of a large number of people (Dawson 2007, pp. 167–8). But herd immunity is also a *public good* (Dawson 2007), in the technical sense of the term: it is non-excludable

Original publication details: Alberto Giubilini, Thomas Douglas, and Julian Savulescu, "The Moral Obligation to be Vaccinated: Utilitarianism, Contractualism and Collective Easy Rescue," pp. 547–560 from *Medicine, Health Care and Philosophy* 21 (2018).

Bioethics: An Anthology, Fourth Edition. Edited by Udo Schüklenk and Peter Singer.

and non-rivalrous. Herd immunity is non-excludable in the sense that it is not possible to exclude someone from benefitting from herd immunity, even if she does not contribute to the good through vaccination; in fact, everybody benefits from herd immunity, even those who are in any case protected against the disease in question due to their vaccination status, because in a society where herd immunity is realised fewer resources need to be directed to care for the sick. More importantly, herd immunity reduces the risk of infection for (1) those who are too young to be safely vaccinated [e.g. the injectable influenza vaccine is not recommended for children younger than 6 months old, (CDC 2016b)]; (2) those who cannot be vaccinated for medical reasons (for example because they are allergic to certain vaccines or are immunosuppressed); and (3) those for whom vaccination is ineffective [for example, the pertussis vaccine is only 70% effective during the first year and only 30–40% effective after 4 years (CDC 2016c)]. Herd immunity is also non-rivalrous, in the sense that anyone benefitting from it does not reduce the extent to which others can benefit as well.

There has recently been considerable discussion (Pierik 2016; Flanigan 2014; Dawson 2011; Luyten et al. 2011; Verweij and Dawson 2004) regarding whether the state should enforce compulsory or mandatory vaccination in order to realise herd immunity. In this paper we address a different, though related, issue, namely whether *individuals* have a *moral* obligation to be vaccinated or to have one's children vaccinated, in spite of the fact that any single vaccination does not make a significant difference to vaccination coverage rates. Thus, the question we aim to answer is the following: how can we justify the existence of an individual moral obligation to be vaccinated or to have one's children vaccinated, if any individual being vaccinated does not significantly affect a community's capacity to achieve herd immunity and therefore to protect its vulnerable members?

Two observations about the scope of our arguments are in order. First, we take our argument to apply only to the case of vaccinations protecting against communicable diseases that pose significant risks to the health or life of at least some of those infected. These include, for example,

vaccines against seasonal influenza, the MMR (measles, mumps, rubella) vaccine, vaccines against pneumococcal and meningococcal infections, the varicella vaccine, and more generally the vaccines against communicable diseases that healthcare systems recommend for children and adults (see e.g. the communicable diseases, and *only* the communicable diseases, listed at CDC 2016d). Our arguments do not apply to vaccines against non communicable infectious diseases, such as tetanus.

Second, our argument for the existence of a collective and of an individual moral obligation to be vaccinated applies both to adults and to children who can be considered moral agents, i.e., who can appreciate and respond to moral reasons. For example, some vaccines, such as vaccines against meningococcal groups A, C, W and Y disease, are usually recommended for 12 year old children, who certainly count as moral agents and are subject to moral obligations; other vaccines, such as the seasonal flu vaccine, are recommended for children and adults of all ages starting from 6 months old, and many of these individuals certainly are moral agents. In the case of young children who cannot be considered moral agents, and therefore who cannot be subject to moral obligations – such as, for example, 3 year old children for whom the MMR vaccine is recommended – our arguments for the existence of an individual moral obligation with regard to vaccination applies to the parents, who are responsible for decisions about their children's vaccination; in such cases, the individual moral obligation in question is not that of being vaccinated, but that of having one's children vaccinated. Now, attributing parents a moral obligation to vaccinate their children might be considered problematic because, whatever the source of such moral obligation, parents also have a moral obligation to act in the best interests of their children. And in certain cases, the obligation to act in the best interest of one's children provides pro tanto moral reasons for not vaccinating the children.[1] For example, it might be in the best interest of a healthy child not to be vaccinated against varicella (chickenpox): since varicella is not a serious or dangerous disease for healthy children, it might be better for the children to avoid the risk of side effects of the varicella vaccine, which range from mild rash to serious anaphylactic reactions (around 1 in 1 million vacci-nated individuals), even at the cost of being exposed to the risk of getting the disease. Or, one might suggest, it might not be in the best interest of a child to be vacci-nated even against more serious diseases, such [as] mea-sles, in those circumstances in which vaccine coverage rate is already very high: the child would be protected anyway through herd immunity without needing to be exposed to the (very small) risks of vaccination (assum-ing for the sake of argument that the child will always remain within an area in which vaccination coverage rate is sufficiently high). In such cases we would have a clash between two pro tanto moral obligations: the moral obligation to vaccinate one's children in order to protect other people (whose justification will be the topic of this paper) and the moral obligation not to vaccinate them in order to pursue their best interest. Therefore, in order to demonstrate that parents have not only a pro tanto, but an all-things-considered moral obligation to vaccinate their children we would have to demonstrate that the moral obligation to protect others by vaccinating one's child outweighs the moral obliga-tion to act exclusively in the best interest of the child. While we will not try to argue for this thesis, we are confident that the arguments we are going to provide are strong enough to make it at least plausible to claim that the pro tanto moral obligation to vaccinate one's children does outweigh the pro tanto moral obligation not to vaccinate them at least in some cases.

It is important to make the question of individual moral obligation to be vaccinated or to have one's children vaccinated central to discussion of the ethics of vaccination. If people were convinced that there is an individual moral obligation to be vaccinated or to have one's children vaccinated and fulfilled this obliga-tion, compulsory vaccination would not be necessary (Dawson 2011, pp. 150–1). Moreover, the existence of a moral obligation is relevant to the justifiability of state-sponsored vaccination programmes. As Marcel Verweij noted with regard to the influenza vaccine, "if citizens have a moral duty to accept vaccination because in this way they will protect others (e.g. the elderly and chronically ill) for whom influenza poses a serious risk, this will give support to a general vaccination policy"

(Verweij 2005, p. 324). The thought here is that it will be easier to justify state-sponsored vaccination pro-grammes if these merely encourage or require individu-als to do what they in any case have a moral obligation to do than if they encourage or require individuals to go beyond their moral obligations. Thus, it is important to provide a solid justification for the existence of an individual moral obligation to be vaccinated or to have one's children vaccinated which could strengthen the justification for such vaccination programmes.

From Collective to Individual Responsibility

The behaviour of a certain number of people is nec-essary and sufficient to realise herd immunity but no one individual's actions make a significant difference to whether the effect obtains for the group. This sug-gests that individuals cannot be morally responsi-ble, in the standard kind of way, for producing herd immunity. However, as we will argue in "Easy rescue, collective obligations, and the individual duty to be vaccinated", it is possible to attribute moral respon-sibility to groups in respect of herd immunity. In the retrospective sense of "responsibility", groups can be *blameworthy* for failing to realise herd immunity, and in the prospective sense of responsibility, groups have a moral *obligation* to realise herd immunity.

Attribution of *individual* responsibility – which is the central issue of this article – is more problematic. Because each individual contribution to the realisa-tion of herd immunity is negligible, it seems prob-lematic to argue that any particular individual has the moral obligation to make her contribution to herd immunity by being vaccinated or by vaccinating their children. Let's consider vaccination for oneself, and let's examine two possible scenarios, one in which herd immunity is realised, and one in which it is not. In the first case, where herd immunity is realised, some have argued that since the risk that other people become infected is very small, the ground for attri-bution of an individual obligation to be vaccinated is weak (Dawson 2007, p. 171). But, as others have observed, one's contribution to vaccine coverage rates also seems virtually irrelevant if herd immunity is not realised: the risk that other people are infected would be high anyway, regardless of whether one vaccinates, and any effect of one's decision on the risk of contagion is likely to be negligible (Verweij 2005, p. 329).

Contrary to what these positions maintain, in this paper we argue that individuals do have a moral obligation to be vaccinated or to vaccinate their children even if their contribution to herd immunity is negligible. For brevity's sake, we will be referring from now on only to the individual moral obligation to be vaccinated, but it is understood that the same arguments apply to the moral obligation to vaccinate one's children. In "The utilitarian approach: group beneficence and imperceptible contributions" we analyse a utilitarian ethical approach based on Derek Parfit's Principle of 'Group Beneficence'; in "The deontological approach", we consider two possible versions of a deontological approach. We argue that both a utilitarian and a deontological contractualist approach do provide support to the idea that individuals have a moral obligation to be vaccinated. In "Duty of easy rescue and fairness: a further argument for an individual moral obligation to be vaccinated", we propose a further ethical approach that can justify attribution of individual responsibility to be vaccinated, and that does not presuppose any contentious comprehensive moral theory: we argue that individuals have a moral obligation to contribute to herd immunity by being vaccinated on the basis of a collective duty of easy rescue and of a principle of fairness in the distribution of the burdens that such collective duty entails.

The Utilitarian Approach: Group Beneficence and Imperceptible Contributions

In *Reasons and Persons*, Derek Parfit discusses the following example:

> a large number of wounded men lie out in the desert, suffering from intense thirst. We are an equally large

number of altruists, each of whom has a pint of water. We could pour these pints into a water-cart. This would be driven into the desert, and our water would be shared equally between all these many wounded men. By adding his pint, each of us would enable each wounded man to drink slightly more water – perhaps only an extra drop. Even to a very thirsty man, each of these extra drops would be a very small benefit. The effect on each man might even be imperceptible" (Parfit 1984, p. 76).

The contribution of an extra drop of water to alleviating the men's thirst may be as imperceptible as the contribution that each individual would make to vaccination rates and to the realisation of herd immunity by being vaccinated. In spite of this imperceptibility, we might still say that each individual has an obligation to be vaccinated in virtue of the same principle whereby Parfit, in his example, attributes to each altruist a moral obligation to make their (imperceptible) contribution to alleviating the wounded men's thirst. The principle is the following:

> When (1) the best outcome would be the one in which people are benefited most, and (2) each of the members of some group could act in a certain way, and (3) they would benefit people if *enough* of them act in this way, and (4) they would benefit people *most* if they *all* act in this way, and (5) each of them both knows these facts and believes that enough of them will act in this way, then (6) each of them ought to act in this way (Parfit 1984, p. 77).

We might call this the Principle of Group Beneficence (Otsuka 1991): each individual member of the collective has a moral obligation to make her contribution to enable the collective to cause the desirable collective effect. The moral obligation of each individual is derived from a principle of utility maximization, since, as per condition (1), the "best" outcome is the one where people are benefited most, and according to Parfit, individuals ought collectively to do what brings about the best outcome. Parfit appeals to an intuition according to which "it is clear" that "each of us should pour his pint into the water-cart" (Parfit 1984, p. 77). If this intuition is veridical, then, given the analogy with the case of vaccination, we should also say that each individual should be vaccinated so as to make one's contribution to herd immunity.

However, one might object that condition (4) creates a problem for any attempt to apply the Principle of Group Beneficence to cases of imperceptible individual contributions to a collective effect. According to that condition, the moral obligation to make one's small contribution to a desirable collective effect exists where a group of individuals would produce the most benefit if *all* the individuals acted in a certain way. The principle might in itself be valid. However, at a first glance it seems to apply neither to Parfit's example nor to the case of individuals' contribution to herd immunity. Recall that in Parfit's example, and also in the case of vaccination, each individual's contribution to the collective effect is imperceptible. Accordingly, it would seem that if all but one of the people (and therefore *not all* individuals) poured their pint into the water-cart, the benefit to the thirsty men would not be significantly smaller than the benefit they would get if all poured their pint. Suppose one of the altruists is also thirsty: it seems that utility would be maximized if this individual drank her pint of water instead of pouring it into the water-cart, because her thirst would be alleviated at no significant cost to the wounded men. In the same way, one might say, if all but one person were vaccinated, vaccination coverage rates would not be significantly lower than they would be if all were vaccinated, since each individual contribution to coverage rates is negligible. Suppose a person is opposed to vaccination: utility would be maximized if this individual was not vaccinated, because she would have her anti-vax preference satisfied without any significant impact on coverage rates or herd immunity. For the same reason, the situation in which all but two people are vaccinated is better, from the point of view of utility maximization, than the one in which all but one are vaccinated; and so forth.

The same reasoning might be iterated also beyond the point at which the non-vaccinated people are so many that herd immunity is lost. In those cases,

herd immunity would not be realised anyway, even if one more individual contributed by being vaccinated. In such cases, one might be tempted to agree with Marcel Verweij that "if most people forgo vaccination against influenza, the effects on public health of my choice for vaccination become negligible" (Verweij 2005, p. 329). Therefore, as far as utility maximization is concerned, "if non compliance is common, my obligation to contribute to prevention will weaken or even fade away" (Verweij 2005, p. 330).

Thus, whether or not herd immunity is realised, any individual might be able to claim that the imperceptibility of her contribution implies that she does not have the moral obligation to be vaccinated.

However, there is more to say in support of Parfit's intuition, and in support of the idea that condition (4) – namely that individuals would benefit people *most* if they *all* contributed through pouring their pint of water in the water tank (or through being vaccinated) – does apply to the case of realisation of herd immunity. An analogy with a relevantly similar case might provide support to Parfit's claim that "each of us should pour his pint into the water-cart" because people would benefit most if all contributed. Parfit's example discussed above is relevantly similar to one in which there is the same amount of water, the same number of potential water-givers, and the same number of water-recipients, but each water-giver's pint, instead of being collected into a water-cart, goes directly to a single thirsty man, and thus makes a significant difference to a single person (for an analogous case, see Glover 1975, pp. 174–5). On this variant of the case, if one person does not pour her pint, then one thirsty man gets no water and dies. In such cases, it seems obvious that each man ought to donate [their] pint of water. But it does not seem that it should make a moral difference whether exactly the same donation is directed to a specific individual (call this "directed donation") or is collected together with other donations and then distributed among all the thirsty individuals (call this "collected donation"). It seems at least plausible to suggest that the difference in the method of delivery of water is morally irrelevant. Therefore, one might continue, if it is wrong not to make your directed donation, and considering that the difference between the directed and the collected donation is morally irrelevant, it is wrong not to make your collected donation either, i.e. not to pour your pint into the water-cart.

Now, one might reply by questioning the moral equivalence between directed and collected types of donation in Parfit's example – after all, one might say, it does make a moral difference, from a consequentialist perspective, whether one's pint of water is given to a specific individual or simply collected in a water cart: a single donation has perceptible consequences in the former but not in the latter case. However, the moral equivalence between directed and collected types of benefit seems less controversial in the case of individual contributions to herd immunity. Although each person who is vaccinated contributes only imperceptibly to vaccination rates – and therefore vaccination is in this respect analogous to collected donation –, vaccination might be decisive in whether or not another person is infected – and therefore vaccination is in this respect analogous to directed donation. Each person who is not vaccinated, although contributing only imperceptibly to herd immunity, might be the one who infects another, in the same way as each person who does not contribute her pint of water is paired with a thirsty person who does not receive any water in the case of directed donation. In the case of vaccination, then, directed and collected types of benefit overlap. Suppose that each individual non-vaccination constitutes a risk of infecting others of, say, 0.1%. This means that, statistically, one in every 1,000 non-vaccinated individuals will infect another person. But anyone can be the non-vaccinated person who infects others. When infection happens, not being vaccinated is to be considered as analogous to not giving one's pint of water in 'directed donation' for the purpose of attribution of moral responsibility: in both cases a person suffers or might even die for an easily preventable cause, and in both cases there is one person who could have prevented the harm and who is paired with the person who suffers the consequences of the first person's choice. Accordingly, we can conclude that, given the risk of infecting others posed by

any non-vaccinated person, given that the cost to each individual of avoiding this risk is small (considering the safety of vaccines), and given that infection can be an extremely negative outcome (which in some cases can cause the death of the infected individual), a utilitarian approach does justify a moral obligation to be vaccinated in spite of the imperceptible contribution of each vaccination to vaccine coverage rates.

The fact that there is only a small risk that infection will occur does not mean that individuals do not have a moral obligation to avoid the risk of being the ones who infect others: to the extent that the expected harm to others of non-vaccination remains larger than the expected harm of vaccination to the vaccinated individual (which seems to be the case, considering the proven safety of vaccines), the expected utility of non-vaccination is negative, and therefore utilitarianism implies that there is a *prima facie* moral obligation to be vaccinated. In fact, the only significant difference between the case of directed water donation and the case of vaccination is that in the former case the harm inflicted on other persons if individuals fail to make their contribution is certain, whereas in the latter case there is only a risk of inflicting harm on any individual. However, this difference is not significant enough to render non-vaccination permissible from a utilitarian point of view. If the harm of infection is large, even a small risk of causing infection due to non-vaccination may be sufficient to generate a significant expected harm.

As Dawson has noted, every single vaccination matters morally, at least where herd immunity does not exist, because without herd immunity any individual non-vaccination increases the risk of a significant harm to others "even if in an infinitely small way" (Dawson 2007, p. 170). Therefore, Dawson claims, "where we can perform an action to reduce the risk of foreseen harm to others through undergoing vaccination (at least where herd protection does not exist), then we may be obligated to do so" (Dawson 2007, p. 171). The analogy with directed water donation provides support for this claim, but also allows us to extend the same consideration to cases in which herd immunity does exist. After all, where the risk is of a very bad outcome and is applied to a large population, the fact that non-vaccination only very slightly increases the risk of infecting others (such as in cases where herd immunity does exist) does not make such risk insignificant.

Thus, a utilitarian approach supports a moral obligation to be vaccinated, *unless the individual cost of being vaccinated would be so great as to outweigh the expected negative contribution of non-vaccination to the aggregate wellbeing of others.* To compare, we can think of a case in which each of the men with the pint of water is also extremely thirsty to the point that they are about to die, and at least as thirsty as any of the wounded men in Parfit's example. In such case, utilitarianism would not ground a moral obligation for him to give away [their] pint of water to relieve another person's thirst. However, as a matter of fact, vaccination does not pose any significant cost to most individuals, and actually it provides significant benefits. Vaccines are very safe and effective, the risks of side-effects or iatrogenic diseases is very small, and there are typically also significant benefits in terms of protection from life-threatening diseases for the vaccinated individual (Andre et al. 2008). For example, the MMR vaccine is very safe when administered to healthy adults who are not allergic to the vaccine: the most common side effects consist at most in pain at the injection site, fever, a mild rash, and temporary pain and stiffness in the joints; the most serious side effect, immune thrombocytopenic purpura (ITP) (a disorder that decreases the body's ability to stop bleeding), has been observed in children, not in adults, and is in any case extremely rare, amounting to 1 case every 40,000 vaccinated children (CDC 2015a). In contrast, mumps, measles, and rubella can have serious and potentially fatal complications, including meningitis, swelling of the brain (encephalitis) and deafness; measles' fatality rate is around 0.2% (CDC 2016e) and acute encephalitis occurs in approximately 0.1% of reported cases; rubella in pregnancy can also result in serious birth defects and miscarriages (NHS 2015).

We can therefore refine the analogy with the case of water donation so as to reflect the fact that the cost to each individual of being vaccinated is small.

We can compare the case of vaccination with a case in which 1,000 people have 5 Ls (instead of 1 L) of water each, and each of 1,000 thirsty men needs only 1 L to alleviate their thirst. In this case, the cost to each individual of pouring 1 L in the water tank or of giving 1 L of water to a specific thirsty man is very small, because each individual can keep 4 Ls for herself. This analogy seems to better reflect the small cost that vaccination poses on each individual.

Thus, in spite of the imperceptible contribution each single vaccination makes to vaccine coverage rates and therefore to herd immunity, a utilitarian approach to vaccination does justify a moral obligation to be vaccinated, at least in cases in which the expected utility of non-vaccination for others is negative (there is a small risk of an extremely bad outcome), and the cost to each individual of preventing the negative outcome is small (we will discuss below in "High cost vaccinations" the case of individuals to whom the cost of vaccination is not small).

While the utilitarian justification for a moral obligation to be vaccinated applies to anyone (except those for whom vaccination would involve high risks), it is particularly compelling for people who are more likely to be exposed to infectious diseases and to infect others, such as health workers.

The Deontological Approach

This section explores two deontological approaches to responsibility for herd immunity: a (non-Kantian) approach based on universalization, or the generalization of a maxim of non-vaccination, and a contractualist theory.

Vaccination and the generalization test

The first deontological approach is based on a particular understanding of the universalizability test, which is often considered as the decisive test for assessing the morality of certain behaviours. According to this view – which is also known as the "generalization test" (Glover 1975, pp. 175–6) – a certain action is wrong if the consequences of everybody acting in that way would be significantly bad, even if the consequences of any one particular person acting in that way are not bad. In other words, according to this account, the question we should ask in order to assess the morality of a certain action is: what if everybody acted in this way? And in particular: what if everybody refused vaccination (for themselves or for their children)? Clearly, universal non-vaccination would have very bad consequences. So one might say that this moral approach renders non-vaccination immoral even if the consequences of any one person not being vaccinated are not bad. There are however two objections – at least one of which is decisive – that can be raised against the generalization test as a valid criterion for moral assessment.

First, one might appeal to the same (act) consequentialist objection that Shelly Kagan offered against the generalization test. The objection is that the generalization test is "in tension with the thought that the rightness or wrongness of a given act should depend upon the consequences of that act" (Kagan 2011, p. 112), rather than on counterfactual considerations about the consequences of hypothetical agents all acting in the same way. If we agree with Kagan's objection, we have to conclude that the generalization test does not represent a reliable method of moral assessment, and therefore that the question "what if everybody refused vaccination?" is irrelevant for a moral assessment of non-vaccination. This objection to the generalization test is however only available to those who subscribe to act consequentialism.

A second – and decisive – objection to the generalization test is based on the idea that, for the purpose of applying the generalization test, a full description of the action in question should include the description of all the circumstances which characterize that action (Glover 1975, pp. 176–7). But refining further the description of the action to be generalized would undermine the generalization test, because "the more complete in the relevant respects the description becomes, the closer the generalization test comes to giving the same answer that one gets to the question "what will happen if *I* do this?" (Glover 1975, p. 176).

Thus, for example, at least in cases where herd immunity is realised, a person who chooses not to be vaccinated because she *knows* that, say, 95% of other people will be vaccinated anyway, could claim that her action is to be described not simply as 'non-vaccination' – whose generalization would have bad consequences – but more specifically as 'non-vaccination on the basis of the knowledge that enough other people around me are vaccinated'. Thus, the answer to the question 'what would happen if everybody were not vaccinated in the circumstances I find myself in?' would be equivalent to the answer to the question 'what would happen if I were not vaccinated?' The generalization test boils down to an act-consequentialist assessment of non-vaccination. Therefore, the generalization test would be redundant: we do not need it to decide the morality of non-vaccination, which would ultimately depend on whether or not we accept act-consequentialism.

Vaccination and contractualism

A second possible deontological approach is contractualism (see Ashford and Mulgan 2012). According to contractualism, people should act upon principles to which all could accede, or would accede under some specified ideal circumstances. Scanlon's (1998) classic formulation holds, more precisely, that

> [a]n act is wrong if its performance under the circumstances would be disallowed by any set of principles for the general regulation of behaviour that no one could reasonably reject as a basis for informed, unforced, general agreement. (Scanlon 1998, p. 153).

Marcel Verweij holds that, when applied to the case of vaccination, contractualism is a very demanding theory. As he writes, "[p]ersons most vulnerable to the disease do not respond optimally to vaccination (. . .) and therefore they will be much better protected if everyone were vaccinated, the old and the young, the ill and the healthy" (Verweij 2005, p. 333). It seems therefore that a person could not justify her decision not to be vaccinated to the vulnerable members of the community who are at risk of contagion, as contractualism would require.

One might reply that the additional risk that any non-vaccinated person would pose to others is negligible, as is the additional contribution of the individual to coverage rates and to herd immunity. Accordingly, it might seem that a person could justify her decision not to be vaccinated to vulnerable people. For example, the principle regulating her behaviour might be something like 'I won't be vaccinated if I know that enough other people in my community are vaccinated anyway', or 'I won't be vaccinated if I know that few people in my community are vaccinated anyway'. In either case non-vaccination would pose only a small additional risk to vulnerable people. However, such a small additional risk does make a difference in terms of the moral assessment of non-vaccination not only in a utilitarian perspective (as seen above), but also within a contractualism framework. It is rational for each person who is at risk of infection to demand that others contribute to keeping this risk of infection to a minimum. When keeping the risk of infection to a minimum comes at a small cost to others, as is the case with vaccination, this demand by persons at risk is not only rational, but also reasonable. We are here defining "reasonable" in such a way that the objective costs one has to bear, such as the risks of side-effects the vaccinated takes on herself, make the option in question reasonable or an unreasonable to reject; thus, the small risks involved make a principle that prescribe to be vaccinated, in this sense, unreasonable to reject. However, some would insist that the psychological or emotive costs of vaccination would remain very high for those who have deeply held religious or moral beliefs against vaccination or who are genuinely scared of the possible side-effects of vaccines. We will address the issue of vaccination that are high cost in psychological or emotive terms in "High cost vaccinations".

Thus, contractualism can ground a moral obligation to be vaccinated, at least as long as vaccination entails a small cost to individuals.

Verweij says that "contractualism requires us to take precautions that seem to be excessive" (Verweij 2005,

p. 334), and more generally some have claimed that contractualism is a too demanding ethical theory (Ashford 2003). Whether or not this is true, contractualism does not seem to be too demanding in the case of vaccination, and therefore this objection is not available to those who wish to reject a contractualist justification of a moral duty to be vaccinated. The precautions that contractualism requires us to take do not seem to be excessive in the case of vaccination, considering the very small individual cost that vaccination entails, at least for the vast majority of individuals (again, we will address the issue of the moral obligation of those for whom vaccination would entail a high cost below in "High cost vaccinations"). Thus, regardless of whether contractualism is in itself a too demanding theory, to the extent that vaccination entails a small cost to individuals we can certainly appeal to contractualism to justify a moral obligation to be vaccinated, in spite of the negligible contribution of each vaccination to the realisation of herd immunity.

Duty of Easy Rescue and Fairness: A Further Argument for an Individual Moral Obligation to be Vaccinated

We have seen that both a utilitarian and a contractualist approach can justify a moral obligation to be vaccinated (or to vaccinate one's children) in spite of the negligible individual contribution to herd immunity, at least if non-vaccination constitutes a small additional risk of infecting others that can be prevented at a very small cost to individuals. One might reply, however, that appealing to utilitarianism or to contractualism is problematic because it requires accepting comprehensive moral theories to which many reasonable people do not subscribe. Both utilitarianism and contractualism are often considered very demanding theories. In fact, they would justify an obligation to be vaccinated even if the cost to individuals were not small, as long as the benefits to others of vaccination remain sufficiently large, and some may reject the theories on this basis. Thus, in this section we seek to offer a more ecumenical justification for a moral obligation to be vaccinated, one that renders it unnecessary to appeal to utilitarianism, contractualism, or any other contested, comprehensive moral doctrine. Our justification appeals to a duty of easy rescue applied to collectives that could be endorsed by proponents of a wide range of such doctrines.

Easy rescue, collective obligations, and the individual duty to be vaccinated

A duty of easy rescue is an almost uncontroversial requirement of morality, i.e. a requirement on which most reasonable people would agree, no matter what moral theory or moral view they subscribe to (with the exception, perhaps, of some libertarians). According to the duty of easy rescue, when I could do something that entails a small cost to me and a significant benefit to others, I have a moral duty to do it. Peter Singer provided perhaps the most famous characterization of the duty of easy rescue in his article *Famine, affluence, and morality*, through the well-known example of the child drowning in a pond. The case is analogous to all the cases in which an agent could easily avoid serious harm to someone else without significant personal costs. According to Singer,

> "if I am walking past a shallow pond and see a child drowning in it, I ought to wade in and pull the child out. This will mean getting my clothes muddy, but this is insignificant, while the death of the child would presumably be a very bad thing" (Singer 1972, p. 231).

The duty of easy rescue as expressed by Singer's example does not presuppose, nor does it support (though it is consistent with), a utilitarian morality. A formulation of the duty of easy rescue has been provided by Tim Scanlon, according to whom, "[i]f we can prevent something very bad from happening to someone by making a slight or even moderate sacrifice, it would be wrong not to do so" (Scanlon 1998, p. 224). Thus, both utilitarians (such as Peter Singer)

and contractualists (such as Tim Scanlon) have endorsed a duty of easy rescue. This is not surprising: we have seen above that both a utilitarian and a contractualist ethical approach support a moral obligation to be vaccinated and to reduce the small additional risk of infecting others at least *as long as this comes at a small cost to individuals*.

Now, considering the small cost to individuals of vaccination, being vaccinated is comparable to getting one's clothes muddy in Singer's example, or to donating one's litre of water in Parfit's example (or perhaps, one could plausibly argue, it is even less costly, given its benefits). However, the desirable outcome – namely herd immunity – cannot be realised individually. Herd immunity is a "collective effect": it requires the contribution of a sufficiently large number of individuals to be realised. Accordingly, if there is a moral duty to realise herd immunity, such moral duty will arguably need to take a collective, rather than an individual form: no individual can realise herd immunity, in the same sense in which no individual can form a circle. Many would take this to imply that no individual can have a duty to realise such immunity, since 'has a duty to' implies 'can'.

As is the case with individuals, one uncontroversial way to justify the collective moral responsibility to realise herd immunity is to say that such responsibility expresses a duty of easy rescue, and more precisely a collective duty of easy rescue: realising herd immunity would be a collective moral obligation if it came at a very small cost to the collective. We can express the principle at the basis of the collective duty of easy rescue in the case of herd immunity as follows:

> If a collective could realise herd immunity, then this collective ought to realise herd immunity, provided that the collective cost is small and can distributed in such a way that the cost borne by each individual is also small (so that the collective cost is small under any plausible understanding of "collective" and that the collective duty is consistent with an individual duty of easy rescue)

It is not difficult to see how the principle grounds a collective moral duty to realise herd immunity: the small individual cost of vaccination entails that the cost to the collective of fulfilling its duty is also very small, because it merely consists of the aggregate individual small costs of vaccination, and there is no additional cost that the collective has to bear; at the same time, the benefits of realising herd immunity are very large. Therefore, there is the collective moral duty, grounded in a collective duty of easy rescue, to realise herd immunity. For the sake of consistency with the terminology used in the relevant literature, we will refer to this collective duty also with the terms "collective responsibility" and "collective obligation": for the purpose of the present discussion, these terms are to be understood as synonymous.

Now, who exactly is the bearer of such responsibility? Is it borne by the collective as a unified agent? Is it somehow distributed across the individuals that comprise the collective? Or both? Here, we need to distinguish two questions: the first is a conceptual question: *what does it mean* to attribute moral responsibility to a loose collection of individuals – understood as a collection without a decisional procedure and an internal structure – like the individuals who together could realise herd immunity? The second question is instead genuinely ethical: what are the *ethical implications* of attribution of collective responsibility to loose collections of individuals for attribution of individual responsibility?

The debate on collective responsibility of loose collectives has focussed mainly on the former question, providing different answers (see e.g. Wringe 2016, 2010; Aas 2015; Pinkert 2014; Björnsson 2014; Collins 2013; Schwenkenbecher 2013; Lawford-Smith 2012; Isaacs 2011). To give just a quick overview of the types of concepts involved, the collective responsibility of loose collection has been conceived as a "joint" responsibility or duty (Pinkert 2014; Schwenkenbecher 2013), or as "shared" responsibility (Björnsson 2014), or as a "putative" collective responsibility (Isaacs 2011 and 2014), or as a form of responsibility attributed to a collective agent (Aas 2015), or as a form of responsibility that "supervenes" on individual responsibilities (Wringe 2016). However, we do not need to go into the details of each of these

positions here, and therefore we are not going to provide a definition of each of these concepts. Rather, here we want to address directly the second, ethical question about what the attribution of a collective obligation to a loose collection of individuals implies, for an ethical point of view, in terms of attribution of individual responsibility.

We suggest that an ethical analysis of collective responsibility can allow the derivation from the existence of a collective duty of easy rescue of an individual *duty to contribute* to the relevant collective outcome, which, in the case of a collective obligation to realise herd immunity, translates into an individual duty to be vaccinated (or to vaccinate one's children). More in particular, the collective obligation to realise herd immunity implies a duty for each individual to contribute to herd immunity – and therefore to be vaccinated – on the basis of a principle of *fairness* in the distribution of the burdens entailed by the collective moral obligation, or, as George Klosko put it, on the basis of a "just distribution of benefits and burdens" (Klosko 2004, p. 34). The burdens consist in people having to pay a visit to the doctor, receive an injection, incur the (very small) risk of side effects of the vaccine and of iatrogenic disease, and, for those who have reservations about the ethics of vaccination, overcome such reservations. A principle of fairness requires that such burdens be distributed fairly across individuals, and therefore that each individual take on herself a fair share of the burdens entailed by the collective obligation by being vaccinated, unless being vaccinated is too burdensome for the individual (we will consider these rare cases in "High cost vaccinations"). This means that the type of collective responsibility that is entailed by the duty of collective easy rescue can be understood in a merely *distributive* sense (Held 1970). We can take the notion of *distributive* collective responsibility to indicate that *all* members of a sufficiently large group have an individual obligation to *contribute* to the realisation of a desirable collective effect, such as herd immunity, and that in virtue of a principle of fairness in the distribution of the burdens entailed by a collective obligation such individual obligation exists in spite of the fact that any individual's contribution to coverage rates and to the realisation of herd immunity is imperceptible.

Notice that our argument is *not* the same as the argument according to which the non-vaccinated would be impermissibly free-riding on herd immunity (Navin 2013, pp. 70–75, 2015, pp. 143–144; van den Hoven 2012; Dawson 2007, pp. 174–176), although the impermissibility of free-riding is an implication of our argument. To use once again George Klosko's words, the problem is not so much that "[i]ndividuals who benefit from the cooperative efforts of others have obligations to cooperate as well" (Klosko 2004, p. 34), and therefore that individuals would violate a requirement of reciprocity. Rather, the unfairness implied by the decision not to contribute to herd immunity is, at a more fundamental level, the unfairness of failing to make one's contribution to fulfilling a collective obligation that is ascribed to the collective of which we are part, i.e. the collective that can realise herd immunity from any disease. The conceptual distinction between the two types of unfairness also has significant practical implications. For example, suppose that in a given community there is herd immunity against measles but not against HPV. In such a context, the unfairness of free-riding on herd immunity implies that a person has a moral obligation to be vaccinated against measles, but not against HPV, given that in the case of HPV there is no herd immunity on which this person can free-ride. However, our argument based on the unfairness of failing to make one's contribution to a collective good like herd immunity implies that a person has a moral obligation to be vaccinated against both, given that herd immunity against both measles and HPV is a valuable societal goal that that community has a moral obligation to realise or to preserve. Or consider the following:[2] sometimes, in polio outbreaks, healthy people who have been already vaccinated with the inactivated polio virus (IPV) are called to take the oral polio vaccine (OPV) as well in order to disseminate it in the benefit of the vulnerable: the attenuated vaccine virus in the OPV replicates in the intestine and is then excreted, which

allows it to spread in the immediate community (WHO 2017). Thus, those taking OPV do not need vaccination for themselves at all if they have already been vaccinated with IPV; they only take OPV in order to benefit their community. Once again, while an argument based on the unfairness of free-riding would not imply that these healthy people have a moral obligation to take the OPV – because, being already vaccinated, they would not "benefit" from herd immunity (except in the broad sense in which everyone benefits from living in a society without polio) – our argument based on a fairness based obligation to make a contribution to a public good does imply that they have such a moral obligation, though it may be a weaker one to the extent that the benefit of the vaccination is smaller in such cases.

Also, our argument can be taken to have some implications for the issue of whether, in case of an infectious disease outbreak, those who refused vaccination for themselves or for their children for non medical reasons should be held accountable, or morally responsible, for the whole outbreak, i.e. even if they have not directly infected anyone or only infected a few people. The answer to this question depends on whether the notion of 'accountability' or 'moral responsibility' we are using presupposes causal responsibility. If we think that accountability or moral responsibility presuppose causal responsibility, i.e., that someone can be accountable, or morally responsible, for outcome x only if they are to some extent causally responsible for x, then of course a non-vaccinated individual is not accountable for the outbreak unless she infects so many people that the number of people infected by her is so great that it constitutes by itself an outbreak (which is unlikely), or unless the chain of infections that spread among the population can all be traced back to her as the one who started the contagion. However, if we think that accountability or moral responsibility do not presuppose causal responsibility, i.e. that someone can be held accountable, or morally responsible, for x even if she does not play any causal role in bringing about x, then our argument does imply that she is accountable, or morally responsible, for the outbreak, because she failed to fulfil her moral duty to make her fair contribution to the prevention of the contagion, regardless of whether her contribution would have made a difference. In the same way we can say, for example, that I am accountable or morally responsible for global warming if I engage in practices that involve unnecessary release of carbon emissions, even if the quantity of my carbon emissions does not make any difference to whether global warming occurs.

Let us address two possible objections to our arguments.

The first objection is that individuals have a right to bodily integrity, which includes a right not to have any external substance injected in their body. This right to bodily integrity could be thought to outweigh any moral obligation to be vaccinated. In this view, making one's fair contribution to herd immunity would be morally different from making one's contribution to any other collective or public good that does not involve the violation of individual rights to bodily integrity. A right to bodily integrity can be understood in either of two senses: either as a right not to undergo any invasive medical procedure without one's consent or as a right not to have external substances introduced in one's body without one's consent. However, on either of these two understandings, this objection misconstrues the nature of the right to bodily integrity. The right to bodily integrity is normally understood – with reference to Hohfeld's analysis of rights – as a claim-right held against others. It is a right that others not interfere with one's body in certain ways, and perhaps also that they provide one with certain forms of assistance required for the minimal functioning of one's body. Understood thus, the right to bodily integrity may imply that others are under a *pro-tanto* duty not to impose vaccination on an individual without their consent. However, the claim-right to bodily integrity held *against others* does not imply that one is under no moral duty to vaccinate oneself: having a claim right to non-x (e.g., to non-vaccination) is quite consistent with having a moral duty to x. In other words, if you have a right to bodily integrity, the right will entail that other people are under a duty not to force

the vaccine on you. But it does not imply anything about what you morally ought to do. Thus, in principle, an appeal to the right to bodily integrity does not constitute a reason against the existence of a moral duty to be vaccinated. Of course, in practice, when vaccination is imposed by parents or medical professionals on children, children may possess a right to bodily integrity that is infringed by this imposition. However, it should be noted that, if the child is competent to consent, their valid consent could be obtained prior to vaccination, and this would prevent the vaccination from infringing the right to bodily integrity. In that case, the parents could still have an obligation to vaccinate their child, conditional on the child consenting to this. If consent cannot be obtained, then whether the *pro-tanto* duty not to impose vaccination that derives from a right to bodily integrity represents an all-things-considered duty not to vaccinate a child without their consent will depend on (I) how weighty the right is relative to the goods that can be achieved by forcible vaccination and the values that can be promoted (e.g., fairness), and (II) whether imposing vaccination involves bodily interference of the sort that infringes the right to bodily integrity, which remains to be established. Thus, parents might still be under a moral obligation to vaccinate their children even if this entails some violation of their right to bodily autonomy. In any case, even if the right to bodily autonomy is very weighty, it does not represent an argument against a duty to be vaccinated or to vaccinate one's children, but only an argument against *the enforcement* of such duty.

The second objection is that, as Pinkert put it in his criticism of Wringe's distributive notion of collective responsibility, moral obligations to *contribute* to a collective outcome, without any further qualification, "imply that you ought to contribute even if not enough others contribute as well"; however, Pinkert continues, "it is implausible that one ought to perform such pointless actions" (Pinkert 2014, p. 189). Admittedly, our distributive notion of collective responsibility grounded in a principle of fairness implies that any individual has a moral obligation to contribute to herd immunity regardless of whether other members of the collective do their part, and therefore even if her contribution is pointless. Requiring everybody to be vaccinated regardless of how many people around them are vaccinated might sound implausible because a principle of utility conflicts with a principle of fairness: fairness would require to choose an option, namely vaccination, that has no utility net, and actually has a (small) cost for the individual. Our reply to this objection is twofold.

First, even if the act of vaccination is "pointless" as a contribution to herd immunity, it is not pointless on a utilitarian assessment. As we saw in the section on utilitarianism, it is simply not true that the utility net of any individual vaccination would be zero, given that any non-vaccinated person has a small chance of infecting others. Therefore, in this perspective, each individual vaccination is not pointless: vaccination might not be morally obligatory as a "contribution" to herd immunity, but it would still be morally required in order to minimize the risk of infecting others. In this sense, vaccination is different from the contribution to any other outcome that requires the imperceptible contribution of each of a large number of individuals, such as filling the water cart in Parfit's example. There is a small chance that any vaccination would make a difference not qua "contribution" to herd immunity but in terms of infection prevention. Therefore, fairness does not conflict with expected utility: they both imply that individuals ought to be vaccinated. Moreover, another consideration in support of the idea that individual vaccination has positive expected utility and therefore that the moral obligation to be vaccinated can be supported on utilitarian grounds is that community efforts to cultivate herd immunity are often projects only of domestic politics; however, the fact that people in the globalized world travel at an unprecedented rate implies that exposure to vaccine-preventable diseases is only a plane trip away. Therefore, individual vaccination provides expected net utility given that, even when there is herd immunity, there still is vulnerability for individuals in the global context.

Second, fairness would still demand that any individual contributed to herd immunity even if the contribution, qua contribution to herd immunity, would be pointless. There are two possible scenarios here: either the individual contribution, qua contribution to herd immunity, is pointless and herd immunity exists, or the individual contribution, qua contribution to herd immunity, is pointless and herd immunity does not exist. In the first case, every individual would be under a moral obligation to be vaccinated to ensure that those who are vaccinated are not unfairly burdened, even if any contribution, qua contribution to herd immunity, is pointless. Compare the case of vaccination with the case of taxation: society would probably be able to tolerate a certain number of free-riders, who enjoy but do not contribute through their taxes to the maintenance of certain public goods; actually, overall utility would probably be maximized if a few individuals were allowed not to pay taxes, because, without their money, certain public goods, e.g., national defense or a good health care system, could still be guaranteed, and they would get to save some money. However, we are not inclined to tolerate tax evasion regardless of the impact that tax evasion has on the capacity of a state to provide certain public goods, because, at least where the vast majority of individuals do pay their own taxes, we expect all individuals to make their fair contribution: if I am under a moral or a legal obligation to pay my fair amount of taxes, we expect that everybody else is or should be, even if this would not maximize utility. The same considerations can be applied to the case of individuals' fair contribution to the public good of herd immunity.

Consider now the second possible scenario – where any contribution qua contribution is pointless and herd immunity does not exist. Admittedly, in this case it is more difficult to argue that everybody has a fairness based moral obligation to be vaccinated. As Navin put it, "I have a duty of fairness to contribute to herd immunity only if most other members of my community act on the basis of this duty. If they do not, then herd immunity will not exist, and, therefore, I will not have a duty of fairness to contribute to it"

(Navin 2015, p. 180). There are two possible replies here, the first of which is probably stronger than the second.

The first reply is that, as we have said above, in such cases considerations of fairness would be replaced by welfarist considerations or considerations of general beneficence: especially where vaccination rate is low, any non-vaccinated individual would significantly increase the risk that others be infected, so any individual would still have a duty to be vaccinated in order to minimize the risk of harming others.

Second, it is not so obvious that where too few people contribute to a public good and the public good is therefore not realised, there is no duty of fairness to nonetheless make one's contribution. One could plausibly argue that even if most people around me did not pay their taxes, I would still have a moral duty to pay my fair share, on condition that what is considered fair is not determined by the fact that others do not make their fair contribution – for example, on condition that I am not requested to pay more taxes to compensate for the fact that many people around me do not pay theirs. This condition however does not apply to the case of vaccination, given that there is nothing more that any individual could do to contribute to herd immunity than to be vaccinated (or to vaccinate her children). Therefore, one could plausibly argue that I have a duty of fairness to be vaccinated even if few people around me are vaccinated in the same way as I have a duty of fairness to pay my fair (but no more than my fair) share of taxes even if many people around me do not. Admittedly, though, if such a moral duty existed, it would be quite a weak duty, and indeed it would be the weaker, the higher the number of people around me who fail to make their contribution. Also, the intuition that there is even a weak moral duty to make one's contribution in such circumstances is probably not widely shared.

High cost vaccinations

Mark Navin holds that one's contribution to herd immunity is fair when the cost is not only roughly the same for everyone, but also "reasonable", i.e. not overdemanding (Navin 2015, p. 142). This restriction seems appropriate in light of a duty of (individual) easy rescue and to the extent that, generally speaking, the cost individuals *normally* have to bear for being vaccinated is small.

But what kind of cost can be considered large enough to outweigh the moral duty to be vaccinated, i.e. to make vaccination supererogatory? One might suppose that it would make a difference whether an individual has health insurance (or is anyway covered by a national healthcare system). Without health insurance, any possible side effect of vaccination could potentially become a great burden. However, we need to consider that, as we said above, side effects of vaccines are very rare, and the most common of these rare side effects are not serious. Thus, the risks of vaccination for the uninsured remain very small, and indeed, though we cannot argue for this point here, we believe they are so small that they are insufficient to undermine the moral obligation to be vaccinated.

Admittedly, though, the cost of vaccination is not always small. Some people are too young or too old to be vaccinated, some people are allergic to vaccines, some people are immunosuppressed. Vaccination would be unsafe for these individuals, and therefore the cost to them of being vaccinated would not be small. Fortunately, our arguments do not imply that individuals have an obligation to undergo *high cost* vaccinations. Indeed, our requirement that the costs of fulfilling the collective duty to realise herd immunity must be distributed fairly could be invoked in support of the view that individuals need not undergo high cost vaccinations. Such high cost vaccinations would be unfair, since these individuals would be required to bear a greater share of the costs of realising herd immunity than others. As noted above, fairness requires that individuals bear similar costs.

Besides, our formulation of the collective duty of easy rescue requires that the costs for all individuals be small. This means that those for whom vaccination would represent a high cost will have to be excluded from the collective that is subject to the collective obligation, in order for the collective to fall under the duty in the first place.

It might be the case that some vaccinations entail high costs of a psychological nature, for example when parents have religion based objections to vaccines that use materials from cell lines derived from aborted foetuses or experience severe psychological distress worrying about potential vaccine complications for their vaccinated child. Perhaps in such cases fairness-based reasons are not strong enough to justify the existence of a duty to vaccinate, given that one might object that vaccinating in such cases is supererogatory. Now, it is not clear whether the moral significance of the psychological costs involved outweighs the strength of fairness-based reasons. But let's assume, for the sake of argument, that it does. Even if that is the case, the problem is not so much with the fairness demand itself, but with what is demanded, namely vaccination. Exactly as is the case with pacifists' exemptions from military duties, fairness would still demand that vaccine refusers make some alternative contribution to public health that could be considered equivalent to one's contribution to herd immunity, as has recently been argued (Giubilini et al. 2017). The important point, for the purposes of the present discussion, is that individuals cannot simply escape a basic fairness demand to contribute to herd immunity; assuming for the sake of argument that for certain people for whom vaccination would entail a high psychological cost such demand of fairness does not translate into a moral obligation to vaccinate, fairness would still demand that these people make up, or compensate for their failure to vaccinate.

Conclusion

We saw earlier that the difficulty with attributing to individuals the moral obligation to be vaccinated is due to the fact that any individual contribution to the realisation of herd immunity is negligible. We have shown that this negligibility is not enough to rule out two arguments for the existence of a moral obligation to be vaccinated, i.e. a utilitarian argument based on Parfit's Principle of Group Beneficence and a contractualist argument.

We have also offered an additional argument for a moral obligation to contribute to herd immunity, an argument that does not require committing to problematic and not universally accepted moral theories. We have argued that there exists a duty of easy rescue – a type of duty on which most reasonable people would agree – that can be applied to collectives to ground a collective obligation to realise herd immunity. A principle of fairness in the distribution of the burdens entailed by such collective obligation allows to derive from it an individual moral obligation to be vaccinated.

Thus, we can conclude that, in spite of the negligible impact of individual vaccinations on vaccine coverage rates and on the realisation of herd immunity, there are at least three types of argument, at least one of which morally uncontroversial, that justify an individual moral obligation to be vaccinated.

Such moral obligation, in turn, strengthens the ethical justification for the imposition of coercive vaccination policies. Examples of such policies include mandatory vaccination, such as making vaccination a requirement for enrolling children in school or daycare; withholding of financial benefits for those who are not vaccinated or do not vaccinate their children; and outright compulsory vaccination. Determining which of these policies would be preferable, both from a pragmatic and from an ethical perspective, would require a separate discussion.

Notes

1 We are grateful to an anonymous reviewer for raising this objection.

2 We are grateful to an anonymous reviewer for having drawn our attention to this implication.

References

Aas, S. 2015. Distributing collective obligation. *Journal of Ethics and Social Philosophy* 9: 3.

Andre, F. E., et al. 2008. Vaccination greatly reduces disease, disability, death, and inequity worldwide. *Bulletin of the World Health Organization*, 86: 2. http://www.who.int/bulletin/volumes/86/2/07-040089/en/. Accessed 17 Aug 2017.

Ashford, E. 2003. The demandingness of Scanlon's contractualism. *Ethics* 113 (2): 273–302.

Ashford, E., and T. Mulgan. 2012. Contractualism. In *Stanford Encyclopedia of Philosophy*, ed. Edward N. Zalta. https://plato.stanford.edu/entries/contractualism/.

Björnsson, Gunnar. 2014. Essentially shared obligations. *Midwest Studies in Philosophy* 38 (1): 103–20.

CDC. 2015a. *Vaccine Safety*. http://www.cdc.gov/vaccinesafety/index.html. Accessed 17 Aug 2017.

CDC. 2015b. *Measles, Mumps, and Rubella (MMR) Vaccines*. https://www.cdc.gov/vaccinesafety/vaccines/mmr-vaccine.html.

CDC. 2016a. *Measles Cases and Outbreaks*. http://www.cdc.gov/measles/cases-outbreaks.html. Accessed 17 Aug 2017.

CDC. 2016b. *Who Should & Who Should Not get vaccinated*. https://www.cdc.gov/flu/prevent/whoshouldvax.htm.

CDC. 2016c. *Long-term Effectiveness of Whooping Cough Vaccines*. http://www.cdc.gov/pertussis/pregnant/mom/vacc-effectiveness.html. Accessed 17 Aug 2017.

CDC. 2016d. *Adult Immunization Schedule*. http://www.cdc.gov/vacci nes/schedules/hcp/imz/adult.html. Accessed 17 Aug 2017.

CDC. 2016e. *Measles*. https://www.cdc.gov/vaccines/pubs/pinkbook/meas.html. Accessed 17 Aug 2017.

Collins, S. 2013. Collectives' duties and collectivisation duties. *Australasian Journal of Philosophy* 91 (2): 231–48.

Dawson, Angus. 2007. Herd protection as a public good: vaccination and our obligations to others. In *Ethics, Prevention, and Public Health*, eds. A. Dawson, and M. Verweij, 160–87. Oxford: Clarendon Press.

Dawson, Angus. 2011. Vaccination ethics. In *Public Health Ethics. Key Concepts and Issues in Policy and Practice*, ed. A. Dawson, 143–53. New York: Cambridge University Press.

ECDC. 2017. *Epidemiological Update: Measles – Monitoring European Outbreaks*, 7 July 2017. https://ecdc.europa. eu/en/news-events/epidemiological-update-measles-monitoring-european-outbreaks-7-july-2017. Accessed 17 Aug 2017.

Fine, Paul, et al. 2011. "Herd immunity": a rough guide. *Clinical Infectious Diseases* 52 (7): 911–6.

Flanigan, Jessica. 2014. A defense of compulsory vaccination. *HEC Forum* 26: 5–25.

Giubilini, A., T. Douglas, and J. Savulescu. 2017. Liberty, fairness, and the 'contribution model' for non-medical vaccine exemption policies: a reply to Navin and Largent. *Public Health Ethics* 10 (3): 235–40.

Glover, Jonathan. 1975. It makes no difference whether or not I do it. In *Proceedings of the Aristotelian Society, Supplementary Volumes*, 49: 171–209.

Harmsen, Irene, et al. 2013. Why parents refuse childhood vaccination: a qualitative study using online focus groups. *BMC Public Health* 13: 1183.

Held, Virginia. 1970. Can a random collection of individuals be morally responsible? *Journal of Philosophy* 67 (14): 471–81.

Isaacs, Tracy. 2011. *Moral Responsibility in Collective Contexts*. New York: Oxford University Press.

Isaacs, Tracy. 2014. Collective Responsibility and Collective Obligation. *Midwest Studies in Philosophy* 38 (1), 40–57.

Kagan, Shelly. 2011. Do I make a difference? *Philosophy and Public Affairs* 39 (2): 105–141.

Klosko, George. 2004 (1992). *The Principle of Fairness and Political Obligation*. Lanham: Rowman and Littlefield.

Lawford-Smith, Holly. 2012. The feasibility of collectives' actions. *Australasian Journal of Philosophy* 90: 453–67.

Luyten, Jeroen, et al. 2011. Vaccination policy and ethical challenges posed by herd immunity, suboptimal uptake, and subgroup targeting. *Public Health Ethics* 4 (3): 280–91.

Navin, Mark. 2013. Resisting moral permissiveness about vaccine refusal. *Public Affairs Quarterly* 27 (1): 69–85.

Navin, Mark. 2015. *Values and Vaccine Refusal: Hard Questions in Ethics, Epistemology, and Health Care*. New York: Routledge.

NHS. 2015, *MMR Vaccine*. http://www.nhs.uk/Conditions/vaccinations/Pages/mmr-vaccine.aspx. Accessed 28 Nov 2016.

Otsuka, Michael. 1991. The paradox of group beneficence. *Philosophy and Public Affairs* 20 (2): 132–49.

Parfit, Derek. 1984. *Reasons and Persons*. Oxford: Oxford University Press.

Pierik, Roland. 2016. Mandatory vaccination: an unqualified defense. *Journal of Applied Philosophy.* https://doi.org/10.1111/japp.12215.

Pinkert, Felix. 2014. What we together can (be required to) do. *Midwest Studies of Philosophy* 23: 187–202.

Scanlon, Tim. 1998. *What We Owe to Each Other.* Cambridge, MA: Harvard University Press.

Schwenkenbecher, Anne. 2013. Joint duties and global moral obligations. *Ratio* 26: 310–28.

Singer, Peter. 1972. Famine, affluence, and morality. *Philosophy and Public Affairs* 1 (3): 229–43.

Smith, Philip, et al. 2011. Parental delay or refusal of vaccine doses, childhood vaccination coverage at 24 months of age, and the health belief model. *Public Health Report* 126: 135–46.

van den Hoven, M. 2012. Why one should do one's bit: Thinking about free riding in the context of public health ethics. *Public Health Ethics* 5 (2): 154–60.

Verweij, Marcel. 2005. Obligatory precautions against infections. *Bioethics* 19 (4): 323–35.

Verweij, Marcel, and A. Dawson. 2004. Ethical principles for collective immunization programs. *Vaccine* 22: 3122–36.

WHO. 2017, What is vaccine-derived polio? http://www.who.int/features/qa/64/en/. Accessed 3 Feb 2018.

Wringe, Bill. 2010. Global obligations and the agency objection. *Ratio* 23 (2): 217–231.

Wringe, Bill. 2016. Collective obligations: their existence, their explanatory power, and their supervenience on the obligations of individuals. *European Journal of Philosophy* 24 (2): 472–97.

72

Taking Responsibility for Responsibility

Neil Levy

Governments, physicians, media and academics have all called for individuals to bear responsibility for their own health. In this article, I argue that requiring those with adverse health outcomes to bear responsibility for these outcomes is a bad basis for policy. The available evidence strongly suggests that the capacities for responsible choice, and the circumstances in which these capacities are exercised, are distributed alongside the kinds of goods we usually talk about in discussing distributive justice, and this distribution significantly explains why people make bad health choices. These facts suggest that we cannot justifiably hold them responsible for these choices. We do better to hold responsible those who determine the ways in which capacities and circumstances are distributed: they are indirectly responsible for these adverse health outcomes and possess the capacities and resources to take responsibility for these facts.

Calls for us to take responsibility for our health, and expressions of blame for those become ill, are common. While the harshest condemnation comes from the popular press, calls for us to take responsibility come from a variety of sources, including physicians themselves and even governments. In this article, I argue that these calls are unjustified. I argue that the capacities for responsibility, and the circumstances in which they are exercised, are themselves distributed: typically, agents can effectively take responsibility for their own health by adopting healthier lifestyles only if they are the beneficiaries of distributive mechanisms that allocate life chances.[1] In this light, calls for us to take responsibility for our health are best understood as responsibility-shifting mechanisms: they serve to shift the burden from those who are best equipped to meet it to those who cannot.

Calls for us to take responsibility come from multiple sources. They are to be found in the popular press (Macrae, 2016), in the academic literature (Callahan, 2013) and in public statements from corporations (Kent, 2009). In this article, I am concerned with these calls only insofar as they might form a basis for public policy. Responsibility is already enshrined in the *NHS Constitution for England* (NHS, 2015) and underlies health policy in other countries. For example, Hungary reportedly uses adherence to dietary recommendations to exclude patients from access to

Original publication details: Neil Levy, "Taking Responsibility for Responsibility," pp. 108–113 from *Public Health Ethics* 12: 2 (July 2019). Oxford University Press / Open access.

some therapies (Hazell, 2012). It is with responsibility in these kinds of contexts that I am principally concerned. While the considerations I will cite have implications that are broader than exhortations to responsibility in these contexts, it is here that their implications are clearest. Responsibility is not a good basis for public policy, I will suggest, because policies should be formulated in ways that are insensitive to fine-grained differences in the capacities that underlie responsibility. While there may be individuals who might appropriately be asked to take responsibility for their health, they form too small a minority, and they are too difficult to identify, for responsibility to be a good basis for policy. Conversely, there is a large group of individuals who might appropriately be asked to take responsibility *for* responsibility. It is both fairer, and better policy, to address such demands to them, and not to those whose health suffers as a consequence of their own choices.

Responsibility for Health

Should agents be expected to take responsibility for their health? Calls for us to do so have arisen in response to the recognition that ill-health is not something that just happens to us. Rather, early mortality and increases in morbidity are often due at least in important part to our behavior. Lifestyle factors are very significantly responsible for the global burden of disease: up to 40 per cent of premature deaths are preventable by changes to lifestyle (Yoon et al., 2014). We are in the midst of what the World Health Organization (2003) described as an *obesity epidemic*, and it is widely held that obesity is a risk factor for cancer, heart disease and stroke (WHO, 2014).[2] Accordingly, WHO has called for changes in lifestyle to halt this epidemic, as well as to reduce or eliminate other risk factors for early mortality and increased morbidity (WHO, 2014). Lack of sufficient exercise, excessive drinking and smoking all contribute to ill-health. Moreover, when disease arises, there is usually a great deal we can do to help to manage it, and patients fail surprisingly often to do these things – only about

half of all prescribed doses of medication are taken by patients, for instance (Nieuwlaat et al., 2014).

In the light of these facts, calls for us to take responsibility for our health therefore make *prima facie* sense (see Brown, 2013; Friesen, 2018 for discussion). Whether or not we fall ill depends, significantly, on what we do, and whether or not we recover depends, significantly, on what we do. They fall within the purview of our agency. We are, partly but significantly, *causally* responsible for our own health and wellbeing, and causal responsibility is widely held to be a necessary condition of moral responsibility (at least of the sort that will be under discussion). If we are causally responsible for some consequence, and that consequence falls within the sphere of facts that are properly moralized, then we may be morally responsible for it as well.

There are multiple senses of the phrase 'moral responsibility'. For instance, on some accounts of moral responsibility attributions of responsibility are justified on consequentialist grounds: an agent is morally responsible for an action just in case it makes sense, on forward-looking grounds, to *hold* her morally responsible (her future behavior can be expected to improve, say, or others will be deterred by the example). In this article, I am concerned with moral responsibility in what has been called the basic desert sense (Pereboom, 2014): to say someone is morally responsible, in this sense, is to say that they *deserve* to be treated better or worse – say by being subjected to blame and condemnation – on backwards looking grounds *alone*.[3] The basic desert sense of moral responsibility is probably the central sense. In fact, ordinary people appear to understand responsibility for actions and for consequences as referring first and foremost to this sense of term (Cushman, 2008). Certainly, it plays an important role in our legal system: while consequentialist considerations matter to our system of fines and imprisonment, for instance, most people appear to believe that serious sanctions should express our condemnation of the offense, independently of any salutary effects condemnation has (indeed, ordinary people are almost entirely insensitive to consequentialist considerations in assessing how severe a punishment should be; Carlsmith and Darley, 2008). When agents are responsible, in this sense, for wrongful actions, they are blameworthy.

Of course, it is controversial what conditions must be satisfied for agents to be morally responsible. In common with most people who work on the topic, I assume that agents can be morally responsibility only if they satisfy control and epistemic conditions (Fischer and Ravizza, 1998; Eshleman, 2014). At minimum, (a) the action or state of affairs for which the agent is supposed to be responsible must be causally sensitive to her actions, and (b) she must understand that this is true, and know how to intervene in it.[4] Of course, there is a very rich debate on how to make these conditions more precise, which I can't hope to do justice to here. It suffices to note that there is a near consensus, among philosophers (Bourget and Chalmers, 2014) and ordinary people (Roskies and Nichols, 2008) that most agents routinely satisfy these conditions. Ordinary people are either compatibilists (Murray and Nahmias, 2014), holding that even if our actions are determined, we may be responsible for them, or they are libertarians (Nichols and Knobe, 2007), holding that our actions are not determined; they are rarely skeptics.

Thus, if agents are responsible (in the relevant sense) for their ill-health, they might deserve to bear the consequences. They might, for example, be assigned a lower priority when it comes to the allocation of health resources. For instance, it has been suggested that those who are responsible for the fact that they need a liver transplant (due to their heavy drinking) should have a lower priority when it comes to the allocation of scarce organs than those whose develop the need through no fault of their own (Glannon, 1998). Public health care resources might be denied to those responsible for their ill-health altogether, or they might be required to contribute more to their care than those who are not responsible, or they might be given a lower standard of care (more expensive medications might be reserved for more deserving cases, for instance).

Of course, the allocation of scarce resources to those who have brought about their own ill-health might be justified on consequentialist grounds. In particular, sometimes attempts are made to justify them on the grounds that the expected benefit to someone who is likely to engage in unhealthy behavior in the future is too small to justify some expenditures of health dollars. Policies that assign responsibility in this kind of way do not rely on the basic desert sense of responsibility. However, it is plausible that intuitions about desert play a subterranean role in motivating these apparently consequentialist policies. Proposals to delay surgery for those who are obese or currently smoking are sometimes justified on these kinds of grounds, but these claims are likely false: the interventions appear to be cost effective (Shaw, 2016). It may be that these proposals pass scrutiny only because many people are eager to ensure that people get what they (putatively) deserve.[5]

One way to resist the conclusion that agents are morally responsible (in the basic desert sense) for their ill-health is to deny that these behaviors or their consequences fall within the sphere of morality. On most accounts, we cannot be morally responsible for the morally neutral or the nonmoral: an agent cannot be morally responsible for the color of their T-shirt or for scratching their ears: not unless it was reasonable to expect that someone might (say) be offended by the color, or they had an obligation not to scratch, and so on. There is a very plausible case for thinking that diet and its consequences (in particular) is moralized in ways that are inappropriate (think of 'fat shaming'). Some of the opprobrium that attaches to those who engage in unhealthy behavior almost certainly stems from such inappropriate moralizing. Other people may have different tastes, and (for example) value sensual pleasure sufficiently to make it rational for them to take the risk of a shortened lifespan or a decrease in quality of life in the future. Nevertheless, the claim that ill-health is not a moral concern at all is implausible.

The very existence of the field of medical ethics testifies to our belief that healthcare is a moral issue. We believe, rightly, that it is morally incumbent on us to treat the ill, and health care budgets are finite. Money spent on one group of patients is not available

for others. Difficult decisions about resource allocation must be made, and these are importantly moral
decisions. *Prima facie*, at least, if people are responsible
for their ill-health, they may be blamed on the grounds
of imposing costs on a health system that must allocate scarce resources.[6] Those people, however numerous they may be, who are rational in preferring to
engage in unhealthy activities do not absolve themselves of responsibility for the consequences of their
behavior, for themselves or for others. If anything, the
opposite seems true: to the extent that they grasp that
they trade off present pleasure for future costs, they
are responsible for the choices and its consequences.

The claim that the allocation of healthcare
resources should be sensitive to the responsibility of
agents is therefore *prima facie* plausible. It is *prima facie*
plausible that some agents *deserve* more than others to
be allocated scarce organs (for instance). If an agent
knowingly and voluntarily engages in an activity that
risks imposing burdens on others, for trivial or self-
interested reasons,[7] that agent is *prima facie* responsible
for the outcome and our response can rightfully take
that fact into account. If you reject this claim, it is
worth noting – if you judge that people cannot be
responsible for their ill-health in virtue of their lifestyle-related behavior – then you are not my target,
because you do not hold the view I aim to criticize:
that a large class of agents can be given lower priority
for healthcare in virtue of their responsibility.

There are, however, other grounds for denying that
most people are responsible for their ill-health. I will
argue that the capacities for responsible agency, *especially* the kind of responsible agency exercised over
health in the kinds of cases mentioned above, are
themselves socially distributed (along with, and in a
way that is highly correlated with, other important
goods and opportunities). Because they are so distributed, those who are (on average) least able to exercise
them are the ones most in need of them. Holding
these agents responsible for bad outcomes is, in this
domain (though perhaps not others), deeply unfair as
a consequence. Moreover, it serves to deflect responsibility from those individuals and institutions responsible for the unfair allocation of burdens and capacities,

and who have the wherewithal to do something
about them, to those to whom they are allocated and
who do not.

I will argue that the best explanation for the social
gradient in health is that capacities and circumstances
are distributed in a way that ensures that those who
face the most temptations have the least capacity to
resist them. In doing so, I build upon, but substantially
go beyond, Brown's (2013) case that psychological
mechanisms might explain the gradient and thereby
undermine responsibility.

The Social Determinants of Health

Let me begin with a striking fact: there is a strong
correlation between chronic disease, increased risk of
morbidity and early mortality, on the one hand, and
socioeconomic status (SES), on the other (Marmot
et al., 2008; Marmot, 2018). There is a social gradient in ill-health: the lower one's level of education
and income, the worse one's health is (on average, of
course). There are a variety of reasons for this correlation, and some factors fall outside the scope of
facts over which individuals might reasonably be
expected to exercise any significant degree of control.
For instance, poorer people may live in environments
that are less healthy (close to pollution-producing
factories, or alongside major roads and therefore in
proximity to exhaust emissions and to noise, both of
which are known to contribute to heart disease; see
Shah et al., 2013 on pollution; Gan et al., 2012 on
noise). They may work in more stressful jobs, and have
less opportunity to exercise because their local neighborhoods lack parks to walk in. These are factors over
which it is not reasonable to expect them to exercise
much control, because doing something about them
requires resources they lack. Secure housing may not
be available in better areas at a price they can afford,
for example.

But causal factors in the social determinants of
health include behaviors that might reasonably be
thought to be within the sphere of control of the individual. For instance, there is a significant correlation

between SES and rates of smoking in many countries (Greenhalgh et al., 2015), but smoking is a voluntary behavior (of course, nicotine is highly addictive, which introduces complications with regard to the extent to which it is voluntary; nevertheless, at the very least beginning to smoke is voluntary). Similarly, in higher income countries (but not lower-income countries) obesity is negatively correlated with SES, and part of the explanation for these differences lies with diet quality (e.g. Darmon and Drewnowski, 2008). While healthier foods can be more expensive than less healthy, cost does not fully explain the differences in diet quality between high and low SES populations (Pechey and Monsivais, 2016).

We might take the evidence that appears to indicate that some, but not all, of the causal factors that underlie health differences between high and low SES groups are within the scope of their potential control to indicate something about the *extent* to which people should be held responsible, or the *scope* of justified responsibility ascriptions. That is, we might conclude, on the basis of the fact that some of the variance in health across demographic groups is the product of agential behavior, that agents are responsible just to the extent to which this is true, or responsible for those behaviors that are sufficiently agential. I will suggest that this response does not go anywhere near far enough. We should think that the group difference is not explained by behavior for which agents might appropriately be held responsible: though some of the social determinants of health are mediated by agential behavior, those agents with worse outcomes have (on average) significantly worse capacities to exercise what is sometimes called 'responsibility-level' control (Haji, 2012).

Social science aims to identify the factors that together explain outcomes. In this case, the outcome we are attempting to explain is the difference in health between high and low SES populations. We have seen that some of the variance in this difference is explained by factors over which low SES individuals (that is, those people whose health is, on average, worse) have insufficient control to justify holding them responsible. But other factors fall within

the scope of their agency: they could eat better, for example. We might therefore conclude that they are somewhat responsible for their ill-health, because it is partially the result of actions of theirs for which they are responsible.

But while it might be true that agential behavior plays a role in explaining health outcomes, these behavioral differences *themselves* cry out for explanation. What explains the fact that members of one group make worse choices than members of another? Citing their free choices is no explanation at all, because it leaves entirely mysterious why there are systematic differences between groups in how choice is exercised.[8] We should think that systematic differences like this can themselves be explained, and we should be open to the possibility that this explanation might be responsibility-undermining (or shifting).

Why would one group of individuals make choices that are worse than another? While there is no general answer to that question, in the context of these choices there are several different factors which together help to explain differences in behavior. Agents face different choices, in different contexts, with different capacities and with different senses of their options and their significance. Looking to the choices that high and low SES agents face, the contexts in which they face them, the capacities for choice they have and the senses they are likely to have of their options together go a long way toward explaining the differences in the choices they make.

I will begin with the capacities agents have. Agential behavior depends on capacities to resist impulses, to plan and to implement these plans. These are capacities that differ across groups. SES affects our brains, as much as it affects our environment (it affects our brains *by* affecting our environments). Most relevantly for our purposes, differences in working memory (the capacity to keep information in mind for a short period of time) and in inhibitory control (the capacity to resist temptations, or to inhibit habituated responses) emerge early in childhood (Lipina et al., 2005; Lipina 2014). These differences increase over development, and implicate other capacities, such as the capacity to focus attention (see Hackman et al., 2010 for review). In every case, lower SES correlates with reduced executive function. These differences in capacity to attend, to resist distraction, to plan and to inhibit impulses are not themselves differences over which agents have control. They develop early, before the person is in a position to make responsible choices. Together, they explain much of the difference in the choices lower SES individuals make, compared to higher.

These differences can be themselves be explained. In part, these differences are adaptive responses to the environment in which lower SES individuals find themselves. Take the capacity to inhibit impulses. This is a capacity that develops through use, and lower SES individuals get fewer opportunities to practice the capacity for inhibition. They face fewer contexts in which they will be rewarded for delaying gratification. Delay of gratification is adaptive in environments that are richer in resources, because in such environments foregoing a reward is not likely to be costly. There will be other opportunities to secure equally valuable goods. But in poorer environments, rewards foregone might be lost forever (Kidd et al., 2012). We are likely sensitive to cues of resource richness, and respond by up- or down-regulating mechanisms for inhibitory control (Levy, 2016). It is in part because we face choices in different contexts that we have different capacities for choice.

Whereas some of these differences represent adaptive responses to contexts, others might be explained in other ways. For instance, some of the observed differences in attentional control are the product of exposure to chronic stress (Liston et al., 2009). Poverty causes stress in a variety of ways: worrying about paying bills, about the security of housing, and so on. But stress does not only undermine capacities: it also makes certain choices more tempting. Part of the reason why lower SES individuals smoke at higher rates, for instance, is that smoking alleviates stress, at least in the short term (McClernon and Gilbert, 2010). Similarly, lower SES individuals may eat tempting but unhealthy foods, in part, to alleviate stress (Adam and Epel, 2007).

Finally, SES correlates with education and therefore with knowledge of which foods are healthy and the long-term consequences of bad food choices. Thus lower SES individuals face more difficult choices – unhealthy foods are likely to be more tempting for them – with reduced capacities for making such choices, in contexts in which they are likely to see less reason for making such choices. Making worse choices is therefore not mysterious at all: it is the expected upshots of these differences in capacities, contexts and knowledge.

One might object these differences do not show that lower SES individuals are not responsible for their lifestyle-related choices. They are responding *rationally* to the circumstances in which they find themselves, and rational choice is (other things equal) responsible choice.[9] Indeed, this point – that responsibility should be understood as centrally involving the capacity to respond, appropriately, to reasons – is at the heart of the reasons-responsiveness account to which many philosophers subscribe (Fischer and Ravizza, 1998 is the locus classicus; I have endorsed a variant of this account in Levy, 2017).

In response to this objection, several things should be emphasized. First, a significant part of the explanation for the choices of lower SES individuals involves mechanisms that are not reasons responsive. A decreased capacity to inhibit impulses is a volitional defect, rather than a cognitive mechanism. Second, the fact that the explanation for the set up of some mechanism cites reasons does not show that the mechanism is, in the relevant sense, reasons-responsive. Evolutionary theorists distinguish *distal* and *proximal* explanation. Distal explanations explain how a mechanism is adaptive: how it functions to increase the organism's fitness. Proximal explanation explain how it is implemented. In many cases, a distal explanation cites reasons, but those reasons need not be reasons *from the organism's perspective*. Thus, the distal explanation for decreased sensitivity to longer term rewards cites reasons: it is adaptive for organisms to prefer immediately available rewards under many conditions. But these reasons may not be reasons *for the person*. Indeed, she may recognize that in her current environment (which differs so dramatically from the environment for which these mechanisms are adaptations), she has better reason to abstain than to consume, but these reasons have reduced motivational power for her due the ways in which these mechanisms are configured.

Finally, and most importantly, the reasons-responsiveness account of moral responsibility should not be understood as simply asserting that agents are responsible for actions when they act on reasons-responsive mechanisms. Rather, the account is more fine-grained than that: an agent is responsible *for violating certain norms* if she acted on a mechanism that is responsive to the set of reasons that apply in the domain of those norms. Thus, non-human animals are arguably reasons-responsive – their behavior is guided by states of affairs that function as reasons for them – but they are not morally responsible because they lack the capacity to respond to moral reasons specifically. Analogously, it would be a mistake to conclude on the basis of the fact that their lifestyle behaviors are often guided by reasons that lower SES individuals may be held responsible for the outcomes in the kinds of way that are relevant here. It is because they have reduced capacities to respond *to the relevant reasons* that they find it difficult to guide their behavior in their light.

None of this entails that lower SES individuals are not capable of responsible choice. Typically, theorists of moral responsibility hold that agents are morally responsible for their behavior if they have *enough* in the way of the relevant capacities to make the relevant choice in the relevant context, and in addition satisfy the epistemic condition on choice sufficiently well. Particularly in the context of criminal behavior, this kind of approach has a great deal to recommend it. While we may want our justice tempered by a mercy that stems from a recognition that some people find it harder to resist temptations to criminal activity or are more likely to behave impulsively than others, most people think that above a certain threshold of capacity, it is reasonable to expect individuals to refrain from seriously immoral actions. Given the stakes, we expect normal individuals to be sufficiently motivated to marshal the resources they need to avoid such behavior.

However, in the much lower stakes contexts with which we are concerned here, the repeated context of choice of one food over another, say, the demand that people somehow find the wherewithal to make the right choices sufficiently often is much less reasonable. There are at least two reasons why it is reasonable to hold people to higher standards in higher-stakes contexts. One is that we reasonably expect that recognition that one is in a high-stakes context is motivating. When someone recognizes that something of great significance is on the line, we expect them to pay attention, to make a great effort, and so on. Thus, we accept 'it was too hard' as an excuse for not bringing in the washing much more easily than we do for not feeding the children, for instance. Second, high-stakes contexts, and thus the need to make an effort and attend, are relatively rare for most of us. If a particular challenge arises repeatedly, we may expect that someone will fail eventually, due to inattention, fatigue or sheer bad luck. But they have no such excuse available when the challenge is rare and high-stakes.

We might bring this out by comparing two kinds of contexts. Most of us have experienced situations in which our executive capacities are impaired (due to tiredness or alcohol consumption, say) and we have experienced a fleeting temptation to engage in clearly immoral behavior. The temptation might be to drive while seriously drunk, or to steal someone's wallet, or even to commit more seriously wrong actions. Most of us have not engaged in the behavior, I hope: even in our impaired state, the high stakes have been sufficient to bring us to pull ourselves together and refrain. But, we cannot say the same thing about much lower stakes contexts in which we have been impaired in executive control and faced temptation. In these contexts, we may have engaged in trivially immoral behavior (not paying for a drink, or insulting someone, say) or prudentially unwise behavior (smoking, drinking more than we should, taking risks that are unjustified). These latter slips seem explicable and forgivable. But low SES individuals find themselves in analogous situations *routinely*. If our lapses are forgivable – not the kind of thing on which it makes sense to hang serious consequences – then so, it seems, are theirs. Whereas we, with our greater capacity to control our behavior in the light of (the relevant) reasons may deserve responsibility if we repeatedly engage in risky or indulgent behavior in these (individually) low stakes context, and therefore be responsible for the outcomes, lower SES individuals may not be responsible for the overall pattern of behavior and therefore for the outcomes, despite the fact that they have the wherewithal to guide their behavior by moral norms in higher-stakes contexts.

If the between-group differences are explained by these factors – factors concerning which agents have no choice, and factors which excuse their choices – then it seems we cannot rightly hold agents responsible for the consequences of their choices. Those low SES individuals who end up with poorer health as a consequence of their behavior will be those who have made poor choices often enough (not necessarily on every occasion, of course; for many such individuals, there will be many instances of successful self-control – but it takes only one slip to render many such instances otiose), and these poor choices are not such that we can reasonably expect them to make better choices.[10]

Of course, many low SES individuals do not exhibit the reduction in executive function characteristic of the group. Some will even have superior executive function. Similarly, many will not face greater temptations to engage in unhealthy behaviors, or will not experience more stressors, or more chronic stress, than those individuals in higher SES groups (equally, we will find individuals in the latter group who exhibit these deficits, are subject to these temptations, experience these stressors). We will even find individuals who suffer from *none* of these problems, internal or external. Many of these individuals will put their good fortune to good use, and engage in healthier behaviors than is typical for their group, but some will choose unhealthy behaviors, and some of this group will suffer adverse health consequences as a result. These individuals do not have the excuses that group membership makes available to others, and therefore might appropriately be held responsible (for all that has been said here).

But in this context, policy is better formulated in ways that are insensitive to these kinds of differences.

For reasons of cost and efficiency, we shouldn't subject individuals to extensive neuropsychological testing and take detailed life histories. While policy in this domain may take individual circumstances into account, it should do so more in the kind of way actuarial tables do: by considering basic demographic information, rather than fine-grained details of individual differences. It will often be difficult to discern when individuals are exceptions to the generalizations we can draw from this kind of information. We have sophisticated tests for cognitive control (e.g. Go/No-go tasks), but they are time consuming and resource intensive, and much more reliable at detecting group than individual differences. Moreover, there are good reasons to think that there is little point in enquiring into such details. Health policies that require individuals to bear responsibility for their own behavior, when it results in adverse outcomes *and* they possess, or possessed at relevant times, unimpaired executive function in propitious circumstances, would apply to a small group of individuals. Most of the people who are causally responsible for ill-health do not satisfy these conditions. Since such a policy would apply to relatively few individuals, the costs of implementing it – requiring, as it would, testing of a large number of individuals to identify the few – would likely be significantly greater than the savings in health care costs. Unless we think that wreaking retribution on these few is a high priority, such an approach is bad policy.

Taking Responsibility for Responsibility

In the previous section, I argued that the correlation between low SES and adverse health outcomes, to the extent it is mediated by agential behavior, is very largely explained by the decreased capacities of members of that group, combined with the more demanding context in which they find themselves. Low SES individuals typically must make choices that are more difficult *and* have reduced capacities to make these choices. While their capacities may be sufficient for the kinds of challenges that fall within the scope of criminal responsibility, the combination of difficult circumstances, reduced capacities and repeated challenges to them makes it hard to hold them responsible for outcomes in the domain of health. We would do well to avoid making assumptions about the responsibility of those whose ill-health arise from lifestyle into our health-related policies.

That is not to say, however, that responsibility is not important from a policy perspective. Policy should strive for efficient and ethical uses of scarce resources, by ensuring that individuals and institutions responsible for outcomes are held to account for them. There are appropriate targets of responsibility ascription. They are the institutions – political, judicial and corporate – and individuals actually responsible for the distribution of responsibility-relevant capacities and the distribution of the circumstances in which choices are made. Exactly how these institutions can be held responsible is a difficult question, of course. There is considerable debate in the literature over whether there are legitimate ascriptions of 'corporate responsibility' (Sverdlik, 1987; Sepinwall, 2016), or whether all such ascriptions are reducible to conjunctions about claims about individuals (Giubilini and Levy, 2018). However that debate is settled, responsibility surely attaches to many individuals: to policy makers, legislators, highly placed businesspeople and perhaps ordinary people (especially higher SES individuals) in their capacity as voters.

The choices of these individuals and institutions play a significant role in the distribution of the capacities other individuals find themselves with. These institutions and individuals have the ability to coordinate their behavior, if they choose, and to ensure that capacities are more evenly distributed, and that a higher proportion of the population have a greater capacity to take responsibility for their behavior. The extent to which some groups of individuals are exposed to serious stressors to a significantly greater extent than others, and the extent to which some grow up in resource-poor environments is a result in very important part of political choices we have made, and the circumstance and capacities of individuals are very significantly within the sphere of our control.

We can begin to address inequality in capacities and circumstances of choices in much the same way as we might address other inequalities. For instance, we can ensure that there is an adequate safety net, so that parents are not highly anxious about getting or keeping their jobs. Equally, we can ensure that jobs are adequately paid, so that parents need only work one job. If we do these kinds of things, we ensure that parental stress levels are lower. That's important, because stress is communicated, advertently or not. Stressed parents have stressed children. Indeed, the stress response begins in utero (O'Donnell et al., 2009): the children of stressed parents have brains preadapted to expect stressors and are hypersensitive to cues for stress. We can ensure that children develop in environments in which they get the opportunity to delay gratification, secure in the knowledge that a reward delayed is not a reward foregone. We can ensure that people are better educated, so that the epistemic conditions on responsibility are better satisfied. We can ensure that people have more opportunities and that the costs of failure are lower. Much of this is familiar, of course: we address responsibility inequalities in much the same ways as we address other inequalities (in fact, social inequality and responsibility inequalities are closely linked: in addressing one, we typically address the other). By doing these things, the individuals and institutions most appropriately held responsible for ill-health would discharge the obligations they have in virtue of being responsible.

Who, precisely, should be responsible for the ways in which the contexts and capacities for choice are distributed is a very difficult question. Making progress on this question will require detailed conceptual and empirical work, for which I have neither the space nor the capacity. Some cases are relatively easy (senior executives at soft drink manufacturers seem to be cases of agents who amply satisfy the control and epistemic conditions; senior politicians, too, are easy cases). Others are much harder (how does one hold voters, an extremely heterogenous group, responsible)? While this is an extremely important question, I cannot address it. I will be content if the arguments given here motivate others to take it seriously enough to carry out the detailed investigation required to assess the issue adequately.

Asking low SES individuals to bear responsibility for adverse health outcomes is asking those with the least capacity to take responsibility to bear it. It is subjecting them to a double dose of unfairness: the unfairness of having to act in unpropitious circumstances with reduced capacities for choice, and the unfairness of being penalized in some way for those choices. We do far better to ask those of us with greater capacities to take responsibility. We bear responsibility, indirectly at least, for *their* health outcomes, because our political and social choices structure the environments which ensures their reduced capacities and their more demanding circumstances. Just as we bear responsibility for how incomes, and opportunities, and statuses, are distributed, so we bear responsibility for how responsibility is distributed.[11]

Notes

1   Sally Haslanger (2020) has recently suggested that work on justice has focused too much on distributive justice, neglecting processes whereby some things come to be seen as valuable in the first place. In addition to expanding work on justice in the way she suggests, I aim to show that we need a broader conception of what gets distributed.

2   While it should be acknowledged that the evidence that obesity causes cancer is mainly correlational, correlational data is (defeasible) evidence for causation. In this case, we have good mechanistic models that make the claim that the correlation is indicative of a causal relation plausible. I thank a reviewer for forcing me to think about this issue more deeply.

3   The basic desert sense is sometimes called the *accountability* sense of responsibility, as opposed to the attributability (or appraisal) and answerability sense. See Shoemaker (2015) for elaboration.

4   As a reviewer for this journal [*Public Health Ethics*] points out, there are philosophers who deny that responsibility requires control. These philosophers instead claim that responsibility requires endorsement or expression of the real self. While it is true that members of this school maintain that agents can be responsible for actions or states of affairs they can't control (see Frankfurt, 1971 for the classic expression of this view), they accept that there is normally a close link between responsibility, at least in the sense at issue (as opposed to the 'appraisal' sense) and control, because we typically express our real selves in the actions we control, and fail to do so in those we do not (see Smith, 2008 for discussion).

5   Further, there is evidence that holding people responsible for their ill-health, whether or not they deserve to be so held, does not in fact produce the consequences that might be hoped for. There appears to be an inverse correlation between willingness to support effective policies and holding people responsible for their health; to that extent, it might actual serve as an obstacle to addressing these challenges (AU).

6   A referee for this journal objects to the claim that healthcare is a domain in which we might have obligations, on the grounds that if resource allocation dilemmas are moral dilemmas, it is easy to obligate others. I am far from confident that we shouldn't accept that it is easy to obligate others: if you reasonably believe that the £5 I offer you would otherwise be spent in a way that is morally better, you may indeed have an obligation to refuse. Whether you have such an obligation depends on whether the domain in which the money would be spent is appropriately moralized.

7   As a reviewer for this journal points out, these kinds of qualifications are needed because we often do not judge agents blameworthy for risking ill-health. The reviewer gives two examples: firefighters and women who intentionally become pregnant. It is worth noting that some people will judge that agents can be responsible for risking ill-health even in these kinds of circumstances, when the conditions mentioned aren't satisfied. The firefighter who risks her life to rescue a pet might be judged responsible and thought to be less deserving of treatment in virtue of her action. The woman who has several children and has been warned that she is at high risk of death (and therefore leaving them orphans) if she attempts to carry a child to term might also be judged responsible in the sense at issue.

8   Two reviewers for this journal worry that this claim begs the question against those who hold that responsible

choice requires indeterminism. While it is true that libertarians are committed to thinking that there are free choices that cannot be explained, they accept that antecedent factors play a very significant role in explaining how we choose. As they sometimes say, such causes incline without necessitating choice. They therefore expect that the overall pattern of choice will reflect prior causal factors (Kane, 2005). Note that this assumption is required to explain the systematic differences in how people choose, such as the correlation with SES.

9   I owe this objection to a reviewer for this journal.

10 It should be acknowledged that the details of the proposed explanation for the differences in the choices that low and high SES individuals make are somewhat

speculative and controversial. However, unless we are prepared to think that such systematic differences are brute facts that cannot be explained, we should acknowledge that some such account is correct. As long as the account explains different choices by reference to social facts that are not themselves chosen by low SES individuals (an extremely plausible suggestion, implementation details aside), we should think that their responsibility is mitigated and that those with more power over these facts are morally and practically better situated to take responsibility for them.

11 I am very grateful to two reviewers and the editors of this journal for helpful comments that enabled me to greatly improve this paper.

References

Adam, T. C. and Epel, E. S. (2007). Stress, Eating and the Reward System. *Physiology & Behavior*, 91, 449–58.

Bourget, D. and Chalmers, D. J. (2014). What do Philosophers Believe? *Philosophical Studies*, 170, 465–500.

Brown, R. C. H. (2013). Moral Responsibility for (un) Healthy Behaviour. *Journal of Medical Ethics*, 39, 695–8.

Callahan, D. (2013). Obesity: Chasing an Elusive Epidemic. *Hastings Center Report*, 43, 34–40.

Carlsmith, K. M. and Darley, J. M. (2008). Psychological Aspects of Retributive Justice. *Advances in Experimental Social Psychology*, 40, 193–236.

Cushman, F. A. (2008). Crime and Punishment: Differential Reliance on Causal and Intentional Information for Different Classes of Moral Judgment. *Cognition*, 108, 353–80.

Darmon, N. and Drewnowski, A. (2008). Does Social Class Predict Diet Quality? *The American Journal of Clinical Nutrition*, 87, 1107–17.

Eshleman, A. (2014). Moral Responsibility. In Edward N. Zalta (ed.), *The Stanford Encyclopedia of Philosophy* (Winter 2016 Edition), available from: https://plato.stanford.edu/archives/win2016/entries/moral-responsibility/ [accessed January 3, 2019].

Fischer, J. M. and Ravizza, M. (1998). *Responsibility and Control: An Essay on Moral Responsibility*. Cambridge: Cambridge University Press.

Frankfurt, H. (1971). Freedom of the Will and the Concept of a Person. *Journal of Philosophy*, 68, 5–20.

Friesen, P. (2018). Personal Responsibility Within Health Policy: Unethical and Ineffective. *Journal of Medical Ethics*, 44, 53–8.

Gan, W. Q., Davies, H. W., Koehoorn, M., and Brauer, M. (2012). Association of Long-Term Exposure to Community Noise and Traffic-Related Air Pollution with Coronary Heart Disease Mortality. *American Journal of Epidemiology*, 175, 898–906.

Glannon, W. (1998). Responsibility, Alcoholism, and Liver Transplantation. *Journal of Medicine and Philosophy*, 23, 31–49.

Greenhalgh, E., Bayly, M., and Winstanley M. (2015). Trends in the Prevalence of Smoking by Socio-economic Status. In Scollo, M. and Winstanley, M. (eds.), *Tobacco in Australia: Facts and Issues*. Melbourne: Cancer Council Victoria, available from: http://www.tobaccoinaustralia.org.au/chapter-1-prevalence [accessed July 17, 2018].

Giubilini, A. and Levy, N. (2018). What in the World is Collective Responsibility? *Dialectica*, 72, 191–217.

Hackman, D. A., Farah, M. J., and Meaney, M. J. (2010). Socioeconomic Status and the Brain: Mechanistic Insights from Human and Animal Research. *Nature Reviews Neuroscience*, 11, 651–9.

Haji, I. (2012). *Reason's Debt to Freedom*. Oxford: Oxford University Press.

Haslanger, S. F. (2020). Cognition as a Social Skill. *Australasian Philosophical Review*, 3:1.

Hazell, K. (2012). Hungary Pledges to Deprive Diabetes Sufferers of Treatment if They Fail Healthy Eating Plan. *Huffington Post*, 24, available from: https://www.huffingtonpost.co.uk/2012/04/24/hungary-deprives-%20diabetics-treatment-punishment_n_1449036.html [accessed September 18, 2018].

Kane, R. (2005). *A Contemporary Introduction to Free Will*. New York: Oxford University Press.

Kent, M. (2009). Coke Didn't Make American Fat. *Wall Street Journal,* October 7.

Kidd, C., Palmeri, H., and Aslin, R. N. (2012). Rational Snacking: Young Children's Decision-Making on the Marshmallow Task is Moderated by Beliefs About Environmental Reliability. *Cognition*, 126, 109–14.

Levy, N. (2016). The Sweetness of Surrender: Glucose Enhances Self-control by Signalling Environmental Richness. *Philosophical Psychology.* 29, 813–25.

Levy, S. N. (2017). Implicit Bias and Moral Responsibility: Probing the Data. *Philosophy and Phenomenological Research*, 94, 3–26.

Lipina, S. J. (2014). Biological and Sociocultural Determinants of Neurocognitive Development: Central Aspects of the Current Scientific Agenda. In Battro, A. M., Potrykus, I. and Sorondo, M. S. (eds.), *Bread and Brain, Education and Poverty.* Vatican: Pontifical Academy of Science, pp. 37–66.

Lipina, S. J., Martelli, M. I., Vuelta, B. and Colombo, J. A. (2005). Performance on the A-not-B Task of Argentinian Infants from Unsatisfied and Satisfied Basic Needs Homes. *Interamerican Journal of Psychology*, 39, 49–60.

Liston, C., McEwen, B. S., and Casey, B. J. (2009). Psychosocial Stress Reversibly Disrupts Prefrontal Processing and Attentional Control. *Proceedings of the National Academy of Sciences*, 106, 912–17.

Macrae, F. (2016). Fat People SHOULD be Told That Their Size is Their Own Fault, Experts Warns. *Daily Mail,* April 9, available from: http://www.dailymail.co.uk/health/article-3530957/Fat-people-toldsize-fault-expert-warns.html [accessed September 18, 2018].

Marmot, M. (2018). Health Equity, Cancer, and Social Determinants of Health. *The Lancet Global Health*, 6, S29.

Marmot, M., Friel, S., Bell, R., Houweling, T. A. J., and Taylor, S. (2008). Closing the Gap in a Generation: Health Equity Through Action on the Social Determinants of Health. *The Lancet*, 372, 1661–9.

McClernon, F. J. and Gilbert, D. G. (2010). Smoking and Stress. In Fink, G. (ed.), *Stress Consequences: Mental, Neuropsychological and Socioeconomic*. San Diego: Academic Press, pp. 214–18.

Murray, D. and Nahmias, E. (2014). Explaining Away Incompatibilist Intuitions. *Philosophy and Phenomenological Research*, 88, 434–67.

NHS. (2015). *The NHS Constitution (for England)*. London: Department of Health.

Nichols, S. and Knobe, J. (2007). Moral Responsibility and Determinism: The Cognitive Science of Folk Intuitions. *Noûs*, 41, 663–85.

Nieuwlaat, R., Wilczynski, N., and Navarro, T. (2014). Interventions for Enhancing Medication Adherence. *Cochrane Database of Systematic Reviews*, 20, CD000011.

O'Donnell, K. J., O'Connor, T. G., and Glover, V. (2009). Prenatal Stress and Neurodevelopment of the Child: Focus on the HPA Axis and Role of the Placenta. *Developmental Neuroscience*, 31, 285–92.

Pechey, R. and Monsivais, P. (2016). Socioeconomic Inequalities in the Healthiness of Food Choices: Exploring the Contributions of Food Expenditures. *Preventive Medicine*, 88, 203–9.

Pereboom, D. (2014). *Free Will, Agency, and Meaning in Life*. Oxford: Oxford University Press.

Roskies, A. and Nichols, S. (2008). Bringing Moral Responsibility Down to Earth. *Journal of Philosophy*, 105, 371–88.

Sepinwall, A. J. (2016). Corporate Moral Responsibility. *Philosophy Compass*, 11, 3–13.

Shah, A. S. V., Langrish, J. P., Nair, H., McAllister, D. A., Hunter, A. L., Donaldson, K., Newby, D. E., and Mills, N. L. (2013). Global Association of Air Pollution and Heart Failure: A Systematic Review and Meta-analysis. *The Lancet*, 382, 1039–48.

Shaw, D. (2016). Delaying Surgery for Obese Patients or Smokers is a Bad Idea. *British Medical Journal*, 355, i5594.

Shoemaker, D. (2015). *Responsibility from the Margins*. Oxford: Oxford University Press.

Smith, A. M. (2008). Control, Responsibility, and Moral Assessment. *Philosophical Studies*, 138, 367–92.

Sverdlik, S. (1987). Collective Responsibility. *Philosophical Studies*, 51, 61–76.

World Health Organization. (2003). Controlling the Global Obesity Epidemic, available from: http://www.who.int/nutrition/topics/obesity/en/ [accessed November 5, 2018].

World Health Organization. (2014). Global Status Report on Noncommunicable Diseases, available from: http://apps.who.int/iris/bitstream/10665/148114/1/9789241564854_eng.pdf?ua=1 [accessed November 5, 2018].

Yoon, P. W., Bastian, B. A., Anderson, R. N., Collins, J. L., and Jaffe, H. W. (2014). Potentially Preventable Deaths from the Five Leading Causes of Death – United States, 2008–2010. *Morbidity and Mortality Weekly Report*, 63, 369–74.

Part IX

Ethical Issues in the Practice of Healthcare

Introduction

In the Hippocratic tradition, it has long been assumed that the first responsibility of doctors is to the health and well-being of each individual patient, rather than to patients as a whole, or to society at large. Another traditional assumption among physicians was that they are entitled to be paternalistic towards their patients. This means that doctors may sometimes – in seeking to protect the physical health and well-being of patients – ignore the wishes of their patients, and deceive them about the state of their health. Today, however, it is widely assumed that respect for patient autonomy, rather than medical paternalism, ought to be the cornerstone of the doctor–patient relationship. It is also commonly accepted that the duties and responsibilities of doctors extend beyond those they owe to their individual patients. But, as the articles in the present Part of the *Anthology* illustrate, the contemporary emphasis on autonomy and patient consent raises some complex ethical issues.

When do Doctors have a Duty to Treat?

During the SARS-CoV-2 pandemic many doctors and other healthcare professionals were reluctant to provide care to COVID-19 patients. They were concerned that personal protective equipment (PPE) was unavailable to them. A significant number of healthcare professionals contracted the disease at work and got sick, some died. In the first chapter of this section Udo Schüklenk argues that, in the absence of PPE, healthcare workers are under no professional obligation to provide care. His main contention is that taxpayers who fund public healthcare systems continued to elect governments who cut back on healthcare services, in return for lower taxes. PPE was relatively inexpensive to purchase prior to the pandemic, and there had been many warnings of pandemics of this kind occurring. Schüklenk maintains that taxpayers-turned-patients have only themselves to blame if cost-cutting policies render healthcare professionals unable to protect themselves, and so render them unable to provide patient care without unreasonable cost to themselves.

Doctors refuse care not only when the risk to their own well-being might be too high, but also for other reasons. Traditionally, medical schools have taught that we should accommodate the conscientious choices of healthcare professionals who refuse to provide a particular medical service, not on clinical grounds, but on grounds of their religious or moral views. Respecting the right to conscientious objection has been seen as a noble response to the moral dilemmas faced by such professionals. Today the issue has become more controversial, mostly as a result of a growing number of jurisdictions introducing medical services such as abortion, euthanasia, or medical aid in dying, and reproductive health services like IVF for same-sex couples.

In "Conscientious Objection in Health Care" Mark R. Wicclair surveys the ethical arguments put forward in influential articles on this controversial topic published in bioethics journals. He notes that two extreme positions exist. On the one hand some writers give conscience claims absolute priority over eligible patients' demands to receive the care to which they would normally be entitled. Other writers assert that medical professionalism is incompatible with accommodating conscientious objection. Wicclair proceeds then to defend an account between these extremes, accepting conscientious objection, but only when health professionals satisfy a set of specific requirements that reduce the burden on patients.

Udo Schüklenk takes a different stance, defending the incompatibilism thesis, in "Conscientious Objection in Medicine: Accommodation versus Professionalism and the Public Good." Healthcare professionals have, he contends, been granted a societal monopoly on the provision of professional services. They joined the professions voluntarily and promised to serve the public good by providing services, within the scope of their practice, reliably and competently to the public. Refusals to provide those monopoly services on grounds other than professional, clinical - judgment grounds are, Schüklenk argues, incompatible with professional conduct.

Confidentiality

One of the pledges in the Hippocratic Oath reads: "What I may see or hear in the course of treatment or even outside of the treatment in regard to the life of men, which on no account must spread abroad, I will keep to myself . . ."

Traditional Western medicine has taken the principle of confidentiality very seriously. But is the principle still relevant today? Patients are often treated by a number of doctors and a range of other healthcare professionals, in large hospitals. Pathology companies perform myriad tests that may reveal sensitive information. Records are stored and transmitted electronically, with many people having access. Record-keeping, the involvement of different healthcare specialists and good communication between them, are essential for the effective delivery of healthcare. While patients are the prime beneficiaries of these contemporary arrangements, Mark Siegler argues that they spell the end of confidentiality in the traditional sense. His view is encapsulated in the title of his essay: "Confidentiality in Medicine: A Decrepit Concept." Rather than invest energy in vainly trying to preserve confidentiality as a whole, Siegler suggests that patients and doctors would be better served if attention were directed toward determining which aspects of the principle are worthy of preservation, and which we can and should do without.

As Siegler notes, there are two reasons for treating medical information as confidential: Firstly, confidentiality might be defended as a corollary of the value of respecting the patient's autonomy and privacy. Secondly, confidentiality might be seen as an important element in the provision of good healthcare. If patients did not trust their doctors and feared disclosure of sensitive medical information to third parties, some would be unlikely to confide in their doctors, thus jeopardizing both diagnosis and treatment. After suggesting that these two functions of confidentiality are as important today as they have been in the past, Siegler proceeds to sketch a number of ways in which "the confidentiality problem" might be overcome.

Kenneth Kipnis, on the other hand, in "A Defense of Unqualified Medical Confidentality", argues that while doctors have professional obligations to prevent public peril, they do not live up to those obligations by breaching patient confidentiality. The doctor–patient relation is essentially a trust-based relationship. Public trust in the profession and its member would be severely eroded if doctors behaved in ways that undermined that trust. Kipnis discusses a case involving an HIV-infected spouse where the doctor is faced with the choice of breaching confidentiality in order to protect the uninfected spouse or maintain confidentiality and face the prospect of the uninfected spouse unwittingly acquiring HIV.

Kipnis discusses the situation in terms of core ethical values like trustworthiness, which requires maintaining confidentiality, and beneficence, which requires a breach of it. He then proceeds to provide a list of professional values, asking again how they would impact on the problem at hand. At issue is the profession's obligation to diminish public perils, as HIV undoubtedly is. Does the harm of the previously uninfected spouse's HIV infection outweigh the cost involved in breaching confidentiality? His conclusion is that once patients understand that confidentiality would be breached under such circumstances, those at risk of HIV-infection would seek to avoid seeing doctors precisely because of concerns about the confidentiality of their diagnosis. The overall damage this would do arguably outweighs the damage done to people like the uninfected spouse in Kipnis' example.

Truth-Telling

Another set of moral problems in healthcare relates to the issue of truth-telling. As we have already noted, in the Hippocratic medical tradition, it used to be regarded as proper for doctors to act paternalistically, if they considered it to be in the best interests of the patient. In line with this thinking, doctors are seen as justified in withholding the truth from patients, or lying to them, if – in the doctor's' view – a patient would be harmed by knowing the truth. The questioning of medical paternalism, and the movement for greater patient autonomy that began in the twentieth century, has led to the widespread rejection of the view that doctors can lie to their patients. But, as with the notion of confidentiality, the question arises whether, and if so when, the principle that doctors should not deliberately deceive patients, may be broken.

Not many philosophers have claimed that it is always wrong to lie. Immanuel Kant is the most notable exception. In his essay "On a Supposed Right to Lie from Altruistic Motives" he defends the principle that we must never lie, even if our doing so could prevent the death of an innocent human being. For Kant, "[t]o be *truthful* . . . is . . . a sacred unconditional command of reason, and not limited by any expediency". Joseph Collins, in his essay "Should Doctors Tell the Truth?" written in 1927, takes a very different view. He argues that many patients do not want to know the truth, and would be harmed by being given bad news. They would often enjoy life less, and sometimes even die earlier than they would if they had been shielded from the truth. Rather than burden patients with this kind of information, there is, Collins argues, merit in "cultivating lying as a fine art".

Roger Higgs ("On Telling Patients the Truth") accepts that the temptation to withhold bad news from patients can be strong. But, he argues, truth is important for trust in the doctor–patient relationship, and is a prerequisite for respect for patient autonomy – for how can patients decide on their treatment if they do not know the truth about their diagnosis and prognosis? While some writers draw a moral distinction between lying and other forms of deliberately withholding or masking the truth, Higgs follows the philosopher Sissela Bok in holding that any statement or omission that is intended to mislead amounts to lying, even if the statement itself is not false. While not ruling out the possibility that there might be occasions when lying is justified, such occasions would, Higgs concludes, be rare. Higgs' position thus lies somewhere between those of Kant and Collins.

Informed Consent and Patient Autonomy

The idea that autonomy or self-determination is valuable is not new. It has been defended by many philosophers on the grounds that without autonomy, liberty, or self-determination, we are not our own persons, deciding on how we shall live, but rather the creatures of others who directly or indirectly impose their will on us. John Stuart Mill, in his essay "On Liberty," an excerpt of which we include here, provides a forceful and eloquent defence of liberty. In a famous sentence, he writes: ". . .the only purpose for which power can be rightfully exercised over any member of a civilized community, against his will, is to prevent harm to others. His own good, either physical or moral, is not a sufficient warrant."

Nevertheless, as Tom L. Beauchamp describes in "Informed Consent: Its History, Meaning and Present Challenges," it was only in second half of the twentieth century that courts began to hold that competent patients have a right not to be treated without their informed consent. US Justice Benjamin N. Cardozo had articulated the general idea already in 1914 when he stated that "[e]very human being of adult years and sound mind has a right to determine what shall be done with his own body . . ." (*Schloendorff v. New York Hospital,* 1914), but it was not until the 1970s that informed consent became part of more mainstream legal thinking, and subsequently found its way into medical practice.

For a patient's consent to a procedure to be valid, "informed consent", it is widely held that at least the following five conditions must be met. The patient must

1. be competent or of "sound mind"
2. be adequately informed.
3. substantially understand the information.
4. make the decision free from coercion or undue influence.
5. intentionally authorize the medical procedure or treatment plan.

If all five conditions are fully observed, we would have what Beauchamp argues is the essence of informed consent as it should be understood: an autonomous authorization for treatment (or for participation in a research project). This is, however, a high standard, and it is not clear how much progress has been made in achieving it.

Part of the problem is that terms like "adequately" and "substantially" are vague. What does it mean for a patient to be "adequately informed"? How do we know whether a patient has "substantially understood" or is subject to "undue influence" – and what kind of influence is "due"? Beauchamp gives one example – a research project involving the Havasupai Indians of the Grand Canyon – where it seems clear that there was no substantial understanding of the purposes for which biological samples would be used.

Should we assume that people from different cultural backgrounds – whether indigenous people like the Havasupai, or people from East Asia, or the Middle East, or parts of Europe – share our view of the importance of informed consent, patients' rights, and autonomy? Some have claimed that the current emphasis in healthcare ethics on autonomy is part of a distinctively North American elevation of the individual over the community. Most other societies around the world, so the criticism goes, place the family, the community or society above the rights or interests of the individual. This is often understood as supporting the argument that ethics is relative and that what is right in one society may be wrong in another. Ruth Macklin discusses this question in "The Doctor–Patient Relationship in Different Cultures." Drawing on a rich array of examples from different parts of the world, Macklin shows that arguments in support of cultural relativism are often confused and simplistic. Cultures are not monolithic, and different members of them may take different views, so the differences between cultures are not as sharp as many assume. Even if they were, however, Macklin argues, it would not necessarily show that it was right for a doctor to tell the patient the truth in North America, and wrong for a doctor to do that in another country.

A quite different problem is discussed in Maura Priest's "Transgender Children and the Right to Transition: Medical Ethics when Parents Mean Well but Cause Harm." She describes the harms that befall many transgender youths during puberty when their bodies evolve in ways not aligning with their identity. This can be addressed by means of reversible puberty blocking treatments; but who should make the decision to have, or not have, such treatments? Are children at the age of puberty old enough to exercise autonomy in such cases? Priest argues that they are, and rejects the view that access to such treatments should be subject to parental consent. Transgender children should be able to autonomously request, and consent to, puberty blocking treatments if that is what they wish. Her contention is that the state ought to protect such children from well-meaning but harm-causing parents who refuse to give authorization to their children receiving such treatments, by legally mandating a right to puberty blocking treatments.

The case of Keira Bell, a former teenage patient in the UK, shows how difficult decision-making in this area is. Bell sued the National Health Service (NHS), because when she was 16, it provided her with puberty blocking drugs. When Bell turned 20, she undertook surgery to remove her breasts, in an effort to fully transition to male. She eventually regretted that choice, and argued that NHS staff should have more aggressively challenged her about her intention to transition from female to male. In the UK, the age of consent for medical procedures is 16.[1] The court agreed with Bell that she had been rushed through gender reassignment, and the NHS Tavistock clinic has stopped using puberty blockers without a court order.[2]

Carl Elliott's "Amputees by Choice" deals with people with what, to most of us, seems a bizarre desire. If someone asks a doctor to amputate a healthy arm or leg, would it ever be appropriate for the doctor to accede to such a request? How far does patient autonomy stretch in these circumstances? Or is the very fact of making such a request sufficient to show that the patient, or would-be patient, is not of sound mind, and that therefore questions of autonomy do not apply?

Elliott writes that he was initially revolted by the idea of amputating healthy limbs as a form of treatment, but his opinion changed after he began talking to people who wanted to have a limb amputated, and understood their condition better. Moreover if their requests for amputation are rejected on the grounds that the conditions of informed consent are not satisfied, or that doctors should not remove healthy tissue, Elliott's account suggests that many other similarly situated patients and a range of accepted surgical procedures would have to be rejected as well. Surgeons already suck fat from people's thighs, lengthen penises, reduce or increase the size of breasts, redesign labia, and split tongues. Why, then, not amputate a limb, particularly if the aim is to alleviate the intense suffering of a patient?

Arguably, if the only thing that will stop me being miserable is the amputation of a healthy limb, then the desire to have that limb amputated is rational. What might be considered irrational, in this situation, is the fact that the presence of a healthy limb is making me miserable. In situations of the kind that Julian Savulescu discusses in his article, "Rational Desires and the Limitation of Life-Sustaining Treatment," however, we may consider a patient's desire to be irrational. It may, for instance, be inconsistent with other stronger or more enduring desires that the patient has. This leads to a broader problem for the notion of informed consent: should we do what a patient desires even if the patient's desire is not rational? Savulescu answers that question in the negative. To defend that answer, we need to be able to distinguish between rational and irrational desires, and then to evaluate whether a specific desire in a particular context is or is not rational. While not downplaying the difficulties inherent in this task, Savulescu argues that it is one we cannot avoid if we are to respect patient autonomy. As Savulescu himself notes, however, such a policy is open to paternalistic abuse. Because of this it might be preferable to have a policy that accepts a competent patient's choices as a matter of course. But in that case the justification is not based, Savulescu suggests, on respect for patient autonomy, but elsewhere – presumably in the desirability of avoiding the harms that can flow from excessive paternalism.

Notes

1 Holt, Alison. 2020. NHS Gender clinic "should have challenged me more" over transition. *BBC News* March 01. https://www.bbc.com/news/health-51676020 [accessed March 2, 2020]

2 The full court judgment can be found here: https://www.judiciary.uk/wp-content/uploads/2020/12/Bell-v-Tavistock-Judgment.pdf

When do Doctors have a Duty to Treat?

What Healthcare Professionals Owe Us

Why Their Duty to Treat During a Pandemic is Contingent on Personal Protective Equipment (PPE)

Udo Schüklenk

Introduction

During the SARS-CoV2 pandemic many doctors and nurses have been reluctant to provide care to COVID-19 patients. The UK's doctors' leaders have warned repeatedly that the lack of appropriate PPE puts doctors' lives at risk.[1] PPE levels in Australia's state of Queensland were very low, noted the state's Clinical Senate Chair Alex Markwell.[2] Bulgaria has seen a wave of doctors and nurses resigning at two hospitals in the country's capital[3] over the lack of access to PPE, Zimbabwean doctors and nurses have reportedly gone on strike over the lack of protective equipment,[4] and nurses across the USA have protested about the lack of PPE.[5] These healthcare workers had every reason to be concerned for their own well-being. At the time of writing 100 doctors who provided care to Italian COVID-19 patients have died as a result of contracting SARS-CoV2 on the job.[6] Many more have fallen very seriously sick. A list of 'Fallen Coronavirus Heroes' maintained by Michael C Gibson, a medical doctor, lists (on 5 April 2020) 136 healthcare professionals who lost their lives as a result of COVID-19 infections they acquired while caring for infected patients.[7] The number is now almost certainly significantly higher, and it is bound to increase daily for some time to come. Despite some effort I have failed to track down a list looking at COVID-19 care-related deaths of other healthcare workers, such as nurses. However, there can be no doubt that the death toll among healthcare professionals caring for COVID-19 patients all over the world will be significant.

In response to concerns about the availability of healthcare professionals during expected COVID-19 case surges, a state government in one of Germany's most populous states, North-Rhine Westphalia, seriously considered introducing a compulsory service obligation for healthcare professionals.[8] Little did doctors know, when they joined the profession, that at some point further down the road, government would be planning to draft them into compulsory

Original publication details: Udo Schüklenk, "What Healthcare Professionals Owe Us: Why Their Duty to Treat During a Pandemic is Contingent on Personal Protective Equipment (PPE)," pp. 432–435 from *Journal of Medical Ethics* 46: 7 (2020).

service, much like soldiers. Desperate governments around the globe have come up with their own policies and ethics documents looking at the question of whether healthcare workers have a professional duty of care under the circumstances. Remarkably, they were haphazardly put together during the pandemic, and there was no preparation in any of the countries mentioned thus far. It is probably a sign of the times that the bar these documents set for a justifiable refusal to work is extraordinarily high. This suits those writing them. In all earnestness the Canadian province of British Columbia issued an ethics document that, while arguably producing conflicting guidance, could be interpreted as the view that healthcare workers do have an obligation to provide care if and only if they do not face 'certain and significant harm'.[9] The guidance is based on a pandemic influenza ethical guidance document[10] that shows a flaw that is replicated in many other documents of this kind.[11] It proffers a collection of disparate ethical values to consider, a vegetable garden equivalent of values, for you to pick and choose the ones that sound nicest. Of course, neither clear action guidance nor action justification can be derived from such documents. Unsurprisingly, while citing the document, and copy-pasting those ethical values, the British Columbia government task force fails to show how it derived its action guidance from said document. In medicine few things are ever certain. Realistically no healthcare workers could demonstrate in advance that they did not just face a risk – even a high risk – of significant harm, but that they would face significant harm with certainty if they were made to work.

What Healthcare Professionals Owe Us

What is it then that healthcare professionals owe us in a crisis like the current one? As patients we depend on doctors and nurses to provide professional care to us, because they have the specialist training, and they have a monopoly on the provision of these kinds of services. It is not as if we could turn around and go

elsewhere if the hospital's intensive care unit has an insufficient number of healthcare workers on call.

Most doctors in their graduation ceremonies take a public oath to serve the public good, oftentimes modelled on the World Medical Association's Declaration of Geneva.[12] The Declaration is arguably a modern-day Hippocratic Oath. Until the 1994 version of that influential document, doctors promised to provide emergency care, without any ifs, ands or buts. However, that promise has not been repeated in subsequent iterations of that document,[13] so that approach does not address the question at hand. Perhaps the world's doctors woke up to the dangers of making promises they did not realistically intend to live up to. What do the traditions of the medical profession look like then? As Ariel R. Schwartz notes, 'the history of medical ethics reveals that the medical community has never come to a consensus on the nature and scope of its responsibilities during an epidemic'.[14] His description of the behaviour of doctors during infectious disease outbreaks from the black plague in the 14th and 15th centuries to the bubonic plague in the 17th century suggests a deeply individualistic response. Many ran away to protect themselves; others stayed behind to care for their patients. The same pattern of behaviour held true during the 2014–16 Ebola virus disease outbreaks in West African countries.

Neither the history of how healthcare professionals responded in the past to pandemic outbreaks, nor their professed values, provide us with much guidance on what the professionals themselves take to be their professional obligations. In any case, why would anyone want to leave decisions on what the profession and its members owe to society to the profession?[15] We have little reason to assume that it won't look after its members first. Medical associations, unlike statutory regulatory bodies, despite protestations to the contrary, are essentially glorified trade unions representing their members' interests. This situation would not be the first where such associations might prioritise their members' interests over the good of society.[16]

One could reasonably argue that there is an implied voluntary consent to risk-taking when healthcare workers accepted the deal their profession cut with society. Monopoly powers, high societal standing and, at least for medical doctors, oftentimes high salaries do not come without a price. Healthcare professionals knew, if they paid attention to the subject in their global health classes, that infections such as severe acute respiratory syndrome (SARS), Middle East respiratory syndrome (MERS), Ebola and others were going to raise their ugly heads during their lifetime, and joining the profession meant accepting a duty to provide care. During the early days of the HIV pandemic, when an infection with that virus meant certain death, regulatory bodies in most countries eventually decreed that healthcare professionals had an obligation to treat.[14] Given COVID-19's much lower mortality risk, this should settle it, or so one might think. That is a mistaken view.

What makes SARS-CoV2 different is that the HIV response was predicated on the availability of PPE to healthcare professionals. In such a reality, if healthcare professionals followed universal precautions and had the right protective equipment, the odds of them picking up HIV would have been negligible. With SARS-CoV2 we are, in most countries, in a very different situation.

Neoliberalism and the Fetishisation of 'Efficiency'

One feature closely linked to the functioning of global capitalism is efficiency. Everybody involved in the value chain aims to avoid the waste of money and resources. There is a virtue in running 'lean' operations. Most countries in the global north, that operate varieties of public or publicly funded healthcare systems, saw the re-election of cost-cutting governments who ran successfully on election campaign platforms promising to 'return money to our back pockets' and away from big government.[17] This claim certainly is an uncontroversial one for governments elected in countries like the UK, France, Germany, and Australia, to name just a few, during the last few decades. And as taxpayers we did get money returned to our back pockets by low tax regimes. As neoliberal election campaign lore

has it, we know best how to spend our hard-earned money. Such policies were anything but cost neutral, as those in need of public services have known for a long time. They succeeded in hollowing out the healthcare delivery infrastructures in most countries. The literature providing evidence to this effect is vast, and it is impossible to do it justice here.[18–21] There are still appreciable differences between countries; for example, Germany has about 29 intensive care unit (ICU) beds available per 100,000 inhabitants, versus 6.5 in the UK.[22] In the UK, since Prime Minister Margaret Thatcher's tenure, citizens have been treated to decades of low-tax, small-state austerity, effectively rendering the National Health Service (NHS) unable to cover regular influenza season patient case loads without great difficulty.[23] In the USA, where publicly funded healthcare delivery is close to non-existent and for-profit operators often dictate the levels of care that will be provided, the results were quite similar, except there the availability of and access to healthcare infrastructure was dictated by profit objectives driving many hospitals, as well as for-profit insurers that pay for-profit and non-profit hospitals alike for particular services.

Implications for Healthcare Professionals' Obligations

The endpoint was the same: democratically elected governments across the global north have left hospitals woefully unprepared for the onslaught of patients, not only in terms of ICU beds and ventilators, but also in terms of PPE. The latter is what matters when we ask ethical questions about healthcare workers' responsibilities during pandemic outbreaks. The unavailability of PPE to efficiently maintain universal precautions while on the job was a foreseeable consequence of the race to the public services bottom that globalisation motivates.

If the lack of available PPE for frontline healthcare professionals would have been due to a natural occurrence, one could reasonably argue that they should be prepared to accept a certain higher degree of risk. The argument in support of such a view could take recourse to the already-mentioned voluntary informed consent argument. Healthcare professionals signed voluntarily a contract with society to provide reliable services, not only when the sun is shining, but also in times of crisis. If there were a situation where, despite society's best efforts at resourcing the protection of its healthcare workers against acquiring life-threatening infections while on the job, their risk would remain high, one could argue that they ought to accept a certain degree of risk. They knew there was a chance such an outbreak could occur during their lifetime, and part of the deal with society was not that they could refuse the provision of professional care. However, there clearly have to be some limits to such a duty. For instance, society cannot afford to lose a very large number of its healthcare workers during a pandemic, because the time will come when the pandemic wave has passed, and doctors will still be needed. It would also be unrealistic to expect doctors to risk their lives if there were a high probability of death, say because the best societal effort at resourcing their protection was still insufficient to protect the workers. Surely then their continuing provision of professional services would constitute a supererogatory kind of action.

In any case, these kinds of arguments have been discussed in the literature for a long time. Whatever one makes of these arguments has no bearing on the current situation. The reason for this is that in the current situation the lack of PPE is truly deliberate, it is by human, cost-cutting design. It is not as if governments and their experts did not know that the occurrence of an agent like SARS-CoV2 or worse was likely. For a specialist audience the US Centers for Disease Control and Prevention issued in 2017 community mitigation guidelines.[24] In fact, during former President George W Bush's presidency the country went to significant lengths in its global pandemic planning.[25] Even lay people were able to read up on the issue, in a multitude of media. Understanding the likelihood of something like this to occur during our lifetime did not require a great deal of specialist knowledge.[26] Given all this, it was quite a remarkable

sight to see on global news programmes the UK Chancellor and Prime Minister standing outside 10 Downing Street, wildly applauding their country's healthcare professionals' heroism.[27] The heroism that they were celebrating, however, was a direct, avoidable consequence of their own government's austerity policies. An adequately resourced NHS would not have required a significant degree of beyond-the-call-of-duty heroism by healthcare professionals. I should note that I am not making an argument here about the rights and wrongs of resourcing healthcare systems with large numbers of ICU beds, ventilators and other equipment, just in case they might be needed as a result of a new virus making its way through a population. That obviously would require a very significant outlay in terms of resources, and it is unclear to me whether that would indeed be a sound way to spend finite healthcare resources. However, PPE does not constitute hi-tech expensive equipment; all of it can be produced relatively cheaply, and it can be stored in large quantities without taxing a given healthcare system unreasonably financially. That at least seems an uncontroversial claim for any country of the global north. The much vaunted N95 respirator – that probably every country on the globe is trying to purchase at the time of writing in large quantities for healthcare workers – could be obtained for US$12 for a box of 20 in home improvement stores in the USA, before the pandemic struck. Healthcare systems would have been able to purchase these at a very significant discount. Unsurprisingly, the price of that kind of equipment during pandemic outbreaks rises significantly.

We live in democracies, and we elected politicians who promised us time and again that we could have our cake and eat it. It turns out, unsurprisingly, we cannot have that. There is no reason why doctors, nurses and other healthcare workers should be seen to be professionally obliged to risk their well-being during pandemic outbreaks, in the global north, because we chose governments that starved the healthcare delivery infrastructure sufficiently of resources to permit them to do their job safely or with minimal increases to their average on-the-job risk. Elections have consequences.

Conclusion

We should be grateful to any healthcare professional willing to care for COVID-19 patients, in the absence of professional-standard PPE, but we have no reason to take for granted that there will be one when needed. No healthcare professional can be expected to accept a higher-than-usual degree of risk to their own well-being, simply because we chose not to provide them with the necessary equipment to protect themselves efficiently.

References

1   Newman M. COVID-19: doctors' leaders warn that staff could quit and may die over lack of protective equipment. *BMJ* 2020; 368.

2   Lynch L. Queensland hospitals 'very low' on gloves, masks, gowns and told to reuse. *Brisbane Times*, 2020. Available:https://www.brisbanetimes.com.au/national/queensland/queensland-hospitals-very-low-on-gloves-masks-gowns-and-told-to-reuse-20200317-p54azh.html [Accessed 2 Apr 2020].

3   Petkova M. Dozens of Bulgarian doctors resign amid COVID-19 crisis. *Aljazeera*, 2020. Available:https://www.aljazeera.com/news/2020/03/dozens-bulgarian-doctors-resign-covid-19-crisis-200318151643933.html [Accessed 2 Apr 2020].

4   Munhende L. Zimbabwe: COVID-19 – Harare hospital closed, patients discharged as doctors, nurses down tools in demand of protective clothing. *AllAfrica*, 2020. Available:https://allafrica.com/stories/202003270832.html [Accessed 2 Apr 2020].

5   McNamara A. Nurses across the country protest lack of protective equipment. *CBS news*, 2020.Available:https://www.cbsnews.com/news/health-care-workers-protest-lack-of-protective-equipment-2020-03-28/ [Accessed 2 Apr 2020].

6   FNOMCeO. Elenco dei Medici caduti nel corso dell'epidemia di COVID-19. *FNOMCeO*, 2020. Available:https://portale.fnomceo.it/elenco-dei-medici-caduti-nel-corso-dellepidemia-di-covid-19/ [Accessed 2 Apr 2020].

7   List *Fallen Coronavirus Heroes (Responses)* is maintained. Available: https://docs.google.com/spreadsheets/d/1pFdoZqjnDRaSzJi0JJJ3f5zdb87Q5tL3zc4nGx1nejI/edit#gid=1744604459 [Accessed 2 Apr 2020].

8   Biermann K. and Gutensohn D. Aerzte und Pfleger warnen vor Zwangsarbeit. *Zeit* 2020. [Epub ahead of print: 2 Apr 2020].

9   British Columbia Ministry of Health Provincial COVID-19 Task Force. *COVID-19 ethics analysis: what is the ethical duty of health care workers to provide care during COVID-19 pandemic?* 2020. Available:https://www2.gov.bc.ca/assets/gov/health/about-bc-s-health-care-system/office-of-the-provincial-health-officer/covid-19/duty_to_care_during_covid_march_28_2020.pdf [Accessed April 3, 2020].

10   University of Toronto Joint Centre for Bioethics Pandemic Influenza Working Group. *Stand on guard for thee: ethical considerations in preparedness for pandemic influenza,* 2005. Available:https://web.archive.org/web/20051130054722/http://www.utoronto.ca/jcb/home/documents/pandemic.pdf [Accessed 3 Apr 2020].

11   Schüklenk U. and Zhang E.Y. Public health ethics and obesity prevention: the trouble with data and ethics. *Monash Bioeth Rev* 2014; 32(1–2):121–40.

12   World Medical Association. *International code of medical ethics,* 1994. Available: https://www.wma.net/wp-content/uploads/2018/07/Decl-of-Geneva-v1994-1.pdf [Accessed 2 Apr 2020].

13   World Medical Association. *Declaration of Geneva,* 2017. Available: https://www.wma.net/policies-post/wma-declaration-of-geneva/ [Accessed 2 Apr 2020].

14   Schwartz A.R. Doubtful duty: physicians' legal obligation to treat during an epidemic. 60 *Stan. L. Rev* 2007; 657.

15   Veatch R.M. Who should control the scope and nature of medical ethics? In: Baker R.B., Caplan A.L., Emanuel L.L., et al., eds. *The American Medical Ethics Revolution: How the AMA's Code of Ethics has Transformed Physicians' Relationship to Patients, Professionals, and Society.* Baltimore: Johns Hopkins University Press, 1999: 158–70.

16   Schüklenk U. Conscientious objection in medicine: accommodation versus professionalism and the public good. *Br Med Bull* 2018; 126(1):47–56 https://academic.oup.com/bmb/article/126/1/47/4955771 (See also Chapter 75 of this *Anthology*.)

17   Jakobsson N. and Kumlin S. Election campaign agendas, government partisanship, and the welfare state. *European Political Science Review* 2017; 9(2):183–208.

18 McGregor S. Neoliberalism and health care. *Int J Consum Stud* 2001; 25(2):82–9.

19 Donelan K., Blendon R.J., Schoen C., et al. The cost of health system change: public discontent in five nations. *Health Aff* 1999; 18(3):206–16.

20 Sakellariou D. and Rotarou E.S. The effects of neoliberal policies on access to healthcare for people with disabilities. *Int J Equity Health* 2017; 16(1):199.

21 Mercille J. Neoliberalism and health care: the case of the Irish nursing home sector. *Crit Public Health* 2018; 28(5):546–59.

22 McCarthy N. The countries with the most critical care beds per capita. *Forbes*, 2020. Available: https://www.forbes.com/sites/niallmccarthy/2020/03/12/the-countries-with-the-most-critical-care-beds-per-capita-infographic/#5daa41ff7f86 [Accessed 2 Apr 2020].

23 Anonymous. NHS winter pressure: hospitals report 99 per cent capacity over festive season as flu season looms. *Independent,* 2018. Available: https://www.independent.co.uk/news/uk/home-news/nhs-winter-pressure-flu-season-capacity-patients-corridors-a-e-vaccine-a8136231.html [Accessed April 2, 2020].

24 Qualls N., Levitt A., Kanade N., et al. Community mitigation guidelines to prevent pandemic influenza. *Morb Mortal Wkly Rep* 2017; 66(1):1–34.

25 Mosk M. George W. Bush in 2005: 'If we wait for a pandemic to appear, it will be too late to prepare'. *ABC News*, 2020. Available:https://abcnews.go.com/amp/Politics/george-bush-2005-wait-pandemic-late-prepare/story?id=69979013 [Accessed 2 Apr 2020].

26 Garrett L. *The coming plague: newly emerging diseases in a world out of balance*. New York: Farrar, Straus and Giroux, 1994.

27 Storyful. Boris Johnson takes part in nationwide applause to support NHS workers. *Yahoo news*, 2020. Available: https://uk.news.yahoo.com/boris-johnson-takes-part-nationwide-205636024.html [Accessed 2 Apr 2020].

74

Conscientious Objection in Health Care

Mark R. Wicclair

Introduction

Until relatively recently, conscientious objection was primarily associated with objections to military service. However, it is now a common phenomenon in health care as well. A significant number of health professionals, including doctors, nurses, pharmacists, and midwives, refuse to provide legal, professionally accepted, and clinically appropriate medical services within the scope of their competence because they claim doing so would be contrary to their moral convictions. Most often, conscientious objection in health care is in relation to reproductive health services and end-of-life care. The former includes abortion, contraception, and assisted reproduction. The latter includes forgoing life-sustaining treatment, especially medically provided nutrition and hydration (MPNH); a procedure for procuring organs for transplant after life support is withdrawn known as donation after cardiac determination of death (DACDD); a procedure for alleviating intractable pain in terminally ill patients that may hasten death referred to as sedation to unconsciousness; and, in jurisdictions in which it is legal, physician-assisted suicide.

Since conscientious objection is an increasingly common occurrence in health care, it is essential to understand when accommodation is warranted. Approaches to accommodation can span a wide spectrum. At one extreme, health professionals are offered broad protections with few, if any, limitations. This approach is aptly designated "conscience absolutism." Two measures, one in the U.S. and the other in the UK, illustrate this approach.

The US Health and Human Services (HHS) Final Rule, "Protecting Statutory Conscience Rights in Health Care; Delegations of Authority" (45 CFR 88), provides broad protection to health professionals who refuse to provide or assist in the performance of services that are contrary to their consciences.[1] "Assist in the performance" is broadly defined: "to take an action that has a specific, reasonable, and articulable connection to furthering a procedure or a part of a health service program or research activity undertaken by or with another person or entity." The following examples are among those identified in the Final Rule: pre- and post-operative support for an abortion procedure; scheduling an abortion or preparing a room and the

Original publication details: Mark R. Wicclair, "Conscientious Objection in Health Care," in Hugh LaFollette (ed.), *Ethics in Practice: An Anthology*, Fifth Edition (Hoboken, NJ: Wiley-Blackwell, 2020). Reproduced with permission of John Wiley & Sons.

instruments for an abortion; driving patients to hospitals or clinics for scheduled abortions; physically delivering abortion inducing drugs; and counseling, referral, training, or "otherwise making arrangements" if "aid is provided by such actions." The Final Rule's broad interpretation of "assist in the performance" would also seem to include ancillary personnel such as file clerks, orderlies, and office staff who object to abortion or other medical services. The following statement in the Final Rule captures its perfunctory concern for patients: "The Department finds that finalizing the rule is appropriate without regard to whether data exists on the competing contentions about its effect on access to services. . .these rights [of conscientious objection] are worth protecting even if they impact overall or individual access to a particular service. . ."

In the UK, a proposed bill in the House of Lords, the Conscientious Objection (Medical Activities) Bill, would give broad protection to health professionals with conscientious objections to withdrawing life-sustaining treatment; IVF and other fertility treatments; and abortion, including "activity required to prepare for, support or perform termination of pregnancy."[2] Similar to the HHS Final Rule, the proposed British bill protects "participation," which is broadly defined to include "any supervision, delegation, planning or supporting of staff" in relation to an activity to which the practitioner objects. The proposed British bill, like its HHS counterpart, also does not include any protections for patients; and neither includes a review mechanism to assess the nature and sincerity of the alleged moral objection.

At the other extreme is the view that conscientious objection has no place in health care. Refusing to provide a legal, professionally approved and clinically appropriate service within the scope of a practitioner's clinical competence is said to be unprofessional conduct. Insofar as this view assumes that conscientious objection in health care is incompatible with professional obligations, it is aptly termed "incompatibilism." Julian Savulescu offers what might well be considered the classic statement of incompatibilism in a 2006 article: "If people are not prepared to offer legally permitted, efficient, and beneficial care

to a patient because it conflicts with their values, they should not be doctors."[3] A more recent article co-authored by Savulescu reiterates this view:

> If society thinks contraception, abortion and assistance in dying are important, it should select people prepared to do them, not people whose values preclude them from participating. Equally, people not prepared to participate in such expected courses of action should not join professions tasked by society with the provision of such services."[4]

"Reasonable accommodation" is an approach between the two extremes. Unlike conscience absolutism, reasonable accommodation includes limits to accommodation designed in part to protect patients. Unlike incompatibilism, reasonable accommodation holds that there is a legitimate place for conscientious objection in health care. An approach known as the "conventional compromise" is a frequently cited conception of reasonable accommodation.[5] It exempts health professionals from providing a medical service that is against their conscience only if the following three conditions are satisfied: 1) health professionals inform patients about the medical service if it is clinically appropriate; 2) health professionals refer patients to another professional willing and able to provide the medical service; and 3) referrals do not impose an unreasonable burden on patients.

This essay critically analyzes conscience absolutism and incompatibilism and argues that even though there is a grain of truth in both, neither approach is justified. Different conceptions of reasonable accommodation are identified and explained. They are distinguished primarily by the requirements health professionals must satisfy to qualify for an accommodation. The essay defends one of these conceptions. First, however, it is necessary to define "conscientious objection."

What is Conscientious Objection?

A health professional's objection to providing a medical service is an instance of conscientious objection only if the objection is conscience-based. There are several different conceptions of conscience.[6] However, for the purposes of analyzing conscientious objection in health care, it suffices to stipulate that an objection is conscience-based only if it is based on the health professional's fundamental *moral* beliefs, which can, but need not be, faith-based. For example, suppose an obstetrician-gynecologist (ob-gyn) refuses to perform abortions. If her refusal is based on her moral belief that abortion is ethically wrong because it involves the unjustified killing of a being with moral standing, her refusal is conscience-based and is an instance of conscientious objection. However, ob-gyns might object to providing abortions for other reasons. For example, in view of the violence and threats directed at abortion providers, an ob-gyn who has no moral objection to abortion might refuse to perform abortions out of a concern for her safety and well-being. Since this refusal is not based on a moral objection to abortion, it is not an instance of conscientious objection. Similarly, if a pharmacist's refusal to dispense emergency contraception (EC) is based on his moral beliefs, his refusal is an instance of conscientious objection. However, if the pharmacist has no moral objection to EC but refuses to dispense it to avoid protests, boycotts, and loss of business, his refusal is not an instance of conscientious objection.

Other examples of refusals that are not instances of conscientious objection include: 1) A physician who is not morally opposed to assisted suicide refuses to provide it to a patient who requests it because the practice is illegal in the state or country in which she practices. 2) A physician who believes the death penalty is ethically justified refuses to participate in executions because it would violate the profession's code of ethics; 3) A physician refuses a patient's request for antibiotics because the physician has determined that the patient has a viral infection and antibiotics are ineffective and not clinically indicated for viral infections. 4) An internist who supports palliative care refuses to provide it to a patient who requests it because she has had no training in palliative care or the proper administration of pain medication.

Generally, conscience-based refusals to provide a medical service occur within a distinctive context:

The service is legal, professionally accepted, clinically appropriate, and within the scope of the clinician's competence; and a health professional refuses to provide it because it is contrary to the practitioner's moral beliefs.

Assessing Approaches to Conscientious Objection in Health Care

Conscience absolutism

A grain of truth in conscience absolutism is the recognition that the exercise of conscience (i.e., an ability to act in accordance with one's fundamental ethical beliefs) is valuable and worth protecting. There are several reasons for accepting this assessment of the exercise of conscience. The primary reason is the connection between the exercise of conscience and moral integrity. To maintain moral integrity, a person must refrain from performing actions that are against her conscience. As Jeffrey Blustein observes, when one acts against one's conscience, "one violates one's own fundamental moral or religious convictions, personal standards that one sees as an important part of oneself and by which one is prepared to judge oneself."[7]

Moral integrity in turn is valuable and worth protecting for several reasons. First, it can be an essential component of a person's conception of a good or meaningful life and can have intrinsic worth or value to a person. Second, a loss of moral integrity can be devastating. It can result in strong feelings of guilt, remorse, and shame, as well as loss of self-respect. It also can be experienced as an assault on one's self-image or identity. Third, although the available evidence is equivocal, it has been claimed that a loss of moral integrity can result in a general decline in a person's moral character. For example, a professor of pharmacy maintains "We would be naive to expect a pharmacist to forsake his or her ethics in one area (e.g., abortion) while applying them for the patient's welfare in every other area."[8]

Finally, it can be claimed that moral integrity generally has intrinsic worth or value. To be sure, insofar as moral integrity can involve a commitment to any ethical or religious beliefs and principles, it does not guarantee ethically acceptable behavior. Nevertheless, similar to courage and honesty, which also can serve immoral ends and produce undesirable consequences, it can be claimed that moral integrity is a virtue and its value is not exclusively a function of ends and consequences.

The exercise of conscience is valuable and worth protecting for several additional reasons. The first derives from the value of autonomy and the associated principle of respect for autonomous agents: "to respect autonomous agents is to acknowledge their right to hold views, to make choices, and to take actions based on their values and beliefs."[9] Second, the value of the exercise of conscience can be said to derive in part from the value of moral/cultural diversity, and protecting its exercise can be defended as a requirement of toleration of moral/cultural diversity. Third, the notion of ethical epistemic modesty or humility can be cited as a basis for respecting and protecting the exercise of conscience. Ethical epistemic modesty is the view that although ethical beliefs can be correct or incorrect and justified or unjustified, we might be mistaken when we think that a particular ethical belief is correct or justified. This recognition suggests "modesty" or "humility" and a rejection of dogmatism in relation to beliefs that we do not accept. A fourth reason applies specifically to health professionals. It can be argued that a failure to accommodate conscience-based refusals to provide a medical service may discourage people who value moral integrity from entering health professions. An unintended consequence might be to pre-select for individuals who are ethically insensitive. Finally, protecting the exercise of conscience by health professionals can promote diversity within the health professions. Conversely, failing to protect the exercise of conscience can discourage religious and ethnic minorities from becoming health professionals. For all these reasons, then, it can be maintained that the exercise of conscience is valuable and worth protecting.

A grain of truth in incompatibilism reveals the primary problem with conscience absolutism: Health care practitioners are professionals and as such, they have professional obligations to patients. Unqualified accommodation exposes patients to burdens and harms and can violate the professional obligations of doctors, nurses, pharmacists and other health care providers. Professional obligations restrict when health care practitioners may justifiably refuse to provide medical services that are legal, professionally accepted, clinically appropriate, and within the scope of their clinical competence. Next, let's consider incompatibilism.

Incompatibilism

A common argument for incompatibilism draws upon a contrast between conscientious objection to performing compulsory military service and conscientious objection to providing specific medical services.[10] Typically, it refers to physicians, but it can be generalized to apply to other health professions. For the sake of assessing incompatibilism, I will focus on the medical profession.

Unlike compulsory military service, it is claimed, becoming a physician is a *voluntary choice*. Military conscripts have not chosen to become soldiers; and if they are assigned combat roles, they have not voluntarily accepted those roles or the corresponding role obligations and responsibilities. Exempting conscientious objectors from combat prevents them from being compelled to act against their conscience. By contrast, it is argued, when individuals enter the medical profession, they do so voluntarily, and in doing so, they explicitly or implicitly agree to accept the obligations of the profession. Individuals who are conscientiously opposed to providing a legal and professionally accepted medical service have no legitimate claim for accommodation because they can avoid acting against their conscience by choosing a profession, medical specialty, or practice location and environment that will not require them to act contrary to their conscience.

This line of argument fails to justify incompatibilism. At most, it supports the claim that insofar as individuals voluntarily decide to enter the medical profession, they are bound by the corresponding professional obligations. To support incompatibilism, it must be shown further that refusing to provide a legal, professionally accepted, clinically appropriate medical service within the scope of a physician's clinical competence because it violates a physician's moral convictions is contrary to his or her professional obligations. Incompatibilists have tended to rely on one or both of two claims: 1) Physicians have an obligation to put patients' interests or well-being above their own self-interest. I will refer to this as the Patients' Interests First Principle (PIFP). 2) Physicians are obligated to provide all services within the scope of professional practice. I will refer to this as the Scope of Professional Practice Principle (SOPPP).

The Patients' Interests First Principle (PIFP)
It is a generally recognized principle that physicians have an obligation to put patients' interests or well-being above their own self-interest. In view of the wide recognition of the PIFP, it is not implausible to claim that individuals explicitly or implicitly agree to accept this principle when they voluntarily enter the medical profession. However, the PIFP is general and needs to be specified. It clearly prohibits physicians from considering their financial interests when making recommendations to patients. But beyond that, what are the scope and implications of the PIFP? Is there no significant ethical difference between a physician's financial interests and his or her interest in maintaining moral integrity? Are there no limits to the sacrifices of their own well-being that physicians are obligated to make for sake of their patients' health or well-being? Surely, there must be limits or physicians would not be able to take vacations, refuse to make house calls, limit their practice hours, refuse to expose themselves to excessive financial losses or extreme risks of harm, and so forth.

What are the implications of the PIFP for conscientious objection? Typically, incompatibilists simply assume, without support, that conscientious objection is incompatible with the PIFP. An article by Ronit Stahl and Ezekiel Emanuel is representative.[11] The authors cite the following statement in Section 1.1.1 of the American Medical Association (AMA) *Code of Medical Ethics*: "physicians' ethical responsibility [is] to place patients' welfare above the physician's own self-interest."[12] However, if the AMA *Code of Medical Ethics* is the basis for interpreting the PIFP, one would have to conclude that conscientious objection is *not* inconsistent with that principle. The same chapter of the *Code of Medical Ethics* (1.1.7) addresses conscientious objection and recognizes its value:

> Preserving opportunity for physicians to act (or to refrain from acting) in accordance with the dictates of conscience in their professional practice is important for preserving the integrity of the medical profession as well as the integrity of the individual physician, on which patients and the public rely. Thus, physicians should have considerable latitude to practice in accord with well-considered, deeply held beliefs that are central to their self-identities.

The *Code* also explicitly denies that conscientious objection is incompatible with the obligations of physicians. It states that, with three specified limitations, "physicians may be able to act (or refrain from acting) in accordance with the dictates of their conscience *without violating their professional obligations* (1.1.7; emphasis added).[13]

Consequently, the AMA *Code* does not appear to support an interpretation of the PIFP that rules out conscientious objection. Elsewhere, I consider several accounts of the professional obligations of physicians and argue that none supports incompatibilism.[14] I will not repeat those arguments here. Suffice it to say that providing a plausible and convincing defense of the claim that conscientious objection is incompatible with the PIFP is a more formidable challenge than its supporters appear to realize.

There is another strategy to show that conscientious objection is incompatible with the PIFP. It is to minimize or even trivialize the interests at stake for physicians. For example, conscience claims are characterized as "essentially arbitrary dislikes"[15] or nothing more than efforts to avoid "personal psychic distress."[16] If a physician's interest in accommodation is characterized in this way, it would not be implausible to claim that physicians who refuse to provide medical services for reasons of conscience violate the PIFP and their fiduciary duty to patients.

Depending on the basis of the objection to providing a medical service, this strategy can unjustifiably devalue an objecting physician's interest in accommodation.[17] The strength and moral weight of an objecting physician's interest in accommodation depends in part on whether the objection is based on peripheral moral beliefs or fundamental moral convictions. The following two cases illustrate the distinction between objections based on peripheral moral beliefs and fundamental moral convictions:

Case 1: An 89-year-old nursing home resident with advanced Alzheimer's is admitted to a hospital ICU after presenting at the emergency department (ED) with pneumonia and kidney failure. An intensivist believes that providing life support would be wasteful and an unjust use of medical resources. Although providing the requested life support would be unjust in the eyes of the intensivist, it would comprise an injustice of a type that he routinely tolerates rather than a perceived grave injustice such as discrimination based on race or sexual orientation. Consequently, the intensivist's objection is based on a peripheral moral belief.

Case 2: An intensivist believes that palliative sedation to unconsciousness is morally equivalent to unjustified killing. The belief that unjustified killing is wrong is among her most deeply held moral convictions. As she explains it, "Offering palliative sedation to unconsciousness is something I simply cannot do. I couldn't live with myself if I were to offer it." The intensivist's objection is based on a fundamental moral conviction.

In Case 1, insofar as the intensivist's objection is based on a peripheral moral belief rather than a fundamental moral conviction, providing life support would not undermine his moral integrity. It might not be unwarranted to claim that, insofar as the objection is based on a peripheral moral belief, it does not rise to the level of a genuine conscientious objection. Nevertheless, it would be unwarranted to characterize

the basis of the objection as "an arbitrary dislike." Even if providing life support would not cause substantial moral harm to the intensivist, he may well experience moral distress. Insofar as the intensivist's moral integrity is not at stake, if he were to request an accommodation, it might be warranted to deny it and pursue other means to address and reduce his moral distress.[18]

In Case 2, insofar as the intensivist's objection is based on her fundamental moral convictions, offering palliative sedation to unconsciousness would undermine her moral integrity. Consequently, if the intensivist in Case 2 were to request an accommodation, given what is at stake, it would be unwarranted to dismiss her request out of hand by claiming that her objection is nothing more than an "arbitrary dislike" or an effort to avoid "personal psychic distress."[19]

The Scope of Professional Practice Principle (SOPPP)
Some defenders of incompatibilism maintain that physicians are obligated to provide all services within the scope of professional practice. It is claimed that individuals who voluntarily become physicians accept an obligation to provide all services that are within the scope of the profession's practice and that society reasonably expects them to provide those services. Doctors who are unwilling to fulfill that obligation, it is concluded, "should be replaced by someone who is willing to undertake the work."[20]

Assessing these claims requires a definition of "the scope of professional practice." It is implausible to maintain that all physicians have a professional obligation to provide all legal and professionally accepted medical services. Medicine includes several recognized specialties and sub-specialties, and physicians are not obligated to provide medical services that are outside the scope of their chosen specialty or sub-specialty. Internists and gynecologists are not obligated to perform cataract surgery. Gastroenterologists and dermatologists are not obligated to offer treatment for pneumonia or schizophrenia. Pediatric oncologists are not obligated to treat adult patients; geriatricians are not obligated to treat infants; and neonatologists are not obligated to provide intensive care for elderly patients.

Physicians can limit the scope of their practice even further within chosen specialties and sub-specialties. Orthopedic surgeons can limit their practice to hip and knee replacement surgery, shoulder surgery, or foot surgery. Dermatologists can limit their practice to cosmetic or therapeutic reconstructive surgery, and internists and neurologists can limit their practice to the diagnosis and treatment of specified diseases. Obstetrician-gynecologists can decide not to deliver babies, and gastroenterologists can decide not to offer bariatric surgery. In short, physicians appear to have wide discretion about the legitimate scope of their professional practice and this would appear to undermine the claim that physicians who refuse to provide a medical service – whether for reasons of conscience or other reasons – are violating an obligation to provide all services within the scope of their professional practice.

In response, Schüklenk and Smalling claim that the discretion to limit the scope of one's professional practice is limited by society: "it is ultimately up to society to determine the scope of professional practice."[21] Although this claim apparently is intended to significantly restrict the discretion of individual physicians to decide which medical services they will offer, it actually undermines the case for incompatibilism. For, insofar as a society accepts (limited) conscientious objection in health care, it could not be claimed that conscience-based refusals are *ipso facto* contrary to an obligation to provide all medical services within the scope of (socially determined) professional practice. For example, since the United States Federal government as well as several individual states protect physicians who conscientiously object to performing abortions and prescribing emergency contraception (EC), it cannot be claimed that physicians who practice in jurisdictions that offer such protection and refuse to perform abortions or prescribe EC for reasons of conscience are failing to fulfill a duty to provide medical services within the scope of (socially determined) professional practice. In addition, insofar as a country or state sanctions (limited) conscientious objection in medicine, patients cannot expect that physicians will never refuse to provide medical services that violate their conscience.[22]

Reasonable accommodation

The primary aim of reasonable accommodation is to accommodate clinicians' claims of conscience without unjustifiably compromising other values and interests (e.g., patient health and well-being). There are different conceptions of reasonable accommodation, and they differ in three major respects: 1) whether they require specified actions by health professionals; 2) whether they require alternative service; and 3) whether they require health professionals to provide a public justification of their refusal.

Are specific actions required?

The "conventional compromise" referred to earlier is representative of approaches that require specified actions (e.g., informing and referring). However, insofar as the primary aim of reasonable accommodation is to accommodate clinicians' claims of conscience without unjustifiably compromising other values and interests, it may not be necessary for *objecting physicians* to inform or refer. Depending on the circumstances, it might be possible for patients and surrogates to receive relevant information and for patients to receive clinically appropriate medical services from non-objecting providers in a timely fashion – and without excessively burdening non-objecting providers or organizations. Insofar as the conventional compromise requires specific actions regardless of the circumstances, it can unnecessarily undermine an objector's moral integrity.

A more satisfactory conception of reasonable accommodation focuses on expected outcomes and protects patients and other third parties (e.g., surrogates, other health care providers and organizations) by accommodating objecting health professionals only if it is not expected to: 1) impede a patient's/surrogate's timely access to relevant information and referral; 2) impede a patient's timely access to clinically appropriate health care services; and 3) impose excessive burdens on other clinicians or organizations. This will be referred to as the *outcome-focused* conception of reasonable accommodation. Insofar as it protects patients and other third parties without unnecessarily limiting objecting health professionals' exercise of conscience, it is preferable to the conventional compromise.

The first two conditions derive from the professional obligations of health professionals. A refusal to provide a legal, professionally accepted, and clinically appropriate medical service within the scope of a clinician's competence that compromises patient health and well-being is a clear violation of the Patients' Interests First Principle. The third condition is justified by considerations of fairness. It is unfair to impose excessive burdens on other health professionals and organizations; and they do not have an obligation to facilitate an accommodation if it is expected to impose excessive burdens on them.

Employing the outcome-focused conception to manage conscientious objection requires decisions about accommodation to be context-dependent. Case 3 illustrates this point.

Case 3: Dr Kramer is a Memorial Hospital emergency department (ED) physician. He conscientiously objects to providing emergency contraception (EC). He believes that it is morally wrong to give EC to patients, including rape victims. He also believes that he will be complicit in a moral wrong if he informs rape victims about EC or refers them to other providers who will dispense it. Offering EC to rape victims who present at a hospital ED is standard of care and required by Memorial Hospital policy.

To determine whether Dr Kramer can be accommodated, the outcome-focused conception requires asking whether it is feasible to implement a process in the Memorial Hospital ED that: 1) assures that all rape victims who present at the Memorial Hospital ED are offered EC (i.e., they will receive information about EC and will receive it if they request it); 2) does not require any participation on the part of Dr Kramer; and 3) does not place an excessive burden on other ED physicians or Memorial Hospital. A process that satisfies these requirements might task triage personnel with the responsibility of assigning rape victims to other ED physicians whenever Dr Kramer is on service. That arrangement would relieve Dr Kramer

of any responsibility to offer EC or refer patients to other physicians who will offer it.

Unfortunately, there is no simple rule for determining when burdens are "excessive," in part because excessiveness is largely context dependent. Whether an accommodation will impose excessive burdens depends on a variety of contextual factors, including the number of staff members whose clinical competencies overlap with those of the clinician who seeks accommodation, the willingness of those clinicians to provide the medical service from which the clinician requests an exemption, the existing responsibilities and work-load of staff and administrators, and the availability of funds to pay overtime or hire additional staff. Moreover, the assessment of burdens is in part subjective insofar as burdensomeness depends on a person's life circumstances. For example, whereas a schedule shift or additional time on service may not be an excessive burden to a clinician who has no partner or children, it might be an excessive burden to a clinician who is a single parent of a young child or a clinician who has other professional responsibilities (e.g., research, consulting, or teaching).

Consequently, the feasibility of a process that can accommodate Dr Kramer depends in part on the staff and institutional resources of Memorial Hospital. If it is a hospital within a major urban academic health care center, accommodation is likely to be more feasible than if it is a small rural community hospital.

As this case suggests, it can be important for health professionals who have a moral objection to a medical service to provide advance notification of their objection. The time for Dr Kramer to disclose his objection to EC is not when a rape victim presents at the ED. To minimize the risk of compromising patient care and to maximize the feasibility of accommodation, Dr Kramer should inform the department head of his moral objection and request an exemption.

Suppose Memorial is a small rural community hospital and due to staff and resource limitations, it is not feasible to accommodate Dr Kramer. Can he legitimately claim that he was unjustifiably denied an accommodation? He cannot insofar as anyone who voluntarily enters a health profession acquires special obligations. Herein is a possible grain of truth in Savulescu's previously cited claim that people who are "not prepared to offer legally permitted, efficient, and beneficial care to a patient because it conflicts with their values. . .should not be doctors."[23] It is too extreme to tell Dr Kramer that he can't complain because he should not have chosen to become a doctor. However, Dr Kramer should understand that it is generally the responsibility of ED physicians to offer EC to rape victims. Hence, he could have reduced the risk that satisfying his professional obligations would require him to provide a medical service that is contrary to his ethical beliefs by choosing another sub-specialty; or, he could have increased the chances that an accommodation would be feasible by seeking a position in a larger urban medical center.

Concerns about timely access within health care institutions (e.g., hospitals and nursing homes) can be addressed by institutional policies that include appropriate constraints to protect patients. But what about concerns about access on a societal level? It has been claimed, for example, that conscientious objection to abortion by physicians in Italy has resulted in limited access to abortion.[24] One proposed solution for countries like Italy that have public health systems is to enact changes that will protect access to abortion and accommodate (some) objecting physicians. Specific recommended changes include eliminating the provision that only obstetricians and gynecologists are permitted to perform abortions and controlling the ratio of conscientious objectors to non-conscientious objectors in hospitals and/or geographic areas.[25]

Since the US does not have a public health care system comparable to that of Italy, some measures that might protect access in Italy and other countries with comparable public health systems (e.g., Canada and the UK) are unavailable currently in the US. However, there are proposed strategies to address the access issue in the US. One of these relies primarily on state medical licensing boards to assure that the supply of physicians in geographic areas will meet the demand for specific medical services.[26] Proponents of this approach maintain that it is the responsibility of the medical profession, not individual physicians, to

ensure that patients have access to a wide range of medical services; and medical licensing boards are said to share the responsibility for ensuring that this obligation is satisfied.

It is worth noting that, unlike Italy, conscience-based refusals to provide abortion may not be among the foremost impediments to women's access to abortion in the US. In many states, laws and regulations that restrict access to abortion may play a more significant role in limiting access to the procedure than conscientious objection.[27] These restrictions include Targeted Regulation of Abortion Providers (TRAP) requirements that are so onerous and demanding that many abortion clinics have been forced to close, leaving women in certain areas of the country without convenient access to abortion.[28] Indeed, in view of legal and institutional constraints on abortion providers, physicians who believe they have a moral obligation to *provide* abortion can facilitate access by engaging in a type of conscientious objection: *conscientious action* or *conscientious commitment*.[29]

Another point to consider is that limited access to legal and professionally accepted medical services due to a shortage of providers in certain geographic areas is a pervasive ethical problem. Addressing it requires systematic solutions that go well beyond prohibiting physicians from refusing to provide medical services that are contrary to their fundamental moral convictions. At most, conscientious objection is only the tip of the iceberg in relation to the general problem of lack of effective access to medical services. This observation is not meant to dismiss a concern about the potential effect of accommodation on access. It is only meant to suggest that singling out limited access due to conscientious objection neglects the big picture and selectively applies an important principle of justice in health care.

Is alternative service required?

Supporters of an alternative service requirement typically appeal to an analogy with conscientious objection to military service.[30] In the case of military service, since conscientious objectors are exempted from an important social obligation, it is said to be fitting to require them to provide public service in some other way. Similarly, it is claimed, physicians who are exempted from providing medical services for reasons of conscience should be willing to provide some alternative form of public service. However, there is a significant disanalogy between conscientious objection to military service and conscientious objection in medicine: Whereas there is no assurance that individuals who are exempted from military service will provide comparable public service unless it is required; physicians who refuse to provide a specific medical service continue to provide other valuable medical services. Whereas conscientious objectors to military service refuse to serve as soldiers, physicians who refuse to provide a medical service for reasons of conscience continue to function as physicians.

Another line of argument appeals to burdens imposed on others. Conscientious objectors who are exempted from military service impose burdens on those who serve. Alternative service is a means of compensating for these burdens and showing respect for those who serve. Similarly, it is claimed physicians who are granted exemptions from providing a medical service for reasons of conscience impose burdens on others (e.g., patients and other physicians who provide the service); and alternative service is a means of compensating for these burdens and showing respect for patients and other physicians. However, insofar as reasonable accommodation includes constraints that protect patients and other physicians from excessive burdens, there is no need for "compensation;" and refusing to provide a medical service is not disrespectful.

Is a public justification required?

Robert Card, a leading advocate of a public justification requirement, maintains that an accommodation should be granted "only if the practitioner makes the objection and its reasoned basis public, and the justification offered for the exemption is subjected to assessment."[31] Three of his criteria for assessing "grounding reasons" seem plausible: 1) they must be genuinely held fundamental moral beliefs; 2) they must be consistent with relevant empirical information; and 3) they may not be based on discriminatory beliefs.

With respect to the first condition, as already noted, one of the main reasons for granting an accommodation is to enable health professionals to maintain their moral integrity, and their moral integrity is at stake only if providing a medical service is contrary to their fundamental moral convictions. Hence, the first condition is justified.

With respect to the second condition, objections based on demonstrably false empirical (factual) beliefs do not merit accommodation. Consider, for example, moral objections to EC. Studies have reported that some pharmacists who object to filling prescriptions for EC misunderstand its mechanism.[32] Some fail to understand the difference between EC, the primary function of which is to prevent or delay ovulation and prevent fertilization, and abortifacients – medications such as mifepristone that terminate pregnancies. Suppose a pharmacist objects to dispensing EC because he believes it can terminate pregnancies after implantation. He is asked whether he would continue to object to EC if, contrary to what he believes, it cannot terminate pregnancies after implantation. He responds that he would no longer object. However, despite conclusive scientific evidence to the contrary, he continues to insist that EC is an abortifacient and can terminate pregnancies after implantation. Insofar as the pharmacist's objection is based on a demonstrably false clinical belief, he does not have a legitimate claim for accommodation.

The third condition also is warranted. It is one thing for health professionals to object to providing a specific medical service (e.g., abortion or EC); and quite another thing to object to providing a medical service to African American or Muslim patients and yet be willing to provide the same medical service to white or Christian patients. Ethical codes of major health professions prohibit discrimination; and it is a settled view – one based on defensible and widely shared conceptions of justice, equality, dignity, and respect – that racial, ethnic, religious and gender-based prejudice or bias are ethically wrong.[33] Even if they are conscience-based (i.e. rooted in fundamental moral beliefs), accommodation for objections based on such discriminatory beliefs is unwarranted.

There is an additional justified condition that Card does not consider: A provider's conscience-based refusal has significant moral weight only if it is not incompatible with the goals of his or her profession. Suppose, for example, after practicing family medicine for several years, a physician converts to Buddhism. Subsequently, she believes that pain is the working out of life's karma. In addition, she believes that interfering in the patient's suffering would only contribute to the patient's continued trials on the wheel of rebirth. Based on these beliefs, she refuses to provide pain medication to patients. As a second example, suppose a nurse refuses to administer pain medication because he believes that pain is God's justified punishment for sin. Arguably, neither practitioner's conscience-based objection to providing pain medication merits any moral weight. A person who has a conscience-based objection to relieving pain should not enter a field such as family medicine or nursing that is committed to that goal.

Card endorses additional conditions that can be challenged. He maintains that grounding reasons must be: 1) reasonable; 2) subject to evaluation in terms of their justifiability; and 3) based on reasonable conceptions of the good. He offers the following justification for requiring this thorough assessment of objectors' reasons:

> Since conscientious objection essentially involves moral beliefs, and the validity of ethical beliefs (and acts based upon them) depends upon critically assessing their justification, then a proper view on conscientious objection must examine the justificatory reasons of objecting providers.[34]

It undoubtedly is desirable for anyone, including health professionals, to have basic critical thinking skills that enable them to reflect on their fundamental moral convictions, critically assess them, and provide a public justification. However, as desirable as it may be, it is unclear whether this ability is an appropriate criterion for accommodation. People can have sincere and deeply held self-defining fundamental moral convictions and yet lack the critical thinking

skills that would enable them to provide a satisfactory justification of their grounding reasons; or they might opt to shield fundamental convictions, especially if they are faith-based, from public scrutiny. It is unclear why an inability (or unwillingness) to provide a satisfactory public justification should disqualify conscientious objectors from being considered for accommodation.

Moreover, unless there are unambiguous and defensible criteria for assessing conscientious objectors' grounding reasons, requiring a justification that satisfies the person or persons conducting the review (e.g., department heads, members of ethics committees, or members of licensing or review boards) is too prone to unjustified bias and subjectivity. Requiring health professionals to convince others of the "reasonableness" of their objections risks thwarting one of the primary aims of reasonable accommodation: to provide health professionals moral space in which they can maintain their moral integrity. Finally, lest it be thought that epistemic requirements such as "reasonableness" are needed to protect patient access to medical care, this objective is more directly and effectively accomplished by constraints on accommodation that explicitly protect patients, such as those endorsed above.

Conscientious Objection vs. Obstruction

Accommodation enables health professionals to refuse to perform actions contrary to their conscience, such as performing abortions and prescribing and dispensing EC. The point is to allow individuals to refrain from performing actions against their conscience and maintain their moral integrity. However, enabling person A to refrain from acting against A's conscience is not to be confused with enabling A to prevent person B from performing actions that are contrary to A's, but not B's, ethical or religious beliefs. To prevent B from performing actions that are contrary to A's, but not B's ethical or religious beliefs can be unjustified obstruction. Case 4, an actual case, is an example of unjustified obstruction.[35]

> *Case 4:* A transgender woman from Fountain Hills, Arizona (a Phoenix suburb) went to a CVS pharmacy to fill her first prescriptions for hormone therapy. The pharmacist refused to fill one of the prescriptions, and he refused to return the script to enable her to fill it at another pharmacy.

There are two reasons for not allowing health professionals to actively block or impede a patient's access to a legal and clinically appropriate good or service. First, such behavior is inconsistent with the obligation to protect and promote the health of patients. Second, that behavior also fails to respect patient autonomy. Health professionals who actively block or impede patient access may only intend to avoid their complicity in the perceived wrong-doing of patients. However, another possible aim is to prevent the patient from engaging in behavior that is contrary to the physician's ethical or religious beliefs. If someone believes that an action is seriously immoral, it is understandable if she also is committed to preventing others from performing the action. Nevertheless, it generally is inappropriate for health professionals to exploit their professional gate-keeping power and authority to impose their ethical or religious beliefs on patients who do not accept them. Even if a health professional's intent is only to avoid his own complicity in a perceived moral wrong, the effect can be to impose his ethical or religious beliefs on a patient who does not accept those beliefs, which is inconsistent with respect for patient autonomy.

The CVS pharmacy in Case 4 appropriately recognized that the pharmacist had engaged in an unjustified act of obstruction. CVS apologized to the woman and stated that the pharmacist violated company policy and was no longer employed at the pharmacy.

Conclusion

Since conscientious objection is an increasingly common occurrence in health care, it is essential to understand when accommodation is warranted. Approaches to accommodation can span a wide spectrum. At one extreme (conscience absolutism), health professionals are offered broad protections with few, if any, limitations. At the other extreme (incompatibilism), there is no place for conscientious objection in health care. Refusing to provide a legal, professionally approved and clinically appropriate service within the scope of a practitioner's clinical competence is said to be unprofessional conduct.

Neither of these two extremes is acceptable. The unqualified accommodation granted by conscience absolutism exposes patients to burdens and harms and can violate the professional obligations of doctors, nurses, pharmacists and other health care providers. Incompatibilism is subject to two major criticisms. First, although doctors, nurses, pharmacists and other health care providers are professionals, they also are moral agents with a legitimate interest in maintaining their moral integrity. Incompatibilism fails to acknowledge the value of moral integrity and the importance of maintaining it. Second, incompatibilism requires an implausible specification of the professional obligations of health care providers.

Reasonable accommodation is an approach between the two extremes. The primary aim is to accommodate clinicians' claims of conscience without unjustifiably compromising other values and interests (e.g., patient health and well-being). There are different conceptions of reasonable accommodation, and they differ in three major respects: 1) whether they require specified actions by health professionals; 2) whether they require alternative service; and 3) whether they require health professionals to provide a public justification of their refusal.

Reasonable accommodation should not require specific actions (e.g., informing and referring). Instead, patients and third parties (e.g., surrogates, other health professionals, and organizations) should be protected by focusing on expected outcomes, such as the effect on timely access to relevant information, referral, and appropriate medical services; and the impact on other clinicians and organizations.

There is insufficient justification for an alternative service requirement. Health professionals who are exempted from providing a medical service for reasons of conscience perform public service by providing other medical services. In addition, since the preferred conception of reasonable accommodation includes constraints that protect patients and other physicians from excessive burdens, there is no need for "compensation;" and refusing to provide a medical service is not disrespectful.

With respect to public justification, an objector's grounding reasons must satisfy the following requirements: 1) they must be genuinely held fundamental moral beliefs; 2) they must be consistent with relevant empirical information; 3) they may not be based on discriminatory beliefs: and 4) they may not be incompatible with the goals of the objector's profession. There are several reasons for rejecting a more stringent requirement to publicly justify one's objection. First, it is unclear why an inability or unwillingness to provide a satisfactory public justification should disqualify conscientious objectors from being considered for accommodation. Second, unless there are unambiguous and defensible criteria for assessing conscientious objectors' grounding reasons, requiring a justification that satisfies the person or persons conducting the review is too prone to unjustified bias and subjectivity. Third, lest it be thought that epistemic requirements such as "reasonableness" are needed to protect patient access to medical care, this objective is more directly and effectively accomplished by constraints on accommodation that explicitly protect patients, such as those endorsed in this essay.

Notes

1 Available at: https://www.govinfo.gov/content/pkg/FR-2019-05-21/pdf/2019-09667.pdf. Accessed August 29, 2019.

2 Available at:https://publications.parliament.uk/pa/bills/lbill/2017-2019/0014/18014.pdf. Accessed August 29, 2019.

3 Julian Savulescu, "Conscientious Objection in Medicine," *British Medical Journal* 332 (2006), p. 294.

4 Julian Savulescu and Udo Schüklenk, "Doctors Have No Right to Refuse Medical Assistance in Dying, Abortion, or Contraception," *Bioethics* 31,3 (2017), p. 165.

5 Dan Brock, "Conscientious Refusal by Physicians and Pharmacists: Who is Obligated to do What, and Why?" *Theoretical Medicine and Bioethics* 29(2008), pp.187–200.

6 For alternative definitions of conscience, see Mark R. Wicclair, "Conscience," in *International Encyclopedia of Ethics*, ed. Hugh LaFollette (Hoboken, NJ: John Wiley & Sons, 2013); John Skorupski, "Conscience," in *The Routledge Companion to Ethics*, ed. John Skorupski (London and New York: Routledge, 2010), pp. 550–61; and Martin Benjamin, "Conscience," in *Encyclopedia of Bioethics*, ed. Stephen G. Post (New York: Macmillan Reference, 2004), pp. 513–17.

7 Jeffrey Blustein, "Doing What the Patient Orders: Maintaining Integrity in the Doctor-Patient Relationship," *Bioethics* 7,4 (1993), p. 295.

8 Charles D. Helper, "Balancing Pharmacists' Conscientious Objections with Their Duty to Serve," *Journal of the American Pharmacists Association* 45, 4 (2005), p. 434.

9 Tom L. Beauchamp and James F. Childress, *Principles of Biomedical Ethics*, Seventh ed. (New York, NY: Oxford University Press, 2013), p. 106.

10 See, for example, Ronit Y. Stahl and Ezekiel J. Emanuel, "Physicians, Not Conscripts – Conscientious Objection in Health Care," *New England Journal of Medicine* 376,14 (2017) pp.1380–5; and Udo Schüklenk and Ricardo Smalling, "Why Medical Professionals have no Moral Claim to Conscientious Objection Accommodation in Liberal Democracies," *Journal of Medical Ethics* 43 (2017), pp. 234–40.

11 Stahl and Emanuel (2017).

12 American Medical Association, *Code of Medical Ethics* (2017). Chapter 1, "Opinions on Patient-Physician Relationships," is available at: https://www.ama-assn.org/sites/default/files/media-browser/code-of-medical-ethics-chapter-1.pdf. Accessed August 25, 2018. The General Medical Council's *Good Medical Practice: Duties of a Doctor* (2014) states that UK physicians have the following obligations: a duty to "make the care of their patients their first concern" and a duty to "protect and promote the health of patients and the public." Available at: https://www.gmc-uk.org/

ethical-guidance/ethical-guidance-for-doctors/good-medical-practice. Accessed August 25, 2018.

13 The three specified limitations are: "Physicians are expected to provide care in emergencies, honor patients' informed decisions to refuse life-sustaining treatment, and respect basic civil liberties and not discriminate against individuals in deciding whether to enter into a professional relationship with a new patient" (1.1.7). The *Code* includes the following additional guideline: "Several factors impinge on the decision to act according to conscience. Physicians have stronger obligations to patients with whom they have a patient-physician relationship, especially one of long standing; when there is imminent risk of foreseeable harm to the patient or delay in access to treatment would significantly adversely affect the patient's physical or emotional well-being; and when the patient is not reasonably able to access needed treatment from another qualified physician" (1.1.7).

14 Mark R. Wicclair, *Conscientious Objection in Health Care: An Ethical Analysis* (Cambridge, England: Cambridge University Press, 2011); and Mark R. Wicclair, "Is Conscientious Objection Incompatible with a Physician's Professional Obligations?" *Theoretical Medicine and Bioethics* 29,3 (2008), pp. 171–85.

15 Udo Schüklenk and Ricardo Smalling (2017), p. 238.

16 Rosamond Rhodes, "The Ethical Standard of Care," *American Journal of Bioethics* 6,2 (2006), p. 78.

17 This strategy also begs the question by assuming that accommodation is incompatible with adequately protecting patients and ensuring that physicians who are accommodated will not violate their fiduciary duty to patients. Specifically, the strategy fails to consider whether enforceable constraints on accommodation, including, but not limited to, those cited in the *Code* can protect patients from harms and excessive burdens. I will consider this issue when I discuss reasonable accommodation.

18 For a discussion of differing institutional responses to conscientious objection and moral distress, see Mithya Lewis-Newby, Mark Wicclair, Thaddeus Pope, Cynda Rushton, Farr Curlin, Douglas Diekema, "An Official American Thoracic Society Policy Statement: Managing Conscientious Objections in Intensive Care Medicine," *American Journal of Respiratory and Critical Care Medicine* 191,2 (2015), pp. 219–27.

19 Martha Nussbaum cites a powerful image that Roger Williams used to defend liberty of conscience: "To impose an orthodoxy upon the conscience is nothing less than what Williams, in a memorable and oft-repeated image, called 'Soule rape.'" Martha C. Nussbaum, *Liberty of Conscience: In Defense of America's Tradition of Religious Equality* (New York, NY: Basic Books, 2008), p. 37. The reference to rape of the soul suggests that this statement was meant primarily as a defense of religious tolerance. Nevertheless, when a failure to accommodate secular fundamental moral convictions results in a loss of moral integrity, it also can be experienced as an assault on one's self or identity.

20 Udo Schüklenk and Ricardo Smalling (2017), p. 238.

21 (2017), p. 238.

22 However, they can protest and seek changes if they believe that the current "social compact" is unjustified.

23 Savulescu (2006), p. 94.

24 Francesca Minerva, "Conscientious Objection in Italy," *Journal of Medical Ethics* 41 (2015), pp. 170–3.

25 Francesca Minerva (2015); and Franesca Minerva, "Conscientious Objection, Complicity in Wrongdoing, and a Not-so-Moderate Approach," *Cambridge Quarterly of Healthcare Ethics* 26 (2017), pp. 109–19.

26 Holly Fernandez Lynch, *Conflicts of Conscience in Health Care: An Institutional Compromise* (Cambridge, MA: The MIT Press, 2008).

27 According to the Guttmacher Institute, As of January 1, 2018, all but 10 states had implemented at least one of the following "major abortion restrictions:" "unnecessary regulations" on abortion clinics, mandated counseling, a mandated waiting period, a "parental involvement" requirement for minors, and a prohibition on the use of state Medicaid funds to pay for medically necessary abortions. Guttmacher Institute, "Induced Abortion in the United States." Available at: https://www.guttmacher.org/fact-sheet/induced-abortion-united-states?gclid=EAIaIQobChMI_fPo5MKc2gIVylYNCh2Z8AYeEAAYASABEgICZfD_BwE. Accessed August 29, 2019.

28 According to the Guttmacher Institute, as of August 1, 2019: 24 states had laws or policies that regulate abortion providers that "go beyond what is necessary to ensure patients' safety;" 17 states had "onerous licensing standards many of which are comparable or equivalent to the state's licensing standards for ambulatory surgical centers;" 18 states had specific requirements for procedure rooms and corridors and required facilities to be near to, and have relationships with, local hospitals; and 13 subjected clinicians who perform abortions to "unnecessary requirements" (e.g., admitting privileges

at a local hospital). Guttmacher Institute, "Targeted Regulation of Abortion Providers." Available at: https://www.guttmacher.org/state-policy/explore/targeted-regulation-abortion-providers. Accessed August 29, 2019.

29 See for example, Lisa H. Harris, "Recognizing Conscience in Abortion Provision," *New England Journal of Medicine* 367 (2012), pp. 981–3; B. M. Dickens and R. J. Cook, "Conscientious Commitment to Women's Health," *International Journal of Gynecology and Obstetrics* 113 (2011), pp. 163–6; and Mark R. Wicclair, "Negative and Positive Claims of Conscience," *Cambridge Quarterly of Healthcare Ethics* 18,1 (2009), pp. 14–22.

30 See, for example, Christopher Meyers and Robert D. Woods, "An Obligation to Provide Abortion Services: What Happens When Physicians Refuse?" *Journal of Medical Ethics* 22 (1996), pp. 115–20; and Hugh LaFollette, "My Conscience May Be My Guide, but You May Not Need to Honor It," *Cambridge Quarterly of Healthcare Ethics* 26 (2017):44–58.

31 Robert F. Card, "The Inevitability of Assessing Reasons in Debates about Conscientious Objection in Medicine," *Cambridge Quarterly of Healthcare Ethics* 26 (2017), p. 82.

32 See, for example, Kristi K. Van Riper and Wendy L. Hellerstedt, "Emergency Contraceptive Pills: Dispensing Practices, Knowledge and Attitudes of South Dakota Pharmacists," *Perspectives on Sexual and Reproductive Health* 37,1 (2005), pp. 19–24; Matthew E. Borrego, Jennifer Short, Naomi House, Gireesh Gupchup, Rupali Naik, and Denise Cuellar, "New Mexico Pharmacists' Knowledge, Attitudes, and Beliefs Toward Prescribing Oral Emergency Contraception," *Journal of the American Pharmacists Association* 46,1 (2006), pp. 33–43.

33 There is considerable agreement that it is wrong to discriminate against members of these "protected classes." However, currently, there is no similar agreement about whether anti-discrimination rules apply to members of other historically marginalized groups. It is beyond the scope of this essay to resolve this issue or to specify the scope of "invidious discrimination." Suffice it to say that however it is specified, invidious discrimination should not be accommodated.

34 Robert F. Card, "Reasons, Reasonability and Establishing Conscientious Objector Status in Medicine," *Journal of Medical Ethics* 43 (2017), p. 222.

35 Julia Jacobs, "Transgender Woman Says CVS Pharmacist Refused to Fill Hormone Prescription," *New York Times*, July 20, 2018.

75

Conscientious Objection in Medicine
Accommodation versus Professionalism and the Public Good

Udo Schüklenk

Introduction

Acts of conscientious objection can occur in at least three quite different contexts, only one of which is relevant to this article. Acts of conscientious objection historically were most prevalent in the context of pacifists' objections to conscription to military service. Objectors would go to great length, including prison, to avoid becoming part of an organization they objected to on religious or ethical grounds. They were prepared to make personal sacrifices to live true to their conscience. Other types of objectors refuse to do certain things because they aim to maintain the professional standards of their profession. This could entail doctors refusing to undertake cost-cutting measures in their for-profit hospital if in their considered judgement these measures are detrimental to patients' best interests. This article is not concerned with either of these cases of conscientious objection.

I will be focusing on the more fundamental question of whether or not health care professionals have morally justifiable claims to see their conscience-based refusals to provide professional services accommodated by regulatory bodies or the state, if eligible patients are demanding those services of them and if those patients are entitled to receive those services.

Patients suffer significant harmful health consequences when access to health services is denied on grounds of provider conscience and alternative access avenues to the required service are unavailable.[1] Chavkin et al.,[1] for example, note that 'in South Africa, widespread conscientious objection limits the number of willing providers and, thus, access to safe care, and the number of unsafe abortions has not decreased since the legalization of abortion'. Minerva describes a similar phenomenon for Italy.[2] There can be little doubt that many, but arguably not all conscience related claims are reflections and consequences of ongoing societal culture wars. NeJaime and Siegel[3] point out that they are a 'transnational phenomenon, and the organizations and activists encouraging these claims work across borders'.

Historically the need to accommodate conscientious objectors in medicine was taken for granted in medical ethics, and certainly among medical doctors'

Original publication details: Udo Schüklenk, "Conscientious Objection in Medicine: Accommodation Versus Professionalism and the Public Good," pp. 47–56 from *British Medical Bulletin* 126 (2018).

associations. The view was held that particular practices in medicine could impact on professionals' individual consciences and potentially constitute a threat to their integrity as moral agents.[4,5]

Unsurprisingly perhaps, the courts in many jurisdictions have addressed various aspects of the conscientious objection issue, among them the question of whether there is a legally relevant difference between conscientiously objecting to the provision of particular health services and transferring an eligible patient to a colleague who would provide such services if one refused to provide them on grounds of conscience, as well as the question of whether health care institutions could reasonably defend their refusal to provide particular health services on grounds of conscience.[6,7]

Much of the legal dispute on conscientious objection in national jurisdictions is foreshadowed in a landmark international human rights document issued by the United Nations. Its International Covenant on Civil and Political Rights states in Article 18(1)1: 'Everyone shall have the right to freedom of thought, conscience and religion. This right shall include freedom to have or to adopt religion or belief of his choice, and freedom, either individually or in community with others and in public or private, to manifest his religion or belief in worship, observance, practice and teaching.' Article 18(3)1 aims to limit the exercise of these freedoms. 'Freedom to manifest one's religion or beliefs may be subject only to such limitations as are prescribed by law and are necessary to protect public safety, order, health or morals or the fundamental rights and freedoms of others.'[8] While health care professionals, like everyone else, have a moral claim to freedom of conscience and religion, these rights are not absolute, they are limited to the extent that they infringe on others' fundamental rights.

Most liberal democracies' constitutional arrangements mirror if not the wording, but certainly the sentiments expressed in the Covenant. How the limitations on 18(1)1 that are introduced in 18(3)1 are realized varies widely among jurisdictions. In a number of US states conscientious objectors among health care professionals are well within their legal rights to even refuse the provision of emergency services.

The European Court of Human Rights, on the other hand, concluded that a pharmacist may not refuse to sell contraceptives on conscience grounds, because 'as long as the sale of contraceptives is legal and occurs on medical prescription nowhere other than in a pharmacy, the applicants cannot give precedence to their religious beliefs and impose them on others as justification for their refusal to sell such products, since they can manifest those beliefs outside the professional sphere'.[9] The view held by this court is essentially that while Article 9 of the European Convention on Human Rights guarantees freedom of conscience, among others, it does not protect 'each and every act or form of behaviour motivated or inspired by a religion or a belief'.[9] That limitation is particularly important 'with regard to the right to behave in public in a manner governed by that belief'.[9] The European Commission of Human Rights noted that the protection for conscience guaranteed by the European Convention on Human Rights extends only to individuals and not to institutions.[6] That matters a great deal, given the large number of religiously affiliated hospitals. Courts in the USA reached the opposite conclusion with regard to that country's Constitution.[7]

Chavkin et al.,[1] in a review article analysing conscientious objection globally in the context of health care professionals' refusal to provide certain contested reproductive health services, conclude that 'objection occurs least when the law, public discourse, provider custom and clinical experience all normalize the provision of the full range of health services'. Of note, in at least one jurisdiction, Sweden, health care professionals' conscientious objection accommodation claims have no legal standing. Munthe explains Sweden's rationale, 'first, deeply entrenched and widely shared views on the importance of public service provision, and of related civic duties to take part in the promotion and not to prevent the production of public goods. Second, strong ideals about the rule of law, equality before the law and non-discrimination.'[10]

This article is primarily focused on the ethical issues involved in the debates on conscientious objection accommodation; however, reference to some relevant court cases will be made in so far as they are instructive. As mentioned, historically conscientious objection has been discussed in the context of 'conscription' to military service. Of course, people 'voluntarily' choose to study medicine and become doctors, hence, care has to be taken not to conflate two very different scenarios. It is noteworthy that today most conscientious objection claims that reach the courts are not the result of conflicts over conscription but the result of the latter scenario. They are lodged by people who volunteer to join particular professions or who choose to become monopoly providers of particular services to the public, and who subsequently object, despite their career choices.

Conscience – What Is It, and Does It Matter?

Perhaps surprisingly, there is no consensus in either the ethics or the legal literature on an uncontroversial definition of 'conscience', or, indeed, on why (and whether at all) it is morally important.[11] At its most basic conscience is often described as a religious or ethical belief or conviction that motivates us to act or omit to act in a particular manner. Conscience itself is unlikely a faculty with an epistemological property, rather, as Childress suggests, it 'emerges after a moral judgement or after the application of moral standards'.[12] Sulmasy[13] probably gets it right when he conceptualizes conscience as the conviction that we should act in accordance with our individual understanding of what morality demands of us, but also as then autonomously acting in accordance with what we consider to be morally good and right.

Typically conflicts or frictions arise in the health care context when a health care professional's conscience and their professional obligations collide. Many a country's constitutions protect individual conscience indirectly, by guaranteeing freedom of religion or, as is sometimes the case in more recent documents, also explicitly freedom of conscience, as for instance, the Canadian Charter or Rights and Freedoms does, when it states 'Everyone has the following fundamental freedoms: (a) freedom of conscience and religion. . ..'[14] Of course, that does not mean that Canadians would have an absolute right to follow the tenets of their conscience convictions or religion, no matter what the consequences, especially for others, might be.[15] However, what is uncontroversial is that in liberal democracies citizen's rights to live their lives by their own values are given a great deal of importance.

Wicclair[16] gives four reasons why the exercise of conscience ought to be protected:

- by protecting conscientious objectors society shows respect for autonomous agents' moral choices and integrity. In this analysis a health care professional's refusal to provide professional services on grounds of conscience is not merely an expression of their moral values (as opposed to their professional judgement), it is also giving notice that their integrity as moral agents is at stake. Pellegrino[17] discusses similar rationales. It is not difficult to appreciate that threats to one's moral integrity or even the perceived loss of one's moral integrity have the potential to cause significant psychological harms to those at the receiving end of those threats. The above mentioned international human rights documents and court decisions suggest that even if one agreed with Wicclair, such accommodation rights are not absolute;
- by protecting conscientious objectors we underline the importance of diversity and toleration in a multi-cultural society;
- by protecting conscientious objectors we acknowledge that our current take on the subject matter of the objection could be mistaken; and
- by protecting conscientious objectors we ensure that members of society that would likely become conscientious objectors are not prevented from joining particular professions.[18]

Similar reasons have been discussed by West-Oram and Buyx[19] and Cowley.[20] I will address the most significant of these arguments in the second half of this article. Support in favour of the accommodation of conscientious objectors cuts across the dividing line of religious[17] and secularist.[21]

Conscience Claims – Should They be Reasonable and Genuine?

Assuming one was swayed by the arguments presented thus far, invariably the question would arise whether conscience claims should be reasonable in terms of the substance of the convictions a claimant reports to hold.

Should there be a minimum reasonability standard with regard to the rationality or coherence of the basis of conscience claims? Indeed, some authors have proposed just that.[22] Card, for instance, proposes that objectors must provide reasons for their objection as opposed to merely claiming their objection. He suggests that the accommodation seeking objector 'must state and explain their putative conscientious objection and the beliefs supporting it, thereby allowing [a regulatory body] to understand the objector's reasoning and assess how its weight compares with the provider's professional duties'.[23] Others have proposed different standards, but the principle that objectors ought to explain themselves, as it were, is supported by numerous authors.[24]

In the USA the courts have put to rest any notion that objectors must provide rationales for their professed conscience convictions. The US Supreme Court writes on this issue, 'what principle of law or logic can be brought to bear to contradict a believer's assertion that a particular act is 'central' to his personal faith? Judging the centrality of different religious practices is akin to the unacceptable 'business of evaluating the relative merits of differing religious claims.'. . . it is not within the judicial ken to question the centrality of particular beliefs or practices to a faith, or the validity of particular litigants' interpretation of those creeds . . . courts must not presume to determine the place of a particular belief in a religion or the plausibility of a religious claim'.[25] The US Supreme Court is not unique in its take on this subject, as Canadian

jurisprudence demonstrates.[26] The views expressed by these courts seem reasonable, given the need for the secular state to remain neutral with regard to the validity or otherwise of these ideologies and individual convictions.

If the reasonableness of a conscientious objector's views cannot be evaluated for the reason mentioned, should a society at least want to ensure that the conscience claims made are genuine? In Canada, for instance, doctors reportedly turn away patients asking for medical aid in dying because they consider the schedule of fees set by government for the delivery of their services to be too low.[27] Is it possible to determine whether objectors hold the conscience views they claim to hold, as opposed to other concerns to do with financial issues, inconvenience, etc.? Some authors have proposed that the evaluative focus should not be on the reasonableness of a conscience claim but on its genuineness. Myers and Woods,[28] for instance, expect conscientious objectors to show that they are sufficiently serious about their objection that the failure to accommodate them would cause significant mental hardship. This does seem similar to Wicclair's concerns about threats to health care professionals' integrity as moral agents. Kantymir and McLeod[24] have rightly pointed out that this standard would require the accommodation of conscientious objectors who are genuine, but who are genuinely racist, sexist or homophobic. MacLure and Dumont[29] note that courts in Canada do 'probe the 'sincerity' of the claimant'. In reality such tests can only investigate how efficient conscience claimants are in terms of persuading a regulatory body or a court that they are genuine. None of that proves sincerity. Genuineness cannot be tested, and as Kantymir and colleague show, even if it could be tested, it is not a plausible standard for determining whether a conscientious objector should be accommodated.

Conscience and Professionalism

A number of authors, including me, have defended the so-called 'incompatibility thesis'.[18] A hallmark of a professional judgement is that it is informed exclusively by specialist technical competencies and professional values. A conscientious objector insists on overriding what they know a professional judgement would demand of them. They place their personal convictions above their professional obligations.[30] Rhodes, for instance, argues that medical practice ought to be understood as a contract between society that grants both a high degree of self-governance as well as a monopoly on the provision of particular specialist services to doctors, and the professions. The profession promises that its members will – in return – provide reliably professional specialist services that are governed by its professional values. In Rhodes' words, this view implies 'First, [. . .] clinician decisions must be informed by professional judgement, not personal judgement. Patients and society rely on physicians to provide treatment according to that standard and, for the most part, they cannot know enough about their doctors' personal values to choose them on any other basis. The second implication is that becoming a doctor is a moral commitment to give priority to 'the ethical standard of care' over personal values. Becoming a doctor is, therefore, also ceding authority to professional judgement over personal preference'.[30] Essentially, as the name suggests, the incompatibility thesis maintains that professionalism and conscientious objection are incompatible.

The opposite view argues that health care professionals have an absolute moral right to object on grounds of conscience, and that they should have an absolute legal right, to abstain from the delivery of professional services that they object to on grounds of conscience. The argument is that compromises that are oftentimes implemented by policy makers and regulators, are not compromises, they are asking too much of the conscientious objector. Proponents of this stance might, for instance, think of the examples of abortion and voluntary euthanasia. Conscientious objectors could consider one or both of these as acts of murder, with terrible punitive consequences for them in the afterlife that they believe in. If someone believes that these professional services are acts of murder, or morally equivalent to acts of murder, they are absolutists who – on their worldview – are rightly objecting to a compromise position that would not

require of them to provide an abortion or euthanasia in response to an eligible patient's request, but that would oblige them to transfer the patient without delay to a colleague who they know will provide these contested services to eligible patients. While it is true, there are degrees of complicity, as for instance, Sulmasy[13] notes, it is also not too difficult to understand that to such a conscientious objector the moral distinction between actively killing and transferring a patient on to a colleague whom they consider a killer, amounts to mere academic hair-splitting. Accordingly, this view holds that health care professionals must have an absolute right to conscientious objection accommodation. This stance is oftentimes taken by doctors' voluntary associations such as the Canadian Medical Association.[31] Typically, but not always, the line drawn in the sand is emergency situations where even doctors' lobby organizations concede that their members have a conscience-overriding professional obligation to provide services.[32] Of note, in a fair number of states in the USA, as NeJaime mentions '. . . health care refusal laws allow doctors or nurses to refuse to treat a patient even in an emergency situation and do so without requiring that health care professionals provide advance notice of their objection to the employer so that the patient receives needed care. In addition, some of these laws allow health care workers and institutions to refuse to provide referrals, counselling, or information that would notify the patient of the availability of alternative care'.[7] This undoubtedly represents the extreme policy end of the spectrum, but it is one that is consistent with the view that conscientious objectors have an absolute right to refuse not only the provision of professional services to eligible patients, but also an absolute right to refuse the participation in the timely transfer of these patients to colleagues who will provide those services.

Voluntariness and Monopoly

Opponents of conscientious objection accommodation point to two features that they argue make a crucial difference to the moral evaluation of accommodation demands, when compared to the military conscription scenario. The first is that health care professionals volunteered to join the profession. Nobody forced them to join a profession the scope of which they object to. They knew that during their lifetime the scope of the profession could and likely would change, as is true for most, if not all career choices. They also knew that they would not be able to control what kind of changes would occur. In most, if not all other professions, professionals unwilling to adapt have the choice to change their careers.[33] Indeed, this is also true for the medical profession. It is unclear why health care professionals and their associations take as a given that they are entitled to practice as they began practicing when they joined the profession.[34]

Professionals also enjoy a societal monopoly on the provision of the kinds of services that lie within the scope of the profession. Societies typically subsidize their training and grant professions a high degree of self-regulation. In return, as Munthe[10] noted, they promise to place the patient interest and the public good above their own sectarian interests. For professionals to accept that kind of special status and the privileges that come with it, and then refuse to provide the services they contracted and promised to provide when they join a particular profession is difficult to justify.

Equality of Opportunity

Some authors have argued that the refusal to accommodate conscientious objectors would unacceptably impact on their equality of opportunity with regard to their job choices and opportunities.[29] That argument suffers from various weaknesses. If a person knows that they would conscientiously object to the provision of the professional scope of practice in a particular specialty, say, gynaecology or palliative care, they would still be free to choose a different area of specialization within medicine.

It is implausible to insist that one's equality of opportunity in the job market and specifically with regard to job choice was violated because one chose to refuse to accept the obligations that are part and parcel of a

particular job. Animal rights activists choosing to apply for and accepting a job offer in a butchery also could not reasonably demand conscientious objection accommodation. The killing of animals is part and parcel of what it means to be a butcher. It does appear strange indeed that anyone would choose to join a profession the scope of practice one objects to in the first place.

Card discusses a somewhat related problem, namely the issue of conscientiously objecting medical students.[35] He notes that the kinds of professionalism based arguments that are usually deployed against conscientious objection accommodation do not apply to medical students, because, while students, they are not professionals. Card is troubled by reports about some Muslim medical students in the UK asking for accommodation during teaching exercises involving the touching (for diagnostic purposes) of persons of the opposite sex. He rightly notes that students refusing to participate in such learning activities will fail to acquire important skill sets that enable them to distinguish between sensual and clinical touching, for instance. While there are a few exceptions, in most countries conscientious objection accommodation is not granted for scenarios involving emergency circumstances. If students such as those described by Card were accommodated, they would be unable to respond appropriately if faced with such emergency situations. It is arguable that medical schools' admissions committees would be well advised to discriminate against prospective students who will object on grounds of conscience to the provision of professional services that are within the scope of professional practice.

The courts, keeping in mind the limitations set out in the earlier cited International Covenant on Civil and Political Rights Article 18(3)1 will have to determine whether this view would be minimally impairing on conscientious objectors. Different jurisdictions will take different views on this question.

Diversity

Another argument cautions against a reduction of diversity in the profession, triggered by expectations of greater uniformity of service delivery by professionals. This view is expressed in different ways. Some warn against automatons taking over, where humanity and subjectivity disappear. Others suggest we ought to show some degree of epistemic humility by permitting diversity of opinion at least on controversial issues such as abortion and euthanasia. After all, as Mill would have it in 'On Liberty' [see Chapter 65 of this *Anthology*], we might be mistaken, and we would never find out if we eliminated all divergence of opinion from the profession.

Of course, what is justifiably considered controversial is in itself a matter of opinion rather than fact. However, Mill was correct, diversity of opinion is important in more than one way, but the question arises what is the proper locus for discussions about controversial practices in medicine. Should it really be at the bedsit, or should it be on the societal level where, once a decision has been made by democratic means, it is the profession's role to implement it. As Savulescu notes, 'the place of reasons and values in medicine is properly located in dialogue with patients, and in attempting to shape policy and law. . ...However, [health care professionals, U. Sch.] are not entitled to impose those values on patients in the delivery of health care and deny treatment when these patients are legally entitled to access that particular service.'[33]

Given that the primary reason for having specialist monopoly provider professions in society is to maximize the public good,[36] it is worth asking whether a possible reduction in the number of professionals refusing to contribute toward achieving that objective is an outcome that is indefensible, in light of the arguable impact on diversity. Depending on one's answer to this question one would arrive at different policy recommendations for members of medical school admissions committees who are reviewing applications by prospective students.

Equal Citizenship

Proponents of conscientious objector accommodation reject the idea set forth in the International Covenant on Civil and Political Rights Article 18(3)1. They do not think the state or any other regulatory agency (in a self-regulated profession this could well be a statutory body such as the UK's General Medical Council) has any role to play with regard to mediating when a conflict arises between doctors and patients. Lyus, for instance, writes in response to critics of conscientious objection accommodation, that their stance 'demands individuals to devolve moral decision-making to a forum separate from that in which the moral act takes place. This forum might be at the level of managers, regulatory bodies or philosophical discourse. . . .I find this proposal concerning.'[37]

The difficulty with this stance, a stance that is held by many doctors' associations, is that if we accept it we must give up on the idea of equal citizenship. In the case Lyus is concerned about, namely access to abortion in a society where abortion is legal, publicly funded, and eligible women are entitled to receive this service, his stance would imply that the doctor, whose profession enjoys a monopoly on the provision of this service, would have the final say on whether an equal citizen is able to enjoy her rights as a citizen. At issue is not only that the doctor refuses to provide a service that the patient cannot receive from someone other than a doctor, but also that the doctor's action ultimately is designed to ensure that the patient lives by the doctor's values, as opposed to their own values. The objective of the conscientious objection is not merely to avoid participating in the provision of a professional service the doctor objects to, it also aims to subvert the patient's ability to enjoy their rights as citizens. Delston[38] describes how doctors in the USA who refuse to provide contraceptives resort to ever more sophisticated means to prevent equal citizens from the enjoyments of their rights, because they disapprove of their choices. Artificial hurdles are mounted, for instance, in front of women seeking access to birth control, such as asking women who never had sex to undergo Pap smears before the prescription of birth control.[39]

Some statutory bodies have tried to address this problem. The College of Physicians and Surgeons of British Columbia, for instance, while claiming a doctor's [. . .] 'right to decide whether or not to perform or be involved in' medical aid in dying, also stresses that objecting doctors must not delay the transfer of information from such patients to administrators who would then be able to assist such patients in finding a non-objecting doctor.[40] Evidently, this policy does involve the objecting doctor in medical aid in dying. Despite myriad efforts such as this, there does not appear to be a reasonable compromise position that accommodates the conscientious objector and guarantees patients' equal citizenship rights. At the time of writing a court in the Canadian province of Ontario supported the provincial statutory body's policy that conscientiously objecting doctors must provide effective referrals.[41]

Peaceful Co-existence

Sulmasy asks us to be tolerant toward conscientious objectors, a claim he has not yet directed toward conscientious objectors whose patients demonstrably suffer hardship due to their doctors' decision to prioritize their ideological commitments over professional patient care.[42,43] Still, it could be argued that there might be no good reasons to accommodate conscientious objectors, but perhaps we should do so regardless, in order to avoid infinite societal strive. Health care systems should try to find a way to work around these objectors who otherwise might be valuable parts of the system. Perhaps, we should put more effort into designing creative ways that ensure that eligible patients asking for particular services receive those in a timely manner, despite the existence of objectors. If we acted accordingly we might be able to avoid the culture wars entering our health care system any more than they already have.

I have doubts that this is as easily possible as some supporters of conscientious objection claim it is. Quite conceivably this could be true for patients seeking access to care in metropolitan areas; alas, the abortion data from Italy that I mentioned earlier strongly suggest that even that might be overly optimistic. Certainly, patients living in rural areas, where doctors are likely to be in limited supply, will find the enjoyment of their citizenship rights subverted by the accommodation of objectors.

Because there is no fact of the matter that can be established, with regard to who objects on grounds of conscience against what kind of service, we are at risk of having to accommodate ever more professionals objecting to ever more services, especially with new medical products entering the market that might assist us in living longer or improving particular dispositional capabilities. It is unclear how a health care system could operate efficiently and reliably that aimed to account for whatever service it is that conscientious objectors might wish to object to at a certain point in time.

It is likely that the continuation of conscientious objection accommodation in our health care systems is lengthening the culture wars rather than contributing toward ending them.

Conclusion

Conscientious objection is undoubtedly always a personal choice, but it is at the same token more than that. Today it is also the peculiar health care profession specific expression of 21st century culture wars. No other profession that professionals voluntarily enter makes similar demands of the society it claims to serve. Arguments ethical, legal and political over conscientious objection accommodation will not disappear any time soon. Health care systems need to consider carefully how reliable service delivery can be guaranteed so that patients, the most vulnerable parts of the system, and the reason for why both the system and the health care professions exist, will be able to receive the services they are entitled to receive in a timely fashion. Patients cannot rely on doctors, doctors' associations or even on statutory bodies, typically made up predominantly of professionals, to take the public good and their rights sufficiently serious to ensure reliable access to care.

References

1 Chavkin W., Leitman L., and Polin K. Conscientious objection and refusal to provide reproductive healthcare: a White Paper examining prevalence, health consequences, and policy responses. *Int J Gynecol Obstet* 2013; 123: 541–56.

2 Minerva F. Conscientious objection in Italy. *J Med Ethics* 2015; 41:170–3.

3 NeJaime D. and Siegel R. Conscience wars in transnational perspective: religious liberty, third-party harm, and pluralism. In: Mancini S, Rosenfeld M. *The Conscience Wars: Rethinking the Balance Between Religion, Identity, and Equality*. Cambridge: Cambridge University Press, 2018.

4 Wicclair M.R. Conscientious objection in medicine. *Bioethics* 2000; 14:205–27.

5 Crigger B.J., McCormick P.W., Brotherton S.L., et al. Report by the American Medical Association's Council on ethical and judicial affairs on physicians' exercise of conscience. *J Clin Ethics* 2016; 27:219–26.

6 Zampas C. and Ximena A.-I. Conscientious objection to sexual and reproductive health services: International Human Rights Standards and European Law and Practice. *Eur J Health Law* 2012; 19:231–56.

7 NeJaime D and Siegel R.B. Conscience wars: complicity-based conscience claims in religion and politics. *Yale Law J* 2015; 124:2516–91.

8 International Covenant on Civil and Political Rights. Adopted December 16, 1966. General Assembly Resolution 2200A(XXI), United Nations GAOR, 21st Session, Supp. No. 16, at 52, U.N. Doc. A/6316 (1966), 999 U.N.T.S. 171.

9 *Pichon and Sajous v France*, 2001-X Eur. Ct. H.R.

10 Munthe C. Conscientious refusal in healthcare: the Swedish solution. *J Med Ethics* 2017; 43:257–9.

11 Wicclair M. Conscience. In: LaFollette H. *The International Encyclopedia of Ethics*. Malden, MA: Wiley Blackwell, 2013; 1009–20.

12 Childress J.F. Appeals to conscience. *Ethics* 1979; 74: 315–35.

13 Sulmasy D.P. What is conscience, and why is respect for it so important? *Theor Med Bioeth* 2008; 29:135–4.

14 Constitution Act 1982. *Charter or Rights and Freedoms*. http://laws-lois.justice.gc.ca/eng/Const/page-15. html (23 September 2017, date last accessed).

15 Smalling R. and Schüklenk U. Against the accommodation of subjective health care providers beliefs in medicine: counteracting supporters of conscientious objector accommodation arguments. *J Med Ethics* 2017; 43: 253–6.

16 Wicclair M. *Conscientious Objection in Health Care: An Ethical Analysis*. Cambridge: Cambridge University Press, 2011.

17 Pellegrino E. The physician's conscience, conscience clauses, and religious belief: a catholic perspective. *Fordham Urban Law J* 2002; 30:221–44.

18 Wicclair M. Conscience and professionals. In: LaFollette H. *The International Encyclopedia of Ethics Malden*. MA: Wiley-Blackwell, 2013; 1021–9.

19 West-Oram P. and Buyx A. Conscientious objection in health care provision: a new dimension. *Bioethics* 2016; 30:336–43.

20 Cowley C. A defence of conscientious objection in medicine: a reply to Schüklenk and Savulescu. *Bioethics* 2016; 30:358–64.

21 Weinstock D. Conscientious refusal and healthcare professionals: does religion make a difference? *Bioethics* 2014; 28:8–15.

22 Liberman A. Wrongness, responsibility, and conscientious refusal in health care. *Bioethics* 2017; 31:495–504.

23 Card R. Reasonability and conscientious objection. *Bioethics* 2014;28:320–6.

24 Kantymir L. and McLeod C. Justification for conscience exemptions in health care. *Bioethics* 2014; 28:16–23.

25 Smith. *Employment Division, Department of Human Resources of Oregon v. Smith*, [1990] 494 US 872.

26 Amselem. *Syndicat Northcrest v Amselem*, [2004] 2 SCR 551 2004 SCC 47, paragraph 43.

27 Grant K. Canadian doctors turn away from assisted dying over fees. *Globe and Mail*. July 03, 2017. https://beta.theglobeandmail.com/news/national/payment-complications-turning-canadian-doctors-away-from-assisted-dying/article35538666/ (26 September 2017, date last accessed).

28 Myers C. and Woods R. Conscientious objection? Yes, but make sure it is genuine. *AJOB* 2007; 7:19–20.

29 Maclure J. and Dumont I. Selling conscience short: a response to Schüklenk and Smalling on conscientious objections by medical professionals. *J Med Ethics* 2017; 43:241–4.

30 Rhodes R. The ethical standard of care. *AJOB* 2006; 6:76–8.

31 Blackmer J. Clarification of the CMA's position concerning induced abortion. *CMAJ* 2007; 176:1310.

32 American Medical Association Council on Ethics and Judicial Affairs. Physician Exercise of Conscience. 2014. https://www.ama-assn.org/sites/ama-assn.org/files/corp/media-browser/public/about-ama/councils/Council%20Reports/council-on-ethics-and-judicial-affairs/i14-ceja-physician-exercise-conscience.pdf at 3. (27 September 2017, date last accessed).

33 Savulescu J. and Schüklenk U. Doctors have no right to refuse medical assistance in dying, abortion or contraception. *Bioethics* 2017; 31:162–70.

34 Schüklenk U. and Smalling R. Why medical professionals have no moral claim to conscientious objection accommodation in liberal democracies. *J Med Ethics* 2017; 43:234–40.

35 Card R. Is there no alternative? Conscientious objection by medical students. *J Med Ethics* 2012; 38:602–4.

36 Freidson E. Theory and the professions. *Indiana Law J* 1989; 64:423–32.

37 Lyus R.J. Response to: 'Why medical professionals have no moral claim to conscientious objection accommodation in liberal democracies' by Schüklenk and Smalling. *J Med Ethics* 2017; 43:250–2.

38 Delston J.B. When doctors deny drugs: sexism and contraception access in the medical field. *Bioethics* 2017; 31:703–10. doi:10.1111/bioe.12373.

39 Saraiya M., Martinez G., Glaser K., et al. Pap testing and sexual activity among young women in the United States. *Obstet Gynecol* 2009; 114:1213–9.

40 College of Physicians and Surgeons of British Columbia. Physicians must not delay or impede access to medical assistance in dying. *College Connector* 2017; 5. https://www.cpsbc.ca/for-physicians/college-connector/2017-V05-05/04 (18 October 2017, date last accessed).

41 Loriggia P. Ontario doctors who object to treatment on moral or religious grounds must provide referral: court. *Toronto Star* 01 Feb 2018. https://www.thestar.com/news/canada/2018/01/31/ontario-doctors-who-object-to-treatment-on-moral-or-religious-grounds-must-give-referral-court.html (1 February 2018, date last accessed).

42 Sulmasy D.P. Tolerance, professional judgement, and the discretionary space of the physician. *Camb Q Healthc Ethics* 2017;26:18–31.

43 Caruk H. and Hoye B. Waiting to die: Winnipeg man says faith-based hospital delayed access to assisted death. *CBC News*. 26 Oct 2017. http://www.cbc.ca/news/canada/manitoba/misericordia-assisted-dying-maid-1.4371796 (4 November 2017, date last accessed).

Confidentiality

76

Confidentiality in Medicine
A Decrepit Concept

Mark Siegler

Medical confidentiality, as it has traditionally been understood by patients and doctors, no longer exists. This ancient medical principle, which has been included in every physician's oath and code of ethics since Hippocratic times, has become old, worn-out, and useless; it is a decrepit concept. Efforts to preserve it appear doomed to failure and often give rise to more problems than solutions. Psychiatrists have tacitly acknowledged the impossibility of ensuring the confidentiality of medical records by choosing to establish a separate, more secret record. The following case illustrates how the confidentiality principle is compromised systematically in the course of routine medical care.

A patient of mine with mild chronic obstructive pulmonary disease was transferred from the surgical intensive-care unit to a surgical nursing floor two days after an elective cholecystectomy. On the day of transfer, the patient saw a respiratory therapist writing in his medical chart (the therapist was recording the results of an arterial blood gas analysis) and became concerned about the confidentiality of his hospital records. The patient threatened to leave the hospital prematurely unless I could guarantee that the confidentiality of his hospital record would be respected.

This patient's complaint prompted me to enumerate the number of persons who had both access to his hospital record and a reason to examine it. I was amazed to learn that at least 25 and possibly as many as 100 health professionals and administrative personnel at our university hospital had access to the patient's record and that all of them had a legitimate need, indeed a professional responsibility, to open and use that chart. These persons included 6 attending physicians (the primary physician, the surgeon, the pulmonary consultant, and others); 12 house officers (medical, surgical, intensive-care unit, and "covering" house staff); 20 nursing personnel (on three shifts); 6 respiratory therapists; 3 nutritionists; 2 clinical pharmacists; 15 students (from medicine, nursing, respiratory therapy, and clinical pharmacy); 4 unit secretaries; 4 hospital financial officers; and 4 chart reviewers (utilization review, quality assurance review, tissue review, and insurance auditor). It is of interest that this patient's problem was straightforward, and he therefore did not require many other technical and

Original publication details: Mark Siegler, "Confidentiality in Medicine: A Decrepit Concept," pp. 1518–1521 from *New England Journal of Medicine* 307: 24 (December 1982). © 1982 Massachusetts Medical Society. Reproduced with permission of Massachusetts Medical Society.

support services that the modern hospital provides. For example, he did not need multiple consultants and fellows, such specialized procedures as dialysis, or social workers, chaplains, physical therapists, occupational therapists, and the like.

Upon completing my survey I reported to the patient that I estimated that at least 75 health professionals and hospital personnel had access to his medical record. I suggested to the patient that these people were all involved in providing or supporting his health-care services. They were, I assured him, working for him. Despite my reassurances the patient was obviously distressed and retorted, "I always believed that medical confidentiality was part of a doctor's code of ethics. Perhaps you should tell me just what you people mean by 'confidentiality'!"

Two Aspects of Medical Confidentiality

Confidentiality and third-party interests

Previous discussions of medical confidentiality usually have focused on the tension between a physician's responsibility to keep information divulged by patients secret and a physician's legal and moral duty, on occasion, to reveal such confidences to third parties, such as families, employers, public-health authorities, or police authorities. In all these instances, the central question relates to the stringency of the physician's obligation to maintain patient confidentiality when the health, well-being, and safety of identifiable others or of society in general would be threatened by a failure to reveal information about the patient. The tension in such cases is between the good of the patient and the good of others.

Confidentiality and the patient's interest

As the example above illustrates, further challenges to confidentiality arise because the patient's personal interest in maintaining confidentiality comes into conflict with his personal interest in receiving the best

possible health care. Modern high-technology health care is available principally in hospitals (often, teaching hospitals), requires many trained and specialized workers (a "health-care team"), and is very costly. The existence of such teams means that information that previously had been held in confidence by an individual physician will now necessarily be disseminated to many members of the team. Furthermore, since health-care teams are expensive and few patients can afford to pay such costs directly, it becomes essential to grant access to the patient's medical record to persons who are responsible for obtaining third-party payment. These persons include chart reviewers, financial officers, insurance auditors, and quality-of-care assessors. Finally, as medicine expands from a narrow, disease-based model to a model that encompasses psychological, social, and economic problems, not only will the size of the health-care team and medical costs increase, but more sensitive information (such as one's personal habits and financial condition) will now be included in the medical record and will no longer be confidential.

The point I wish to establish is that hospital medicine, the rise of health-care teams, the existence of third-party insurance programs, and the expanding limits of medicine all appear to be responses to the wishes of people for better and more comprehensive medical care. But each of these developments necessarily modifies our traditional understanding of medical confidentiality.

The Role of Confidentiality in Medicine

Confidentiality serves a dual purpose in medicine. In the first place, it acknowledges respect for the patient's sense of individuality and privacy. The patient's most personal physical and psychological secrets are kept confidential in order to decrease a sense of shame and vulnerability. Secondly, confidentiality is important in improving the patient's health care – a basic goal of medicine. The promise of confidentiality permits people to trust (i.e., have confidence) that information revealed to a physician in the course of a medical encounter will not be disseminated further. In this way patients are encouraged to communicate honestly and forthrightly with their doctors. This bond of trust between patient and doctor is vitally important both in the diagnostic process (which relies on an accurate history) and subsequently in the treatment phase, which often depends as much on the patient's trust in the physician as it does on medications and surgery. These two important functions of confidentiality are as important now as they were in the past. They will not be supplanted entirely either by improvements in medical technology or by recent changes in relations between some patients and doctors toward a rights-based, consumerist model.

Possible Solutions to the Confidentiality Problem

First of all, in all nonbureaucratic, noninstitutional medical encounters – that is, in the millions of doctor–patient encounters that take place in physicians' offices, where more privacy can be preserved – meticulous care should be taken to guarantee that patients' medical and personal information will be kept confidential.

Secondly, in such settings as hospitals or large-scale group practices, where many persons have opportunities to examine the medical record, we should aim to provide access only to those who have "a need to know." This could be accomplished through such administrative changes as dividing the entire record into several sections – for example, a medical and financial section – and permitting only health professionals access to the medical information.

The approach favored by many psychiatrists – that of keeping a psychiatric record separate from the general medical record – is an understandable strategy but one that is not entirely satisfactory and that should not be generalized. The keeping of separate psychiatric records implies that psychiatry and medicine are different undertakings and thus drives deeper the wedge between them and between physical and

psychological illness. Furthermore, it is often vitally important for internists or surgeons to know that a patient is being seen by a psychiatrist or is taking a particular medication. When separate records are kept, this information may not be available. Finally, if generalized, the practice of keeping a separate psychiatric record could lead to the unacceptable consequence of having a separate record for each type of medical problem.

Patients should be informed about what is meant by "medical confidentiality." We should establish the distinction between information about the patient that generally will be kept confidential regardless of the interest of third parties and information that will be exchanged among members of the health-care team in order to provide care for the patient. Patients should be made aware of the large number of persons in the modern hospital who require access to the medical record in order to serve the patient's medical and financial interests.

Finally, at some point most patients should have an opportunity to review their medical record and to make informed choices about whether their entire record is to be available to everyone or whether certain portions of the record are privileged and should be accessible only to their principal physician or to others designated explicitly by the patient. This approach would rely on traditional informed-consent procedural standards and might permit the patient to balance the personal value of medical confidentiality against the personal value of high-technology, team health care. There is no reason that the same procedure should not be used with psychiatric records instead of the arbitrary system now employed, in which everything related to psychiatry is kept secret.

Afterthought: Confidentiality and Indiscretion

There is one additional aspect of confidentiality that is rarely included in discussions of the subject. I am referring here to the wanton, often inadvertent, but avoidable exchanges of confidential information that occur frequently in hospital rooms, elevators, cafeterias, doctors' offices, and at cocktail parties. Of course, as more people have access to medical information about the patient the potential for this irresponsible abuse of confidentiality increases geometrically.

Such mundane breaches of confidentiality are probably of greater concern to most patients than the broader issue of whether their medical records may be entered into a computerized data bank or whether a respiratory therapist is reviewing the results of an arterial blood gas determination. Somehow, privacy is violated and a sense of shame is heightened when intimate secrets are revealed to people one knows or is close to – friends, neighbors, acquaintances, or hospital roommates – rather than when they are disclosed to an anonymous bureaucrat sitting at a computer terminal in a distant city or to a health professional who is acting in an official capacity.

I suspect that the principles of medical confidentiality, particularly those reflected in most medical codes of ethics, were designed principally to prevent just this sort of embarrassing personal indiscretion rather than

to maintain (for social, political, or economic reasons) the absolute secrecy of doctor–patient communications. In this regard, it is worth noting that Percival's Code of Medical Ethics (1803) includes the following admonition: "Patients should be interrogated concerning their complaint in a tone of voice which cannot be over-heard." We in the medical profession frequently neglect these simple courtesies.

Conclusion

The principle of medical confidentiality described in medical codes of ethics and still believed in by patients no longer exists. In this respect, it is a decrepit concept. Rather than perpetuate the myth of confidentiality and invest energy vainly to preserve it, the public and the profession would be better served if they devoted their attention to determining which aspects of the original principle of confidentiality are worth retaining. Efforts could then be directed to salvaging those.

77

A Defense of Unqualified Medical Confidentiality

Kenneth Kipnis

It is broadly held that confidentiality may be breached when doing so can avert grave harm to a third party. This essay challenges the conventional wisdom. Neither legal duties, personal morality nor personal values are sufficient to ground professional obligations. A methodology is developed drawing on core professional values, the nature of professions, and the justification for distinct professional obligations. Though doctors have a professional obligation to prevent public peril, they do not honor it by breaching confidentiality. It is shown how the protective purpose to be furthered by reporting is defeated by the practice of reporting. Hence there is no conflict between confidentiality and the professional responsibility to protect endangered third parties.

The Case of the Infected Spouse

The following fictionalized case is based on an actual incident.

1982: After moving to Honolulu, Wilma and Andrew Long visit your office and ask you to be their family physician. They have been your patients ever since.

1988: Six years later the two decide to separate. Wilma leaves for the Mainland, occasionally sending you a postcard. Though you do not see her professionally, you still think of yourself as her doctor.

1990: Andrew comes in and says that he has embarked upon a more sophisticated social life. He has been hearing about some new sexually transmitted diseases and wants to be tested. Testing reveals that he is positive for the AIDS virus, and he receives appropriate counseling.

1991: Visiting your office for a checkup, Andrew tells you Wilma is returning to Hawaii for reconciliation with him. She arrives that afternoon and will be staying at the Moana Hotel. Despite your best efforts to persuade him, Andrew leaves without giving you assurance that he will tell Wilma about his infection or protect her against becoming infected.

Do you take steps to see that Wilma is warned? If you decide to warn Wilma, what do you say to Andrew when, two days later, he shows up at your office asking how you could reveal his confidential test results?

Original publication details: Kenneth Kipnis, "A Defense of Unqualified Medical Confidentiality," pp. 7–18 from *American Journal of Bioethics* 6: 2 (2006). Reproduced with permission of Taylor & Francis.

If you decide not to warn Wilma, what do you say to her when, two years later in 1993, she shows up at your office asking how you, her doctor, could possibly stand idly by as her husband infected her with a deadly virus. She now knows she is positive for the virus, that she was infected by her husband, and that you – her doctor – knew, before they reconciled, that her husband would probably infect her.

The ethical challenges here emerge from an apparent head-on collision between medical confidentiality and the duty to protect imperiled third parties. Notwithstanding Andrew's expectation of privacy and the professional duty to remain silent, it can seem unforgivable for anyone to withhold vital assistance in such a crisis, let alone a doctor. The case for breaching confidentiality is supported by at least five considerations: First, the doctor knows, to a medical certainty, that Andrew is both infected with HIV and infectious. Second, knowing Wilma as a patient, let us suppose the doctor reasonably believes that she is not infected. (Wilma cannot be at risk of contracting the disease if she is infected already.) Third, Wilma's vulnerability is both serious and real. HIV infection is both debilitating and, during those years, invariably fatal. The couple's sexuality makes eventual infection highly likely. Fourth, assuming that preventing Wilma's death is the goal, it is probable that, were Wilma to be told of Andrew's infection, she would avoid exposing herself to the risk. This is not a trivial condition: many people knowingly risk illness and injury out of love and other honorable motivations. Molokai's Father Damien contracted and died from Hansen's disease while caring for patients he knew might infect him. Soldiers, police, and firefighters commonly expose themselves to grave risk. It is not enough that a warning would discharge a duty to Wilma, merely so she could make an informed choice. Plainly, the paramount concern has to be to save Wilma's life. Finally, Wilma is not a mere stranger. Instead she has an important relationship with you – her doctor – that serves as a basis for special obligations: You have a special duty to look out for her health.

In the light of these five considerations, it should not be a surprise that the conventional wisdom in medical ethics overwhelmingly supports either an ethical obligation to breach confidentiality in cases like this one or, occasionally and less stringently, the ethical permissibility of doing so (Lo 1995). Notwithstanding this consensus, it is my intention to challenge the received view. I will argue in what follows that confidentiality in clinical medicine is far closer to an absolute obligation than it has generally been taken to be; doctors should honor confidentiality even in cases like this one. Although the focus here is on the *Case of the Infected Spouse,* the background idea is that, if it can be demonstrated that confidentiality should be scrupulously honored in this one case where so many considerations support breaching it, the duty of confidentiality should be taken as unqualified in virtually all other cases as well (Kottow 1986). I shall not, however, defend that broader conclusion here.

Although this essay specifically addresses the obligations of doctors, its approach applies more broadly to all professions that take seriously the responsibility to provide distressed practitioners with authoritative guidance (Kipnis 1986, 63–79; Wicclair 1985). With its focus narrowly on "professional obligations," the methodology used below also represents something of a challenge to much of the conventional thinking in medical ethics.

Clearing the Ground: What Professional Obligations Are Not

Among philosophers, it is commonplace that if people are not asking the same questions, they are unlikely to arrive at the same answers. It may be that the main reason doctors have difficulty reaching consensus in ethics is that, in general, systematic discussion about professional responsibility is commonly confused with at least three other types of conversation. When one asks whether one should call the hotel to warn Wilma, one can be asking: 1) what the law requires; 2) what one's personal morality requires (e.g., as an Orthodox Jew, a Roman Catholic, etc.); or 3) what is required by one's most deeply held personal values (e.g., preventing deaths or scrupulously honoring other obligations). Discussions can meander mindlessly over all three areas without attending to boundary crossings. More to the point, effective deliberation about professional obligations, as I will try to show, differs importantly from all three of these discussions. Accordingly, it is necessary to identify and bracket these other perspectives in order to mark off the intellectual space within which practitioners can productively reflect on questions of professional responsibility. Let us examine these different conversations.

Law

The conventional wisdom on the ethics of medical confidentiality has been largely shaped by a single legal case: *Tarasoff v. Regents of the University of California* (Supreme Court of California; 529 p. 2d 553, Cal. 1974). In 1969, Prosenjit Poddar, a student at UC Berkeley, told a university psychologist he intended to kill a Ms Tatiana Tarasoff, a young woman who had spurned his affections. The psychologist dutifully reported him to the campus police, who held him briefly and then set him free. Shortly afterwards, Poddar did as he said he would, stabbing the young woman to death. The Tarasoff family sued the University of California for their daughter's death, finally prevailing in their contention that the psychologist (and, by implication, the University) had failed in their duty to protect, since neither Tatiana nor those able to apprise her of danger were warned. The University was found liable and had to compensate the family for its loss. Today it is hard to find discussions of the ethics of confidentiality that do not appeal to this legal parable and, occasionally, to its California Supreme Court moral: "The protective privilege ends where the public peril begins."

Taking its cue from *Tarasoff*, the prevailing standard in medical ethics now holds that the obligation of confidentiality will give way when a doctor is aware that a patient will seriously injure some identified other person. (One might ask why disclosure is not required when a patient will seriously injure many unidentified persons. Under the narrower standard, there is no duty to alert others about an HIV-infected prostitute who neither informs nor protects a large

number of anonymous at-risk clients.) We assume that the physician knows Andrew is seropositive, that Wilma is likely seronegative, that the two will likely engage in activities that transmit the virus, and that breaching confidentiality will probably result in those activities not occurring and Wilma's not becoming infected. Thus, a physician's warning in the *Case of the Infected Spouse* will mean that Wilma is very likely to remain infection-free, and a failure to warn her is very likely to result in her eventual death from AIDS.

Focusing on the legal standard, it is useful to distinguish between "special" and "general" legal duties. Special duties can apply to individuals occupying certain roles. A parent, but not a bystander, has a special duty to rescue a drowning daughter; firefighters and police officers have special duties to take certain occupational risks, and doctors have many special duties toward their patients: confidentiality is a good example. In contrast, virtually everyone has a general duty to be scrupulously careful when handling explosives, to pay taxes on income, to respect others' property, and so on. It is notable that the duty to warn in *Tarasoff* is a special duty, applicable only to those occupying special roles. So if my neighbor casually assures me he is going to kill his girlfriend tomorrow, the *Tarasoff* ruling does not require me to warn her.

It is surprising to many that the default standard in Anglo-American jurisprudence is that there is no general duty to improve the prospects of the precariously placed, no legal obligation to undertake even an easy rescue. As first-year law students discover, one can stand on a pier with a lifeline in hand and, with complete impunity, allow a stranger to drown nearby. Although we will pass over it, it is notable that, in general, the parties who are legally obligated to warn are those who are otherwise ethically obligated not to disclose. One should reflect on the absence of a general duty to warn.

The easy transition from law to ethics reflects a common error. The mistake is to move from the premise that some action is legally required (what the *Tarasoff* opinion establishes in the jurisdictions that have followed it) to the conclusion that the same action is ethically required. But ethical obligations can conflict with legal ones. Journalists, for example, are sometimes ordered by the courts to reveal the identities of their confidential sources. Although law demands disclosure, professional ethics requires silence. Reporters famously go to jail rather than betray sources. Journalists can find themselves in a quandary: while good citizens obey the law and good professionals honor their professional codes, laws requiring journalists to violate their duties to confidential sources force a tragic choice between acting illegally and acting unethically. Conscientious persons should not have to face such decisions.

Similarly in pediatrics, statutes may require doctors to report suspicions of child abuse. But where protective agencies are inept and overworked and foster care is dangerous or unavailable, a doctor's report is more likely to result in termination of therapy and further injury to the child instead of protection and care. To obey the law under these appalling, but too common, circumstances is most likely to abandon and even cause harm to the minor patient, both of which are ethically prohibited in medicine. To assume that legal obligations always trump or settle ethical ones is to blind oneself to the possibility of conflict. Professions have to face these dilemmas head-on instead of masking them with language that conflates legal standards and ethical ones. They must conceive professional ethics as separate from the law's mandate. When law requires what professional responsibility prohibits (or prohibits what professional responsibility requires), professional organizations must press the public, legislatures, and the courts to cease demanding that conscientious practitioners dishonor the duties of their craft. This is an important responsibility of professional organizations. It is a mistake to configure professional obligations merely to mirror the law's requirements. Rather the law's requirements must be configured so that they do not conflict with well-considered professional obligations. Law is a human artifact that can be crafted well or badly. In a well-ordered society no one will have to choose between illegality and immorality. Since the law can require conduct that violates ethical standards (and ethical standards can require conduct that violates the law), it cannot be the case that legal

obligations automatically create ethical obligations. As the tradition of civil disobedience shows, it can be ethically permissible or obligatory (though not legal) to violate an unjust law.

Even though laws cannot create ethical obligations by fiat, professions need to distinguish between the state's reasonable interests in the work of doctors (e.g., preventing serious harm to children) and the specific legal mandates a state imposes (e.g., requiring doctors to report suspicion of child abuse to an incompetent state agency). Just as patients can make ill-considered demands that should not be satisfied, so too can the state and its courts.

Accordingly, it is assumed that the state has a legitimate interest in preventing harm to people, and that doctors have an ethical obligation to further that important public objective. The focus in this essay is on the shape of the resulting ethical obligation as it applies narrowly to cases like those involving Wilma Long and Tatiana Tarasoff. Because they introduce complexities that will carry us far afield, we set aside cases involving: (a) children brought in by parents (Kipnis 2004); (b) patients referred for independent medical evaluation; (c) mentally ill or [intellectually disabled] patients in the custody of health care institutions; (d) health care that is the subject of litigation; (e) gunshot, knife wounds, and the like; (f) workers' compensation cases; and a few others. While a much longer discussion could cover these areas, many readers can extend the analysis offered here to discern much of what I would want to say about those other cases.

Though I will not discuss them, institutional policies (hospital rules, for example) function very much like laws. Both involve standards that can be imposed externally upon practitioners. Both can be formulated knowledgeably and wisely or with a disregard for essential professional responsibilities.

Personal morality

We will understand a "morality" as a set of beliefs about obligations. There are plainly many such sets of beliefs: the morality of Confucius has little in common with the moralities of George W. Bush and Thomas Aquinas. For most of us, morality is uncritically absorbed in childhood, coming to consciousness when we encounter others whose moral beliefs differ.

There are still parts of the world in which virtually all members of a community are participants in a common morality. But moral pluralism now seems a permanent part of the social order. Consider a Jehovah's Witness physician who is opposed, on religious grounds, to administering blood transfusions. If this doctor were the only physician on duty when his patient needed an immediate transfusion, a choice would have to be made between being a good Jehovah's Witness and being a good doctor. The doctor's personal moral convictions are here inconsistent with professional obligations. It follows that clarity about personal morality is not the same as clarity about medical ethics. Professionalism can require that one set aside one's personal morality or carefully limit one's exposure to certain professional responsibilities. Here the rule has to be that doctors will not take on responsibilities that might conflict with their personal morality. Problems could be sidestepped if the Jehovah's Witness doctor specialized in a field that didn't involve transfusion (e.g., dermatology) or always worked with colleagues who could administer them. If I am morally against the death penalty, I shouldn't take on work as an executioner. If I am deeply opposed to the morning-after pill, I shouldn't counsel patients at a rape treatment center. To teach medical ethics in a pluralistic professional community is to try to create an intellectual space within which persons from varied backgrounds can agree upon responsible standards for professional conduct. Participants in such a conversation may have to leave personal morality at the door. For some, it may be a mistake to choose a career in medicine.

If ethics is a critical reflection on our moralities, then the hope implicit in the field of medical ethics is that we might some day reach a responsible consensus on doctors' obligations. While medicine has dozens of codes, it is not hard to observe commonalities: the standards for informed consent, for example. At a deeper level, there can also be consensus on the justifications for those standards. One role for the philosopher is, as in this essay, to assess carefully the soundness of those arguments. A major task for professions is to move beyond the various personal moralities embraced by practitioners and to reach a responsible consensus on common professional standards.

Personal values

Values are commonly a part of an explanation of personal conduct. It is always reasonable to ask of any rational action: what good was it intended to promote? While some wear shoes to avoid hurting their feet (embracing the value of comfort), others think they look better in shoes (embracing aesthetic values). Where we have to make personal decisions, often we consider how each option can further or frustrate our values, and try to decide among the good and bad consequences.

This strategy can serve when the question is "What should I do?" But the question "What should a good doctor do?" calls for a different type of inquiry. For while I have many personal values, the "good doctor" is an abstraction. She is neither Protestant nor Buddhist, doesn't prefer chocolate to vanilla, and doesn't care about money more than leisure time. Questions about professional ethics cannot be answered in terms of personal values.

A second difficulty appears when we consider that one can give perfect expression to one's most deeply held personal values and still act unethically. Hannibal Lecter in *Silence of the Lambs* and Mozart's Don Giovanni are despicable villains who give vigorous effect to deeply held if contemptible personal values. While personal values can determine action, they do not guarantee that the favored actions are ethical.

Accordingly, we cannot appeal to our personal values to inquire about what physicians in general ought to do. Medicine has no personal values, only individual physicians do. When a physician must decide whether or not to resuscitate a patient, personal values should have nothing to do with the issue. Whether you like the patient or detest him, whether you are an atheist or a fundamentalist believer in a joyous hereafter, should not weigh in the balance. A key part of professionalism involves being able to set personal values aside. While medical students have much to gain by becoming clear about their personal values, that clarity is not the same as responsible certainty about professional obligations.

To summarize the argument so far, discussion about professional obligations in medicine is not the same as discussion about legal and institutional obligations, personal morality or personal values. If a responsible ethical consensus is to be achieved by a profession, it is necessary for physicians to learn to bracket their personal moral and value commitments and to set aside, at least temporarily, their consideration of legal or institutional rules and policies. The practical task is to create an intellectual space within which responsible consensus can be achieved on how physicians, as professionals, ought to act. I will now describe one way in which this might be done.

The Concept of a Professional Obligation

Professional ethics involves disciplined discussion about the obligations of professionals. One place to begin is with a distinction between personal values, already discussed, and what can be called "core professional values." A physician can prefer (1) pistachios to Brazil nuts, and (2) confidentiality to universal candor. While the preference for pistachios is merely personal, the preference for confidentiality is a value all doctors ought to possess. The distinction between personal values and "core professional values" is critical here. There is what this flesh-and-blood doctor happens to care about personally, and what the good doctor ought to care about. This idea of a "good doctor" is a social construction, an aspect of a determinate social role, an integral element of medical professionalism. Our idea of a good doctor includes a certain technical/intellectual mastery coupled with a certain commitment to specific professional values. As with the Jehovah's Witness doctor, personal and professional values may be in conflict. As part of an appreciation

of the ethical claims of professionalism, physicians must be prepared to set aside their personal values and morality, to set aside what the legal system and their employers want them to care about, and to take up instead the question of what the responsible physician ought to care about. The profession's core values inform those purposes that each medical professional should have in common with colleagues. In discussing the professionally favored resolution of ethically problematic cases (the *Case of the Infected Spouse,* for example) physicians can ask – together – how medicine's core professional values ought to be respected in those circumstances.

We have alluded to some of these core professional values. Trustworthiness needs to be on the list. Beneficence toward the patient's health needs is essential. Respect for patient autonomy is a third. Others might be collegiality (duties to colleagues), and perhaps a few others: nondiscrimination and a certain deference to families are among the most commonly mentioned candidates. If we were to leave out that doctors should care about the wellbeing of the public, the argument for confidentiality would be easy. But it too properly goes on the list. Anyone seeing no point in furthering and securing these values would be ill-suited for the practice of medicine.

Each of these professional values has two dimensions. Along one vector, they define the shared aspiration of a profession. At any time, medicine's ability to benefit patients will be limited. But it is a part of the profession's commitment to push its envelope, to enlarge its collective competency and draw upon its knowledge and skill. Those who master and extend the profession's broadest capabilities are exemplary contributors, but practitioners do not discredit themselves by failing to serve in this estimable way.

Along the second vector, values define a bottom line beneath which practitioners shall not sink. Paraphrasing Hippocrates, although you may not always be able to benefit your patients, it is far more important that you take care not to harm them. Knowingly to harm a patient (on balance) is not merely a failure to realize the value of beneficence. It is a culpable betrayal of that value, a far more serious matter.

All the values above can be understood in this second way. Trustworthiness entails that I not lie to patients, or deliberately withhold information they have an interest in knowing. Respect for patient autonomy can require that I not use force or fraud upon them. And the concern for the well-being of the public requires that that interest somehow appear prominently upon every practitioner's radar screen, that doctors not stand idly by in the face of perils the profession can help to avert and, as a lower limit, that they not do anything to increase public peril. Consider that the overutilization of antibiotics, resulting in drug-resistant infectious agents, is professional misconduct that increases public peril.

Ethical problems can arise, first, when core values appear to be in conflict, as with the *Case of the Infected Spouse*. At issue are trustworthiness toward Andrew on one side, and beneficence toward Wilma and a concern for the well-being of the public on the other. If the conflict is real, what is required is a priority rule. For example, the concept of decisional capacity is part of a priority rule resolving the well-studied conflict between beneficence and autonomy: when do physicians have to respect a patient's refusal of life-saving treatment? There is what the patient wants and what the patient needs. But when a patient is decisionally capacitated and informed, his or her refusal trumps the doctor's recommendation.

Second, ethical problems can also arise when it is unclear what some core professional value requires one to do. Though we can all agree that doctors should avoid harming their patients, there is no professional consensus on whether deliberately causing the deaths of certain unfortunate patients – those experiencing irremediable and intense suffering – is always a betrayal of beneficence. Likewise, although doctors may be in a position to prevent harm to third parties, it is not well understood what they must do out of respect for that value. When core values conflict, what is required is a priority rule. When they are unclear, what is required is removal of ambiguity: what philosophers call "disambiguation." These two tasks – prioritizing and disambiguating core professional values – need to be carried out with a high degree of intellectual responsibility.

The above list of medicine's core values is not controversial. Propose a toast to them at an assemblage of physicians and all can likely drink with enthusiasm. What is less clear is why such a consensus should obligate professionals. A criminal organization can celebrate its shared commitment to the oath of silence. But it doesn't follow that those who cooperate with the police are unethical. In addition to organizational "celebratability," three additional elements are required to establish a professional obligation.

The first element is that attention to core values has to be a part of professional education. Most medical education is aimed at beneficence. The procedures used in informed consent express a commitment of respect for patient autonomy and trustworthiness. If the profession wholly fails to equip its novices to further its core values, it can be argued that it is not serious about those professed values. Its public commitments will begin to look like they are intended to convey an illusion of concerned attention. In replicating itself, a profession must replicate its commitment. Students of medicine must come to care about the goods that doctors ought to care about. Because justice is rarely explored as a topic in medical education, I do not think it can be counted as a core professional value. However some parts of justice – nondiscrimination, for example – are routinely covered.

The second element is critical. The core values are not just goods that doctors care about and that doctors want other doctors to care about. They are also goods that the rest of us want our doctors to care about. I want my doctor to be trustworthy, to be intent on benefiting my health, to take my informed refusals seriously, and so on. And we want our doctors to look out for the wellbeing of the public. The core professional values are also social values. (Consider that it is not reasonable to want our mobsters to respect their oaths of silence.)

The third element flows from the second: an exclusive social reliance upon the profession as the means by which certain matters are to receive due attention. We mostly respect medical competence. But it is precisely because, as a community, we have also come to accept that doctors are reliably committed to their values (our values), that we have, through state legislatures, granted the medical profession an exclusive monopoly on the delivery of medical services. The unauthorized practice of medicine is a punishable crime. If, like the medical profession, one were to make a public claim that, because of unique skills and dedication, some important social concern ought to be exclusively entrusted to you, and the public believes you and entrusts those important matters to you, incidentally prohibiting all others from encroachment upon what is now your privilege, you would have thereby assumed an ethical obligation to give those important matters due attention. Collectively, the medical profession has done exactly this in securing its monopoly on the delivery of certain types of health care. Accordingly the profession has a collective obligation to organize itself so that the shared responsibilities it has assumed in the political process of professionalization are properly discharged by its membership.

A sound code of ethics consists of a set of standards that, if adhered to broadly by the profession's membership, will result in the profession as a whole discharging its responsibilities. Where physician behavior brings about a public loss of that essential trust, society may have to withdraw the monopolistic privilege and seek a better way of organizing health care. Professionalization is but one way of organizing an essential service. There are others.

In summary, the medical profession has ethical obligations toward patients, families, and the community because of its public commitment to secure and further certain critical social values and because of society's exclusive reliance on the profession as its means of delivering certain forms of health care. With the professional privilege comes a reciprocal collective responsibility (Kipnis 1986, 1–14). We can now turn our attention to medicine's responsibility to diminish public perils.

The Duty to Diminish Risks to Third Parties

There is an implication for the way in which we must now understand the problem in the *Case of the Infected*

Spouse. The opening question "Do you take steps to warn Wilma?" has to be understood as a question about medical ethics and not about "you." We want to know what the "good doctor" should do under those circumstances. Each doctor is ethically required to do what a responsible doctor ought to do: in order to properly respect the core values of the profession. To become a doctor without a proper commitment to respect the profession's values is to be unfit for the practice of medicine. So how are trustworthiness and confidentiality to be understood in relationship to medicine's commitment to diminish risks to third parties?

In the *Case of the Infected Spouse* the ethical question is posed in 1991, after the doctor–family relationship has been in place for a decade. The dilemma arises during and immediately after a single office visit, forcing a choice between calling Wilma either you will have to explain to Andrew, in two days, why you disclosed his infection to his wife, or you will have to explain to Wilma, in two years, why you did not disclose his infection to her. Each option has a bad outcome: the betrayal of Andrew's trust or the fatal infection of Wilma. Either way, you will need to account for yourself.

Infection seems a far worse consequence for Wilma than betrayal is for Andrew. Much of the literature on confidentiality has been shaped by this fact, and perhaps the standard strategy for resolving the problem calls attention to the magnitude and probability of the bad outcomes associated with each option. While predictions of harm can sometimes be wrong, it can be evident that Tatiana Tarasoff and Wilma Long are at grave risk and, accordingly, it can seem honorable to diminish the danger to vulnerable parties like them. Justice Tobriner appeals to a version of this consequentialist argument in *Tarasoff*:

> Weighing the uncertain and conjectural character of the alleged damage done the patient by such a warning against the peril to the victim's life, we conclude that professional inaccuracy in predicting violence [or deadly infection] cannot negate the therapist's duty to protect the threatened victim.

Beauchamp and Childress, in their widely read *Principles of Biomedical Ethics* (2001, 309), urge clinicians to take into account "the probability that a harm will materialize and the magnitude of that harm" in any decision to breach confidentiality. (While they also urge that clinicians take into account the potential impact of disclosure on policies and laws regarding confidentiality, they are not very clear about how this assessment is to be carried out.) In brief, the very bad consequences of not disclosing risk to Wilma – disease and death and the betrayal of her trust – outweigh the not-all-that-bad consequence of breached confidentiality to Andrew. Your explanation to Andrew could cover those points.

The preferred argument would go something like this: The state's interest in preventing harm is weighty. Medicine has an obligation to protect the well-being of the community. Because the seriousness of threatened grave injury to another outweighs the damage done to a patient by breaching confidentiality, the obligation of confidentiality must give way to a duty to prevent serious harm to others. Accordingly, despite confidentiality, warning or reporting is obligatory when it will likely avert very bad outcomes in this way. Of course clinicians should try to obtain waivers of confidentiality before disclosure, thereby avoiding the need to breach a duty. But the failure to obtain a waiver does not, on this argument, affect the overriding obligation to report.

A Defense of Unqualified Confidentiality

As powerful as the above justification is, there are problems with it. Go back to 1990, when Andrew comes in to be tested for sexually transmitted diseases. Suppose he asks: "If I am infected, can I trust you not to disclose this to others?" If, following the arguments set out in the previous paragraphs, we are clear that confidentiality must be breached to protect third parties like Wilma, then the only truthful answer to Andrew's question is "No. You can't trust me." If the profession accepts that its broad promise of confidentiality must sometimes be broken, then any unqualified assurances are fraudulent and the profession should stop making them. If there are exceptions, clinicians have a duty to be forthcoming about what they are and how they work. Patients should know up front when they can trust doctors, and when they can't. To withhold this important information is to betray the value of trustworthiness.

Accordingly, the argument for breaching confidentiality has to be modified to support a qualified confidentiality rule, one that carves out an exception from the very beginning, acknowledging an overriding duty to report under defined circumstances. (In contrast, an unqualified confidentiality rule contemplates no exceptions.) Instead of undertaking duties of confidentiality and then violating them, doctors must qualify their expressed obligations so they will be able to honor them. Commentators who have walked through the issues surrounding confidentiality have long understood the ethical necessity of "Miranda warnings" (Bok 1983; Goldman 1980): A clinician would have to say early on, "Certain things that I learn from you may have to be disclosed to . . . under the following circumstances . . .; and the following things might occur to you as a result of my disclosure: . . . " If doctors are ethically obligated to report, they need to say in advance what will be passed along, when, to whom, and what could happen then. They should never encourage or accept trust only to betray their patients afterwards. To do so is to betray the value of trustworthiness.

But now a second problem emerges. If prospective patients must understand in advance that a doctor will report evidence of a threat to others, they will only be willing to disclose such evidence to the doctor if they are willing to accept that those others will come to know. If it is important to them that the evidence not be reported, they will have a weighty reason not to disclose it to those who are obligated to report it.

Some have questioned this proposition, arguing that there is no empirical evidence that prospective patients will avoid or delay seeking medical attention or conceal medically relevant information if confidentiality is qualified in this way. Despite widespread reporting practices, waiting rooms have not emptied and no one really knows if people stop talking openly to their doctors when confidentiality is breached.

Three responses are possible regarding this claim. First, there is a serious difficulty doing empirical research in this area. How, for example, do we determine the number of abusive parents who have not brought their injured children to doctors out of a fear that they will get into trouble with the authorities? How many HIV+ patients avoid telling their doctors all about their unsafe sexual practices? How many of us would volunteer unflattering truthful answers to direct questions on these and other shameful matters? It is notoriously difficult to gather reliable data on the embarrassing, criminal, irresponsible things people do, and the steps they take to avoid exposure, especially if those are wrongful too. I don't want to suggest that these problems are insurmountable (Reddy et al. 2002), but they are decidedly there and they often make it hard to study the effects of these betrayals.

Second, despite the problems, certain types of indirect evidence can occasionally emerge. Here are two anecdotal examples from Honolulu. There was a time, not long ago, when military enlistees who were troubled by their sexual orientation knew that military doctors and psychologists would report these problems to their officers. Many of these troubled soldiers therefore obtained the services of private psychologists and psychiatrists in Honolulu, despite the fact that free services were available in military clinics. The second example emerged from the failure of the Japanese medical system to keep diagnoses of HIV infection confidential. Many Japanese who could afford it traveled to Honolulu for diagnosis and treatment, avoiding clinics in Japan. At the same time, Japanese data on the prevalence of HIV infection were unrealistically low, especially considering the popularity of Japanese sex tours to the HIV-infected brothels of Thailand. Evidence of this sort can confirm that the failure to respect confidentiality can impair the ability of doctors to do their job.

And third, there is an argument based on the motivational principle that if one strongly desires that

event E does not occur, and one knows that doing act A will bring about event E, then one has a weighty reason not to do act A. The criminal justice system is based on this idea. We attach artificial and broadly unwelcome consequences (imprisonment and other forms of punishment) to wrongful, harmful conduct with the expectation that, even if inclined, most people will decide against the conduct in order to avoid the unwelcome consequence. If I don't want to go to prison, and a career in burglary will likely result in my going to prison, then I have a weighty reason to choose a different career. Likewise, if I don't want my marriage to be destroyed by my wife's discovery that I am HIV+, and I know that telling my doctor about reconciliation will result in her discovering just that, then I have a weighty reason not to tell my doctor. The presumption must be in favor of the truth of this seemingly self-evident principle. If critics allege that it is false or otherwise unworthy of endorsement, it seems the burden of disproof belongs to them. It is their responsibility to come up with disconfirming evidence.

It can be argued, in rebuttal, that people still commit burglary and, despite reporting laws, people still go to doctors for HIV testing, even knowing that confidentiality has its limits. But no one would maintain that punishing convicted criminals totally prevents crime and that breaching confidentiality results in all people avoiding or delaying medical treatment, or concealing aspects of their lives. The situation is more complicated.

Consider that Andrew belongs to one of two groups of prospective patients. Members of the first group are willing enough to have reports made to others. Members of the second are deterred from disclosure by the fear of a report. Of course we can't know in advance which type of patient Andrew is, but if both groups are treated alike, uncertainty will not be a problem. (While this division into two groups may be oversimplified, working through the qualifications would take us too far afield.)

Consider the first group: patients who would be willing to have a report made. Recall that the physician in the *Case of the Infected Spouse* tried to obtain assurance that Wilma would be protected. Under an unqualified confidentiality rule – no exceptions – if the patient were willing to have reports made to others, the doctor should be able to obtain a waiver of confidentiality and Wilma could then be informed. Once permission to report is given, the ethical dilemma disappears. Notice that for this group of patients an exceptionless confidentiality rule works just as well as a rule requiring doctors to override confidentiality when necessary to protect endangered third parties. At-risk parties will be warned just the same, but with appropriate permission from patients. In these cases there is no need to trim back the obligation of confidentiality since patients in this first group are, by definition, willing to have a report made.

Difficulties arise with the second type of patient: those who will not want credible threats reported. Notice that these prospective patients are in control of the evidence doctors need to secure protection for parties at risk. If a patient cannot be drawn into a therapeutic alliance – a relationship of trust and confidence – then doctors will not receive the information they need to protect imperiled third parties (at least so long as patients have options). As a result, doctors will not be able to mobilize protection. When one traces out the implications of a reporting rule on what needs to be said in 1990 (when Andrew asked to be tested and the doctor disclosed the limits to confidentiality), it becomes evident that Wilma will not be protected if Andrew (a) does not want her to know, and (b) understands that disclosure to his doctor will result in her knowing. Depending on his options and the strength of his preferences, he will be careful about what he discloses to his doctor, or will go without medical advice and care, or will find another physician who can be kept in ignorance about his personal life.

We began by characterizing the *Case of the Infected Spouse* as an apparent head-on collision between the doctor's duty of confidentiality and the duty to protect imperiled third parties. But if the argument above is sound, there is no collision. The obligation to warn third parties does not provide added protection to those at-risk. In particular, a no-exceptions confidentiality rule has a better chance of getting the facts on

the table, at least to the extent that honest promises of confidentiality can make it so. To be sure, clinicians would have to set aside the vexing "Should I report?" conundrum and search for creative solutions instead. These strategies will not always prevent harm, but they will sometimes. The nub of the matter is that these strategies can never work if they can't be implemented. And they can't be implemented if the fear of reporting deters patients from disclosure. Accordingly there is no justification for trimming back the obligation of confidentiality since doing so actually reduces protection to endangered third parties, increasing public peril.

The argument advanced here is that – paradoxically – ethical and legal duties to report make it less likely that endangered parties will be protected. Depending on the prospective patient, these duties are either unnecessary (when waivers can be obtained) or counterproductive (when disclosure to the doctor is deterred and interventions other than disclosure are prevented).

In part, the conventional wisdom on confidentiality errs in focusing on the decision of the individual clinician at the point when the choice has to be made to disclose or not. The decision to violate confidentiality reaches backwards to the HIV test administered years earlier and, as we shall see, even before. Perhaps little will be lost if one doctor betrays a single patient one time, or if betrayals are extremely rare. But medical ethics is not about a single decision by an individual clinician. The consequences and implications of a rule governing professional practice may be quite different from those of a single act. Better to ask, what if every doctor did that?

While it is accepted here that doctors have an overriding obligation to prevent public peril, it has been argued that they do not honor that obligation by breaching or chipping away at confidentiality. This is because the protective purpose to be furthered by reporting is defeated by the practice of reporting. The best public protection is achieved where doctors do their best work and, there, trustworthiness is probably the most important prerequisite. Physicians damage both their professional capabilities and their communities when they compromise their trustworthiness.

If the argument above is sound and confidentiality must be respected in this case, we must now return to the question of what the doctor must say to Wilma when, now infected, she returns to the office two years after the reconciliation. Though this question has finally to be faced in 1993, it is on the table before her return to Honolulu. It is there even before Andrew asks to be tested in 1990, and you then have to decide whether to live out the trust he has placed in you or disabuse him of it. In fact, the problem is on the table in 1982, when the couple first enters your office and asks you to be their physician. As a doctor, you have obligations of beneficence and confidentiality and you owe both to each. But now – having read this far – you are aware that something can happen that you cannot control; and, if it does happen, you will face those apparently conflicting obligations. You can only provide what you owe to one if you betray your obligation to the other. That is the choice you will have to make in 1993, unless you (and the medical profession) contour professional responsibilities now.

If, in choosing a governing ethical principle, the end-in-view is to protect vulnerable third parties; and if this can be done best, as I have tried to show, by honoring confidentiality and doing one's best to protect imperiled third parties within that framework; then what you must say to both Wilma and Andrew, when they enter your office in 1982, should be something like this:

> There is an ethical problem physicians sometimes face in taking on a married couple as patients. It can happen that one partner becomes infected with a transmissible disease, potentially endangering the other. If the infected partner won't share information with me because he or she fears I will warn the other, there will be no protection at all for the partner at risk. There may, however, be things I can do if I can talk with the infected partner. What I promise both of you is, if that were to happen, I will do everything I possibly can to protect the endangered partner, except for violating confidentiality, which I will not do. You both need to remember that you should not count on me to guarantee the wholesomeness of your spouse, if doing this means betrayal.

It is in these words that the final explanation to Wilma can be found. If Wilma understands from the beginning that medical confidentiality will not be breached; if she (and the public generally) understand that the precariously placed are safer under unqualified confidentiality, she will understand she has final responsibility for her choices. If you are clear enough about it, she will grasp that she can't depend on you to protect her at the cost of betrayal, and that she is better off because of that. Both the doctor and the medical profession collectively need to work through these issues and fully disclose the favored standard to prospective patients before the occasion arises when a doctor must appeal to it. The view defended here is that the profession should continue to make an unqualified pledge of confidentiality, and mean it.

It is also appropriate to consider what should be said to Andrew as he is about to leave your office in 1991 to prepare for a romantic dinner with Wilma. I once spent part of an afternoon with a healthcare professional who had served in Vietnam. He had counseled married enlistees who had returned from visits with their wives and had been diagnosed with a venereal disease that was probably contracted before they left Vietnam. It is likely that these men may have infected their wives. This clinician had learned how to persuade these men to agree to disclosure. He stressed that their wives would likely find out eventually and that the emotional and medical consequences would be far more severe because of the delay. More importantly – given the soldiers' tentative decisions not to let their at-risk spouses know – he would ask whether this was a marriage they really wanted to preserve? I recall that he claimed a near perfect record in obtaining permission to notify the at-risk spouses. It would be useful if there were skilled allied caregivers, bound by confidentiality, who could routinely conduct these specialized counseling sessions. While this is not the place to set out the full range of options for a profession reliably committed to trustworthiness, it will suffice to point out a direction for professional and institutional development.

Concluding Remarks

Even if the forgoing is accepted, what may trouble doctors still is a fear that they will learn about an endangered person and be barred by this no-exceptions confidentiality rule from doing anything. Actually, there is only one thing they cannot do: disclose. All other paths remain open. Even if a reporting rule keeps many prospective patients out of the office, or silences them while they are there, the rule protects doctors from the moral risk of having to allow injury to third parties when a simple disclosure would prevent it. This distress is significant and has to be faced.

Here we must return to an error discussed earlier: the conflation of personal morality and professional ethics. Like law, personal morality can also conflict with professional responsibility. We considered a Jehovah's Witness surgeon, morally prohibited from administering blood transfusions to patients needing them. Likewise a Catholic doctor may be unable to discuss certain reproduction-related options. And despite understandable moral misgivings, doctors everywhere must be prepared to administer high-risk treatments they know will cause the deaths of some of their patients. Paradoxically, a personal inability to risk killing patients can disqualify one for the practice of medicine. While personal morality can play a decisive role in career choice, it shouldn't play a decisive role within medical ethics.

Many enter medicine believing that good citizens must prevent serious injury to others, even if that means violating other obligations. But the task of professional ethics in medicine is to set out principles that, if broadly followed, will allow the profession to discharge its collective responsibilities to patients and society. Confidentiality, I have argued, is effective at getting more patients into therapeutic alliances more quickly, it is more effective in bringing about better outcomes for more of them and – counter-intuitively – it is most likely to prevent serious harm to the largest number of at-risk third parties. Now it is ethically praiseworthy for honorable people to belong to a profession that, on balance, diminishes the amount of harm to others, even though these same professionals must sometimes knowingly allow (and sometimes even cause) harm to occur. Although doctors may feel guilty about these foreseeable consequences of their actions and inactions, they are not guilty of anything. They are acting exactly as it is reasonable to want doctors to act.

It is hard enough to create therapeutic alliances that meet patients' needs. But if doctors take on the added duty to mobilize protective responses without waivers of confidentiality, their work may become impossible in too many important cases. And all of us will be the worse for that. The thinking that places the moral comfort of clinicians above the well-being of patients and their victims is in conflict with the requirements of professional responsibility, properly understood. While it will be a challenge for many honorable physicians to measure up to this standard, no one ever said it was easy to be a good doctor.

References

Beauchamp, T. L., and J. F. Childress. 2001. *Principles of biomedical ethics*. New York: Oxford University Press.

Bok, S. 1983. *Secrets*. New York: Pantheon Books.

Goldman, A. 1980. *The philosophical foundations of professional ethics*. Totowa, NJ: Rowman & Littlefield.

Kipnis, K. 1986. *Legal ethics*. Englewood Cliffs, NJ: Prentice-Hall.

Kipnis, K. 2004. Gender, sex, and professional ethics in child and adolescent psychiatry. *Child and Adolescent Psychiatric Clinics of North America*. 13(3): 695–708.

Kottow, M. 1986. Medical confidentiality: An intransigent and absolute obligation. *Journal of Medical Ethics*. 12: 117–22.

Lo, B. 1995. *Resolving ethical dilemmas: A guide for clinicians*. Baltimore: Williams and Wilkins.

Reddy, D. M., R. Fleming, and C. Swain. 2002. Effect of mandatory parental notification on adolescent girls' use of sexual health care services. *Journal of the American Medical Association*. 288: 710–14.

Wicclair, M. 1985. A shield right for reporters vs. the administration of justice and the right to a fair trial: Is there a conflict? *Business & Professional Ethics Journal*. 4(2): 1–14.

Truth-Telling

78

On a Supposed Right to Lie from Altruistic Motives

Immanuel Kant

In the work called *France*, for the year 1797, Part VI., No. 1, on Political Reactions, by *Benjamin Constant*, the following passage occurs, p. 123: –

"The moral principle that it is one's duty to speak the truth, if it were taken singly and unconditionally, would make all society impossible. We have the proof of this in the very direct consequences which have been drawn from this principle by a German philosopher, who goes so far as to affirm that to tell a falsehood to a murderer who asked us whether our friend, of whom he was in pursuit, had not taken refuge in our house, would be a crime."

The French philosopher opposes this principle in the following manner, p. 124: – "It is a duty to tell the truth. The notion of duty is inseparable from the notion of right. A duty is what in one being corresponds to the right of another. Where there are no rights there are no duties. To tell the truth then is a duty, but only towards him who has a right to the truth. But no man has a right to a truth that injures others." The πρῶτον ψεῦδος here lies in the statement that "*To tell the truth is a duty, but only towards him who has a right to the truth.*"

It is to be remarked, first, that the expression "to have a right to the truth" is unmeaning. We should rather say, a man has a right to his own *truthfulness* (*veracitas*), that is, to subjective truth in his own person. For to have a right objectively to truth would mean that, as in *meum* and *tuum* generally, it depends on his *will* whether a given statement shall be true or false, which would produce a singular logic.

Now, the *first* question is whether a man – in cases where he cannot avoid answering Yes or No – has the *right* to be untruthful. The *second* question is whether, in order to prevent a misdeed that threatens him or some one else, he is not actually bound to be untruthful in a certain statement to which an unjust compulsion forces him.

Truth in utterances that cannot be avoided is the formal duty of a man to everyone, however great the disadvantage that may arise from it to him or any other; and although by making a false statement I do no wrong to him who unjustly compels me to speak, yet I do wrong to men in general in the most essential point of duty, so that it may be called a lie (though not in the jurist's sense), that is, so far as in me lies I cause

Original publication details: Immanuel Kant, "On a Supposed Right to Lie from Altruistic Motives," pp. 361–363 from *Critique of Practical Reason and Other Works on the Theory of Ethics*, 6th edition, trans. T. K. Abbott (London, 1909). Public domain. This essay was first published in a Berlin periodical in 1797.

that declarations in general find no credit, and hence that all rights founded on contract should lose their force; and this is a wrong which is done to mankind.

If, then, we define a lie merely as an intentionally false declaration towards another man, we need not add that it must injure another; as the jurists think proper to put in their definition (*mendacium est falsiloquium in praejudicium alterius*). For it always injures another; if not another individual, yet mankind generally, since it vitiates the source of justice. This benevolent lie *may*, however, by *accident (casus)* become punishable even by civil laws; and that which escapes liability to punishment only by accident may be condemned as a wrong even by external laws. For instance, if you have *by a lie* hindered a man who is even now planning a murder, you are legally responsible for all the consequences. But if you have strictly adhered to the truth, public justice can find no fault with you, be the unforeseen consequence what it may. It is possible that whilst you have honestly answered Yes to the murderer's question, whether his intended victim is in the house, the latter may have gone out unobserved, and so not have come in the way of the murderer, and the deed therefore have not been done; whereas, if you lied and said he was not in the house, and he had really gone out (though unknown to you), so that the murderer met him as he went, and executed his purpose on him, then you might with justice be accused as the cause of his death. For, if you had spoken the truth as well as you knew it, perhaps the murderer while seeking for his enemy in the house might have been caught by neighbours coming up and the deed been prevented. Whoever then *tells a lie*, however good his intentions may be, must answer for the consequences of it, even before the civil tribunal, and must pay the penalty for them, however unforeseen they may have been; because truthfulness is a duty that must be regarded as the basis of all duties founded on contract, the laws of which would be rendered uncertain and useless if even the least exception to them were admitted.

To be *truthful* (honest) in all declarations is therefore a sacred unconditional command of reason, and not to be limited by any expediency.

79

Should Doctors Tell the Truth?

Joseph Collins

This is not a homily on lying. It is a presentation of one of the most difficult questions that confront the physician. Should doctors tell patients the truth? Were I on the witness stand and obliged to answer the question with "yes" or "no," I should answer in the negative and appeal to the judge for permission to qualify my answer. The substance of this article is what that qualification would be.

Though few are willing to make the test, it is widely held that, if the truth were more generally told, it would make for world-welfare and human betterment. We shall probably never know. To tell the whole truth is often to perpetrate a cruelty of which many are incapable. This is particularly true of physicians. Those of them who are not compassionate by nature are made so by experience. They come to realize that they owe their fellow-men justice, and graciousness, and benignity, and it becomes one of the real satisfactions of life to discharge that obligation. To do so successfully they must frequently withhold the truth from their patients, which is tantamount to telling them a lie. Moreover, the physician soon learns that the art of medicine consists largely in skillfully mixing falsehood and truth in order to provide the patient with an amalgam which will make the metal of life wear and keep men from being poor shrunken things, full of melancholy and indisposition, unpleasing to themselves and to those who love them. I propose therefore to deal with the question from a pragmatic, not a moral standpoint.

"Now you may tell me the truth," is one of the things patients have frequently said to me. Four types of individuals have said it: those who honestly and courageously want to know so that they may make as ready as possible to face the wages of sin while there is still time; those who do not want to know, and who if they were told would be injured by it; those who are wholly incapable of receiving the truth. Finally, those whose health is neither seriously disordered nor threatened. It may seem an exaggeration to say that in forty years of contact with the sick, the patients I have met who are in the first category could be counted on the fingers of one hand. The vast majority who demand the truth really belong in the fourth category, but there are sufficient in the second – with whom my concern chiefly is – to justify considering their case.

Original publication details: Joseph Collins, "Should Doctors Tell the Truth?" pp. 320–326 from *Harper's Monthly Magazine* 155 (August 1927).

Bioethics: An Anthology, Fourth Edition. Edited by Udo Schüklenk and Peter Singer.

One of the astonishing things about patients is that the more serious the disease, the more silent they are about its portents and manifestations. The man who is constantly seeking assurance that the vague abdominal pains indicative of hyperacidity are not symptoms of cancer often buries family and friends, some of whom have welcomed death as an escape from his burdensome iterations. On the other hand, there is the man whose first warning of serious disease is lumbago who cannot be persuaded to consult a physician until the disease, of which the lumbago is only a symptom, has so far progressed that it is beyond surgery. The seriousness of disease may be said to stand in direct relation to the reticence of its possessor. The more silent the patient, the more serious the disorder.

The patient with a note-book, or the one who is eager to tell his story in great detail, is rarely very ill. They are forever asking, "Am I going to get well?" and though they crave assistance they are often unable to accept it. On the other hand, patients with organic disease are very chary about asking point blank either the nature or the outcome of their ailment. They sense its gravity, and the last thing in the world they wish to know is the truth about it; and to learn it would be the worst thing that could happen to them.

This was borne in upon me early in my professional life. I was summoned one night to assuage the pain of a man who informed me that he had been for some time under treatment for rheumatism – that cloak for so many diagnostic errors. His "rheumatism" was due to a disease of the spinal cord called locomotor ataxia. When he was told that he should submit himself to treatment wholly different from that which he had been receiving, the import of which any intelligent layman would have divined, he asked neither the nature nor the probable outcome of the disease. He did as he was counselled. He is now approaching seventy and, though not active in business, it still engrosses him.

Had he been told that he had a disease which was then universally believed to be progressive, apprehension would have depressed him so heavily that he would not have been able to offer the resistance to its encroachment which has stood him in such good stead. He was told the truth only in part. That is, he was told his "rheumatism" was "different"; that it was dependent upon an organism quite unlike the one that causes ordinary rheumatism; that we have preparations of mercury and arsenic which kill the parasite responsible for this disease, and that if he would submit himself to their use, his life would not be materially shortened, or his efficiency seriously impaired.

Many experiences show that patients do not want the truth about their maladies, and that it is prejudicial to their well-being to know it, but none that I know is more apposite than that of a lawyer, noted for his urbanity and resourcefulness in Court. When he entered my consulting room, he greeted me with a bonhomie that bespoke intimacy but I had met him only twice – once on the golf links many years before, and once in Court where I was appearing as expert witness, prejudicial to his case.

He apologized for engaging my attention with such a triviality, but he had had pain in one shoulder and arm for the past few months, and though he was perfectly well – and had been assured of it by physicians in Paris, London, and Brooklyn – this pain was annoying and he had made up his mind to get rid of it. That I should not get a wrong slant on his condition, he submitted a number of laboratory reports furnished him by an osteopath to show that secretions and excretions susceptible of chemical examinations were quite normal. His determination seemed to be to prevent me from taking a view of his health which might lead me to counsel his retirement. He was quite sure that anything like a thorough examination was unnecessary but he submitted to it. It revealed intense and extensive disease of the kidneys. The pain in the network of nerves of the left upper-arm was a manifestation of the resulting autointoxication.

I felt it incumbent upon me to tell him that his condition was such that he should make a radical change in his mode of life. I told him if he would stop work, spend the winter in Honolulu, go on a diet suitable to a child of three years, and give up exercise, he could look forward confidently to a recovery that would permit of a life of usefulness and activity in his profession. He assured me he could not believe that one who felt no worse than he did should have to make such a radical change in his mode of life. He impressed upon me that I should realize he was the kind of person who had to know the truth. His affairs were so diversified and his commitments so important that he *must* know. Completely taken in, I explained to him the relationship between the pain from which he sought relief and the disease, the degeneration that was going on in the excretory mechanisms of his body, how these were struggling to repair themselves, the procedure of recovery and how it could be facilitated. The light of life began to flicker from the fear that my words engendered, and within two months it sputtered and died out. He was the last person in the world to whom the truth should have been told. Had I lied to him, and then intrigued with his family and friends, he might be alive today.

The longer I practice medicine the more I am convinced that every physician should cultivate lying as a fine art. But there are many varieties of lying. Some are most prejudicial to the physician's usefulness. Such are: pretending to recognize the disease and understand its nature when one is really ignorant; asserting that one has effected the cure which nature has accomplished, or claiming that one can effect cure of a disease which is universally held to be beyond the power of nature or medical skill; pronouncing disease incurable which one cannot rightfully declare to be beyond cessation or relief.

There are other lies, however, which contribute enormously to the success of the physician's mission of mercy and salvation. There are a great number of instances in support of this but none more convincing than that of a man of fifty who, after twenty-five years of devotion to painting, decided that penury and old age were incompatible for him. Some of his friends had forsaken art for advertising. He followed their lead and in five years he was ready to gather the first ripe fruit of his labor. When he attempted to do so he was so immobilized by pain and rigidity that he had to forgo work. One of those many persons who assume responsibility lightly assured him that if he would put himself in the hands of a certain osteopath

he would soon be quite fit. The assurance was without foundation. He then consulted a physician who without examining him proceeded to treat him for what is considered a minor ailment.

Within two months his appearance gave such concern to his family that he was persuaded to go to a hospital, where the disease was quickly detected, and he was at once submitted to surgery. When he had recovered from the operation, learning that I was in the country of his adoption, he asked to see me. He had not been able, he said, to get satisfactory information from the surgeon or the physician; all that he could gather from them was that he would have to have supplementary X-ray or radium treatment. What he desired was to get back to his business which was on the verge of success, and he wanted assurance that he could soon do so.

He got it. And more than that, he got elaborate explanation of what surgical intervention had accomplished, but not a word of what it had failed to accomplish. A year of activity was vouchsafed him, and during that time he put his business in such shape that its eventual sale provided a modest competency for his family. It was not until the last few weeks that he knew the nature of his malady. Months of apprehension had been spared him by the deception, and he had been the better able to do his work, for he was buoyed by the hope that his health was not beyond recovery. Had he been told the truth, black despair would have been thrown over the world in which he moved, and he would have carried on with corresponding ineffectiveness.

The more extensive our field of observation and the more intimate our contact with human activity, the more we realize the finiteness of the human mind. Every follower of Hippocrates will agree that "judgment is difficult and experience fallacious." A disease may have only a fatal ending, but one does not know; one may know that certain diseases, such as general paresis, invariably cause death, but one does not know that tomorrow it may no longer be true. The victim may be reprieved by accidental or studied discovery or by the intervention of something that still must be called divine grace.

A few years ago physicians were agreed that diabetes occurring in children was incurable; recently they held that the disease known as pernicious anemia always ended fatally; but now, armed with an extract from the pancreas and the liver, they go out to attack these diseases with the kind of confidence that David had when he saw the Philistine approach.

We have had enough experience to justify the hope that soon we shall be able to induce a little devil who is manageable to cast out a big devil who is wholly out of hand – to cure general paresis by inoculating the victim with malaria, and to shape the course of some varieties of sleeping sickness by the same means.

I am thankful for many valuable lessons learned from my early teachers. One of them was an ophthalmologist of great distinction. I worked for three years in his clinic. He was the most brutally frank doctor I have known. He could say to a woman, without the slightest show of emotion, that she was developing a cataract and would eventually be blind. I asked a colleague, who was a co-worker in the clinic at that time and who has since become an eminent specialist, if all these patients developed complete opacity of the crystalline lens.

"Not one half of them," said he. "In many instances the process is so slow that the patient dies before the cataract arrives; in others it ceases to progress. It is time enough for the patient to know he has cataract when he knows for himself that he is going blind. Then I can always explain it to him in such a way that he does not have days of apprehension and nights of sleeplessness for months while awaiting operation. I have made it a practice not to tell a patient he has cataract."

"Yes, but what do you tell them when they say they have been to Doctor Smith who tells them they have cataract and they have come to you for denial or corroboration?"

"I say to them, 'You have a beginning cloudiness of the lens of one eye. I have seen many cases in which the opacity progressed no farther than it has in your case; I have seen others which did not reach blindness in twenty years. I shall change your glasses, and I think you will find that your vision will be improved.'"

And then he added, "In my experience there are two things patients cannot stand being told: that they have cataract or cancer."

There is far less reason for telling them of the former than the latter. The hope for victims of the latter is bound up wholly in early detection and surgical interference. That is one of the most cogent reasons for bi-yearly thorough physical examination after the age of forty-five. Should we ever feel the need of a new law in this country, the one I suggest would exact such examination. The physician who detects malignant disease in its early stages is never justified in telling the patient the real nature of the disease. In fact, he does not know himself until he gets the pathologist's report. Should that indicate grave malignancy no possible good can flow from sharing that knowledge with the patient.

It is frequently to a patient's great advantage to know the truth in part, for it offers him the reason for making a radical change in his mode of life, sometimes a burdensome change. But not once in a hundred instances is a physician justified in telling a patient point blank that he has epilepsy, or the family that he has dementia præcox, until after he has been under observation a long time, unless these are so obvious that even a layman can make the diagnosis. We do not know the real significance of either disease, or from what they flow – we know that so many of them terminate in dementia that the outlook for all of them is bad. But we also know that many cases so diagnosticated end in complete recovery; and that knowledge justifies us in withholding from a patient the name and nature of his disorder until we are beyond all shadow of doubt.

Patients who are seriously ill are greedy for assurance even when it is offered half-heartedly. But those who have ailments which give the physician no real concern often cannot accept assurance. Not infrequently I have been unable to convince patients with nervous indigestion that their fears and concern were without foundation, and yet, years later when they developed organic disease, and I became really concerned about them, they assured me that I was taking their ailments too seriously.

There was a young professor whose acquaintance I made while at a German university. When he returned he took a position as professor in one of the well-known colleges for women. After several years he consulted me for the relief of symptoms which are oftentimes associated with gastric ulcer. It required no elaborate investigation to show that in this instance the symptoms were indicative of an imbalance of his nervous system. He refused to be assured and took umbrage that he was not given a more thorough examination each time that he visited me. Finally he told me that he would no longer attempt to conceal from me that he understood fully my reasons for making light of the matter. It was to throw him off the track, as it were. No good was to be accomplished from trying to deceive him; he realized the gravity of the situation and he was man enough to confront it. He would not show the white feather, and he was entitled to know the truth.

But the more it was proffered him, the greater was his resistance to it. He gave up his work and convinced his family and friends that he was seriously ill. They came to see me in relays; they also refused to accept the truth. They could understand why I told the patient the matter was not serious, but to them I could tell the facts. It was their right to know, and I could depend upon them to keep the knowledge from the patient and to work harmoniously with me.

My failure with my patient's friends was as great as with the patient himself. Fully convinced his back was to the wall, he refused to be looked upon as a lunatic or a hypochondriac and he decided to seek other counsel. He went from specialist to naturopath, from electrotherapist to Christian Scientist, from sanatorium to watering place and, had there been gland doctors and chiropractors in those days, he would have included them as well. Finally, he migrated to the mountains of Tennessee, and wooed nature. Soon I heard of him as the head of a school which was being run on novel pedagogic lines; character-building and health were the chief aims for his pupils; scholastic education was incidental. He began writing and lecturing about his work and his accomplishments, and soon achieved considerable notoriety. I saw him occasionally when he came north and sometimes referred to his long siege of ill-health and how happily it had terminated. He always made light of it, and declared that in one way it had been a very good thing: had it not been for that illness he would never have found himself, never have initiated the work which was giving him repute, happiness, and competency.

One summer I asked him to join me for a canoe trip down the Allegash River. Some of the "carrys" in those days were rather stiff. After one of them I saw that my friend was semi-prostrated and flustered. On questioning him, I learned that he had several times before experienced disagreeable sensations in the chest and in the head after hard manual labor, such as chopping trees or prying out rocks. He protested against examination but finally yielded. I reminded myself how different it was fifteen years before when he clamored for examination and seemed to get both pleasure and satisfaction from it, particularly when it was elaborate and protracted. He had organic disease of the heart, both of the valve-mechanism and of the muscle. His tenure of life depended largely on the way he lived. To counsel him successfully it was necessary to tell him that his heart had become somewhat damaged. He would not have it. "When I was really ill you made light of it, and I could not get you interested. But now, when I am well, you want me to live the life of a dodo. I won't do it. My heart is quite all right, a little upset no doubt by the fare we have had for the past two weeks, but as soon as I get back to normal I shall be as fit as you are, perhaps more so."

We returned to New York and I persuaded him to see a specialist, who was no more successful in impressing him with the necessity of careful living than I was. In despair, I wrote to his wife. She who had been so solicitous, so apprehensive, and so deaf to assurance during the illness that was of no consequence wrote, "I am touched by your affectionate interest, but Jerome seems so well that I have not the heart to begin nagging him again, and it fills me with terror lest he should once more become introspective and self-solicitous. I am afraid if I do what you say that it might start him off again on the old tack, and the memory of those two years frightens me still."

He died about four years later without the benefit of physician.

No one can stand the whole truth about himself; why should we think he can tolerate it about his health, and even though he could, who knows the truth? Physicians have opinions based upon their own and others' experience. They should be chary of expressing those opinions to sick persons until they have studied their psychology and are familiar with their personality. Even then it should always be an opinion, not a sentence. Doctors should be detectives and counsellors, not juries and judges.

Though often it seems a cruelty, the family of the patient to whom the truth is not and should not be told are entitled to the facts or what the physician believes to be the facts. At times, they must conspire with him to keep the truth from the patient, who will learn it too soon no matter what skill they display in deception. On the other hand, it is frequently to the patient's great advantage that the family should not know the depth of the physician's concern, lest their unconcealable apprehension be conveyed to the patient and then transformed into the medium in which disease waxes strong – fear. Now and then the good doctor keeps his own counsel. It does not profit the family of the man whose coronary arteries are under suspicion to be told that he has angina pectoris. If the patient can be induced to live decorously, the physician has discharged his obligation.

I recall so many instances when the truth served me badly that I find it difficult to select the best example. On reflection, I have decided to cite the case of a young man who consulted me shortly after his marriage.

He was sane in judgment, cheerful in disposition, full of the desire to attract those who attracted him. Anything touching on the morbid or "unnatural" was obviously repellent to him. His youth had been a pleasant one, surrounded by affection, culture, understanding, and wealth. When he graduated he had not made up his mind what he wanted to do in the world. After a year of loafing and traveling he decided to become an engineer. He matriculated at one of the technical schools, and his work there was satisfactory to himself and to his professors.

He astonished his intimates shortly after obtaining a promising post by marrying a woman a few years older than himself who was known to some of them as a devotee of bohemian life that did not tally with the position in society to which she was entitled by family and wealth. She had been a favorite with men but she had a reputation of not being the "marrying kind."

My friend fell violently in love with her, and her resistance went down before it. His former haunts knew him no more, and I did not see him for several months. Then, late one evening, he telephoned to say that it was of the greatest importance to him to consult me. He arrived in a state of repressed excitement. He wanted it distinctly understood that he came to me as a client, not as a friend. I knew, of course, that he had married. This, he confessed, had proved a complete failure, and now his wife had gone away and with another woman, one whom he had met constantly at her home during his brief and tempestuous courtship.

I attempted to explain to him that she had probably acted on impulse; that the squabbles of early matrimony which often appeared to be tragedies, were adjustable and, fortunately, nearly always adjusted.

"Yes," said he, "but you don't understand. There hasn't been any row. My wife told me shortly after marrying me that she had made a mistake, and she has told me so many times since. I thought at first it was caprice. Perhaps I should still have thought so were it not for this letter." He then handed me a letter. I did not have to read between the lines to get the full significance of its content. It set forth briefly, concretely, and explicitly her reasons for leaving. Life without her former friend was intolerable, and she did not propose to attempt it longer.

He knew there were such persons in the world, but what he wanted to know from me was, Could they not, if properly and prudently handled, be brought to feel and love like those the world calls normal? Was it not possible that her conduct and confession were the result of a temporary derangement and that indulgent handling of her would make her see things in the right light? She had not alienated his love even though she had forfeited his respect; and he did not attempt to conceal from me that if the tangle could not be straightened out he felt that his life had been a failure.

I told him the truth about this enigmatic gesture of nature, that the victims of this strange abnormality are often of great brilliancy and charm, and most companionable; that it is not a disease and, therefore, cannot be cured.

In this instance, basing my opinion upon what his wife had told him both in speech and in writing,

I was bound to believe that she was one of the strange sisterhood, and that it was her birthright as well as her misfortune. Such being the case, I could only advise what I thought might be best for their mutual and individual happiness. I suggested that divorce offered the safest way out for both. He replied that he felt competent to decide that for himself; all that he sought from me was enlightenment about her unnatural infatuation. This I had only too frankly given him.

Two days later his body with a pistol wound in the right temple was found in a field above Weehawken.

That day I regretted that I had not lied to him. It is a day that has had frequent anniversaries.

80

On Telling Patients the Truth

Roger Higgs

That honesty should be an important issue for debate in medical circles may seem bizarre. Nurses and doctors are usually thought of as model citizens. Outside the immediate field of health care, when a passport is to be signed, a reference given, or a special allowance made by a government welfare agency, a nurse's or doctor's signature is considered a good warrant, and false certification treated as a serious breach of professional conduct. Yet at the focus of medical activity or skill, at the bedside or in the clinic, when patient meets professional there is often doubt. Is the truth being told?

Many who are unfamiliar with illness and its treatment may well be forgiven for wondering if this doubt has not been exaggerated. It is as if laundry-men were to discuss the merits of clean clothes, or fishmongers of refrigeration. But those with experience, either as patients or professionals, will immediately recognize the situation. Although openness is increasingly practised, there is still uncertainty in the minds of many doctors or nurses faced with communicating bad news; as for instance when a test shows up an unexpected and probably incurable cancer, or when meeting the gaze of a severely ill child, or answering the questions of a mother in mid-pregnancy whose unborn child is discovered to be badly disabled. What should be said? There can be few who have not, on occasions such as these, told less than the truth. Certainly the issue is a regular preoccupation of nurses and doctors in training. Why destroy hope? Why create anxiety, or something worse? Isn't it 'First, do no harm'?[1]

The concerns of the patient are very different. For many, fear of the unknown is the worst disease of all, and yet direct information seems so hard to obtain. The ward round goes past quickly, unintelligible words are muttered – was I supposed to hear and understand? In the surgery the general practitioner signs his prescription pad and clearly it's time to be gone. Everybody is too busy saving lives to give explanations. It may come as a shock to learn that it is policy, not just pressure of work, that prevents a patient learning the truth about himself. If truth is the first casualty, trust must be the second. 'Of course they wouldn't say, especially if things were bad,' said the elderly woman just back from out-patients, 'they've got that Oath, haven't they?' She had learned to expect from doctors, at the

Original publication details: Roger Higgs, "On Telling Patients the Truth," pp. 186–202 and 232–233 from Michael Lockwood (ed.), *Moral Dilemmas in Modern Medicine* (Oxford: Oxford University Press, 1985). Reproduced with permission of Oxford University Press.

best, silence; at the worst, deception. It was part of the system, an essential ingredient, as old as Hippocrates. However honest a citizen, it was somehow part of the doctor's job not to tell the truth to his patient. . .

It is easier to decide what to do when the ultimate outcome is clear. It may be much more difficult to know what to say when the future is less certain, such as in the first episode of what is probably multiple sclerosis, or when a patient is about to undergo a mutilating operation. But even in work outside hospital, where such dramatic problems arise less commonly, whether to tell the truth and how much to tell can still be a regular issue. How much should this patient know about the side effects of his drugs? An elderly man sits weeping in an old people's home, and the healthy but exhausted daughter wants the doctor to tell her father that she's medically unfit to have him back. The single mother wants a certificate to say that she is unwell so that she can stay at home to look after her sick child. A colleague is often drunk on duty, and is making mistakes. A husband with venereal disease wants his wife to be treated without her knowledge. An outraged father demands to know if his teenage daughter has been put on the pill. A mother comes in with a child to have a boil lanced. 'Please tell him it won't hurt.' A former student writes from abroad needing to complete his professional experience and asks for a reference for a job he didn't do.[2] Whether the issue is large or small, the truth is at stake. What should the response be?

Discussion of the apparently more dramatic situations may provide a good starting-point. Recently a small group of medical students, new to clinical experience, were hotly debating what a patient with cancer should be told. One student maintained strongly that the less said to the patient the better. Others disagreed. When asked whether there was any group of patients they could agree should never be told the truth about a life-threatening illness, the students chose children, and agreed that they would not speak openly to children under six. When asked to try to remember what life was like when they were six, one student replied that he remembered how his mother had died when he was that age. Suddenly the student who had advocated non-disclosure became animated. 'That's extraordinary. My mother died when I was six too. My father said she'd gone away for a time, but would come back soon. One day he said she was coming home again. My younger sister and I were very excited. We waited at the window upstairs until we saw his car drive up. He got out and helped a woman out of the car. Then we saw. It wasn't mum. I suppose I never forgave him – or her, really.'[3]

It is hard to know with whom to sympathize in this sad tale. But its stark simplicity serves to highlight some essential points. First, somehow more clearly than in the examples involving patients, not telling the truth is seen for what it really is. It is, of course, quite possible, and very common in clinical practice, for doctors (or nurses) to engage in deliberate deceit without actually *saying* anything they believe to be false. But, given the special responsibilities of the doctor, and the relationship of trust that exists between him and his patient, one could hardly argue that this was morally any different from telling outright lies. Surely it is the *intention* that is all important. We may be silent, tactful, or reserved, but, if we intend to deceive, what we are doing is tantamount to lying. The debate in ward or surgery is suddenly stood on its head. The question is no longer 'Should we tell the truth?' but 'What justification is there for telling a lie?' This relates to the second important point, that medical ethics are part of general morality, and not a separate field of their own with their own rules. Unless there are special justifications, health-care professionals are working within the same moral constraints as lay people. A lie is a lie wherever told and whoever tells it.

But do doctors have a special dispensation from the usual principles that guide the conduct of our society? It is widely felt that on occasion they do, and such a dispensation is as necessary to all doctors as freedom from the charge of assault is to a surgeon. But, if it is impossible to look after ill patients and always be open and truthful, how can we balance this against the clear need for truthfulness on all other occasions? If deception is like a medicine to be given in certain doses in certain cases, what guidance exists about its administration?

My elderly patient reflected the widely held view that truth-telling, or perhaps withholding, was part of the tradition of medicine enshrined in its oaths and codes. Although the writer of the 'Decorum' in the Hippocratic corpus advises physicians of the danger of telling patients about the nature of their illness '. . . for many patients through this cause have taken a turn for the worse',[4] the Oath itself is completely silent on this issue. This extraordinary omission is continued through all the more modern codes and declarations. The first mention of veracity as a principle is to be found in the American Medical Association's 'Principles of Ethics' of 1980, which states that the physician should 'deal honestly with patients and colleagues and strive to expose those physicians deficient in character or competence, or who engage in fraud and deception'.[5] Despite the difficulties of the latter injunction, which seems in some way to divert attention from the basic need for honest communication with the patient, here at last is a clear statement. This declaration signally fails, however, to provide the guidance that we might perhaps have expected for the professional facing his or her individual dilemma.

The reticence of these earlier codes is shared, with some important exceptions, by medical writing elsewhere. Until recently most of what had been usefully said could be summed up by the articles of medical writers such as Thomas Percival, Worthington Hooker, Richard Cabot, and Joseph Collins, which show a wide scatter of view points but do at least confront the problems directly.[6] There is, however, one widely quoted statement by Lawrence Henderson, writing in the *New England Journal of Medicine* in 1935.[7] 'It is meaningless to speak of telling the truth, the whole truth and nothing but the truth to a patient. . .because it is. . .a sheer impossibility. . .Since telling the truth is impossible, there can be no sharp distinction between what is true and what is false.'. . .

But we must not allow ourselves to be confused, as Henderson was, and as so many others have been, by a failure to distinguish between truth, the abstract concept, of which we shall always have an imperfect grasp, and *telling* the truth, where the intention is all important. Whether or not we can ever fully grasp or express the whole picture, whether we know ultimately what the truth really is, we must speak truthfully, and intend to convey what we understand, or we shall lie. In Sissela Bok's words, 'The moral question of whether you are lying or not is not *settled* by establishing the truth or falsity of what you say. In order to settle the question, we must know whether you *intend your statement to mislead*.'[8]

Most modern thinkers in the field of medical ethics would hold that truthfulness is indeed a central principle of conduct, but that it is capable of coming into conflict with other principles, to which it must occasionally give way. On the other hand, the principle of veracity often receives support from other principles. For instance, it is hard to see how a patient can have autonomy, can make a free choice about matters concerning himself, without some measure of understanding of the facts as they influence the case; and that implies, under normal circumstances, some open, honest discussion with his advisers.[9] Equally, consent is a nonsense if it is not in some sense informed. . .

Once the central position of honesty has been established, we still need to examine whether doctors and nurses really do have, as has been suggested, special exemption from being truthful because of the nature of their work, and if so under what circumstances. . .It may finally be decided that in a crisis there is no acceptable alternative, as when life is ebbing and truthfulness would bring certain disaster. Alternatively, the moral issue may appear so trivial as not to be worth considering (as, for example, when a doctor is called out at night by a patient who apologizes by saying, 'I hope you don't mind me calling you at this time, doctor', and the doctor replies, 'No, not at all.'). However. . .occasions of these two types are few, fewer than those in which deliberate deceit would generally be regarded as acceptable in current medical practice, and should regularly be debated 'in public' if abuses are to be avoided.[10] To this end it is necessary now to examine critically the arguments commonly used to defend lying to patients.

First comes the argument that it is enormously difficult to put across a technical subject to those with little technical knowledge and understanding, in a situation where so little is predictable. A patient has bowel cancer. With surgery it might be cured, or it might recur. Can the patient understand the effects of treatment? The symptom she is now getting might be due to cancer, there might be secondaries, and they in turn might be suppressible for a long time, or not at all. What future symptoms might occur, how long will she live, how will she die – all these are desperately important questions for the patient, but even for her doctor the answers can only be informed guesses, in an area where uncertainty is so hard to bear.

Yet to say we do not know anything is a lie. As doctors we know a great deal, and *can* make informed guesses or offer likelihoods. The whole truth may be impossible to attain, but truthfulness is not. 'I do not know' can be a major piece of honesty. To deprive the patient of honest communication because we cannot know everything is, as we have seen, not only confused thinking but immoral. Thus deprived, the patient cannot plan, he cannot choose. If choice is the crux of morality, it may also, as we have argued elsewhere, be central to health. If he cannot choose, the patient cannot ever be considered to be fully restored to health.[11]

This argument also raises another human failing – to confuse the difficult with the unimportant. Passing information to people who have more restricted background, whether through lack of experience or of understanding, can be extremely difficult and time-consuming, but this is no reason why it should be shunned. Quite the reverse. Like the difficult passages in a piece of music, these tasks should be practised, studied, and techniques developed so that communication is efficient and effective. For the purposes of informed consent, the patient must be given the information he needs, as a reasonable person, to make a reasoned choice.

The second argument for telling lies to patients is that no patient likes hearing depressing or frightening news. That is certainly true. There must be few who do. But in other walks of life no professional would normally consider it his or her duty to suppress information simply in order to preserve happiness. No accountant, foreseeing bankruptcy in his client's affairs, would chat cheerfully about the Budget or a temporarily reassuring credit account. Yet such suppression of information occurs daily in wards or surgeries throughout the country. Is this what patients themselves want?

In order to find out, a number of studies have been conducted over the past thirty years.[12] In most studies there is a significant minority of patients, perhaps about a fifth, who, if given information, deny having been told. Sometimes this must be pure forgetfulness, sometimes it relates to the lack of skill of the informer, but sometimes with bad or unwelcome news there is an element of what is (perhaps not quite correctly) called 'denial'. The observer feels that at one level the news has been taken in, but at another its validity or reality has not been accepted. This process has been recognized as a buffer for the mind against the shock of unacceptable news, and often seems to be part of a process leading to its ultimate acceptance.[13] But once this group has been allowed for, most surveys find that, of those who have had or who could have had a diagnosis made of, say, cancer, between two-thirds and three-quarters of those questioned were either glad to have been told, or declared that they would wish to know. Indeed, surveys reveal that most *doctors* would themselves wish to be told the truth, even though (according to earlier studies at least) most of those same doctors said they would not speak openly to their patients – a curious double standard! Thus these surveys have unearthed, at least for the present, a common misunderstanding between doctors and patients, a general preference for openness among patients, and a significant but small group whose wish not to be informed must surely be respected. We return once more to the skill needed to detect such differences in the individual case, and the need for training in such skills.

Why doctors have for so long misunderstood their patients' wishes is perhaps related to the task itself. Doctors don't want to give bad news, just as patients don't want it in abstract, but doctors have the choice of withholding the information, and in so doing protecting themselves from the pain of telling and from the blame of being the bearer of bad news. In addition it has been suggested that doctors are particularly fearful of death and illness. Montaigne suggested that men have to think about death and be prepared to accept it, and one would think that doctors would get used to death. Yet perhaps this very familiarity has created an obsession that amounts to fear. Just as the police seem over-concerned with violence, and firemen with fire, perhaps doctors have met death in their professional training only as the enemy, never as something to come to terms with, or even as a natural force to be respected and, when the time is ripe, accepted or even welcomed.

Undeniably, doctors and nurses like helping people and derive much satisfaction from the feeling that the patient is being benefited. This basic feeling has been elevated to major status in medical practice. The principle of beneficence – to work for the patient's good – and the related principle of non-maleficence – 'first do no harm' – are usually quoted as the central guiding virtues in medicine. They are expanded in the codes, and underlie the appeal of utilitarian arguments in the context of health care. 'When you are thinking of telling a lie,' Richard Cabot quotes a teacher of his as saying, 'ask yourself whether it is simply and solely for the patient's benefit that you are going to tell it. If you are sure that you are acting for his good and not for your own profit, you can go ahead with a clear conscience.'[14] But who should decide what is 'for the patient's benefit'? Why should it be the doctor? Increasingly society is uneasy with such a paternalistic style. In most other walks of life the competent individual is himself assumed to be the best judge of his own interests. Whatever may be thought of this assumption in the field of politics or law, to make one's own decisions on matters that are central to one's own life or welfare and do not directly concern others would normally be held to be a basic *right*; and hardly one to be taken away simply on the grounds of illness, whether actual or merely potential.

Thus if beneficence is assumed to be the key principle, which many now have come to doubt, it can easily ride roughshod over autonomy and natural justice. A lie denies a person the chance of participating in choices concerning his own health, including that

of whether to be a 'patient' at all. Paternalism may be justifiable in the short term, and to 'kid' someone, to treat him as a child because he is ill, and perhaps dying, may be very tempting. Yet true respect for that person (adult or child) can only be shown by allowing him allowable choices, by granting him whatever control is left, as weakness gradually undermines his hold on life. If respect is important then at the very least there must be no acceptable or effective alternative to lying in a particular situation if the lie is to be justified. . .

However, a third argument for lying can be advanced, namely, that truthfulness can actually do harm. 'What you don't know can't hurt you' is a phrase in common parlance (though it hardly fits with concepts of presymptomatic screening for preventable disease!). However, it is undeniable that blunt and unfeeling communication of unpleasant truths can cause acute distress, and sometimes long-term disability. The fear that professionals often have of upsetting people, of causing a scene, of making fools of themselves by letting unpleasant emotions flourish, seems to have elevated this argument beyond its natural limits. It is not unusual to find that the fear of creating harm will deter a surgical team from discussing a diagnosis gently with a patient, but not deter it from performing radical and mutilating surgery. Harm is a very personal concept. Most medical schools have, circulating in the refectory, a story about a patient who was informed that he had cancer and then leapt to his death. The intended moral for the medical student is, keep your mouth shut and do no harm. But that may not be the correct lesson to be learned from such cases (which I believe, in any case, to be less numerous than is commonly supposed). The style of telling could have been brutal, with no follow-up or support. It may have been the suggested treatment, not the basic illness, that led the patient to resort to such a desperate measure. Suicide in illness is remarkably rare, but, though tragic, could be seen as a logical response to an overwhelming challenge. No mention is usually made of suicide rates in other circumstances, or the isolation felt by ill and warded patients, or the feelings of anger uncovered when someone takes such precipitate and forbidden action against himself. What these cases do, surely, is argue, not for no telling, but for better telling, for sensitivity and care in determining how much the patient wants to know, explaining carefully in ways the patient can understand, and providing full support and 'after-care' as in other treatments.

But even if it is accepted that the short-term effect of telling the truth may sometimes be considerable psychological disturbance, in the long term the balance seems definitely to swing the other way. The effects of lying are dramatically illustrated in 'A Case of Obstructed Death?'[15] False information prevented a woman from returning to healthy living after a cancer operation, and robbed her of six months of active life. Also, the long-term effect of lies on the family and, perhaps most importantly, on society, is incalculable. If trust is gradually corroded, if the 'wells are poisoned', progress is hard. Mistrust creates lack of communication and increased fear, and this generation has seen just such a fearful myth created around cancer.[16] Just how much harm has been done by this 'demonizing' of cancer, preventing people coming to their doctors, or alternatively creating unnecessary attendances on doctors, will probably never be known.

There are doubtless many other reasons why doctors lie to their patients; but these can hardly be used to justify lies, even if we should acknowledge them in passing. Knowledge is power, and certainly doctors, though usually probably for reasons of work-load rather than anything more sinister, like to remain 'in control'. Health professionals may, like others, wish to protect themselves from confrontation, and may find it easier to coerce or manipulate than to gain permission. There may be a desire to avoid any pressure for change. And there is the constant problem of lack of time. But, in any assessment, the key issues remain. Not telling the truth normally involves telling lies, and doctors and nurses have no *carte blanche* to lie. . .

If the importance of open communication with the patient is accepted, we need to know when to say what. If a patient is going for investigations, it may be possible at that time, before details are known, to have a discussion about whether he would like to know the details. A minor 'contract' can be made. 'I promise to tell you what I know, if you ask me.' Once that time is past, however, it requires skill and sensitivity to assess what a patient wants to know. Allowing the time and opportunity for the patient to ask questions is the most important thing, but one must realize that the patient's apparent question may conceal the one he really wants answered. 'Do I have cancer?' may contain the more important questions 'How or when will I die?' 'Will there be pain?' The doctor will not necessarily be helping by giving an extended pathology lesson. The informer may need to know more: 'I don't want to avoid your question, and I promise to answer as truthfully as I can, but first. . .' It has been pointed out that in many cases the terminal patient will tell the doctor, not vice versa, if the right opportunities are created and the style and timing is appropriate. Then it is a question of not telling but listening to the truth.[17]

If in spite of all this there still seems to be a need to tell lies, we must be able to justify them. That the person is a child, or 'not very bright', will not do. Given the two ends of the spectrum of crisis and triviality, the vast middle range of communication requires honesty, so that autonomy and choice can be maintained. If lies are to be told, there really must be no acceptable alternative. The analogy with force may again be helpful here: perhaps using the same style of thinking as is used in the Mental Health Act, to test whether we are justified in removing someone's liberty against their will, may help us to see the gravity of what we are doing when we consider deception. It also suggests that the decision should be shared, in confidence, and be subject to debate, so that any alternative which may not initially have been seen may be considered. And it does not end there. If we break an important moral principle, that principle still retains its force, and its 'shadow' has to be acknowledged. As professionals we shall have to ensure that we follow up, that we work through the broken trust or the disillusionment that the lie will bring to the patient, just as we would follow up and work through bad news, a major operation, or a psychiatric 'sectioning'. This follow-up may also be called for in our relationship with our colleagues if there has been major disagreement about what should be done.

In summary, there are *some* circumstances in which the health professions are probably exempted from society's general requirement for truthfulness. But not telling the truth is usually the same as telling a lie, and a lie requires strong justification. Lying must be a last resort, and we should act as if we were to be called upon to defend the decision in public debate, even if our duty of confidentiality does not allow this in practice. We should always aim to respect the other important principles governing interactions with patients, especially the preservation of the patient's autonomy. When all is said and done, many arguments for individual cases of lying do not hold water. Whether or not knowing the truth is essential to the patient's health, telling the truth is essential to the health of the doctor–patient relationship.

Notes

1   *Primum non nocere* – this is a Latinization of a statement which is not directly Hippocratic, but may be derived from the *Epidemics* Book 1 Chapter II: 'As to diseases, make a habit of two things – to help, or at least do no harm.' *Hippocrates*, 4 vols (London: William Heinemann, 1923–31), vol. I, trans. W. H. S. Jones.

2   Cases collected by the author in his own practice.

3   Case collected by the author.

4   Quoted in Reiser, Dyck, and Curran (eds), *Ethics in Medicine, Historical Perspectives and Contemporary Concerns* (Cambridge, MA: MIT Press, 1977).

5   American Medical Association, 'Text of the American Medical Association New Principles of Medical Ethics', *American Medical News* (August 1–8 1980), 9.

6   To be found in Reiser et al., *Ethics in Medicine*.

7   Lawrence Henderson, 'Physician and Patient as a Social System', *New England Journal of Medicine*, 212 (1935).

8   Sissela Bok, *Lying: Moral Choice in Public and Private Life* (London: Quartet, 1980).

9   Alastair Campbell and Roger Higgs, *In That Case* (London: Darton, Longman and Todd, 1982).

10   John Rawls, *A Theory of Justice* (Cambridge, MA: Harvard University Press, Belknap Press, 1971).

11   See Campbell and Higgs, *In That Case*.

12   Summarized well in Robert Veatch, 'Truth-telling I' in *Encyclopaedia of Bioethics*, ed. Warren T. Reich (New York: Free Press, 1978).

13   The five stages of reacting to bad news, or news of dying, are described in *On Death and Dying* by Elizabeth Kubler-Ross (London: Tavistock, 1970). Not everyone agrees with her model. For another view see a very stimulating article 'Therapeutic Uses of Truth' by Michael Simpson in E. Wilkes (ed.), *The Dying Patient* (Lancaster: MTP Press, 1982). 'In my model there are only two stages – the stage when you believe in the Kubler-Ross five and the stage when you do not.'

14   Quoted in Richard Cabot, 'The Use of Truth and Falsehood in Medicine; an experimental study', *American Magazine*, 5 (1903), 344–9.

15   Roger Higgs, 'Truth at the Last – A Case of Obstructed Death?' *Journal of Medical Ethics*, 8 (1982), 48–50, and Roger Higgs, 'Obstructed Death Revisited', *Journal of Medical Ethics*, 8 (1982), 154–6.

16   Susan Sontag, *Illness as Metaphor* (New York: Farrar, Straus and Giroux, 1978).

17   Cicely Saunders, 'Telling Patients', *District Nursing* (now *Queens Nursing Journal*) (September 1963), 149–50, 154.

Informed Consent and Patient Autonomy

81

On Liberty

John Stuart Mill

The object of this essay is to assert one very simple principle, as entitled to govern absolutely the dealings of society with the individual in the way of compulsion and control, whether the means used be physical force in the form of legal penalties, or the moral coercion of public opinion. That principle is, that the sole end for which mankind are warranted, individually or collectively, in interfering with the liberty of action of any of their number, is self-protection. That the only purpose for which power can be rightfully exercised over any member of a civilized community, against his will, is to prevent harm to others. His own good, either physical or moral, is not a sufficient warrant. He cannot rightfully be compelled to do or forbear because it will be better for him to do so, because it will make him happier, because, in the opinions of others, to do so would be wise, or even right. These are good reasons for remonstrating with him, or reasoning with him, or persuading him, or entreating him, but not for compelling him, or visiting him with any evil in case he do otherwise. To justify that, the conduct from which it is desired to deter him must be calculated to produce evil to someone else. The only part of the conduct of anyone, for which he is amenable to society, is that which concerns others. In the part which merely concerns himself, his independence is, of right, absolute. Over himself, over his own body and mind, the individual is sovereign.

It is perhaps hardly necessary to say that this doctrine is meant to apply only to human beings in the maturity of their faculties. We are not speaking of children, or of young persons below the age which the law may fix as that of manhood or womanhood. Those who are still in a state to require being taken care of by others, must be protected against their own actions as well as against external injury. For the same reason, we may leave out of consideration those backward states of society in which the race itself may be considered as in its nonage. The early difficulties in the way of spontaneous progress are so great, and there is seldom any choice of means for overcoming them; and a ruler full of the spirit of improvement is warranted in the use of any expedients that will attain an end, perhaps otherwise unattainable. Despotism is a legitimate mode of government in dealing with barbarians, provided the end be their improvement, and the means justified by

Original publication details: John Stuart Mill, "On Liberty," first published in 1859. Public domain.

Bioethics: An Anthology, Fourth Edition. Edited by Udo Schüklenk and Peter Singer.
Editorial material and organization © 2022 John Wiley & Sons, Inc. Published 2022 by John Wiley & Sons, Inc.

actually effecting that end. Liberty, as a principle, has no application to any state of things anterior to the time when mankind have become capable of being improved by free and equal discussion. Until then, there is nothing for them but implicit obedience to an Akbar or a Charlemagne, if they are so fortunate as to find one. But as soon as mankind have attained the capacity of being guided to their own improvement by conviction or persuasion (a period long since reached in all nations with whom we need here concern ourselves), compulsion, either in the direct form or in that of pains and penalties for non-compliance, is no longer admissible as a means to their own good, and justifiable only for the security of others.

It is proper to state that I forgo any advantage which could be derived to my argument from the idea of abstract right, as a thing independent of utility. I regard utility as the ultimate appeal on all ethical questions; but it must be utility in the largest sense, grounded on the permanent interests of a man as a progressive being. Those interests, I contend, authorized the subjection of individual spontaneity to external control, only in respect to those actions of each which concern the interest of other people. If anyone does an act hurtful to others, there is a *prima facie* case for punishing him, by law, or, where legal penalties are not safely applicable, by general disapprobation. There are also many positive acts for the benefit of others, which he may rightfully be compelled to perform: such as to give evidence in a court of justice; to bear his fair share in the common defense, or in any other joint work necessary to the interest of the society of which he enjoys the protection; and to perform certain acts of individual beneficence, such as saving a fellow-creature's life, or interposing to protect the defenseless against ill usage, things which whenever it is obviously a man's duty to do, he may rightfully be made responsible to society for not doing. A person may cause evil to others not only by his actions but by his inaction, and in either case he is justly accountable to them for the injury. The latter case, it is true, requires a much more cautious exercise of compulsion than the former. To make anyone answerable for doing evil to others is the rule; to make him answerable for not preventing evil

is, comparatively speaking, the exception. Yet there are many cases clear enough and grave enough to justify that exception. In all things which regard the external relations of the individual, he is *de jure* amenable to those whose interests are concerned, and, if need be, to society as their protector. There are often good reasons for not holding him to the responsibility; but these reasons must arise from the special expediencies of the case: either because it is a kind of case in which he is on the whole likely to act better, when left to his own discretion, than when controlled in any way in which society have it in their power to control him; or because the attempt to exercise control would produce other evils, greater than those which it would prevent. When such reasons as these preclude the enforcement of responsibility, the conscience of the agent himself should step into the vacant judgment seat, and protect those interests of others which have no external protection; judging himself all the more rigidly, because the case does not admit of his being made accountable to the judgment of his fellow-creatures.

But there is a sphere of action in which society, as distinguished from the individual, has, if any, only an indirect interest; comprehending all that portion of a person's life and conduct which affects only himself, or if it also affects others, only with their free, voluntary, and undeceived consent and participation. When I say only himself, I mean directly, and in the first instance; for whatever affects himself, may affect others through himself; and the objection which may be grounded on this contingency, will receive consideration in the sequel. This, then, is the appropriate region of human liberty. It comprises, *first*, the inward domain of consciousness; demanding liberty of conscience in the most comprehensive sense; liberty of thought and feeling; absolute freedom of opinion and sentiment on all subjects, practical or speculative, scientific, moral, or theological. The liberty of expressing and publishing opinions may seem to fall under a different principle, since it belongs to that part of the conduct of an individual which concerns other people; but, being almost of as much importance as the liberty of thought itself, and resting in great part on the same reasons, is practically inseparable from it.

Secondly, the principle requires liberty of tastes and pursuits; of framing the plan of our life to suit our own character; of doing as we like, subject to such consequences as may follow: without impediment from our fellow-creatures, so long as what we do does not harm them, even though they should think our conduct foolish, perverse, or wrong. *Thirdly*, from this liberty of each individual, follows the liberty, within the same limits, of combination among individuals; freedom to unite, for any purpose not involving harm to others: the persons combining being supposed to be of full age, and not forced or deceived.

No society in which these liberties are not, on the whole, respected, is free, whatever may be its form of government; and none is completely free in which they do not exist absolute and unqualified. The only freedom which deserves the name, is that of pursuing our own good in our own way, so long as we do not attempt to deprive others of theirs, or impede their efforts to obtain it. Each is the proper guardian of his own health, whether bodily, or mental and spiritual. Mankind are greater gainers by suffering each other to live as seems good to themselves, than by compelling each to live as seems good to the rest.

82

From *Schloendorff v. New York Hospital*

Justice Benjamin N. Cardozo

Every human being of adult years and sound mind has a right to determine what shall be done with his own body; and a surgeon who performs an operation without his patient's consent commits an assault, for which he is liable in damages. (*Pratt* v. *Davis*, 224 Ill. 300; *Mohr* v. *Williams*, 95 Minn. 261.) This is true except in cases of emergency where the patient is unconscious and where it is necessary to operate before consent can be obtained.

Original publication details: Justice Benjamin N. Cardozo, Judgment from *Schloendorff* v. *New York Hospital* (1914), p. 526 from Jay Katz (ed.), *Experimentation with Human Beings: The Authority of the Investigator, Subject, Professions, and State in the Human Experimentation Process* (New York: Russell Sage Foundation, 1972). Reproduced with permission of Russell Sage Foundation.

83

Informed Consent

Its History, Meaning, and Present Challenges

Tom L. Beauchamp

The practice of obtaining informed consent has its history in, and gains its meaning from, medicine and biomedical research. Discussions of disclosure and justified nondisclosure have played a significant role throughout the history of medical ethics, but the term "informed consent" emerged only in the 1950s. Serious discussion of the meaning and ethics of informed consent began in medicine, research, law, and philosophy only around 1972. In the mid-1970s medical and research ethics gradually moved from a narrow focus on the physician's or the researcher's obligation to disclose information to an emphasis on the quality of a patient's or subject's understanding of information and right to authorize or refuse a biomedical intervention. This shift was the real beginning of a meaningful notion of informed consent. However, it may be doubted that this notion has ever been put into real-world contexts of practice. Put another way, the bulk of consents given still today may not be sufficiently informed to qualify as *informed* consents.

I first discuss the early history of informed consent, including its critical landmarks. I argue that its arrival was sudden and impressive, but the path thereafter to high-quality consents has been rocky. I then explore two different meanings of "informed consent" at work in literature on the subject. The most established meaning derives from institutional and regulatory rules, although I give reasons to think that this meaning is morally suspicious. Finally, in the third part I discuss several contemporary challenges to informed consent that suggest we still have unresolved problems about whether, when, and how to obtain informed consents.

The Historical Foundations of Informed Consent

Classic documents in the history of medicine such as the Hippocratic writings (fifth to fourth century BC) and Thomas Percival's *Medical Ethics* (1803)[1] present an extremely disappointing history from the perspective of the right to give informed consent. The central concern in these writings was how to avoid making disclosures that might harm or upset patients. Physician ethics was traditionally a nondisclosure

Original publication details: Tom L. Beauchamp, "Informed Consent: Its History, Meaning, and Present Challenges," pp. 515–523 from *Cambridge Quarterly of Health Care Ethics* 20: 4 (2011). © 2011 Royal Institute of Philosophy. Reproduced with permission of Cambridge University Press and Tom L. Beauchamp.

Bioethics: An Anthology, Fourth Edition. Edited by Udo Schüklenk and Peter Singer.
Editorial material and organization © 2022 John Wiley & Sons, Inc. Published 2022 by John Wiley & Sons, Inc.

ethics with virtually no appreciation of a patient's right to consent. The doctrine of informed consent was imposed on medicine through nonmedical forms of authority such as judges in courts and government officials in regulatory agencies.

During the 1950s and 1960s the duty to obtain consent in a few medical fields, such as surgery, evolved through the courts into an explicit duty to disclose certain forms of information and to obtain consent in both practice and research. This development needed a new term, and so the word "informed" was tacked onto the word "consent," creating the expression "informed consent." This expression appeared publicly for the first time in the landmark decision in *Salgo v. Leland Stanford, Jr. University Board of Trustees* (1957).[2] The *Salgo* court said – prophetically, but probably incorrectly – that the duty to disclose the risks and alternatives of treatment was not a new duty, only a logical extension of the already-established duty to disclose the treatment's nature and consequences. In fact, *Salgo* not only introduced new elements into the law but initiated the history of informed consent. The *Salgo* court was not merely interested in whether a recognizable consent had been given. The court latched tenaciously onto the problem of whether the consent was itself *adequately informed*.

This development initiated a series of court cases that step-by-step added requirements into the doctrine of informed consent. For 15 years after *Salgo*, these changes came slowly and incrementally in courts of law. Then, suddenly, in 1972 there came down three court decisions in three separate state courts in the United States that would solidify the place of informed consent and advance to prominence the importance of its moral demands. The three landmark cases were *Canterbury v. Spence*, *Cobbs v. Grant*, and *Wilkinson v. Vesey*.[3] *Canterbury* had a particularly massive influence in demanding a more patient-oriented standard of disclosure. Judge Spottswood Robinson held that "[t]he patient's right of self-decision shapes the boundaries of the duty to reveal. That right can be effectively exercised only if the patient possesses enough information to enable an intelligent choice."[4] Informed consent would never thereafter lose its place as a significant

legal doctrine, but it would soon be considerably expanded through discussions of the ethical demands of consent in both medicine and research.

Numerous articles in the medical literature on issues of consent were soon published, largely on the significance of the precedent cases. Doctors were fearful, and their articles functioned to alert physicians to informed consent as a worrisome new legal development with the potential to increase malpractice risk. A study done in the mid-1960s, conducted by a lawyer-surgeon team, showed that *consent forms* were not yet a ubiquitous feature even of the practice of surgery – let alone elsewhere in medicine.[5] This would change rapidly after the 1972 court decisions. During the years between 1972 and 1978, there was a dramatic solidification of the view that both physicians and biomedical researchers have a moral and legal duty to obtain consent for certain procedures. These developments prompted an explosion of largely negative commentary on informed consent in the medical literature of the mid-1970s. Physicians saw the demands of informed consent as impossible to fulfill and, at least in some cases, inconsistent with good patient care.[6]

We might ask why informed consent became so important and the focus of so much attention in case law, ethics, and biomedicine in the next few years. The most likely explanation is that law, ethics, medicine, and research were all affected by issues of individual liberty and social equality in the wider society. These issues were made dramatic by an increasingly technological and impersonal medical care. Informed consent was swept along with this tide of social concerns, which broadly propelled the new bioethics throughout the 1970s. As it happened, the arrival of informed consent and the birth of bioethics occurred at exactly the same time.

These developments, as thus far traced, tell us little about physicians' and researchers' actual consent practices or opinions, or about how informed consent was viewed or experienced by patients and subjects. The empirical evidence on this subject during the late 1970s and early 1980s is mixed. Perhaps the best and most interesting data on the subject are the findings of a national survey conducted by Louis Harris and Associates for a US President's Commission on bioethics in 1982. Almost all of the physicians surveyed indicated that they obtained written consent from their patients before inpatient surgery or the administration of general anesthesia. Approximately 85 percent said they usually obtain consent – written or oral – for minor office surgery, setting of fractures, local anesthesia, invasive diagnostic procedures, and radiation therapy. Only blood tests and prescriptions appear to have proceeded frequently without some form of patient consent.[7]

This survey indicates that the explosion of interest in informed consent in the 1970s had an enormously powerful impact on medical practice by the early 1980s. However, evidence from the Harris survey and other sources also questions the quality and meaningfulness of this consent-related activity. The overwhelming impression from the available empirical literature and from reported clinical experience is that the process of soliciting informed consent often fell far short of a show of respect for the decisional authority of patients. As the authors of one empirical study of physician-patient interactions put it, "[D]espite the doctrine of informed consent, it is the physician, and not the patient, who, in effect, makes the treatment decision."[8]

To conclude this section, the history of informed consent indicates that medicine quickly experienced widespread changes under the influence of legal requirements of informed consent, setting in motion an evolving process in our understanding of informed consent and the moral demands involved in obtaining it. The 1970s framers of the rules wanted genuine informed consent, but that goal has been more difficult to achieve than was the impressive body of rules, court decisions, and books on informed consent that soon followed the early history. Practice has been slow to conform to abstract theory.

The Concept of Informed Consent

Accordingly, the claim that a signed consent form is evidence of an informed consent cannot always be

taken at face value. Before we can legitimately infer that what is called an informed consent is truly an informed consent, we need to know what to look for. If one uses overly demanding criteria of informed consent – such as full disclosure and complete understanding – then an informed consent can hardly ever be obtained. Conversely, if underdemanding criteria such as a signed consent form are used, an informed consent becomes too easy to obtain, and the term loses its moral significance. Although a physician's or a research investigator's truthful disclosure to a patient has often been declared the essence of informed consent in legal and medical literature, mere disclosure is seldom evidence of an informed consent.

The question "What is an informed consent?" is complicated because at least two common, entrenched, and irreducibly different meanings of "informed consent" have been at work in its history. In the first sense, an informed consent is an *autonomous authorization* by individual patients or subjects. A person gives an informed consent in this first sense if and only if the person, with substantial understanding and in substantial absence of control by others, intentionally authorizes a health professional to do something. Here informed consent is fundamentally a matter of autonomous or self-determining choice.

In the second sense, informed consent is analyzable in terms of *institutional and policy rules of consent* that collectively form the social practice of informed consent in institutional contexts. Here "informed consent" refers only to a legally or institutionally effective approval given by a patient or subject. An approval is therefore "effective" or "valid" if it conforms to the rules that govern specific institutions. In this sense, unlike the first, conditions and requirements of informed consent are relative to the social and institutional context and need not be truly autonomous authorizations. Informed consent in the second sense has been the mainstream conception in the regulatory rules of US federal agencies as well as in healthcare institutions, and this situation is not likely to change.[9]

However, literature in bioethics has increasingly maintained, as I would, that any justifiable analysis of informed consent must be rooted in autonomous choice by patients and subjects, because otherwise there is no truly informed consent. The first sense captures the morally best standard, because the whole point of the practice of informed consent is to protect and enable meaningful choice. Although living up to this standard has proved to be difficult in contexts of practice, informed consent as autonomous authorization arguably provides a model standard for fashioning institutional and policy requirements of informed consent. That is, truly autonomous choice can and should serve as the benchmark against which the moral adequacy of prevailing rules and practices are to be evaluated.

Current Challenges to Informed Consent

I turn next to some of the challenges we face today in the theory and practice of informed consent, with an emphasis on challenges in practice.

The limits of the law in biomedical ethics

A first challenge is how to understand the way the law should shape our understanding of informed consent. I maintained previously that the law has been more influential historically than any other field of thought in the United States. The doctrine of informed consent *is* the legal doctrine, and informed consent has often been treated as synonymous with this legal doctrine, which is centered almost entirely on *disclosure* and on *liability for injury*. This basis is unduly narrow for thinking about both research and medical practice, which is to say that the law is ill-equipped to help us in our thinking about informed consent beyond the restricted limits within which the law operates. Those limits can and often have misled us about our responsibilities to patients and subjects. American legal scholar and psychiatrist Jay Katz was appropriately unrelenting, throughout his career, in criticizing court decisions and the legal model. He regarded the declarations of courts as filled with overly optimistic

and often morally empty and evasive rhetoric. The problem, in his view, is that the law has little to do with fostering morally required forms of communication in the clinic and in the research environment.[10]

The theory of liability under which a case is tried in American law determines the duty that must be fulfilled. In classic informed consent cases, negligence is the reigning theory of liability. This approach is itself a misleading and uninformative basis for thinking about informed consent in contexts of clinical practice and research. Negligence may be good for understanding what has gone wrong in some cases, but this rationale provides an inadequate framework for determining what we ought to be doing in soliciting consent or in waiving consent in institutions.

In the end, legal standards are not of major assistance in formulating a conception of informed consent for medicine and research. These standards do as much to distract us from an appropriate model as to contribute to the model, because they focus on illegal rather than unethical treatment. The heart of issues about informed consent is moral, not legal.[11]

The quality of consent

In discussing both meaningful choice and the limits of law, I have noted that problems about the quality and adequacy of consent probably cannot be resolved unless conventional disclosure rules are refocused so that we look instead at the quality of understanding in a consent as well as the rights of patients and their needs for information. This approach centers attention on the need for effective communication and genuine understanding by patients and subjects. Without a proper climate of exchange in the consent context, a request from a professional that the patient or subject ask for information is as likely to result in silence as to elicit the desired result of a meaningful informational exchange and consent. However, it is not clear how much progress has been made on this front in the last 20 years, and it is a good guess that relatively little educating and communication that conform to this model occur at present in either clinical practice or research. Achieving informed consent under the first of the two senses of informed consent discussed previously is still the principal challenge that we confront.

Problems of broad consent

A third set of challenges derives from contemporary concerns about broad consent. In Europe there is currently an active discussion of broad consent in settings in which obtaining consent is difficult or in which risk is extremely low. Although it is not as active, this topic haunts US discussions as well. There has been a pervasive view in US bioethics that if we must get consent, then it should be an *adequately informed* consent and that a broad consent is not an adequately informed consent. However, this view is now under pressure. I will approach the problem primarily through questions of the banking of biological samples.

The banking of samples   Certain advances in science have made efficiently promoting scientific advances while protecting the rights of donors ever more problematic. Samples collected for future – not merely present – research may not be adequately described in a protocol or consent form when sample collection occurs. How shall we understand what constitutes an adequately informed consent under these circumstances? The content of the consent will be roughly dictated by current and anticipated future uses of the samples. In giving consent, research subjects should be assured that sensitive personal information and data will be protected in a way that will not cause stigma or harm their dignity, will not violate privacy and confidentiality, and will not lead to discriminatory treatment.[12]

This challenge cannot be met merely by internal protections when obtaining consent. Biological samples and data from samples are often obtained from external sources such as industry, government, universities, or nonprofits. Here it must be ascertained whether samples were collected under valid consent policies. Surplus biological material that is often described as waste raises similar concerns. The use of a sample for purposes other than those specifically stated in the consent process is a violation of the trust that bonds the subject–investigator relationship and the original consent situation. If an investigator seeks to use a sample for purposes not originally stated in an informed consent form, the subject likely would have to be re-contacted and re-consented. However, there are exceptions to this rule – for example, when only minor departures are made from the original protocol and consent form and (in some cases) when samples cannot be linked with a donor. However, there seems to be only a narrow range of such valid exceptions. Even making samples anonymous is not a valid exception, because it may well violate the investigator–subject trust relationship.

These are just some of the problems that need to be addressed about the notion of broad consent. I will not try to resolve these issues here. However, I will follow up the challenges thus far noted with analysis of a case in which broad consent was used with disastrous consequences. This case beautifully exemplifies how morally complicated the informed consent process can be.

The Havasupai Indians and diabetes research   This case involves research conducted at the Arizona State University using as research subjects the Havasupai Indians of the Grand Canyon. Matters did not go well both because a broad consent was used by investigators when it was inappropriate and because university committee review of the research was ineffective. The case starts in 1990, when members of the fast-disappearing Havasupai tribe gave DNA samples to university researchers at Arizona State with the goal of providing genetic information about the tribe's rate of diabetes. Dating from the 1960s, the Havasupai had experienced a surprisingly high incidence of type 2 diabetes, which led to amputations and had forced many tribal members to leave their village in the Grand Canyon for dialysis.

The tribe's diabetes was examined in the research, but the blood samples that had been donated were then put to additional uses in genetics research, and here the trouble began. One use of the samples was to study mental illness (one professor had a special interest in schizophrenia). Another use was to study the tribe's geographical origins, which cast doubt on cherished tribal views about their historical origins. Approximately two dozen scholarly articles were published on the basis of research on the samples. Some of this research was judged by the Havasupai to be offensive, insulting, and provocative. For example, one study reported a high degree of inbreeding in the tribe.

A geneticist responsible for some of the research reported that she had obtained an adequate informed consent for wide-ranging genetic studies and defended her actions as late as 2009 as ethically justified. The problem was the use of broad consent. From 1990 to 1994, about 100 members of the tribe signed a broad consent that said the research was to "study the causes of behavioral/medical disorders." The consent form was intentionally confined to clear, simply written, basic information, because English is a second language for many Havasupai, and few of the tribe's remaining 650 members had graduated from high school. From the researchers' perspective, tribe members had consented to collecting the blood and to its use in genetic research well beyond the research on their particular disease. The Havasupai, however, adamantly deny that they gave permission for any non-diabetes research or that they were given an adequate understanding of the risks of the research before they agreed to participate.[13]

This case presents paradigmatic problems of human rights and informed consent. One reading of the case is that it is essentially about researchers' responsibility to communicate what might happen with the samples. The case also raises classic questions of whether scientists had taken advantage of a vulnerable population, and in this respect the case raises questions about exploitation that preys on ignorance.

Both the researchers and the review committee at the university overlooked the serious risks involved. One scholarly article eventually published by investigators theorized that the tribe's ancestors had crossed the frozen Bering Sea to arrive in North America. This directly contradicted the tribe's traditional stories and cosmology, which have quasi-religious significance for the Havasupai. Their history has it that they originated in the Grand Canyon and that the tribe had been assigned to be the canyon's guardian.

To be told that the tribe was instead of Asian origin and that this was learned from studies on their blood, which has a special significance to the Havasupai, is to them disorienting and abhorrent. The account also introduced legal alarm. The Havasupai had argued that their origin in the canyon was the legal basis of their entitlement to the land, which is otherwise US federal land.

Finally, in retrospect, there were significant risks for the university in the conduct of this research and in allowing a broad consent. In the end the university's Board of Regents agreed to pay $700,000 to 41 of the tribe's members, while acknowledging that the payment was to "remedy the wrong that was done." The university spent $1.7 million fighting lawsuits by tribe members. The university had worked for years to establish good relationships with Native American tribes in Arizona. The reservoir of trust that had been established was seriously threatened by this case.[14]

This tragic case apparently happened with virtually no appreciation, during the course of ethics review, that obtaining a broad consent, under the circumstances, was an ethically dubious practice.

The regulation of consent and the research–treatment distinction

A fourth type of challenge to informed consent requirements comes in how we should alter the ways in which consent is regulated.

I start with a basic distinction in bioethics, viz., that between clinical research and medical practice. This distinction has dominated how we think about biomedical ethics, including informed consent. Since the early 1970s it has been thought that research is risky, whereas accepted practice is aimed at the best interests of the patient. This belief is probably traceable to the history of abuses of subjects in biomedical research, and so there arose in the 1970s the assumption that research using human subjects is dangerous, exists for the benefit of future patients, and is aimed at scientific knowledge, not benefit for immediate subjects.

Accordingly, it has been thought that the need for consent is more pervasive and the threshold of an adequate informed consent higher in research than in medical practice. But do we have good reasons to warrant this sharp distinction between research and practice – and the different levels of consent requirements that co-travel with it? And should the distinction between research and practice make any difference to requirements of informed consent? Perhaps today patients are underprotected, and research subjects overprotected, by our moral arrangements for consent. This matter will likely receive close inspection in upcoming years, and it presents an important challenge to current consent practices.

One central question will be whether we should have a moral system in which there is an intense, close ethical review of consent forms in research protocols and no close parallel attention given to consent forms in medical practice. One dimension of the problem is whether we should have government regulatory systems for research, but no comparable systems for the regulation of practice. In America, the vast differences

in our systems rest on doctors' desires to not be regulated in the practice of medicine. But from the perspective of genuine informed consent, the US system sometimes seems irrational, especially if there are dangers and risks in medical practice comparable to those in research. If so, then is it time for us to have comparable oversight systems in both research and practice?

Conclusion

I have been critical of various practices in the obtaining of and the failure to obtain informed consents. However, before we too sternly condemn defects in the judgments and practices of the past, we should remember that the history of informed consent is still unfolding and that current failures may be no less apparent to future generations than are the failures that I have found in the past and the present. Clearly we still face unresolved and critical moral challenges.

Notes

1 Percival T. *Medical Ethics; or a Code of Institutes and Precepts, Adapted to the Professional Conduct of Physicians and Surgeons.* Manchester: S. Russell; 1803.

2 *Salgo v. Leland Stanford Jr. University Board of Trustees,* 317 P.2d 170 (1957).

3 *Canterbury v. Spence,* 464 F.2d 772 (D.C. Cir. 1972); *Cobbs v. Grant,* 104 Cal. Rptr. 505, 502 P.2d 1 (1972); *Wilkinson v. Vesey,* 295 A.2d 676 (R.I. 1972).

4 See *Canterbury v. Spence,* at 786.

5 Hershey N. and Bushkoff S.H. *Informed Consent Study.* Pittsburgh: Aspen Systems Corporation; 1969:4.

6 National Library of Medicine, 272 citations on informed consent in the period from January 1970 to April 1974, in Medical Literature Analysis and Retrieval System (MEDLARS), NLM Literature Search No. 74–16 (1974); Kaufmann C.L. Informed consent and patient decision making: Two decades of research. *Social Science and Medicine* 1983; 17:1657–64.

7 Louis Harris and Associates. Views of informed consent and decisionmaking: Parallel surveys of physicians and the public. In: President's Commission for the Study of Ethical Problems in Medicine and Biomedical and

Behavioral Research. *Making Health Care Decisions.* Washington: US Government Printing Office; 1982: vol. 2:302.

8 Siminoff L.A. and Fetting J.H. Factors affecting treatment decisions for a life-threatening illness: The case of medical treatment for breast cancer. *Social Science and Medicine* 1992; 32:813–8, at 817.

9 Faden R.R. and Beauchamp T.L. *A History and Theory of Informed Consent.* New York: Oxford University Press; 1986: 276–87.

10 Katz J. *The Silent World of Doctor and Patient.* New York: Free Press; 1984.

11 For an example of how the legal doctrine is still today used by prominent authors in bioethics as a foundational starting point for theory and practice, see Appelbaum P.S., Lidz C.W., and Klitzman R. Voluntariness of consent to research: A conceptual model. *Hastings Center Report* 2009; 39(1):30–9.

12 Buchanan A. An ethical framework for biological samples policy. In: National Bioethics Advisory Commission. *Research Involving Human Biological Materials: Ethical Issues and Policy Guidance,* vol. II: *Commissioned Papers.*

Rockville: National Bioethics Advisory Commission; January 2000; Pentz R.D., Billot L., and Wendler D. Research on stored biological samples: Views of African American and White American cancer patients. *American Journal of Medical Genetics.* 2006 Mar 7; available at http://onlinelibrary.wiley.com/doi/10.1002/ajmg.a.31154/full (accessed 14 Sept 2010).

13 Harmon A. Indian tribe wins fight to limit research of its DNA. *New York Times.* 2010 Apr 21; available at http://www.nytimes.com/2010/04/22/us/22dna.

html; Harmon A. Havasupai case highlights risks in DNA research. *New York Times.* 2010 Apr 22; available at http://www.nytimes.com/2010/04/22/us/22dnaside.html (last accessed 14 Sept 2010).

14 Harmon A. Where'd you go with my DNA? *New York Times.* 2010 Apr 25; available at http://www.nytimes.com/2010/04/25/weekinreview/25harmon.html (accessed 14 Sept 2010). Also see Harmon, Indian tribe wins fight to limit research of its DNA; Harmon, Havasupai case highlights risks in DNA research.

84

The Doctor–Patient Relationship in Different Cultures

Ruth Macklin

When bioethicists from the United States call for recognition of the rights of patients, are they simply expressing their unique American adherence to individualism? The familiar charge of "ethical imperialism" is leveled against proposals that patients in other countries, where individualism is not a prominent value, should nevertheless be granted a similar right to informed consent. While it is true that the doctrine of informed consent focuses on the rights of individual patients, it is not rooted solely in the cultural value of individualism. Rather, it stems from a value many cultures recognize, especially those that aspire to democracy and a just social order: the notion that powerful agents, be they from governmental or nongovernmental organizations, may not invade the personal lives, and especially the bodies, of ordinary citizens.

The prominent American sociologist Renée Fox accurately describes the early focus of American bioethics: "From the outset, the conceptual framework of bioethics has accorded paramount status to the value-complex of individualism, underscoring the principles of individual rights, autonomy, self-determination, and their legal expression in the jurisprudential notion of privacy."[1] Critics of mainstream bioethics within the United States and abroad have complained about the narrow focus on autonomy and the concept of individual rights. Such critics argue that much – if not most – of the world embraces a value system that places the family, the community, or the society as a whole above that of the individual person. But we need to ask: What follows from value systems that accord the individual a lower priority than the group? It hardly follows that individual patients should not be granted a right to full participation in medical decisions. Nor does it follow that individual doctors need not be obligated to disclose information or obtain their patients' voluntary, informed consent. It surely does not follow that the needs of society or the community for organs, bone marrow, or blood should permit those bodily parts or products to be taken from individuals without their permission. What might follow, however, is that patients' families may be fuller participants in decision-making than the patient autonomy model ordinarily requires.

Perhaps we need to be reminded just why American bioethics began with such a vigorous

Original publication details: Ruth Macklin, "The Doctor–Patient Relationship in Different Cultures," pp. 86–107 from *Against Relativism: Cultural Diversity and the Search of Ethical Universals in Medicine* (New York: Oxford University Press, 1999). © 1999 by Oxford University Press, Inc. Reproduced with permission of Oxford University Press, USA.

Bioethics: An Anthology, Fourth Edition. Edited by Udo Schüklenk and Peter Singer. Editorial material and organization © 2022 John Wiley & Sons, Inc. Published 2022 by John Wiley & Sons, Inc.

defense of autonomy. It is because patients tradi- tionally had few, if any, rights of self-determination: Doctors neither informed patients nor obtained their consent for treatment or for research. In a country founded on conceptions of liberty and freedom, it was at least odd that the self-determination Americans so highly prized in other areas of life was largely absent from the sphere of medical practice. An evolution took place in the United States over a period of many years, from an early court ruling in 1914 that required surgeons to obtain the consent of patients through a series of informed consent cases in the 1950s and 1970s. By the time bioethics became an international field of study, paternalistic medicine had been largely transformed in the United States and patients' rights had been solidly established. The same developments are occurring today in the many developing countries where bioethics has more recently become a topic of interest and study. Although most of these countries lack the tradition of individualism that marks North American culture, the legal guarantee of certain rights of the individual has in the past few decades been one of the goals of social and political reformers.

Cross-cultural misunderstandings can affect the way people in one country perceive a situation in another. Participating in a workshop in the Philippines,[2] I encountered an example of a common cross-cultural misunderstanding about informed consent. The dis- cussion focused on the ethical principle of respect for persons and its role in justifying the need to inform patients and obtain their permission to carry out therapeutic or research procedures. A Filipino physi- cian in the audience objected that informed consent may be needed in the United States, where people do not trust their doctors, but, he said, in the Philippines patients place great trust in their physicians. Doctors do not need to protect themselves against lawsuits by having patients sign a consent form.

Throughout the world (and even at times in the United States), people confuse informed consent with the informed consent document. The Filipino physician misunderstood two things: first, the ethical basis for informed consent; and second, the differ- ence between the *process* of informing and obtaining

permission and the piece of paper (the documenta- tion) attesting that the process took place. The ethi- cal judgment that patients should be full participants in their treatment decisions is the ethical justification for the doctrine of informed consent. It is not the protection of the doctor, as the Filipino physician believed, that serves as an ethical basis for the practice. Although it is true that the number of medical mal- practice lawsuits in the United States far exceeds that in other countries, especially in the developing world, that phenomenon bears little relation to whether patients lack trust in their doctors.

"Physicians Treat Patients Badly"

"Physicians treat patients badly" was a constant theme in virtually all of the developing countries I visited. Unfortunately, many of the shortcomings in the physician–patient relationship that are all too common in many countries continue to exist in the United States, as well. A major difference is that patients in this country are more aware of their legal and moral rights and are consequently more assertive. An Egyptian physician said that in Egypt there is no process by which consent is obtained in clinical prac- tice. She complained that there is no physician–patient communication, in part because doctors do not have the time. Patients are not told about complications, about medical errors, or anything that transpires in the course of treatment. Patients can get no information whatsoever from doctors about their diagnosis, prog- nosis, or proposed treatment. Before surgical proce- dures, papers are signed. But those papers say nothing at all. Patients who ask questions are viewed by the doctors as "impolite," and in any case doctors do not like to answer questions posed by patients.

This Egyptian physician did not seek to defend the customary practices of doctors in her country or to argue that they were reflections of cultural val- ues in Egypt. On the contrary, she was attempting in her work to introduce reforms into medical practice in order to bring about better treatment of patients. When I asked what possible remedies there could be for all these ethical shortcomings, she replied by describing two broad strategies. The first is to document abuses – violations of patients' rights, failures to obtain proper informed consent, and the like; the second is to mount a campaign by lobbying, bringing these issues before the public, and putting cases into court. I asked whether these steps are likely to be effective, and she replied that they can succeed in raising consciousness and awareness and further that people have received some compensation when their cases have reached the courts. Gathering cases and making them public can be used to mount campaigns. By this means reforms might be accomplished. The Egyptian physician's criticism of practices in her own country and the specific reforms she sought to introduce show that, however different in other ways the culture of Egypt may be from that of Western nations, the ethical ideal that requires physicians to treat their patients with respect is widely acknowledged, if not always honored.

A colleague in Mexico gave a similar account of the lack of recognition of patients' rights in her country.[3] One example was a story told to her by the doorman of her building. His wife was in labor and went to the public hospital. She remained in labor for 2 days, during which time neither the woman nor her husband were told anything about her condition. Eventually she gave birth and was discharged from the hospital while the baby had to remain there for a while longer. Still the couple was told nothing. My colleague expressed her outrage at this situation, blaming the doctors in public hospitals for their unwillingness to disclose information to patients, much less to obtain properly informed consent.

While I agreed that this was an outrage, I noted that things were not so very different years ago in the United States. It is a mere 40 years since the concept of informed consent to treatment was introduced into the legal domain and probably only about 25 years since the practice of obtaining informed consent took root. Still, my Mexican colleague insisted, there are cultural differences. As an example, she cited the pervasive corruption in Latin America as a difference between that region and the North. "What, no

corruption in the United States or in Europe?" was my surprised reaction. Of course there is, but we have a much lower tolerance for official corruption, we make strenuous efforts to root it out, and we probably succeed more often in punishing instances that are discovered.

In India I heard more stories about how doctors treat patients badly. One physician described the efforts he and others have been making to inform and enlist the public in opposing unethical medical practices.[4] He recounted a long list of horrors: incompetent doctors practicing poorly or negligently; untrained and unlicensed doctors practicing medicine; physicians overcharging patients; and more. The array of unethical behavior ranged from genuine malpractice to arrogance and indifference to patients. I asked about legal recourse, and here the situation is just as bleak. There exists a body called the Medical Council of India, which is supposed to be responsible for monitoring and dealing with the standard of care delivered by physicians. But this is a peer review system in which doctors protect other doctors. When cases of blatant malpractice are brought before this council, they fail to find the physician at fault. As a result, nothing is done to remedy instances of actual malpractice or the behavior of incompetent physicians. Patients can, in principle, bring suits against doctors. However, doctors win most of the cases brought to court in spite of their having committed actual malpractice, and judicial appeals take many years.

A different group of doctors repeated the same list of horror stories that I had heard from the first Indian physician, and more. When they mentioned the "kickback" system, I naively though they were referring only to money paid to the referring doctor by the surgeon or specialist to whom the referral was made. But they meant much more by "kickbacks," including demands by the referring doctor that the surgeon perform unnecessary procedures, charge the patient for them, and then give a percentage of the take to the referring doctor. Surgeons and other specialists who rely on referrals for their practice have to play the game or else they are not sent a single patient. Thus even doctors who begin by being ethical and idealistic end up getting caught up in a system in which they must play or fail to make a living.

All these accounts of bad behavior of physicians toward patients have little to do with cultural differences or with ethical relativism. They simply remind us that arrogance, corruption, greed, and indifference are universal character flaws that can be found in human beings throughout the world, wherever they live and whatever their profession. The chief difference between these countries and the United States lies not in a divergence in the cultural acceptance of such behavior by physicians but, rather, in the existence of laws and other forms of social control to root out and punish doctors who violate universally acknowledged ethical norms and standards of good clinical practice. The efforts of the Egyptian physician and the Indian doctors to bring about reforms in their countries are evidence of a widespread cross-cultural identification of the same ethical values that ought to govern the doctor–patient relationship everywhere. Respect for persons – in this case, individual patients – was the principle invoked implicitly or explicitly by people from Latin America, Asia, and North Africa in my visits to those regions.

Similarities and Differences

Even in those parts of the world where the cultural traditions differ radically from those in the West, certain values in the doctor–patient relationship are overarching. I participated in a meeting in Nigeria that included several non-English speaking tribal chiefs and native healers. One chief was asked for his views about helping a woman to have an abortion. (Abortion is illegal in Nigeria as in many other countries, but legal prohibitions have never succeeded anywhere in eliminating requests for or performance of the procedure.) Suppose a woman came to him, a traditional healer, asking for an abortion. What would he do? His reply was translated from his native tongue as follows: "If a client comes to me, as a professional, I will help the woman because I have the knowledge to do so." He added, however, that "the community would not be happy."

Here was a medical person – a traditional healer – referring to his "professional" obligation to his patient. He invoked precisely the same consideration most Western physicians would appeal to as a reason why they should help a woman to have an abortion despite the community's disapproval of abortion. Although the cultures may differ in significant ways, the obligations of healers to those who come to them for help remain a cultural universal, one that exists in virtually all societies.

Not every customary practice is properly termed a *tradition*. Values inherent in a social institution such as medical practice may be a reflection of a value in the culture at large, or they may be specific to that particular institution. Lack of recognition and respect for the decision-making autonomy of patients has been a feature of Western medicine throughout most of history and even today remains prominent in other parts of the world. There is a difference, however, between the professional norm in which doctors decide for their patients and a cultural norm that gives family members complete control of another's freedom of decision and action.

Similarly, not every set of norms deserves to be called a *culture*. Although phrases like "the culture of Western medicine" are tossed around, medicine is not a culture in the genuine sense of the term, as anthropologists define it. To refer to "the culture of medicine" is to speak metaphorically rather than anthropologically. As one commentator observes: "Used metaphorically, *culture* is everywhere these days. . . .Today the press is full of stories about the 'culture' of the Defense Department, the Central Intelligence Agency. . ., Congress. . ., and any large corporation that happens to be in the news. GQ even describes opera as being characterized by 'the culture of booing.'"[5]

Rural areas in many parts of the world still maintain many features of traditional culture in the true sense of the term. Women's health advocates in Mexico reported that in some areas the husband or mother-in-law of a woman decides whether she may visit a physician or whether she may use a method of birth control.[6] This behavior prevails today in rural areas and among indigenous groups and is sanctioned by certain beliefs and values regarding women. For example, women are believed incapable of making their own decisions; or, even if they are capable, they must remain subordinate to men; or the role of women is to reproduce and therefore they should not be permitted to choose to control their own fertility. Control by husbands and mothers-in-law of a woman's fertility is based on the traditional culture and has little to do with the social institution of medicine. Although these sorts of beliefs and values have deep cultural roots they, too, may change over time, as women's health advocates work at the grassroots level and expose women in rural and indigenous communities to the ideas of the global women's movement. Defenders of traditional culture condemn these activists in Mexico and elsewhere as intrusive purveyors of Western feminism who seek to destroy traditional cultural values.

Interestingly, some women's health advocates worry about the effect of introducing values such as autonomy and independence to the women they work with. One social scientist used the example of women with whom they work in a traditional Mexican setting. These women have to ask permission from their mothers-in-law to visit a physician. A mother-in-law may question that decision or refuse to grant permission. The woman then asks the researcher for help. This poses a problem for the researcher: Can the researcher provide some assistance without causing the research subject further psychological damage or harm to her interests? The woman might actually be expelled from her home if the mother-in-law finds out she has gone to a physician without her permission.

While it is no doubt true that some customary practices are rooted in cultural traditions, others may simply have been passed down from one generation to the next as ways of behaving that no one questioned or sought to change. The medical profession has a long history of customary practices, but few qualify as "cultural" traditions. The custom of physicians withholding information from patients and talking, instead, to family members is probably a good example. Everyone from Western anthropologists to

physicians in non-Western cultures remark on the difference between the nature of communications between doctors and patients in North America and other parts of the world as if this represents a deep-seated difference in cultural traditions. These commentators probably do not realize, or may have forgotten, that it is only a few decades since physicians in the United States began disclosing diagnoses of fatal illnesses directly to patients. One may call these norms of truth-telling a "tradition," but that would be to distort the more prevalent meaning of "tradition." That meaning is related to the concerns of the ethical relativist – that different societies have distinct and possibly incommensurate ethical values stemming from their cultural diversity.

One commentator suggests that cross-cultural differences in the physician–patient relationship are attributable to different systems of biomedical ethics. Diego Gracia, a professor of public health and history of science in Spain, distinguishes between Mediterranean biomedical ethics and the Anglo-American variety. Gracia notes that patients in Southern European nations are generally less concerned with matters related to informed consent and respect for autonomy than with trust in their physician. Mediterranean bioethics emphasizes virtues rather than rights. Accordingly, the virtue of trustworthiness is more crucial to patients than the right to information.[7]

But Gracia also points to a recent trend in Mediterranean countries, a trend that once again shows the evolution of the physician–patient relationship and the introduction of new ethical values. Gracia notes that, in all Mediterranean countries, respect for patients' autonomy and the right of patients to participate in medical decisions have grown extensively in the last decades. Coming some decades after the patients' rights movement began in the United States, this new trend in the Mediterranean countries also includes complaints about health care workers' failure to provide information and for nonconsensual touching.

This phenomenon is one of historical evolution of the doctor–patient relationship rather than a cross-cultural difference between individualistic American culture and the more communitarian or virtue-based value systems in other countries. If the "culture" of medicine has evolved in this way first in the United States and shortly thereafter in some European countries, it is reasonable to suppose that the wider culture – society as a whole – may undergo other changes. No country today is so isolated from the rest of the world that it can remain aloof from and immune to cross-cultural influences.

Conceptions of Autonomy: East and West

A Japanese physician, Noritoshi Tanida, describes sharp differences between features of Japanese and Western culture related to the role of the individual.[8] Tanida says that tradition has left little room for the individual or for individualism in Japan; yet he acknowledges that, since the opening of Japan to the West about 130 years ago, Western individualism was introduced into the country. Nevertheless, most Japanese are much less individualistic than are Westerners, a feature that is evident in the decision-making process. In general, Tanida notes, there is no open discussion or clear responsibility, but rather a process of mutual dependency. As a result, the person most affected by a decision may not be informed of what is happening and is not always a part of the decision-making process. The clearest example of this, Tanida holds, is concealing the truth from cancer patients in the practice of clinical medicine.

Another East Asian, Ruiping Fan, puts forth an even stronger view of the difference between East and West with regard to the individual's role in medical decision-making.[9] Fan argues that the Western concept of autonomy, which demands self-determination on the part of the individual, is incommensurable with the East Asian principle of autonomy, which requires family determination. In contending that these two notions of autonomy are incommensurable, Fan insists that there is no shared abstract content between the

Western and Eastern principles of autonomy; the two are separate and distinct.

One conclusion that can be drawn from the contrast between East and West is that there simply is no universal ethic regarding disclosure of information, informed consent, and decision-making in medical practice. Not only do these practices differ as a matter of fact in different societies, but they are incompatible. This conclusion is obviously true for the descriptive thesis of ethical relativism: Truth-telling, informed consent, and decision-making about medical treatment vary in different cultures. Furthermore, if we accept Fan's account, a conceptual variation exists as well; autonomy means something different in East Asia from what it signifies in the West.

The East Asian principle of autonomy holds that "Every agent should be able to make his or her decisions and actions harmoniously in cooperation with other relevant persons."[10] Thus, when patients and family are in harmony, they decide together. That situation probably prevails most of the time in Western medical practice as well. However, it is the family who has the final authority to make clinical decisions in accordance with the East Asian principle. According to Ruiping Fan, if a patient requests or refuses a treatment while a relevant family member disagrees with that decision, the doctor should not simply follow the patient's wish but should urge the patient and the family to negotiate and come to an agreement before the physician will act. It is the family that constitutes the autonomous social unit, and the physician may not act contrary to their decision.

This example of cultural diversity raises the enduring question of normative ethical relativism: Has Western bioethics arrived at the ethically right position with regard to respecting the individual autonomy of the patient? Is the practice in other cultures of deferring to the patient's family, or leaving the decision in the hands of the physician, right in those cultures although it would be wrong in the United States?

The emphasis on autonomy, at least in the early days of bioethics in the United States, was never intended to cut patients off from their families by insisting on an obsessive focus on the patient. Rather, it was intended to counteract the predominant mode of paternalism on the part of the medical profession. In fact, there was little discussion of where the family entered in and no presumption that a family-centered approach to sick patients was somehow a violation of the patient's autonomy. Most patients want and need the support of their families whether or not they seek to be autonomous agents regarding their own care. Respect for autonomy is perfectly consistent with recognition of the important role that families play when a loved one is ill. Autonomy has fallen into such disfavor among some ethicists in the United States that the pendulum has begun to swing in the direction of families, with urgings to "take families seriously"[11] and even to consider the interests of family members equal to those of the competent patient.[12]

Fan says that some people may deny that what he refers to as the "East Asian principle of autonomy" can even be characterized as a principle of autonomy. He nevertheless defends his use of the term, noting that the word for autonomy in the Chinese language is often used not only for individuals, but also for units like a family or a community. The same is true in the English language: In its political sense, *autonomy* means "self-rule" and can therefore apply to communities, countries, and, as in Mexico, universities.

Fan demonstrates that the East Asian principle of autonomy has significant implications for truth-telling, informed consent, and advance directives in the East Asian clinical setting. If a physician directly informs a patient about a diagnosis of a terminal disease instead of first telling a member of the family, that would be extremely rude and inappropriate. Interestingly, however, while East Asian custom allows the family to choose a treatment on behalf of a competent patient, the family may not readily refuse a treatment on behalf of a competent patient. This is evidently because of the underlying assumption that a treatment recommended by a physician will be beneficial to the patient, whereas it is at least questionable whether a withholding or withdrawing of treatment is in the interests of a competent patient.

So when it comes to actually making medical decisions, who should decide? Should it be patients themselves in the West, in accordance with the principle of autonomy as "self-determination," and families of patients in the East, in accordance with the "family-determination-oriented" principle? There is little doubt at this point that in the United States the patient with decisional capacity holds the moral and legal right to decide, with very rare exceptions. Those exceptions include some cases in which a pregnant woman's refusal of an intervention is deemed harmful to the life or health of the fetus (forced cesarean sections are the clearest example of this) and the situation in which physicians judge a treatment to be "medically futile" and take the decision-making out of the patient's hands. But these exceptions are contested by those who contend that pregnant women should have all the rights of other competent patients and that a physician's assessment that a treatment is "medically futile" should not replace the patient's wish for the treatment, which may have psychological value.

So we are left with ethical relativism. As Ruiping Fan puts it: "Which principle is more true: the Western principle of autonomy or the East Asian principle of autonomy? Who should give up their own principle and turn to the principle held by the other side?"[13] Fan's own solution is to adopt the procedural principle of freedom, allowing both Western and East Asian people to follow their respective and incommensurable principles of autonomy. Interestingly, Fan's solution appeals to a higher principle, that of freedom or liberty. He acknowledges as much and articulates the principle of freedom commonly associated with Western philosophical and political thought: "Every group of people as well as every single individual has freedom to act as they see appropriate, insofar as their action does not harm other people."[14] That sounds remarkably like something John Stuart Mill might have written.

Application of this principle appears to grant to an individual patient the right to reject the cultural custom of family autonomy in favor of individual decision-making. But would it really? If East Asian patients insisted on their freedom to act as they deem appropriate, doing so might damage family harmony, so perhaps other people would be harmed after all. Ruiping Fan does not raise the explicit question of what individual patients or physicians might do, but refers only to "Western and East Asian people" being free to follow their respective principles of autonomy. It leaves ambiguous the status of the individual patient in East Asia and possibly also the role of a family in the West that seeks to follow the family-determination notion of autonomy.

Is this a relativist solution? Fan says no, it is not to surrender to ethical relativism, "but to secure the most reasonable in a peaceful way in this pluralist world."[15] This reply embraces tolerance and is a practical accommodation to cross-cultural diversity. If not a surrender to relativism, how can we characterize Fan's position? Fan himself describes this type of thought as a "transcendental argument for a content-less principle that ought to be employed in a secular pluralist society."[16] This merely replaces the puzzling with the obscure. Philosophy should seek to explain and clarify, not to obfuscate and muddy. We have to do better.

Truth-Telling

In the Western world the custom of withholding information from patients goes back at least as far as Hippocrates. Hippocrates admonished physicians to perform their duties

> calmly and adroitly, concealing most things from the patient while you are attending to him. Give necessary orders with cheerfulness and sincerity, turning his attention away from what is being done to him; sometimes reprove sharply and emphatically, and sometimes comfort with solicitude and attention, revealing nothing of the patient's future or present condition.[17]

Does this ancient practice represent a tradition of some cultural group? If so, which one? Ancient Greek tradition, carried down through the Greco-Roman empire? That would not have been a likely influence on Asian medical practice. If it is part of any "culture"

at all, it is that of the medical profession (speaking metaphorically), renowned throughout the ages for its paternalism. Medical paternalism remains the rule rather than the exception in Asia and Latin America, and it persists to a somewhat lesser extent in some parts of Western Europe, as well.

The shift in attitude toward disclosing the diagnosis to cancer patients began to occur in the United States in the late 1960s, a millennial moment since the time of Hippocrates. Although often portrayed as a cultural tradition, one in which many countries diverge from the preeminence accorded to the individual in the United States, nondisclosure by physicians to patients appears rather to have been a nearly universal customary practice dictated by medical professionals throughout the world.

But things change. Attitudes and practices of physicians in the United States have undergone a striking reversal in the past three decades. A study conducted in 1961 revealed that 90% of physicians did not inform their patients of the diagnosis of cancer.[18] When that study was redone in 1977, it revealed that 98% of doctors usually informed patients of the diagnosis of cancer.[19] It is entirely possible that such changes will begin to occur in other countries as well. Evidence suggests that this has already begun to happen.

These changes do not require us to impugn the motives of physicians who have thought it best not to tell patients they have cancer, nor is it to condemn the benevolence that undergirds medical paternalism in general. Now, as in the past, most justifications for withholding information from patients have rested implicitly or explicitly on an appeal to the principle of beneficence. If the behavior of doctors in the United States has changed in the past three decades or so, it is not because the principle of beneficence no longer serves as a justification or that physicians no longer act from benevolent motives. It is simply that the competing ethical principle of respect for autonomy has taken priority over the principle of beneficence in motivating and justifying physicians' behavior. Once it became evident that patients wished to know their diagnoses (or already knew they had cancer in spite of families and physicians conspiring to keep the news from them), and once physicians came to realize that disclosing a diagnosis of cancer did not typically cast the patient into a deep depression and very rarely, if ever, led to documented cases of patients committing suicide, then benevolent paternalism could no longer be sustained on ethical grounds.

From the earliest moments of modern bioethics, some people worried about the alleged requirement always to "tell the truth." In response to the claim that patients have "a right to know" their diagnosis and prognosis, challengers replied: what about "the right not to know?" Of course, there is no inconsistency here. People have a right to receive information, if they want it, and also the right to refuse to receive that information. That is precisely what "respect for persons" supports: respect for the wishes and values of the individual patient.

This is the point at which the philosophical distinction between ultimate moral principles and specific rules of conduct becomes critical. "Respect for persons" is a fundamental, or ultimate, ethical principle. The imperative "tell patients the truth about their condition" is a specific rule of conduct. Moreover, respecting a particular patient's wish not to know is perfectly consistent with the general obligation to disclose to patients their diagnosis. This also demonstrates the distinction between ethical universals and moral absolutes. "Always tell patients the truth about their condition" would be the moral absolute in this case, clearly a different imperative from one that mandates respect for the wishes of patients.

On this analysis, the answer to the question of how the case of truth-telling to patients fits into the debates over ethical relativism is simple (relatively speaking). No universal ethical mandate exists to tell patients the truth about their terminal illness. Nor is it the case that telling the patients the truth is right in some countries or cultures and wrong in others. Moreover, to contend that the principle of autonomy mandates disclosure misinterprets how that ethical principle should be applied. Respect for autonomy means, among other things, acting in a way that respects the values of individuals. Individuals' values often mirror the predominant values of their country

or culture, but they do not always do so. When they do, we must be sensitive to those values and respectful of the people who hold them.

A lingering problem, however, is that doctors often do not know or do not take the time or trouble to find out the patient's values. They take the family's word for whether the patient "can handle" the information. Or they simply honor the family's wish not to tell the patient. Here is where the practice in the United States is most likely to diverge from that in other countries. Because respect for the patient's autonomy has become entrenched in American medical practice, most physicians will probably not automatically comply with the family's wish not to reveal a diagnosis of cancer or other fatal or terminal illness.

It is clear from published reports in the medical and bioethical literature that doctors in other countries do readily honor a family's request not to tell the patient a diagnosis of cancer or other terminal illness. I believe that behavior is as much a reflection of the still dominant paternalism of physicians as it is an expression of a cultural value. When respect for autonomy is not recognized as an ethical principle in medical practice, physicians see no need to find out whether a patient wants to know the diagnosis of cancer or terminal illness. Medicine has always been paternalistic and hierarchical. In some ways, the culture of medicine remains paternalistic in the United States, as anyone can attest who has heard physicians urge the omission of "scary" items from consent forms.

A medical oncologist from Italy, who had practiced for a while in the United States, reported what she had learned in medical school.[20] The Italian Deontology Code, written by the Italian Medical Association, included the following statement: "A serious or lethal prognosis can be hidden from the patient, but not from the family."[21] That was in the late 1970s. The Deontology Code was revised in 1989, with this statement: "The physician has the duty to provide the patient – according to his cultural level and abilities to understand – the most serene information about the diagnosis, the prognosis and the therapeutic perspectives and their consequences. Each question asked by the patient has to be accepted and answered clearly." The code goes on to grant to physicians the well-known "therapeutic privilege" of withholding information if disclosure would be harmful to the patient, and in that case the information must be communicated to the family. But the revised code still represents a sharp reversal from the presumption of nondisclosure in the code of a mere decade earlier.

The Italian oncologist who wrote about this shift stated her belief that ethics is connected to cultural values and varies in different societies. She rejected a belief in "absolute values" in favor of respecting the pluralism of different cultures. This was by way of background to her contention that "the Italian society is not prepared for the American way." She explained further, saying that even today Italians believe that patients will never acquire enough knowledge to enable them to understand what physicians tell them and therefore to participate in their own care. Italians still believe that protecting an ill family member from painful information prevents the sick person from suffering alone, from isolation, and is essential for keeping the family together.

Is it reasonable to expect that these attitudes will gradually be transformed, just as similar attitudes were in the United States several decades ago? The Italian oncologist waffled a bit on this point. On the one hand, she stated her belief that "Italians should not borrow the American way." On the other hand, she urged Italians to learn from Americans and "try to find a better Italian way." As examples of changes taking place within the medical profession, she noted courses in bioethics in universities and medical meetings on truth-telling and communicating with patients. In the end, she reached the conclusion that "the only way to respect both Italian ethical principles and the patient's autonomy and dignity is to let the patient know that there are no barriers to communication and to the truth."[22] What is most peculiar is the reference to "Italian ethical principles." Withholding information from patients is not a function of ethnic traditions but rather of how the medical profession has historically conducted its practice in most places in the world. It is also a class phenomenon, since doctors are typically better educated than most of their

patients and question the ability of patients to fully understand what they have been told.

A mere 5 years after its 1989 revision, the Italian code of medical ethics was revised once again. The revision reflected the "constantly changing relationship between the medical profession and society, and between physicians and patients."[23] In the newly revised code, the "Italian way" has come very close to the "American way." Article three of the new code adds to the physician's obligation expressed in the 1989 code "to respect the dignity of the human being" the additional obligation to respect the patient's freedom of choice. Article four of the new code adds the physician's obligation to respect the rights of the individual, and extensive revisions of the doctrine of informed consent are in conformity with other modern codes of ethics. The code mandates respect for the decisional autonomy of the patient, even in cases in which the life of the patient is threatened.[24]

Equally striking are revisions on the topic of confidentiality. Whereas the earlier Italian code permitted doctors to conceal the truth from the patient and disclose it to the next of kin, the new code essentially prohibits nondisclosure to the patient and disclosure to a third party. Two exceptions to this rule are, first, when the patient specifically authorizes disclosure to others and, second, when there is potential for harm to a third party.[25] It would be absurd to conclude that "Italian ethical principles" have changed in this brief interlude between the 1989 code and the more recent revisions. Instead, as the authors of an article describing the new code observe, "from a paternalistic attitude in which the physician, for the good of the patient, felt authorised and justified to set aside the personal requests of the patient and even to violate his wishes, a therapeutic alliance has evolved, in which the two partners together try to decide on the clinical choices that best promote the patient's wellbeing."[26]

Changes are also occurring in Asia, a region of the world often cited as adhering to family and group values almost to the exclusion of recognizing the importance of the individual. A Japanese physician observes that the concept of informed consent has recently been recognized in his country, yet he acknowledges that most Japanese physicians withhold information about diagnosis and prognosis from their patients who have cancer.[27] It is reasonable to wonder whether "informed consent" means the same thing in Japan as it does in the West. One report notes that the Bioethics Council of the Japanese Medical Association introduced the idea of "Japanese informed consent," which was to be carried out in accordance with the prevailing medical paternalism in that country.[28] A survey in Japan showed that 67% of physicians would disclose the diagnosis to patients with early cancer, but only 16% would tell those with advanced cancer. Studies from other countries show that many patients do want to be informed of a diagnosis of cancer, but a discrepancy exists between patients' preferences and physicians' attitudes.[29]

A physician speaking at an international conference about truth-telling in Japanese medicine[30] described a number of cultural features that help to explain physicians' reluctance to disclose a bad prognosis. That reluctance stems from patients' unwillingness to receive such information, which in turn is based on deeper cultural roots. Patients want to have an "edited" version of the truth. They enter a tacit conspiracy with their family and the physician to avoid a difficult subject. This results in the family taking over all responsibility and decisions for the patient's illness. Although many patients will guess and come to know the truth eventually, they still will not ask directly. This behavior is rooted in the Japanese ethos in which silent endurance is a virtue. The aim is to make dying easier, not to invoke a dogma of telling patients the truth. Patients want to die as calmly and peacefully as possible, and that goal is more readily achieved if they remain ignorant of their prognosis. Relatives assume the burden of making an intuitive judgment of whether the patient wants to know the diagnosis and can handle it. Not to accept one's death gallantly is worse than death itself. Physicians, patients, and families all want to avoid a "disgraceful upset" that conveying bad new could produce. The physician who explained all this echoed what others discussing medicine in Japan have said: Despite powerful influences from Western countries, Japan is not totally Westernized, yet the Japanese do not want to stick to their old traditions completely. The physician ended by saying that the Japanese people must achieve a new type of death education, with more ethical emphasis, closer to the Western style of dealing with death.

But let us assume that a cultural gap does exist between North American practices of disclosing bad news to patients and different customs in other parts of the world. What should we conclude about whether one cultural practice is "right" and the other "wrong"? How does this example fit into the debates over ethical relativism?

The answer depends entirely on how the question is framed and how the situation is described. Consider the following alternative descriptions.

1   Doctors and patients in the United States believe that patients should be told the truth about a diagnosis of terminal illness. Doctors and patients in other countries believe that doctors should tell the family but not the patient. The ethical principle of "respect for autonomy" mandates that doctors treat patients as autonomous individuals and so must inform them about their illness. The truth-telling practice in the United States conforms to this principle and is ethically right, whereas the nondisclosure practice in other countries violates this practice and is ethically wrong.

2   Autonomy is the predominant value in North American culture. Doctors and patients in the United States adhere to an autonomy model of disclosure in medical practice. Family-centered values are more prominent than individual autonomy in other cultures. Doctors and patients in these cultures adhere to a family-centered practice of disclosure of terminal illness. Therefore, it is right to disclose to a patient a diagnosis of terminal cancer in the United States and wrong to make that same disclosure in the other countries.

3   Autonomy is the predominant value in North American culture, but disclosure of terminal illness by doctors to patients is nevertheless a fairly recent practice. The US population comprises many recent immigrants, and some cultural groups adhere to

family-centered values from their country of origin, especially in specific matters such as disclosure of terminal illness. Family-centered values predominate in other countries, but practices such as disclosure of a diagnosis of terminal illness have begun to change in those places. "Respect for persons" requires that in any country or culture, doctors should discuss with their patients whether they want to receive information and make decisions about their medical care or whether they want the physician to discuss these matters only with the family.

The third description is obviously the "right" answer. What is wrong with the other two descriptions shows what is frequently amiss in debates over ethical relativism. Description 1 has two main flaws. The first is the common failing of distorting or misusing the principle of respect for autonomy. The principle does not require inflicting unwanted information on people; rather, it requires first finding out how much and what kind of information they want to know and then respecting that expressed wish. When the principle of autonomy is interpreted in that way, nothing automatically follows regarding whether patients should be told the truth about their diagnosis. The second flaw is the assumption that all people in a country or culture have the same attitudes and beliefs toward the values that

predominate in that culture. In a Los Angeles study of senior citizens' attitudes toward disclosure of terminal illness, in no ethnic group did 100% of its members favor disclosure or nondisclosure to the patient. Forty-seven percent of Korean-Americans believed that a patient with metastatic cancer should be told the truth about the diagnosis, 65% of Mexican-Americans held that belief, 87% of European-Americans believed patients should be told the truth, and 89% of African-Americans held that belief. If physicians automatically withheld the diagnosis from Korean-Americans because the majority of people in that ethnic group did not want to be told, they would be making a mistake almost 50% of the time.[31]

Description 2 is flawed for one of the same reasons that description 1 is flawed: It presupposes that all people in a country or culture have the same attitudes and beliefs toward the values that predominate in that culture. That assumption is clearly false, as the Los Angeles study just cited demonstrates. In a multicultural society such as the United States, ethical relativism poses an array of problems not likely to arise in countries that enjoy a common cultural heritage (if any such countries still remain). "Multiculturalism is good," its proponents contend.[32] Whether or not that is true, it surely causes difficulties for doctors and patients.

Notes

1 Renée C. Fox, "The Evolution of American Bioethics: A Sociological Perspective," in George Weisz (ed.), *Social Science Perspectives on Medical Ethics* (Philadelphia: University of Pennsylvania Press, 1990), p. 206.
2 The workshop, part of my Ford Foundation project, took place in Davao, Mindanao, in December 1995.
3 This interview took place in February 1996 during my second Ford Foundation project.
4 This interview took place in April 1994 in Bombay.
5 Christopher Clausen, "Welcome to Postculturalism," *The Key Reporter*, Vol. 62, No. 1 (1996), p. 2.
6 This meeting took place during my Ford Foundation visit to Mexico in February 1993.

7 Diego Gracia, "The Intellectual Basis of Bioethics in Southern European Countries," *Bioethics*, Vol. 7, No. 2/3 (1993), pp. 100–1.
8 Noritoshi Tanida, "Bioethics Is Subordinate to Morality in Japan," *Bioethics*, Vol. 10 (1996), pp. 202–11.
9 Ruiping Fan, "Self-Determination vs. Family-Determination: Two Incommensurable Principles of Autonomy," *Bioethics*, Vol. 11 (1997), pp. 309–22.
10 Fan, p. 316.
11 James Lindemann Nelson, "Taking Families Seriously," *Hastings Center Report*, Vol. 22 (1992), pp. 6–12.
12 John Hardwig, "What About the Family?" *Hastings Center Report*, Vol. 20 (1990), pp. 5–10.

13 Fan, p. 322.

14 Fan, p. 322.

15 Fan, p. 322.

16 Fan quotes this phrase from H. Tristram Engelhardt, Jr., *The Foundations of Bioethics*, 2nd edition (New York: Oxford University Press, 1996).

17 Citation from President's Commission for the Study of Ethical Problems in Medicine and Biomedical and Behavioral Research, *Making Health Care Decisions* (Washington, DC: Government Printing Office, 1982), Vol. 1, p. 32.

18 D. Oken, "What To Tell Cancer Patients: A Study of Medical Attitudes," *Journal of the American Medical Association*, Vol. 175 (1961), pp. 1120–8.

19 Dennis H. Novack, Robin Plumer, Raymond L. Smith, Herbert Ochitill, Gary R. Morrow, and John M. Bennett, "Changes in Physicians' Attitudes Toward Telling the Cancer Patient," *Journal of the American Medical Association*, Vol. 341 (1979), pp. 897–900.

20 Antonella Surbone, "Truth-Telling to the Patient," *Journal of the American Medical Association*, Vol. 268 (1992), pp. 1661–2.

21 Surbone, p. 1661.

22 Surbone, p. 1662.

23 Vittorio Fineschi, Emanuela Turillazzi, and Cecilia Cateni, "The New Italian Code of Medical Ethics," *Journal of Medical Ethics*, Vol. 23 (1997), p. 238.

24 Fineschi, Turillazzi, and Cateni, pp. 241–2.

25 Fineschi, Turillazzi, and Cateni, p. 243.

26 Fineschi, Turillazzi, and Cateni, p. 241.

27 Atsushi Asai, "Should Physicians Tell Patients the Truth?" *Western Journal of Medicine*, Vol. 163 (1995), pp. 36–9.

28 Tanida, p. 208.

29 Asai, p. 36.

30 Shin Ohara, "Truth-Telling and We-Consciousness in Japan: Some Biomedical Reflections on Japanese Civil Religion," unpublished paper presented at the conference, "Ethics Codes in Medicine and Biotechnology," Freiburg, Germany, October 12–15, 1997.

31 Leslie J. Blackhall, Sheila T. Murphy, Gelya Frank, Vicki Michel, and Stanley Azen, "Ethnicity and Attitudes Toward Patient Autonomy," *Journal of the American Medical Association*, Vol. 274, No. 10 (1995), pp. 820–5.

32 Blaine J. Fowers and Frank C. Richardson, "Why Is Multiculturalism Good?" *American Psychologist*, Vol. 51, No. 6 (1996), pp. 609–21.

85

Transgender Children and the Right to Transition
Medical Ethics When Parents Mean Well But Cause Harm

Maura Priest

1   Introduction

Most of us that live in liberal democracies agree that parents have the right to raise their own children. Most, however, also agree that there are limits to parental authority. Arguably, these limits have grown stronger and more expansive throughout the 20th century.[1] Consider, for instance, that several states and counties have outlawed programs which attempt to change the sexual orientation of homosexual youth.[2] Not too long ago, it would have been unimaginable that a religious program which threatens no physical harm to children would be legally prohibited.

Outlawing the above mentioned, "gay reform camps" suggests not only that we are taking youth rights more seriously, but that we are taking the notion of *psychological harm* more seriously. While we have long accepted that mental states arise from brain states, there remains a lingering tendency for experts and lay persons alike to think of psychological harm in a distinct and less important category than physical harm. This is despite the evidence that points to psychological abuse being every bit as harmful as physical and sexual abuse (Spinazzola et al., 2014).

Yet the tide is turning. Not only are gay reform camps now illegal in some states, but laws against bullying and harm via cyber space are increasingly becoming a matter of legislative prohibition. Along similar lines, therapy and psychiatric drugs are used much more frequently than ever before.[3] Both of these moves suggest a growing concern with mental ailments that fall upon children and adolescents.

As we continue to move in the direction of seeing psychological harm in the same light as we see physical harm, we should expect to see an increase in the ways in which the state intervenes with parental authority. After all, for most of the history of liberal democratic societies, parents "psychologically" harming their children was not considered a matter for the state to deal with at all. There are hence large gaps in appropriate measures to protect those not of age to protect themselves. In the United Kingdom, for instance, new "Cinderella" legislation (formally, *Serious Crime Act of 2014*) was recently ratified and is aimed at protecting emotionally abused youth and

Original publication details: Maura Priest, "Transgender Children and the Right to Transition: Medical Ethics When Parents Mean Well But Cause Harm," pp. 45–59 from *American Journal of Bioethics* 19 (2019). Reproduced with permission of Taylor & Francis.

Bioethics: An Anthology, Fourth Edition. Edited by Udo Schüklenk and Peter Singer.

punishing their perpetrators. Parliament member Robert Buckland had this to say about the legislation: "Our criminal law has never reflected the full range of emotional suffering experienced by children who are abused by their parents or caretakers. The sad truth is that, until now, the wicked stepmother would have got away scot free" (Chorley, 2014). Buckland's statement well exemplifies the legal gap when it comes to protecting minors from non-physical forms of abuse.

This paper discusses one area of psychological harm that is worthy of new attention: harm to transgender youth who have non-supportive parents (by "non-supportive" I do not mean parents who do not love or care for their children. I rather mean parents who do not support, aid, and/or approve of the transition process.) In particular, I will argue that transgender adolescents have a fundamental right to PBT (puberty-blocking treatment) *even if* their parents disapprove. The need for this type of state protection is serious. The World Professional Association of Transgender Health (WPATH) warns us that, "refusing timely medical interventions for adolescents might prolong gender dysphoria and contribute to an appearance that could provoke abuse and stigmatization" (Coleman et al., p.78: 2012). A child is transgender if he or she identifies with a gender other than their biological sex. A child has gender dysphoria if such atypical identification causes distress.[4] Being transgender itself does not necessarily mean one suffers from gender dysphoria. Transgender youth who lack supportive families, for instance, are far more likely to experience gender dysphoria (Olson et al., 2016; Gorin-Lazard et al., 2012; and de Vries et al., 2014.)

Sadly, youth suffering from gender dysphoria often face more than just psychological harm, but all too often the ultimate physical harm. Transgender youth are ten times as likely to attempt suicide when compared to their cisgender peers (Haas et al., 2010). Even more, suicide has recently moved up the list from the third leading cause of death amongst teenagers to the second. From the words of the American Academy of Pediatrics, "With suicide rising to the second-leading cause of death among adolescents, the American Academy of Pediatrics (AAP) is publishing updated

guidelines advising pediatricians how to identify and help teens at risk" (AAP, 2016). If suicide is already a serious risk amongst adolescents, and this risk is magnified by 10-fold when it comes to transgender youth, this is nothing other than a serious mental health crisis. These statistics suggest that not only should pediatricians be especially concerned with psychological harm that befalls marginalized youth such as transgender children, but arguably so should the state. The formal argument runs as follows:

1. The state has a duty to protect minors from serious harm inflicted by their caretakers.
2. Harm which leads to suicide is a serious harm.
3. Transgender youth with non-supportive parents are at a high risk of psychological harm leading to suicidal tendencies.
4. Therefore the state should pay special attention to, and has a duty to protect, transgender minors from psychological harm inflicted via their caretakers.

Admittedly, the above argument, even if persuasive, leaves much vague. The remainder of this paper will attempt to fill in those details.

My strategy for defending the formal argument above revolves around arguing in favor of two normative claims:

1. Transgender youth should have access to treatment which is not dependent upon parental approval.
2. There should be state-sponsored publicly available information regarding gender dysphoria, transgender identification, and means of appropriate treatment.

The next section offers an overview of gender dysphoria and the use of PBT. Section 3 describes the particular *psychiatric* problems that befall transgender youth in the absence of PBT. Section 4 focuses on the *physical* harms that result from the absence of PBT. Section 5 argues that the harms described in Sections 3 and 4 indeed justify state intervention into the life of transgender minors and their families. Section 6 argues that the state has not only a role to play in legally mandating the right to PBT, but also in using government institutions to educate the public about transgender issues and treatment. In Section 7, I respond to potential objections. Section 8 reviews the paper's main argument and offers concluding remarks.

2   Gender Dysphoria and Treatment for Transgender Youth

2.1   Gender dysphoria and its consequences

Gender dysphoria, the feeling of disconnect and unease at the difference between one's biological gender and one's sense of gender identity, often begins at a surprisingly young age.[5] Many parents, knowing nothing about what it means to be transgender, are baffled by toddlers who insist that they are the gender opposite the one on their birth certificate. A dad might be horrified when his little boy comes downstairs in a tutu. A mother might be exasperated that her 6-year-old daughter insists on calling herself a "big brother" rather than a big sister.[6] And two Christian parents might cry themselves to sleep because their preschooler insists on playing with girl toys and has already been labeled "gay" by his peers.[7] While all parents understandably feel stressed in such situations, different parents often handle these situations in polarizing fashions. Not only do some parents not accept their transgender children, but sadly more than a few have forced their children out of the home, leaving them homeless. Indeed, being transgender is one of the leading risk factors for homelessness.[8]

While many parents are unaware of how to address their transgender child's expressions of dysphoria, the earliest treatment requires neither medication nor any intervention that is irreversible. Rather, specialists recommend that parents of young transgender children offer support in at least two ways. First, because their child is likely to go through psychological stress unlike

that of their gender conforming peers, counseling of some sort is often helpful (Ettner et al., p. 101, 2016, and Krieger, p. 40, 2011). Or, to put things more starkly, "It is recommended that all transgender adolescents be involved in psychological therapy, even those who are functioning well, to ensure that they have the necessary support they need and a safe place to explore identities and consider the transitioning experience" (Levine, p. 308, 2013). In addition, parents wishing to help their children maintain a healthy psychological state should be supportive and non-judgmental of their children's gender expression (Olson et al., 2016). Indeed, perhaps nothing speaks to the importance of parental support more than the disparity in the suicide rate of transgender teens without supportive parents compared to those who do have support. A recent *Huffington Post* article notes the following,

> Transgender people who are rejected by their families or lack social support are much more likely to both consider suicide, and to attempt it. Conversely, those with strong support were 82% less likely to attempt suicide than those without support, according to one recent study. Another study showed that transgender youth whose parents reject their gender identity are 13 times more likely to attempt suicide than transgender youth who are supported by their parents. (Tannehill, 2016).[9]

Parents who have mixed feelings about their children's transgender expressions are wise to keep this statistic in mind. It is fine for parents to have internal questions, but parents who want to protect their kids should outwardly express support and love to young persons already prone to feelings of isolation and rejection.

The transgender child who cannot dress or express oneself genuinely will likely face an insufferable sense of gender dysphoria (Burgess, 1999; de Vries et al., 2014 and 2012; Durso and Gates, 2012; Frisch, 2016; Garofalo et al., 2006; Watson et al., 2017). When a child is accepted by their family and allowed to express their gender identity, they remain transgender but may experience little to no gender dysphoria.[10] However, a child who is not accepted and not allowed to express their gender identity is likely to struggle with the mismatch between their physical body and their gender identity (Olson et al., 2016; Gorin-Lazard et al., 2012; and de Vries et al., 2014).

2.2 Do children own their bodies?

Philosopher John Locke argued that our bodies are our property; in his words, ". . .every man has a Property in his own Person" (John Locke, *Second Treatise*, Ch. 5, book 27). This idea has been foundational to liberal democracies ever since: members of liberal democracies should have the liberty to do with their body what they want, when they want to, and with whom they choose. Yet for transgender youth approaching puberty, their bodies do not feel like their property at all. Indeed, such puberty induced changes create a body they would rather disown than own. In the words of Irwin Krieger, "When transgender kids reach puberty, their bodies begin to betray them. They develop the physical characteristics that are typical of their biological sex but not in accord with their deeply felt gender. . . . As puberty progresses, many begin to feel hopeless about their future" (p. 20, 2011). If transgender youth are truly the owners of their bodies, they should have the right to prevent them from going through changes of which they disapprove. What these adolescents would like to do with their bodies is clear: they want to take steps to make the puberty induced changes stop. And indeed, the standard of care for transgender adolescents lines up with their wants. The recommendation for adolescents beginning puberty up until age 16 is to undergo PBT. According to the Standards of Care for transgender persons, "withholding puberty suppression and subsequent feminizing or masculinizing hormone-therapy is not a neutral option for adolescets" (Coleman et al., 2012). This does not mean every gender dysphoric child should go forward with PBT, but that those adolescents who (after an evaluation) are deemed good candidates should have the option available. PBT freezes the child in time physiologically. Hence, a transgender boy need not go through the horrors of developing breasts nor a transgender girl look in the mirror and see facial hair. With this treatment, the development of these secondary-sex characteristics is put on hold.

In spite of their children's struggles, parents understandably might worry that their child, at such a young age, does not know what they want, especially not for the rest of their life. Indeed, these parents might point out that they (the parents) are the true owners of their children's bodies, at least until they become legal adults. Before that time, it is the job of the parents to protect the bodies of their children in ways they see fit. Or so one might argue. However, even if parents are worried that their child might change their mind regarding their gender identity; the comforting news is that PBT is reversible (Cohen-Kettenis et al., p. 1894, 2008, and Delemarre-van de Waal and Cohen-Kettenis, 2006). Puberty-blockers give youth time to be sure that they really do identify with their non-biological gender. The WPATH makes a recommendation for puberty-suppressing treatment with the following justification:

> Two goals justify intervention with puberty suppressing hormones: (i) their use gives adolescents more time to explore their gender nonconformity and other developmental issues; and (ii) their use may facilitate transition by preventing the development of sex characteristics that are difficult or impossible to reverse if adolescents continue on to pursue sex reassignment. Puberty suppression may continue for a few years, at which time a decision is made to either discontinue all hormone therapy or transition to a feminizing/masculinizing hormone regimen (Coleman et al., p. 177, 2012).

Most adolescents who use puberty-blockers do later choose to continue throughout life with a transgender identification (de Vries et al., 2014). However, it is always possible some will not, and for these youth it is a great relief that their body has not been changed permanently. Again, from the WPATH, "Pubertal suppression does not inevitably lead to social transition or to sex reassignment" (Coleman et al., p.177, 2012).

Following treatment with puberty suppressants, the next step in care involves taking cross-sex hormones so the transgender youth might experience the puberty of their identified gender (to the closest extent possible.) According to Endocrine Society Guidelines, "We recommend treating transsexual adolescents (Tanner stage 2) by suppressing

puberty with GnRH analogues until age 16 years old, after which cross-sex hormones may

be given" (Hembree et al., p. 3133, 2009). And as the WPATH notes, "Feminizing/masculinizing hormone therapy – the administration of exogenous endocrine agents to induce feminizing or masculinizing changes – is a medically necessary intervention for many transsexual, transgender, and gender nonconforming individuals with gender dysphoria" (Coleman et al., p.187, 2012, and Gorin-Lazard et al., 2012). At this stage of cross-sex hormone-treatment, unlike the stage of PBT some of the bodily changes enacted are irreversible (Ettner et al., p. 201, 2016).

Although this stage of cross-sex hormone intervention is clearly important, it is not the focus of this paper. One reason is that I believe that the thesis *I am arguing for* (the need for PBT), is an issue worthy of a paper on its own. In addition, when youth reach the appropriate age for cross-sex hormone-treatment, in many countries they have already reached the age of medical consent or they are very close to doing so. In comparison, when youth reach the apt age for PBT most are too young to make legal medical decisions. Therefore, it seems that PBT is a more pressing issue than is cross-sex hormone-treatment.

2.3 Persisting and desisting

It is not only parents that might worry about transgender children simply going through a "phase." There has also been a series of studies about "persisters" and "desisters" that suggest many transgender children do not become transgender adults (see Steensma et al., 2011 and 2013; Drummond et al., 2008; `ien and Cohen-Kettenis, 2008.) These studies label transgender children who maintain their transgender identity into adulthood "persisters," and those who revert back to their natal gender as "desisters." Taken as a whole, this literature suggests that most transgender children do not go on to become transgender adults, but rather cisgender homosexuals.

So why recommend PBT if evidence suggests that most seemingly transgender children are going to desist? Four points explain why PBT remains the best option:

1. The empirical work on persisters and desisters is controversial, leaving much room for doubt.
2. Most of the work on persisters and desisters focuses on childhood; however, the stage at which PBT is recommended is adolescence.
3. Regardless of the literature on persisters and desisters, and regardless of some disagreement among experts, PBT is the standard of care consistent with the opinion of the collective body of experts in the field of transgender medicine and endocrine studies.
4. Even assuming a significant number of youth who receive PBT do not go on to be transgender adults, this treatment risks far less harm than the absence of PBT.

Let us discuss each of the above in turn. A series of articles has offered compelling criticism of the literature on persisters and desisters (a non-exhaustive list includes Temple Newhook et al., 2018; Olson and Durwood, 2016; Olson, 2016; Pyne, 2014; Serano, 2016; Winters, 2014; Ehrensaft et al., 2018). It will be helpful to briefly summarize some of these criticisms here. One suggested difficulty with the desisting literature is that those who "desisted" might not have met criteria for having gender dysphoria in the first place. The criteria used for diagnosing children with *gender identity disorder* (the diagnosable condition at the time) would not meet today's standards for *gender dysphoria* (the revised diagnosable condition). In the words of Temple et al.,

> Due to such shifting diagnostic categories and inclusion criteria . . . these studies included children who, by current DSM-5 standards, would not likely have been categorized as transgender (i.e., they would not meet the criteria for gender dysphoria) and therefore, it is not surprising that they would not identify as transgender at follow-up. (p. 4, 2018).

This (subjects not meeting criteria for gender dysphoria) is arguably the most serious problem for these studies, for it leaves open the possibility that children *who are* diagnosed with gender dysphoria indeed persist in their identities. Concerning still, as Temple et al. explain further, in one particular study 40% of the subjects did not even meet the criteria for gender identity disorder (p. 5, 2018). Let us look at this piece by piece. In one study 40% of children did not meet standards for gender identity disorder. Of the remaining 60% of subjects who did meet gender identity disorder standards, many of these would not have met the standards for gender dysphoria. Looking at those two statistics together, it is unclear what percentage of the subjects provide evidential relevance for today's transgender youth diagnosed with gender dysphoria.

A different difficulty with the desisting studies was the high attrition rate of participants, and even in one case, classifying those who left the study as desisting, with the justification that, ". . .the Amsterdam Gender Identity Clinic for children and adolescents is the only one in the country . . . we assumed that their gender dysphoric feelings had desisted..." (Steensma et al., p. 501, 2011). So in this case it was actually unknown whether subjects desisted, but simply assumed that they did. While it *might* be true that participants who did not return desisted, there are many other explanations for these participants not returning. Other criticisms of the studies include the fact that the numbers of children in the study were small and confined to two specific cultures (The Netherlands and Canada), the age at the follow-up was relatively young, and the fact that one of the clinics in the study actively worked to discourage persisting (Temple et al., 2018).

When the above criticisms are taken into consideration, one is likely to walk away with considerable doubt over whether most transgender children are desisters. Moreover, even the desisting literature suggests that when children *explicitly state they are the gender opposite of their natal birth*, (as opposed to simply showing gender non-conforming behaviors or claiming they "wished" they were the other gender) we have strong reason to believe these children will be persisters. In the words of Steensma et al., "Persisters

indicated that they felt they were the 'other' sex and the desisters indicated they wished they were the 'other' sex . . . explicitly asking gender dysphoric children with which sex they identify seems to be of great value in predicting a future outcome for both gender dysphoric boys and girls" (p. 588, 2013). Hence this criterion (openly stating their transgender identity) can be used to help diagnose adolescents who are good candidates for PBT.

My point in bringing up this discussion, is to make clear that the commonly heard claim that "most transgender children do not become transgender adults" is far from settled. Notwithstanding, as I will argue below, *even if* most transgender children *were* desisters, there remains strong reason to believe that gender dysphoric youth deserve access to PBT.

2.4   PBT is the best route, regardless

Suppose that for whatever reason a clinician is convinced by the desisting literature, and believes many transgender children do not become transgender adults. There are still three reasons to think PBT is the best medical route. The first is that much of the desisting and persisting literature concerns children. It is at *adolescence*, however, that PBT is recommended. As noted by Coleman et al., "In contrast (to childhood), the persistence of gender dysphoria into adulthood appears to be much higher for adolescents" (p. 172, 2012). While the field of transgender health is still emerging, and while there are many areas where researchers have disagreements, puberty suppression at early adolescence is suggested both by the World Professional Association of Transgender Health and the Endocrine Society. As stated earlier in the paper, according to Endocrine Society Guidelines, "We recommend treating transsexual adolescents (Tanner stage 2) by suppressing puberty with GnRH analogues until age 16 years old, after which cross-sex hormones may be given" (Hembree et al., p. 3133, 2009). And as the WPATH notes, "Feminizing/masculinizing hormone therapy – the administration of exogenous endocrine agents to induce feminizing or masculinizing changes – is a medically necessary intervention for many transsexual, transgender, and gender nonconforming individuals with gender dysphoria" (Coleman et al., p.187, 2012). As said in the abstract of the 7th edition of the Standards of Care for the Health of Transsexual, Transgender, and Gender-Nonconforming People, "The Standards of Care are based on the best available science and expert professional consensus" (Coleman et al., 2012).

We can see that despite the controversy surrounding persisting and desisting literature, experts have managed to agree on standards of care for transgender youth, and such standards are consistent with PBT at early adolescence (Coleman et al., pp. 177–9, 2012). Now this, of course, is not to say that every gender dysphoric child should receive PBT. There are a number of other criteria that make gender dysphoric adolescents appropriate candidates for PBT, and an extensive medical evaluation by a medical and/or psychological professional is an important part of the process. This paper only contends that parental approval need not be an important part of this process.

Some might still worry that over-ruling parental decisions is going too far. It is *possible*, after all, that any given transgender adolescent will not become a transgender adult. No medical test guarantees that a youth who claims to be transgender will carry that identity into adulthood. Said differently, there is no way to know that any given transgender youth will turn out to be a "persister" rather than a "desister." With other types of medical treatment, one might argue, we have blood tests or X-rays which can confirm a diagnosis. This is not so with gender dysphoria.

It is true that PBT comes with risks. However, let us recall that there are risks on both sides. The risks of *not treating* with PBT are very serious: gender dysphoric youth forced to go through puberty of their natal gender are likely to suffer from especially strong dysphoric feelings. They are also unlikely to feel a sense of support from their families or physicians. Such factors put transgender minors at high risk for mental health problems and potentially suicide (Burgess, 1999; de Vries et al., 2014 and 2012; Durso and Gates, 2012; Frisch 2016; Garofalo et al., 2006; and Watson et al., 2017). Even more, those transgender

adolescents who *do* persist in their identities, and have not been given PBT, enter adulthood with a body they reject. Their first years as an independent autonomous agent might be spent worrying about physical features which are either impossible, expensive, or dangerous to change (Taylor, 2015). Let us compare this to an adolescent who takes PBT but then desists. Fortunately for these young persons, PBT is reversible and hence desisters can experience the normal (albeit delayed) puberty process with little physical risk, resulting in the adult body the desister desires (Cohen-Kettenis et al., 2011). When we compare these risks against each other, the riskier, more dangerous, and more permanent option *is not* the option of using PBT and desisting. It is rather bypassing PBT and persisting.

3   Psychological Harm and Epistemic Barriers

In spite of the serious harms facing transgender youth, one reason society, parents, and clinicians might be disinclined to take this harm seriously is that much of the harm is psychological. Ethically speaking, this distinction is irrelevant: we are psychological selves every bit as much as we are physical selves, and harm to either one of these parts is real and ethically significant. Yet one (perhaps legitimate) reason that to be less inclined to take action against psychological harm (in comparison to physical harm) is that we frequently lack the evidential manifestations present with physical harm.

Psychological harm leaves no visible bruises. Even when we can identify the presence of extreme psychological harm, we rarely can be sure that harm was caused by the parent rather than siblings or the stress of school, sports, or other stress points. These epistemic difficulties in establishing the cause and true consequence of psychological ailments explains and justifies hesitancy in state meddling. While these reasons are perhaps justified, they have nothing to do with psychological harm being *intrinsically* less wrong or damaging than physical harm. Given that such justifications are epistemic, when we *do* have an epistemic hold over certain kinds of mental ailments, there is every bit as much reason for the state to intervene as in cases of *physical* abuse.

The harm transgender youth suffer is importantly different from typical instances of psychological harm, and for at least three reasons. First, we have clear and specific evidence that going through puberty of their natal gender imposes serious psychological harm on a transgender child. Second, we have evidence that this harm is often long-term and potentially irreversible. Third, we know exactly what causes this harm (the distressing experience of going through puberty of the "wrong" gender) (Coleman et al., 2012; Tannehill, 2016; Olson et al., 2014 and 2016; Gorin-Lazard et al., 2012; and de Vries et al., 2012, 2014, and 2016; Murad et al., 2010, and Kids Pay the Price, 2017). In all these ways, harm to transgender children is unlike other kinds of psychological harms where important variables are epistemically suspect. Thus, whatever epistemic concerns we may have about psychological harms in other contexts, these should not factor into the topic of consideration in this paper.

4   The Physical Risks

Although many of the notable harms that a transgender child suffers are psychological, there also are risks of physical harm. The increased risk of the ultimate physical harm: death by suicide, has already been stated. But in addition, we should consider the physical realities of what happens when a transgender child is forced to go through the puberty process of their natal sex. This process will result in the secondary-sex physical characteristics that the transgender child so dearly wants to avoid, i.e. breasts, hips, and feminized voice and face for transgender men and facial hair, height, muscle development, and masculine voice and face transgender women. While it is possible to change many of these features through surgery as an adult, this is anything but a simple process. It is important to note that if the youth was denied recommended treatment according to the WPATH transition stages,

the surgical operations needed to fully transition as an adult are much more expensive and complex (Taylor, 2015).

A second physical risk of avoiding recommended puberty-blocking treatment is that transgender children sometimes seek to self-medicate (Garofalo et al., 2006; Clark et al., 2008; Schmid et al., 2005; Rosioreanu et al., 2004). Let us remember that many transgender youths are homeless, having been abandoned by their family for their identity (Burgess, 1999; Keuroghlian et al., 2014; Durso and Gates, 2012). Homelessness is of course a physical risk on its own. But whether the transgender child is homeless or not, they might seek puberty-blockers that can be found on the street or via questionable internet websites. Some transgender adolescents attempt to access this treatment after they are denied it through sanctioned means. Not only is the child not under medical supervision – and hence more at risk of dosage errors – but the medication can be counterfeit, i.e., either not really puberty-blockers at all, or synthetic PBT mixed with dangerous substances. This can, in turn, lead to infection and sadly even death (Garofalo et al., 2006; Clark et al., 2008; Schmid et al., 2005, and Rosioreanu et al., 2004).

Transgender children seeking puberty-blockers via their own means is clearly not an outcome any decent parent would want, even parents who disapprove of puberty-blockers in general. We might compare this to parents who disapprove of their children having sex but would never wish that their children contract an STD if they did. Indeed, one of the justifications behind having sexual education in school is that even if it is "best" for adolescents to wait, many will have sex anyway. This puts teens in grave risk if not taught to take proper precautions. Currently, many teens not only receive sexual education in school, but have access to both private and public health clinics to get access to sexually related treatment (much like sexual education, minors' access to sexual healthcare via public clinics varies by state and jurisdiction). See Klein et al., 2018, for an in-depth look at a state law in Arizona that afforded minors special rights related to sexual health).

I propose that we expand traditional sexual preventative health education to cover transgender health. We should include education relevant to transgender persons and transgender care, as well as have such care available at public and private health clinics. Admittedly, this wish might have better chances of becoming a reality in some parts of the United States than in other parts. Sexual education is not uniform throughout the US, and schools that insist on abstinence only education are unlikely to implement curriculum concerning transgender health. Notwithstanding, we should work toward implementing transgender health education where possible, and further work toward expanding these programs as conditions permit.

5   Justifying Intervention

5.1   A child's right to their body

The first stages of puberty (and hence the approximate time to begin puberty-blockers) begins far younger than the age of legal majority (Selva, 2017). Hence, we run into a dilemma if parents are insistent against such treatment. One potential solution, at least in the United States, is to appeal to what is known as *the mature minor doctrine*. This doctrine recognizes that some adolescents are wise beyond their years, and hence leaves room for these precocious children to make their own medical decisions when deemed sufficiently mature by the courts (Coleman and Rosoff, 2013). However, this is not the solution I want to defend. While I have no issue with using this justification in some cases, I believe that transgender children have a right to treatment apart from any use of the mature minor doctrine, a right that is both universal and not dependent on the transgender child possessing a specific level of maturity. After all, not all transgender youth meet the requirements of a mature minor. Hence, if *all* transgender youth deserve access to PBT, it is best that we do so on different grounds. The justifying principles fit for this task are similar to principles used in the following two types of cases:

1. Principles that justify taking a neglected child away from the home.
2. Principles that justify performing a blood transfusion on children of Jehovah's Witnesses.

Notice that in neither of the cases above is the mature minor doctrine the justification for state action. And while the justifications for these two interventions are not identical, the relevance of each is important. The comparison to negligence explains why the state must help even if the parents have no intention to harm their child. Just as is the case with negligent parents, transgender children should not suffer due to their parents' unintentional mistakes.

Sometimes parental decisions against PBT might be motivated from religious belief, i.e., parents might believe that God made people biologically the gender that they were "meant" to be. While there is a strong presumption supporting parental rights to raise their child according to the parents' religious values, like most rights, this one is limited. As bioethical cases concerning Jehovah's Witnesses have taught us, children should not be destined to suffer because of the religious beliefs of their parents (Guichon and Mitchell, 2007; Woolley, 2005; and Press Association, 2014). Children's future autonomy, autonomy which includes making their own religious choices as adults, is arguably as important as a parent's right to religion and hence must be preserved. While most religious choices made by parents do not interfere with a child making different choices when they reach adulthood, some do. Religious choices which prevent a child from ever reaching adulthood, or reaching adulthood in a healthy state, are problematic. And whether the parents fully understand or not, transgender children going through puberty of the "wrong" gender is harmful in this way. As we have seen, refusing PBT first presents immediate and intense psychological harm. And second, it causes lasting and *irreversible* physical harm (Bauer et al., 2015; Brill and Pepper, 2008; Burgess, 1999; Cohen-Kettenis et al., 2008; de Vries et al., 2012 and 2014; Delemarre-van de Waal et al., 2006; Krieger 2011; Zucker 2012).

We can compare the parents of transgender children opposed to physician-recommended treatment to "naturalist" parents, i.e., parents who mistrust traditional Western medicine. Regardless of whether these parents have good intentions, these children are often at risk of harm. In various cases the courts have ruled that not only are these "naturalist" parents required to treat their children with Western medicine, but also that they are criminally liable if their children are harmed due to lack of treatment.

Just as it is the state's duty to step in when naturalist parents are refusing insulin to their diabetic son or antibiotics to their daughter sick with meningitis, so is it the state's duty to step in when the parents of gender dysphoric children are avoiding medically-recommended treatment. Whatever genuine mistrust parents might have of traditional treatment for gender dysphoria, as soon as their behavior threatens serious and irreversible harm to their child (and we can reliably identify as much), the state has a duty to intervene and protect the child. In this circumstance, this duty entails legally mandating that transgender children have a right to puberty-blockers.

Should we worry that my theoretical argument might have problematic and far-reaching implications? There are a number of conditions and activities, after all, that might put a child at risk of serious and irreversible harm. A few examples are refusing to give children certain vaccinations (consider HPV) or even refusing to spend quality-time with a child. There are two replies to those worried about the implications of my view. The first is that I am only advocating that the state takes action if there is clear evidence that a youth faces a high risk of irreversible, serious, harm. Depending on what potential harm is at issue, the risk might be low, or we might lack proper evidence, or the harm might not be serious. Any one of the aforementioned (low risk, lack of evidence, lack of seriousness) justifies the state staying out of parental affairs. However, supposing all of these conditions are met (serious harm, high likelihood, evidence), state intervention seems a blessing rather than a curse. Why would anyone want children to be at serious risk of irreversible harm? While state intervention into

parental authority must be justified, when it is justified, it is an ethically positive rather than negative state of affairs.

5.2 Putting rights into practice

For the sake of argument, suppose we have determined that transgender children have a right to PBT and the state has a duty to help enforce this right. How exactly, one might wonder, should the state intervene? Given that we are indeed entering new terrain when it comes to the state protecting children from psychological harm, it is important that the state not be perceived to be overstepping certain boundaries. If this interference is viewed as an unreasonable government intrusion, it might negatively influence the chances that the state could ever play a role in psychologically protecting minor children. For these reasons, the children themselves have an important part to play as a self-advocate.

The first step is for transgender children to seek help outside of the home. This could be possible to facilitate at school (as the next section argues), privately funded public health clinics like Planned Parenthood, or publicly funded health clinics. A healthcare worker can then counsel the child through the process of applying for PBT, a process which adolescents should be allowed to conduct without parental permission. At some point in the process, perhaps the parents would be notified that their child is seeking this type of treatment and has a right to receive it. Parental notification has its pluses and minuses. In this particular situation, not notifying might result in confusion from parents who notice their child is not going through the normal puberty process. Notification would also open the door to therapy for child and parents together. Lastly, notification would likely make mandatory PBT easier to pass by legislatures. On the other hand, some children might face serious harm if parents are notified, and the risk of harm might be a reason to have an exception to any notification demands, if we are to have them at all.

There are many variations of the scenario I just described, and it requires a separate paper to discuss the specific details at length. Notwithstanding, what matters is that transgender children may apply for PBT in a way that makes them feel safe and empowered. One way to make the process easier is to have a state-sponsored website where a transgender child could apply for both a health mentor and puberty-blocking treatment. Another way is to have applicable services available in public schools. And this is the topic of the next section.

6   Spreading the Word and the Role of Schools

Even if we come to agreement regarding the right of transgender children to receive PBT, that is just one step of the process. The other is some sort of collective effort to articulate and publicize a public conception of transgender identity and the relevant recommended treatment for those seeking to transition. There are many moral reasons, of course, to support this second step of the process. But for the purposes of this essay, the primary reason is to facilitate transgender adolescents' understanding of who they are and what medical interventions are available to help. It is only once adolescents understand this that they can seek PBT. Moreover, the less supportive their parents, the less likely the youth fully understands what it means to be transgender. Because of religious beliefs, parents might not allow their children to express their gender identity. Given the harm that can befall transgender young persons without proper information, there is a moral duty for all of us to help communicate the issue and a duty for the state to make efforts to protect this vulnerable population.

The best place to provide information about gender identity and treatment for transgender adolescents is public schools. The reasons are both pragmatic and moral. The pragmatic justification is that there is perhaps no other place where such a large number of children are gathered together. It has already been accepted that schools have a role to play in youth healthcare. Schools are commonly where children

are screened for eye problems, scoliosis, and hearing issues. In addition, schools are places of learning: what it means to be transgender and potential treatment is just one more thing to learn. The most obvious place to include this lesson is part of sex education. Earlier lessons are also a good idea. But a refresher course that begins around the same time as sexual education is the perfect place to teach about PBT. Sexual education, after all, usually occurs right before most children start puberty.

For children who lack supportive homes, a lesson at school is not enough. If these adolescents asked their parents for PBT, the parents would likely refuse. Thus, each school should have a trusted counselor, with whom students know they can discuss gender dysphoria issues (and schools already should have a counselor trained to assist with the various psychological problems that arise with adolescents) (Levine, p. 308, 2013). Lastly, whether it be directly connected to the school or not, advocates for transgender children should be publicly provided. Adolescents are unlikely to be resourceful enough to confront and negotiate with unsupportive parents themselves. They need help, not only with receiving the puberty-blockers, but with counseling and emotional support. These children, after all, will likely be experiencing a tough situation at home going against their parents' wishes. Hence, for children who do proceed with PBT sans parental approval, a support system should be in place to help these children through an emotionally difficult situation.

Obviously, not all minors attend public school. In fact, one might argue that children with less supportive parents are more likely to attend a private religious school. As such, much of the effort to inform other families will need to be performed by private persons and organizations, perhaps through websites, videos, and testimonials from transgender youth and their families. Indeed, these types of activities are already fostering greater public awareness (Craig et al., 2015; Mehra et al., 2004; Land, 2014). We should hope that transgender children will take the initiative and search for information online. Yet there still remains a small but important role for the state.

Large cities with sufficient budgets could and should fund either healthcare centers for transgender youth, or they should integrate transgender youth healthcare services at existing community health centers. Such healthcare services can offer free information about PBT and other issues relevant to transgender healthcare. Counselors could be available to talk to those who need help. Public service announcements can broadcast over the internet, television, and radio. Consider that today very few people are unaware of the dangers of smoking. Public service information campaigns played an important role in public awareness and helping smokers quit (Siegel and Biener, 2000; Warner, 1977; Wakefield et al., 2008, and Brook, 2004). Young persons are often savvier than we think, and many (but not all) are likely to find their way. It is impossible to inform everyone, but the state has an obligation to make reasonable efforts to help those minors who are not yet of age to fully help themselves.

7   Objections and How to Answer Them

Here I respond in detail to two objections that I suspect will be common lines of argument against my proposal. (Such suspicions are based on discussions with academics, physicians, therapists, and lay persons.)

7.1   Parental rights to raise their children

One objection to my proposal is simply a concern about the intrusion it imposes on the autonomy of the family. Imagine that parents have religious values against children expressing transgender dress and behavior. Are not parents allowed to raise their kids according to their own religious values? And if so, how can I argue that parents must be forced not only to accept, but to facilitate, transition?

The mistake here is in thinking that parents have rights to raise their children according to their religious values, *full stop*. Like nearly all rights, the right of parents to raise children according to their own values is not absolute. Rather, parents have such authority up and until the point at which a given decision or practice threatens serious harm. According to some religious sects, after all, girls who are raped should be put to death. Obviously, parents have no right to do this regardless of whether doing so accords with their religion. Requiring that transgender adolescents have access to PBT is simply an instance of preventing parents from imposing harmful values against their children's will. The reason we may be disinclined to see things this way is that (1) much of the harm is psychological, and (2) some of the harm will occur in the future. But when we think about it, neither of these are sufficient grounds. The first reverts back to our bias that physical harm is worse than psychological (even though the latter often leads to death via suicide), while the second is ethically irrelevant. A parent who encouraged their toddler to smoke would be abusing the child, even if the harmful effects would not be present for decades to come.

7.2   Funding issues

The legal right to PBT is not the only barrier that transgender youth face in accessing PBT. How to pay for it is another issue (Khan, 2011; Reisner et al., 2015 and 2014; Macapagal et al., 2016; Shipherd et al., 2010). Some transgender adolescents with non-supportive parents have insurance that would cover PBT, others do not (Baker, 2017; Stevens et al., 2015; Khan, 2011; and Stroumsa 2014). Some reside in states where PBT treatment would be covered via state-sponsored healthcare schemes, others do not (Green, 2014; Sheets 2014; Reisner et al., 2015). Still other transgender teens would have access to charitable sources to pay for PBT while others would lack this option (Wylie and Wylie, 2016). Regardless, even if transgender adolescents have the legal right to seek PBT without parental permission, it does not follow that they would be able to access PBT. It might sadly be the case that a transgender adolescent has no means of funding expensive PBT treatment.

While I acknowledge funding PBT is an important issue, it is simply a separate issue from the one addressed in this paper. If funding was available to all transgender youth who desired PBT, transgender youth without supportive parents would still lack the treatment they need. Parental permission and funding are two separate obstacles that transgender youth face in receiving PBT. Because they are separate obstacles, (i.e. these obstacles are not conceptually linked: adolescents can run into one obstacle but not the other) they require distinct scholarly investigations. This paper attempts to fill a distinct gap in the literature while in no way minimizing the importance of tackling healthcare funding for transgender youth.

7.3   Why not take it further?

I have argued for a rather narrow proposition – namely, that transgender adolescents have a right to PBT without parental approval. I have also argued that the state should play a role in providing information to transgender youth who might not have supportive families. Some might think I should go further and argue, for instance, that transgender youth should be able to get cross-sex hormone-treatment without parental approval or that young children should be able to dress in accordance with their gender identification. Let me start with the latter first. It is important to keep the reach of the law to what it can enforce. Having unenforceable laws creates a false sense of security. It is also important to not overuse the power of the state since laws that help a just cause can quickly lead to other laws which work against it. I worry that trying to legally enforce how parents allow transgender children to dress is unenforceable, or if enforced, would stretch the appropriate powers of the state. Another concern with such regulation is that the harms imposed do not threaten the same irreversibility as the absence of PBT. Once an adolescent turns 18, they may dress as they wish. Being forced to dress a certain way as a youth does not impair their ability to dress as one wants as an adult. With PBT, however, the absence of this treatment not only has consequences for the youth's body while they are a

youth, but also when they are an adult. The feasibility concerns, alongside the lack of permanent harm, explains why it is a mistake for the state to enforce a dress code, but apt to enforce PBT. There remains the potential, of course, for scholars to argue otherwise. Yet for the purposes of this paper, the ethical reach is constrained to a few issues that can currently be advocated with confidence.

Unlike enforcing dress requirements, requiring that underage transgender teens have a right to cross-sex treatment is plausibly enforceable. Yet I restrain my paper to arguing only for PBT latter for a few reasons. I want to make the strongest argument I can in favor of something that can have a real impact in the life of marginalized young persons. My argument for PBT is stronger than any argument for cross-sex hormones might be. Hence, I want to devote a paper entirely to making this strong case, without the risk that other issues bring my whole argument into doubt.

The case for PBT is stronger than cross-sex hormones for a few reasons. First, cross-sex hormones (unlike PBT) induce irreversible changes (Coleman et al., 2012). It is more plausible to argue that minors should have access to reversible treatment than treatment that causes permanent changes. Second, as mentioned, in many parts of the world, minors reach the medical age of consent, or even the full age of majority, at 16 or younger, which is already the recommended age to begin cross-sex hormone-treatment (de Vries and Cohen-Kettenis, 2016; Hembree, 2009).

8   Review and Concluding Remarks

This paper argued that (1): transgender adolescents should have the legal right to access puberty-blocking treatment (PBT) without parental approval; and (2), the state has a role to play in publicizing information about gender dysphoria, appropriate treatment, and leading gender dysphoric youth to appropriate healthcare resources. First let me review my main argument for the former. There is now well-documented evidence that transgender youth who lack access to PBT suffer both physically and emotionally (Coleman et al., p. 178, 2012; Olson et al., 2016; Gorin-Lazard et al., 2012; de Vries et al., 2014). Emotional harm can be long term, and might even result in suicide (Haas et al., 2010). Certain physical changes which transgender youth experience during puberty are irreversible (Bauer et al., 2015; Brill and Pepper, 2008; Burgess 1999; Cohen-Kettenis et al., 2008; de Vries et al., 2012 and 2014; Delemarre-van de Waal et al., 2006; Krieger 2011; Zucker 2012). For the transgender person these permanent physical changes are harms that prevent one from living a satisfying life (Burgess 1999; Cohen-Kettenis et al., 2011; de Vries et al., and 2014; Frisch 2016). In addition, transgender youth who lack support in the home are at an unusually high risk of homelessness, and might even end up seeking PBT through non-medically secure fashions (Burgess, 1999; Keuroghlian et al., 2014, and Durso and Gates, 2012; Garofalo et al., 2006; Clark et al., 2008; Schmid et al., 2005; Rosioreanu et al., 2004).

Not only are transgender youth harmed psychologically and physically via lack of access to PBT, but PBT is an established standard of care. Given that we generally think that parental authority should not go so far as to, (1) severely and permanently harm a child, and (2) prevent a child from access to standard physical care, then it follows that parental authority should not encompass denying gender dysphoric children access to PBT.

Implementing the above policy only is half the battle. Transgender youth without supportive parents are not helped unless they access healthcare clinics and counseling that will help with the transition. Hence there is an additional duty of the state to help facilitate sharing this information with vulnerable youths. I argued that one of the first places this should be done is in public schools. In addition, information should be available at publicly funded health clinics.

While it is implausible that the state will stop all forms of parental abuse, especially all forms of psychological abuse, transgender youth seeking puberty-blocking treatment is a special case. It is special because the need for the treatment and the treatment itself are identifiable and accessible, respectively. As such, it is sensible and legitimate for the state to take action via legislation. More specifically, the law should clearly state that transgender youth (after having met appropriate diagnostic criteria) have a legal right to PBT regardless of parental approval. In addition to these legal parameters, the state should play a role in publicizing information about gender dysphoria and treatment via public schools, government sponsored websites, and public service announcements.

Notes

1 One landmark case that comes to mind is *Prince vs. Massachusetts* where the court ruled that a child's welfare can justify overruling parental rights, even parental rights regarding a child being raised according to parental religious beliefs (https://www.law.cornell.edu/supremecourt/text/321/158). But what is a child's welfare? Generally, we have seen this ruling bear out in laws against neglect and abuse which generally (but not exclusively) override parental authority in cases in which a child faces *physical* harm.

2 As of August, 2019, 17 US states have banned conversion therapy, with the most recent being Colorado (Taylor: 2019). In alphabetical order, the remaining 16 states are: California, Connecticut, Delaware, Hawaii, Illinois, Maryland, Massachusetts, Nevada, New Hampshire, New Jersey, New Mexico, New York, Oregon, Rhode Island, Vermont, and Washington (Leins: 2019). Counties with laws prohibiting conversion therapy include (but are not limited to) Pima County, AZ; Westminster, CO; Bay Harbor Islands, FL; Boynton Beach, FL; Delray Beach, FL; El Portal, FL; Greenacres, FL; Key West, FL; Lake Worth, FL; Miami, FL; Miami Beach, FL; Riviera Beach, FL; Tampa, FL; Wellington, FL; West Palm Beach, FL; Wilton Manors, FL; Athens, OH; Cincinnati, OH; Columbus, OH; Dayton, OH; Toledo, OH; Allentown, PA; Philadelphia, PA; Pittsburgh, PA; and Seattle, WA. (See, Kids Pay the Price: 2017).

3 Every US state now has a law against bullying. Admittedly, the definition of "bullying" varies by district. The extent of the penalty for violating bullying laws also varies. Notwithstanding, the fact that these laws are common place speaks to a growing concern for the psychological health of adolescents ("Specific State Laws Against Bullying": 2017). Another sign that we are taking psychological harm more seriously is the increasing use of psychiatric medication. According to a 2013 report from the CDC, "Approximately 6.0% of U.S. adolescents aged 12–19 reported psychotropic drug use in the past month" (See Jonas et al.: 2013). Please note this is in reference to all youth, not just transgender youth. We are taking psychological harm more seriously across the board, and transgender youth deserve special attention in this regard, for they face increased risk of these mental harms.

4 "Gender dysphoria is usually experienced from childhood on, and it is not based on any cultural preference but on a person's innate sense of self: it is characterized by persistent discomfort and distress about one's assigned sex or gender. . ." (Brill and Pepper: p. 200: 2008). And similarly, ". . .gender dysphoria refers to discomfort or distress that is caused by a discrepancy between a person's gender identity and that person's sex assigned at birth (and the associated gender role and/or primary and secondary sex characteristics)" (Coleman et al.: 2012).

5 "During the last decade, more children have made a social gender role transition, sometimes as early as 4 or 5 years of age" (de Vries and Cohen-Kettenis 2016). And similarly, "Children as young as age two may show features that could indicate gender dysphoria" (Coleman et al., 2012). See also, Brill and Pepper, 2008.

6 These examples are taken from the experience of real families. The first can be found in Nutt, 2017 and the second in Whittington and Gasbarre, 2016.

7 Of course, gender nonconforming behavior does not alone mean that a child is transgender (nor does its absence mean a child is cisgender.) Plenty of cisgender children enjoy games and dress that is traditionally considered typical of the opposite gender. Nonetheless, gender nonconforming behavior is often listed as one of the many "signs" that a child might be transgender. For example, in *Principles of Transgender Medicine and Surgery*, Walter Bockting (Professor of Medical Psychology) and Eli Coleman (Professor of Family Medicine and Community Health) describe one "vignette" in the early stages of the coming-out process (coming out as transgender) in the following fashion, "His parents expressed concern about Ben's gender nonconformity. People regularly mistook him for a girl. Ben identified with Dorothy from The Wizard of Oz. At Christmas, he asked for ruby slippers" (Ettner et al., p. 140, 2016).

8 For information on transgender youth and homelessness, see Burgess, 1999; Keuroghlian et al., 2014, and Durso and Gates, 2012. Seaton and Durso and Gates contain specific information about the risk factors for transgender homelessness.

9 The studies mentioned include Bauer et al., 2015 and Travers et al, 2012. In addition, Olson et al., 2016 show that transgender children who do have supportive parents have average levels of depression. In these studies support was measured via surveys where transgender teens described the level of support they received from their parents.

10 Throughout this paper, I will use the term "they" as a singular gender-neutral pronoun. The term "they" is becoming increasingly used (and advocated) as a singular gender-neutral pronoun, especially amongst the LGBT community. For instance, see Dembroff and Wodak, 2018, and McKenzie and Dembroff, 2018.

References

AAP. "With suicide now teens' second leading cause of death pediatricians urged to ask about its risks." *American Academy of Pediatrics*. June 27, 2016. Accessed November 21, 2017. https://www.aap.org/en-us/about-the-aap/aap-press-room/pages/With-suicide-Now-Teens%E2%80%99-Second-Leading-Cause-of-Death-Pediatricians-Urged-to-Ask-About-its-Risks.aspx.

Baker, Kellan E. "The future of transgender coverage." *New England Journal of Medicine* 376, no. 19 (2017): 1801–4.

Bauer, Greta R., Ayden I. Scheim, Jake Pyne, Robb Travers, and Rebecca Hammond. "Intervenable factors associated with suicide risk in transgender persons: a respondent driven sampling study in Ontario, Canada." *BMC Public Health* 15, no. 1 (2015): 525.

Brill, Stephanie A., and Rachel Pepper. *The Transgender Child: A Handbook for Families and Professionals*. San Francisco, CA: Cleis, 2008

Brook, Stephen. "Anti-smoking ads help 1 million quit." *The Guardian*. November 03, 2004. Accessed December 04, 2017. https://www.theguardian.com/media/2004/nov/03/advertising.society.

Burgess, Christian. "Internal and external stress factors associated with the identity development of transgendered youth." *Journal of Gay & Lesbian Social Services* 10, no. 3–4 (1999): 35–47.

Chorley, Matt. "'Cinderella Law' to stop emotional abuse of children: parents who fail to show love could face prison." *Daily Mail Online*. March 31, 2014. Accessed November 23, 2017. http://www.dailymail.co.uk/news/article-2593042/Cinderella-Law-stop-emotional-abuse-children-Parents-fail-love-face-prison.html.

Clark, Richard F., F. Lee Cantrell, Adam Pacal, William Chen, and David P. Betten. "Subcutaneous silicone injection leading to multi-system organ failure." *Clinical Toxicology* 46, no. 9 (2008): 834–7.

Cohen-Kettenis, Peggy T., Henriette A. Delemarre-van de Waal, and Louis J.G. Gooren. "The treatment of adolescent transsexuals: changing insights." *The Journal of Sexual Medicine* 5, no. 8 (2008): 1892–7.

Cohen-Kettenis, Peggy T., Sebastiaan E.E. Schagen, Thomas D. Steensma, Annelou L.C. de Vries, and Henriette A. Delemarre-van de Waal. "Puberty suppression in a gender-dysphoric adolescent: a 22-year follow-up." *Archives of Sexual Behavior* 40, no. 4 (2011): 843–7.

Coleman, Doriane Lambelet, and Philip M. Rosoff. "The legal authority of mature minors to consent to general medical treatment." *Pediatrics* 131, no. 4 (2013): 786–93.

Coleman, Eli, Walter Bockting, Marsha Botzer, Peggy Cohen-Kettenis, Griet DeCuypere, Jamie Feldman, Lin Fraser, et al. "Standards of care for the health of transsexual, transgender, and gender-nonconforming people, version 7." *International Journal of Transgenderism* 13, no. 4 (2012): 165–232

Craig, Shelley L., Lauren McInroy, Lance T. McCready, and Ramona Alaggia. "Media: a catalyst for resilience in lesbian, gay, bisexual, transgender, and queer youth." *Journal of LGBT Youth* 12, no. 3 (2015): 254–75.

Delemarre-van de Waal, Henriette A., and Peggy T. Cohen-Kettenis. "Clinical management of gender identity disorder in adolescents: a protocol on psychological and paediatric endocrinology aspects." *European Journal of Endocrinology* 155, no. suppl 1 (2006): S131–S137.

Dembroff, Robin, and Daniel Wodak. "He/She/They/Ze." *Ergo, an open access journal of philosophy* 5 (2018).

Drummond, Kelley D., Susan J. Bradley, Michele Peterson-Badali, and Kenneth J. Zucker. "A follow-up study of girls with gender identity disorder." *Developmental psychology* 44, no. 1 (2008): 34.

Durso, Laura E., and Gary J. Gates. "*Serving our youth: findings from a national survey of services providers working with lesbian, gay, bisexual and transgender youth who are homeless or at risk of becoming homeless.*" (2012).

de Vries, Annelou, and Peggy Cohen-Kettenis. "Gender dysphroia in children and adolescents." Edited by Randi Ettner, Stan Monstery, and Eli Coleman. In *Principles of Transgender Medicine and Surgery*. Frankfurt Am Main: Taylor & Francis, 2016.

de Vries, Annelou L.C., Jenifer K. McGuire, Thomas D. Steensma, Eva C.F. Wagenaar, Theo A.H. Doreleijers, and Peggy T. Cohen-Kettenis. "Young adult psychological outcome after puberty suppression and gender reassignment." *Pediatrics* 134, no. 4 (2014): 696–704.

de Vries, Annelou L.C., and Peggy T. Cohen-Kettenis. "Clinical management of gender dysphoria in children and adolescents: the Dutch approach." *Journal of Homosexuality* 59, no. 3 (2012): 301–20.

Ehrensaft, Diane, Shawn V. Giammattei, Kelly Storck, Amy C. Tishelman, and Colton Keo-Meier. "Prepubertal social gender transitions: what we know; what we can learn – a view from a gender affirmative lens." *International Journal of Transgenderism* (2018): 1–18.

Ettner, Randi, Stan Monstrey, and Eli Coleman, eds. *Principles of Transgender Medicine and Surgery*. Second ed. Frankfurt Am Main: Taylor & Francis, 2016.

Frisch, Ian. "Transgender women are heading to South Korea for vocal surgery." Bloomberg.com. July 25, 2016. Accessed November 22, 2017. https://www.bloomberg.com/features/2016-voice-feminization/

Garofalo, Robert, Joanne Deleon, Elizabeth Osmer, Mary Doll, and Gary W. Harper. "Overlooked, misunderstood and at-risk: exploring the lives and HIV risk of ethnic minority male-to-female transgender youth." *Journal of Adolescent Health* 38, no. 3 (2006): 230–6.

Gorin-Lazard, Audrey, Karine Baumstarck, Laurent Boyer, Aurélie Maquigneau, Stéphanie Gebleux, Jean-Claude Penochet, Dominique Pringuey et al. "Is hormonal therapy associated with better quality of life in transsexuals? A cross-sectional study." *The Journal of Sexual Medicine* 9, no. 2 (2012): 531–41.

Green, Jamison. "Transsexual surgery may be covered by Medicare." *LGBT Health* 1, no. 4 (2014): 256–8.

Guichon, Juliet, and Ian Mitchell. "Medical emergencies in children of orthodox Jehovah's Witness families: three recent legal cases, ethical issues and proposals for management." *Paediatrics & Child Health* 11, no. 10 (2007): 655–8.

Haas, Ann P., Mickey Eliason, Vickie M. Mays, Robin M. Mathy, Susan D. Cochran, Anthony R. D'Augelli, Morton M. Silverman, et al. "Suicide and suicide risk in lesbian, gay, bisexual, and transgender populations: review and recommendations." *Journal of Homosexuality* 58, no. 1 (2010): 10–51.

Hembree, Wylie C., Peggy Cohen-Kettenis, Henriette A. Delemarre-Van De Waal, Louis J. Gooren, Walter J. Meyer III, Norman P. Spack, Vin Tangpricha, and Victor M. Montori. "Endocrine treatment of transsexual persons: an Endocrine Society clinical practice guideline." *The Journal of Clinical Endocrinology & Metabolism* 94, no. 9 (2009): 3132–54.

Jonas, Bruce S., Qiuping Gu, and Juan R. Albertorio-Diaz. "Psychotropic medication use among adolescents: United States, 2005–2010." *NCHS Data Brief* 135 (2013): 1–8.

Keuroghlian, Alex S., Derri Shtasel, and Ellen L. Bassuk. "Out on the street: a public health and policy agenda for lesbian, gay, bisexual, and transgender youth who are homeless." *American Journal of Orthopsychiatry* 84, no. 1 (2014): 66.

Khan, Liza. "Transgender health at the crossroads: legal norms, insurance markets, and the threat of healthcare reform." *Yale J. Health Policy L. & Ethics* 11 (2011): 375.

"Kids Pay the Price." Movement Advancement Project | Conversion Therapy Laws. Accessed October 29, 2017. http://www.lgbtmap.org/equality-maps/conversion_therapy.

Klein, D. A., Paradise, S. L., and Goodwin, E. T. Caring for transgender and gender-diverse persons: what clinicians should know. *American Family Physician* 98 no. 11 (2018): 645–53.

Krieger, Irwin. *Helping Your Transgender Teen: A Guide for Parents*. London: Jessica Kingsley Publishers, 2011.

Land, Abbe. "Recognizing Transgender Awareness Week." *The Huffington Post*. November 19, 2014. Accessed November 27, 2017. https://www.huffingtonpost.com/abbe-land/recognizing-transgender-awareness-week_b_6188542.html.

Leins, Casey. "States that have banned conversion therapy." *U.S. News World Report.*, April 11, 2019. https://www.usnews.com/news/best-states/articles/2019-04-11/these-states-have-banned-conversion-therapy.

Levine, David A. "Office-based care for lesbian, gay, bisexual, transgender, and questioning youth." *Pediatrics* 132, no. 1 (2013): e297–e313.

Locke, John, and Richard Howard Cox. *Second Treatise of Government*. Arlington Heights, IL: H. Davidson, 1982.

Macapagal, Kathryn, Ramona Bhatia, and George J. Greene. "Differences in healthcare access, use, and experiences within a community sample of racially diverse lesbian, gay, bisexual, transgender, and questioning emerging adults." *LGBT Health* 3, no. 6 (2016): 434–42.

McKenzie, Katherine, and Robin Dembroff. "He, she, they: pediatricians should ask kids about gender identity." Broad Jurisdiction of U.S. Border Patrol Raises Concerns About Racial Profiling | *WBUR News*. May 2, 2018. Accessed May 31, 2018. http://www.wbur.org/cognoscenti/2018/05/02/gender-atypical-youth-health-robin-dembroff-katherine-mckenzie.

Mehra, Bharat, Cecelia Merkel, and Ann Peterson Bishop. "The internet for empowerment of minority and marginalized users." *New Media & Society* 6, no. 6 (2004): 781–802.

Murad, Mohammad Hassan, Mohamed B. Elamin, Magaly Zumaeta Garcia, Rebecca J. Mullan, Ayman Murad, Patricia J. Erwin, and Victor M. Montori. "Hormonal therapy and sex reassignment: a systematic review and meta-analysis of quality of life and psychosocial outcomes." *Clinical Endocrinology* 72, no. 2 (2010): 214–31.

Nutt, Amy Ellis. *Becoming Nicole*. Bloomsbury: Atlantic Books, 2017.

Olson, Kristina R. "Prepubescent transgender children: what we do and do not know." *Journal of the American Academy of Child & Adolescent Psychiatry* 55, no. 3 (2016): 155–6.

Olson, Kristina R., Lily Durwood, Madeleine DeMeules, and Katie A. McLaughlin. "Mental health of transgender children who are supported in their identities." *Pediatrics* (2016): 2015.

Olson, J., Schrager, S. M., Clark, L. F., Dunlap, S. L., and Belzer, M. "Subcutaneous testosterone: an effective delivery mechanism for masculinizing young transgender men." *LGBT Health* 1 no. 3 (2014): 165–7.

"*Prince v. Massachusetts*." LII / *Legal Information Institute*, www.law.cornell.edu/supremecourt/text/321/158.

Press Association. "Judge rules Jehovah's Witness boy can receive blood transfusion." *The Guardian*. December 08, 2014. Accessed December 05, 2017. https://www.theguardian.com/world/2014/dec/08/judge-rules-jehovahs-witness-boy-blood-transfusion.

Pyne, J. "*Health and wellbeing among gender independent children: a critical review of the literature.*" Supporting transgender and gender creative youth: Schools, families, and communities in action. New York: Peter Lang (2014).

Reisner, Sari L., Judith Bradford, Ruben Hopwood, Alex Gonzalez, Harvey Makadon, David Todisco, Timothy Cavanaugh, et al. "Comprehensive transgender healthcare: the gender affirming clinical and public health model of Fenway Health." *Journal of Urban Health* 92, no. 3 (2015): 584–92.

Reisner, Sari L., Jaclyn M. White, Judith B. Bradford, and Matthew J. Mimiaga. "Transgender health disparities: comparing full cohort and nested matched-pair study designs in a community health center." *LGBT Health* 1, no. 3 (2014): 177–84.

Rosioreanu, Alex, Geraldine T. Brusca-Augello, Qanta A.A. Ahmed, and Douglas S. Katz. "CT visualization of silicone-related pneumonitis in a transsexual man." *American Journal of Roentgenology* 183, no. 1 (2004): 248–9.

Schmid, Andreas, Assaf Tzur, Lidiya Leshko, and Bruce P. Krieger. "Silicone embolism syndrome: a case report, review of the literature, and comparison with fat embolism syndrome." *CHEST Journal* 127, no. 6 (2005): 2276–81.

Selva, Karin. "PBT and puberty inhibitors." TransActive Gender Center. Accessed December 05, 2017. https://www.transactiveonline.org/resources/youth/puberty-blockers.php.

Serano, Julia. "Detransition, desistance, and disinformation: a guide for understanding transgender children..." *Medium*, Augmenting Humanity, 2 Aug. 2016, medium.com/@juliaserano/detransition-desistance-and-disinformation-a-guide-for-understanding-transgender-children-993b7342946e.

Sheets, Debra. "Transgender Tuesdays: a clinic in the tenderloin, by Mark Freeman." *Journal of Gerontological Social Work* 57, no. 2–4 (2014): 413–15.

Shipherd, Jillian C., Kelly E. Green, and Sarah Abramovitz. "Transgender clients: identifying and minimizing barriers to mental health treatment." *Journal of Gay & Lesbian Mental Health* 14, no. 2 (2010): 94–108.

Siegel, Michael, and Lois Biener. "The impact of an anti-smoking media campaign on progression to established smoking: results of a longitudinal youth study." *American Journal of Public Health* 90, no. 3 (2000): 380.

"Specific state laws against bullying." *Findlaw* Accessed October 29, 2017. http://education.findlaw.com/student-conduct-and-discipline/specific-state-laws-against-bullying.html.

Spinazzola, Joseph, Hilary Hodgdon, Li-Jung Liang, Julian D. Ford, Christopher M. Layne, Robert Pynoos, Ernestine C. Briggs, Bradley Stolbach, and Cassandra Kisiel. "Unseen wounds: the contribution of psychological maltreatment to child and adolescent mental health and risk outcomes." *Psychological Trauma: Theory, Research, Practice, and Policy* 6, no. S1 (2014): S18.

Steensma, Thomas D., Roeline Biemond, Fijgje de Boer, and Peggy T. Cohen-Kettenis. "Desisting and persisting gender dysphoria after childhood: a qualitative follow-up study." *Clinical Child Psychology and Psychiatry* 16, no. 4 (2011): 499–516.

Steensma, Thomas D., Jenifer K. McGuire, Baudewijntje P.C. Kreukels, Anneke J. Beekman, and Peggy T. Cohen-Kettenis. "Factors associated with desistence and persistence of childhood gender dysphoria: a quantitative follow-up study." *Journal of the American Academy of Child & Adolescent Psychiatry* 52, no. 6 (2013): 582–90.

Stevens, Jaime, Veronica Gomez-Lobo, and Elyse Pine-Twaddell. "Insurance coverage of puberty blocker therapies for transgender youth." *Pediatrics* 136, no. 6 (2015): 1029–31.

Stroumsa, Daphna. "The state of transgender health care: policy, law, and medical frameworks." *American Journal of Public Health* 104, no. 3 (2014): e31–e38.

Tannehill, Brynn. "The truth about transgender suicide." *The Huffington Post*. November 14, 2016. Accessed December 04, 2017. https://www.huffingtonpost.com/brynn-tannehill/the-truth-about-transgend_b_8564834.html.

Taylor, Chris. "Doing the transgender math: the costs of transition." *Reuters*. October 29, 2015. Accessed November 27, 2017. https://www.reuters.com/article/us-transgender-costs/doing-the-transgender-math-the-costs-of-transition-idUSKCN0SN1UA20151029.

Taylor, Derrick Bryson. "Colorado bans 'conversion therapy' for minors." *The New York Times*, June 1, 2019. https://www.nytimes.com/2019/06/01/us/gay-conversion-therapy-colorado.html.

Temple Newhook, Julia, Jake Pyne, Kelley Winters, Stephen Feder, Cindy Holmes, Jemma Tosh, Mari-Lynne Sinnott, Ally Jamieson, and Sarah Pickett. "A critical commentary on follow-up studies and "desistance" theories about transgender and gender-nonconforming children." *International Journal of Transgenderism* (2018): 1–13.

Travers, Robb, Greta Bauer, and Jake *Pyne. Impacts of strong parental support for trans youth: a report prepared for Children's Aid Society of Toronto and Delisle Youth Services.* Trans Pulse, 2012.

Wakefield, Melanie A., Sarah Durkin, Matthew J. Spittal, Mohammad Siahpush, Michelle Scollo, Julie A. Simpson, Simon Chapman, Victoria White, and David Hill. "Impact of tobacco control policies and mass media campaigns on monthly adult smoking prevalence." *American Journal of Public Health* 98, no. 8 (2008): 1443–50.

Wallien, Madeleine S.C., and Peggy T. Cohen-Kettenis. "Psychosexual outcome of gender-dysphoric children." *Journal of the American Academy of Child & Adolescent Psychiatry* 47, no. 12 (2008): 1413–23.

Warner, Kenneth E. "The effects of the anti-smoking campaign on cigarette consumption." *American Journal of Public Health* 67, no. 7 (1977): 645–50.

Watson, Ryan J., Jaimie F. Veale, and Elizabeth M. Saewyc. "Disordered eating behaviors among transgender youth: probability profiles from risk and protective factors." *International Journal of Eating Disorders* 50, no. 5 (2017): 515–22.

Whittington, Hillary, and Kristine Gasbarre. *Raising Ryland: Our Story of Parenting a Transgender Child with No Strings Attached*. New York, NY: William Morrow, an Imprint of HarperCollins Publishers, 2016.

Winters, Kelley. "Methodological questions in childhood gender identity 'desistence' research." In *23rd World Professional Association for Transgender Health Biennial Symposium*. 2014.

Woolley, Sarah. "Children of Jehovah's Witnesses and adolescent Jehovah's Witnesses: what are their rights?" *Archives of Disease in Childhood* 90, no. 7 (2005): 715–19.

Wylie, Kevan, and Rebecca Wylie. "Supporting trans people in clinical practice." *Trends in Urology & Men's Health* 7, no. 6 (2016): 9–13.

Zucker, Kenneth J., Hayley Wood, Devita Singh, and Susan J. Bradley. "A developmental, biopsychosocial model for the treatment of children with gender identity disorder." *Journal of Homosexuality* 59, no. 3 (2012): 369–97.

86

Amputees by Choice

Carl Elliott

> I get glimpses of the horror of normalcy.
> Arturo Binewski in *Geek Love*

In January 2000 British newspapers began running articles about Robert Smith, a surgeon at Falkirk and District Royal Infirmary, in Scotland. Smith had amputated the legs of two patients at their request, and he was planning to carry out a third amputation when the trust that runs his hospital stopped him. These patients were not physically sick. Their legs did not need to be amputated for any medical reason. Nor were they incompetent, according to the psychiatrists who examined them. They simply wanted to have their legs cut off. In fact, both the men whose limbs Smith amputated have declared in public interviews how much happier they are, now that they have finally had their legs removed.[1]

Healthy people seeking amputations are not nearly as rare as one might think. In May 1998 a seventy-nine-year-old man from New York traveled to Mexico and paid $10,000 for a black-market leg amputation; he died of gangrene in a motel. In October 1999 a mentally competent man in Milwaukee severed his arm with a homemade guillotine, and then threatened to sever it again if surgeons reattached it. That same month a legal investigator for the California state bar, after being refused a hospital amputation, tied off her legs with tourniquets and began to pack them in ice, hoping that gangrene would set in, necessitating an amputation. She passed out and ultimately gave up. Now she says she will probably have to lie under a train, or shoot her legs off with a shotgun.[2]

For the first time that I am aware of, we are seeing clusters of people seeking voluntary amputations of healthy limbs and performing amputations on themselves. The cases I have identified are merely those that have made the newspapers. On the Internet there are enough people interested in becoming amputees to support a minor industry. One discussion listserv has over 3,200 subscribers.

"It was the most satisfying operation I have ever performed," Smith told a news conference in February 2000. "I have no doubt that what I was doing was the

Original publication details: Carl Elliott, "Amputees by Choice," pp. 208–210, 210–215, 219–223, 227–231, 234–236, 323–326 from *Better Than Well: American Medicine Meets the American Dream* (New York and London: W.W. Norton, 2003). © 2003 by Carl Elliott. Reproduced with permission of W.W. Norton & Company, Inc.

Bioethics: An Anthology, Fourth Edition. Edited by Udo Schüklenk and Peter Singer.
Editorial material and organization © 2022 John Wiley & Sons, Inc. Published 2022 by John Wiley & Sons, Inc.

correct thing for those patients."[3] Although it took him eighteen months to work up the courage to do the first amputation, Smith eventually decided that there was no humane alternative. Psychotherapy "doesn't make a scrap of difference in these people," psychiatrist Russell Reid, of Hillingdon Hospital in London, said in a BBC documentary on the subject, called "Complete Obsession."[4] "You can talk till the cows come home; it doesn't make any difference. They're still going to want their amputation, and I know that for a fact." Both Smith and Reid pointed out that these people may unintentionally harm or even kill themselves trying to amputate their own limbs. As retired psychiatrist Richard Fox observed in the BBC program, "Let's face it, this is a potentially fatal condition."

Yet the psychiatrists and the surgeon were all baffled by the desire for amputation. Why would anyone want an arm or a leg cut off? Where does this sort of desire come from? Smith has said that the request initially struck him as "absolutely, utterly weird." "It seemed very strange," Reid told the BBC interviewer. "To be honest, I couldn't quite understand it."

In 1977, mental health professionals published the first modern case histories of what Johns Hopkins University psychologist John Money termed "apotemnophilia" – an attraction to the idea of being an amputee.[5] Money distinguished apotemnophilia from "acrotomophilia," a sexual attraction to amputees. The suffix -philia is important here. It places these conditions in the group of psychosexual disorders called paraphilias, often referred to outside medicine as perversions. Fetishes are fairly common sorts of paraphilias. In the same way that some people are turned on by, say, shoes or animals, others are turned on by amputees. Not by blood or mutilation – pain is not usually what they are looking for. The apotemnophile's desire is to be an amputee, whereas the acrotomophile's desire is turned toward those who happen to be amputees. In the *Bulletin of the Menninger Clinic* that same year, another group of researchers described a patient who would have qualified as both an apotemnophile and an acrotomophile: a twenty-eight-year-old man who was sexually attracted to female amputees, and who intensely wished to be handicapped himself.[6] [. . .]

Reviewing the medical literature, it is easy to conclude that apotemnophilia and acrotomophilia are extremely rare. Fewer than half a dozen articles have been published on apotemnophilia, most of them in arcane journals.[7] Most psychiatrists and psychologists I have spoken with – even those who specialize in paraphilias – have never heard of apotemnophilia. On the Internet, however, it is an entirely different story. Acrotomophiles are known on the Web as "devotees," and apotemnophiles are known as "wannabes." "Pretenders" are people who are not disabled but use crutches, wheelchairs, or braces, often in public, in order to feel disabled. Various Web sites sell photographs and videos of amputees, display stories and memoirs, recommend books and movies, and provide chat rooms, meeting points, and electronic bulletin boards. Much of this material caters to devotees, who seem to be far greater in number than wannabes. It is unclear just how many people out there actually want to become amputees, but there exist numerous wannabe and devotee listservs and Web sites.

Like Robert Smith, I have been struck by the way wannabes use the language of identity and selfhood in describing their desire to lose a limb. "I have always felt I should be an amputee." "I felt, this is who I was." "It is a desire to see myself, be myself, as I 'know' or 'feel' myself to be." This kind of language has persuaded many clinicians that apotemnophilia has been misnamed – that it is not a problem of sexual desire, as the -philia suggests, but a problem of body image. What true apotemnophiles share, Smith said in the BBC documentary, is the feeling "that their body is incomplete with their normal complement of four limbs." Smith has elsewhere speculated that apotemnophilia is not a psychiatric disorder but a neuropsychological one, with biological roots.[8] Perhaps it has less to do with desire than with being stuck in the wrong body.

Yet what exactly does it mean to be stuck in the wrong body? Even people who use more conventional enhancement technologies often use the language of self and identity to explain why they want these interventions: a woman who says she is "not herself" unless she is on Prozac; a bodybuilder who says he took anabolic steroids because he wants to look on the outside the way he feels on the inside; a transsexual who describes her experience as "being trapped in the wrong body." The image is striking, and more than a little odd. In each case the true self is the one produced by medical science.

Some people are inclined to think of this language as a literal description. Maybe some people really do feel as if they have found their true selves on Prozac. Maybe they really did feel incomplete without cosmetic surgery. Yet it may be better to think of these descriptions not as literally true but as expressions of an ambivalent moral ideal – a struggle between the impulse toward self-improvement and the impulse to be true to oneself. Not that I can see no difference between a middle-aged man rubbing Rogaine on his head every morning and a man whose discomfort in his own body is so all-consuming that he begins to think of suicide. But we shouldn't be surprised when any of these people, healthy or sick, use phrases like "becoming myself" and "I was incomplete" and "the way I really am" to describe what they feel, because the language of identity and selfhood surrounds us. This is simply the language we use now to describe the way we live.

Perhaps the question to be answered is not only why people who want to be amputees use the language of identity to describe what they feel, but also what exactly they are using it to describe. One point of contention among clinicians is whether apotemnophilia is, as John Money thought, really a paraphilia. "I think that John Money confused the apotemnophiles and the acrotomophiles," Robert Smith wrote to me from Scotland. "The devotees I think are paraphilic, but not the apotemnophiles." The question here is whether we should view apotemnophilia as a problem of sexual desire – a variety of the same genre of conditions that includes pedophilia, voyeurism, and exhibitionism. Smith, in agreement with many of the wannabes I have spoken with, believes that apotemnophilia is closer to gender-identity disorder, the diagnosis given to people who wish to live as the opposite sex. Like these people, who are uncomfortable with their identities and want to change sex, apotemnophiles are uncomfortable with their identities and want to be amputees.

But deciding what counts as apotemnophilia is part of the problem in explaining it. Some wannabes are also devotees. Others who identify themselves as wannabes are drawn to extreme body modification. There seems to be some overlap between people who want finger and toe amputations and those who seek piercing, scarring, branding, genital mutilation, and such. Some wannabes, Robert Smith suggests, want amputation as a way to gain sympathy from others. And finally, there are "true" apotemnophiles, whose desire for amputation is less about sex than about identity. "My left foot was not part of me," says one amputee, who had wished for amputation since the age of eight. "I didn't understand why, but I knew I didn't want my leg."[9] Another says, "My body image has always been as a woman who has lost both her legs."[10] A woman in her early forties wrote to me, "I will never feel truly whole with legs." Her view of herself has always been as a double amputee, with stumps of five or six inches.

Many devotees and wannabes describe what Lee Nattress, an adjunct professor of social work at Loma Linda University, in California, calls a "life-changing" experience with an amputee as a child. "When I was three years old, I met a young man who was completely missing all four of his fingers on his right hand," writes a twenty-one-year-old woman who says she is planning to have both her arms amputated. "Ever since that time, I have been fascinated by all amputees, especially women amputees who were missing parts of their arms and wore hook prostheses." Hers is not an unusual story. Most wannabes trace their desire to become amputees back to before the age of six or seven, and some will say that they cannot remember a time when they didn't have the desire. Nattress, who surveyed fifty people with acrotomophilia (he prefers the term "amelotasis") for a 1996 doctoral dissertation, says that much the same is true for devotees. Three quarters of the devotees he surveyed were aware of their attraction by the age of fifteen, and about a quarter wanted to become amputees themselves.[11]

Many of the news reports about the case at the Falkirk and District Royal Infirmary identified Smith's patients as having extreme cases of body dysmorphic disorder. Like people with anorexia nervosa, who believe themselves to be overweight even as they become emaciated, people with body dysmorphic disorder are preoccupied with what they see as a physical defect: thinning hair, nose shape, facial asymmetry, the size of their breasts or buttocks. They are often anxious and obsessive, constantly checking themselves in mirrors and shop windows, or trying to disguise or hide the defect. They are often convinced that others find them ugly. Sometimes they seek out cosmetic surgery, but frequently they are unhappy with the results and ask for more surgery. Sometimes they redirect their obsession to another part of the body.[12] But none of this really describes most of the people who are looking for amputations – who, typically, are not convinced they are ugly, do not imagine that other people see them as defective, and are usually focused exclusively on amputation (rather than on, say, a receding hairline or bad skin). Amputee wannabes more often see their limbs as normal, but as a kind of surplus. Their desires frequently come with chillingly precise specifications: for instance, an above-the-knee amputation of the right leg.

Like many conditions, it is not clear whether the desire to be an amputee is new, or whether it is merely taking a new shape in response to changing cultural conditions. The psychiatrist Douglas Price has unearthed and translated a 1785 text by the French surgeon and anatomist Jean-Joseph Sue that describes an Englishman who may have been both a wannabe and a devotee. The Englishman was in love with a woman who was an amputee, and wanted to become an amputee himself. He offered 100 guineas to a French surgeon to amputate his healthy leg. The surgeon refused, protesting that he did not have the proper equipment. But he changed his mind when the Englishman produced a gun, and then he proceeded to amputate the Englishman's leg under threat of death. Later he received a letter in the mail, along with payment for the amputation. "You have made me the happiest of all men," explained the Englishman,

"by taking away from me a limb which put an invincible obstacle to my happiness."[13]

When John Money designated apotemnophilia a "paraphilia," he placed it in a long and distinguished lineage of psychosexual disorders. The grand old man of psychosexual pathology, Richard von Krafft-Ebing, cataloged an astonishing range of paraphilias in his 1906 classic *Psychopathia Sexualis*, from necrophilia and bestiality to fetishes for aprons, handkerchiefs, and kid gloves. Some of his cases involve an attraction to what he called "bodily defects." One was a twenty-eight-year-old engineer who had been excited by the sight of women's disfigured feet since the age of seventeen. Another had pretended to be lame since early childhood, limping around on two brooms instead of crutches. The philosopher René Descartes, Krafft-Ebing noted, was partial to cross-eyed women.[14]

Yet the term "sexual fetish" could be a misleading way to describe the fantasies of wannabes and devotees, if what is on the Web is any indication (and, of course, it might well not be). Many of these fantasies seem almost presexual. This is not to suggest that there is any shortage of amputee pornography on the Internet. *Penthouse* has published in its letters section many of what it terms "monopede mania" letters, purportedly from devotees, and *Hustler* has published an article on amputee fetishism. But many other amputee Web sites have an air of thoroughly wholesome middle-American hero worship, and perhaps for precisely that reason they are especially disconcerting, like a funeral parlor in a shopping mall. Some show disabled men and women attempting nearly impossible feats – running marathons, climbing mountains, creating art with prostheses. It is as if the fantasy of being an amputee is inseparable from the idea of achievement – or, as one of my correspondents put it, from an "attraction to amputees as role models." "I've summed it up this way," John Money said, a little cruelly, in a 1975 interview: "Look, Ma, no hands, no feet, and I still can do it."[15] One woman, then a forty-two-year-old student and housewife whose history Money presented in a 1990 research paper, said one of the appeals of being an amputee was "coping heroically."[16] A man told Money that his fantasy was that of "compensating or overcompensating, achieving, going out and doing things that one would say is unexpectable."[17] One of my wannabe correspondents wrote that what attracted him to being an amputee was not heroic achievement so much as "finding new ways of doing old tasks, finding new challenges in working things out and perhaps a bit of being able to do things that are not always expected of amputees." [. . .]

But how should the shared desire [of wannabes] be characterized? Some argue that the desire to have a limb amputated is no different in principle from the desires motivating other enhancement technologies, like cosmetic surgery. In the same way that a person might want to have healthy tissue removed through breast-reduction surgery, so an amputee wannabe wants to have healthy tissue removed through amputation. Cosmetic surgery is certainly not prohibited by law, and the courts have even allowed healthy organs and other tissue to be removed for medical purposes deemed worthwhile, such as the transplantation of a kidney, bone marrow, or a liver lobe from a healthy donor into a needy recipient. (Courts have allowed such transplantations even when the donor is a child or a mentally impaired adult.)[18] But others believe that the desire to have a limb amputated qualifies, at least in some cases, as a psychiatric illness, for which surgery is a potentially effective treatment. On purely pragmatic grounds, this second strategy may be the best way for wannabes to get surgeons to cooperate with them – to have the desire for amputation recognized as a mental disorder, codified in the forthcoming *DSM-V*, reported on in respected medical journals, and legitimated with diagnostic instruments, reimbursement codes, and specialty clinics.

Some clinicians do not like to admit it, but even wannabes who describe the desire for amputation as a wish for completeness will often admit that there is a sexual undertone to the desire. "For me having one leg improves my own sexual image," one of my correspondents wrote. "It feels 'right,' the way I should always have been and for some reason in line with what I think my body ought to have been like." When I asked one wannabe (who also happens to be a psychologist) if he experiences the wish to lose a limb as a matter of sex or a matter of identity, he disputed the very premise of the question. "You live sexuality," he told me. "I am a sexual being twenty-four hours a day." Even ordinary sexual desire is bound up with identity, as I was reminded by Michael First, a psychiatrist at Columbia University, who was an editor of the fourth edition of the American Psychiatric Association's *Diagnostic and Statistical Manual*. First is undertaking a study that will help determine whether apotemnophilia should be included in the fifth edition of the *DSM*. "Think of the fact that, in general, people tend to be more sexually attracted to members of their own racial group," he pointed out. What you are attracted to (or not attracted to) is part of who you are.

It is clear that for many wannabes, the sexual aspect of the desire is much less ambiguous than many wannabes and clinicians have publicly admitted. A man described seventeen years ago in the *American Journal of Psychotherapy* said that he first became aware of his attraction to amputees when he was eight years old. That was in the 1920s, when the fashion was for children to wear short pants. He remembered several boys who had wooden legs. "I became extremely aroused by it," he said. "Because such boys were not troubled by their mutilation and cheerfully, and with a certain ease, took part in all the street games, including football, I never felt any pity towards them." At first he nourished his desire by seeking out people with wooden legs, but as he grew older, the desire became self-sustaining. "It has been precisely in these last years that the desire has gotten stronger, so strong that I can no longer control it but am completely controlled by it." By the time he finally saw a psychotherapist, he was consumed by the desire. Isolated and lonely, he spent some of his time hobbling around his house on crutches, pretending to be an amputee, fantasizing about photographs of war victims. He was convinced that his happiness depended on getting an amputation. He desperately wanted his body to match his self-image: "Just as a transsexual is not happy with his own body but longs to have the body of another sex, in the same way I am not happy with my present body, but long for a peg-leg."[19]

The comparison of limb amputation to sex-reassignment surgery comes up repeatedly in discussions of apotemnophilia, among patients and among clinicians. "Transsexuals want healthy parts of their body removed in order to adjust to their idealized body image, and so I think that was the connection for me," psychiatrist Russell Reid stated in the BBC documentary "Complete Obsession." "I saw that people wanted to have their limbs off with equally as much degree of obsession and need and urgency."[20] The comparison is not hard to grasp. When I spoke with Michael First, he told me that his group was considering calling it "amputee identity disorder," a name with obvious parallels to the gender-identity disorder that is the diagnosis given to prospective transsexuals. The parallel extends to amputee pretenders, who, like cross-dressers, act out their fantasies by impersonating what they imagine themselves to be.

But gender-identity disorder is far more complicated than the "trapped in the wrong body" summary would suggest. For some patients seeking sex-reassignment surgery, the wish to live as a member of the opposite sex is itself a sexual desire. Ray Blanchard, a psychologist at the University of Toronto's Center for Addiction and Mental Health, has studied men being evaluated for sex-reassignment surgery. He has found an intriguing difference between two groups: men who are homosexual and men who are heterosexual, bisexual, or asexual. The "woman trapped in a man's body" tag fit the homosexual group relatively well. As a rule, these men had no sexual fantasies about being a woman; only a small percentage say they are sexually excited by cross-dressing, for example. Their main sexual attraction is to other men.[21]

Not so for the men in the other group: almost all are excited by fantasies of being a woman. Three-quarters of them are sexually excited by cross-dressing. Blanchard coined the term "autogynephilia" – "the propensity to be sexually aroused by the thought or image of oneself as a woman" – as a way of designating this group. Note the suffix -philia. Blanchard thought that a man might be sexually excited by the fantasy of being a woman in more or less the same way that people with paraphilias are sexually excited

by fantasies of wigs, shoes, handkerchiefs, or amputees. But here sexual desire is all about sexual identity – the sexual fantasy is not about someone or something else, but about yourself. Anne Lawrence, a transsexual physician and a champion of Blanchard's work, calls this group "men trapped in men's bodies."[22]

If sexual desire, even paraphilic sexual desire, can be directed toward one's own identity, then perhaps it is a mistake to try to distinguish pure apotemnophilia from the kind that is contaminated with sexual desire. Reading Blanchard's work, I was reminded of a story that Peter Kramer tells in his introduction to *Listening to Prozac*. Kramer describes a middle-aged architect named Sam who came to him with a prolonged depression set off by business troubles and the deaths of his parents. Sam was charming, unconventional, and a sexual nonconformist. He was having marital trouble. One of the conflicts in his marriage was his insistence that his wife watch hard-core pornographic videos with him, although she had little taste for them. Kramer prescribed Prozac for Sam's depression, and it worked. But one of the unexpected side-effects was that Sam lost his desire for hard-core porn. Not the desire for sex: his libido was undiminished. Only the desire for pornography went away.[23]

Antidepressants like Prozac have long been used to treat compulsive desires, and some clinicians are also starting to use them for patients with paraphilias and sexual compulsions.[24] Can an antidepressant selectively knock out an aberrant or unwanted sexual desire, while leaving ordinary sexual desire intact? Even more interesting, though, is the way in which Sam came to view his desire. Before treatment he had thought of his taste for porn simply as part of who he was – an independent, sexually liberated guy. Once it was gone, however, it seemed as if it had been a biologically driven obsession. "The style he had nurtured and defended for years now seemed not a part of him but an illness," Kramer writes. "What he had touted as independence of spirit was a biological tic." Does this suggest that erotic desire is simply a matter of biology? Not necessarily. What it suggests is that an identity can be built around a desire. The person you have become may be a consequence of the things you desire. This may be as true for wannabes as it was for Sam, especially if their desires have been with them for as long as they can remember. [. . .]

Even if we assume that the obsessive desire for amputation is evidence of a psychiatric disorder, it is unclear why such a desire should be growing more common just now. Why do certain psychopathologies arise, seemingly out of nowhere, in certain societies and during certain historical periods, and then disappear just as suddenly? Why did young men in late-nineteenth-century France begin lapsing into fugue states, wandering the continent with no memory of their past, coming to themselves months later in Moscow or Algiers with no idea how they got there? What was it about America in the 1970s and 1980s that made it possible for thousands of Americans and their therapists to come to believe that two, ten, even dozens of personalities could be living in the same head? One does not have to imagine a cunning cult leader to envision alarming numbers of desperate people asking to have their limbs removed. One has only to imagine the right set of historical and cultural conditions.

So, at any rate, suggests the philosopher and historian of science Ian Hacking, who has attempted to explain just how "transient mental illnesses" such as the fugue state and multiple-personality disorder arise.[25] A transient mental illness is by no means an imaginary mental illness, though in what ways it is real (or "real," as the social constructionists would have it) is a matter for philosophical debate. A transient mental illness is a mental illness that is limited to a certain time and place. It finds an "ecological niche," as Hacking puts it. In the same way that the idea of an ecological niche helps to explain why the polar bear is adapted to the Arctic ecosystem, or the chigger to the South Carolina woods, Hacking's ecological niches help to explain the conditions that made it possible for multiple-personality disorder to flourish in late-twentieth-century America and the fugue state to flourish in nineteenth-century Bordeaux. If the niche disappears, the mental illness disappears along with it.

Hacking does not intend to rule out other kinds of causal mechanisms, such as traumatic events in childhood and neurobiological processes. His point is that a single causal mechanism isn't sufficient to explain psychiatric disorders, especially those contained within the boundaries of particular cultural contexts or historical periods. Even schizophrenia, which looks very much like a brain disease, has changed its form, outlines, and presentation from one culture or historical period to the next. The concept of a niche is a way to make sense of these changes. Hacking asks: What makes it possible, in a particular time and place, for this to be a way to be mad?

Hacking's books *Rewriting the Soul* and *Mad Travelers* are about "dissociative" disorders, or what used to be called hysteria. He has argued, I think very persuasively, that psychiatrists and other clinicians helped to create the epidemics of fugue in nineteenth-century Europe and multiple-personality disorder in late-twentieth-century America simply by the way they viewed the disorders – by the kinds of questions they asked patients, the treatments they used, the diagnostic categories available to them at the time, and the way these patients fit within those categories. He points out, for example, that the multiple-personality-disorder epidemic rode on the shoulders of a perceived epidemic of child abuse, which began to emerge in the 1960s and which was thought to be part of the cause of multiple-personality disorder. Multiple personalities were a result of childhood trauma; child abuse is a form of trauma. It seemed to make sense that, if there were an epidemic of child abuse, we would see more and more multiples.

Sociologists have made us familiar with the idea of "medicalization," which refers to the way that a society manages deviant behavior by bringing it under the medical umbrella.[26] A stock example of medicalization is the way that homosexuality was classified by the American Psychiatric Association as a psychiatric disorder until the 1970s. Many enhancement technologies become popular only when they are conceptualized as treatments for medicalized conditions, such as Ritalin and Adderall for Attention Deficit Disorder (medicalized distractibility) or Paxil and Nardil for social phobia (medicalized shyness). Many technologies (including some of those used to treat medicalized conditions) are also used as "normalizing" procedures. Normalizing procedures bring a deviant behavior, characteristic, or personality type back within a range considered normal, or at least aesthetically acceptable. Cosmetic facial surgery for children with Down's syndrome is a normalizing procedure, in that it is performed not for medical reasons but to make the child look more like an ordinary child. Both "normalization" and "medicalization" are related to the processes that Hacking describes, but Hacking is onto something slightly different. By "transient mental illnesses" he does not have in mind new descriptions of old conditions so much as conditions that look new in themselves.[27]

Crucial to the way that transient mental illnesses arise is what Hacking calls "looping effects," by which he means the way a classification affects the thing being classified. Unlike objects, people are conscious of the way they are classified, and they alter their behavior and self-conceptions in response to their classification. Look at the concept of "genius," Hacking says, and the way it affected the behavior of people in the Romantic period who thought of themselves as geniuses. Look also at the way in which their behavior in turn affected the concept of genius. This is a looping effect: the concept changes the object, and the object changes the concept. To take a more contemporary example, think about the way that the concept of a "gay man" has changed in recent decades, and the way this concept has looped back to change the way that gay men behave. Looping effects apply to mental disorders too. In the 1970s, Hacking argues, therapists started asking patients they thought might be multiples if they had been abused as children, and patients in therapy began remembering episodes of abuse (some of which may not have actually occurred). These memories reinforced the diagnosis of multiple-personality disorder, and once they were categorized as multiples, some patients began behaving as multiples are expected to behave. Not intentionally, of course, but the category "multiple-personality disorder" gave them, as Hacking provocatively puts it, a new way to be mad.

I am simplifying a very complex and subtle argument, but the basic idea should be clear. By regarding a phenomenon as a psychiatric diagnosis – treating it, reifying it in psychiatric diagnostic manuals, developing instruments to measure it, inventing scales to rate its severity, establishing ways to reimburse the costs of its treatment, encouraging pharmaceutical companies to search for effective drugs, directing patients to support groups, writing about possible causes in journals – psychiatrists may be unwittingly colluding with broader cultural forces to contribute to the spread of a mental disorder.

Suppose doctors started amputating the limbs of wannabes. Would that contribute to the spread of the desire? Could we be faced with an epidemic of people wanting their limbs cut off? Most people would say, Clearly not. Most people do not want their limbs cut off. It is a horrible thought. The fact that others are getting their limbs cut off is no more likely to make these people want to lose their own limbs than state executions are to make people want to be executed. And if by some strange chance more people did ask to have their limbs amputated, that would be simply because more people with the desire were encouraged to "come out" rather than suffer in silence.

I'm not so sure. Clinicians and patients alike often suggest that apotemnophilia is like gender-identity disorder, and that amputation is like sex-reassignment surgery. Let us suppose they are right. Fifty years ago the suggestion that tens of thousands of people would someday want their genitals surgically altered so that they could change their sex would have been ludicrous. But it has happened. The question is, Why? One answer would have it that this is an ancient condition, that there have always been people who fall outside the traditional sex classifications, but that only during the past forty years or so have we developed the surgical and endocrinological tools to fix the problem.

But it is possible to imagine another story, that our cultural and historical conditions have not just revealed transsexuals but created them. That is, once "transsexual" and "gender-identity disorder" and "sex-reassignment surgery" became common linguistic currency, more people began conceptualizing and interpreting their experience in these terms. They began to make sense of their lives in a way that hadn't been available to them before, and to some degree they actually became the kinds of people described by these terms.

I don't want to take a stand on whether either of these accounts is right. It may be that neither is. It may be that there are elements of truth in both. But let us suppose that there is some truth to the idea that sex-reassignment surgery and diagnoses of gender-identity disorder have helped to create the growing number of cases we are seeing. Would this mean that there is no biological basis for gender-identity disorder? No. Would it mean that the term is a sham? No. Would it mean that these people are faking their dissatisfaction with their sex? Again, no. What it would mean is that certain social and structural conditions – diagnostic categories, medical clinics, reimbursement schedules, a common language to describe the experience, and, recently, a large body of academic work and transgender activism – have made this way of interpreting an experience not only possible but more likely. [. . .]

I will confess that my opinions about amputation as a treatment have shifted since I began talking to wannabes. My initial thoughts were not unlike those of a magazine editor I approached about writing a piece on the topic, who replied, "Thanks. This is definitely the most revolting query I've seen for quite some time." Yet there is a simple, relentless logic to these people's requests for amputation. "I am suffering," they tell me. "I have nowhere else to turn." They realize that life as an amputee will not be easy. They understand the problems they will have with mobility, with work, with their social lives; they realize they will have to make countless adjustments just to get through the day. They are willing to pay their own way. Their bodies belong to them, they tell me. The choice should be theirs. What is worse: to live without a leg or to live with an obsession that controls your life? For at least some of them, the choice is clear – which is why they are talking about chain saws and shotguns and railroad tracks.

And to be honest, haven't surgeons made the human body fair game? You can pay a surgeon to suck fat from your thighs, lengthen your penis, augment your breasts, redesign your labia, even (if you are

a performance artist) implant silicone horns in your forehead or split your tongue like a lizard's. Why not amputate a limb? At least Robert Smith's motivation was to relieve his patients' suffering.

It is exactly this history, however, that makes me worry about a surgical "cure" for apotemnophilia. Psychiatry and surgery have had an extraordinary and very often destructive collaboration over the past seventy-five years or so: clitoridectomy for excessive masturbation, cosmetic surgery as a treatment for an "inferiority complex," intersex surgery for infants born with ambiguous genitalia, and – most notorious – the frontal lobotomy. It is a collaboration with few unequivocal successes. Yet surgery continues to avoid the kind of ethical and regulatory oversight that has become routine for most areas of medicine. If the proposed cure for apotemnophilia were a new drug, it would have to go through a rigorous process of regulatory oversight. Investigators would be required to design controlled clinical trials, develop strict eligibility criteria, recruit subjects, get the trials approved by the Institutional Review Board, collect vast amounts of data showing that the drug was safe and effective, and then submit their findings to the US Food and Drug Administration. But this kind of oversight is not required for new, unorthodox surgical procedures. (Nor, for that matter, is it required for new psychotherapies.) New surgical procedures are treated not like experimental procedures but like "innovative therapies," for which ethical oversight is much less uniform.

The fact is that nobody really understands apotemnophilia. Nobody understands the pathophysiology; nobody knows whether there is an alternative to surgery; and nobody has any reliable data on how well surgery might work. Many people seeking amputations are desperate and vulnerable to exploitation. "I am in a constant state of inner rage," one wannabe wrote to me. "I am willing to take that risk of death to achieve the needed amputation. My life inside is just too hard to continue as is." These people need help, but, when the therapy in question is irreversible and disabling, it is not at all clear what that help should be. Many wannabes are convinced that amputation is the only possible solution to their problems, yet they have never seen a psychiatrist or a psychologist, have never tried medication, have never read a scientific paper about their problems. More than a few of them have never even spoken face to face with another human being about their desires. All they have is the Internet, and their own troubled lives, and the place where those two things intersect. "I used to pretend as a child that my body was 'normal' which, to me, meant short, rounded thighs," one wannabe wrote to me in an e-mail message. "As a psychology major, I have analyzed and reanalyzed, and re-reanalyzed just why I want this. I have no clear idea."

Editors' Note

Various passages have been deleted. Readers interested in following up specific issues may want to consider the original publication.

Notes

1 P. Taylor, "'My Left Foot Was Not Part of Me,'" *The Guardian*, February 6, 2000, 14; Tracey Lawson, "Therapist Praises Doctor's Bravery," *The Scotsman*, February 1, 2000; Clare Dyer, "Surgeon Amputated Healthy Legs," *British Medical Journal* 320 (February 5, 2000): 332.

2 J. H. Burnett, "Southside Man Uses Homemade Guillotine to Sever Arm," *Milwaukee Journal Sentinel*, October 7, 1999; Stephen McGinty and Sue Leonard, "Secret World of Would-Be Amputees," *Sunday Times*, February 6, 2000; Michelle Williams, "Murder Trial Opens for Fetish M.D.," *Associated Press*, September 29, 1999.

3 Cherry Norton, "Disturbed Patients Have Healthy Limbs Amputated," *The Independent*, February 1, 2000.

4 BBC2 Horizon, "Complete Obsession," Transcript of television documentary, screened in United Kingdom Feb 17, 2000; http://www.bbc.co.uk/science/horizon/1999/obsession.shtml. More recently, the Australian radio program "Soundprint" broadcast a documentary on amputee wannabes, available on-line at: http://soundprint.org/radio/display_show/ID/87/name/Wannabes.

5 J. Money, R. Jobaris, and G. Furth, "Apotemnophilia: Two Cases of Self-Demand Amputation as a Paraphilia," *Journal of Sex Research* 13:2 (May 1977): 114–25.

6 P. L. Wakefield, A. Frank, and R. W. Meyers, "The Hobbyist: A Euphemism for Self-mutilation and Fetishism," *Bulletin of the Menninger Clinic* 41 (1977): 539–52.

7 W. Everaerd, "A Case of Apotemnophilia: a Handicap as a Sexual Preference," *American Journal of Psychotherapy* 37:2 (April 1983): 285–93; J. Money, "Paraphilia in Females: Fixation on Amputation and Lameness: Two Personal Accounts," *Journal of Psychology and Human Sexuality* 3:2 (1990): 165–72; R. L. Bruno, "Devotees, Pretenders and Wannabes: Two Cases of Factitious Disability Disorder," *Sexuality and Disability* 15:4 (Winter 1997): 243–60; Wakefield, Frank, and Meyers, "The Hobbyist." On acrotomophilia, see Grant Riddle, *Amputees and Devotees* (New York: Irvington Publishers, 1989).

8 Keren Fisher and Robert Smith, "More Work Is Needed to Explain Why Patients Ask for Amputation of Healthy Limbs," letter, *British Medical Journal* 320 (April 22, 2000): 1147. Smith and Gregg Furth also recently published a book titled *Amputee Identity Disorder: Information, Questions, Answers, and Recommendations About Self-Demand Amputation* (Portland, Ore.: 1st Books Library, 2000).

9 Taylor, "'My Left Foot Was Not Part of Me.'"

10 Helen Rumbelow and Gillian Harris, "Craving That Drives People to Disability," *The Times* (London), February 1, 2000.

11 L. E. Nattress, "Amelotasis: A Descriptive Study." Unpublished doctoral dissertation, Walden University, 1996.

12 Katherine A. Phillips, *The Broken Mirror: Understanding and Treating Body Dysmorphic Disorder* (New York: Oxford University Press, 1996). Phillips is a psychiatrist at Brown University who has also published extensively on body dysmorphic disorder in the medical literature. The patients she describes generally do not much resemble amputee wannabes, but she does briefly mention a man who asked a surgeon to remove his nose (p. 289).

13 J.-J. Sue, *Anecdotes Historiques, Littéraires et Critiques, sur la Médecine, la Chirurgie, & la Pharmacie* (Paris: Chez la Bocher, 1785). I am indebted to Dr Price, who wrote to me about this text and generously sent me his translation, along with other materials on amputation.

14 Richard von Krafft-Ebing, *Psychopathia Sexualis* (New York: Putnam, 1906; originally published in 1898), 234–8.

15 B. Taylor, "Amputee Fetishism: An Exclusive Journal Interview with Dr John Money of Johns Hopkins," *Maryland State Medical Journal* (March 1976): 35–8.

16 John Money, "Paraphilia in Females: Fixation on Amputation and Lameness, Two Personal Accounts," *Journal of Psychology and Human Sexuality* 3:2 (1990): 165–72.

17 Money, Jobaris, and Furth, "Apotemnophilia."

18 Josephine Johnston has written about the legal aspects of healthy limb amputation for her master's dissertation at the University of Otago. She and I have also written about the issue in a forthcoming article in *Clinical Medicine*. For a comprehensive review of moral and legal aspects of organ and tissue donation by children, see Robert Crouch, "The Child as Tissue and Organ Donor" (Master's Dissertation, McGill University, Department of Philosophy, 1996); also R. Crouch and C. Elliott, "Moral Agency and the Family: The Case of Living Related Organ Transplantation," *Cambridge Quarterly of Healthcare Ethics* 8:3 (1999), 257–87. See also Sally Sheldon and Stephen Wilkinson, "Female Genital Mutilation and Cosmetic Surgery: Regulating Non-Therapeutic Body Modification," *Bioethics* 12:4 (1998): 263–85.

19 Everaerd, "A Case of Apotemnophilia," 286–7.

20 BBC2 Horizon, "Complete Obsession."

21 R. Blanchard, "The Concept of Autogynephilia and the Typology of Male Gender Dysphoria," *Journal of Nervous and Mental Disease* 177:10 (October 1989): 616–23; R. Blanchard, "Clinical Observations and Systematic Studies of Autogynephilia," *Journal of Sex and Marital Therapy* 17:4 (Winter 1991): 235–51; R. Blanchard, "Nonmonotonic Relation of Autogynephilia and Heterosexual Attraction," *Journal of Abnormal Psychology* 101:2 (May 1992): 271–76.

22 See Anne Lawrence's Web site at: http://www.annelawrence.com. Blanchard has also found that a subset of autogynephiles is sexually aroused by the thought of themselves not as complete women, but as having a mixture of male and female sex characteristics. He calls this group "partial autogynephiles." See R. Blanchard, "The She-Male Phenomenon and the Concept of Partial Autogynephilia," *Journal of Sex and Marital Therapy* 19:1 (Spring 1993): 69–76.

23 Peter D. Kramer, *Listening to Prozac* (London: Fourth Estate, 1993), ix–xi.

24 M. P. Kafka and J. Hennen, "Psychostimulant Augmentation during Treatment with Selective Serotonin Reuptake Inhibitors in Men with Paraphilias and Paraphilia-Related Disorders: A Case Series," *Journal of Clinical Psychiatry* 61:9 (September, 2000): 664–70; A. Abouesh and A. Clayton, "Compulsive Voyeurism and Exhibitionism: A Clinical Response to Paroxetine," *Archives of Sexual Behavior* 28:1 (February, 1999): 23–30; V. B. Galli, N. J. Raute, B. J. McConville, S. L. McElroy, "An Adolescent Male with Multiple Paraphilias Successfully Treated with Fluoxetine," *Journal of Child and Adolescent Psychopharmacology* 8:3 (1998): 195–7; R. Balon, "Pharmacological Treatment of Paraphilias with a Focus on Antidepressants," *Journal of Sex and Marital Therapy* 24:4 (October–December, 1998): 241–54; M. P. Kafka, "Sertraline Pharmacotherapy for Paraphilias and Paraphilia-Related Disorders: An Open Trial," *Annals of Clinical Psychiatry* 6:3 (September 1994): 189–95.

25 See especially Ian Hacking, *Mad Travelers: Reflections on the Reality of Transient Mental Illness* (Charlottesville: University Press of Virginia, 1998) and Ian Hacking, *Rewriting the Soul: Multiple Personality and the Sciences of Memory* (Princeton, NJ: Princeton University Press, 1995).

26 Ivan Illich, *Limits to Medicine* (London: Marion Boyars, 2002); Peter Conrad and Joseph W. Schneider, *Deviance and Medicalization: From Badness to Sickness* (Philadelphia, PA.: Temple University Press, 1992); Allan V. Horwitz, *Creating Mental Illness* (Chicago: University of Chicago Press, 2002).

27 What looks like an entirely new condition may on closer examination turn out to be a new variation on previously existing conditions. Hacking suggests, for instance, that some of the young men characterized as having fugue states would, in the terms of today, be characterized as having epilepsy or traumatic head injuries.

87

Rational Desires and the Limitation of Life-Sustaining Treatment

Julian Savulescu[1]

That suicide may often be consistent with interest and with our duty to ourselves, no one can question, who allows that age, sickness or misfortune may render life a burden, and make it worse even than annihilation. I believe that no man ever threw away life, while it was worth keeping. For such is our natural horror of death, that small motives will never be able to reconcile us to it.[2]

Two hundred years after Hume wrote these words, society has begun to accept that continued life can be worse than "annihilation" and that it is not necessary, nor even desirable, to prolong all lives as long as is biologically possible. "Quality of life", we now realize, is important too. "Living wills", "advance directives", "respect for autonomy", "shared decision-making" and "the right to die" help to ensure, we hope, that the days are over when a person is compelled to live a life which has become a burden.

But there is naive optimism in Hume's second belief "that no man ever threw away life, while it was worth keeping". There are good reasons to believe that normal people, when evaluating whether it is worth living in a disabled state in the future, will undervalue that existence, even in terms of what they judge is

best. I will examine the evidence for this claim and look at the implications for the limitation of life-sustaining treatment of formerly competent but now incompetent patients, and, more briefly towards the end, of competent patients.

It has been argued that life-sustaining treatment ought to be limited when such treatment limitation shows respect for a patient's autonomy or promotes a patient's best interests. I will examine what constitutes autonomy and, more briefly, best interests. My point is that being autonomous involves making a certain kind of judgement about how one would like one's life to go over time. It involves making some quite complex evaluations. Which of a person's desires are expressions of her autonomy may not be transparent to casual observation. Indeed, some expressed desires actually prevent a person achieving what she judges to be best for herself. We need to look more carefully and critically at a person's desire to die before we can say that the satisfaction of it shows respect for her autonomy.

Questions of treatment limitation can be considered from many perspectives: that of the patient,

Original publication details: Julian Savulescu, "Rational Desires and the Limitation of Life-Sustaining Treatment," pp. 191–222 from *Bioethics* 8: 3 (1994). Reproduced with permission of John Wiley & Sons.

his family or society. I will consider only the patient perspective. I use the term "treatment limitation" to cover all cases of withdrawal, with-holding or other limitation of treatment. Within the following sets, I use the terms interchangeably: "preference" and "desire", "autonomy" and "autonomous desire" as a desire which is a reflection of a person's autonomy.

The President's Commission Report

The President's Commission Report argues that treatment of incompetent patients ought to be limited if the patient in question would now desire to have treatment limited, if he were competent. This, it is said, shows respect for the patient's former autonomy. If there is no evidence concerning what the patient would desire, treatment can be limited if it is not in the best interests of the patient.

> [D]ecisionmaking for incapacitated patients should be guided by the principle of substituted judgement which promotes the underlying values of self-determination and well-being better than the best interests standard does.[3]

This is based on the guiding principle of the Commission that "a competent patient's self-determination is and should be given greater weight than other people's views of that individual's well-being."[4]

How are we to determine what a person "would now desire"? It has been claimed that a patient's past preference on a related issue or an advance directive constitute sufficient evidence for what a patient would now desire. I will argue that this sense of "what a patient would now desire" is insufficient to determine whether life-sustaining treatment should be limited. It reflects a superficial understanding of what constitutes autonomy. In order to respect former autonomy, we must ask not, "What would the patient now desire if she were competent?" but rather, "What would she now rationally desire if she were competent?" I will argue that self-determination is reflected by a person's own rational hypothetical desire.

Part I. What is Autonomy?

The word, "autonomy", comes from the Greek: *autos* (self) and *nomos* (rule or law).[5] Autonomy is self-government or self-determination.[6] "Self-determination" entails forming a plan for how one's life is to go through time, choosing a course according to what one judges is best for oneself. Autonomous choice fundamentally involves evaluation. It is not mere desiring; rather, it is the weighing and evaluation of alternatives by a person, and the selection of that alternative which best suits that person's judgement for how she wants her life to go.

Self-determination thus entails forming desires for how one's life is to go through time. These desires constitute what has been called a "life-plan". As Robert Young puts it, "[t]he term 'plan' here is intended to refer merely to whatever it is that a person broadly wants to do in and with his or her life – thus covering career, life-style, dominant pursuits and the like."[7]

Consider the simple case of a person, P, faced with only two options: A and B. Imagine that A is suffering from a painful cancer of the knee and B is having one leg amputated. For P's preference for, say, A over B to be a reflection of his autonomy, it must be the result of an evaluation which judges that A is better for P than B. I will argue that being self-determining entails that this evaluation must involve at least three elements: (1) knowledge of relevant, available information concerning each of the states of affairs A and B, (2) no relevant, correctable errors of logic in evaluating that information, and (3) vivid imagination by P of what each state of affairs would be like for P. Call those desires which satisfy these three conditions, rational desires. That is,

> P rationally desires some state of affairs, that q, iff (if and only if) P desires that q while in possession of all relevant, available information, without making relevant, correctable error of logic and vividly imagining what each state of affairs would be like for P.[8]

I will argue that:

> One necessary condition for a desire to be an expression of a person's autonomy is that it is a rational desire or that it satisfies a rational desire.

An argument for rational desiring

The paradigm of P autonomously choosing between A and B entails that, having appreciated the nature of A and B, P judges that one is better for her, fits better her "life-plan", than the other. Why is appreciation of the nature of A and B important? It will not do when imagining what A is like, to imagine some state of affairs which is more like B, or some other state of affairs. If P were to choose A under these circumstances, what P would really want is B, or something else entirely.

To appreciate A and B as they are, P must know what each is like. P must have relevant, available information. If the cancer will cease to be painful after a certain stage, or if amputation means that P can still get around with an artificial leg, it is relevant for P to know these facts.

In processing this information, it is important not to make any errors of logic. P is trying to decide whether to have the amputation. Suppose that P is provided with information and reasons in the following way.

1. There is a risk of dying from anaesthesia. (true)
2. I will require an anaesthetic if I am to have an amputation. (true)
   Therefore, if I have an amputation, I will die. (false)

Logic is important so that P can utilize available facts properly. False beliefs which arise from correctable errors of logic corrupt P's appreciation of the nature of the options, and so reduce the autonomy of his choice.

Not all false beliefs corrupt P's appreciation of the alternatives in a way that matters. If P falsely believes that the anaesthetic will be a gas, when it will be an intravenous infusion with the same risks and benefits, then this false belief is irrelevant to her evaluation of the anaesthetic.[9]

What if P desires to not use all the information available or to commit errors of logic? What if P wants only to know whether an operation will cause pain or not? P does not want to know what its likely benefits are. Should these be presented to her?

The default answer is that such a person should be compelled to confront available information and any errors of logic. It is only then that she can be self-determining and get what she really wants.

However, there is one exception. Some people really do not want to know all the facts. They might not want to know the risk of death which an operation entails. That desire ought to be respected *if it has been evaluated in the right way*. Has the person stood back and imagined the possible implications of such a stance? If she has, then this desire may inherit autonomy from the parent evaluation. If, however, such a reaction is driven only by fear or dread, then it is not an expression of autonomy.

In addition to the provision and logical evaluation of information, the evaluative sense of the concept of self-determination requires that alternative states of affairs be "vividly imagined". What constitutes "vivid imagination"?

The concept of choice entails that at least two alternatives are available. But it is necessary to distinguish between subjectively and objectively available alternatives. Two objective alternatives may exist with only one subjective alternative.

Consider the converse of Locke's case.[10] A person in a room is led to believe that the room is locked, when in fact one door is open. This person has two objective alternatives (leave or stay) but only one subjective alternative (stay).

It is only after a person has presented herself with subjective alternatives that she can choose the one which she judges is best. One cannot logically be self-determining if one believes that the path one sets upon is the only path available. As far as demonstrating that a choice is autonomous, it is not enough to show that objective choices exist. There must be some evidence that subjective choice exists.[11]

In order to be self-determining, then, it is necessary to present at least two alternatives to oneself. However, being autonomous requires more than this. Imagine that P wants to do A. P believes that she could also do B. However, it is A that P wants to do, and P does not think about B. In one sense, it can be said that P has *chosen* to do A, but is doing A an expression of P's *self-determination*? Self-determination is an active process of actually determining the path of one's life. In order to judge what is best for herself, P must think and imagine what it would be like for her if A and B obtained, and what the consequences, at least in the short term, of each of these would be for her. Thus, not only must P know what A and B are like, but she must also imagine what A and B would be like *for her*. I call this vivid imagination.

Depression is one condition which may reduce one's capacity to be autonomous. The depressive loses the ability to "live life". At the level of decision-making, this manifests itself as an inability to present alternatives in the vivid colours of reality. Once depression has lifted, some describe the experience as being one where a "veil" descended on their life. Such people may be cognizant of facts, but they are unable to engage in the process of vivid imagination which brings meaning to our choices.[12]

Two objections to vivid imagination

1 *Uncertainty and the unknown*   It might be argued that my requirement for vivid imagination is too strong. We do not require that our choices be made with knowledge of what the outcome will be. Such knowledge may not be available. The paradigm case is that of explorers such as Captain Cook or Columbus. These men could not have vividly imagined the outcome of their explorations, but surely their decision to explore the unknown could have been autonomous?[13]

I am not suggesting that one must vividly imagine what an alternative is like before one can autonomously choose that alternative; I am only suggesting that one must imagine it *as far as is possible*. These explorers were faced with many different courses of action. The results of some of these were clearly imaginable (like staying at home and reading a book), while the results of others were largely unpredictable (like exploring the Pacific). One can autonomously choose to explore the unknown. However, one must gather as many facts as possible about the unknown, if one is to choose to explore it autonomously.

We are in some ways like these explorers. There are various courses of action open to us, and various outcomes are possible with each course of action. Under conditions of uncertainty, we must present to ourselves a "reasonable range of alternatives" for each course of action entertained. A "reasonable range of alternatives" is that range defined by P's rational beliefs about what courses of action are open to P (and their probabilities of producing various outcomes).[14] P's beliefs are rational if they are based on an appreciation of all relevant facts available at the time to P, evaluated by P without any errors of logic being committed. We must vividly imagine these alternatives, as far as is possible.

Contrast this with an example of non-autonomously choosing the unknown. Imagine that John is considering setting out to explore an uncharted part of the interior of Africa. Although this area has not been mapped, it is known from natives who have been there that it is infested with tsetse flies. These flies cause a fatal sleeping sickness. John knows this fact, but does not vividly imagine what it would be like to be in a dense jungle infested with tsetse flies. It is not that he wants to die. He is merely a person who can't be bothered thinking carefully about the consequences of his actions. John's desire to explore the interior of Africa without appropriate precautions frustrates what he really wants: to chart the interior of Africa and stay alive.

2 *Impulsiveness and choosing to ignore available facts*   It might be objected that we are in many ways like John. We often choose impulsively and choose to ignore available facts, yet we do not believe that the impulsiveness of our choice precludes it from being autonomous.[15] If this is so, then vivid imagination of the alternatives is not necessary.

It is true that a person can autonomously choose to lead an impulsive life. What matters is whether she evaluates the impulsive life, whether she imagines in broad and general strokes, what it is to live an impulsive life, and what other lives are like. She can only then *autonomously* choose to live the impulsive life.

The impulsive explorer comes in two versions. In one version, at some prior point she stands back from her life and evaluates it as the best overall for her.

She sees people living their lives like accountants, or crude short-sighted utilitarians, scrutinizing the value of every possible option. She decides that spontaneity is more important. This impulsive explorer is autonomous. Autonomy of choice can be inherited if the parent choice was autonomous.

In the second version, the impulsive explorer never stands back and engages in vivid imagination of the alternatives. She never evaluates her life. She is not self-determining.

Two senses of rational desiring

A rational desire can be described in an actual (non-counterfactual) sense: (1) as a desire which *does* satisfy or *has* satisfied the three evaluative conditions, or in a hypothetical (counterfactual) sense: (2) as a desire which *would* satisfy the three conditions. I favour the actual (non-counterfactual) reading.

Consider the happy follower. This person is happy simply being one of the herd. She passively does as others do, lets her friends and family decide for her, leads the most unoriginal of existences. This person can be autonomous, if she has chosen her life for a reason. Such a person may find choice burdensome, or realize that she is a bad chooser. Or perhaps she enjoys the pleasure others feel in choosing for her. If she stands back and evaluates her life as good for one of these reasons, she may be autonomous in being a follower. But if there has been no such reflection, no such deliberate choice, no such conscious planning, then her life is the paradigm of lack of autonomy.

It may be true of this latter person that, *if* she had confronted her life, she would have endorsed it. However, it is necessary for self-determination that she *determine* her life, that she *actually* chooses a certain life according to what she judges best, not that she would have chosen that life under certain ideal conditions.

It might be objected that few people have rational desires. Clearly, we hardly ever go through the process of collecting information, logically evaluating it and vividly imagining the alternatives in a formal, overt and organized way. Evaluation is often fractured

over time, and in the background of our minds. Yet I believe that we do engage in this kind of evaluation. We do form considered judgements about what is best for ourselves.

Autonomy as a dispositional concept

It is important to recognize that to be autonomous it is not necessary that we are *always* evaluating states of affairs rationally, in the way I have described. Firstly, as I have shown, a desire can inherit autonomy if it springs from an overall plan or desire which is itself rational and autonomous.

However, there is a second way in which we are often autonomous at a certain time in the absence of having a rational desire at that time. Autonomy is a dispositional concept.[16] When we say that P is autonomous, we mean that P has a disposition to behave (under certain conditions[17]) in a certain way. That is, P is autonomous if P *would* behave in way A if circumstances C were present. More specifically, P is autonomous if, under certain conditions, P would bring about what she rationally evaluates to be best for herself. That is, P would act, and perhaps also form other desires, so as to realize her rational desires for how she would like her life to go. Thus, while it is necessary that a person rationally evaluate states of affairs *at some point* in order to be autonomous, it is not true that she is only autonomous when she is actually rationally desiring some end.

Being autonomous thus requires both: (1) forming a rational desire for what is best for ourselves, and (2) having a disposition to realize our rational desires, that is, having a disposition (or tendency) to bring about what we judge to be best for ourselves.

The account of rational desiring I have provided is like some accounts of valuing.[18] However, valuing is a dispositional concept.[19] (I still value freedom when I am anaesthetized, yet I may have no desires at that time. So values must not necessarily be actual desires.) The relationship between valuing and rational desiring can be put this way:

P values that q iff P would rationally desire that q in C.

"To value" is the dispositional verb to which the corresponding occurrent or episodic verb is "to rationally desire". Valuing captures the dispositional sense of being autonomous.

Ulysses and the Sirens: an example of obstructive desire

I have argued that a rational desire is a desire formed under conditions of awareness of available information, evaluated without error of logic and after engaging in a process of vivid imagination. Call a desire which does not satisfy these three conditions, a non-rational desire. Some non-rational desires frustrate the satisfaction of our rational desires, that is, obstruct the expression of our autonomy. Call these irrational or obstructive desires.

An example of obstructive desire is seen in the case of Ulysses and the Sirens. Ulysses was to pass "the Island of the Sirens, whose beautiful voices enchanted all who sailed near. [They]. . .had girls' faces but birds' feet and feathers. . .[and] sat and sang in a meadows among the heaped bones of sailors they had drawn to their death," so irresistible was their song. Ulysses desired to hear this unusual song, but also wanted to avoid the usual fate of sailors who succumbed to this desire. So he contrived to plug his men's ears with beeswax and instructed them to bind him to the mast of his ship. He told them: "if I beg you to release me, you must tighten and add to my bonds." As he passed the island, "the Sirens sang so sweetly, promising him foreknowledge of all future happenings on earth." Ulysses shouted to his men to release him. However, his men obeyed his previous orders and only lashed him tighter. They passed safely.[20]

Before sailing to the Island of the Sirens, Ulysses made a considered evaluation of what he judged was best. His order that he would remain shackled was an expression of his autonomy. In the grip of the Sirens' song, Ulysses' strongest desire was that his men release him. This may have been his only desire. But it was an irrational desire. Moreover, this desire obstructed the expression of his autonomy.

We see in this case how it is necessary to frustrate some of a person's desires if we are to respect his autonomy.

One objection

How, it might be objected, can Ulysses' desire to be released obstruct his autonomy when he has no other desire at the time of hearing the Sirens?

Ulysses did rationally desire to live and he will rationally desire to live, but he now irrationally desires to move closer to the Island. This last desire entails dying.[21] His past and future rational desires are reflections of a settled disposition to stay alive. Ulysses has this disposition at the time of hearing the Sirens, though it fails to issue in a present desire. It is out of respect for autonomy in its dispositional sense that we believe Ulysses ought to be lashed tighter to the mast.[22] It is out of respect for Ulysses' values that we restrain him.

Part II. "No Man Ever Threw Away Life, While It Was Worth Keeping"

It is difficult for a person to evaluate future states in which she suffers a significant physical disability. In such cases, there are several hurdles to forming a desire which expresses our autonomy. Obstructive desires often arise. I will now review the evidence for these claims.

Consider the following case.

Mrs X was a woman in her mid-forties with severe diabetes, and many complications of that disease, including severe vascular disease. She was admitted to hospital with pain in her foot. The circulation of blood to her foot was so poor that it required amputation. The necessity of amputation was explained to her. She, however, refused to have an amputation. She did not want to be bed-or wheelchair-bound and dependent on her husband, she said. It was carefully explained to her that most amputees were able to walk independently on an artificial leg. She did not believe that she would be able to walk on a prosthesis. She would, she said, rather die. Amputees were brought in to the ward to show that it was possible to independently ambulate with an artificial leg. Other attempts were made to dispel any false belief about amputation. She, however, remained unmoved. She was discharged home. Sometime later, she was rushed to hospital. Gangrene had developed in her foot. She was in septic shock. She became delirious. It became obvious that she would die without amputation. On death's door, the medical staff cajoled her into "consenting" to an above knee amputation, though it appeared clear to all that this was not what she had wanted and that she was at the time incompetent to consent to operation. Her amputation went well (from a medical point of view), her infection cleared and she went to a rehabilitation hospital. When one of her doctors saw her a year later, she had had a second amputation. Remarkably, she was walking on bilateral prostheses. He asked her how she was going with the amputations. "Fine," she remarked to his astonishment. "But you never even wanted the first amputation." "Yes," she replied, "but that was because I never believed that *I* would be able to walk with an amputation. It was being stuck in a wheelchair that I dreaded. But now I can get around by myself and it's not so bad."

Why did this woman refuse amputation?

The problem was not merely one of lack of information, although information could have been more effectively presented. Let us assume that all the facts had been made available. Mrs X had at least one relevantly false belief: that *she* would not be independent after an amputation. This belief was not supported by the information available to her. However, she made a second evaluative error: she failed to vividly imagine what life as an amputee would be like for her.[23]

Before I address why these evaluative errors might have occurred, I will show that in some respects Mrs X is not an unusual case. Many people ultimately adapt to disability following life-threatening illness.

Adaptation to disability

People suffering painful or disabling illnesses often adapt to a significant decrement in function. Following a large review of the medical literature, De Haes and Van Knippenberg conclude:

> It is commonly assumed that cancer and cancer treatment have a severe, negative impact on the QOL [quality of life] of patients. . .However, no differences were found with respect to most QOL indicators: satisfaction with family, friends, work, income, values, activities, community, local government, health, the overall quality of life; psychological functioning; anxiety, depression, positive well-being, general mental well-being; daily activities; and work satisfaction. Interestingly, survived cancer patients have reported more satisfaction with care from their partner and others than have healthy controls.[24]

There were no differences between normal and mastectomy, chemotherapy or melanoma patients over a wide range of subjective indicators of quality of life. Cancer patients judged their situation more positively and more like "normals" than patients with skin disease.[25] Patients with chronic renal failure on dialysis subjectively rank their life quality only 6% below the average of the normal population.[26] Kidney transplant recipients rank their subjective quality of life more highly than the general population rates theirs.[27] Brickman, Coates and Janoff-Bulman found that recent lottery winners were no happier than control groups. Paraplegics were less happy, though still above the midpoint of the scale.[28]

Some victims of personal tragedy even derive something positive from their experience. One polio victim remarked:

> Far away from the hospital experience, I can evaluate what I have learned. . .I know my awareness of people has deepened and increased, that those who are close to me can want me to turn all my heart and mind and attention to their problems. I could not have learned *that* dashing all over the tennis court.[29]

Interviews with women with breast cancer revealed similar experiences:

> I have much more enjoyment of each day, each moment. I am not so worried about what is or isn't or what I wish

I had. All those things you get so entangled with don't seem to be part of my life right now.

You take a long look at your life and realize that many things you thought were important before are totally insignificant. . .What you do is put things in perspective. You find out things like relationships are really the most important things you have – the people you know and your family – everything is just way down the line. It's very strange that it takes something serious to make you realize that.[30]

Taylor concludes:

victims of life-threatening attacks, illness, and natural disaster sometimes seem from their accounts. . .to have benefited from it. . .Studies of chronic illness or conditions, such as cancer, diabetes, severe burns, cystic fibrosis, or hemophilia, and investigations of coping with the loss of a child or a spouse reveal that most people experiencing such events are able to say that their lives are as good as or better than they were before the events.[31]

It is possible to portray an overly rosy picture of serious illness. Many people do not find meaning in their illness. But many at least appear to adapt.[32]

Hurdles to evaluation: loss aversion and contrast

If it is true that many people, like Mrs X, will ultimately adapt to their disability, is there any reason to believe that they will, like Mrs X, fail to rationally evaluate those states of disability? The psychological coding mechanisms of *contrast* and *loss aversion* tend to prevent rational evaluation.

Maintenance of a state and frequent repetition of a stimulus result in adaptation. Exposure to repeated stimulation thus tends to produce a neutral subjective state, or null state. Contrasting states become the primary determinants of experience.[33] The principle of contrast states that the experience of a given stimulus or state is determined to a significant extent by its contrast to the null or present adapted state (size and rate of change of difference are important).

Consider an example. In one experiment, subjects were asked to describe the facial expression of a woman seen in a photograph. The face was "enigmatically unemotional". Before viewing this photograph, however, subjects were shown another photograph which expressed a strong emotion. The target face was judged by subjects to express a moderately intense *contrasting* emotion.[34] Tversky and Griffin have shown that perceived levels of happiness behave in a similar way.[35]

Thus, it is not the level of a person's function, but the change from whatever level she has adapted to which is important in determining a person's evaluation of that state. Although many paraplegics ultimately adapt to their level of function, becoming a paraplegic is a terrible event because one moves rapidly from a normal state to a paralysed state. One paraplegic stated in a television interview, "You probably think that I am unhappy but you are wrong. And I used to think that I knew what suffering was, but I was wrong."[36]

The phenomenon of *loss aversion* also distorts the evaluative experience. This is the psychological phenomenon where "losses loom larger than gains." The dread Mrs X had of dependency may be one example.

Consider another example. Participants in an experiment were indifferent between the following prospects: (1) equal chances to win $20 or lose $5, with a 0.5 chance to win or lose nothing and (2) equal chances to win $60 or lose $15, and a 0.5 chance to win or lose nothing. "Here, a chance to win $60 rather than $20 was needed to compensate for the risk of losing $15 rather than $5 – a ratio of 4:1 between matched differences of losses and gains."[37]

From experiments such as these, it has been concluded that "[w]hen left to their own devices. . .decision makers focus myopically at problems one at a time, and their choices appear to be dominated by the anticipated emotional consequences of individual losses."[38]

People often also focus on the present and near future, and discount the more distant future. They are biased to the present and near future.[39]

It would be expected, then, that people, prior to injury, will concentrate "myopically" on the loss of becoming disabled, and ignore the value of their adapted state. Kahneman and Varey conclude:

> In dealing with unfamiliar states, however, most people probably have a more accurate view of the utility of the transition than of the steady state. As a consequence, adaptation will tend to be neglected or underestimated and differences between states correspondingly exaggerated.[40]

This is in agreement with Tversky and Griffin's conclusions:

> A common bias in the prediction of utility is a tendency to overweight one's present state or mood. . .A related source of error is the failure to anticipate our remarkable ability to adapt to new states. . .People generally have a reasonable idea of what it is like to lose money or to have a bad cold, but they probably do not have a clear notion of what it means to go bankrupt, or to lose a limb.[41]

The implication here is that people may have a good idea about treatment decisions relating to familiar problems, like having a cold, a sprained or broken limb. But, as treatment decisions pertain to more unfamiliar states, people will have more difficulty in imagining what these states will be like. The evidence is that, prior to experiencing them, they will systematically underrepresent their utility. The President's Commission appears to fail to appreciate the difficulty facing patients who make decisions concerning unfamiliar states:

> The Commission has found no reason for decisions about life-sustaining therapy to be considered differently from other treatment decisions. A decision to forego such treatment is awesome because it hastens death, but that does not change the elements of decision-making capacity and need not require greater abilities on the part of the patient.[42]

While the Commission is right that such decisions are not different to other decisions about unfamiliar states (such as those involving serious disability), they

are different to the everyday health care decisions which people make about familiar health problems.

Mrs X failed to vividly imagine what it would be like to adapt to a disabled state. Loss aversion, contrast and discounting of the future prejudice appreciation of future life with disability. Importantly, false beliefs about dependency may persist even after presentation of evidence to the contrary. Kahneman and Miller describe the "well-documented" phenomenon of "the perseverance of discredited beliefs".[43] "The message. . .is that traces of an induced belief persist even when its evidential basis has been discredited."[44]

In conclusion, the process of vivid imagination so necessary for evaluation is no easy or straight-forward process to engage in. It involves not only the provision of much information, but the overcoming of several innate psychological hurdles.

Part III. Limitations of Treatment of Incompetent Patients

Should Mrs X's leg have been amputated when she was incompetent?

The President's Commission Report argues that the limitation of treatment of formerly competent but now incompetent patients should attempt to achieve two goals: promotion of well-being and respect for autonomy.[45] Respect for self-determination becomes embodied in the notion of "substituted judgement". Substituted judgement attempts to arrive at a hypothetical or counter-factual preference – what the patient would prefer, were she competent now. Treatment is only to be in accordance with the best interests standard if we cannot form a substituted judgement.

How are we to determine what a patient would prefer?

Buchanan and Brock claim that there must be "sufficient evidence". Exactly what constitutes sufficient evidence is left somewhat unclear. They seem to equate it with the expression of a past preference for a related issue (including an advance directive).

The manner in which they restrict the use of substituted judgement provides support for this contention. Substituted judgements do *not* represent "a surrogate exercise of the right of self-determination" if: (1) individuals "have not clearly expressed the relevant preferences prior to the onset of incompetence or because they have expressed relevant but contradictory preferences" and (2) patients have never been competent.[46]

Which desires will count as reflecting a patient's autonomy according to the President's Commission? Firstly, the principal (person making the directive) should be legally competent. Secondly, "[a] statute might require evidence that the person has the capacity to understand the choice embodied in the directive when it is executed." This capacity will be assessed in lay terms by lay people. "Furthermore, the standard they are asked to attest to may be as low as that used in wills, unless specified differently." The principal should also understand the seriousness of the step being taken. The Commission recommends that the principal "have had a discussion with a health care professional about a directive's potential consequences".[47]

The loaded concept in these accounts is "competence". If competence to make a life and death choice means that the patient must be in possession of the available facts, without committing relevant errors of logic and vividly imagining the relevant states of affairs, then it is *ex hypothesi* true that a competent patient will make an autonomous choice.[48] However, the notions of competence and autonomy, although related, are generally though[t] to be separate.[49] I will not address the notion of competence. It suffices to say that unless the notions of competent choice and autonomous choice are collapsed, it will be possible that a competent person will express a non-autonomous desire.

If this is right, it will not do to look only to a past competent preference if we wish to respect an incompetent patient's former autonomy. Some desires, even some competent desires, frustrate a person's autonomy. We need also to ask: was the desire obstructive?

Consider the case of Mrs X. She rationally desired to live independently (let us assume). Amputation and a prosthetic leg would have allowed her to live independently. Her false belief (that she would be dependent after an amputation) led her to desire to die. This desire prevented her from getting what she rationally desired (and valued). Her expressed desire to die was obstructive.

Moreover, it would be wrong to conclude from this expressed past desire that she would now, at the time of being incompetent, rationally desire to die if she were competent. She would now rationally desire to be treated.

False belief is not always present. But other evaluative failings are equally important. If Mrs X had failed to vividly imagine what it would be like to adapt to life with a prosthetic leg, her previous desire to die would have been irrational and quite possibly obstructive.

The important question, then, is: was Mrs X's past desire an expression of her *autonomy*? Buchanan and Brock claimed that "acting in accordance with a patient's prior preferences" shows "a respect for the patient's former autonomy".[50] This claim is not necessarily true. Some preferences, and even some preferences of competent persons, frustrate autonomy. In order to determine whether a desire is rational or obstructive requires considerable evaluation, and certainly more than that suggested by the President's Commission.

In order to form a substituted judgement, we must ask not what would the patient desire, but what *would* the patient *rationally desire*? A person's past rational desires give us a clue as to what this person's "life-plan" is, and so to what she would now rationally prefer.

In the case where a past desire to die now is obstructive, and it is clear that the patient would now *rationally* desire to live, then respect for autonomy requires that we treat the patient.

In many cases, it will not be possible to clarify whether a past desire was an expression of a person's autonomy. In health care, there is often a presumption of competence: a person is presumed to be competent until proven otherwise. What will *not* do is to presume that a competent person's desire is autonomous, in so far as treatment limitation decisions are concerned.

There are too many factors operative which can interfere with the required evaluation.

Moreover, it is possible that some people have never rationally evaluated their lives and lack entirely a rational life plan. Without a plan, without making certain evaluations, a person cannot be autonomous.

What ought to be done, then, when it is not clear what the patient would now rationally desire or if the patient lacks the relevant rational desires?

The following principle is reasonable: in the case that a person has no relevant rational desires or as we become more unclear what the patient would now rationally desire, treatment should promote that patient's best interests.

These principles apply to advance directives. If there are reasons to believe that such a directive was not an expression of the patient's autonomy, then it is appropriate to disregard such a directive and assess the situation afresh.

Consider an example from The *Hastings Center Report*.[51] A 32-year-old, HIV-positive man presented with shortness of breath. He was diagnosed as having *Pneumocystis* pneumonia. Upon being told his diagnosis, the man produced a living will forbidding artificial ventilation "under any circumstances" and endowing his friend with Enduring Power of Attorney (or equivalent). The friend left. Upon commencement of antibiotic treatment, the patient had an unexpected anaphylactic reaction, rendering him incompetent. The doctor, who "believe[d] strongly in patient autonomy", was faced with a dilemma: the patient required immediate intubation or he would die. He was likely to require such intubation only until the anaphylaxis resolved. However, such intubation had been expressly forbidden by the patient. His proxy was not contactable. What should the doctor do?

This is a case where the meaning of the past desire is unclear. It is likely that the patient did not intend to forbid artificial ventilation in a case of drug-related anaphylaxis. Indeed, it is likely that he would rationally desire to be ventilated in these circumstances.

I am arguing for something stronger. I am arguing that there is still a case for artificial ventilation to be given even if the patient has expressly forbidden that

"artificial ventilation in cases of anaphylaxis" be instituted *if* that desire was based on inadequate information, either about artificial ventilation or anaphylaxis and their consequences, or inadequate imagination or feeble reflection. I am claiming that such deficiencies may be common. It is necessary then to go beyond what people have said, or written, to how they have lived their lives, what they have thought important, what their goals and rational desires are, that is, to what they have rationally evaluated is the best life for themselves. It is important to know what they value.

When is limitation of treatment in a patient's best interests?

If we do not know what this person values or if she has no values, then she ought to be treated according to her best interests. But how are we to define interests?

The President's Commission defines "interests" in terms of "more objective, societally shared criteria" of "welfare". The following factors are important:

> the relief of suffering, the preservation or the restoration of functioning, and the quality as well as the extent of life sustained. An accurate assessment will encompass consideration of present desires, the opportunities of future satisfactions, and the possibility of developing or regaining the capacity for self-determination.[52]

This is all rather superficial. What precisely is meant by "quality of life"? More rigorous accounts are available. Derek Parfit has distinguished three theories of well-being: Hedonistic Theories, Desire-Fulfilment Theories and Objective List Theories.[53]

The classical doctrine of Hedonism describes only one valuable mental state – happiness or pleasure – and one negative mental state – unhappiness or pain. More recent accounts argue that there are many mental states aside from pleasure which are valuable.

Desire-Fulfilment Theories claim that a person's life goes well when her desires are satisfied.

The Objective List approach to well-being claims that certain activities are objectively good. Parfit argues that being morally good, engaging in rational activity, developing one's abilities, having children and being a good parent (and presumably engaging in other meaningful human relationships), gaining knowledge and being aware of "true" beauty are examples of such activities.[54]

Each of these theories has problems.[55] Parfit argues that, while each of these three elements (desire satisfaction, happiness, valuable activity) is necessary for a good life, no one in isolation is sufficient for a valuable life. What makes a life go well is to have all three together.[56] On this approach, an example of what is good for someone is to be engaged in fulfilling, meaningful human relationships, wanting to be so engaged and gaining pleasure from these relationships.

There are problems still with this account. However, the aim of this paper is to show when a person's interests ought to be invoked, and not how we should construe interests.

Two points are important. Firstly, the account makes clear that there is a difference between a person's (narrowly construed) medical interests. Restoring the hearing of a member of the deaf community may make him better off medically (from the point of view of his health), but, if it will alienate him from his community and he strongly desires not to have the operation, the operation may not be in his overall best interests.

Secondly, one item missing from Parfit's list of objectively valuable activities is that activity which is an expression of a person's autonomy. Promoting a person's interests is thus interconnected with respecting her autonomy.[57] However, even if autonomous activity is valuable, the account makes clear that autonomous activity is only *a part* of what makes a person's life go well. A person's interests ought not be equated with satisfaction of autonomous desires. A person can autonomously choose a way of life which makes her life go less well overall than it could. Satisfaction of autonomous desire is not the only good in life.

Consider an example. A Jehovah's Witness refuses a blood transfusion and suffers serious brain damage which fundamentally impairs her ability to get what she wants, to carry on social relations, etc. She has made her life go badly. If her choice is to be justified, it will have to be in terms of her autonomy, not in terms of her interests.

When should treatment be limited in a person's best interests? On this account, life would be not worth living when it fell below a certain threshold where a person could no longer engage in a reasonable spectrum of valuable activity, could no longer gain happiness from that life and no longer satisfy her desires to engage in worthwhile activity.

There are lives which are so bad. A life with late stage Huntington's Chorea is one example. However, from empirical studies of patients with paraplegia, it appears that such people are able to lead fulfilling lives.[58]

Limitation of Treatment of Competent Patients

> An advance directive does not, however, provide self-determination in the sense of active moral agency by the patient on his or her behalf. . .[A]lthough self-determination is involved when a patient establishes a way to project his or her wishes into a time of anticipated incapacity, it is a sense of self-determination lacking in one important attribute: active, contemporaneous personal choice. Hence a decision not to follow an advance directive may sometimes be justified when it is not acceptable to disregard a competent patient's contemporaneous choice. Such a decision would most often rest on a finding that the patient did not adequately envision and consider the particular situation within which the actual medical decision must be made.[59]

The point made here by the President's Commission is that an advance directive which was formed by a person who failed to adequately envision the situation at hand does not provide self-determination. It can be disregarded *because it is not an instance of active, contemporaneous choice*. Implied, then, is that (competent) active, contemporaneous choice ought to be respected, *even when* that choice is the result of evaluation which does not adequately envision the situation at hand. I will argue that we ought not to respect all competent contemporaneous choices. Consider an example.

J is a man in a situation very like that of Mrs X. He, however, has no false beliefs. He believes that he will be able to walk independently on an artificial leg. He finds this abhorrent. An attempt is made to bring in amputees to talk to him about their lives. He refuses to see them. He has made his decision, he says, and we do not have the right to interfere.

J's wife subsequently reveals that J was involved in a car accident 10 years ago. As a result, J was critically ill. At the time, it was clear that if he was treated, he would be left a paraplegic. J desired to die. However, his doctors treated him against his will. He was left a paraplegic. Initially, J was depressed and continued to want to die, but gradually he adapted. He came to find life very fulfilling, participating in the "Para-Olympics". Some years later, a new surgical technique involving the use of a "nerve growth factor" was developed for conditions of spinal injury. After being operated on, J was able to regain the use of his legs. J's wife claims that he is now deliberately suppressing this information. He is an attention-seeker, she claims, and always tries to make his situation look as bad as possible to manipulate the sympathy of others. "He pulled the same stunt last time," she says. "He doesn't really want to die. He just wants you all running around after him, like I do every day."

A person's evaluation of what is best for himself can change. A person can judge that p is best now, but later judge that not-p is best.[60] But imagine that J's wife can give us good reasons why she believes that J would now rationally desire to live, that J values life as a paraplegic more than death. (His past behaviour provides valuable clues.) J's desire to die is then obstructive.[61]

What ought to be done when a competent person's desire obstructs the expressions of his autonomy?

If a person's expressed desire is obstructive, steps should be taken to facilitate the expression of his rational desires. Exactly how this can be done is a matter for psychological investigation.

In some cases, it will not be possible to set the conditions which will facilitate autonomous choice. A young trauma victim, rushed to hospital, may refuse to have some urgent, life-saving operation, like having a bleeding spleen removed. She may not believe that, if her spleen is removed, she will completely recover. Or she might claim to "not like operations". There may not be time to present enough information in a way that promotes adequate evaluation. It is reasonably to operate on this young person if there is a reasonable expectation that, with appropriate information and reflection, she would consent. In some cases, we ought to satisfy a person's rational, hypothetical desire (her values), rather than her actual desire. If we wish to respect autonomy, it is more important to respect a person's values than satisfy an obstructive actual desire.

The situation becomes more complicated when an obviously obstructive desire is resistant to change, even after considerable counselling and provision of information. My own feeling is that, if we wish to respect autonomy, such desires ought to be overridden. This is contentious.

Another difficult situation arises when we suspect, but do not know, that an expressed desire is obstructive. Or we may believe that this person has never formed a rational life-plan, that she has failed entirely to rationally evaluate *anything*. Such a person is not autonomous. One possible solution is to treat her according to her interests.

It might be objected that such a policy is liable to paternalistic abuse. We may, in these cases, abide by competent persons' desires *as a matter of policy*. But the justification for this lies not necessarily with respect for this patient's autonomy, but elsewhere.

Two Objections

1. Respect only articulated desires?

It might be agreed that in cases like that of Ulysses, where a person has expressed two conflicting desires, the desire which better promotes autonomy ought to be respected. However, it might be argued that if a competent person, like J, expresses a desire to die, and there is *no contrary desire articulated*, then that desire ought to be presumed to be autonomous.

There are two reasons why we ought not to respect only articulated desires.

Firstly, being autonomous does not entail that one has a rational desire at the moment. Being autonomous does entail having a certain disposition, but this disposition will not always be "momentarily actualized", as Ryle put it,[62] in the form of a desire. Assume that, when I am deeply asleep, I have no desires. *A fortiori*, at that time I do not desire my freedom. But if I were awoken by the gunshots of a revolution, I *would* desire my freedom. When I am asleep, I still value my freedom, but I do not at that time rationally desire it.

The less my valuing of, say, freedom manifests itself in an actual desire, the less chance there is for someone to witness my desiring freedom. I may still value freedom, but few may ever have heard me *articulate* that value.

Secondly, some of a person's desires are *never* articulated. Some rational desires remain unarticulated. Is this claim plausible?

What determines whether a person articulates her desires or not? A lot depends on what sort of person she is: is she the kind of person who articulates her thoughts and beliefs to others? Is she the sort of person who thinks in terms of words, sentences and "propositions"? Or is she a person who does not verbalize in her own mind her experiences? Moreover, articulation of desire has nothing necessarily to do with whether the desire is rational or not. There is no reason to believe that rational desires will necessarily be articulated. There is no reason to believe that all people who value freedom will have articulated this value at some point in time.

A related objection can be levelled at articulated desires: how do we *know* that Mrs X *rationally desired* living independently?[63] Why wasn't *this* desire obstructive? The answer turns on how we can come to know whether the three evaluative conditions were satisfied. There is not space to address this important issue. I suspect that the answer is, in part, in the realm of the psychologist. However, we *can* know that some of a person's desires are rational. Ulysses' men, confronted with two conflicting desires, knew what he judged was best, what he rationally desired. It was

clear, without him *fully articulating* it, what Ulysses' *plan* was. Though his instructions were brief, his intentions were clear. Our plans may not be so clear, but they are, I believe, intelligible. And they are often intelligible to a greater extent than we articulate them.

It is of course possible that Mrs X has not rationally evaluated her life at any stage. I think this unlikely, but, if so, she ought to be treated according to her interests.

2. Autonomy and false beliefs

> Every creature that lives and moves shall be food for you. . .But you must not eat the flesh with life, which is the blood, still in it. (Gen. 9:3–5)
>
> Abstain from. . .fornication, from anything that has been strangled and from blood. (Acts 15:19–21)

Jehovah's Witnesses interpret these passages as forbidding blood transfusion.

A Jehovah's Witness (JW) is involved in a car accident. He requires a blood transfusion if he is to live. He refuses to have the blood transfusion. He would prefer to die. Should his desire be respected?

I have argued that Mrs X's false belief distorts her appreciation of treatment options available to her. It precludes her choice to die from being autonomous. However, not giving blood to JW is said to respect his autonomy. Yet JW (let us assume) holds a false belief: if he receives a blood transfusion, he'll go to Hell. Why is the refusal of treatment of JW an expression of his autonomy, and that of Mrs X not? Aren't they both under a misapprehension as to a matter of relevant fact? Why does "If I have an amputation, I'll be confined to a wheelchair" make Mrs X's refusal non-autonomous, whereas "If I get blood, I'll be confined to Hell" doesn't make the Witness' refusal non-autonomous?[64]

a. *Instrumental irrationality* JW may be instrumentally irrational, that is, mistaken about the appropriate means to his ends. Assume that the Bible only forbids the consumption of animal blood. Assume also that JW rationally desires (in the narrow sense in which I have defined it) to live in accordance with the dictates of the Bible. JW mistakenly believes that the Bible forbids blood transfusion, when the Bible is only referring to certain dietary practices. His desire not to receive blood is the result of false belief about what the Bible says. His desire will cause him to die. It is thus an obstructive desire. It prevents him achieving what he judges is best: *living* in accordance with the Bible. His *instrumental* irrationality frustrates his autonomy. This kind of JW is like Mrs X.[65]

b. *Instrumentally valuable false beliefs*   A person can rationally (in both my sense and a broader sense) choose to hold false beliefs. Knowing that I must fight courageously in battle to survive, I might form the false belief that I am the incarnation of a great Hindu Warrior. Or I may be dying of some disease. In order to put on a brave face for my family, I cause myself to believe that death will not be the end. Indeed, a person can rationally cause himself to act irrationally.[66] Desire based on false belief is often instrumentally irrational; however, it is not *necessarily* instrumentally irrational.

If it is the case that JW's false belief serves some useful purpose, then this provides some reason to hold this belief. For instance, the belief that Witnesses have in bodily purity sets them apart from other sects. If holding this false belief is necessary for their identity as members of this discrete sect, and being a member confers great advantages not easily found elsewhere (feelings of solidarity, uniqueness, camaraderie, loyalty, etc.), then each person would have a reason to hold the false belief.

As I argued before, autonomy can be inherited from a parent evaluation. If JW autonomously chose to be a member of this sect, having appreciated what it entails, including the risk of death from blood loss, and holding this false belief is *necessary* if one is to be a member of this sect, then holding this false belief is an expression of his autonomy.

To what degree the false belief is necessary in either of these two senses is an open question.

c. *Descriptive and non-descriptive beliefs*   One can have beliefs about descriptive and non-descriptive statements or claims. Descriptive statements are pure statements of fact. Non-descriptive statements are not pure statements of fact, but may in part be "expressions of attitudes, prescriptions or something else non-descriptive".[67] A belief about a descriptive statement is meant to describe the way the world is. Examples might be "I believe that the cat is on the mat" or "I believe that Rome is further north than Athens." Beliefs about descriptive statements are verifiable by empirical investigation of the world. That is, my belief is false if the cat is *not* on the mat, and so on.

I will call beliefs about descriptive statements, descriptive beliefs. One way to interpret religious belief is as descriptive belief, that is, as representing the way the world is. This would include the belief that there *is* a place, Heaven and another, Hell, there *is* a being, God, and so on. On this interpretation, JW is expressing a descriptive belief: if he gets a blood transfusion, he will actually go to Hell, which is supposed to be a place of fire and eternal torment, inhabited by beings with horns on their heads and tails, holding small pitch-forks.

As far as being an empirical hypothesis about the way the world is, there is no good reason to believe that such descriptions of the world represent true propositions. Available evidence suggests that there is no Hell of any description. If held in this descriptive manner, religious belief distorts one's grasp on the nature of the world. In this case, the JW's belief would be like that of Mrs X; his desire to die would not be autonomous.

Compare the following statements: (1) I ought to hand in the money I found. (2) The painting is beautiful. (3) God exists.

(1) represents a moral statement. There is division about whether moral statements are descriptive or non-descriptive. I will not enter that debate. A non-descriptive account of (1) is that the statement expresses in part some attitude on the part of the speaker. The meaning of the statement is not fixed by properties of actions, the world or other descriptive criteria.[68]

It seems to me that if non-descriptivism is a coherent account of the meaning of moral statements, then it may also be a coherent account of other statements. I have in mind statements like (2). It is possible to agree on all the facts concerning a painting: what colours it employs, the type of brush strokes, the subject, the quality of the canvas, and so on, and yet disagree about whether it is beautiful. The expression that something is beautiful is, at least in part, the expression of a certain attitude.

But, if this is right, it is possible that religious statements, although ostensibly purporting to report some property or fact about the world, may be non-descriptive statements.[69] Statements "reporting" religious fact may be like statements "reporting" aesthetic fact. (3) may be like (2). Statement (3) may represent, not a mere statement of fact or the description of a property, but an expression of an attitude, a commitment to a way of life, an adherence to an ideal. On this reading, religion is a construct which gives meaning to people's lives, rather than an empirical statement about the nature of the world. JW's belief, B, that if he receives blood, he'll go to Hell, can thus be viewed as a belief about a non-descriptive statement. The following statements all represent a similar attitude or commitment about which we can have beliefs: "If I receive blood, it will be very bad," "If I receive the blood, I'll go to Hell," "I ought not to receive the blood."

Since non-descriptive statements do not describe properties of the world, they cannot be assessed for their truth or falsehood by empirical examination of the world or of the people in it.

Just as there is no property of descriptive criterion of a painting that will establish that the painting is beautiful, so too there is no property of the world that will establish that God exists. To say to JW that B is false is like saying to a small clique of painters that their paintings are ugly. They might reply, "But we think that they are beautiful." There is no fact of the matter which will settle that the paintings are "truly beautiful". Beauty is in the eye of the beholder, at least for the non-descriptivist.

Nor is there any necessary irrationality or failure of rational evaluation in dying for a non-descriptive construct. It is no more non-autonomous to die for one's religion than it is to die for one's country.

There is, then, not one kind of Jehovah's Witness, but many. Some are irrational and non-autonomous, while others are as autonomous as the next man, or woman. What respect for autonomy requires depends on how a particular Witness holds his belief.

Conclusion

The President's Commission, along with many contemporary bioethicists, accepts that treatment of previously competent but now incompetent patients can be limited if that is what the patient would desire, if she were now competent. If this hypothetical desire cannot be determined, then treatment can be limited if it is not in the patient's best interests. On this approach, a past preference on a related issue or an advance directive constitutes sufficient evidence of what a patient would now desire, if she were competent.

I have distinguished between desiring and rational desiring. One necessary condition for a desire to be fully autonomous is that it is a rational desire or that it satisfies a rational desire. A person rationally desires a state of affairs if that person desires that state of affairs while being in possession of all available relevant facts, without committing relevant error of logic, and vividly imagining what a reasonable range of states of affairs associated with each course of action would be like for him or her.

Not all desires are expressions of a person's autonomy. Some competent, expressed desires obstruct one's autonomy. In evaluating a life of suffering and disability, there are several psychological mechanisms which tend to prevent adequate evaluation of those states. The process of vivid imagination so necessary for rational evaluation is no easy or straightforward process to engage in. When deciding whether to live or die, there are many hurdles to forming a desire which is an expression of our autonomy.

In relation to limitation of treatment of incompetent patients, I conclude: (1) If past desires (including those expressed in advance directives) are to be full expressions of a person's former autonomy, they must have been formed by a person who was in possession of all relevant, available information, who did not commit relevant logical errors and who was vividly acquainted with the lives on offer. (2) In the realm of decisions about states of significant disability, it ought not to be presumed that past competent desires (including advance directives) were necessarily autonomous. (3) Past competent desires (including advance directives) ought to be evaluated to examine whether they were the expression of a person's autonomy. (4) In order to respect a now incompetent patient's former autonomy, it is not enough to know what a patient would now desire if she were competent. We must know what she would rationally desire. (5) Treatment of an incompetent person ought to be limited if limitation is what she would rationally desire. Evidence of what a patient would now rationally desire is what she did rationally desire. (6) If it is clear that allowing a patient to die is a violation of his former autonomy (as reflected by what he or she rationally desired), then he or she ought not be allowed to die. This may entail acting contrary to an expressed past preference (including an advance directive), if that preference was irrational (obstructive). (7) As our degree of belief that a past expressed desire (including an advance

directive) was not autonomous increases, and we are not confident that we know what the patient would now rationally desire, treatment should promote an incompetent patient's best interests.

My arguments have implications for the limitation of treatment of competent patients. My conclusions in this regard are: (1) Care providers ought to ensure that the conditions under which a patient can choose autonomously are secured. This includes provision of information, purging of errors of logic and facilitation of imagination of options on offer. (2) When it is clear that a competent desire is obstructive, and what the person would rationally desire can be confidently estimated, then it is best if we wish to respect autonomy to override the obstructive desire in favour of what the patient would rationally desire. (3) Cases where an obstructive desire persists, or where a person has failed to rationally evaluate the relevant states of affairs, or it is unclear whether the expressed desire is obstructive are complex. If we elect to obey a competent desire, we must recognize that we may not be respecting, and may even be frustrating, this patient's autonomy.

Notes

1   Thanks to two anonymous referees who reviewed an earlier draft. Their detailed comments greatly improved the paper. I am also indebted to Helga Kuhse, Justin Oakley, Cora Singer, Robert Young, Professor R. M. Hare, Hilary Madder and, most of all, to Peter Singer, for their pains and the many invaluable comments which they gave me. This paper was written with the support of a National Health and Medical Research Council of Australia Medical Scholarship.

2   David Hume, "Of Suicide", in P. Singer (ed), *Applied Ethics* (Oxford: Oxford University Press, 1986), p. 26.

3   President's Commission for the Study of Ethical Problems in Medicine and Biomedical and Behavioral Research, *Deciding to Forgo Life-Sustaining Treatment: A Report on the Ethical, Medical and Legal Issues in Treatment Decisions* (March 1983), p. 136.

4   Ibid., p. 27.

5   G. Dworkin, *The Theory and Practice of Autonomy* (Cambridge: Cambridge University Press, 1988), p. 12.

6   R. Young, *Personal Autonomy: Beyond Negative and Positive Liberty* (London: Croom Helm, 1986), p. 8.

7   Ibid., p. 8. The term "life-plan" is used on p. 78.

8   This account is like Brandt's account of rational desires (*A Theory of the Good and the Right* (Oxford: Clarendon Press, 1979), pp. 111ff). One important difference is that Brandt's is a counterfactual account. Young also appeals to a similar notion of rational desire (*Personal Autonomy*, p. 10 and pp. 43–5).

9   I assume she does not have an intrinsic distaste for intravenous infusions.

10 In Locke's case, the person believes the door is open when in fact it is locked (J. Locke, *An Essay concerning Human Understanding*, ed. A. S. Pringle-Pattinson (Oxford: Clarendon Press, 1924), Book II, Chapter xxi, sec. 10).

11 Kahneman and Varey note: "A basic tenet of psychological analysis is that the contents of subjective experience are coded and interpreted representations of objects and

events. An objective description of stimuli is not adequate to predict experience because coding and interpretation can cause identical physical stimuli to be treated as identical." (D. Kahneman and C. Varey, "Notes on the psychology of utility", in J. Elster and J. E. Roemer, *Interpersonal Comparisons of Well-Being* (Cambridge: Cambridge University Press, 1991), p. 141.)

12 If the reader does not accept the preceding argument, then his or her favoured account of autonomous desiring should be inserted.

13 This formulation of the objection is Robert Young's.

14 I will not discuss the more complex problem of which of all the possible courses of action open to an agent ought to be entertained for a choice to be autonomous.

15 This formulation of the objection is again Robert Young's. Dan Brock puts the problem in the form of "impetuous Adam". (See D. Brock, "Paternalism and Autonomy", *Ethics*, 98 (April 1988), 550–65.) My response is similar to that of Feinberg (*Harm to Self* (New York: Oxford University Press, 1986), p. 109).

16 Professor Hare convinced me of this (personal communication). I use "dispositional concept" in Ryle's sense (G. Ryle, *The Concept of Mind* (Harmondsworth: Penguin, 1963), pp. 43, 113–20). Young also argues that autonomy has an important dispositional sense (*Personal Autonomy*, p. 8).

17 I will not discuss these in detail. Examples might be that the person is not asleep, not under anaesthesia, not in the grip of psychotic illness, not under the influence of certain drugs, not being coerced by others, etc.

18 See, for example, G. Watson, "Free Agency", *Journal of Philosophy*, 72 (1975) and D. Gauthier, *Morals by Agreement* (Oxford: Clarendon Press, 1986).

19 P desires that q iff P would desire that q under conditions C. See: M. Smith, "Valuing: Desiring or Believing?" in D. Charles and D. Lennon (eds), *Reduction, Explanation and Realism* (Oxford University Press, 1995).

20 R. Graves, *The Greek Myths*, vol. 2 (Harmondsworth: Penguin, 1960), p. 361.

21 One editor asked whether Ulysses knows that he will die at the time he commands his men to move closer to the Island. If he does, his desire is more clearly irrational. But let us assume that he does not know this at the time. Let us assume that the Sirens' song removes this belief or makes it inaccessible. It might be objected that Ulysses is not then irrational because he does not know that he will die in moving closer to the Sirens. However, Ulysses' desire is still irrational because it

has not been made by vividly imagining the relevant alternatives. The Sirens' song causes Ulysses' mind to be dominated by one alternative.

22 I thank Professor Hare for this objection and for drawing to my attention this crucial distinction between disposition and desire.

23 I will not address the relationship between these two errors. It may be that the false belief caused the failure of imagination *or* that the failure in imagination caused the false belief. Her *dread* of amputation may have prevented her believing she would walk.

24 J. C. J. M. De Haes and F. C. E. Van Knippenberg, "Quality of life of cancer patients: a review of the literature" in N. K. Aaronson and J. Beckmann (eds), *The Quality of Life of Cancer Patients* (New York: Raven Press, 1987), p. 170. These results represent the cumulation of a series of studies – see De Haes and Van Knippenberg for specific references.

25 Ibid. for specific references.

26 P. Menzel, *Strong Medicine* (Oxford: Oxford University Press, 1990), p. 82. Menzel also shows that these patients will prefer to shorten their lives by 50% to be cured of their disease, p. 81. These findings together may suggest that these patients value normality more than normal people do.

27 Ibid., p. 82, n. 11.

28 P. Brickman, D. Coates, and R. Janoff-Bulman, "Lottery winners and accident victims: is happiness relative?" *Journal of Personality and Social Psychology*, 36(8) (1978), 917–27 as quoted in D. Kahneman and C. Varey, "Notes on the psychology of utility", in J. Elster and J. E. Roemer, *Interpersonal Comparisons of Well-Being* (Cambridge: Cambridge University Press, 1991).

29 From Heinrich and Kriefel cited in E. Goffman, *Stigma: Notes on the Management of Spoiled Identity* (Englewood Cliffs, NJ: Prentice-Hall, 1963) as cited in S. E. Taylor, *Positive Illusions* (Basic Books, 1989), p. 161.

30 All quotations are from S. E. Taylor, "Adjustment to threatening events: A theory of cognitive adaptation", *American Psychologist*, 38 (1983), 1161–73 as quoted in Taylor, *Positive Illusions*, pp. 195–6.

31 Ibid, p. 166. She quotes from several different sources (see text for full references).

32 Kahneman and Varey ("Psychology of Utility", pp. 136–7) argue that adaptation is a normal phenomenon.

33 Ibid., pp. 136–7.

34 J. A. Russell, and B. Fehr, "Relativity in the perception of emotion in facial expressions", *Journal of Experimental*

Psychology: General, 116(3) (1987), 223–37, as quoted in Kahneman and Varey, "Psychology of Utility", p. 139.

35 For more recent experiments illustrating the significance of contrast effects, see A. Tversky and D. Griffin, "Endowment and contrast in judgements of well-being" in F. Strack, M. Argyle and N. Schwarz (eds), *Subjective Well-Being* (Oxford: Pergamon, 1991), pp. 101–18.

36 Kahneman and Varey, "Psychology of Utility", p. 144.

37 Ibid., p. 149.

38 Ibid., p. 149.

39 See D. Parfit, *Reasons and Persons* (Oxford: Clarendon Press, 1984), Part III for a discussion of the rationality of this bias. I am not arguing that these attitudes or psychological responses *necessarily* preclude autonomy. I am not arguing that one cannot be autonomously loss or risk-averse, or "live for the moment". But, to be autonomous and hold these attitudes and biases, they must at some point have been evaluated in the right way and endorsed. Most people have not evaluated their biases.

40 "Psychology of Utility", p. 144.

41 "Endorsement", pp. 113–14.

42 President's Commission, p. 45.

43 D. Kahneman and D. T. Miller, "Norm Theory: Comparing Reality to Its Alternatives", *Psychological Review*, 93(2), (1986), 136–53. The quote is on p. 148.

44 Ibid., p. 148.

45 President's Commission, p. 132.

46 A. Buchanan and D. Brock, "Deciding for Others", *Milbank Quarterly*, 64(Suppl. 2), (1986), 17–94.

47 President's Commission, p. 149.

48 I here assume that a desire's being rational is *sufficient* for its being autonomous. This is an oversimplification. Other necessary conditions must be satisfied for a desire to be autonomous.

49 T. L. Beauchamp and J. F. Childress, *Principles of Biomedical Ethics* (New York: Oxford University Press, 1989), p. 83. Beauchamp and Childress describe a competent person as one who possesses certain abilities or capacities, pp. 79–85. They claim that it "seems a plausible hypothesis that an autonomous person is necessarily a competent person", p. 83. The more relevant question for me is: is a competent person *necessarily* autonomous?

50 Buchanan and Brock, "Deciding for Others", p. 70.

51 L. M. Silverman, et al., "Whether No Means No", *Hastings Center Report*, (May–June 1992), 26–7.

52 President's Commission, p. 135.

53 See D. Parfit, *Reasons and Persons*, pp. 493–502 and J. Griffin, *Well-Being* (Oxford: Clarendon Press, 1986).

54 Parfit, *Reasons and Persons*, p. 499.

55 See Parfit (*Reasons and Persons*) and Griffin (*Well-Being*).

56 Parfit, *Reasons and Persons*, p. 502.

57 A point forcefully made by Robert Young.

58 Clearly not all paraplegics later find life worth living. There is some uncertainty about whether *this* person's life will be worth living as a paraplegic. This issue is dealt with in my "Treatment Limitation Decisions under Uncertainty: the Value of Subsequent Euthanasia", *Bioethics*, 8(1), (Jan. 1994).

59 President's Commission, p. 137.

60 Better than vivid imagination is actual experience. Still, there are factors which can interfere with rational evaluation based on experience. We may focus on only one aspect of that experience or unjustifiably generalize from one aspect, and so on.

61 Third party evaluations of what a patient values raise problems. There is a suggestion of antipathy between J and his wife. She may want him to be punished. We must keep clear that our aim is to determine what the patient values. Third party evaluations constitute just one line of evidence.

62 *Concept of Mind*, p. 84.

63 Another related question is: if one can rationally desire death, then one must have vividly imagined what death is like. Is this possible? Imagination of what being dead is like ought only to occur to the extent that it can occur. One way in which being dead can be imagined is as the absence of certain states of affairs.

64 This objection is Peter Singer's.

65 The importance of the instrumentality, and the example given, was raised by one referee.

66 See Derek Parfit's "Could It Be Rational to Cause Oneself to Act Irrationally?" in *Reasons and Persons*, pp. 12–13.

67 R. M. Hare, *Moral Thinking* (Oxford: Clarendon Press, 1981), p. 208.

68 Ibid., p. 70.

69 Professor Hare gives a detailed non-descriptivist interpretation of religious statements in "The Simple Believer", "Appendix: Theology and Falsification" and "Religion and Morals" in his *Essays on Religion and Education* (Oxford: Clarendon Press, 1992). I thank Professor Hare for very valuable discussion on these points.

Part X

Disability

Introduction

In recent years, issues relating to disability have become more prominent in bioethics. As we shall see, some of the writing on this topic probes fundamental questions about what makes a life worth living, and whether it is possible to compare the quality or desirability of different lives. Moreover, these questions are raised, not only for the sake of exploring deep philosophical issues, interesting as that may be, but in practical contexts where people are facing some of the most important choices they will ever make. A woman may be considering whether to terminate a pregnancy or allow it to continue until a child is born. A healthcare team may consult with a couple about whether to withdraw life support from their newborn child. A deaf couple may wish to use in vitro; fertilization and preimplantation genetic diagnosis to ensure that their child will also be deaf. All of these issues are discussed either in Part X below or in readings in the "Newborns" section of Part IV: Life and Death Issues, some of which also relate to questions about disability, and which may be read in conjunction with this Part.

In "Valuing Disability, Causing Disability," Elizabeth Barnes asks the broadest question about disability: is being disabled bad for you? Most of us take it for granted that it is. Isn't it obvious that it is better to see, hear, and walk than to be blind, deaf, or in a wheelchair? No, some disability activists say. They concede that life can be worse for people with disabilities when people discriminate against them, or fail to accommodate their need for access to buildings, or for forms of communication that are suitable for them. But in a society that was fully accepting of people with disabilities, the difference between being disabled and not being disabled would, they say, be a "mere difference," like the difference between being male or female, or gay or straight, rather than a "bad difference" like the difference between being well and having a chronic and painful illness.

One common argument for the bad-difference view is that if being disabled does not make you worse off, it would not be wrong to cause someone to become disabled. But surely it is wrong to cause someone to become blind, deaf, or unable to walk. Therefore these disabilities must be bad differences, not mere differences. Barnes seeks to meet this argument by offering an explanation of why it is wrong to cause someone to be disabled that is compatible with the mere-difference view.

Greg Bognar asks, in response to Barnes: "Is Disability Mere Difference?" He also considers several other arguments for the view that disability is a mere difference rather than a bad difference. None of these arguments, he concludes, succeeds in showing that disability is not a harm.

Bioethics: An Anthology, Fourth Edition. Edited by Udo Schüklenk and Peter Singer.
Editorial material and organization © 2022 John Wiley & Sons, Inc. Published 2022 by John Wiley & Sons, Inc.

Adrienne Asch, who died in 2013, was born prematurely and became blind soon afterwards, as a result of an excess of oxygen in her incubator. Her article "Prenatal Diagnosis and Selective Abortion," first published in 1999, is a pioneering critique of the assumption that disability is bad and hence that pregnant women should be encouraged to have prenatal diagnosis, followed by abortion if the test detects a disability. Asch argues that our assumptions about life with disability rest on misinformation. Obstetricians, midwives, nurses, and genetic counselors are often poorly informed about the extent to which having a disability adversely affects the quality of a person's life. To become better informed, Asch suggests, people facing a decision about whether to terminate a pregnancy to avoid having a disabled child should consult with an organization of people with the disability in question, or of the parents of people with the disability.

The next two articles in this section, both published in the *Washington Post*, present opposite sides of the most common circumstance in which women or couples choose whether to abort a fetus after prenatal testing: when the test has shown that the child will have Down syndrome. Renate Lindeman's description of her feelings after her first child was born supports Asch's view. Lindeman's initial negative response to the knowledge that her child had Down syndrome was, she says, based on outdated information. By the time she was pregnant again, and prenatal testing showed that her second child would also have Down syndrome, her attitudes were entirely different. She outlines the reasons for her present, much more positive, view of the condition, and why she sees systematic screening for Down syndrome as a violation of human rights.

Ruth Marcus, a political commentator and journalist, acknowledges that many parents cherish their children with Down syndrome, and that those with the syndrome often live happy lives. Nevertheless, she tells her readers, she would have aborted a fetus with Down syndrome, as two-thirds of American women do. (In the United Kingdom, Australia, and several other countries, the figure is over 90%.) She defends women's rights to have abortions, and argues that it is absurd to assert that women have a right to abortion for any reason, *except* because the fetus has Down syndrome.

88

Valuing Disability, Causing Disability

Elizabeth Barnes

Disability rights activists often claim that being disabled isn't something that's bad for you. Disability is, rather, a natural part of human diversity – something that should be valued and celebrated, rather than pitied and ultimately "cured." But though this view is common among disability rights activists, many (perhaps most) philosophers find it implausible and radical. A major objection to such views of disability – one which tries to reinforce the idea that the position is deeply implausible – is this: were they correct, they would make it permissible to cause disability and impermissible to cause nondisability (or impermissible to "cure" disability, to use the value-laden term). The aim of this article is to show that these twin objections don't succeed. We can appeal to neither the permissibility of causing disability nor the impermissibility of causing nondisability to undermine the disability-positive position.

In what follows, I first attempt to clarify the position being objected to. To do this, I unpack the distinction between what I call "mere-difference" views of disability (like those often favored by disability rights advocates) and the more familiar "bad-difference"

views of disability (Sec. I). I then discuss the objection to mere-difference views of disability based on causing disability (Sec. II). I look at different ways one could cause disability and discuss what defenders of a mere-difference view can say about them (Secs. III, IV, and V), and then address the potential discrepancies between causing and "curing" disability (Sec. VI).

But first a note on terminology. In what follows, I attempt to characterize the distinction between mere-difference and bad-difference views of disability, and discuss the implications of the mere-difference view. I make no attempt, however, to define "disability." For present purposes, I want to understand "disability" as a term introduced by ostension.[1] Think of paradigm cases of disability – mobility impairments, blindness, deafness, rheumatoid arthritis, achondroplasia, and so forth. I am interested in what follows if we say that *these kind of things* – whatever they may be – are mere-difference rather than bad-difference. Would it follow that it is permissible to cause people to have these kinds of features? Would it follow that it is impermissible to seek to remove or prevent these features?

Original publication details: Elizabeth Barnes, "Valuing Disability, Causing Disability," pp. 88–113 from *Ethics* 125 (2014). Reproduced with permission of University of Chicago Press.

I　The Bad-Difference/Mere-Difference Distinction

Disability rights activists often adopt a "disability-positive" position: disability is not, by itself, something bad, harmful, or suboptimal. I'm arguing that causation-based objections to this view don't succeed. But I first need to briefly make clearer what the disability-positive position is.[2]

Let's call views that maintain that disability is by itself something that makes you worse off "bad-difference" views of disability. According to bad-difference views of disability, not only is having a disability bad for you, having a disability would still be bad for you even if society was fully accommodating of disabled people. In contrast, let's call views that deny this "mere-difference" views of disability. According to mere-difference views of disability, having a disability makes you nonstandard or different, but it doesn't by itself make you worse off. This rough-and-ready distinction highlights the basic ideas, but it needs to be explained more thoroughly if it is going to be put to work.

Unfortunately, though, there isn't a single best way of characterizing this distinction. The difference between mere-difference and bad-difference views of disability is best understood as a difference in the interaction between disability and well-being. But there are many different – and quite disparate – theories of well-being. There isn't a way of characterizing the mere-difference/bad-difference distinction that cuts neatly across all these different views of well-being – or at least if there is one I haven't been able to come up with it.

First, let me explain why it is complicated. The mere-difference view isn't simply the view that, on average, disabled people aren't any worse off than nondisabled people. It is perfectly consistent with the mere-difference view that the actual well-being of disabled people is, on average, lower than that of nondisabled people, simply because of how society treats disabled people. The mere-difference view also needn't deny that disability involves the loss of intrinsic goods

or basic capabilities (and, mutatis mutandis, needn't deny that disability is, in a restricted sense, a harm – a harm with respect to particular features or aspects of life). It is perfectly consistent with the mere-difference view that disability always involves the loss of some goods. It's just that, according to the mere-difference view, disability can't be merely a loss or a lack. The mere-difference view can maintain that the very same thing which causes you to lose out on some goods (unique to nondisability) allows you to participate in other goods (perhaps unique to disability). For example, a defender of the mere-difference view can grant that the ability to hear is an intrinsic good. And it is an intrinsic good that Deaf people lack. But there might be other intrinsic goods – the unique experience of language had by those whose first language is a signed rather than spoken language, the experience of music via vibrations, and so on – experienced by Deaf people and not by hearing people. Deafness can involve the lack of an intrinsic good without being merely the lack of an intrinsic good.[3]

So the mere-difference view can't simply be the view that disability doesn't involve the loss of goods, nor the view that disability doesn't in fact reduce well-being. But nor can the mere-difference view be characterized simply as the view that disability is not intrinsically bad for you, or intrinsically something that makes you worse off. Suppose, for example, that your view of well-being is a strong form of hedonism – one which maintains that the only thing that's intrinsically good for you is pleasure and the only thing that's intrinsically bad for you is pain. Disability doesn't make you intrinsically worse off on this view. But suppose you further think that disability always or almost always leads to a net loss of pleasure and that this loss of pleasure would persist even in the absence of ableism. In that case, your view of disability sounds like a bad-difference view – even though disability isn't something that's intrinsically bad for you.

In light of these sorts of complexities, I think the best thing to do is to give several different, nonequivalent ways of characterizing the mere-difference/

bad-difference distinction. Hopefully, at least one of them will be adequate, whatever your theory of well-being. To begin with, we have the simple:

i. Disability is something that is an automatic or intrinsic cost to your well-being.

Broadly Aristotelian or "objective list" views of well-being often view disability in a way that supports (i).[4] There is, on these views, some norm of human flourishing or set of basic capabilities from which disability detracts. This is one way of holding a bad-difference view of disability. But it is certainly not the only way. A claim like (i) will be rejected by those who favor desire-satisfaction or hedonistic theories of well-being, for example – though one can easily maintain a bad-difference view on such theories of well-being. An alternative characterization of the bad-difference view, more amenable to such views of well-being would be:

ii. Were society fully accepting of disabled people, it would still be the case that for any given disabled person x and arbitrary nondisabled person y, such that x and y are in relevantly similar personal and socioeconomic circumstances, it is likely that y has a higher level of well-being than x.

That is, even if we eradicated ableism, disability would still have a negative impact on well-being. If you compared two people who were relatively similar in their socioeconomic and personal circumstances but who differed in whether they were disabled, the disabled person would likely be worse off than the nondisabled person – society's acceptance notwithstanding. Suppose, for example, that you hold some version of a desire-satisfaction theory of well-being and further think that disability is strongly correlated with the frustration of desires. Your view of disability wouldn't support (i), but it would support (ii). You think that, even in the absence of ableism, a disabled person is likely to have more unfulfilled desires than a nondisabled person in relatively similar

circumstances – and so you think a disabled person in relatively similar circumstances is likely to be worse off. But some subjectivists about well-being might be unhappy with the interpersonal comparisons of well-being required in (ii), so instead we could characterize the bad-difference view as:

iii. For any arbitrary disabled person x, if you could hold x's personal and socioeconomic circumstances fixed but remove their disability, you would thereby improve their well-being.

Almost no one – however committed to a bad-difference view of disability she may be – thinks that being disabled always makes your life go worse for you. Someone might have been a lonely shut-in, with no friends and no community, before she became disabled. She then goes to a rehabilitation center, where she makes a lot of friends, becomes involved in sports or the arts, and so forth. This person's life has, on balance, gone better for her in a way that's causally related to becoming disabled. But it hasn't gone better for her in virtue of being disabled. If she could keep her friends, her interests, and her community but lose her disability most people think she would be better off. There are caveats, of course. If a person makes her living from disability theater or is a star in the paralympics, it isn't obvious she'd be better off without her disability. But if we could hold fixed most of her external circumstances but remove her disability, a standard interpretation of the bad-difference view says we've thereby made her better off. And that's the idea (iii) tries to capture.

Claim (iii) is very strong, however: it is saying that removing someone's disability (provided you could hold other things fixed) will automatically make them better off. There are other options (like [ii]) which are weaker but which still count as bad-difference views. For example, a desire-satisfaction theorist could maintain that you don't automatically make someone better off if you can hold their circumstances fixed but remove their disability. After all, you have to leave room for odd desires. And similar points apply, mutatis mutandis, for the hedonist who wants to leave room for unusual sources of pleasure. Still, many such people would want to say that it is incredibly likely that you make someone better off by removing their disability, even in the absence of ableism. That claim is weaker than (iii) but still in the spirit of bad-difference views.[5]

To sum up: none of (i)–(iii) is necessary for maintaining a bad-difference view. But maintaining any of (i)–(iii) is sufficient for a bad-difference view of disability. Mere-difference views of disability must deny all of (i)–(iii). But the mere-difference view is not simply the denial of (i)–(iii). Mere-difference views must also deny the converse claims (the "good-difference" view of disability that says that disability makes you better off). Traditionally, mere-difference views are also further associated with various positive claims about disability, including:

a. Disability is analogous to features like sexuality, gender, ethnicity, and race.
b. Disability is not a defect or departure from "normal functioning."
c. Disability is a valuable part of human diversity that should be celebrated and preserved.
d. A principal source of the bad effects of disability is society's treatment of disabled people, rather than disability itself.

None of (a)–(d) are essential to maintaining a mere-difference view of disability. The mere-difference view can be understood simply as the denial of claims like (i)–(iii), and of their good-difference converses. But something along the lines of (a)–(d) is characteristic of the view of disability that at least most mere-difference views maintain. Commitment to (d) is of course not unique to mere-difference views; bad-difference views can agree that social prejudice causes harm to disabled people. But bad-difference views and mere-difference views often disagree over how much weight they place on (d) and likewise on to what extent the bad effects of disability are caused by society, rather than by disability itself.

II   A Problem for the Mere-Difference View?

Notably, some combination of (i)–(iii) is generally taken to be the "common sense" or "intuitive" view of disability. Likewise, many philosophers react to claims like (a)–(d) with incredulity. The reasons for such incredulity are no doubt complex and varied. But I am here concerned with a specific argument – given in, inter alia, McMahan, Harris, Kahane, and Singer – which is often supplied in its support.[6] If disability were mere-difference rather than bad-difference, it would be permissible to cause disability; it is obviously impermissible to cause disability; therefore, disability is not mere-difference; it is bad-difference. And it is also argued that the mere-difference view is implausible because it would make it impermissible to remove disability.[7]

It is worth emphasizing the philosophical importance of these arguments. The bad-difference view is often assumed rather than argued for: we are meant to have the intuition that it is correct, or simply take it as obvious. But the bad-difference view is a characterization of disability which is not obvious to many disabled people. And relying on brute intuition can offer little in the way of dialogue for those who simply don't share the intuition (and who might be skeptical that the intuitions of the majority offer particularly good insight into the well-being of the minority). The causation-based objections are an attempt to do better – to get some independent traction on the mere-difference/bad-difference debate. They try to show that the mere-difference view has implausible, impermissible consequences, even by the lights of its defenders. In what follows, I argue that these causation-based objections do not succeed: they do not in fact give this sort of independent traction on the mere-difference/bad-difference debate.

In order to make this argument, I am going to proceed on the assumption that disability is, in relevant respects, analogous to features like sexuality, gender, and race. That is, I am going to assume that being disabled is relevantly similar to other features we standardly treat as mere-difference features. I'm not going to argue for this assumption. And that's because the objection I am opposing takes the form of a conditional: *if* disability is mere-difference, *then* it is permissible to cause disability (and likewise impermissible to remove or prevent disability). I am arguing that this inference is mistaken: it is not the case that if disability is mere-difference we can thereby infer that it is permissible to cause disability. To make this point, I consider other features which we standardly consider mere-differences – being gay, being female, and so on – and consider what we say about causation in those cases. I argue that in general the inference from "*x* is mere-difference" to "causing *x* is permissible" isn't one we accept, and thus that we shouldn't accept the inference from "disability is mere-difference" to "causing disability is permissible."

III   Causing a Nondisabled Person to Become Disabled

There are many different ways one can cause disability. In what follows, I certainly don't take myself to be giving an exhaustive account of causing disability; but I think the cases I consider are illustrative more generally of the kinds of things mere-difference views can say about causing disability. For some cases, treating disability as mere-difference rather than bad-difference does not entail the permissibility of causing disability. For other cases, it plausibly does allow such permissions, but in ways which are unobjectionable. Either way, the issue of causing disability is not one which undermines mere-difference views.

Let's begin by considering perhaps the most straightforward case of causing disability: an autonomous adult causes another autonomous adult to become disabled. That is what happens in this case:

Light Show: Amy and her nondisabled friend Ben work in a lab. After hours one day, they are playing around with lasers. Ben is not wearing any protective eyewear, and Amy knows that if she directs the laser beam at his eyes he is at risk of permanent vision loss. Nevertheless,

Amy does not take any precautions to avoid directing the beam at Ben's eyes. Ben becomes permanently blind. When Ben confronts Amy angrily about what she has done, Amy explains that she hasn't done anything wrong. It's not any worse to be disabled than to be nondisabled. So while she has made Ben a minority with respect to sight, she hasn't made him any worse off.

In response to this case, I'll wager that most of us share the following two reactions:

i. Amy has done something wrong or blameworthy (and perhaps more strongly, she has wronged Ben).
ii. Amy's reaction to Ben's anger is problematic/ confused/misguided/etc.

Moreover, many of us would persist in these reactions regardless of how Ben ultimately reacts to his disability. Even if Ben becomes a happy, well-adjusted disabled person who is proud of his blindness, Amy's conduct still seems bad.

Does the view that disability is mere-difference rather than bad-difference have a problem justifying reactions (i) and (ii), or their persistence in the face of positive adaptation? No. And it is easy to see why not.

The first and most obvious thing to say about a case like Light Show is simply that it involves unjustified interference in another person's life. Most of us think you shouldn't go around making substantial changes to people's lives without their consent (even if those changes don't, on balance, make them worse off). We'd be inclined to say that Amy does something wrong if she carelessly (and permanently) turns Ben's hair from brown to blond, if she carelessly (and permanently) changes Ben's height by a few inches, and so forth. Such changes aren't particularly substantial and aren't likely to make Ben worse off in the long run. But we have a basic reaction that Amy shouldn't alter Ben in any of these ways without his consent – regardless of the overall effect of such alterations on Ben's well-being. Amy just shouldn't mess with people like that.

But for those who don't find this sort of noninterference principle compelling, the defender of the mere-difference view can address Amy's treatment of Ben more specifically, and perhaps more strongly. First, Amy's action is risky. Ben may well end up a flourishing disabled person. But he may not (many people adapt very well to disability, but not everyone does).[8] And Amy isn't in a position to know which will happen. But suppose that Amy were in a position to know – suppose she has a crystal ball that tells her that Ben will adapt very well to disability. Most of us would still be inclined to say that Amy has done something wrong. That is, Amy does something wrong regardless of whether Ben winds up adapting well to his disability and regardless of what she knows about his ability to so adapt.

The mere-difference view can accommodate this. Advocates of the mere-difference view think that being disabled is not, by itself, a harm. But there's a big difference between being disabled and becoming disabled. Many people find being disabled a rewarding and good thing. But there is an almost universal experience for those who acquire disability – variously called adaptive process or transitions costs – of great pain and difficulty associated with becoming disabled. However happy and well-adjusted a disabled person ends up, the process of becoming disabled is almost universally a difficult one.

The advocate of mere-difference can appeal to transition costs to explain why Amy's reaction to Ben's disability is misguided – and, indeed, why Amy has done something wrong and harmful to Ben.[9] Let's assume that Ben is a perfectly happy, well-adjusted nondisabled person. If Amy is careful with her laser beam, Ben will continue his happy, well-adjusted life without incident or interruption. If Amy is careless with her laser beam, Ben's happiness, his lifestyle, and perhaps even his self-conception will be radically, drastically interrupted. He will have to reshape his life around his new disability. If Ben is like most people, this will be a deeply painful process. It may be a deeply painful process that ends with Ben as a perfectly happy, well-adjusted disabled person. But even if Ben adapts perfectly well to his blindness, he can justifiably say that what Amy did was wrong. Amy – carelessly, thoughtlessly – caused him great pain. On most any theory of morality, that's wrong.

So it simply does not follow from holding a mere-difference view that it is permissible to cause someone to become disabled in a case like Amy and Ben's. Even if being disabled is not a harm, becoming disabled is still a difficult and painful process – a process that the mere-difference view can happily say is wrong to inflict on someone against their will.[10]

IV   Causing a Nondisabled Person to Become Disabled Without Transition Costs

Not all cases of causing disability, however, are like Light Show. It is possible to cause someone to become disabled without any associated transition costs. The most obvious such case is where the person who becomes disabled is an infant (or even a fetus, if you think there's personal identity between a late-stage fetus and the child it becomes). Consider this case:

> **Disabled Baby:** Cara has a six-month-old baby, Daisy. Cara values disability and thinks that disability is an important part of human diversity. Moreover, she thinks that increasing the number of happy, well-adjusted, well-educated disabled people is an important part of combating ableism (and has a justified belief that any child she raises has a good chance of ending up happy, well adjusted, and well educated). With all this in mind Cara has Daisy undergo an innovative new pro-disability procedure. Daisy doesn't endure any pain from this, and she won't remember it. But as a result, Daisy will be disabled for the rest of her life.

Just as in Light Show, most people will judge that Cara has done something wrong. And more specifically, they will judge that she has wronged Daisy. But here the wrongness can't be explained by transition costs. Daisy won't suffer a painful transition as she adjusts to disability, because all her formative experiences will include her disability.

Again, the mere-difference view has no difficulty accommodating this. And again, the easiest way to see this is to consider relevant analogies. Suppose, for the sake of argument, a strong biological view of sexuality according to which sexuality is wholly or largely determined by genetics. Further suppose that a procedure was developed which allowed us to alter the genes that determine sexuality in an infant. Now replace disability in the case above with sexuality:

Baby Genes: Cara values gayness, and thinks that gayness is an important part of human diversity, Moreover, she thinks that increasing the number of happy, well-adjusted, well-educated gay people is an important part of combating homophobia (and she has a justified belief that any child she raises has a good chance of ending up happy, well adjusted, and well educated). With all this in mind Cara puts Daisy through a gene-alteration program. Daisy doesn't endure much pain from this, and she won't remember it. But as a result, Daisy will grow up to self-identify as gay rather than straight.

Most of us, I think, would be inclined to say that Cara does something wrong – that she shouldn't put Daisy through such a procedure. Moreover, we don't think that we're thereby committed to saying it is worse to be gay than to be straight. (It might be equally wrong for Cara to alter Daisy's genes such that Daisy grows up straight rather than gay.) And the same holds if we replace sexuality with sex – even if it were possibly to painlessly and harmlessly perform a sex-alteration procedure on an infant, I suspect most of us would think this is something we shouldn't do – not because one sex is superior to the other, but simply because we're uncomfortable with the idea of making such drastic changes to a child's life.

We again seem guided, in such cases, by strong noninterference principles. Ceteris paribus, we tend to think you should refrain from drastically altering a child's physical development. (Perhaps this is just an instance of a wider phenomenon – just as, in Light Show, we tend to think you should refrain from drastically altering a person's body without their consent.) Our reaction to Disabled Baby can be justified by (and explained as a species of) these noninterference principles, rather than anything specific to disability.

It is difficult, of course, to say what these sorts of noninterference principles amount to. We think it is perfectly permissible – indeed, we think it is morally required – for parents to interfere with their children's development, including their physical development. Parents make choices about education, diet, health care – all sorts of things that have a dramatic effect on a child's development. And we think that they're perfectly justified in doing so. Indeed, parenthood can seem like one long series of interferences. So perhaps our noninterference judgments in cases like Baby Genes are simply unprincipled. Or perhaps, more sympathetically, our noninterference judgments are tracking something like a distinction between traits which are identity-determining[11] and those which are not. To choose where your child goes to school, what they eat, where they live, and so on is to make decisions about how that person grows up. But to choose to make your straight child gay or your male child female is to, in a sense, make it the case that your child grows up to be a different person than they would otherwise have been. And it may be that we find the former sort of interferences acceptable, but not the latter.[12]

Let me be clear: I am not attempting to give an account of what these noninterference judgments are, nor am I arguing that they are justified. What I am arguing is that, absent further argument, commitment to the impermissibility of causing feature x doesn't by itself entail – or even suggest – that x is somehow bad or suboptimal. And it doesn't entail – or even suggest – this even in the absence of transition costs. There are plenty of cases in which we think it's impermissible to cause some feature x in another person (even a baby, even your own baby), although we by no means think it is suboptimal to be x. We think that causing another person (even a baby, even your own baby) to be x would somehow amount to unjustified interference. Whether or not we're right about this, and whatever such noninterference principles ultimately consist in, the distance between thinking some feature x is a perfectly good way to be and thinking it is permissible to cause another person (even a baby, even your own baby) to be x is enough to show that there's no obvious entailment from a mere-difference view of disability to the permissibility of causing another person (even a baby, even your own baby) to be disabled.

But the advocate of the bad-difference can try to press a disanalogy here. It is wrong for Cara to cause her nondisabled infant to become disabled. But suppose the case was reversed, and Daisy was born disabled:

> **Reverse Disabled Baby:** Cara has a six-month-old baby, Daisy, who is disabled. Cara values Daisy's happiness and well-being. Moreover, she thinks that Daisy will have a better chance of being happy, well adjusted, and well educated if she is nondisabled. With all this in mind Cara puts Daisy through a radical new treatment for infant disability. Daisy doesn't endure much pain from this, and she won't remember it. But as a result, Daisy will grow up nondisabled.

Most of us would think that Cara does something good in this case. It would not be wrong, most people assume, for Cara to cause Daisy to become nondisabled. (It might even be morally obligatory.) That there is such a discrepancy supports a bad-difference view of disability, rather than a mere-difference view.[13]

In response to this proposed disanalogy, two main lines of response are open to the defender of the mere-difference view: she can agree that there is such a discrepancy between cases of causing disability and causing nondisability but argue that this discrepancy does not undermine the mere-difference view; or she can deny that there is any such discrepancy and try to explain away intuitions to the contrary. I'll explain the former response, because I think it is important to note that adopting a mere-difference view of disability does not entail a specific stance on the cause/remove discrepancy. But I ultimately think this milder response doesn't work. The defender of a mere-difference view, I'll argue, should maintain that Disabled Baby and Reverse Disabled Baby are on a par.

Suppose that the defender of a mere-difference view wanted to preserve a discrepancy between causing disability in an infant and causing nondisability

in an infant – with the latter permissible but the former impermissible. How might such a discrepancy be maintained if disability is no worse than nondisability? To address this puzzle, the advocate of the mere-difference view can appeal to the idea of potential risk.

If Cara causes Daisy to be disabled, Daisy may well grow up to be a happy, well-adjusted disabled person. But she may not. She may resent her disability, wish to be nondisabled, and be unhappy as a result. Conversely, if Cara causes Daisy to be nondisabled, Daisy is unlikely to grow up resenting her lack of disability or wishing to be disabled. And if Cara refrains from causing Daisy to be nondisabled, Daisy may well resent that choice. Causing Daisy to be disabled is riskier than causing Daisy to be nondisabled (though, again, we can't assume a priori that causing Daisy to be nondisabled is without risk – see note 8).[14]

The thinking here is simple. Suppose that the disability in question is blindness. It is unlikely that Daisy, if she grows up sighted, will be frustrated by her sight and wish to be blind. It is not unlikely that Daisy, if she grows up blind, will be frustrated by her blindness and wish to be sighted. Many blind people are perfectly happy with their blindness, but not all of them are. Sight is much less likely to make Daisy unhappy than blindness.[15] And so on, mutatis mutandis, for other, relevantly similar examples of disability. It is hard to think of a disability that – given the way the world is now – is more likely to have a positive effect on a person's well-being than is the absence of that disability.

But it can't be quite that simple. Being gay is a greater risk to well-being than being straight. There are more people who regret being gay or suffer from being gay than (at least consciously) regret or suffer from being straight.[16] But again, consider the case in which we can alter a child's sexuality:

> **Reverse Baby Genes:** Cara has a six-month-old baby, Daisy, who will grow up to self-identify as gay. Cara values Daisy's happiness and well-being. Moreover, she thinks that Daisy will have a better chance of being happy, well adjusted, and well educated if she is straight. With all this in mind Cara puts Daisy through a radical

new gene therapy program. Daisy doesn't endure much pain from this, and she won't remember it. But as a result, Daisy will grow up to self-identify as straight.

Most of us would balk at the idea that it is permissible to change a child in this way. (Indeed, making such a change strikes many of us as homophobic.)[17] We tend to think such alteration is impermissible, regardless of whether being gay is in some sense riskier than being straight.

Perhaps the mere-difference view of disability can press a disanalogy here. Perhaps it would be wrong to cause a child to become straight (instead of gay) because such an action would always communicate homophobia. But in the relevantly similar case of causing someone to be nondisabled, you might argue that the action doesn't always communicate ableism – though the explanation of why it doesn't communicate ableism would need to be spelled out.[18]

Or perhaps the issue is one of degree of risk. Any gay person will have to deal with homophobia, and any disabled person will have to deal with ableism. But the parents of a gay child can make proactive efforts to mediate the bad effects of homophobia. They can make choices about what they say, where they live, where they send their child to school, and so on – to make sure their children grow up in an environment that is as gay friendly as possible. The parents of a disabled child can make similar efforts, of course. But it's not clear that those efforts can have as much effect – since in the case of disabilities the issues facing their child will be access to basic services and navigation of basic social interaction.[19] Our society is very unaccepting of disabled people.[20] And there is a limited amount that individual parents can do to mediate this. They can tell their child that she's valued just the way she is, but they can't make buildings accessible and they can't make people less awkward around her.

So perhaps there's a case to be made that, given the way the world currently is, it is in many cases riskier to have a disabled child than to have a gay child – at least in some contexts and environments. And that elevated risk is why there's a discrepancy between Disabled Baby and Reverse Disabled Baby, whereas

there's no such discrepancy between Baby Genes and Reverse Baby Genes. Such discrepancies, however, are highly contingent and circumstantial. If we lived in a society that was more accommodating and accepting of disabled people, the discrepancy could easily disappear.[21] Likewise, if we lived in a society where gay people were even more heavily discriminated against (as they are in some eastern European and African countries, for example) a similar discrepancy might be created.

I present the above line of thought as an avenue that could be explored by the defender of a mere-difference view who wants to maintain that there is a discrepancy between Disabled Baby and Reverse Disabled Baby, but I ultimately don't think it's what a defender of a mere-difference view should say. I worry that comparing the amount and severity of risk (and thus, by proxy, the amount and severity of prejudice) is a shaky foundation on which to motivate a discrepancy between Disabled Baby and Reverse Disabled Baby. It would be difficult to say how much of a difference in risk would be enough difference to motivate such discrepancy. And, more importantly, it would be difficult – and deeply problematic – to argue that one minority (disabled people) are somehow more disadvantaged than another (gay people).

I think the defender of a mere-difference view should instead say that, in fact, there is no discrepancy between the cases of causing an infant to be disabled and causing an infant to be nondisabled. Disabled Baby and Reverse Disabled Baby are on a par. This response is not entailed by commitment to a mere-difference view – as the availability of the above line of response shows. But I think it is both more plausible and less extreme than it may appear on the surface.

In order to argue this point, the mere-difference advocate needs to say – contra the response just discussed – that the potential risk associated with disability isn't enough to warrant interfering with the development of a child who would otherwise be disabled in order to make them nondisabled. That is, if noninterference principles are a good guide to action in the case of causing disability, they should likewise be a good guide to action in the case of causing nondisability. (The general issue of causing vs. curing will be discussed further in Sec. VI.)

We wouldn't want to cause a child who would otherwise grow up to be gay to instead grow up to be straight (as in Reverse Baby Genes). Doing so would be unjustified interference and could reasonably be said to communicate homophobia. That the child is more likely to regret being gay than being straight and more likely to suffer from being gay than from being straight doesn't affect this. Likewise, we shouldn't cause a child who would otherwise grow up to be disabled to instead grow up to be nondisabled. Doing so would be unjustified interference and could reasonably be said to communicate ableism. That the child is more likely to regret being disabled than being nondisabled and more likely to suffer from being disabled than being nondisabled doesn't affect this.

A similar, real-world case is that of children who are born intersex. Standard procedure is to perform binary-sex-assignment operations on these children when they are very young (procedures which are often invasive, painful, and have long-term side effects). The justification is that the best outcomes for such procedures require them to be performed on infants and young children – so if the procedures aren't done when the children are very young, those children might grow up to regret the lost opportunity for "normal" sex characteristics or sex assignments. And that's no doubt true – many people probably would regret it if the procedures weren't performed. Yet there are a growing minority who feel that they were wronged by having been subjected to these procedures without consent. They strongly identify as intersex and feel that their sex characteristics have been unacceptably interfered with. They argue that we should change society's assumptions about sex binaries (and the relationship between sex and gender) rather than changing children who are born intersex.[22]

If she takes this line of response, the advocate of the mere-difference view takes a position that conflicts with common intuitions about such cases (and with common practice). Is this conflict a problem for the mere-difference view? No – it's exactly what should be expected if (as most defenders of the mere-difference view contend) much of our reasoning about disability is clouded by implicit ableism and a poor understanding of the lives of disabled people. That is, if much of the way we think about disability is shaped by ableism, then simply using intuition as a guide to cases like Reverse Disabled Baby is a bad methodology. If "common sense" is affected by ableist bias, then we should expect that our intuitions aren't a particularly good guide to thinking about disability. And we should likewise expect that the mere-difference view will be committed to things that most will find counterintuitive. This point is a simple and familiar one: the intuitions of the (privileged) majority don't have a particularly good track record as reliable guides to how we should think about the minority, especially when the minority is a victim of stigma and prejudice. Just consider how common it was, historically, to find it intuitive that homosexuality was some sort of perversion or aberration, to find it intuitive that nonwhite races were innately inferior, to find it intuitive that women were less rational than men. The mere-difference view claims that what most people find to be "common sense" or intuitive about disability (some version of a bad-difference view) is incorrect. We should thus expect such a view to challenge the received wisdom about disability and to make some claims that most people find "counterintuitive." That doesn't mean that the mere-difference view is utterly unconstrained. When its commitments are counterintuitive, it needs to be able to show how those commitments are nevertheless principled and consistent. Conflict with standard intuition in cases like Reverse Disabled Baby isn't a problem for the mere-difference view, so long as it is a principled and explicable conflict. And I think the analogy to relevantly similar cases shows that it is both.[23]

Insistence on a cause/remove discrepancy is doubtless motivated by the simple fact that most people assume that it is worse, ceteris paribus, to be disabled than to be nondisabled. But the mere-difference view rejects this assumption outright. What more can be said, then, to support the claim that there is obviously a cause/remove discrepancy? Perhaps the discrepancy has to do with available options. In Disabled Baby,

Daisy's options are permanently restricted. Again, suppose the disability in question is blindness. If Daisy is blind, she will never be able to see colors, experience visual art, visually perceive the faces of her loved ones, and so forth. There are goods and experiences that being blind permanently prevents Daisy from participating in. But, mutatis mutandis, there are goods and experiences that Daisy will permanently miss out on in Reverse Disabled Baby. She will never have the auditory or sensory experiences unique to those who have been blind from infancy.[24]

The mundane point here is that lack of interference constrains options, just as interference does. Everyone is constrained by the way their bodies work. If you're biologically male, you can't become pregnant. Most of us will agree that being able to grow a new person inside your body is an impressive ability – and it is one that you miss out on if you lack female reproductive organs. But suppose it was possible – as it may someday be – to change a child's sex in infancy. It wouldn't follow that someone wrongs a male baby – in virtue of constraining its options – if they fail to perform a sex reassignment operation on it when it is a baby. Similarly, it doesn't follow from the fact that disabilities constrain options that it is wrong not to remove disabilities. Being nondisabled also constrains options. (Indeed, having a physical body that is in any specific way a body can constrain options.) It is simply that being nondisabled constrains options in a way we're more comfortable and familiar with. To support the claim that there's an obvious cause/remove discrepancy, you'd need the further claim that the constraints imposed by disability are somehow worse than those imposed by nondisability. And that's precisely the claim that the mere-difference view rejects.

V Causing a Disabled Person to Exist Instead of a Nondisabled Person

Perhaps the most familiar discussion of causing disability in the literature, however, is not a case in which a single person is caused to become disabled, but rather a case in which a disabled person is caused to exist instead of (in some sense) a nondisabled person. This is, for example, the structure of Derek Parfit's famous "handicapped child" case:[25]

Child Now: A woman, Ellen, knows that if she becomes pregnant now the child she conceives will be born disabled. If she waits six months to become pregnant, however, the child she conceives will be born nondisabled. Ellen prefers not to wait, so she becomes pregnant right away. She gives birth to a daughter, Franny, who is disabled.

Parfit's case is meant to be a puzzle for person-affecting ethics. The starting assumption is that Ellen does something wrong by choosing to get pregnant now, but there is no one such that Ellen does something wrong to that person. (She doesn't do something wrong to Franny, because Franny is better off existing than not existing, and had Ellen waited six months to conceive she would – presumably – have had a different child.)

The worry is that the mere-difference view cannot get the puzzle off the ground in the first place. It is supposed to be wrong for Ellen to choose to have a disabled child – that is, to cause a disabled person to exist rather than a nondisabled person to exist, when she could easily have done the reverse. But if being disabled is no worse than being non-disabled – if it is mere-difference rather than bad-difference – then why should we think Ellen's action is wrong?

We shouldn't. If disability is a mere-difference and not a bad-difference, then we should reject the background assumption meant to guide our intuitions in cases like Child Now. It isn't wrong to knowingly cause a disabled child to exist rather than a nondisabled child to exist.[26]

Does this commitment pose a problem for the mere-difference view? No – at least not any sort of additional problem not already present in the view itself. The idea that it is wrong to cause a disabled person to exist rather than a nondisabled person to exist is predicated on the idea that it is worse to be disabled than nondisabled. This is something that the mere-difference view explicitly rejects. So it is certainly no argument against the mere-difference view that they cannot vindicate the intuition that Child Now is a case of wrongdoing, given that this intuition relies on the falsity of the mere-difference view.

But perhaps the intuitive reaction to Child Now can be strengthened. McMahan gives this amplified version as part of his argument that the mere-difference view licenses unacceptable permissions:

The Aphrodisiac: Suppose there is a drug that has a complex set of effects. It is an aphrodisiac that enhances a woman's pleasure during sexual intercourse. But it also increases fertility by inducing ovulation. If ovulation has recently occurred naturally, this drug causes the destruction of the egg that is present in one of the fallopian tubes but also causes a new and different egg to be released from the ovaries. In addition, however, it has a very high probability of damaging the new egg in a way that will cause any child conceived through the fertilization of that egg to be disabled. The disability caused by the drug is not so bad as to make life not worth living, but it is a disability that many potential parents seek to avoid through screening. Suppose that a woman takes this drug primarily to increase her pleasure – if it were not for this, she would not take it – but also with the thought that it may increase the probability of conception; for she wants to have a child. She is aware that the drug is likely to cause her to have a disabled child, but she is eager for pleasure and reflects that, while there would be disadvantages to having a disabled child, these might be compensated for by the special bonds that might be forged by the child's greater dependency. She has in fact just ovulated naturally, so the drug destroys and replaces the egg that was already present but also damages the new egg, thereby causing the child she conceives to be disabled.[27]

Intuitions that there is wrongdoing in cases like Aphrodisiac are arguably stronger than those in the basic Parfit-style cases. As McMahan says, "most of us think that this woman's action is morally wrong. It is wrong to cause the existence of a disabled child rather than a normal child in order to enhance one's own sexual pleasure."

Do cases like Aphrodisiac pose a problem for the mere-difference view? Before proceeding further, it is worth noting that when we're considering the merits of the mere-difference view, our intuitions about a case like Aphrodisiac may not be the best place to start. Aphrodisiac involves, as its central elements, both the actions of a potential mother and female sexual pleasure. It is not too much of a stretch to think that our reactions to such a case might not be guided by the light of pure moral reason alone.

That being said, there may well cases like Aphrodisiac that involve wrongdoing. But that doesn't mean that they involve wrongdoing simply because they involve causing a disabled rather than a nondisabled person to exist. Perhaps it is wrong to "cause the existence of a disabled child rather than a normal child in *order to enhance one's own sexual pleasure*" (my italics). More plausibly, it may well be wrong to cause the existence of a disabled child in order to make yourself seem more interesting, to claim social benefits, and so on. It can, familiarly, be wrong to do x for reason Φ, even if it is not wrong to do x simpliciter. More generally, the mere-difference view maintains that disability itself isn't a bad thing; but that's compatible with many of the things which can cause disability being bad things. Malnutrition is a bad thing. War is a bad thing. Car crashes are bad things. A positive take on disability doesn't in any way involve a positive take on all the ways we can cause disability.

If the defender of the mere-difference view wants to agree that the woman in Aphrodisiac does something wrong, she can. And she can do so without committing herself to the claim that it is wrong to cause a disabled person to exist when one could easily have caused a nondisabled person to exist instead. Perhaps Aphrodisiac shows an unacceptable casualness about reproductive decisions or implies that the mother undervalues the extent to which being disabled will make her child's life harder, even if it does not automatically make it worse. And so on. There's no entailment from the general permissibility of causing a disabled person to exist to the permissibility of any and all instances of causing a disabled person to exist.

In Child Now, the advocate of a mere-difference view of disability should simply resist the idea that there is any wrongdoing. It is not wrong to cause a disabled rather than a nondisabled person to exist. The intuitive reaction that there is wrongdoing in Child Now can be strengthened, but the ways in which it can be strengthened introduce a lot of noise. In these amped-up versions of the basic case – like Aphrodisiac – we can say that there is wrongdoing without claiming that there is wrongdoing in virtue of causing a disabled person rather than a nondisabled person to exist.

VI Causing and "Curing"

Here is a line of thought that may look tempting at this point. Let's abstract away from actions aimed at individuals and simply consider the case of finding a prevention (a "cure," to use the value-laden term) for a given disability. It is a good thing, most people would say, to "cure" disability. This makes disability importantly different from features like sexuality. It would not be a good thing to "cure" minority sexualities. This undermines both the tenability of the mere-difference view and the type of argument that proponents of the mere-difference view tend to use in its defense.

If a scientist is working hard to develop a "cure" for blindness, we say she is doing something good and praiseworthy. We give her grant money and government support. We hope she succeeds. But if a scientist is working hard on a "cure" for gayness, we think she is doing something dystopian and horrible. We shun her from the academic community and take away her support infrastructure. We hope she fails miserably.

This discrepancy arises because we think it is a good thing to cause someone to be nondisabled. We think that we should work toward the ability to cause non-disability. In contrast, it is not a good thing to cause someone to alter their sexuality. We shouldn't work toward the ability to cause changes in sexuality. But if this is the case, then there is a fundamental difference between causing changes to a person's disability status and causing changes to a person's sexuality. And any such fundamental difference undermines the plausibility of the mere-difference view.

But why do we think it's a bad thing to develop "cures" for homosexuality? Perhaps our reaction is in part again due to noninterference principles – we shouldn't alter the sexuality that a person "naturally" has (whatever that means). But I suspect that most, if not all, of our aversion comes from the bad effects we assume would go along – quite contingently – with the development of any such "cure."

The very language of "cure" is, of course, pejorative – it implies a change for the better. But let's assume that what's being researched is simply a drug that can alter sexuality. That is, imagine that scientists are developing a drug that can change gay people into straight people and straight people into gay people. Most of us would, I'll wager, think that this is a bad idea. And that's simply because we can easily imagine what would happen if such a drug were available. Young gay people would be pressured, even coerced, into taking the drug by prejudiced parents. Gay people from prejudiced backgrounds could simply take the drug and become straight, rather than learning to accept their sexuality. There would be immense social pressure, at least in many communities, for anyone who self-identified as gay to "cure themselves." In a situation where either the majority can change to accommodate the minority, or the minority can change to be like the majority, the minority isn't likely to fare very well.

But these consequences are only contingently associated with a drug that alters sexuality. It's not that there's anything intrinsically wrong with such a drug – it's that given the way our world actually is, with all its prejudices and social pressure toward conformity, such a drug would in fact have bad consequences. But the same drug wouldn't have bad consequences in a world that was fully accepting of gay people. In fact, insofar as choice and self-determination are to be valued, it could easily be said to have good consequences. It might be nice for people to be able to determine their own sexuality as they saw fit (and even change back and forth, as desired). The drug only has bad effects when it can be used as a way of undermining gay rights and depopulating the gay community.

Likewise, insofar as choice and self-determination are good things, it's good for people to be able to determine their own physicality. And so there's nothing intrinsically wrong with "cures" for disability – at least if they are understood nonpejoratively simply as a mechanism for causing nondisability. The mere-difference view doesn't maintain that everyone who is disabled likes being disabled. And it is perfectly compatible with the mere-difference view that, even in an ableism-free society, some disabled people would still want to be nondisabled. There's nothing wrong with – and much that's good about – a mechanism that allows such disabled people to become nondisabled if they wish (and allows, vice versa, nondisabled people to become disabled if they wish).[28]

But we should worry about what effects a concerted effort to develop such "cures" for disability will have in the actual, ableist world. There's nothing wrong with disabled people wanting to be nondisabled. And there's nothing wrong with those disabled people who want to be nondisabled seeking the means to make themselves nondisabled. But there is something wrong with the expectation that becoming nondisabled is the ultimate hope in the lives of disabled people and their families. Such an expectation makes it harder for disabled people – who in other circumstances might be perfectly happy with their disability – to accept what their bodies are like, and it makes it less likely that society's ableism will change. It is hard to accept and be happy with a disabled body if the expectation is that you should wish, hope, and strive for some mechanism to turn that disabled body into a nondisabled body. And it is unlikely that society will change its norms to accommodate disability if society can instead change disabled people in a way that conforms them to its extant norms.

As an example, the documentary *The Kids Are All Right* – about people with muscular dystrophy who were featured as "Jerry's Kids" in the famous annual Jerry Lewis telethon, only to grow up to become protesters against the telethon – highlights exactly these problems. Many of the people with muscular dystrophy profiled in the film strongly object to the relentless focus on "the cure" that was a feature of the yearly telethon and are frustrated at how much of the money brought in by the Muscular Dystrophy Association is spent researching these magical "cures." It's not that they object to the existence of – or the search for – treatments which remove or prevent disability. It's rather that they think that focus on such treatments is distracting and unhelpful. What they want are things like: research on how to extend the life span of persons with Duchenne Muscular Dystrophy, better wheelchair technology, focus on helping people with muscular dystrophy find accessible jobs, more public awareness about accessibility, and so forth. These issues – far more than treatments which could make them nondisabled, they argue – are what matter to the day-to-day lives of people like themselves. Research "for a cure" doesn't help them, and pronounced focus on such research further stigmatizes them (by communicating the assumption that "a cure" is something they want or need).

Laura Hershey, a former "Jerry's Kid," addresses the same issues in her now-famous article "From Poster Child to Protestor."[29] Hershey objects to the massive amount of funding and research devoted to "finding the cure" for her disability (rather than in developing assistive technology or helping disabled people find employment, for example). The "search for the cure," she argues, is both practically and ideologically problematic. She writes:

> I've encountered people who, never having tried it, think that living life with a disability is an endless hardship. For many of us, it's actually quite interesting, though not without its problems. And the majority of those problems result from the barriers, both physical and attitudinal, which surround us, or from the lack of decent support services. These are things that can be changed, but only if we as a society recognize them for what they are. We'll never recognize them if we stay so focused on curing individuals of disability, rather than making changes to accommodate disability into our culture.

She continues:

> Sure, some people with muscular dystrophy do hope and dream of that day when the cure is finally found. As people with disabilities, we're conditioned just like everyone else to believe that disability is our problem. . . . When so many of us feel so negative about our disabilities and our needs, it's difficult to develop a political agenda to get our basic needs met. The cure is a simple, magical, non-political solution to all the problems in a disabled person's life. That's why it's so appealing, and so disempowering. The other solutions we have to work for, even fight for; we only have to dream about the cure.
>
> To draw a parallel, when I was a child and first learned about racial discrimination, I thought it would be great if people could all be one color so we wouldn't have problems like prejudice. What color did I envision for this one-color world? White, of course, because I'm white. I didn't bear black people any malice. I just thought they'd be happier, would suffer less, if they were more like me.

There may in fact be a discrepancy between how we view attempts to remove or eliminate disability and attempts to remove or eliminate gayness. But it is not obvious that there should be any stark discrepancy between the cases. Does this mean that the defender of a mere difference is committed to thinking that large swaths of medical research are morally corrupt? No. Much disability-related medical research aims to make life easier for disabled people – not to turn disabled people into nondisabled people. And, again, there's nothing wrong per se with research that aims to allow disabled people to become nondisabled. The point is simply that it is complicated. Given the way the world actually is, such research isn't the obvious and unequivocal good that many take it to be. Nor should it be looked to as the ultimate dream and wish of disabled people and their families, or the ultimate solution to the problems faced by disabled people.

VII Conclusion

I have argued that mere-difference views of disability do not license the permissibility of causing disability

(and conversely, the impermissibility of removing disability) in any way that undermines the tenability of the mere-difference position. In some cases of causing disability, the mere-difference view can agree that causing disability is impermissible. In other cases, the mere-difference view can say that causing disability is permissible – but unproblematically so. And likewise, mutatis mutandis, for causing nondisability. There is no direct route from adoption of a mere-difference view of disability to objectionable (im)permissibilities.

Notably, though, the explanation for why at least some cases of causing disability are impermissible is interestingly different for mere-difference views than it is for bad-difference views. A defender of a mere-difference view can easily say that many cases of causing disability are impermissible. But it is never the case that causing a nondisabled person to be disabled is wrong simpliciter. That is, many cases of causing disability are wrong, but they aren't wrong in virtue of the causing of disability. They are, rather, wrong for reasons separable from disability in particular: they involve unjustified interference or unjustified risk taking, for example. And I suspect it is this point that may be causing a lot of the confusion about what, exactly, mere-difference views are committed to. They can't say that a case of causing disability is wrong in virtue of the fact that the action causes disability – whereas bad-difference views can. But that by itself doesn't generate permission to go around causing disability. Lots of standard cases of causing disability can be wrong, according to mere-difference views, without being wrong in virtue of causing disability.

The most important thing to emphasize, in closing, is this. These causation-based arguments are intended to strengthen the case against the mere-difference view and to provide evidence in favor of the bad-difference view. They cannot do this. The various cases of causing disability – and the diverging viewpoints given by mere-difference and bad-difference views on these cases – give us no independent traction on the question of whether disability is a mere difference or a bad difference.

Notes

1 If you accept a terminological distinction between "disability" and "impairment," with "disability" referring to the socially mediated effects of impairments, then you should reinterpret what follows as talk of causing impairments.

2 For a much more detailed discussion of this distinction, see Elizabeth Barnes, *The Minority Body* (Oxford: Oxford University Press, 2016).

3 Furthermore, it doesn't seem like the mere-difference view can only allow that disabilities involve the absence of some intrinsic goods if the lack of those goods is somehow "compensated for" by other, disability-specific goods. Consider a different case. We might think that the ability to be pregnant and give birth – to grow a new person in your own body – is an intrinsic good, at least insofar as any ability is an intrinsic good. People who are biologically male lack this ability. Nor is there any obvious man-specific ability we can point to which compensates men for this lack. But we don't tend to think that people who are biologically male are automatically worse off than people who are biologically female, simply because they lack an ability we might count as an intrinsic good.

4 Again, just because they often do support this characterization of the bad-difference view doesn't mean that they have to. Nor is commitment to a mere-difference view in any way commitment to a rejection of objective list theories of well-being. It's perfectly consistent for an objective list view of well-being to simply leave out nondisability from their list of things which are objectively good for you. Likewise, it's perfectly consistent for them to maintain that disability always incurs a loss of some objective good but can also create opportunities for experiencing other, different objective goods.

5 For those not happy with (ii), some of these issues with (iii) could be addressed by adding everyone's favorite counterexample avoider: a ceteris paribus clause.

6 Jeff McMahan, "Causing Disabled People to Exist and Causing People to Be Disabled," *Ethics* 116 (2005): 77–99; John Harris, "One Principle and Three Fallacies of Disability Studies," *Journal of Medical Ethics* 27 (2001): 383–7; Guy Kahane, "Non-identity, Self-Defeat, and Attitudes to Future Children," *Philosophical Studies* 145 (2009): 193–214; Peter Singer, "Ethics and Disability: A Response to Koch," *Journal of Disability Policy Studies* 16 (2001): 130–3.

7 See, especially, Allan Buchanan, Dan W. Brock, Norman Daniels, and Daniel Winkler, *From Chance to Choice: Genetics and Justice* (Cambridge: Cambridge University Press, 2000).

8 It is worth pointing out that this is the same for removing disability: many people adapt well to the removal of disability, but not everyone does. Jonathan Glover discusses the case of S.B., a man who had been blind from infancy but then had his vision restored by a surgical procedure. S.B. fell into a deep depression after his blindness was removed and died less than two years after his operation. Jonathan Glover, *Choosing Children* (Oxford: Oxford University Press, 2006), 19–23.

9 Similar points will allow the mere-difference view to uphold the idea that becoming disabled is a misfortune and a harm, even if being disabled is – by itself – neither.

10 See, for example, McMahan, "Causing Disabled People to Exist and Causing People to Be Disabled."

11 In the looser sense of "identity" (traits that determine self-conception) rather than in the stricter sense of "identity" (traits that determine numerical identity).

12 If this is the case, then to make the analogy to gayness or femaleness the mere-difference view would need to maintain that disability is similarly identity determining. But this tends to be what advocates of the mere-difference view think in any case.

13 Versions of this argument are explored in, for example, S. D. Edwards, "Disability, Identity, and the 'Expressivist' Objection," *Journal of Medical Ethics* 30 (2004): 418–20; Elizabeth Harman, "'I'll Be Glad I Did It' Reasoning and the Significance of Future Desires," *Philosophical Perspectives: Ethics* 23 (2009): 177–99.

14 This line of argument is explored – for the case of "procreative beneficence" – in Guy Kahane and Julian Savulescu, "The Moral Obligation to Create Children with the Best Chance of the Best Life," *Bioethics* 23 (2009): 274–90.

15 Note that in pointing out the comparative risks of blindness and sightedness, the advocate of the mere-difference view doesn't tacitly endorse the idea that it is better to be sighted. The greater risk to well-being associated with blindness could be largely or entirely due to how we treat blind people.

16 The most telling evidence for this is the suicide rate among gay teens. A recent meta-analysis of nineteen studies of suicide in gay teens showed that gay teens are

three times more likely than heterosexual teens to report a history of suicidal thoughts, plans, or intent. See Mark Moran, "Data Sounds Alarm on Gay Teens' Heightened Suicide Risk," *Psychiatric News* 46 (2011): 9–28.

17 I realize it might not strike everyone as homophobic. For those who disagree, the main point is simply this: the permissibility of the two cases – Reverse Disabled Baby and Reverse Baby Genes – should stand or fall together. If you're happy to grant that both cases are permissible, then it will be easy for you to allow that there is a cause/remove discrepancy for disability.

18 It is not obvious why it wouldn't, or why the case is importantly different from that of sexuality. Many disability rights activists argue that cases like Reverse Disabled Baby are exactly the sorts of cases that communicate ableism. See, for example, Lennard J. Davis, *Enforcing Normalcy: Disability, Deafness, and the Body* (London: Verso Books, 1995).

19 The effects of social ostracism on persons with visible disabilities is often profound. There's a vast literature on the topic, but one of the most telling examples is the effect of service dogs for people in wheelchairs. Service dogs perform many helpful assistive tasks, but their owners often report that the most substantial effect of the dog's presence is a mediation of social exclusion. Research shows that strangers will smile or speak to a person in a wheelchair if that person is accompanied by a dog, whereas wheelchair users standardly receive little or no social acknowledgment (eye contact, smiles, etc.). Bonnie Mader and Lynnette Hart, "Social Acknowledgement for Children with Disabilities: The Effect of Service Dogs," *Child Development* 60 (1989): 1529–34; Lynette Hart, Benjamin Hart, and Bonita Bergin, "Socializing Effects of Service Dogs for People with Disabilities," *Anthrozoos* 1 (1987): 41–4.

20 For example: according to the 2011 World Health Organization Report on Disability, disabled people are more than three times more likely than their non-disabled peers to report lack of access to health care; in "developed" countries the employment rate for disabled people is 44 percent (compared to around 75 percent for nondisabled people); disabled children are significantly more likely than nondisabled children to drop out of school (http://www.who.int/disabilities/world_report/2011/report/en/index.html).

21 It might also, of course, vary from disability to disability.

22 The fascinating BBC documentary *Me, My Sex, and I* profiles some of these pro-intersex campaigners.

See especially H. F. L. Meyer-Bahlburg, C. J. Migeon, G. D. Berkovitz, J. P. Gearhart, C. Dolezal, and A. B. Wisniewski, "Attitudes of Adult 46, XY Intersex Persons to Clinical Management Policies," *Journal of Urology* 171 (2004): 1615–19.

23 But wait – haven't I been appealing to intuition (especially certain "noninterference" intuitions)? Yes, I have. But I haven't been appealing to intuition about disability. The argument structure has gone like this: (i) if the mere-difference view is correct, then disability is analogous to features like sexuality and gender; (ii) think about how we reason (sometimes based on intuition) about cases involving sexuality and gender; (iii) absent further argument to the contrary, if the mere-difference view is correct then it predicts that we should reason about disability in similar ways. Much of what the mere-difference view says about disability is counterintuitive – and intentionally so. But the upshot is not skepticism about moral intuition. It is instead the admission that moral intuition can be affected by prejudice and false belief and that in cases where we have good reason to think our intuitions are unreliable, we should look for principled ways of revising and reconsidering that aren't based purely on intuitions.

24 It would be a mistake, furthermore, to think that the only potential good effects of blindness come from the (well-documented) sensory uniqueness of the blind. For example, blind storyteller and disability awareness campaigner Kim Kilpatrick runs a blog called "Great Things about Being Blind!", where she documents positive everyday experiences associated with her blindness. Her list includes: not being able to judge people based on what they look like, having no sense of self-consciousness about personal appearance and no temptation to "check the mirror," a love of and facility with Braille, and the deep, profound relationship she has formed with her guide dog (http://kimgia3.blogspot.com). Consider also the Mission Statement from the National Federation of the Blind: "The mission of the National Federation of the Blind is to achieve widespread emotional acceptance and intellectual understanding that the real problem of blindness is not the loss of eyesight but the misconceptions and lack of information which exist" (https://nfb.org/).

25 Derek Parfit, *Reasons and Persons* (Oxford: Clarendon, 1984). Another famous case discussed at length in the literature is that of embryo selection in in vitro; fertilization and the permissibility of selecting for disability.

I'm not going to discuss this case, simply because I think the ethics of embryo selection introduce a lot of noise and might well include complications that cut across the issue of whether we can permissibly cause disability. At the very least, it is important to note that there is clearly no obvious entailment from a mere-difference view of x to the permissibility of selecting for x. Most people think there's no moral difference between being female and being male. And yet many people are uncomfortable with the idea of sex-based embryo selection. The permissibility of sex-based embryo selection isn't settled simply by the fact that it is no better or worse to be male than to be female, and vice versa.

26 A similar line on the nonidentity problem is taken in David Wasserman, "Ethical Constraints on Allowing or Causing the Existence of People with Disabilities," in *Disability and Disadvantage*, ed. Kimberley Brownlee and Adam Cureton (Oxford: Oxford University Press, 2009), 319–51. Wasserman, however, bases his case on the role morality of prospective parents and the "ideal of unconditional welcome." I'm sympathetic to much of what Wasserman says, but I make no positive claims here about role morality. My claim is much simpler: the defender of a mere-difference view of disability should reject the background assumptions of cases like Child Now.

27 McMahan, "Causing Disabled People to Exist and Causing People to Be Disabled," 90.

28 It is very difficult, of course, for most people to imagine anyone wanting to be disabled (or more strongly – wanting to become disabled). But most people associate disability merely with lack of ability. In a society with less ableism, it would be the case not only that many of the bad effects of disability would be lessened but also that many of the good effects of disability would be more widely recognized.

29 Laura Hershey, "From Poster Child to Protestor," *Spectacle* (1997), http://www.cripcommentary.com/frompost.html.

89

Is Disability Mere Difference?

Greg Bognar

Introduction

Some philosophers and disability advocates argue that disability is not bad for you. Rather than treated as a harm, it should be considered and even celebrated as just another manifestation of human diversity. Disability is mere difference. To most of us, these are extraordinary claims. Can they be defended?

Disability and Quality of Life

What do people mean when they claim that disability is mere difference? This is not always clear. Surely, they cannot mean that *all* disabilities are mere differences. There are some disabilities that are so bad that life with them is plainly not worth living. Jonathan Glover reports the case of an infant born with a severe case of dystrophic epidermolysis bullosa, a genetic condition due to which any contact with the skin causes severe blisters and scarring. The condition can extend to the patient's digestive and respiratory tracts, resulting in constant, unbearable pain. Having to live with such

a condition is worse than non-existence. Since death can be a benefit for someone in this condition, having this disability must be a harm.[1]

Or suppose there was a disability that causes no pain but cuts life short. Other than causing premature death, this imagined condition does not have any negative impact on quality of life. (Real *progeroid syndromes* also cause morbidity.) Surely, a person who has this imaginary disability and who wants to go on living would be harmed when she dies early because of it. And if dying prematurely when you want to live on does not harm you, then it is hard to see what does. Therefore, the claim that disability is mere difference cannot apply across the board. It must apply only to *some* disabilities.

One problem is that those who make the claim that disability is mere difference almost never add any qualifications. They do not seem to mean, for instance, that all disabilities are mere differences except for sufficiently severe cases of those disabilities — such that, for instance, short-sightedness could be considered a mere difference but complete blindness should count as a disability. Neither do they classify conditions

Original publication details: Greg Bognar, "Is Disability Mere Difference," pp. 46–49 from *Journal of Medical Ethics* 42 (2016). Reproduced with permission of BMJ Publishing Group Ltd.

according to whether they are disabilities or mere differences – such that, for instance, paraplegia could be considered a mere difference but multiple sclerosis that causes the same limitation should count as a disability. In defences of the mere difference view, there is usually no attempt to clarify which conditions the author has in mind. Typically, only some paradigmatic cases are discussed. Under the circumstances, the best that sceptics of the mere difference view can do is to focus on these paradigmatic cases in order to grant their opponents the strongest form of their argument. I will follow this practice. If there are good reasons to think that disability is harmful in the paradigmatic cases, then there is surely no reason to accept the mere difference view in more extreme cases.

There are different reasons why someone might hold that disability is no harm. The following list introduces some of the arguments that may be used to defend the mere difference view.

One argument might be that people who live with disability do not consider their condition a disadvantage. Those who have no experience of disability are mistaken to believe that it is a harm to be disabled. They simply make an erroneous value judgement.

This argument rests on an empirical claim about how people with disabilities evaluate their condition. Evidently, it needs to be supported by social science showing that a sufficiently high proportion of those who have a particular disability evaluate the burden of that disability in a particular way. This needs to be shown for all relevant disabilities. I am unaware of such scientific findings. To be sure, there is a lot of evidence that people with a particular kind of disability evaluate the burden of that disability differently from others – often (but not always) considering it less bad.[2] But that is not the same as not considering it a burden at all. The best I can tell, there is no evidence for this more radical claim.

But even if there were corroborating results in social science, a problem would remain: it may be that it is the people with disabilities who do not consider their condition a harm that make the erroneous value judgement. On most plausible accounts of well-being, you can be mistaken about your own well-being.[3] So even if every person with disability considered their disability no harm, that would still not get you to the mere difference view – unless you also assumed that their evaluations are to be trusted. In the parlance of the social sciences, it would have to be the case that their evaluations are both reliable and valid.

This leads to a different argument. Perhaps the advocates of the mere difference view have some particular theory of well-being in mind – one that entails the proposition that disability is no harm. For instance, they might accept a simple version of hedonism, on which well-being consists in feelings of pleasure or happiness. On this sort of view, if other things being equal a person with a disability is just as happy as a person who is identical in all relevant respects except that she does not have the disability, then the disability is no harm. It is merely a difference between the two people.

I doubt that proponents of the mere difference view would want to defend their position merely as a by-product of some theory of well-being – let alone one that is as implausible as simple hedonism.[4] I suspect they want to argue that it is independent of philosophical theories of well-being and it is compatible with the range of the most plausible theories. (In any case, the fact that a theory of well-being entails the mere difference view, arguably, constitutes an argument against it – unless of course an independent argument is available for the mere difference view).

There are other arguments about well-being and disability that might be thought to provide a defence for the mere difference view. For example, it is a well-known phenomenon that many people who become disabled are able to adapt to their disability. Adaptation may take some time, and there may be conditions to which it is not possible to adapt. Nevertheless, after the adaptation process, many people consider their condition less bad than others do. In addition, people who are born with disabilities often evaluate their lives similarly to those who are not disabled.[5]

Therefore, perhaps an argument can be made that disability is not a harm because, at least after an adjustment period, people are able to adapt to it and lead lives that are no worse than those without the disability. Call this the *adaptation argument*.

Setting aside the worry that I noted above about the reliance on people's own evaluations, the problem with the adaptation argument is straightforward: adaptation is not always desirable or admirable. You can adapt to adverse circumstances by selecting new worthwhile aims and activities, by learning new skills, by developing effective coping strategies. Or you can adapt to adverse circumstances by giving up your aims and activities and by learning to find satisfaction in whatever is readily available. Adaptation by itself does not make life better. And it certainly does not support the idea that disability is no harm: even successful adaptation does not guarantee a good life.

A related claim that is often made in discussions of disability is this: being disabled enables you to develop abilities that other people lack, and hence on balance it does not cause any disadvantage. For instance, people who are deaf or blind may have other senses that are exceptionally acute; people who have limited mobility may excel in intellectual or artistic pursuits.

The idea is that any shortcoming caused by a disability may be compensated by advantages that are present only because of that very disability. People without the disability in question are unlikely to have similarly acute senses, artistic sensibilities or intellectual skills. As a consequence, the lives of people with the disability are no worse than the lives of those without it, even though the sources of their well-being are different. This is the *compensation argument*.

The compensation argument suffers from many problems. For one thing, it does not seem to be supported by empirical evidence. Even if some people can develop abilities to compensate for the harm of disability, this is unlikely to be true of most people; at least, the argument is undermined by the everyday, commonsense experience of disability that most people have. This claim, opponents will rush to point out, may simply reflect 'ableist' prejudice. Perhaps – but this objection cuts both ways: there is a notable lack of sound social scientific generalisations in this debate, and an abundance of reliance on single, anecdotal cases.[6] But anecdotal evidence is just that. If proponents of the mere difference view want to convince others, they need to do more than just to point to a few cases, ignoring the possibility that they may be unrepresentative.

But set all of these worries aside. Can the compensation argument provide the necessary support for the mere difference view? Plainly, it cannot. The mere difference view says that disability is no harm; the compensation argument makes the claim that the harm of disability can be compensated by benefits that being disabled makes possible. The argument accepts that disability is a harm, it just insists it need not be a harm all things considered. This contradicts the mere difference view.

Disability and Society

There is another approach that might be taken to defend the mere difference view. You might start from the argument that people with disabilities are more than just a collection of individuals who share some characteristics. They form their own unique culture. They might have shared interests, their own history (all too often, a history of discrimination and prejudice), their own language, their own institutions, and so on. These days, for instance, it is no longer controversial that there exists a unique deaf culture (or more precisely several deaf cultures).[7]

But from the fact that a group of people with a particular kind of disability constitute a unique culture, it does not follow that having that particular kind of disability is no harm. People who share some form of disadvantage can and often do participate in a unique culture within the broader society. There is no connection between the existence of disability culture and the mere difference view.

It might be thought that the connection between the mere difference view and the social aspects of disability is more complex. One view of disability has it that the causes of disadvantage for people with disabilities are primarily or perhaps entirely social. It is not the impairment or functional limitation, but the lack of inclusion and accommodation, as well as prejudice and other negative attitudes that are disabling people. This sort of view has become known as the *social model* of disability.[8]

It is not obvious what kind of connection there might be between the social model and the mere difference view. On the one hand, it seems that those who accept the mere difference view must be committed to a strong version of the social model: if disability is no harm in itself, yet people with disability are disadvantaged, then the disadvantages must have social causes. On the other hand, accepting the social model does not necessarily commit you to the mere difference view: you might accept that the impairment or functional limitation underlying disability is a harm, yet maintain that the disadvantages that turn an impairment into a disability are primarily social.

Thus, you can take a stronger view about the connection – one on which the social model is an implication of the mere difference view. In this case, you cannot defend the mere difference view by appealing to the social model of disability since the implication runs the other way. And if you take the weaker view about the connection, then you have conceded from the start that the social model provides no support for the mere difference view.

The Indirect Strategy

Here is a pair of arguments commonly used against the mere difference view. If it was true that disability in itself is no harm, then it would be permissible to cause disability, and, similarly, it would be impermissible to prevent or remove disability. Since it is surely impermissible to cause someone to be disabled, and it is surely permissible to have someone's disability prevented or removed, disability cannot be a mere difference. Hence, the mere difference view is false.[9][10]

In response, defenders of the mere difference view can try to show that even if disability is mere difference it does not follow that it is permissible to cause disability, and it does not follow that it is impermissible to prevent or remove disability. The mere difference view does not have these implications. Rather, it is impermissible to cause disability, and permissible to prevent and remove disability, for other reasons. This indirect line of argument is developed by Elizabeth Barnes.[11]

This is the first argument in the pair of arguments:

1. If disability is mere difference, then you do not make a person worse off by causing her to be disabled.
2. If you do not make a person worse off by causing her to be disabled, then it is permissible to cause her to be disabled.
3. But it is not permissible to cause a person to be disabled.
4. Therefore, disability is not mere difference.

The problem with this argument is that there is a hidden premise:

(1′) If you do not make a person worse off by doing something Φ to them, then it is permissible to Φ.

Needless to say, (1′) is false. Even if you would not make a person worse off by doing Φ to them, it might still be impermissible to Φ for some other reason. For instance, to Φ would be to violate their autonomy. Or to Φ would be impermissible because even if *being* disabled is no harm, *becoming* disabled is. Or, more plausibly, it would be impermissible because causing someone to be disabled is *unjustified interference* with that person's life.

This reply is plausible because it accords with the way most of us regard differences that *are* mere differences: differences in gender, race, sexual orientation, and so on. If you set aside disadvantages that are socially caused, it is clear that being a man or a woman, black or white, straight or gay are no harms in themselves. They are mere differences. But even though they are mere differences, it does not follow that it is permissible to cause a woman to become a man, a black person to become a white person, or a gay person to become straight. To do so would be unjustified interference with the person's life. And, according to the indirect strategy, the same applies to disability.

Two remarks are in order at this point. First, strictly speaking this line of argument falls short of providing a defence of the mere difference view. For even if causing disability is impermissible because it is unjustified interference, it does not follow that this is the only reason for which it is impermissible. It might be that, in addition, it is impermissible because causing someone to be disabled is to cause them harm. So the argument is not conclusive, even if it can go some way towards defending the mere difference view.

Second, suppose that someone consents to your acting in a way that will disable that person. In this case, you have their permission to cause them to be disabled. Your acting in this way is not unjustified interference. Yet even in this case many of us would hesitate to agree that causing disability is permissible. At the very least, we would want more details. And our hesitation may reflect the fact that causing disability is to cause someone serious harm, and therefore requires further justification even in the presence of consent.

But let us set these considerations aside. Let us suppose that the indirect strategy succeeds in undermining the objection that if disability is mere difference then it is permissible to cause disability. Mere differences are not harmful, yet it is impermissible to cause them. If disability is mere difference, it may have the same feature.

What about the second argument in the pair of arguments? This is the objection that if disability is mere difference then it is impermissible to prevent or remove it. But it is clearly permissible to prevent or remove disability. Hence, it is not mere difference.

In the case of mere differences like gender, race or sexual orientation, most of us would agree that it would be unjustified interference to remove or prevent the development of one or the other characteristic. Even if it was possible, it would be impermissible to prevent a child from growing up to be straight or gay, or to remove some feature (whatever it might be) that is responsible for their sexual orientation later in life. The same would be true of choices (were they possible) that interfere with other characteristics that are mere differences. While there may be very few actual possibilities to prevent or remove characteristics in the paradigmatic cases of mere differences, we do seem to have the moral intuition that it would be wrong to do so.

And this is where the indirect strategy breaks down. No such intuition is available in the case of disability. Other things being equal, it would not be *unjustified*

interference to remove or prevent a disability. Of course, doing so might be wrong for other reasons – perhaps you do not have the person's consent, when it is both possible and required to obtain it. But the indirect strategy aims to provide a readily available, alternative general explanation for the permissibility of preventing or removing disability. It aims to show that there is another way to account for the moral intuitions that people have. But the problem is that there is no such alternative when it comes to the case of preventing and removing disability.

An example may help. Suppose you are a surgeon and an unconscious accident victim is brought in to the emergency room where you work. Unless you operate on her, she will become disabled. Surely, you ought to operate on her, even in the absence of consent. What explains this? Most of us would say that it is the moral belief that other things being equal it is wrong not to prevent disability.

Now suppose that the accident victim is conscious and does not give you her consent. She says she wants to become disabled. Even in this case, the lack of consent does not automatically make operating on her impermissible. At the very least, it raises an issue about her competence. What explains this? The moral belief that other things being equal, it is wrong not to prevent disability.

The indirect strategy does not reject this moral belief. What its proponents must do, instead, is to provide an alternative justification for it – one that does not appeal to the idea that disability is harm. But as far as I can tell, no such justification has been given. Barnes, astoundingly, simply gives up the indirect strategy halfway through the argument. She suggests that defenders of the mere difference view should simply dig in their heels and insist that preventing and removing disability would be unjustified interference. To deny this, she adds, is 'ableism'. But this is begging the question. It is like trying to have your cake and eat it too. If you want to defend the mere difference view by using the indirect strategy, you should not abandon it halfway through the argument.

The second of the pair of arguments, therefore, stands. If disability in itself is no harm, then it would be impermissible to prevent or remove disability. Since it is surely permissible to prevent or remove disability, and given that there is no readily available alternative explanation of this moral intuition, it follows that disability cannot be mere difference. It is a harm.

Conclusion

Defenders of the mere difference view argue that disability is not unlike gender, race or sexual orientation. Just as these other differences have been the object of

bigotry and prejudice, disability has often been the object of 'ableist' discrimination and prejudice.

There is undoubtedly still a lot of prejudice and discrimination towards people with disabilities. There is undoubtedly still a great deal more that societies could and should do to accommodate and to support people with disabilities. None of what I have said in this paper should be taken as a defence of prejudice or discrimination. What I have tried to show is that no argument has been put forward so far that can successfully defend the mere difference view. There is no reason to give up just yet the view that disability is harm.

References

1 Glover J. Future people, disability, and screening. In: Laslett P. and Fishkin J.S., eds. *Justice between age groups and generations*. New Haven: Yale University Press, 1992: 127–43.

2 Daniels N., Rose S., and Zide E.D. Disability, adaptation and inclusion. In: Brownlee K. and Cureton A., eds. *Disability and disadvantage*. Oxford: Oxford University Press, 2009: 54–85.

3 Bognar G. The concept of quality of life. *Soc Theory Pract* 2005; 31:561–80.

4 Feldman F. *What is this thing called happiness?* Oxford: Oxford University Press, 2010.

5 Menzel P., Dolan P., Richardson J., et al. The role of adaptation to disability and disease in health state valuation: a preliminary normative analysis. *Soc Sci Med* 2002; 55:2149–58.

6 Goering S. 'You Say You're Happy, but. . .': Contested quality of life judgments in bioethics and disability studies. *Bioet Inq* 2008; 5:125–35.

7 Sparrow R. Defending deaf culture: the case of cochlear implants. *J Polit Philos* 2005; 13:135–52.

8 Shakespeare T. The social model of disability. In: Davis L.J., ed. *The disability studies reader*. New York: Routledge, 2013: 214–21.

9 Harris J. One principle and three fallacies of disability studies. *J Med Ethics* 2001; 27:383–7.

10 McMahan J. Causing disabled people to exist and causing people to be disabled. *Ethics* 2005; 116:77–99.

11 Barnes E. Valuing disability, causing disability. *Ethics* 2014; 125:88–113.

90

Prenatal Diagnosis and Selective Abortion
A Challenge to Practice and Policy

Adrienne Asch

> Although sex selection might ameliorate the situation of some individuals, it lowers the status of women in general and only perpetuates the situation that gave rise to it. . . .If we believe that sexual equality is necessary for a just society, then we should oppose sex selection.
>
> Wertz and Fletcher[1] (pp. 242–3)

> The very motivation for seeking an "origin" of homosexuality reveals homophobia. Moreover, such research may lead to prenatal tests that claim to predict for homosexuality. For homosexual people who live in countries with no legal protections these dangers are particularly serious.
>
> Schüklenk et al.[2] (p. 6)

The tenor of the preceding statements may spark relatively little comment in the world of health policy, the medical profession, or the readers of this journal [*American Journal of Public Health*], because many recognize the dangers of using the technology of prenatal testing followed by selective abortion for the characteristic of fetal sex. Similarly, the medical and psychiatric professions, and the world of public health, have aided in the civil rights struggle of gays and lesbians by insisting that homosexuality is not a disease. Consequently, many readers would concur with those who question the motives behind searching for the causes of homosexuality that might lead scientists to develop a prenatal test for that characteristic. Many in our society, however, have no such misgivings about prenatal testing for characteristics regarded as genetic or chromosomal diseases, abnormalities, or disabilities:

> Human mating that proceeds without the use of genetic data about the risks of transmitting diseases will produce greater mortality and medical costs than if carriers of potentially deleterious genes are alerted to their carrier

Original publication details: Adrienne Asch, "Prenatal Diagnosis and Selective Abortion: A Challenge to Practice and Policy," pp. 1649–1657 from *American Journal of Public Health* 89: 11 (1999). Reproduced with permission of American Public Health Association.

status and *encouraged* to mate with noncarriers or to use other reproductive strategies [emphasis added].[3 (p. 84)]

Attitudes toward congenital disability per se have not changed markedly. Both premodern as well as contemporary societies have regarded disability as undesirable and to be avoided. Not only have parents recognized the birth of a disabled child as a potentially divisive, destructive force in the family unit, but the larger society has seen disability as unfortunate (p. 89). . . .

Our society still does not countenance the elimination of diseased/disabled people; but it does urge the termination of diseased/disabled fetuses. The urging is not explicit, but implicit (p.90).[4]

Writing in the *American Journal of Human Genetics* about screening programs for cystic fibrosis, A. L. Beaudet acknowledged the tension between the goals of enhancing reproductive choice and preventing the births of children who would have disabilities:

Although some would argue that the success of the program should be judged solely by the effectiveness of the educational programs (i.e., whether screenees understood the information), it is clear that prevention of [cystic fibrosis] is also, at some level, a measure of a screening program, since few would advocate expanding the substantial resources involved if very few families wish to avoid the disease.[5 (p. 603)]

Prenatal tests designed to detect the condition of the fetus include ultrasound, maternal serum α-fetoprotein screening, chorionic villus sampling, and amniocentesis. Some (ultrasound screenings) are routinely performed regardless of the mother's age and provide information that she may use to guide her care throughout pregnancy; others, such as chorionic villus sampling or amniocentesis, do not influence the woman's care during pregnancy but provide information intended to help her decide whether to continue the pregnancy if fetal impairment is detected. Amniocentesis, the test that detects the greatest variety of fetal impairments, is typically offered to women who will be 35 years or older at the time they are due to deliver, but recently commentators have urged that the age threshold be removed and that the test

be available to women regardless of age.[6] Such testing is increasingly considered a standard component of prenatal care for women whose insurance covers these procedures, including women using publicly financed clinics in some jurisdictions.

These tests, which are widely accepted in the field of bioethics and by clinicians, public health professionals, and the general public, have nonetheless occasioned some apprehension and concern among students of women's reproductive experiences, who find that women do not uniformly welcome the expectation that they will undergo prenatal testing or the prospect of making decisions depending on the test results.[7] Less often discussed by clinicians is the view, expressed by a growing number of individuals, that the technology is itself based on erroneous assumptions about the adverse impact of disability on life. Argument from this perspective focuses on what is communicated about societal and familial acceptance of diversity in general and disability in particular.[8–17] Like other women-centered critiques of prenatal testing, this article assumes a pro-choice perspective but suggests that unreflective uses of testing could diminish, rather than expand, women's choices. Like critiques stemming from concerns about the continued acceptance of human differences within the society and the family, this critique challenges the view of disability that lies behind social endorsement of such testing and the conviction that women will, or should, end their pregnancies if they discover that the fetus has a disabling trait.

If public health frowns on efforts to select for or against girls or boys and would oppose future efforts to select for or against those who would have a particular sexual orientation, but promotes people's efforts to avoid having children who would have disabilities, it is because medicine and public health view disability as extremely different from and worse than these other forms of human variation. At first blush this view may strike one as self-evident. To challenge it might even appear to be questioning our professional mission. Characteristics such as chronic illnesses and disabilities (discussed together throughout this article) do not resemble traits such as sex, sexual orientation, or race, because the latter are not in themselves perceived as inimical to a rewarding life. Disability is thought to be just that – to be incompatible with life satisfaction. When public health considers matters of sex, sexual orientation, or race, it examines how factors in social and economic life pose obstacles to health and to health care, and it champions actions to improve the well-being of those disadvantaged by the discrimination that attends minority status. By contrast, public health fights to eradicate disease and disability or to treat, ameliorate, or cure these when they occur. For medicine and public health, disease and disability is the problem to solve, and so it appears natural to use prenatal testing and abortion as one more means of minimizing the incidence of disability.

In the remainder of this article I argue, first, that most of the problems associated with having a disability stem from discriminatory social arrangements that are changeable, just as much of what has in the past made the lives of women or gays difficult has been the set of social arrangements they have faced (and which they have begun to dismantle). After discussing ways in which the characteristic of disability resembles and differs from other characteristics, I discuss why I believe the technology of prenatal testing followed by selective abortion is unique among means of preventing or ameliorating disability, and why it offends many people who are untroubled by other disease prevention and health promotion activities. I conclude by recommending ways in which health practitioners and policymakers could offer this technology so that it promotes genuine reproductive choice and helps families and society to flourish.

Contrasting Medical and Social Paradigms of Disability

The definitions of terms such as "health," "normality," and "disability" are not clear, objective, and universal across time and place. Individual physical characteristics are evaluated with reference to a standard of normality, health, and what some commentators term "species-typical functioning."[18, 19] These

commentators point out that within a society at a particular time, there is a shared perception of what is typical physical functioning and role performance for a girl or boy, woman or man. Boorse's definition of an undesirable departure from species-typicality focuses on the functioning of the person rather than the cause of the problem: "[A] condition of a part or process in an organism is pathological when the ability of the part or process to perform one or more of its species-typical biological functions falls below some central range of the statistical distribution for that ability."[18] [(p. 370)] Daniels writes, "Impairments of normal species functioning reduce the range of opportunity open to the individual in which he may construct his plan of life or conception of the good."[19] [(p. 27)]

Chronic illness, traumatic injury, and congenital disability may indeed occasion departures from "species-typical functioning," and thus these conditions do constitute differences from both a statistical average and a desired norm of well-being. Certainly society prizes some characteristics, such as intelligence, athleticism, and musical or artistic skill, and rewards people with more than the statistical norm of these attributes; I will return to this point later. Norms on many health-related attributes change over time; as the life span for people in the United States and Canada increases, conditions that often lead to death before 40 years of age (e.g., cystic fibrosis) may become even more dreaded than they are today. The expectation that males will be taller than females and that adults will stand more than 5 feet in height leads to a perception that departures from these norms are not only unusual but undesirable and unhealthy. Not surprisingly, professionals who have committed themselves to preventing illness and injury, or to ameliorating and curing people of illnesses and injuries, are especially attuned to the problems and hardships that affect the lives of their patients. Such professionals, aware of the physical pain or weakness and the psychological and social disruption caused by acute illness or sudden injury, devote their lives to easing the problems that these events impose.

What many scholars, policymakers, and activists in the area of disability contend is that medically oriented understandings of the impact of disability on life contain 2 erroneous assumptions with serious adverse consequences: first, that the life of a person with a chronic illness or disability is forever disrupted, as one's life might be temporarily disrupted as a result of a back spasm, an episode of pneumonia, or a broken leg; second, that if a disabled person experiences isolation, powerlessness, unemployment, poverty, or low social status, these are inevitable consequences of biological limitation. Body, psyche, and social life do change immediately following an occurrence of disease, accident, or injury, and medicine, public health, and bioethics all correctly appreciate the psychological and physical vulnerability of patients and their families and friends during immediate medical crises. These professions fail people with disabilities, however, by concluding that because there may never be full physical recovery, there is never a regrouping of physical, cognitive, and psychological resources with which to participate in a rewarding life. Chronic illness and disability are not equivalent to acute illness or sudden injury, in which an active disease process or unexpected change in physical function disrupts life's routines. Most people with conditions such as spina bifida, achondroplasia, Down syndrome, and many other mobility and sensory impairments perceive themselves as healthy, not sick, and describe their conditions as givens of their lives – the equipment with which they meet the world. The same is true for people with chronic conditions such as cystic fibrosis, diabetes, hemophilia, and muscular dystrophy. These conditions include intermittent flare-ups requiring medical care and adjustments in daily living, but they do not render the person as unhealthy as most of the public – and members of the health profession – imagine.

People with disabilities are thinking about a traffic jam, a disagreement with a friend, which movie to attend, or which team will win the World Series – not just about their diagnosis. Having a disability can intrude into a person's consciousness if events bring it to the fore: if 2 lift-equipped buses in a row fail to stop for a man using a wheelchair; if the theater ticket agent insults a patron with Down syndrome by refusing

to take money for her ticket; if a hearing-impaired person misses a train connection because he did not know that a track change had been announced.

The second way in which medicine, bioethics, and public health typically err is in viewing all problems that occur to people with disabilities as attributable to the condition itself, rather than to external factors. When ethicists, public health professionals, and policymakers discuss the importance of health care, urge accident prevention, or promote healthy lifestyles, they do so because they perceive a certain level of health not only as intrinsically desirable but as a prerequisite for an acceptable life. One commentator describes such a consensual view of types of life in terms of a "normal opportunity range": "The normal opportunity range for a given society is the array of life plans reasonable persons in it are likely to construct for themselves."[19 (p. 33)] Health care includes that which is intended to "maintain, restore, or provide functional equivalents where possible, to normal species functioning."[19 (p. 32)]

The paradigm of medicine concludes that the gaps in education, employment, and income that persist between adults with disabilities and those without disabilities are inevitable because the impairment precludes study or limits work. The alternative paradigm, which views people with disabilities in social, minority-group terms, examines how societal arrangements – rules, laws, means of communication, characteristics of buildings and transit systems, the typical 8-hour workday – exclude some people from participating in school, work, civic, or social life. This newer paradigm is expressed by enactment of the Individuals with Disabilities Education Act and the Americans with Disabilities Act and is behind the drive to ensure that employed disabled people will keep their access to health care through Medicaid or Medicare. This paradigm – still more accepted by people outside medicine, public health, and bioethics than by those within these fields – questions whether there is an inevitable, unmodifiable gap between people with disabilities and people without disabilities. Learning that in 1999, nine years after the passage of laws to end employment discrimination, millions of people with disabilities are still out of the work force, despite their readiness to work,[20] the social paradigm asks what remaining institutional factors bar people from the goal of productive work. Ethical and policy questions arise in regard to the connection that does or should exist between health and the range of opportunities open to people in the population.

Commitments to alleviate the difficulties arising from chronic illness and disability and efforts to promote healthy lifestyles throughout the population need not lead to a devaluation of the members of society who do not meet our typical understanding of health, but people with disabilities have indeed been subject to systematic segregation and second-class treatment in all areas of life. It is possible to appreciate the norm of 2 arms without being repelled by a woman with 1 arm; yet social science, autobiography, legislation, and case law reveal that people with both visible and "invisible" disabilities lose opportunities to study, work, live where and with whom they choose, attend religious services, and even vote.[21-27]

The Americans with Disabilities Act, signed into law in 1990, is a ringing indictment of the nation's history with regard to people with disabilities:

> Congress finds that. . .(3) discrimination against individuals with disabilities persists in such critical areas as employment,. . .education, recreation,. health services,. . .and access to public services; (7) individuals with disabilities are a discrete and insular minority who have been faced with restrictions and limitations, subjected to a history of purposeful unequal treatment, and relegated to a position of political powerlessness in our society, based on characteristics that are beyond the control of such individuals and resulting from stereotypic assumptions not truly indicative of the individual ability of such individuals to participate in, and contribute to, society.[28]

Eight years after the passage of the Americans with Disabilities Act, disabled people reported some improvements in access to public facilities and that things are getting better in some areas of life, but major gaps between the disabled and the nondisabled still exist in income, employment, and social participation. To dramatically underscore the prevalence of social stigma and discrimination: "fewer than half (45%) of adults with disabilities say that people generally treat them as an equal after they learn they have a disability."[20]

It is estimated that 54 million people in the United States have disabilities, of which impairments of mobility, hearing, vision, and learning; arthritis; cystic fibrosis; diabetes; heart conditions; and back problems are some of the most well-known.[20] Thus, in discussing discrimination, stigma, and unequal treatment for people with disabilities, we are considering a population that is larger than the known gay and lesbian population or the African American population. These numbers take on new significance when we assess the rationale behind prenatal diagnosis and selective abortion as a desirable strategy to deal with disability.

Prenatal diagnosis for disability prevention

If some forms of disability prevention are legitimate medical and public health activities, and if people with disabilities use the health system to improve and maintain their own health, there is an acknowledgment that the characteristic of disability may not be desirable. Although many within the disability rights movement challenge prenatal diagnosis as a means of disability prevention, no one objects to public health efforts to clean up the environment, encourage seatbelt use, reduce tobacco and alcohol consumption, and provide prenatal care to all pregnant women. All these activities deal with the health of existing human beings (or fetuses expected to come to term) and seek to ensure their well-being. What differentiates prenatal testing followed by abortion from other forms of disability prevention and medical treatment is that prenatal testing followed by abortion is intended not to prevent the disability or illness of a born or future human being but to prevent the birth of a human being who will have one of these undesired characteristics. In reminding proponents of the Human

Genome Project that gene therapy will not soon be able to cure disability, James Watson declared,

> [W]e place most of our hopes for genetics on the use of antenatal diagnostic procedures, which increasingly will let us know whether a fetus is carrying a mutant gene that will seriously proscribe its eventual development into a functional human being. By terminating such pregnancies, the threat of horrific disease genes contributing to blight many family's prospects for future success can be erased.[29] (p.19)

But Watson errs in assuming that tragedy is inevitable for the child or for the family. When physicians, public health experts, and bioethicists promote prenatal diagnosis to prevent future disability, they let disability become the only relevant characteristic and suggest that it is such a problematic characteristic that people eagerly awaiting a new baby should terminate the pregnancy and "try again" for a healthy child. Professionals fail to recognize that along with whatever impairment may be diagnosed come all the characteristics of any other future child. The health professions suggest that once a prospective parent knows of the likely disability of a future child, there is nothing else to know or imagine about who the child might become: disability subverts parental dreams.

The focus of my concern here is not on the decision made by the pregnant woman or by the woman and her partner. I focus on the view of life with disability that is communicated by society's efforts to develop prenatal testing and urge it on every pregnant woman. If public health espouses goals of social justice and equality for people with disabilities, as it has worked to improve the status of women, gays and lesbians, and members of racial and ethnic minorities, it should reconsider whether it wishes to continue endorsing the technology of prenatal diagnosis. If there is an unshakable commitment to the technology in the name of reproductive choice, public health should work with practitioners to change the way in which information about impairments detected in the fetus is delivered.

Rationales for prenatal testing

The medical professions justify prenatal diagnosis and selective abortion on the grounds of the *costs* of childhood disability – the costs to the child, to the family, and to the society. Some proponents of the Human Genome Project from the fields of science and bioethics argue that in a world of limited resources, we can reduce disability-related expenditures if all diagnoses of fetal impairment are followed by abortion.[30]

On both empirical and moral grounds, endorsing prenatal diagnosis for societal reasons is dangerous. Only a small fraction of total disability can now be detected prenatally, and even if future technology enables the detection of predisposition to diabetes, forms of depression, Alzheimer disease, heart disease, arthritis, or back problems – all more prevalent in the population than many of the currently detectable conditions – we will never manage to detect and prevent most disability. Rates of disability increase markedly with age, and the gains in life span guarantee that most people will deal with disability in themselves or someone close to them. Laws and services to support people with disabilities will still be necessary, unless society chooses a campaign of eliminating disabled people in addition to preventing the births of those who would be disabled. Thus, there is small cost-saving in money or in human resources to be achieved by even the vigorous determination to test every pregnant woman and abort every fetus found to exhibit disabling traits.

My moral opposition to prenatal testing and selective abortion flows from the conviction that life with disability is worthwhile and the belief that a just society must appreciate and nurture the lives of all people, whatever the endowments they receive in the natural lottery. I hold these beliefs because – as I show throughout this article – there is abundant evidence that people with disabilities can thrive even in this less than welcoming society. Moreover, people with disabilities do not merely take from others, they contribute as well – to families, to friends, to the economy. They contribute neither in spite of nor because of their disabilities, but because along with their disabilities come other characteristics of personality, talent, and humanity that render people with disabilities full members of the human and moral community.

Implications for People with Disabilities

Implications for children and adults with disabilities, and for their families, warrant more consideration. Several prominent bioethicists claim that to knowingly bring into the world a child who will live with an impairment (whether it be a "withered arm," cystic fibrosis, deafness, or Down syndrome) is unfair to the child because it deprives the child of the "right to an open future" by limiting some options.[31] Green's words represent a significant strand of professional thinking: "In the absence of adequate justifying reasons, a child is morally wronged when he/she is knowingly, deliberately, or negligently brought into being with a health status likely to result in significantly greater disability or suffering, or significantly reduced life options relative to the other children with whom he/she will grow up."[32(p10)] Green is not alone in his view that it is irresponsible to bring a child into the world with a disability.[33,34]

The biology of disability can affect people's lives, and not every feature of life with a disability is socially determined or mediated. People with cystic fibrosis cannot now expect to live to age 70. People with type I diabetes can expect to have to use insulin and to have to think carefully and continuously about what and how much they eat and about their rest and exercise, perhaps more than typical sedentary people who are casual about the nutritional content of their food. People who use a wheelchair for mobility will not climb mountains; people with the intellectual disabilities of Down syndrome or fragile X chromosome are not likely to read this article and engage in debate about its merits and shortcomings. Yet, as disability scholars point out, such limitations do not preclude a whole class of experiences, but only certain instances in which these experiences might occur. People who

move through the world in wheelchairs may not be able to climb mountains, but they can and do participate in other athletic activities that are challenging and exhilarating and call for stamina, alertness, and teamwork. Similarly, people who have Down syndrome or fragile X chromosome are able to have other experiences of thinking hard about important questions and making distinctions and decisions. Thus, they exercise capacities for reflection and judgment, even if not in the rarified world of abstract verbal argument (P. Ferguson, e-mail, March 5, 1999).

The child who will have a disability may have fewer options for the so-called open future that philosophers and parents dream of for children. Yet I suspect that disability precludes far fewer life possibilities than members of the bioethics community claim. That many people with disabilities find their lives satisfying has been documented. For example, more than half of people with spinal cord injury (paraplegia) reported feeling more positively about themselves since becoming disabled.[35 (p.83)] Similarly, Canadian teenagers who had been extremely-low-birthweight infants were compared with nondisabled teens and found to resemble them in terms of their own subjective ratings of quality of life. "Adolescents who were [extremely-low-birthweight] infants suffer from a greater burden of morbidity, and rate their health related quality of life as significantly lower than control teenagers. Nevertheless, the vast majority of the [extremely-low-birthweight] respondents view their health-related quality of life as quite satisfactory and are difficult to distinguish from controls."[36 (p. 453)]

Interestingly, professionals faced with such information often dismiss it and insist that happy disabled people are the exceptions.[37] Here again, James Watson expresses a common view when he says,

Is it more likely for such children to fall behind in society or will they through such afflictions develop the strengths of character and fortitude that lead. . .to the head of their packs? Here I'm afraid that the word handicap cannot escape its true definition – being placed at a disadvantage. From this perspective seeing the bright side of being handicapped is like praising the virtues of extreme poverty. To be sure, there are many individuals who rise out of its inherently degrading states. But we perhaps most realistically should see it as the major origin of asocial behavior.[29] (p. 19)

I return to the points made earlier regarding how many of the supposed limits and problems associated with disability are socially, rather than biologically, imposed. The 1998 survey of disabled people in the United States conducted by Louis Harris Associates found gaps in education, employment, income, and social participation between people with disabilities and people without disabilities and noted that fewer disabled than nondisabled people were "extremely satisfied" with their lives. The reasons for dissatisfaction did not stem from anything inherent in the impairments; they stemmed from disparities in attainments and activities that are not inevitable in a society that takes into account the needs of one sixth of its members.[20] Only 29% of people with disabilities work full- or part-time, yet of disabled working-age people surveyed who were unemployed, more than 70% would prefer to work, and most did not perceive their disability as precluding them from productive employment. Unemployment, and thus inadequate income, coupled with problems in obtaining health insurance or in having that insurance pay for actual disability-related expenses, accounts for the problems most commonly described by disabled people as diminishing life satisfaction.[20]

For children whose disabling conditions do not cause early degeneration, intractable pain, and early death, life offers a host of interactions with the physical and social world in which people can be involved to their and others' satisfaction. Autobiographical writings and family narratives testify eloquently to the rich lives and the even richer futures that are possible for people with disabilities today[22,38] (also P. Ferguson, e-mail, March 5, 1999).

Nonetheless, I do not deny that disability can entail physical pain, psychic anguish, and social isolation — even if much of the psychological and social pain can be attributed to human cruelty rather than to biological givens. In order to imagine bringing a child with a disability into the world when abortion is possible,

prospective parents must be able to imagine saying to a child, "I wanted you enough and believed enough in who you could be that I felt you could have a life you would appreciate even with the difficulties your disability causes." If parents and siblings, family members and friends can genuinely love and enjoy the child for who he or she is and not lament what he or she is not; if child care centers, schools, and youth groups routinely include disabled children; if television programs, children's books, and toys take children with disabilities into account by including them naturally in programs and products, the child may not live with the anguish and isolation that have marred life for generations of disabled children.

Implications for Family Life

Many who are willing to concede that people with disabilities could have lives they themselves would enjoy nonetheless argue that the cost to families of raising them justifies abortion. Women are seen to carry the greatest load for the least return in caring for such a child. Proponents of using the technology to avoid the births of children with disabilities insist that the disabled child epitomizes what women have fought to change about their lives as mothers: unending labor, the sacrifice of their work and other adult interests, loss of time and attention for the other children in the family as they juggle resources to give this disabled child the best available support, and uncertain recompense in terms of the mother's relationship with the child.[39]

Writing in 1995 on justifications for prenatal testing, Botkin proposed that only conditions that impose "burdens" on parents equivalent to those of an unwanted child warrant society-supported testing.

> The parent's harms are different in many respects from the child's, but include emotional pain and suffering, loss of a child, loss of opportunities, loss of freedom, isolation, loneliness, fear, guilt, stigmatization, and financial expenses. . . .Some conditions that are often considered severe may not be associated with any experience of harm for the child. Down syndrome is a prime example. Parents

in this circumstance are not harmed by the suffering of a child. . .but rather by their time, efforts, and expenses to support the special needs of an individual with Down syndrome. . . .It might also be added that parents are harmed by their unfulfilled expectations with the birth of an impaired child. In general terms, the claim is that parents suffer a sufficient harm to justify prenatal testing or screening when the severity of a child's condition raises problems for the parents of a similar magnitude to the birth of an unwanted child. . . .[P]arents of a child with unwanted disability have their interests impinged upon by the efforts, time, emotional burdens, and expenses added by the disability that they would not have otherwise experienced with the birth of a healthy child.[40] (pp. 36–7)

I believe the characterizations found in the writings of Wertz and Fletcher[39] and Botkin[40] are at the heart of professionals' support for prenatal testing and deserve careful scrutiny. Neither Wertz and Fletcher nor Botkin offer citations to literature to support their claims of family burden, changed lifestyle, disappointed expectations, or additional expenses, perhaps because they believe these are indisputable. Evaluating the claims, however, requires recognizing an assumption implied in them: that there is no benefit to offset the "burden," in the way that parents can expect rewards of many kinds in their relationship with children who do not have disabilities. This assumption, which permeates much of the medical, social science, and bioethics literature on disability and family life and disability in general, rests on a mistaken notion. As rehabilitation psychologist Beatrice Wright has long maintained,[41,42] people imagine that incapacity in one arena spreads to incapacity in all – the child with cystic fibrosis is always sick and can never play; the child who cannot walk cannot join classmates in word games, parties, or sleepovers; someone who is blind is also unable to hear or speak. Someone who needs assistance with one activity is perceived to need assistance in all areas and to contribute nothing to the social, emotional, or instrumental aspects of family life.

Assuming for a moment that there are "extra burdens" associated with certain aspects of raising children with disabilities, consider the "extra burdens" associated with raising other children: those with

extraordinary (above statistical norm) aptitude for athletics, art, music, or mathematics. In a book on gifted children, Ellen Winner writes,

[A]ll the family's energy becomes focused on this child. . . .Families focus in two ways on the gifted child's development: either one or both parents spend a great deal of time stimulating and teaching the child themselves, or parents make sacrifices so that the child gets high-level training from the best available teachers. In both cases, family life is totally arranged around the child's needs. Parents channel their interests into their child's talent area and become enormously invested in their child's progress.[43] (p. 187)

Parents, professionals working with the family, and the larger society all value the gift of the violin prodigy, the talent of the future Olympic figure skater, the aptitude of a child who excels in science and who might one day discover the cure for cancer. They perceive that all the extra work and rearrangement associated with raising such children will provide what people seek in parenthood: the opportunity to give ourselves to a new being who starts out with the best we can give, who will enrich us, gladden others, contribute to the world, and make us proud.

If professionals and parents believed that children with disabilities could indeed provide their parents many of the same satisfactions as any other child in terms of stimulation, love, companionship, pride, and pleasure in influencing the growth and development of another, they might reexamine their belief that in psychological, material, and social terms, the burdens of raising disabled children outweigh the benefits. A vast array of literature, both parental narrative and social science quantitative and qualitative research, powerfully testifies to the rewards – typical and atypical – of raising children with many of the conditions for which prenatal testing is considered de rigeur and abortion is expected (Down syndrome, hemophilia, cystic fibrosis, to name only some).[44–50] Yet bioethics, public health, and genetics remain woefully – scandalously – oblivious, ignorant, or dismissive of any information that challenges the conviction that disability dooms families.

Two years before the gene mutation responsible for much cystic fibrosis was identified, Walker et al. published their findings about the effects of cystic fibrosis on family life. They found that mothers of children with cystic fibrosis did not differ from mothers of children without the condition on measures of

> . . .Child Dependency and Management Difficulty, Limits on Family Opportunity, Family Disharmony, and Financial Stress. The difference between the two groups of mothers almost reached statistical significance on a fifth subscale, Personal Burden, which measured the mother's feeling of burden in her caretaking role. . . .The similarities between mothers of children with cystic fibrosis and those with healthy children were more apparent than the differences. Mothers of children with cystic fibrosis did not report significantly higher levels of stress than did the control group mothers of healthy children. Contrary to suggestions that mothers of children with cystic fibrosis feel guilty and inadequate as parents, the mothers in this study reported levels of parenting competence equal to those reported by the mothers of healthy children.[50] (pp. 242–3)

The literature on how disability affects family life is, to be sure, replete with discussions of stress; anger at unsupportive members of the helping professions; distress caused by hostility from extended family, neighbors, and strangers; and frustration that many disability-related expenses are not covered by health insurance.[44–51] And it is a literature that increasingly tries to distinguish why – under what conditions – some families of disabled children founder and others thrive. Contrary to the beliefs still much abroad in medicine, bioethics, and public health, recent literature does not suggest that, on balance, families raising children who have disabilities experience more stress and disruption than any other family.[52]

Implications for Professional Practice

Reporting in 1997 on a 5-year study of how families affected by cystic fibrosis and sickle cell anemia viewed genetic testing technologies, Duster and Beeson learned to their surprise that the closer the relationship between the family member and the affected individual, the more uncomfortable the family member was with the technology.

> [The] closer people are to someone with genetic disease the more problematic and usually unacceptable genetic testing is as a strategy for dealing with the issues. . . .The experience of emotional closeness to someone with a genetic disease reduces, rather than increases, the acceptability of selective abortion. A close relationship with an affected person appears to make it more difficult to evaluate the meaning or worth of that person's existence solely in terms of their genetic disease. Family members consistently affirm the value of the person's life in spite of the disorders, and see value for their family in their experiences with [and] of this member, and in meeting the challenges the disease poses.[53] (p. 43)

This finding is consistent with other reports that parents of children with disabilities generally reject the idea of prenatal testing and abortion of subsequent fetuses, even if those fetuses are found to carry the same disabling trait.[54, 55]

Professionals charged with developing technologies, offering tests, and interpreting results should assess their current assumptions and practice on the basis of the literature on disability and family life generally and data about how such families perceive selective abortion. Of the many implications of such data, the first is that familiarity with disability as one characteristic of a child one loves changes the meaning of disability for parents contemplating a subsequent birth. The disability, instead of being the child's sole, or most salient, characteristic, becomes only one of the child's characteristics, along with appearance, aptitudes, temperament, interests, and quirks. The typical woman or couple discussing prenatal testing and possible pregnancy termination knows very little about the conditions for which testing is available, much less what these conditions might mean for the daily life of the child and the family. People who do not already have a child with a disability and who are contemplating prenatal testing must learn considerably more than the names of some typical impairments and the odds of their child's having one.

To provide ethical and responsible clinical care for anyone concerned about reproduction, professionals themselves must know far more than they now do about life with disability; they must convey more information, and different information, than they now typically provide. Shown a film about the lives of families raising children with Down syndrome, nurses and genetic counselors – but not parents – described the film as unrealistic and too positive a portrayal of family life.[56] Whether the clinician is a genetics professional or (as is increasingly the case) an obstetrician promoting prenatal diagnosis as routine care for pregnant women, the tone, timing, and content of the counseling process cry out for drastic overhaul.

Many discussions of genetic counseling suggest that counselors (even graduates of master's-level genetic counseling programs, who now provide a minority of the information that surrounds the testing process and the decisions following results) are ill equipped by their own training and norms of practice to provide any insights into disability in today's society. Most graduate programs in genetic counseling do not include courses in the social implications of life with disability for children and families; do not include contact between counselor trainees and disabled children and adults outside clinical settings; and do not expose counselors to the laws, disability rights organizations, and peer support groups that constitute what is described as the disability rights and independent living movement. Often, if providers seek a "consumer" perspective on genetic issues, they consult the Alliance of Genetic Support Groups. This organization, however, has focused on genetic research and cure and has not concentrated on improving life for people with genetic disabilities; it is not currently allied in activity or ideology with the disabled community and the social paradigm of disability. Reviews of medical school curricula suggest that medical students do not receive formal instruction on life with disability, which would remind them that the people with disabilities they see in their offices have lives outside those offices.

Until their own education is revamped, obstetricians, midwives, nurses, and genetics professionals cannot properly counsel prospective parents. With broader exposure themselves, they would be far more likely to engage in discussions with their patients that would avoid problems such as those noted by Lippman and Wilfond in a survey of genetic counselors. These researchers found that counselors provided far more positive information about Down syndrome and cystic fibrosis to parents already raising children diagnosed with those conditions than they did to prospective parents deciding whether to continue pregnancies in which the fetus had been found to have the condition.

> At the least, we must recognize that every description of a genetic disorder is a story that contains a message. The story is the vehicle through which complex and voluminous information is reduced for the purposes of communication between health-care provider and health-care seeker. The message is shaped as the storyteller selects what to include and what to exclude to reduce the amount of information. . . . Should we strive to tell the same story to families considering carrier testing and prenatal diagnosis and to families who receive a postnatal diagnosis?. . .Is telling the same story required if we are to provide sufficiently balanced information to allow potential parents to make fully informed family-planning decisions?[57]

Lippman and Wilfond question the disparity in information provided; I call for change to ensure that everyone obtaining testing or seeking information about genetic or prenatally diagnosable disability receives sufficient information about predictable difficulties, supports, and life events associated with a disabling condition to enable them to consider how a child's disability would fit into their own hopes for parenthood. Such information for all prospective parents should include, at a minimum, a detailed description of the biological, cognitive, or psychological impairments associated with specific disabilities, and what those impairments imply for day-to-day functioning; a discussion of the laws governing education, entitlements to family support services, access to buildings and transportation, and financial assistance to disabled children and their families; and literature by family members of disabled children and by disabled people themselves.

If prenatal testing indicates a disabling condition in the fetus, the following disability-specific information should be given to the prospective parents: information about services to benefit children with specific disabilities in a particular area, and about which of these a child and family are likely to need immediately after birth; contact information for a parent-group representative; and contact information for a member of a disability rights group or independent living center. In addition, the parents should be offered a visit with both a child and family and an adult living with the diagnosed disability.

Although some prospective parents will reject some or all of this information and these contacts, responsible practice that is concerned with genuine informed decision making and true reproductive choice must include access to this information, timed so that prospective parents can assimilate general ideas about life with disability before testing and obtain particular disability-relevant information if they discover that their fetus carries a disabling trait. These ideas may appear unrealistic or unfeasible, but a growing number of diverse voices support similar versions of these reforms to encourage wise decision making. Statements by Little People of America, the National Down Syndrome Congress, the National Institutes of Health workshop, and the Hastings Center Project on Prenatal Testing for Genetic Disability all urge versions of these changes in the process of helping people make childbearing decisions.[58–61]

These proposals may be startling in the context of counseling for genetically transmitted or prenatally diagnosable disability, but they resonate with the recent discussion about childbearing for women infected with the HIV virus:

> The primary task of the provider would be to engage the client in a meaningful discussion of the implications of having a child and of not having a child for herself, for the client's family and for the child who would be born. . . .Providers would assist clients in examining what childbearing means to them. . . .Providers also

would assist clients in gaining an understanding of the factual information relevant to decisions about childbearing. . .however, the conversation would cover a range of topics that go far beyond what can be understood as the relevant *medical* facts, and the direction of the conversation would vary depending on each person's life circumstances and priorities [emphasis added].[62 (pp. 453–4)]

This counseling process for women with HIV who are considering motherhood demonstrates that information in itself is not sufficient. As Mary White, Arthur Caplan, and other commentators on genetic counseling have noted, the norm of nondirectiveness, even when followed, may leave people who are seeking help with difficult decisions feeling bewildered and abandoned.[63,64] Along with others who have expressed growing concern about needed reforms in the conduct of prenatal testing and counseling, I urge a serious conversation between prospective parents and clinicians about what the parents seek in childrearing and how a disabling condition in general or a specific type of impairment would affect their hopes and expectations for the rewards of parenthood. For some people, any mobility, sensory, cognitive, or health impairment may indeed lead to disappointment of parental hopes; for others, it may be far easier to imagine incorporating disability into family life without believing that the rest of their lives will be blighted.

Ideally, such discussions will include mention of the fact that every child inevitably differs from parental dreams, and that successful parenting requires a mix of shaping and influencing children and ruefully appreciating the ways they pick and choose from what parents offer, sometimes rejecting tastes, activities, or values dear to the parents. If prospective parents cannot envision appreciating the child who will depart in particular, known ways from the parents' fantasy, are they truly ready to raise would-be athletes when they hate sports, classical violinists when they delight in the Grateful Dead? Testing and abortion guarantee little about the child and the life parents create and nurture, and all parents and children will be harmed by inflated notions of what parenting in an age of genetic knowledge can bring in terms of fulfilled expectations.

Public health professionals must do more than they have been doing to change the climate in which prenatal tests are offered. Think about what people would say if prenatal clinics contained pamphlets telling poor women or African American women that they should consider refraining from childbearing because their children could be similarly poor and could endure discrimination or because they could be less healthy and more likely to find themselves imprisoned than members of the middle class or than Whites. Public health is committed to ending such inequities, not to endorsing them, tolerating them, or asking prospective parents to live with them. Yet the current promotion of prenatal testing condones just such an approach to life with disability.

Practitioners and policymakers can increase women's and couples' reproductive choice through testing and counseling, and they can expend energy and resources on changing the society in which families consider raising disabled children. If families that include children with disabilities now spend more money and ingenuity on after-school care for those children because they are denied entrance into existing programs attended by their peers and siblings,[65] public health can join with others to ensure that existing programs include *all* children. The principle of education for all, which is reforming public education for disabled children, must spread to incorporate those same children into the network of services and supports that parents count on for other children. Such programs, like other institutions, must change to fit the people who exist in the world, not claim that some people should not exist because society is not prepared for them. We can fight to reform insurance practices that deny reimbursement for diabetes test strips; special diets for people with disabilities; household modifications that give disabled children freedom to explore their environment; and modifications of equipment, games, and toys that enable disabled children to participate in activities comparable to those of their peers. Public health can fight to end the catch-22 that removes subsidies for life-sustaining personal assistance services once disabled people enter the workforce, a policy that acts as a powerful disincentive to productivity and needlessly perpetuates poverty and dependence.

Laws such as the Individuals with Disabilities Education Act and the Americans with Disabilities Act chart a course of inclusion for disabled people of all ages. In 1980, Gliedman and Roth, who pioneered the development of the minority-group paradigm that infuses much of the critique of current genetic technology, wrote a blueprint for the inclusive society that public health should strive to create:

Suppose that somewhere in the world an advanced industrial society genuinely respected the needs and the humanity of handicapped people. What would a visitor from this country make of the position of the disabled individual in American life?. . .To begin with, the traveler would take for granted that a market of millions of children and tens of millions of adults would not be ignored. He would assume that many industries catered to the special needs of the handicapped. Some of these needs would be purely medical. . .but many would not be medical. The visitor would expect to find industries producing everyday household and domestic appliances designed for the use of people with poor motor coordination. . . .He would anticipate a profusion of specialized and sometimes quite simple gadgets designed to enhance control of a handicapped person over his physical world – special hand tools, office supplies, can openers, eating utensils, and the like. . . .

As he examined our newspapers, magazines, journals and books, as he watched our movies, television shows, and went to our theaters, he would look for many reports about handicap,. . . cartoon figures on children's TV programs, and many characters in children's stories who are handicapped. He would expect constantly to come across advertisements aimed at handicapped people. He would expect to find many handicapped people appearing in advertisements not specifically aimed at them.

The traveler would explore our factories, believing that handicapped people were employed in proportion to their vast numbers. . . .He would walk the streets of our towns and cities. And everywhere he went he would expect to see multitudes of handicapped people going about their business, taking a holiday, passing an hour with able-bodied or handicapped friends, or simply being alone. . . .

He would explore our manmade environment, anticipating that provision was made for the handicapped in our cities and towns. . . .He would expect the tiniest minutiae of our dwellings to reflect the vast numbers of disabled people. . . .

He would assume that disabled individuals had their share of elected and appointive offices. He would expect to find that the role played by the disabled as a special interest group at the local and national levels was fully commensurate with their great numbers.[66 (pp. 13–15)]

Despite the strides of the past few decades, our current society is far from the ideal described by Gliedman and Roth, an ideal toward which the disability community strives. Medicine, bioethics, and public health can put their efforts toward promoting such a society; with such efforts, disability could become nearly as easy to incorporate into the familial and social landscape as the other differences these professions respect and affirm as ordinary parts of the human condition. Given that more than 50 million people in the US population have disabling traits and that prenatal tests may become increasingly available to detect more of them, we are confronting the fact that tests may soon be available for characteristics that we have until now considered inevitable facts of human life, such as heart disease.

In order to make testing and selecting for or against disability consonant with improving life for those who will inevitably be born with or acquire disabilities, our clinical and policy establishments must communicate that it is as acceptable to live with a disability as it is to live without one and that society will support and appreciate everyone with the inevitable variety of traits. We can assure prospective parents that they and their future child will be welcomed whether or not the child has a disability. If that professional message is conveyed, more prospective parents may envision that their lives can be rewarding, whatever the characteristics of the child they are raising. When our professions can envision such communication and the reality of incorporation and appreciation of people with disabilities, prenatal technology can help people to make decisions without implying that only one decision is right. If the child with a disability is not a problem for the world, and the world is not a problem for the child, perhaps we can diminish our desire for prenatal testing and selective abortion and can comfortably welcome and support children of all characteristics.

References

1 Wertz D.C. and Fletcher J.C. Sex selection through prenatal diagnosis. In: Holmes H.B. and Purdy L.M., eds. *Feminist Perspectives in Medical Ethics*. Bloomington: Indiana University Press; 1992: 240–53.

2 Schüklenk U., Stein E., Kerin J., and Byne W. The ethics of genetic research on sexual orientation. *Hastings Center Rep.* 1997; 27(4):6–13.

3 *Mapping Our Genes*. Washington, DC: US Congress, Office of Technology Assessment; 1988.

4 Retsinas J. Impact of prenatal technology on attitudes toward disabled infants. In: Wertz D. *Research in the Sociology of Healthcare*. Westport, Conn: JAI Press; 1991: 75–102.

5 Beaudet A.L. Carrier screening for cystic fibrosis. *Am J Hum Genet.* 1990; 47:603–5.

6 Kuppermann M., Goldberg J.D., Nease R.F., and Washington A.E. Who should be offered prenatal diagnosis? The thirty-five-year-old question. *Am J Public Health.* 1999; 89:160–3.

7 Rothenberg K.H., Thompson E.J., eds. *Women and Prenatal Testing: Facing the Challenges of Genetic Technology*. Columbus: Ohio State University Press; 1994.

8 Miringoff M.L. *The Social Costs of Genetic Welfare*. New Brunswick, NJ: Rutgers University Press; 1991.

9 Hubbard R. *The Politics of Women's Biology*. New Brunswick, NJ: Rutgers University Press; 1990: chap 12–14.

10 Lippman A. Prenatal genetic testing and screening: constructing needs and reinforcing inequities. *Am J Law Med.* 1991; 17(1–2):15–50.

11 Field M.A. Killing "the handicapped" – before and after birth. *Harvard Womens Law J.* 1993; 16:79–138.

12 Fine M. and Asch A. The question of disability: no easy answers for the women's movement. *Reproductive Rights Newsletter.* 1982; 4(3):19–20.

13 Minden S. Born and unborn: the implications of reproductive technologies for people with disabilities. In: Arditti R., Duelli-Klein R., Mindin S., eds. *Test-Tube*

Women: What Future for Motherhood? Boston, Mass: Pandora Press; 1984: 298–312.

14 Finger, A. *Past Due: Disability, Pregnancy and Birth.* Seattle, Wash: Seal Press; 1987.

15 Kaplan D. Prenatal screening and diagnosis: the impact on persons with disabilities. In: Rothenberg K.H. and Thompson E.J., eds. *Women and Prenatal Testing: Facing the Challenges of Genetic Technology.* Columbus: Ohio State University Press; 1994: 49–61.

16 Asch A. Reproductive technology and disability. In: Cohen S. and Taub N. *Reproductive Laws for the 1990s.* Clifton, NJ: Humana Press; 1989: 69–124.

17 Asch A. and Geller G. Feminism, bioethics and genetics. In: Wolf S., ed. *Feminism and Bioethics: Beyond Reproduction.* New York, NY: Oxford University Press; 1996: 318–50.

18 Boorse C. Concepts of health. In: Van de Veer D. and Regan T., eds. *Health Care Ethics.* Philadelphia, Pa: Temple University Press; 1987: 359–93.

19 Daniels N.L. *Just Health Care: Studies in Philosophy and Health Policy.* Cambridge, England: Cambridge University Press; 1985.

20 National Organization on Disability's 1998 Harris Survey of Americans With Disabilities. See http://nod.org/research_publications/surveys_research and http://www.socio.com/rad43.php.

21 Schneider J. and Conrad P. *Having Epilepsy: The Experience and Control of Illness.* Philadelphia, PA: Temple University Press; 1983.

22 Brightman A.J. *Ordinary Moments: The Disabled Experience.* Baltimore, MD: Paul H. Brookes Publishing Co; 1984.

23 Goffman E. *Stigma: Notes on the Management of Spoiled Identity.* Englewood Cliffs, NJ: Prentice-Hall; 1963.

24 Gartner A. and Joe T. *Images of the Disabled, Disabling Images.* New York, NY: Praeger; 1987.

25 Hockenberry J. *Moving Violations: War Zones, Wheelchairs, and Declarations of Independence.* New York, NY: Hyperion; 1996.

26 Russel M. *Beyond Ramps: Disability at the End of the Social Contract.* Monroe, ME: Common Courage Press; 1998.

27 Bickenbach J.E. *Physical Disability and Social Policy.* Toronto, Ontario: University of Toronto Press; 1993.

28 Americans with Disabilities Act (Pub L No. 101–336, 1990, § 2).

29 Watson J.D. President's essay: genes and politics. *Annual Report Cold Springs Harbor.* 1996: 1–20.

30 Shaw M.W. Presidential address: to be or not to be, that is the question. *Am J Human Genetics.* 1984; 36:1–9.

31 Feinberg J. The child's right to an open future. In: Aiken W, LaFollette H, eds. *Whose Child? Children's Rights, Parental Authority, and State Power.* Totowa, NJ: Rowman & Littlefield; 1980: 124–53.

32 Green R. Prenatal autonomy and the obligation not to harm one's child genetically. *J Law Med Ethics.* 1996; 25(1):5–16.

33 Davis D.S. Genetic dilemmas and the child's right to an open future. *Hastings Cent Rep.* 1997; 27(2):7–15.

34 Purdy L. Loving future people. In: Callahan J., ed. *Reproduction, Ethics and the Law.* Bloomington: Indiana University Press; 1995: 300–27.

35 Ray C. and West J. Social, sexual and personal implications of paraplegia. *Paraplegia.* 1984; 22:75–86.

36 Saigal S., Feeny D., Rosenbaum P., Furlong W., Burrows E., and Stoskopf B. Self-perceived health status and health-related quality of life of extremely low-birth-weight infants at adolescence. *JAMA.* 1996; 276:453–9.

37 Tyson J.E. and Broyles R.S. Progress in assessing the longterm outcome of extremely low-birth-weight infants. *JAMA.* 1996; 276:492–3.

38 Turnbull H.R. and Turnbull A.P., eds. *Parents Speak Out: Then and Now.* Columbus, Ohio: Charles E. Merrill Publishing Co; 1985.

39 Wertz D.C. and Fletcher J.C. A critique of some feminist challenges to prenatal diagnosis. *J Womens Health.* 1993; 2:173–88.

40 Botkin J. Fetal privacy and confidentiality. *Hastings Cent Rep.* 1995; 25(3):32–9.

41 Wright B.A. Attitudes and the fundamental negative bias: conditions and correlates. In: Yuker H.E., ed. *Attitudes Toward Persons With Disabilities.* New York, NY: Springer; 1988: 3–21.

42 Wright B.A. *Physical Disability: A Pyscho-Social Approach.* New York, NY: Harper & Row; 1983.

43 Winner E. *Gifted Children: Myths and Realities.* New York, NY: Basic Books; 1996.

44 Massie R. and Massie S.. *Journey.* New York, NY: Alfred A. Knopf; 1975.

45 Berube M. *Life As We Know It: A Father, a Family and an Exceptional Child.* New York, NY: Pantheon; 1996.

46 Beck M. *Expecting Adam: A True Story of Birth, Rebirth and Everyday Magic.* New York, NY: Times Books/Random House; 1999.

47 Turnbull A.., Patterson J.M., Behr S.K., Murphy D.L., Marquis J.G., and Blue-Banning J, eds. *Cognitive Coping,*

Families, and Disability. Baltimore, MD: Paul H. Brookes Publishing Co; 1993.

48 Taanila A., Kokkonen J., and Jarvelin M.K. The long-term effects of children's early-onset disability on marital relationships. *Dev Med Child Neurol.* 1996; 38:567–77.

49 Van Riper M., Ryff C., and Pridham K. Parental and family well-being in families of children with Down syndrome: a comparative study. *Res Nurs Health.* 1992; 15:227–35.

50 Walker L.S., Ford M.B., and Donald W.D. Cystic fibrosis and family stress: effects of age and severity of illness. *Pediatrics.* 1987; 79:239–46.

51 Lipsky D.K. A parental perspective on stress and coping. *Am J Orthopsychiatry.* 1985; 55:614–17.

52 Ferguson P., Gartner A., and Lipsky D.K. The experience of disabilities in families: a synthesis of research and parent narratives. In Parens E. and Asch A., eds. *Prenatal Testing and Disability Rights.* Washington, DC: Georgetown University Press; 2000.

53 Duster T. and Beeson D. *Pathways and Barriers to Genetic Testing and Screening: Molecular Genetics Meets the "High Risk" Family.* Final report. Washington, DC: US Dept of Energy; October 1997.

54 Wertz D.C. How parents of affected children view selective abortion. In: Holmes H.B., ed. *Issues in Reproductive Technology.* New York, NY: New York University Press; 1992: 161–89.

55 Evers-Kiebooms G., Denayer L., and van den Berghe H. A child with cystic fibrosis, II: subsequent family planning decisions, reproduction and use of prenatal diagnosis. *Clin Genet.* 1990; 37:207–15.

56 Cooley W.C., Graham E.S., Moeschler J.B., and Graham J.M. Reactions of mothers and medical professionals to a film about Down syndrome. *Am J Dis Child.* 1990; 144:1112–16.

57 Lippman A. and Wilfond B. Twice-told tales: stories about genetic disorders. *Am J Human Genet.* 1992; 51: 936–7.

58 Little People of America, Position Statement on Genetic Discoveries in Dwarfism. See http://www.lpaonline.org/.

59 National Down Syndrome Congress. *Position Statement on Prenatal Testing and Eugenics: Families' Rights and Needs.* Prepared for and approved by the Professional Advisory Committee. August 1994. See http://www.ndsccenter.org/issue-position-statements/.

60 Appendix: Reproductive genetic testing: impact on women. National Institutes of Health workshop statement. In: Rothenberg K.H. and Thompson E.J., eds. *Women and Prenatal Testing: Facing the Challenges of Genetic Technology.* Columbus: Ohio State University Press; 1994: 295–300.

61 Parens E. and Asch A. The disability rights critique of prenatal genetic testing: reflections and recommendations. *Hastings Cent Rep.* 1999; 29(5, suppl): S1–S22.

62 Faden R.R., Kass N.E., Acuff K.L., et al. HIV infection and childbearing: a proposal for public policy and clinical practice. In: Faden R. and Kass N., eds. *HIV, Aids and Childbearing: Public Policy, Private Lives.* New York, NY: Oxford University Press; 1996: 447–61.

63 Caplan A.L. Neutrality is not morality. In: Bartels D., Leroy B., and Caplan A.L., eds. *Prescribing Our Futures: Ethical Challenges in Genetic Counseling.* New York, NY: Aldine De Gruyter; 1993.

64 White M.T. Making responsible decisions: an interpretive ethic for genetic decisionmaking. *Hastings Cent Rep.* 1999; 29:14–21.

65 Freedman R.I, Lichfield L., and Warfield M.E. Balancing work and family: perspectives of parents of the children with developmental disabilities. *Fam Soc J Contemp Hum Serv.* October 1995: 507–14.

66 Gliedman J. and Roth W. *The Unexpected Minority: Handicapped Children in America.* New York, NY: Harcourt Brace Jovanovich; 1980.

91

Down Syndrome Screening Isn't about Public Health

It's about Eliminating a Group of People

Renate Lindeman

Upon delivering my first child 11 years ago, I heard the words "Down syndrome," and my world collapsed. Visions of children sitting passively in a corner watching life go by, not participating, kept me awake those first nights as a mom.

It didn't take me long, though, to figure out that my ideas were based on negative, outdated information that had nothing to do with the reality of life with Down syndrome today. My daughter April is an active, outgoing girl. She's my nature child, wildly passionate about anything with four legs. Although April uses few words, she's a master communicator. Through her, I've learned that Down syndrome is not the scary, terrible condition it's made out to be.

But while governments (rightly) ban gender selection, selective abortion continues to be encouraged for children with Down syndrome. In the United States and abroad, screenings are a routine part of healthcare programs, and the result is the near-elimination of these children.

When pregnant with my daughter Hazel, tests showed she, too, would be born with Down syndrome. I was shocked when an acquaintance asked me why I did not choose abortion — as if she were a mistake that could be easily erased. Although my personal prejudices have radically changed since the birth of my first daughter with Down syndrome, I realized that negative attitudes about the condition remain deeply rooted. To many, my children and their cohort are examples of avoidable human suffering, as well as a financial burden. Knowing that individuals look at my daughters this way hurts, but seeing governments and medical professionals worldwide reinforce these prejudices by promoting selection is horrendous.

Denmark was the first European country to introduce routine screening for Down syndrome in 2006 as a public health-care program. France, Switzerland and other European countries soon followed. The unspoken but obvious message is that Down syndrome is something so unworthy that we would not want to wish it for our children or society. With the level of screening among pregnant Danish women as high as 90 percent, the Copenhagen Post reported in 2011 that Denmark "could be a country without a single citizen with Down syndrome in the not too distant future."

Original publication details: Renata Lindeman, "Down Syndrome Screening Isn't About Public Health. It's About Eliminating a Group of People," from *Washington Post*, June 16, 2015. Reproduced courtesy of Renata Lindeman.

In 2011, the newest feat in prenatal testing was introduced: the NIPT (Non Invasive Prenatal Test). This DNA test can, with reasonable accuracy, detect Down syndrome in early pregnancy from a single drop of blood taken from the mother. Hailed by medical professionals as the holy grail in prenatal testing, the NIPT has quickly spread across the globe.

Recent research in Britain indicates that introducing the NIPT leads to a higher uptake of screening. With termination rates varying around the world from about 67 percent in the United States to an average of 92 percent in Europe, this will promote even more intensive de-selection of fetuses with Down syndrome, which in turn will negatively affect their position in society.

I don't judge the women who make the choice to terminate. It must be hard to withstand the bias of medical professionals, people you trust most with your health and well-being, when you're pregnant and vulnerable. A 2013 study reports that parents are 2.5 times more likely to have a negative experience on receiving the initial Down syndrome diagnosis than to have a positive one. One in four participants said they had been encouraged by a medical professional to abort, and many received inadequate information and little compassion.

With DNA tests called MaterniT21 being popularly referred to as the "Down test," the primary aim of testing needs no further explanation. I detest the fear that is cultivated by medical professionals, the medical industry and politicians about giving birth to a child with Down syndrome. Down syndrome does not cause human suffering. The real danger lies in voices that claim our children need to be tested before we can decide who is worthy of life. Women are not incubators of socially preferable descendants.

As a mom, former president of a Down syndrome society and spokesperson for Downpride, a grass-roots parent group, I find most people with Down syndrome possess an enormous zest for life, making them very pleasant company, and there are many firsthand accounts describing the ability of people with Down syndrome to bring simplicity and openness to communities. But these aspects of the condition remain understudied. One 2011 study did show that the brothers and sisters of people with Down syndrome overwhelmingly feel love and pride toward their siblings; participants also credited having a sibling with Down syndrome with enhancing their lives and increasing their empathy.

Nevertheless, like other European governments, the Netherlands is currently considering permanently including the NIPT, primarily aimed at Down syndrome, in its prenatal screening program. An American-European-Canadian study on DNA screening for Down syndrome was published in the New England Journal of Medicine this year. Dick Oepkes, chairman of the Dutch NIPT consortium, called results "positive," stating in a recent interview: "Surveys show women experience waiting for test results arduous. Offering the DNA test as a first step will allow women who consider terminating the pregnancy to make their choice before they have felt the fetus move."

The irony is that for a baby with Down syndrome born today, the outlook has never been better. Medical and social advances have radically changed what it means to live with Down syndrome. Most people with Down syndrome are included in schools and communities. They live healthier, longer lives, and many adults live independently, have jobs and enjoy a rich social life. In 2013 a young woman with Down syndrome became Spain's first councilor. One study showed that the majority of people with Down syndrome report being happy and fulfilled, regardless of their functional skills. This is why Downpride is calling on the United Nations High Commissioner for Human Rights to stop systematic screening for Down syndrome as part of public-health programs and to regulate the introduction of prenatal genetic testing – testing should be used to enhance health and human well-being instead of discriminating against people based on their genetic predisposition.

Screening and selection say nothing about the inherent worth of people with Down syndrome. They say everything about the elevation of the capacity for economic achievement above other human traits. My children are fascinating, demanding, delightful, present, annoying, dependent, loving, cuddly, different, unpredictable and completely human, just like other children. They are not a mistake, a burden or a reflection of my "personal choice," but an integral part of society.

If we allow our governments to set up health programs that result in the systematic elimination of a group of people quite happy being themselves, under the false pretense of women's rights, then that *is* a personal choice — one we have to face honestly.

92

I Would've Aborted a Fetus with Down Syndrome
Women Need that Right

Ruth Marcus

There is a new push in antiabortion circles to pass state laws aimed at barring women from terminating their pregnancies after the fetus has been determined to have Down syndrome. These laws are unconstitutional, unenforceable – and wrong.

This is a difficult subject to discuss because there are so many parents who have – and cherish – a child with Down syndrome. Many people with Down syndrome live happy and fulfilled lives. The new Gerber baby with Down syndrome is awfully cute.

I have had two children; I was old enough, when I became pregnant, that it made sense to do the testing for Down syndrome. Back then, it was amniocentesis, performed after 15 weeks; now, chorionic villus sampling can provide a conclusive determination as early as nine weeks. I can say without hesitation that, tragic as it would have felt and ghastly as a second-trimester abortion would have been, I would have terminated those pregnancies had the testing come back positive. I would have grieved the loss and moved on.

And I am not alone. More than two-thirds of American women choose abortion in such circumstances. Isn't that the point – or at least inherent in the point – of prenatal testing in the first place?

If you believe that abortion is equivalent to murder, the taking of a human life, then of course you would make a different choice. But that is not my belief, and the Supreme Court has affirmed my freedom to have that belief and act accordingly.

I respect – I admire – families that knowingly welcome a baby with Down syndrome into their lives. Certainly, to be a parent is to take the risks that accompany parenting; you love your child for who she is, not what you want her to be.

But accepting that essential truth is different from compelling a woman to give birth to a child whose intellectual capacity will be impaired, whose life choices will be limited, whose health may be compromised. Most children with Down syndrome have mild to moderate cognitive impairment, meaning an IQ between 55 and 70 (mild) or between 35 and 55 (moderate). This means limited capacity for independent living and financial security; Down syndrome is life-altering for the entire family.

I'm going to be blunt here: That was not the child I wanted. That was not the choice I would have made. You can call me selfish, or worse, but I am in good company. The evidence is clear that most women

Original publication details: Ruth Marcus, "I Would've Aborted a Fetus with Down Syndrome: Women Need That Right," *Washington Post*, March 9, 2018. Reproduced with permission of Washington Post / PARS.

confronted with the same unhappy alternative would make the same decision.

Which brings us to the Supreme Court. North Dakota, Ohio, Indiana and Louisiana passed legislation to prohibit doctors from performing abortions if the sole reason is because of a diagnosis of Down syndrome; Utah's legislature is debating such a bill.

These laws are flatly inconsistent with the Supreme Court's *Roe v. Wade* ruling, reaffirmed in 1992, that "it is a constitutional liberty of the woman to have some freedom to terminate her pregnancy." *Of the woman.* As U.S. District Judge Tanya Walton Pratt concluded in striking down the Indiana law in September, the high court's determination "leaves no room for the state to examine, let alone prohibit, the basis or bases upon which a woman makes her choice."

Think about it. Can it be that women have more constitutional freedom to choose to terminate their pregnancies on a whim than for the reason that the fetus has Down syndrome? And, to the question of enforceability, who is going to police the decision-making? Doctors are now supposed to turn in their patients – patients whom they owe confidentiality – for making a decision of which the state disapproves?

In an argument worthy of "The Handmaid's Tale," the state of Indiana suggests precisely that scenario. The right to abortion, its lawyer argued before a federal appeals court last month, protects only the "binary" decision of whether to bear a child – not which child you must carry to term once you choose to become pregnant. In other words, though he didn't put it in these exact words, the state can hijack your body.

Technological advances in prenatal testing pose difficult moral choices about what, if any, genetic anomaly or defect justifies an abortion. Nearsightedness? Being short? There are creepy, eugenic aspects of the new technology that call for vigorous public debate. But in the end, the Constitution mandates – and a proper understanding of the rights of the individual against those of the state underscores – that these excruciating choices be left to individual women, not to government officials who believe they know best.

Part XI

Neuroethics

Introduction

As Neil Levy points out at the start of his article "Neuroethics: Ethics and the Sciences of the Mind," "neuroethics" could mean two quite distinct things. It could refer to the *ethics of neuroscience,* that is, the ethics of applying the findings of neuroscience to human beings; or it could refer to the *neuroscience of ethics,* that is, using neuroscience to help us understand ethics, and the brain processes behind our ethical judgments. Levy's main focus in the extract we reprint here is the ethics of neuroscience, and more specifically, the ethics of weakening memories that cause post-traumatic stress disorder (PTSD), though he also raises the broader issue of cognitive enhancement. We too, in this Part, will be concerned with the ethics of neuroscience, rather than the neuroscience of ethics, because strictly speaking, only the former falls within the field of bioethics. Yet the two fields are not entirely unrelated. When Levy turns his attention to drugs shown to have memory and attention-enhancing capacity, he considers objections made by philosophers and bioethicists who argue that such drugs would likely increase the risk of some or many of our actions becoming inauthentic. In response, Levy asks why these writers, along with a significant proportion of the general public, object more to the use of drugs that enhance our cognitive abilities than to other techniques that seek the same goals. To explain this, Levy draws on findings from neuroscientific research on underlying factors that affect our ethical judgments, both in general, and on the specific issue of dualism, or the relationship between our minds and our brains. He then uses these findings to debunk the objections and argue that we should be more accepting of the use of psychopharmaceuticals.

The use of drugs that affect not only our thoughts, but our deepest feelings and most important relationships, is the subject of our next article, aptly entitled "Engineering Love." Julian Savulescu and Anders Sandberg suspect that it may not be within our biological nature to live – happily – in relationships lasting much longer than 10 or 15 years. Given that loving relationships contribute significantly to our well-being, and that we are learning more about the neuroscience of love and even of faithfulness in love, they ask whether we should use this newfound knowledge to design drugs that would a promote or enable loving life-long relationships, and thus make our lives better than our nature, unaided, is likely to do.

Francesca Minerva also writes about "the medicalization of love," but this time in the context of dealing with the pain that unrequited love can cause. In "Unrequited Love Hurts: Should Doctors Treat Broken Hearts?" she refers to research on the neurological correlates of being abandoned by someone you continue to love, and to the possibilities of relieving the pain caused by such abandonment. After discussing two objections to the idea that doctors should become involved in treating heartbreak, she gives an affirmative answer to the question posed in her subtitle, arguing that medical intervention in this painful situation should be regarded as a form of therapy, not enhancement. (As the acknowledgement at the end of her article indicates, she writes from personal experience.)

Walter Glannon takes up a different kind of intervention in "Stimulating Brains, Altering Minds." Deep brain stimulation, or DBS, involves implanting electrodes in the brain. When a battery is connected to the electrodes, the electrical current stimulates activity in the areas of the brain where the electrodes have been placed. DBS can enable patients with Parkinson's disease to regain control over their limbs, and may be useful for some other psychiatric disorders; but it can also bring about disturbing side-effects, including personality changes, such as more impulsive behavior.

Glannon discusses a case in which DBS for Parkinson's disease impaired the patient's decision-making capacity to such an extent that he had to be committed to a psychiatric hospital. Yet when the stimulation was stopped, and his decision-making capacity restored, his loss of motor control was so severe that he was confined to bed and completely dependent on others. Given the choice, the patient chose to restore his own motor control, and, as the lesser evil, give up the decision-making capacity that is essential to being an autonomous agent. Glannon defends the view that doctors should act on a patient's autonomous choice of the option he considers will give him a better quality of life, even if that decision is to give up one's autonomy.

Felicitas Kraemer discusses the same case in her essay "Authenticity or Autonomy? When Deep Brain Stimulation Causes a Dilemma," but she disputes Glannon's interpretation of the patient's choice. Drawing on studies of different patients, she speculates that the patient described by Glannon may not have been choosing a better quality of life for himself, but rather the form of life in which he felt he was his authentic self. Whereas some may see intervention in the brain as changing who we are, Kraemer's interpretation suggests that in some cases it is the disease that changes who we are, and the brain intervention that restores a lost sense of authenticity. This leads Kraemer to ask what weight we should give to the feeling of authenticity. Is it an important intrinsic value, or only a preference that is valuable because people generally have a higher quality of life when they feel that they are living authentically? Whichever answer we give, interventions that restore a feeling of authenticity may be desirable.

Over the past century, as knowledge in the biological and medical sciences has progressed with increasing rapidity, ethics has often struggled to keep up. In the final article in this section, Sara Goering and Rafael Yuste look towards a future in which we develop more sophisticated neurotechnologies that will, as they say, "provide access to the core mechanisms that underlie human identity, memories, emotions, personality and, more generally, our minds." Some of these technologies sound like the stuff of science fiction, but Goering and Yuste believe that it is high time to prepare for them. Their title – "On the Necessity of Ethical Guidelines for Novel Neurotechnologies" – indicates what they think we need to do. Once again, the prospect of a different world is opening up, and neuroscientists, philosophers, lawyers, and social scientists will need to work together to draw up a framework that enables the new technologies to do the good they are capable of doing without threatening values we wish, after reflection, to preserve.

93

Neuroethics

Ethics and the Sciences of the Mind

Neil Levy

The spectacular growth of applied ethics over the past several decades has been spurred, in important part, by the growth in medical knowledge and associated technologies. As our powers over life and death have expanded, so have the potential for these powers to be misused; accordingly, high quality ethical reflection on the nature and limits of these powers has come to seem necessary. As a consequence, a whole new subdiscipline was born, called bioethics. More recently, we have seen an equally dramatic expansion in our knowledge of the workings of the mind/brain. Our increasing powers over the mind have led to a similar demand for ethical reflection, and thus the birth of another new subfield of applied ethics: *neuroethics*. Neuroethics is to the sciences of the mind as bioethics is to the medical sciences.

In one central respect, however, neuroethics is significantly different to bioethics in its scope and ambitions. Whereas bioethics could be described as applying the tools of philosophers to a new set of issues, neuroethics is as much concerned with the nature of the tools it uses as with the problems to which it seeks to apply them. Since the tools of philosophers are cognitive, and the sciences of the mind are concerned with the nature

of cognition (broadly understood), the sciences of the mind are concerned with our tools: with their nature, their strengths and weaknesses and with their reliability. Hence the neuroethicist is adrift on Neurath's boat to an even greater extent than most philosophers: she must address first-order ethical issues using tools whose very reliability is one of her concerns

Given the dual focus of neuroethics, on first-order ethical questions arising from the sciences of the mind, and on the tools the neuroethicist uses in addressing these questions, neuroethics might be said to have two distinct branches. Roskies calls these two branches the *ethics of neuroscience* and the *neuroscience of ethics*. The ethics of neuroscience is concerned with first-order ethical issues; the neuroscience of ethics with normative ethics, meta-ethics and moral psychology insofar as these branches of philosophy are illuminated by the sciences of the mind.

The Ethics of Neuroscience

The sciences of the mind offer us a range of apparently unprecedented powers to intervene in the

Original publication details: Neil Levy, "Neuroethics: Ethics and the Sciences of the Mind," pp. 69–74 (extract) from *Philosophy Compass* 4: 10 (2009). Reproduced with permission of John Wiley & Sons.

mind of human beings, some actual, some just over the horizon, and some very distant (it is a matter of lively dispute which technologies are distant and which imminent). These powers arouse a great deal of unease in many people, prompting philosophers to reflect upon the permissibility of their use. These actual or potential powers include the ability to *enhance cognition*, to *modify memories and emotions*, and to *control or insert beliefs*.[1] Each of these has been the focus of sustained ethical reflection. For reasons of space, I shall consider only the first two topics (see Levy, *Neuroethics* for discussions of the ability to control or insert beliefs).

Memory Modification and Enhancement

Existing techniques to modify memories are relatively crude and weak. These techniques have been developed with therapeutic goals in mind: either to slow the progress of dementia, in the case of techniques that might improve memory, or to treat post-traumatic stress disorder (PTSD) in the case of techniques aimed at weakening specific memories.

Post-traumatic stress disorder is a relatively common, very debilitating psychiatric illness. It is especially common in emergency services personnel and soldiers (Kessler et al.). Since it is burdensome for sufferers and for their families, the treatment of PTSD is prima facie laudable. Obviously, the best way to deal with the problem is to prevent its occurrence, by preventing exposure to potentially traumatic events. Given, however, that the jobs of emergency services personnel and perhaps soldiers are indispensable, the next best option is to prevent PTSD from arising as a result of such exposure.

There is now a promising technique in development which might serve to prevent PTSD. Post-traumatic stress disorder is apparently caused by the over-consolidation of traumatic memories, as a result of the misfiring of a mechanism designed to ensure effective recall of survival-relevant events. Since

endogenous epinephrine plays a crucial role in the over-consolidation cycle, Pitman et al. hypothesized that the development of the syndrome could be prevented by blocking the effect of the stress hormone on the amygdala. Clinical trials using the beta-blocker Propranolol (widely used for the treatment of hypertension) have yielded promising results. Subjects administered Propranolol after involvement in auto accidents were less likely to develop PTSD than controls (Pitman and Delahanty; Vaiva et al.).

Obviously the prevention of PTSD is a laudable goal, yet the research outlined above has been surprisingly controversial. Much of the worry has focused on the potential for abuse of a successful treatment for PTSD. It is plausible to think that painful memories are often both instrumentally valuable and intrinsically significant. Painful memories ought sometimes to be treasured by us, not eliminated: the person who erases, or even just significantly dampens, the memory of the death of a beloved child does not improve her life thereby; instead she strips it of elements central to its meaning. But it might be that developing the kind of emotional maturity needed to appreciate this fact takes time and exposure to pain. Thus, a culture in which drugs are available that have these kinds of effects might be much less conducive to the development of the requisite maturity. The availability of these drugs might therefore contribute to what many people fear is an increasing shallowness characteristic of Western culture. Moreover, Leon Kass, formerly the head of the President's Council of Bioethics, worries that Propranolol might be used to facilitate wrongdoing. For most of us, even for most habitual criminals, the sting of conscience is a genuine and aversive phenomenon. Kass worries that Propranolol might effectively erase that sting, providing a 'morning-after pill for just about anything that produces regret, remorse, pain, or guilt' (Baard).

The worries just sketched focus on the *misuse* of Propranolol and its probable successors; their proponents accept that preventing PTSD is a valuable goal, but worry about the availability of a particular means to that goal. Others have questioned the desirability of treating PTSD at all. Ethicists have worried that treating or preventing PTSD might deny access to the meaning of traumatic events (Hurley; Evers) or deny people access to opportunities for personal growth (Warnick).

Some of these worries are relatively easily dispensed with, especially insofar as they seem to suggest – falsely – that PTSD is, on balance, a good thing for the sufferer (see Levy and Clarke for discussion). Others are worth taking seriously. One question we must ask ourselves whenever we discuss new technologies and their possible problems is the extent to which the problem is genuinely new. Will Propranolol really give us greater powers to dampen the emotional powers of memories than, say, alcohol? Given that the latter has high costs beyond the effects on the emotional life of the subject via memory dampening, perhaps the availability of the former is, on balance, a good thing, allowing people to pursue emotional oblivion at a lower cost; on the other hand, the lower cost might encourage greater use of Propranolol than of alcohol to this end. This question is largely an empirical one; philosophers have no special expertise when it comes to predictions about such matters as to whether people are more likely to use Propranolol than alcohol.

It is probable, however, that some of the anxiety surrounding the use of Propranolol comes from an exaggerated sense of how effective it is likely to be. It has, for instance, the potential to cut us from the emotional significance of events only if it is relatively powerful: if it does not simply prevent *over*-consolidation of memories, but also the normal degree of consolidation. Given that Propranolol has been taken by many thousands of people over an extended period of time, it seems unlikely that its effects will be dramatic. Propranolol has some, relatively subtle, effects on cognition: subjects exhibit a conservative bias on certain memory tasks, compared to controls (Corwin et al.; Callaway et al.). But these effects simply seem too subtle to give cause for alarm.

While much of the debate in the recent neuroethical literature has focused on the use of memory dampeners, far more scientific attention has been focused on means to *improve* memory. The reason is

not far to seek: far more people are affected by dementia than by PTSD, and aging populations ensure that these numbers will only rise. Though to my knowledge no one has objected to the use of medication to treat dementia – it is difficult to see how progressive memory loss could be conducive to any human good – many ethicists have expressed concerns about 'off label' use of such medication, to enhance memory beyond normal. Related concerns have focused on cognitive enhancers – psychopharmaceuticals used to enhance human intelligence beyond its normal limits – more generally.

When considering these kinds of issues, it is necessary to deal separately with questions about the potential unforeseen harms of cognitive or memory enhancers and the more general question: is cognitive enhancement permissible in principle? The former is, once again, largely an empirical question. However, there are certainly some philosophical questions here. For instance, the claim that improvements in some aspects of memory or cognition are likely to come at the cost of deterioration in other aspects, because our memory systems are the product of evolution and therefore likely to be optimal (Glannon 108), seem[s] to me to rest on an implausibly strong adaptationism: evolution is a satisficing process, not an optimising process. Similarly, philosophical expertise (amongst others kinds) is needed to assess the oft-repeated claim that widespread availability of enhancements will cause or exacerbate inequality.

Here I will set aside these important questions, in order to focus on in principle objections to enhancements. Some philosophers have suggested that we ought to reject all such enhancements because they promote attitudes that are incompatible with the virtues, with authenticity or with an attitude to the world which is obligatory. For Michael Sandel, the use of enhancements is incompatible with the gratitude we ought to feel toward the unforced products of nature. Carl Elliott worries that enhancement, especially *affective* enhancement, runs the risk of inauthenticity, as we lose contact with the emotional significance of events, while Carol Freedman worries that the use of such enhancements risks mechanizing ourselves inappropriately. I do not think that any of these concerns are significant enough to warrant serious disquiet regarding the development of cognitive or affective enhancements.

Sandel's concern is to my mind the weakest. It is simply false that there is any interesting sense in which human powers and achievements are currently a gift for which we ought to feel grateful but would no longer be such a gift were cognitive enhancement to become widespread. Our phenotypic traits have never been an unforced gift from nature. Phenotypic traits are always the product of the interaction of the genome (and other developmental resources) and the environment, and *homo sapiens* is a niche constructing animal, an animal who shapes the environment that shapes it in turn (Sterelny). We are deeply and essentially cultural animals; deeply and essentially because it is not just our social organization, but our intrinsic capacities and traits that are shaped by our culture. There is simply no sense in which our current capacities and traits are a gift of nature; at least, there is no sense in which they would not equally be a gift of nature were they also the product of cognitive enhancing pharmaceuticals.

Concerns about authenticity are almost as easily dismissed. As David DeGrazia has pointed out, Elliott's claim that we ought to be true to ourselves, in some sense incompatible with using psychopharmaceuticals, entails the notion of a pregiven self. Deep and persistent changes in an agent's traits or dispositions can be inauthentic only if there is an underlying self apart from these merely accidental properties, with which our traits ought to harmonize. But the self is a creation: we are always in the process of remaking ourselves. There is no essence to which we are required to conform, on pain of inauthenticity. Freedman's worry about inappropriate mechanism of the self is harder to dismiss. We should recognize, first, that there is a sense in which we *are* machines, or, more exactly, built out of machines; our minds emerge from or are realized by myriad mechanisms, each of which is itself mindless. But it certainly doesn't follow from the fact that we are built out of machines that it is appropriate to treat us as machines; we, unlike the machines out of

which we are built, are *not* mindless. Human beings live in the space of reasons: it is this fact that motivates Freedman's concern. If we respond to ourselves or to others as though our emotions and thoughts are merely mechanical reactions, we do not show the proper respect due to agents. Worse, Freedman worries, treat ourselves mechanically and we might actually threaten our status as rational beings.

Still, we must be careful not to overdraw the worry. It does not seem objectionable to treat oneself mechanically, on occasion and to some extent. Some effective treatments for mild depression that do not involve psychopharmaceuticals, such as sun lamps for the treatment of Seasonal Affective Disorder, or the use of exercise to lift mood, are equally mechanistic. They do not give us *reasons* to be happier; they *cause* our mood to improve. Intuitively, these means are acceptable (whether they lift someone out of depression or elevate mood above the normal level). Why should any greater suspicion fall upon psychopharmaceuticals?

By way of transition to a consideration of the neuroscience of ethics, it is worth reflecting further on this question. Given that in many ways the enhancements in question seem to be relevantly similar to existing techniques of increasing cognitive ability – from ensuring adequate nutrition to choosing better schools – why is the use of psychopharmaceuticals, transcranial magnetic stimulation, or what have you so widely regarded with suspicion? It might be that these intuitions have causes that do not reflect good reasons. Jonathan Haidt has argued that very often the reasons people offer for their moral judgments have nothing to do with their actual causes. Together with Thalia Wheatley, moreover, he has shown that the causes of moral judgments can be morally irrelevant. For instance, invoking a disgust response in subjects intensifies their judgments of moral wrongness: it can even cause subjects to judge an entirely innocuous action to be morally wrong (Wheatley and Haidt). It is therefore possible that the causes motivating the judgment that cognitive enhancement is distinctively wrong are morally irrelevant: since a feeling of unease is capable of being mistaken for or generating a moral intuition, evidence that cognitive enhancement would generate such a feeling of unease due to morally irrelevant factors is evidence that the intuition ought to be discounted.

There are, I suggest, good reasons to suggest that the negative response to cognitive enhancement is produced via a morally irrelevant route. The feeling of unease may well be a response to the fact that cognitive enhancement is a violation of implicit dualism. There is evidence that dualism is the cognitive default (Bering; Bering and Bjorklund). Moreover, reaction time studies suggest that it is a default that

is not *replaced* by physicalist convictions but merely *displaced*: that is, we continue to have dualist intuitions which we must effortfully override in order to express a physicalist judgment. Now, there is an obvious sense in which cognitive enhancement is a violation of implicit dualism: it produces alterations in the mind via its physical substrate, which ought to be impossible if dualism is true. Hence it is likely that contemplating the mere possibility of such alterations produces a feeling of unease in us, which is easily mistaken for a moral intuition.

Note

1 There is an ongoing debate whether it is possible to draw a treatment/enhancement distinction that is capable of doing the work that bioethicists typically demand of it (usually distinguishing between permissible and impermissible interventions). Rather than enter into this debate, I use 'enhancement' here simply to refer to interventions that elevate functioning above the statistically normal level. For an argument that no interesting treatment/enhancement distinction is defensible, see Levy, *Neuroethics*.

References

Baard, E. 'The Guilt-Free Soldier'. *Village Voice* January 2003. At https://www.villagevoice.com/2003/01/21/the-guilt-free-soldier/

Bering, J. M. 'Intuitive Conceptions of Dead Agents' Minds: The Natural Foundations of Afterlife Beliefs as Phenomenological Boundary'. *Journal of Cognition and Culture* 2 (2002): 263–308.

Bering, J. M. and D. F. Bjorklund. 'The Natural Emergence of Reasoning about the Afterlife as a Developmental Regularity'. *Developmental Psychology* 40 (2004): 217–33.

Callaway, E., et al. 'Propranolol and Response Bias: An Extension of Findings Reported by Corwin et al.'. *Biological Psychiatry* 30 (1991): 739–42.

Corwin, J., et al. 'Disorders of Decision in Affective Disease: An Effect of β-Adrenergic Dysfunction?'. *Biological Psychiatry* 27 (1990): 813–33.

DeGrazia, D. 'Prozac, Enhancement, and Self-Creation'. *Hastings Center Report* 30 (2000): 34–40.

Elliott, C. 'The Tyranny of Happiness: Ethics and Cosmetic Psychopharmacology'. *Enhancing Human Traits: Ethical and Social Implications*. Ed. Erik Parens. Washington, DC: Georgetown University Press, 1998. 177–88.

Evers, K. 'Perspectives on Memory Manipulation: Using Beta-Blockers to Cure Post-Traumatic Stress Disorder'. *Cambridge Quarterly of Healthcare Ethics* 16 (2007): 138–46.

Freedman, C. 'Aspirin for the Mind? Some Ethical Worries about Psychopharmacology'. *Enhancing Human Traits: Ethical and Social Implications*. Ed. Erik Parens. Washington, DC: Georgetown University Press, 1998. 135–50.

Glannon, W. *Bioethics on the Brain*. Oxford: Oxford University Press, 2007.

Haidt, J. 'The Emotional Dog and Its Rational Tail: A Social Intuitionist Approach to Moral Judgment'. *Psychological Review* 108 (2001): 814–34.

Hurley, E. A. 'The Moral Costs of Prophylactic Propranolol'. *AJOB* 7.9 (2007): 35–6.

Kessler, R. C., et al. 'Posttraumatic Stress Disorder in the National Comorbidity Survey'. *Archives of General Psychiatry* 52 (1996): 1048–60.

Levy, N. *Neuroethics*. Cambridge: Cambridge University Press, 2007.

Levy, N. and S. Clarke. 'Neuroethics and Psychiatry'. *Current Opinion in Psychiatry* 21 (2008): 568–71.

Pitman, R. K. and D. L. Delahanty. 'Conceptually Driven Pharmacologic Approaches to Acute Trauma'. *CNS Spectrum* 10 (2005): 99–106.

Pitman, R. K., et al. 'Pilot Study of Secondary Prevention of Posttraumatic Stress Disorder with Propanolol'. *Biological Psychiatry* 51 (2002): 189–92.

Roskies, A. 'Neuroethics for the New Millennium'. *Neuron* 35 (2002): 21–3.

Sandel, M. *The Case against Perfection: Ethics in the Age of Genetic Engineering*. Cambridge, MA: Belknap Press, 2007.

Sterelny, K. *Thought in a Hostile World: The Evolution of Human Cognition*. Oxford: Blackwell, 2003.

Vaiva, G., et al. 'Immediate Treatment with Propranolol Decreases Posttraumatic Stress Disorder Two Months after Trauma'. *Biol Psychiatry* 54 (2003): 947–9.

Warnick, J. E. 'Propranolol and Its Potential Inhibition of Positive Post-Traumatic Growth'. *AJOB* 7.9 (2007): 37–8.

Wheatley, T. and J. Haidt. 'Hypnotic Disgust Makes Moral Judgments More Severe'. *Psychological Science* 16 (2005): 780–4.

94

Engineering Love

Julian Savulescu and Anders Sandberg

It's easy to forget that we humans are animals too. After all, our relatively large cortices have enabled us to create advanced technology, megacities, nuclear weapons, art, philosophy – in short, a radically different environment to the African savannah we inhabited for most of our history. To top that, we have developed an extraordinarily complex medical system capable of doubling the human lifespan.

Yet in many ways we are stuck with the psychology and drives of our hunter-gatherer ancestors. We are not made for the world and institutions we have created for ourselves, including that of life-long marriage.

Throughout most of our history, people survived for a maximum of 35 years. Staying alive was a full-time job, and most pair-bonds ended with one partner dying. Given this lifespan, at least 50 per cent of mating alliances would have ended within 15 years. This figure is surprisingly close to the current global median duration of marriage, 11 years. It seems unlikely that natural selection equipped us to keep relationships lasting much more than a decade.

The fact is that in the US divorce has surpassed death as the major cause of marital break-up. This has significant consequences, especially for children. As law professor Katherine Spaht of Louisiana State University in Baton Rouge wrote in the *Notre Dame Law Review*: "In comparison with children of intact first marriages, children of divorce suffer in virtually every measure of well-being."

On the other side of the coin, stable, loving relationships are good for us, improving both parent and child welfare through the social support they provide. Most research confirms that successful marriages boost physical and emotional health, self-reported happiness and even longevity. So how can we make up the gap between the health-giving ideal of "till death do us part" and the heartbreaking reality and harms of widespread divorce? And do parents have a special responsibility to do so, given those harms?

One promising route is to consider the advances in neurobiology and see how we might use science. Some of the latest research suggests we could tweak the chemical systems involved to create a longer-lasting love.

Helen Fisher, an evolutionary psychologist at Rutgers University in New Brunswick, New Jersey,

Original publication details: Anders Sandberg and Julian Savulescu, "Love Machine: Engineering Lifelong Romance," pp. 28–29 from *New Scientist* 2864. © 2012 Reed Business Information. Reproduced with permission of Tribune Content Agency.

argues that human love is constructed on top of a set of basic brain systems for lust, romantic attraction and attachment that evolved in all mammals. Lust promotes mating with any appropriate partner, attraction makes us choose and prefer a particular partner, while attachment allows pairs to cooperate and stay together until parental duties are complete.

Human love, of course, is complex. While there is no single "love centre" in the brain, neuroimaging studies of people experiencing romantic love have shown patterns of activation in areas linked to the hormones oxytocin and vasopressin, as well as the brain's reward centres. These findings fit with research into the mating habits of monogamous prairie voles (*Microtus ochrogaster*) and their cousins the polygamous montane voles (*Microtus montanus*).

The receptors for these hormones are distributed differently in monogamous and polygamous voles. Infusing oxytocin into the brains of female prairie voles and vasopressin into the brains of males encouraged pair-bonding activity such as spending time together exclusively and driving away sexual competitors, even in the absence of mating, while the hormones did not affect the non-monogamous montane voles.

In one striking experiment, researchers introduced a vasopressin receptor gene from the faithful prairie vole into the brain of its promiscuous cousin. The modified voles became monogamous (*Neuroscience*, vol 125, p 35).

This gene controls a part of the brain's reward centre. In humans, differences in this gene have been associated with changes in the stability of relationships and in partner satisfaction. If human and vole brains share similar wiring, as research suggests, we might be able to modify our mating behaviour biologically as well.

Tapping into the power of oxytocin could prove useful in other ways. Oxytocin is released during physical contact such as touching, massage or sex, and is involved in nursing behaviour, trust and "mind-reading" – our attempts to work out what our partners think and feel – as well as in counteracting stress and fear. Taking oxytocin in the form of a nasal spray would promote unstressed, trusting behaviours that might reduce the negative feedback in some relationships and help strengthen the positive sides. It could also be used alongside marital therapy to open up communication and encourage bonding.

What of testosterone, the hormone that helps to control sexual desire in men and women? People who have been given the hormone report an increase in sexual thoughts, activity and satisfaction – though not in romantic passion or attachment. But since levels of sexual interest in men and women diverge as a relationship continues, and since this disparity strongly affects its stability, synchronising levels of desire by altering levels of testosterone might help.

It also looks likely that the strong dopamine and oxytocin signals elicited during the early romantic phase of a relationship and during sex help to imprint details of the partner and create positive emotional associations to the relationship. So it may be possible to trigger this imprinting by giving the right drugs while someone is close to their partner.

The stick rather than the carrot in the maintenance of a pair bond is that love is linked to fear and the sadness of separation. This may be due to corticotropin releasing hormone. Carefully boosting it or, rather, the processes behind the "stick" effect, might be useful as a deterrent from straying.

So what of the future? We already modify sexual behaviour, for example, by offering paedophiles chemical castration to squash their sex drive. And given the growing knowledge of the cognitive neuroscience of love and its chemical underpinning, we should expect far more precise interventions to become available soon.

Whether we should do any of this is another matter. Love and relationships are among the most potent contributors to our collective well-being so there are strong moral reasons to make relationships better. But the use of neuroenhancements leads to many questions. Will they render relationships inauthentic, the product of pharmaceutical design? Could we become addicted to love? And could such drugs and chemicals be used to imprison people in bad relationships? So should we change our institutions or stick with modifying our behaviour using counselling and therapy instead?

On balance, no. We argue we need all the help we can get to liberate ourselves from evolution. It has not created us to be happy, but offers enough transient happiness to keep us alive and reproducing. Yet from our human perspective, happiness and flourishing are primary goals. In a conflict between human values and evolution we might well ignore what evolution promotes. "Love drugs" are not a silver bullet, but in a regulated, professional environment and with an informed public, they could help overcome some of biology's obstacles. Why not use all the strategies we can to give us the best chance of the best life?

95

Unrequited Love Hurts
Should Doctors Treat Broken Hearts?

Francesca Minerva

> Amputees suffer pains, cramps, itches in the leg that is no longer there.
> That is how she felt without him,
> feeling his presence where he no longer was
> Gabriel García Márquez, *Love in the Time of Cholera*

Romantic relationships are a big part of human life, both when they work well and when they are the cause of sadness and pain.

In recent years, there has been a debate about the possibility of using so called "love drugs" to enhance romantic relationships in order to make them last "till death do us part."[1] Perhaps unsurprisingly, the suggestion that one could use love drugs (such as oxytocin) to enhance romantic relationship has prompted criticism. Some of these objections are based on the assumption that love is too special an experience to be analyzed, medicalized and pharmaceuticalized. In some cases, opposition to using drugs to "enhance" romantic relationships (that is, to *pharmaceuticalize*) – which could also mean to diminish lust, attraction or attachment in cases where such feelings are harmful – is founded on the assumption that love and romance are different from other human experiences (which, conversely, might be enhanced through drugs and not only through psychotherapy). For instance, Evans has suggested that critics of medicalization would argue that we should *not* accept the medicalization of love, because "there are, or should be, experiences that use an older logic, which are under the jurisdiction of another profession or under no jurisdiction at all. *We can all fear the medicalization of love.*"[2]

In this article, I argue that we should not fear the medicalization of (at least) one particular kind of love: that is unrequited love. I argue that, because (1) unrequited love can be – and often is – a very painful experience, and (2) people are entitled to avoid pain (if they wish to), medicalization and pharmaceuticalization of broken hearts should be an available option. I also argue that it should be considered a form of therapy rather than a form of enhancement.

Original publication details: Francesca Minerva, "Unrequited Love Hurts: The Medicalization of Broken Hearts is Therapy, Not Enhancement," pp. 479–485 from *Cambridge Quarterly of Healthcare* Ethics 24: 4 (2015). Reproduced with permission of Cambridge University Press.

Unrequited Love Hurts

Falling in love and being in a romantic relationship with someone who loves us back is one of the most exhilarating experiences in life. Most of us know how it feels to be in love and to have that love reciprocated. The world, to put it simply, looks like a friendlier and much nicer place. There are, of course, biological reasons why it is so. Aron and colleagues observed that

> Romantic love is also associated, particularly in early stages, with specific physiological, psychological, and behavioral indices that have been described and quantified by psychologists and others. . . These include emotional responses such as euphoria, intense focused attention on a preferred individual, obsessive thinking about him or her, emotional dependency on and craving for emotional union with this beloved, and increased energy.[3]

Unfortunately, not all romances have a happy ending. Nor do all relationships last until both parties mutually agree they are no longer interested in each other. Very often, at the end of all the happiness, the butterflies in the stomach and rose-coloured lenses, there is excruciating pain. Not uncommonly, such pain comes with obsessive thoughts about the now lost object of that love. Research has shown that obsession is a component of unrequited love as well as of the happier, reciprocated kind. Just as the brain in love releases "good" chemicals that make us feel good, the rejected lover's brain also produces chemicals; except these chemicals make us feel miserable, if not desperate.

In a 2010 study published in the *Journal of Neurophysiology*, Fisher and colleagues used fMRI [functional magnetic resonance imaging] to examine the cortical systems of 15 people who had recently been abandoned by their partners but who were still intensely in love with them.[4] The participants were alternately shown a picture of their beloved and a picture of some other person familiar to them. These pictures were also interspersed by a task designed to distract the participants' attention. The responses reported by participants while looking at their rejecter

included love, despair, good and bad memories, and wondering what had gone wrong.

The study was aimed at testing four predictions:

1. Romantic rejection activates subcortical reward systems that mediate motivation and reward.
2. Romantic rejection activates subcortical and cortical areas associated with drug craving.
3. Romantic rejection engages forebrain areas activated by losses and gains and gain anticipation.
4. Romantic rejection activates brain regions associated with the autonomic nervous system because the subjects show a range of intense emotions.

All four of these hypotheses were confirmed by the study. Researchers concluded that

> Forebrain activations associated with motivational relevance, gain/loss, cocaine craving, addiction, and emotion regulation suggest that higher-order systems subject to experience and learning also may mediate the rejection reaction. The results show activation of reward systems, previously identified by monetary stimuli, in a natural, endogenous, negative emotion state. Activation of areas involved in cocaine addiction may help explain the obsessive behaviors associated with rejection in love."[5]

Consistent with these results, other studies suggest that romantic love and cocaine addiction share survival system activation in the brain, demonstrating the strength of the obsession.[6,7]

Many people, during some point in their lives, will experience the obsession and the excruciating pain that the subjects of the above mentioned study experienced when rejected and abandoned.

During the pre-scanning interview in the Fisher et al. study, the participants were asked to talk about the person who had rejected them. Their responses included: "I think about him constantly" (all of the subjects reported thinking of the beloved for more than the 85% of the day), and "I want a letter from him, or a phone call; I want some respect" (all the subjects showed anger as well as the need to understand why the relationship hadn't worked). When attempting to describe their pain, responses from the participants included: "It hurts so much. I crumble. I just start crying" and "I hate what he did to me, but I still love him", as well as "I kept thinking, I love you, I hate you; how could you do this".

Out of the suffering for being rejected by his beloved Lesbia, the Latin poet Catullus composed the famous verses: *"odi et amo, quare id faciam fortasse requiris: nescio, sed fieri sentio, et excrucior"* (I hate and I love. You might ask why: I don't know, but that's how I feel and it is an excruciating pain). Unfortunately, very rarely does a break up produce "side-effects" as beautiful as a song or a poem. More often, unrequited love brings tragic effects. Sometimes people even kill themselves and/or the object of their unrequited love. Even leaving aside such extreme cases, those who are rejected in love frequently experience deep sadness and outright depression.

At the end of the study the authors concluded that "the perspective that rejection in love involves sub-cortical reward gain/loss systems critical to survival helps to explain why feelings and behaviours related to romantic rejection are difficult to control and lends insight into the high cross-cultural rates of stalking, homicide, suicide, and clinical depression associated with rejection in love."[8]

If unrequited love can have such a negative impact on both the people who have been rejected and also – in some extreme cases – on the rejecter, then we should ask ourselves whether there are reasons not to intervene pharmaceutically to speed the process of healing and recovering from such pain.

In the next paragraphs, I consider some objections to the idea of medicalizing love. I will also examine the question of whether pharmaceuticalization of broken hearts is a form of enhancement or a therapeutic option.

Two Arguments Against the Medicalization of Unrequited Love

There are two likely objections to the idea that broken-hearted people should be given the option to receive pharmaceutical treatment for their suffering.

The first objection (which I shall call "the peculiarity of heartbreak objection") is based on the argument that the anguish we experience from a broken heart is of a special kind. Moreover, the anguish is of a kind that does not benefit from quick fixes, but rather through a long period of endurance, because something important is learnt in the process of recovering.

The second objection (which I shall call "the arts objection") is based on the idea that love, and especially unrequited love, motivates people to write poems, books, songs, and to produce art in general, and that such motivation, as well as their products, have a positive value both for the authors and for those who appreciate the resultant artwork.

The peculiarity-of-heartbreak objection

The suffering caused by social rejection, including unrequited love, has often been overlooked as a more endurable and somehow less care-deserving form of pain, as one that is less deserving of being ameliorated, especially by "medical" means. There seems to be a common assumption that a broken limb hurts significantly more, and in a different way, than a broken heart.

New research gives us reasons to question this assumption. According to research published in *PNAS* by Kross and colleagues in 2011, from a neurobiological point of view social pain and physical pain are much more similar than we usually assume. The researchers discovered that "experiences of social rejection, when elicited powerfully enough, recruit brain regions involved in both the affective and sensory components of physical pain."[9] The authors noticed that "social rejection and physical pain are similar not only in that they are both distressing, they share a common representation in somatosensory brain systems as well. These findings offer new insight into how rejection experiences may lead to various physical pain disorders (e.g., somato-form disorders; fibromyalgia), highlighting the role that somatosensory processing may play in this process".

Another study by DeWall and colleagues confirmed an overlap between the body's responses to social and physical pain.[10] Moreover, the researchers discovered that daily doses of 2,000 mg of acetaminophen (paracetamol) can reduce psychological pain due to social rejection by also decreasing neural activity in response to social rejection in brain regions that are associated with the experience of both social and physical pain. Researchers therefore concluded that "an over-the-counter painkiller normally used to relieve physical aches and pains can also at least temporarily mitigate social-pain-related distress."[11]

If both a broken heart and a broken limb hurt, what is wrong with using drugs to ease the pain?
The results of the research just presented suggest that people with broken hearts and people experiencing purely physical pain (such as the one resulting from a broken limb) are not experiencing something significantly different with regard to neural activity. It is noteworthy, for example, that paracetamol can alleviate both kinds of pain. It seems, therefore, that those who oppose the pharmaceuticalization of unrequited love on the basis that it is a *sui generis* kind of pain are wrong as, from a neurobiological point of view, the pain is not dissimilar (at least in terms of the neural activity concerned).

However, perhaps one might oppose pharmaceutical treatment of heartbreak because the pain of a love lost differs from physical pain not in a neurological sense but in a *cognitive* sense. In other words, it might be argued that there is some wisdom to gain in the process of recovering from a broken heart. This is one of the points made by McArthur. He argues that there is a difference between physical and emotional pain, because "emotional suffering is arguably integral to the healing process in a way that physical pain is not" and "learning to make the pain go away is precisely what it is to heal". Besides, he adds, "without the pain of heartsickness, we would be much less motivated to actually learn and mature. People could find themselves trapped in the same endless, destructive cycles throughout their various relationships."[12]

Sometimes people learn something important when they suffer for love, and sometimes they don't learn anything at all. The existence of a link between

suffering and knowledge is still an open empirical issue, not a philosophical certainty. However, even if it were true that people often – or even always – learn something from their heartache, it is not obvious that they should be forced to choose knowledge over relief from pain. Some people might want to live in a pain-free, happy and less self-conscious way, and the fact that some other individuals don't agree with this approach to life is no reason to prevent them from doing so.

One would also have to assess whether all people experience pain in the same way. As is the case with physical pain, some people have a lower threshold of pain, and lower resilience. So it may be that for them it is harder to recover from a break up or that they experience a higher level of suffering. All these questions are open to empirical investigation, but the similarity between physical and psychological pain caused by social rejection ought to be taken into account.

A brief example will help to make my point clearer: suppose that John is in pain because the person he loves has left him, and suppose that Colin is in pain because during his karate training a friend punched him in the nose. Suppose that both John and Colin go to their doctor to ask for pain-relief treatment. Would it be morally justifiable for the doctor to refuse to recommend John a daily dose of 2,000 mg of paracetamol, but to recommend Colin to use the same dose of the same medication to relieve the pain from his swollen nose? Most people would, of course, consider it unacceptable for the doctor to advise Colin – whose nose has been punched – to think about the appropriateness of engaging in karate training. However, those who object to the medicalization of love would consider the same type of behaviour appropriate in the case of John, whose heart has been broken.

This double standard in the treatment of pain would be hardly justifiable through sound arguments. Besides, given that there is no relevant difference (in terms of neurological effects on the individual and in terms of suggested treatment) in the cases of a broken heart and a swollen nose, medicalization of a broken heart should not be considered a form of enhancement (rather, it should be considered a form of therapy), as long as giving paracetamol to Colin cannot be considered a form of enhancement either.

Social rejection and physical pain activate same areas in the brain and the pain caused by social rejection and pain caused by physical trauma can both be relieved through painkillers. Given that considerations about the potential benefits that may result from heartbreak (e.g. pieces of art or lessons about life) are not relevant when making medical decisions, it follows that there are sound reasons to allow the use of drugs to treat social rejection pain, just as we do in the case of physical trauma.

The arts objection

Neil McArthur argued that the medicalization of unrequited love would have a devastating effect on our society's artistic life. As he writes

> The pain of heartache has given us some of our greatest masterworks, in a variety of fields. It would be impossible to present a complete list, but notable examples include the many great poems W. B. Yeats wrote for Maud Gonne (as well as some to her daughter), Goethe's novel The Sorrows of Young Werther, and Eric Clapton's anguished rock classic "Layla".[13]

I agree with McArthur that broken-hearted artists have produced some great pieces of art. And, perhaps, had Catullus been happy, he would never have written those beautiful poems alluded to earlier. But such hypotheses do not take us anywhere: Perhaps Catullus would have written different, happier poems; or perhaps he would have simply enjoyed his romance with Lesbia and not written anything. Perhaps he would have found other sources of unhappiness and dissatisfaction to translate into pieces of art. It is impossible to know how many poems, songs and novels we would lose if the anguish caused by rejection could be fixed quickly with a drug. On the other hand, it is worth noting that it is also impossible to know how many happy poems we are currently missing out on because of the pain caused by heartbreak.

At any rate, let us assume for the sake of argument that medicalization of unrequited love would have a negative effect on our society's artistic life, and that people who enjoy the artistic by-products of suffering would be somehow worse off by the development of a quick fix for broken hearts. It is a reasonable contention that people who enjoy these by-products of suffering derive their enjoyment from the way the suffering being portrayed resonates with their own sadness. The broken-hearted may feel that the poems or songs were written by someone who was experiencing the same pain they are experiencing, and that the poet or singer can express perfectly how broken-hearted people are feeling. In being able to relate to the artist through their music or verse, broken-hearted people may in some cases feel better about themselves. Of course, appreciation for the artistic by-products of unrequited love is not limited to the broken-hearted, and the satisfaction such works generate in us doesn't lie exclusively in our ability to relate to the emotions expressed in the novel or song or poem.

However, it seems quite cruel to prevent people from pharmaceutically recovering from their bad break-up because we want them to write songs and poems, especially if one considers: (1) that there are already many great artworks for us to enjoy; (2) that it is unlikely that all great artists would use such drugs, or perhaps they would only turn to drug therapy after their suffering ceases to be a source of inspiration; and, finally, (3) that not everyone is an artist. Although there are some people in the world who are as good as Shakespeare, Catullus, Goethe and Garcia-Marquez, the majority of people are not artists, or not good ones, and their heartbreak just makes them suffer without leading them to produce (beautiful) works. In such cases, giving them the possibility to reduce their suffering or to not suffer at all should be an acceptable option.

It might be argued that very talented artists at least have a *prima facie* moral obligation to refrain from drug therapy in order to produce art that would bring pleasure to others. But this doesn't imply that artists should be denied the option of pharmaceutical treatment if they wish it, only that talented artists have a stronger moral reason than bad artists or non-artists to refuse such treatments.

Conclusions

In this article, I have shown that unrequited love is a form of love that deserves special consideration in the debate over love-enhancing drugs. I consider the medicalization and pharmaceuticalization of unrequited love to be a form of therapy rather than a form of enhancement because it aims at alleviating pain. Furthermore, the suffering caused by heartbreak is neurologically similar to purely physical pain. If alleviating pain that is caused by physical injuries is not commonly considered a form of enhancement, then pain alleviation for suffering caused by social rejection (that is the same as unrequited love) should not be considered a form of enhancement either.

Acknowledgment

The author would like to thank all the men who broke her heart for giving her food for thought and inspiration for this paper. However, coherently with what is argued here, she would have been even more grateful to them if they had made her happy instead.

Notes

1 Savulescu, J. and Sandberg, A., Engineering love. Chapter 94 in this volume.
2 Quoted in Parens, E. On good and bad forms of medicalization. *Bioethics*, 2013, *27*(1): 28–35 – 33.
3 Aron, A., Fisher, H., Mashek, D. G., Strong, G., Haifang, L., and Brown, L. L. Reward, motivation, and emotion systems associated with early-stage intense romantic love, *Journal of Neurophysiology*, 2005, *94*(1): 327–3 at 327.
4 Fisher H. E., Brown, L. L., Aron, A., Strong, G., and Mashek, D.G., Reward, addiction, and emotion regulation systems associated with rejection in love. *Journal of Neurophysiology*, 2010, *104*: 51–6 at 51.
5 See note 4, Fischer et al. 2010, at 75.
6 Fisher H. E. Lust, attraction, and attachment in mammalian reproduction. *Human Nature*, 1998, *9*: 23–52.
7 Frascella J., Potenza, M. N., Brown, L. L., and Childress, A. R. Shared brain vulnerabilities open the way for non-substance addictions: Craving addiction at a new joint? *Annals of the National Academy of Sciences* 2010; *1187*: 294–315.
8 See note 4 Fischer et al. 2010, at 58.
9 Kross, E., Berman, M. G., Mischel, W., Smith, E. E., and Wager, T. D. Social rejection shares somatosensory representations with physical pain. *Proceedings of the National Academy of Sciences USA*, 2011, *108*: 6270–5, at 6270.
10 DeWall, C. N., MacDonald, G, Webster, G.,D., Masten, C. L, Baumeister, R. F., Powell, C., et al. Acetaminophen reduces social pain: Behavioral and neural evidence. *Psychological Science*, 2010, *21*(7): 931–7. doi: 10.1177/0956797610374741
11 See note 10, DeWall et al. 2010, at 935.
12 McArthur, N. The heart outright: A comment on "If I Could Just Stop Loving You." *The American Journal of Bioethics*, 2013, *13*(11): 24–5, at 25. doi:10.1080/15265161.2013.839773
13 See note 12, McArthur, at 25.

96

Stimulating Brains, Altering Minds

Walter Glannon

Electrical and magnetic stimulation of the brain has shown considerable therapeutic promise for a range of neurological and psychiatric disorders. This includes techniques such as electroconvulsive therapy, transcranial magnetic stimulation (TMS), transcranial direct current stimulation, vagus nerve stimulation and deep-brain stimulation (DBS). The most widely used and effective brain-stimulating technique is DBS. Unlike the other techniques just mentioned, DBS involves direct intervention in the brain and thus entails more risks to the patient. Electrodes are surgically implanted in one or more brain regions. The electrodes are connected to a battery-driven stimulator implanted in the chest near the collarbone that can be switched on and off remotely through the skin. Activation of the electrodes stimulates the relevant sites in the brain.

Most neurological and psychiatric disorders involve dysregulation in cortical, limbic and subcortical regions of the brain. The effects of TMS, for example, are limited because it stimulates only the cortex, and the strength of the magnetic field it generates falls off sharply beyond a few centimetres from the stimulated site. DBS is superior to TMS and other forms of stimulation for neurological and psychiatric disorders because of its modulating effects on cortical-thalamic and cortical-limbic circuits in the three general brain regions. This explains why it has been medically indicated for and used with varying degrees of success to treat Parkinson disease (PD), essential tremor, depression, chronic pain, obsessive-compulsive disorder and Tourette syndrome.[1] Although DBS involves more risks than non-invasive or less invasive forms of brain stimulation, it has fewer risks than ablative neurosurgery, where any damage to the brain can be permanent. Unlike the surgical lesions made to correct dysfunctional brain circuits, DBS is adjustable and reversible. The settings of the electrodes and the stimulator can be changed. Alternatively, the stimulator can be turned off, and the implanted electrodes can be removed from the brain. Nevertheless, because DBS is brain-invasive and does have risks, it is and likely will continue to be offered only to patients with the most severe and intractable disorders that have not responded to any other treatments. The purpose of all forms of neurostimulation is to

Original publication details: Walter Glannon, "Stimulating Brains, Altering Minds," pp. 289–292 from *Journal of Medical Ethics* 35 (2009). Reproduced with permission of BMJ Publishing Group Ltd.

modulate underactive or overactive brain regions mediating motor control and mental states associated with cognition and emotion.

Stimulating the brain may improve physiological and psychological symptoms of some conditions. Yet it may alter a range of mental states critical to thought, personality and behaviour. This can disrupt the integrity and continuity of the psychological properties that constitute the self and one's experience of persisting through time as the same person. As an interdisciplinary group of European neuroscientists, philosophers and legal theorists led by Reinhard Merkel point out:

> Practically no intervention in the structure or functioning of the human brain can be undertaken in complete certainty that it will not affect mental processes, some of which may come to play a key role in a person's self-concept.[2]

The uncertainty is a function of the fact that it is not known exactly how electrical or magnetic stimulation alters brain activity. It is not known which targets in the brain are optimal for producing salutary effects on motor, cognitive and affective functions. Nor is it known at what frequency the stimulation should be delivered to produce these effects, which can vary among different patients.

I discuss actual effects of DBS on the mind and how they influence decisions by patients and physicians about whether to have, forgo, continue or discontinue this treatment. I present a case involving a neurological disorder to generate and frame discussion of the psychological and ethical aspects pertinent to three related questions: how do patients and their physicians weigh the potential benefit against the potential harm of this intervention in the brain? How much alteration of one's thought and personality in treating a neurological or psychiatric disorder with DBS would be consistent with a patient's rational choice to undergo the procedure? How much alteration of the patient's mind would be consistent with a neurologist's or psychiatrist's duty of care to the patient?

Empirical Evidence: Benefits and Risks

DBS has been effective in controlling motor symptoms associated with advanced PD. Its target is two subcortical structures in the basal ganglia critical for motor function, the globus pallidus interna and the subthalamic nucleus. DBS is now considered standard of care for treating PD in some medical centres. It can enable patients to have more control of their condition, not only because the device can improve motor function, but also because patients can operate the device on their own outside of a clinical setting. For some patients, the procedure has a more favourable benefit-risk profile and thus is preferable to drugs such as dopamine agonists, which can cause addiction and other types of compulsive behaviour.[3] The drugs can overcompensate for dopamine depletion in the basal ganglia, which has been implicated as one cause of the disease.

DBS is not without risks, however. In one study, this technique caused symptoms in patients similar to those associated with dopamine agonists. They became impulsive in their decision-making, displaying impairment in their capacity to consider all options before choosing and acting.[4] One explanation of this phenomenon is that stimulating the basal ganglia interferes with the functions of prefrontal cortical areas of the brain, which ordinarily regulate deliberative behaviour. Drugs such as levodopa may control some motor symptoms but may also cause motor fluctuations, dyskinesias and impair some forms of learning. Yet alternatives such as DBS can inappropriately accelerate decision-making in some patients and interfere with their autonomy. This is just one example of the trade-offs between physiological benefit and psychological harm in treating PD.[5] There are physiological risks as well, including haemorrhage and infection at the site where the electrodes are implanted and stimulated.[6] DBS also has significant risks when used for psychiatric disorders. A recent study of subthalamic nucleus stimulation for severe obsessive-compulsive disorder involving

18 patients resulted in 15 severe adverse effects over-all.[7] These included one intracerebral haemorrhage and two infections. The main psychiatric adverse event was hypomania, which resolved after adjustment of the stimulator. This indicated that the stimulation was causing this psychiatric state. In a study using DBS targeting the subcallosal cingulate gyrus for treat-ment-refractory depression, 12 out of 20 patients had significant improvement in their symptoms, effectively going into remission for one year.[8] Yet an earlier study of this technique targeting the subgenual cingulate for depression indicated that it could cause hypomania and amplification of the effects of antidepressants.[9] There were also reports of rebound depression when the stimulator was turned off.

Given that DBS can result in both beneficial and harmful effects in individuals with PD, how do we weigh these different effects in determining whether the procedure can be justified? Because the adverse effects on the mind can be significant, and because these effects are not predictable from one patient to the next, a full complement of medical profession-als should be involved in deliberating these questions with the patient. These would include neurologists, neurosurgeons and anesthesiologists directly involved in the procedure, as well as psychiatrists, psycholo-gists, social workers and family members to explore the potential impact of the procedure on the patient. This involves not only deliberating whether to offer the procedure, but also monitoring its effects in deter-mining whether it should be continued.[10] Whether medical professionals should offer DBS for this dis-order depends on their assessment of benefit and risk. But ultimately it is the mentally competent patient who has to decide whether the effects of DBS would be acceptable and whether he or she should have it.

On one level, the decision hinges on a comparison between the physical benefit of motor control and the potential psychological harm of an adverse change in thought, personality and behaviour. On a deeper level, the decision hinges on a question involving a com-parison between two psychological states: whether the emotional suffering from loss of motor control is worse than changes in other states of mind. The

key factor is the patient's quality of life and whether DBS yields a net benefit in this respect. The medical trade-offs between the positive physical and negative cognitive and emotional effects of drugs versus elec-trical stimulation, or stimulation versus no treatment, also involve ethical trade-offs between different types and degrees of psychological harm.

A Case Study

We can gain insight into this problem by consider-ing a case of a patient from The Netherlands who received DBS for advanced PD.[11] Three years after the implantation of electrodes in the subthalamic nucleus and the start of DBS, a 62-year-old male was admit-ted to a psychiatric hospital for a manic state caused by the stimulation. A mood stabiliser failed to control his symptoms, which included megalomania and cha-otic behaviour that resulted in serious financial debts. He became mentally incompetent. Adjustment of the stimulator resolved the mania and restored his cogni-tive capacity for insight and rational judgment. Yet this resulted in a return of his motor symptoms, which were so severe that the patient became bedridden. This left the patient and his healthcare providers with a choice between two mutually exclusive options: to admit the patient to a nursing home because of a serious physical disability, despite intact cognitive and affective capacities; or to admit the patient to a chronic psychiatric ward because of a manic state, despite restoration of good motor function.

In this case, DBS produced the desired effect of motor control. But it also had the adverse effect of a significant alteration of the patient's state of mind. When his brain was not being stimulated, he was considered competent to decide about his own treat-ment, and he chose the second option. In accord with his competent expressed wish, he was legally committed to a chronic ward in a regional psychi-atric hospital. This clearly was a choice between two undesirable options, a choice that he made on qual-ity-of-life grounds. Assuming that he had the capac-ity to compare the two states, loss of motor control was worse than mania. He chose to continue DBS because the net benefit of being on the stimulator was greater than being off it. Or more accurately, the net harm of stimulation was less than the net harm of stopping it. It was the lesser of two evils. The psychological effect of stimulating the brain in this case is more extreme than the impulsivity mentioned earlier. Yet both cases illustrate how DBS can modulate some brain circuits only to overexcite others and result in psychopathology.

This case raises three main questions. First, by choosing an option that would leave him in a manic and thus mentally incompetent state, would he be waiving his autonomy, specifically regarding his capacity to consent to continuation or discontinuation of DBS and thus the ability to change his mind? Second, given that his choice would radically alter his state of mind, should this influence the decision of the medical team to continue stimulating his brain? Third, if his thought and behaviour significantly changed as a result of brain stimulation, then how could be benefit from it? Each of these ethical questions hinges on the differences between positive physiological and negative psychological effects of a medically indicated treatment

Autonomy and Identity

The patient's decision in this case seems similar in some respects to an advance directive made by a competent patient regarding subsequent medical treatment decisions that will have to be made when he or she is no longer competent to make them. This occurs most commonly in cases of dementia such as Alzheimer disease and usually pertains to end-of-life care. Advance directives allow competent individuals to state the interests they will have over the course of their lives. They can foresee how their bodies and minds will deteriorate over time, which medical interventions would be consistent with their interests, and which surrogate decision-makers would best respect these interests.[12] Formulating an advance directive also gives one control over one's life by limiting decisions

and actions by others that can affect one when no longer competent.

The PD case at issue here is different from the loss of decisional capacity in a typical application of an advance directive in at least two respects. Because the stimulator causes the patient to experience mania when it is turned on, the loss of decisional capacity is not a gradual or subsequent development but immediate. He autonomously and knowingly chooses an option that immediately makes him mentally incompetent and devoid of decisional capacity. The immediate loss of agency distinguishes this case from the gradual loss of agency in Alzheimer disease.[13] Moreover, unlike the demented patient, whose condition in irreversible, this patient's mental incompetence is reversible because the mania can be stopped by turning off the stimulator. While the patient's decision has the effect of binding him to state of mental incompetence, it is not his intention in opting for stimulation. The mania is an undesirable but acceptable side effect of the realisation of his intention to relieve the suffering he experiences in his loss of motor control. Yet his decision would have the effect of precluding any possibility of changing his mind. Paradoxically, an autonomous decision to consent to a medical treatment would make him lose his autonomy and capacity to subsequently choose to continue this treatment and to have or forego others.

Some might question whether the patient is competent enough to make an autonomous decision.[14] His affective state in response to his loss of motor control may impair his capacity to rationally consider the implications of his decision to continue with the stimulation. Antonio Damasio has shown that cognitive and affective capacities are interdependent and sustained by interacting cortical and limbic pathways in the brain. Impairment in either of these capacities may interfere with practical and moral reasoning and decision-making.[15] Yet there is no obvious affective impairment in the PD patient when he decides to resume the stimulation. Even if he were slightly depressed, this by itself would not imply that he lacked decisional capacity. As Paul Appelbaum has convincingly argued, depression by itself does not undermine decisional capacity.[16] A depressed patient may retain a sufficient degree of decisional capacity to understand the consequences of having or forgoing DBS. Nor would any feeling of desperation necessarily mean that the patient's decision was irrational or not sufficiently informed.

Although the patient has exercised his autonomy in consenting to the continuation of DBS for his disease, he need not be so constrained by his decision. Before initiating the procedure, his physicians would be obligated to discuss options that would not foreclose possible future actions that could benefit him. Changing the settings of the stimulator might resolve the mania problem. In the light of this possibility, when the patient made his decision the medical team caring for him would be obligated to offer to revisit the question of whether to continue or discontinue DBS at a later time. This would mean stopping the stimulation so that mental competence could be restored and the patient and his treating physicians could discuss treatment options. In this way, the medical team would be providing conditions allowing the patient the fullest expression of his autonomy in consenting to or refusing an intervention consistent with his own all-things-considered best interests. All of these steps would fall within the medical team's obligation to monitor the patient's condition over an extended period of time. Yet if the patient competently refused the future option of discontinuing stimulation in order to reassess whether to continue or discontinue this treatment, his decision would have to be respected.

The psychological continuity in virtue of which one persists as the same person over time can accommodate some changes in one's mental states.[17] It can accommodate some degree of change in the integrated set of experiences and memories that form one's identity. The concept of identity at issue here is not numerical identity, the idea that an individual at a later time T2 is the same as an individual at an earlier time T1. This condition can be satisfied by a minimal set of physical and psychological properties. Rather, the relevant concept of identity in this case is narrative identity. This consists of the characteristics and experiences that

make up the distinctive autobiography of a person.[18] These characteristics include the set of dispositional traits we refer to as personality. But how much change in one's mental states can an individual undergo and remain the same person? How much disruption can one's life narrative accommodate without threatening the integrity of the whole? Is there a threshold of continuity and integrity below which alteration of the psyche is substantial enough to alter the identity of the person? (Merkel 2007, chpt 5).[2] Gradual and subtle changes in personality are less likely to disrupt the necessary degree of integration of mental states to retain identity. But this may not be the case when there is a sudden radical change between earlier and later mental states. If the mania alters the general content and disrupts the integrity and continuity of his desires, beliefs, intentions and emotions, then the PD patient seems to become a different person once the stimulator is turned on. The mania produced by the DBS may put this patient below the threshold. So even when a medical procedure is effective, can it be justified if it radically alters one's life narrative and effectively turns one into a different person?

Neurosurgery generally involves more risks in altering thought and behaviour than DBS. Resecting a diffuse brain tumour is a delicate procedure that may damage healthy brain tissue and result in loss of language ability, memory, vision or significant changes in personality. Different surgeons and patients will be prepared to accept different degrees of risk. How much risk both parties are willing to accept depends on the probability of biological survival and the patient's quality of life with or without surgery. Although biological survival is not a factor in deciding whether to continue stimulating the brain for advanced PD, the risk of substantial changes to the psyche is. The trade-off is between acceptable quality of life regarding motor control and alteration of the mind. One comes at the cost of the other. The question of justifiability in the case under discussion is significant because the mania that alters identity is not just a probable but a certain result of stimulation.

For the patient, an alteration of his self resulting in less suffering is preferable to a self with more suffering. To be sure, not every patient would have this same preference. Freud had a painful oral cancer for many years that required a series of mouth and jaw operations. Yet he refused to take anything stronger than aspirin until the very end. He reportedly said, "I prefer to think in torment than not to be able to think clearly". Retaining a state of mind that allowed him to remain aware of his surroundings and to interact with others was more important than relief of his pain with narcotics, which would have altered this state.[19] The contrast between Freud and the PD patient illustrates how weighing the positive and negative effects of a drug or procedure on the psyche can be quite different from one person to the next.

One might question how an individual could benefit from a treatment if his or her identity changes as a result of it. If the alteration of mental states is substantial, then it is unclear who the beneficiary of the treatment would be. The individual experiencing the positive effects of the treatment would appear to be a different person from the one who requested the treatment. Still, the manic state of the PD patient does not entail a complete disruption of psychological continuity. This mental abnormality would appear to disrupt the thematic unity of the total set of his mental states over time and thus disrupt his narrative identity. But mania alone would not necessarily preclude his capacity to recall what it was like to lose motor control and to experience the positive effect of restoring this control. In spite of the change from a non-manic to a manic state, there may be enough psychological continuity and narrative integrity for him to retain a weaker yet sufficient sense of identity to remain the same person. Even if there is a substantial change in his identity following the brain stimulation, the moment he experiences relief from his suffering is enough to plausibly say that he benefits from it. The stimulation satisfies his interest in restoring motor control.[20] This point shows that metaphysical and psychological questions of identity cannot be separated from the normative question of benefit versus harm. The possibility of changes to the patient's psyche must be contextualised by the goal of relieving his suffering. Applying Ronald Dworkin's distinction,

the patient's experiential interests supersede his critical interests. The satisfaction he experiences in regaining motor control outweighs any interest he may have had in pursuing more general values and commitments in his life.[21]

The Benelux Neuromodulation Society recommends that

DBS of STN (subthalamic nucleus) for Parkinson disease should not be abandoned because of potential risks for behaviour and cognition. For the time being, extensive preoperative psychiatric and neuropsychological screening and special attention for cognitive and behavioural changes during follow-up seems to be warranted.[10]

The discussion of the case of the 62-year-old with PD suggests that we can go even further and make a stronger claim. Some individuals with neurological disorders suffer from them and desire symptom relief to such a degree that they would be willing to undergo or continue treatment entailing the risk of significant unwanted side effects on the psyche. Indeed, some individuals would be willing to make this choice when these effects were not just probable but certain. Some degree of desperation may motivate their decision. But desperation by itself does not mean that a patient lacks mental competence and decisional capacity, or that this would be an irrational choice for the patient. If the upshot of discussion of treatment options by the patient and the medical team is that the net benefit of DBS outweighs the net harm, then the decision to continue stimulation can be in the patient's best interests and accordingly ethically justified.

Conclusion

Electrical stimulation of subcortical regions of the brain can control and relieve physical and psychological symptoms of a number of neurological and psychiatric disorders. For many patients, however, this involves trade-offs between positive and negative effects on the mind. The technique may effectively treat symptoms associated with a disorder only to cause adverse psychological effects, which may not be predictable. More controlled studies can help to get a clearer sense of the general safety and efficacy of DBS. On this basis, researchers and clinicians can better inform patients with these disorders, or their surrogates, about the relative benefits and risks. Yet no two persons' brains are alike, and no two persons' minds respond in the same way to treatments affecting the brain. A physiological improvement does not always translate into a psychological benefit for a person undergoing an intervention in the brain. What counts as a successful medical treatment for a neurologist or psychiatrist does not necessarily mean that the patient is better off as a result of it. Medical professionals and patients together need to consider the effects of DBS on the brain and the mind. In the end, though, it is the competent patient who has to decide whether the trade-offs in any given treatment would be acceptable and whether he or she should have or continue to have it.

References

1   Benabid A.L. What the future holds for deep-brain stimulation. *Expert Rev Med Devices* 2007; 4:895–903.

2   Merkel R., Boer G., Fegert J., et al. *Intervening in the brain: changing psyche and society.* Berlin: Springer, 2007: 6.

3   Dodd M.L., et al. Pathological gambling caused by drugs used to treat Parkinson disease. *Arch Neurol* 2005; 62:579–83.

4   Frank M., et al. Hold your horses: impulsivity, deep brain stimulation, and medication in Parkinsonism. *Science* 2007; 318:1309–12.

5   Piasecki S.D. and Jefferson J.W. Psychiatric complications of deep-brain stimulation for Parkinson's disease. *J Clin Psychiatry* 2004; 65:845–9.

6   Weaver F., Follet K., Stern M., et al. Bilateral deep-brain stimulation vs best medical therapy for patients with advanced Parkinson disease. *JAMA* 2009; 301:63–73.

7   Mallet L., et al. Subthalamic nucleus stimulation in severe obsessive-compulsive disorder. *N Engl J Med* 2008; 359:2121–34.

8   Lozano A., et al. Subcallosal cingulate gyrus deep-brain stimulation for treatment-resistant depression. *Biol Psychiatry* 2008; 64:461–7.

9   Mayberg H., et al. Deep-brain stimulation for treatment-resistant depression. *Neuron* 2005; 45:651–60.

10 Merkel R., Rosahl S., Nuttin B., et al. Ethical and legal aspects of neuromodulation: on the road to guidelines. *Neuromodulation* 2007; 10:177–86.

11 Leentjens A.F., et al. Manipulation of mental competence: an ethical problem in a case of electrical stimulation of the subthalamic nucleus for severe Parkinson's disease. *Ned Tijdschr Geneesk* 2004; 148:1394–8.

12 Buchanan A. and Brock D. *Deciding for others: the ethics of surrogate decision making.* New York: Cambridge University Press, 1989.

13 Jaworska A. Ethical dilemmas in neurodegenerative disease: respecting patients at the twilight of agency. In: Illes J., ed. *Neuroethics: defining the issues in theory, practice and policy.* Oxford: Oxford University Press, 2006: 87–101.

14 Beauchamp T. and Childress J. *Principles of Biomedical Ethics,* 6th edn, New York: Oxford University Press, 2009: Chpt 4.

15 Damasio A. Neuroscience and ethics: intersections, *AJOB–Neuroscience* 2007; 7:3–7.

16 Appelbaum P. Assessment of patients' competence to consent to treatment. *N Engl J Med* 2007; 357:1834–40.

17 Parfit D. *Reasons and persons.* Oxford: Clarendon Press, 1984: Part 3.

18 Schechtman M. *The Constitution of selves.* Ithaca: Cornell University Press, 1997.

19 Griffin J. *Well-being: its meaning, measurement, and moral importance.* Oxford: Clarendon Press, 1986:8.

20 Feinberg J. *Harm to others.* New York: Oxford University Press, 1986.

21 Dworkin R. *Life's dominion.* New York: Knopf, 1993.

97

Authenticity or Autonomy? When Deep Brain Stimulation Causes a Dilemma

Felicitas Kraemer

Introduction: Feelings of Authenticity and Alienation under Deep Brain Stimulation

Deep brain stimulation (DBS) is a treatment used mainly for patients with Parkinson's disease that helps control Parkinson symptoms. It involves the implantation of a device called a 'brain pacemaker', which connects electrodes implanted in a patient's brain to an electronic pulse generator that controls those electrodes, located beneath the patient's keybone. The electrodes stimulate the thalamus or other parts of the patient's brain and thereby help control Parkinson symptoms. Worldwide, numerous patients are currently treated via DBS, and a considerable number of them experience psychosocial side effects.[1] While the literature in neuroethics has tended to focus on side effects involving personality changes and problems relating to autonomy and accountability, there are also problems relating to what could philosophically be described as feelings of authenticity and alienation.[2] As a recent study by Schüpbach *et al* (2006) reveals,

these feelings emerge in different ways in different patients: some patients report that after having undergone DBS they feel as if they are their 'true selves'; others, however, say that after treatment they no longer recognise themselves and feel alienated. This and other evidence suggests that the patients' subjective experience of feeling authentic or alienated is normatively significant in the context of DBS; however, it has not yet received close enough attention in the neuroethics debates about DBS.[3]

Yet, though the concept of authenticity has not played a major role in debates about DBS, it has become increasingly important in neuroethics more generally and has even started competing with the well established ethical concept of autonomy. This is evident in the debates over the ethics of psychopharmacological neurointerventions. The fact that numerous patients under treatment with the antidepressant Prozac, say they feel 'like themselves' for the first time in their lives has ignited considerable ethical discussion.[4-6] Here, the probably most well known work is Peter Kramer's study *Listening to Prozac*.[5] The present article attempts to show that these sorts of considerations are also relevant in the

Original publication details: Felicitas Kramer, "Authenticity or Autonomy? When Deep Brain Stimulation Causes a Dilemma," pp. 757–760 from *Journal of Medical Ethics* 39 (2013). Reproduced with permission of BMJ Publishing Group Ltd.

context of DBS. In order to bring this to light, I will discuss a recent case study that reveals how feelings of authenticity can play an important role in a patient's experience of DBS; indeed, these feelings can potentially cause patients to face a dilemma in which they have to choose between authenticity and autonomy. My interpretation of this case will, in turn, point toward the most pressing questions that arise from the issues surrounding authenticity and alienation in relation to DBS. I will describe the case, offer an overlooked interpretation that is an alternative to the one supported in the literature and defend it. I will then use my interpretation to raise and discuss general issues about possible conflicts between autonomy and authenticity and why they are ethically important. This will be done in the hope that these concerns will facilitate future discussion of this issue in the ethical discussion of DBS.

A Patient's Dilemma: Choosing between Mental Competence and Well-Being

In a recent article in the Dutch medical journal *Nederlandse Tijdschrift voor Geneeskunde*, Leentjens *et al*[7] report a case study, which I shall refer to as 'the case of the Dutch patient', in which a 62-year-old patient with Parkinson's disease faced a dilemma as a result of DBS. The patient who had a brain pacemaker implant and was under treatment with DBS, developed, along with other psychological and social problems, a permanent manic state that could not be controlled via medication. This case study is paradigmatic of the frequent personality-changing side effects that patients experience as a result of DBS implants. It raises the issues of autonomy, accountability, personal identity and quality of life as they have been discussed in the literature.[8–11] But, significantly for our purposes, it also points toward the importance of the notion of authenticity in our considerations of DBS.

When the patient's mania became so severe that he ran up excessive debts, had an altercation with the police and eventually faced hospitalisation in a psychiatric

clinic, his physicians decided to ask the patient whether they should deactivate his implant. When the device was in the switched-on mode, the patient was in a manic state. In this mode, he was not believed to be accountable and rational, meaning, unable to give informed consent. In the terminology of medical ethics, he was considered to be mentally incompetent and not legally accountable, that is, he was *not an autonomous agent*. In what follows, I will use the term 'autonomous' as a synonym to 'mentally competent' in terms of decision making and the ability to give informed consent. By contrast, when the device was in the switched-off mode, the patient was believed to be 'normal', meaning, he possessed a rational and accountable state of mind in which he was able to autonomously make rational decisions. At the same time, however, in this state, he was physically disabled, bedridden and dependent on others; he was severely depressed and suffered physically and mentally from the burden of his disease.[7]

Eventually, the physicians agreed to ask the patient while he was in the *switched-off mode* (the autonomous mode in which he was believed to be accountable and rational), whether the device should be deactivated. Additionally, he was asked to fill out an advance directive about the future, stating that he agreed to be kept under psychiatric care for the rest of his life if he kept the device activated.

The patient decided to have his implant permanently left switched on, and to spend the rest of his life in a psychiatric clinic – in a decent bodily condition, but in a permanent manic state.[7]

In what follows, I will provide an interpretation of the Dutch case study. In doing so, I will draw inferences from other case studies that I regard as analogous to this one in relevant respects: the aforementioned Schüpbach cases, a study by Munhoz *et al* (ref.[12], cit. in ref.[13]) and the autobiography by Helmut Dubiel, an academic who gets treated by DBS and reports about his feelings of alienation under treatment.[14] I use the content of the patients' statements in these other case studies to shed light on the Dutch case, primarily resorting to Schüpbach's material.

Prima facie, the Dutch case seems to warrant the following interpretation. The patient opted for the switched-on mode for two reasons: first, being under stimulation improved his bodily state and allowed him to avoid physical suffering and dependence on the care of others. Second, the manic state presumably provided the patient with pleasant feelings. In the switched-on mode, he could avoid the depression he experienced in the switched-off mode, whereas in the switched-off state he would have had to endure not only physical but also mental suffering for the rest of his life. In his article 'Stimulating brains, altering minds', Walter Glannon discusses the example of the Dutch patient as well. In his interpretation, the patient made his choice on 'quality of life grounds' (ref.[15], p 290). Glannon writes: 'Assuming that he had the capacity to compare his two states, loss of motor control was worse than mania. He chose to continue DBS because the net benefit of being on the stimulator, was greater than being off it. . . It was the lesser of two evils' (ref.[15], p 290; cf. also ref.[16], p 3).

Understood in this way, the patient faced a dilemma: he had to choose between feeling well and being mentally competent. And, ultimately, *by deciding for his well-being, the patient sacrificed his mental competence and autonomy.*

We know little about the Dutch case, and cannot fully decide whether Glannon's interpretation is the correct one or not. However, there is considerable independent evidence suggesting that the interpretation that I will provide in what follows is at least equally plausible. This interpretation has so far been overlooked, because there is a tendency to focus on quality of life at the expense of autonomy and authenticity. Moreover, this interpretation raises neglected general issues about possible conflicts between autonomy and authenticity in DBS patients. More generally, these issues are of interest even independently of this particular case.

Authenticity or Autonomy? A Philosophical Reinterpretation

One could wonder whether Walter Glannon is right in stating that the Dutch patient faces a dilemma between mental competence and quality of life

(ref.[15], p 290; cf. also ref.[16], p 3). In his interpretation, the Dutch patient opts for permanent stimulation on qualify-of-life grounds – sacrificing his mental competence for his well-being.

However, Glannon's interpretation is contested by cases where people choose authenticity even at a cost to hedonic well-being. For instance, take Peter Kramer's patient Philip, in his *Listening to Prozac.*[5] Philip's mood improves under the intake of Prozac, but he feels inauthentic in the pleasant state and therefore stops the treatment. This is one example that shows that a person's preferences for authenticity can even be more fundamental than hedonic ones. In some cases, people are willing to sacrifice wellbeing in order to remain authentic.

In light of this, it seems likely that a more weighty counterconsideration was behind the Dutch patients' choice as well. A closer look reveals that there is another philosophical interpretation of this case available that runs deeper than a *prima facie* reading focused on quality of life, an interpretation that emphasises the patient's experience of authenticity. This interpretation is guided by other case studies that I regard as analogous to this one in relevant respects.[3 12 14] In these studies, we find numerous patients under stimulation using the language of authenticity and alienation (refs.[3],[6], cf. also ref.[16], p 2).

For instance, one of the patients in the Schüpbach study made it clear that he feels authentic under stimulation and regards his switched-off mode as alienating.[2] Further evidence in the literature can be found where patients describe their switched-on modes under DBS as authentic. For instance, Carter *et al* (2010),[13] with reference to a study by Munhoz *et al*,[12] report on a patient treated with dopamine replacement therapy (DRT) that works on the dopaminergic system in a similar way as DBS does, who under medication indulged in sexual practices that he had not pursued before. Once the medication was stopped, the patient reported that he had these desires prior to DRT treatment, but had been 'too embarrassed to act on them'. As the authors put it, the medication allowed the patient to 'realise these desires'. As they write, 'after a change in his medication', he 'later on expressed regret at his behaviour'. Nevertheless, according to them, this exemplifies a case 'in which DRT induces behaviour that individuals claim are authentic'.[12]

This evidence together with the cases of Prozac-induced felt authenticity described by Peter Kramer,[5] makes one wonder whether these results might be relevant to the Dutch patient. One could ask: might the Dutch patient have felt authentic in the switched-on mode and alienated when switched off, similar to the other cases just considered?

Maybe it was even this felt authenticity that motivated the Dutch patient to stay on stimulation? It is at least a possibility that he could have decided to stay switched-on *because* he felt authentic in the stimulated state and *because* he regarded his unstimulated life as alienating. The authors of the Dutch study do not report any account of the patient's feelings; so here we can only speculate. In one of Schüpbach's cases, a DBS patient says: 'During all these years of illness, I was asleep. Now I am stimulated, stimulated to lead a different life'.[3] Imagine that, in the same vein, the Dutch patient had said or thought something like the following: 'The person that drives his car too fast, that leads a promiscuous life and that runs into debts is really me! In my previous life, before stimulation, I did not dare to do such unreasonable things. I lived a well-adapted life – a life which I now see was never really mine. But now, I have the chance to be who I really am'.

If one, still on the basis of an assumed analogy with the Schüpbach cases, accepts this as a possible narrative for the Dutch patient, a new interpretation of his dilemma arises. On the *prima facie* reading, the patient had to choose between bodily and psychological well-being on the one hand, and autonomy, understood as mental competence, on the other. If, however, he really felt authentic under stimulation, he faced a different dilemma: he had to choose between being autonomous, that is, mentally competent in the switched-off mode, and feeling authentic, albeit being manic, in the switched-on mode. To be both autonomous *and* authentic was not possible for him. In the authentic state, he is no longer able to make

any mentally competent, autonomous decisions in the future, and vice versa, when being mentally competent, he does not feel authentic. In this light, one could redescribe his dilemma as a *dilemma between autonomy and authenticity*.

Having said this, it is important to note that 'authenticity' is not used as an ontological term here, such as, for example, 'authenticity proper' or 'actual authenticity', but rather in the sense of 'felt authenticity'. In this, I follow Kraemer[17] who has argued that in the case of patients taking the antidepressant Prozac, we should primarily focus on subjectively felt authenticity rather than on 'ontological' concepts. This is to avoid resorting to unprovable metaphysical assumptions in the discourse about authenticity.[6]

Is 'Authenticity' the New 'Autonomy' in Neuroethics?

The Dutch case, as construed on the authenticity interpretation, raises at least three ethical questions. Is authenticity as ethically relevant as autonomy? Are there any patients' rights and, accordingly, any duties for healthcare professionals that can be inferred from patients' feelings of authenticity under DBS? In the case of a conflict between authenticity and autonomy, is authenticity always overriding?

Even if one recognises that authenticity is important for some patients, a patient's mental competence, and thus his or her autonomy is still a key capacity when it comes to decision making and informed consent. In the Dutch case, this is presumably why the doctors have the patient make his decision in the switched-off mode in which he is mentally competent. In the Kantian as well as in the utilitarian tradition, autonomy counts as a value. One can conclude that when it comes to decision making, such as in the case of the Dutch patient, then healthcare professionals should primarily focus on autonomy and give less weight to questions of authenticity. Otherwise, the patient's consent would not be ethically valid. In this sense, the answer to the question raised in the heading of the section is 'no': authenticity is not the new autonomy in neuroethics, at least not in the assessment of a patient's decision-making capacities. Under these circumstances, it is still autonomy that is of primary value, not authenticity.

However, on the interpretation of the Dutch case I offered above, felt authenticity seems to play a pre-eminent role *for the patient*. It is his felt preference and a paramount value. Here, the value of authenticity competes with the value of autonomy in the sense that the patient has to decide between them. In a mentally competent state, the patient decides to remain in a mentally incompetent state for the rest of his life in which he feels authentic. For the Dutch patient, the value of authenticity seems to outweigh the one of autonomy.

The second question is whether there are any patients' rights and, accordingly, any duties for healthcare professionals that can be inferred from patients' feelings of authenticity under DBS. From what has been said, it becomes clear that patients' felt authenticity deserves respect as a felt preference. It is a value that some patients may give the preference to over autonomy. However, it would be too fast to infer any general claims from a single case, even if it is backed up by other studies. With respect to the normative status of feelings of authenticity as felt preferences, no immediate normative consequences arise. Accordingly, no special patient rights and duties of healthcare professionals can be derived from them right away. The insight that authenticity matters for some patients seems to be primarily of *heuristic value*: understanding feelings of authenticity is of importance for healthcare professionals in order to better understand their patients' decisions (cf. ref.[2]). Additionally, it is crucial for medical ethicists in order to enable them to develop new theories about what matters in a future ethics of DBS.

The third question is whether, in the case of a conflict between authenticity and autonomy, authenticity is practically overriding? What should we do if someone feels authentic in a mental state that we as a society find problematic? As we saw in the case of the Dutch patient, sometimes feeling authentic is connected with asocial behaviour, which puts the

patient and others at risk. Especially in cases such as the Dutch one, healthcare professionals might be justified in weighing the value of *safety* higher than the one of authenticity. Whenever a patient runs the risk of severely damaging others and himself, healthcare professionals must restrict his or her drive for authenticity. Understood this way, felt authenticity is not everything, that is, it is not necessarily of pre-eminent significance when it clashes with other basic values, such as, for example, safety.

Conclusions

As is evidenced by this discussion, questions surrounding authenticity and alienation should play an important role in our considerations of the ethics of DBS. DBS can change a patient's mental state in a groundbreaking way. In cases like that of the Dutch patient (at least as it is construed in this paper), patients can be faced with a choice between the values of autonomy and authenticity. Healthcare professionals and medical ethicists need to determine which of them should be given more normative weight (cf. ref.[2]).

In the Dutch case, authenticity seems to be of great value for the patient. In the end, he even opts for authenticity against autonomy. The conclusion the current paper draws from this interpretation is twofold. First, feelings of authenticity that can arise under treatment deserve respect as central preferences of some DBS patients, because they are closely connected to their self-understanding and are therefore of paramount value for them. Getting insight into their patients' feelings of authenticity and alienation under treatment is of considerable heuristic value for healthcare professionals and ethicists. It can provide them with a better understanding of the motivation and treatment decisions of a patient and with a better basis for a more elaborate ethics of DBS (cf. also ref.[18]).

Second, however, this does not imply that authenticity should be given equal weight or even more weight than autonomy by caregivers in all contexts. Rather, when it comes to the assessment of a patient's capacity for rational decision making, it is certainly autonomy understood as mental competence rather than feelings of authenticity that should be given more weight. In situations in which the patient endangers herself and others, the significance of autonomy as a guarantor of reasonable behaviour certainly normatively outweighs the one of a patient's feelings of authenticity.

These and similar problems that can arise in the context of DBS will become even more pressing in the future, as countries such as the USA have allowed the use of DBS for psychiatric disorders, such as depression, dystonia, and obsessive-compulsive disorders.[19] One day DBS may even be used for enhancement purposes.[20] In the past, problems relating to authenticity and alienation have been discussed in the context of psychopharmacological neurointerventions. Now it is time to raise them in the context of DBS as well.

References

1   Merello M. Deep brain stimulation of the subthalamic nucleus for the treatment of Parkinson's disease. In: Tarsy D., Vitek J.L., Starr P., and Okun M., eds. *Deep brain stimulation in neurological and psychiatric disorders.* New York: Humana Press, 2008: 253–76.

2   Kraemer F. Me, myself and my brain implant: deep brain stimulation raises questions of personal authenticity and alienation. *Neuroethics* 2013; 6: 483–97.

3   Schüpbach M., Cargiulo M., Welter M.L., et al. Neurosurgery in Parkinson disease: a distressed mind in a repaired body? *Neurology* 2006; 66:1811–16.

4   Elliott C. *Better than well, American medicine meets the American dream.* New York: W.W. Norton & Company, 2003.

5   Kramer P. *Listening to Prozac. A psychiatrist explores antidepressant drugs and the remaking of the self.* New York: Penguin, 1997.

6   Kraemer F. Authenticity Anyone? The Enhancement of Emotions via Neuro-Psychopharmacology. *Neuroethics* 2011; 4:51–64.

7   Leentjens A.F.G., Visser-Vandewalle V., Temel Y., et al. Manipuleerbare wilsbekwaamheid: een ethisch probleem bij elektrostimulatie van de nucleus subthalamicus voor ernstige ziekte van Parkinson. *Nederlandse Tijdschrift voor Geneeskunde* 2004; 148:1394–8.

8   Klaming L. and Haselager P. Did my brain implant make me do it? Questions raised by DBS regarding psychological continuity, responsibility for action and mental competence. *Neuroethics* 2013; 6:527–39.

9   Müller O., Bittner U., and Krug H.. [Narrative identity and therapy with 'brain pacemaker': reflections on the integration of patients' self-descriptions in the ethical assessment of deep brain stimulation.] *Ethik Med* 2011; 22:303–15 (German).

10 Schechtman M. Philosophical reflections on narrative and deep brain stimulation. *Journal of Clinical Ethics* 2010; 21:133–9.

11 Schermer M. Health, happiness and human enhancement – dealing with unexpected effects of deep brain stimulation. *Neuroethics* 2013 ;6:435–45.

12 Munhoz R.P., Fabiani G., Becker N., et al. Increased frequency and range of sexual behavior in a patient with Parkinson's disease after use of pramipexole: a case report. *J Sex Med* 2009; 6:1177–80.

13 Carter A. Ambermoon P., and Hall W.D. Drug-induced impulse control disorders: a prospectus for neuroethical analysis. *Neuroethics* 2010; 4:91–102.

14 Dubiel H. *Deep in the brain: living with Parkinson's disease.* New York: Europa Editions, 2009.

15 Glannon W. Stimulating brains, altering minds. *J Med Ethics* 2009; 35:289–92. [See also Chapter 96 in this *Anthology.*]

16 Bailys F. "I am who I am": on the perceived threats to personal identity from deep brain stimulation. *Neuroethics* 2013; 6:513–26.

17 Kraemer F. Authenticity anyone? The enhancement of emotions via neuro-pharmacology. *Neuroethics* 2011; 4:51–64.

18 Meynen G. Psychiatrie en neuromodulatie. Welke wilsbekwame keuze moet de arts volgen? *Nieuwsbrief Bioethiek* 2011; 18:9–11.

19 Kopell B.H., Greenberg B., and Rezai A.R. Deep brain stimulation for psychiatric disorders. *J Clin Neurophysiol* 2004; 21:51–67.

20 Synofzik M. and Schlaepfer T.E. Stimulating personality: ethical criteria for deep brain stimulation in psychiatric patients and for enhancement purposes. *Biotechnol J* 2008; 3:1511–20.

98

On the Necessity of Ethical Guidelines for Novel Neurotechnologies

Sara Goering and Rafael Yuste

The Brain Research through Advancing Innovative Neurotechnologies (BRAIN) Initiative, as well as other such large-scale projects around the world, is poised to revolutionize our capacity for recording and manipulating large-scale neuronal activity. These methods could spur a new era in the scientific understanding of neural circuits and also enable powerful novel therapeutic approaches to mental and neurological diseases. At the same time, these methods will provide access to the core mechanisms that underlie human identify, memories, emotions, personality and, more generally, our minds. As such, they could have profound consequences for human identity and society.

Spurred by a recent workshop that brought together neurotechnologists and bioethicists, in this Commentary we highlight the need for strong advocacy toward developing and funding neuroethical work to accompany these advances in neuroscience and to guide the development of neurotechnologies. We think that the time is ripe, given that neural interventions currently being studied in many animal models already demonstrate the capacity to decode imagery and intentions, stimulate or alter sensory perceptions, enhance and combine brain processing power, and

alter animal behavior. Even scientists working directly in these areas can recognize the rich opportunities to better understand neural processing while still expressing some trepidation about the kind of future we may be bringing about. This situation calls for the development of a clear set of guidelines, similar to the Belmont Commission Report, to integrate the development and use of these technologies with our core societal and human values. These guidelines could be developed by multidisciplinary panels, composed of scientific, medical, bioethical, and legal experts, as well as representatives of the citizenry at large. Such panels would help to ensure that neurotechnology is developed in ways that are sensitive to some of the profound qualities that serve as the condition of human experience: private mental life, agential action on the world, and an understanding of individuals as bounded by their bodies.

Novel Neurotechnologies and Their Future Use

The BRAIN initiative, sponsored by the White House in 2013, is a large-scale, 12-year-long project aimed at

Original publication details: Sara Goering and Rafael Yuste, "On the Necessity of Ethical Guidelines for Novel Neurotechnologies," pp. 882–885 from *Cell* 167 (2016). Reproduced with permission of Elsevier.

Bioethics: An Anthology, Fourth Edition. Edited by Udo Schüklenk and Peter Singer.

creating tools to interrogate and alter neural circuits in experimental animals and humans with unprecedented detail (https://obamawhitehouse.archives.gov/BRAIN). Similar initiatives are now underway in the European Union, Japan, Korea, Canada, Australia, Israel, and China. As a consequence of these projects, more than two hundred laboratories around the world are now funded to systematically develop new methods for recording and manipulating the activity of neural circuits, including awake behaving animals or human subjects. These methods use optical, electrical, or chemical platforms, aided by novel computational tools that help decipher this trove of neural activity.

While we are still far from properly "breaking the code" that any nervous system uses to generate behavior or mental states, decoding efforts are progressing swiftly. For example, using the relatively low spatio-temporal resolution method of fMRI [functional magnetic resonance imaging], researchers can start to predict the activity patterns associated with complex visual stimuli that a human subject has been exposed to (Kay et al., 2008), and the ability to access high-quality recordings of neural activity will make these efforts more powerful. Once encoding models are accurate, researchers may be able to decode visual imagery from active human subjects, enabling a technology-based kind of "mind reading." Visual imagery is just one of many possibilities for decoding: other scenarios such as the decoding of speech, thoughts (including lies), and dreams, or even the decoding of internal states of animals, can be envisioned. Brain decoding could become ubiquitous. Human subjects using portable decoders could also perhaps covertly communicate with each other without the need to speak, sign, or type their thoughts.

In addition, powerful methods can start to manipulate neuronal activity with single-cell precision. In experimental animals, such as worms, *Drosophila,* zebra fish, or mice, optogenetics is routinely used to alter behavior (Yizhar et al., 2011), including triggering of memories (Ramirez et al., 2013). Two-photon optogenetics enables researchers to implant, and later replay, patterns of activity into the cerebral cortex of awake mice (Carrillo-Reid et al., 2016). While optogenetics is unlikely to be applied to humans in the near future because it involves genetic manipulation, other optical

stimulation methods using optochemical compound or nanoparticles do not require any genetic manipulation and could be more easily adaptable to humans. Such interventions offer considerable promise for managing unwanted patterns of thought and behavior in human patients but also raise daunting possibilities for control.

Manipulating neural circuits to alter behavior in human subjects is not new. Deep brain stimulation (DBS) devices are routinely used as treatment for many neurological diseases with some success, though, in some cases, they lead to changes in personality and behavior. In others cases, subjects report feeling the need to use DBS in order to "become themselves" (Vlek et al., 2012). In addition, brain computer interfaces (BCI) are routinely used in a wide variety of clinical applications to record neuronal activity and connect it via computer systems to control robotic or prosthetic limbs or devices. With BCIs, subjects can be trained to operate robotic prostheses with their thoughts. Such interfaces have provided the ability for paralyzed patients to move prosthetic limbs (Hochberg et al., 2006). Again, once high-quality recordings on neural activity become routine, BCI will become much more powerful. In particular, if neural recordings are performed in a non-invasive fashion, BCI could become widely used to augment the physical or intellectual capabilities of humans. In addition, several human subjects could jointly train connected BCIs to perform a joint task, blurring the identity (and responsibility) of individual users.

Ethical and Societal Issues Raised by Novel Neurotechnologies

While some would say that these scenarios are still in the realm of science-fiction, we believe that they are coming down the pipeline, given ongoing research. Thus, they warrant the question of how the application of novel neurotechnologies to humans should be properly guided and regulated. This problem is not novel, since humankind has been experimenting with methods to alter and manipulate brain activity for thousands of years, for example with alcohol, recreational drugs, or pharmacology. But while those methods normally affect the brain in a relatively coarse fashion, the more we learn about neural processing and the more powerful neuromodulation methods become, the more profound will be the effect of these manipulations on mental states and behavior.

Ethical, legal, and societal issues arising from novel neurotechnologies are many and could unfold progressively: some issues may arise in the very near term, whereas others are farther out and will depend on how research in the intervening period proceeds. Here, we review just a few issues on the horizon, given topics within currently funded neuroscientific research.

One of the more important ethical and philosophical issues ahead is the possibility of substantial changes in the concept of self. While at present we tend to identify ourselves as relatively separate, private entities bounded by our bodies (and even on more dynamic, relational views, like Baylis [2013], we still have private consciousness and distinct agency), the use of novel neurotechnologies may lead to a partial dissolution of traditional ideas of self. Access to neural activity will also call into the question the privacy of our internal lives (Farah and Wolpe, 2004), while the capacity to neuromodulate that activity may alter our sense of agency (Haselager, 2013), along with issues of moral and legal responsibility for our thoughts and actions (Farahany, 2012). If our neural activity can control devices beyond our bodies through thought alone (via BCI devices), our internal body schemas may stretch to encompass the devices under our immediate conscious control, essentially extending our sense of self beyond the boundaries of our bodies. BCI users can already learn to control a robotic arm just by thinking; what if they could send it out of the room to collect a needed item? *Where* is the user in this scenario?

In the other direction, we can also envision changes to our sense of self through the possibility of collecting multiple BCI users into a shared task in a way that results in a common action. Brain-to-brain interface experiments (Stocco et al., 2015), while still primitive in many respects, demonstrate the possibility of sending neural activity from one person's brain directly into another person's brain. Some experiments have demonstrated the capacity to connect neural activity of even three different experimental animals for a common purpose (Pais-Vieira et al., 2015). In these

scenarios, assignments of responsibility and understandings of self and agency will be complicated. The boundary of self (as body) becomes permeable to another's consciousness and control.

These issues are philosophically profound and morally and legally momentous. Traditional understandings of who (and where) we are and what we are responsible for are foundational for our legal systems and our moral interactions with each other. Proper protections for private internal spaces and agential identity will need to be integrated into our understandings of human rights. The use of methods that may substantially alter one's personality, thoughts, and sensorimotor experience requires attention to individual and societal protections.

In addition, the ability to augment one's physical or mental performance raises a host of issues about fairness and justice regarding how those augmenting technologies should be accessed or regulated. Are they intended for mass consumption, or should they be restricted to human users who have identifiable impairments (Aas and Wasserman, 2016)? How should we think about the standards of "normal functioning" and ability expectation (Wolbring and Diep, 2016) in the context of technologies that suggest a kind of ability revolution? If such technology is expensive, as it is bound to be at the beginning, it could generate or exacerbate societal divisions among the population or among inhabitants of different countries.

Pertinent to this discussion are the mobile "smart" devices, such as cell phones, that are increasingly part of our decision making and that could be interpreted as a basic, low-tech BCI devices. The current generation of smart phones is the precursor of future, more powerful prosthetic devices, which could be worn or implanted. The profound impact that smart phones have had in our society and culture over the last decade presages an even larger effect that brain-controlled wearable electronics devices may have. Importantly, in addition to enhancing our access to information, these interactive neural devices incorporate machine-learning algorithms (e.g., in the service of facial recognition software) that may incorporate and reproduce implicit bias, reinforcing negative stereotypes among racial groups or minorities.

Although many of the novel neurotechnologies are currently being explored in the context of medical research and patient care, or in the frame of assistive devices, as with all technology, they are also likely to have commercial applications that would, of necessity, involve different forms of regulation and oversight. Furthermore, one can easily envision military or security applications. As with issues such as chemical, biological, or nuclear weapons or, more recently, cyber warfare, this raises the concern as to the rules under which novel neurotechnologies should be used, if at all, in human conflagrations.

Developing Ethical Principles for Neurotechnologies

We think it is fair to say that, to date, we lack any agreed-upon guidelines to responsibly shape the development and application of these novel neurotechnologies. How could one approach the task of building such ethical guidelines? One possibility is to follow the case of medicine as a natural example, given that medical technology also represents a set of methods that interfere with the function of the human body. Indeed, in medicine, the use of technologies to monitor and alter the capabilities of the human body has always been guided by a common humanistic goal: to help patients in need or, more generally, to promote, without borders, the health of the entire population of the world. Over millennia, at least since the Hippocratic Oath, medicine has developed a corpus of ethical rules that have formed a deontology. These medical ethics principles are taught in medical schools and adhered to closely by practitioners of medicine throughout much of the world and across history. Principles of medical ethics are also respected by society as a whole, including scientists, governments, the private sector, and the military. After the Second World War, modern medical ethics were institutionalized by the Belmont Report, a document generated by the National Commission for the Protection of Human Subjects of Biomedical and Behavioral Research in the US (http://www.hhs.gov/ohrp/regulations-and-policy/belmont-report/index.html). This report proposed ethical principles

and guidelines for research involving human subjects under three core principles: respect, beneficence, and justice. Issues such as informed consent, assessment of risks and benefits, and selection of subjects are dealt with in a practical fashion. The Belmont report is widely respected and constitutes the core set of values underlying modern medical practice.

We think that the time is ripe for a similar set of principles, a Belmont report for neuroethics. These principles should offer guidelines for the effective protection of human subjects and values in conjunction with the ongoing research in this new area. But who should generate such a set of ethical and societal guidelines for the new technologies? Scientific experts who are developing these methods should be involved, given that they know better than anyone the current and likely future capabilities of the technologies. In addition, medical practitioners can contribute their experience interacting with patients seeking help for neurologically related disorders and people interested in assistive devices. Bioethicists, who work at the interface between ethical issues and biomedicine, are also clearly needed. Legal experts can provide important insights regarding human rights protections and approaches to the integration of these technologies in the legal codes of society. Finally, we think that representatives of the citizenship at large should also be involved, including of disabled people who are members of the likely early target populations for BCI and neuromodulation experiments designed to address impairments or offer assistive devices. The progress of science, while it should be freely pursued for curiosity's sake as the best way of enhancing knowledge, should also be informed by the needs and circumstances of the society that, after all, funds and supports all scientific work (Kitcher, 2011). Representatives of the citizens could also play a critical role in translating to the wider society the importance of these methods and discussions and the guidelines that are recommended. Given the amount of hype that abounds in the press and in science-fiction literature and movies, it is of great importance that citizens clearly understand, without any exaggeration, the potential benefits of these technologies, as well as their potential dystopian outcomes.

To complement and sustain the work of these panels, we recommend robust funding of neuroethics in order to develop it further as a subfield of bioethics. This could enable a vigorous academic and societal debate regarding the meaning and consequences of this technology and ensure that the guidelines reflect the best ideas generated by the community. The current NIH BRAIN initiative program to fund neuroethics work (https://grants.nih.gov/grants/guide/notice-files/NOT-MH-16-014.html), together with the recent creation of a Neuroethics working group [https://www.braininitiative.nih.gov/about/neuroethics-working-group], is a good start but still small steps relative to the significance of the issues at hand.

The Importance of Novel Neurotechnology for the Progress of Humankind

In closing, our aim here is not to contribute to or feed fear for doomsday scenarios but to ensure that we are reflective and intentional as we prepare ourselves for the neurotechnological future, which we believe can be a momentous positive change in our history. Indeed, novel neurotechnologies could serve as a liberating force for humankind. Humans have been defined by our tool making, and new technologies and the knowledge accumulated through them have enabled us to free ourselves from some of the tyrannies of prejudice and, in a way, of space and time. Scientific progress has enabled impressive opportunities for health and well-being, communication, and trade. Similar benefits probably lie ahead with the incorporation of novel neurotechnologies to our society. But these advances should be shared equitably, and a responsible society should aim to develop them in ways that are both broadly beneficial and sensitive to individual rights and needs. As we turn our impressive powers of investigation to the task of exploring and understanding the brain – the organ central to the physiological processes that make us who we are – we ought to think hard about the kinds of beings we might want to become and the kind of society we are building for our children. Public confidence in science should be anchored on responsible deployment of scientific advances. Technological advances must be shaped by our collective moral sensibilities in order to ensure that these advances are smoothly incorporated into our culture and indeed contribute to the common good.

References

Aas, S. and Wasserman, D. (2016). *J. Med. Ethics*. 42, 37–40

Baylis, F. (2013). *Neuroethics* 6, 513–26.

Carrillo-Reid, L., Yang, W., Bando, Y., Peterka, D.S., and Yuste, R. (2016). *Science* 353, 691–4.

Farah, M.J. and Wolpe, P.R. (2004). *Hastings Cent. Rep.* 34, 35–45.

Farahany, N. (2012). *Stanford Law Rev.* 64, 351–408.

Haselager, P. (2013). *Minds Mach.* 23, 405–18.

Hochberg, L.R., Serruya, M.D., Friehs, G.M., Mukand, J.A., Saleh, M., Caplan, A.H., Branner, A., Chen, D., Penn, R.D., and Donoghue, J.P. (2006). *Nature* 442, 164–71.

Kay, K.N., Naselaris, T., Prenger, R.J., and Gallant, J.L. (2008). *Nature* 452, 352–5.

Kitcher, P. (2011). Science in a Democratic Society (Prometheus Books).

Pais-Vieira, M., Chiuffa, G., Lebedev, M., Yadav, A., and Nicolelis, M.A. (2015). *Sci. Rep.* 5, 11869.

Ramirez, S., Liu, X., Lin, P.-A., Suh, J., Pignatelli, M., Redondo, R.L., Ryan, T.J., and Tonegawa, S. (2013). *Science* 341, 387–91.

Stocco, A., Prat, C.S., Losey, D.M., Cronin, J.A., Wu, J., Abernethy, J.A., and Rao, R.P. (2015). *PLoS ONE* 10, e0137303. http://dx.doi.org/10.1371/journal.pone.0137303.

Vlek, R.J., Steines, D., Szibbo, D., Kübler, A., Schneider, M.J., Haselager, P., and Nijboer, F. (2012). *J. Neurol. Phys. Ther.* 36, 94–9.

Wolbring, G. and Diep, L. (2016). Cognitive/Neuro-enhancement Through an Ability Studies Lens. In *Cognitive Enhancement: Ethical and Policy Implications in International Perspectives*, F. Jotterand and V. Dubljevic, eds. (Oxford University Press), pp. 57–75.

Yizhar, O., Fenno, L.E., Davidson, T.J., Mogri, M., and Deisseroth, K. (2011). *Neuron* 71, 9–34.

Index

abortion 11–66, 101
  after-birth 269–274
  alleged justification as non-
    intentional killing 47–51
  alternative proposals 21–23
  arguments against 13, 42–53,
    55–56, 57
    alleged immorality 12, 42, 54–66
    critique by pro-choice proponents
     31–41
    denying the innocent a right to
     life 33, 34
    desire account 61–62
    discontinuation account 61, 62
    embryo/fetus complete, if
     immature, human 42–43
    extreme view 32–34
    future-like-ours theory 59–65
    loss of victim's future 58–60
    no-person arguments 43–47
    perceived as homicide 11
    potentiality principle and loss of
     victim's future 11, 24–25, 27,
     45, 46, 58–60

    unjust treatment 36
    wrongness of killing 12, 59–65
  conservative position 15, 23–28
  cutoff points 21–23, 28
  defenders/pro-choice advocates,
    11–13, 22, 31–41, 43, 45,
    51n3 55, 56, 57, 62
    ailing violinist example and
     bodily rights argument 32–38
    critiqu000e of opponents'
     arguments 31–41
    Good Samaritan versus
     Minimally Decent Samaritan
     argument 38–40
    harm to/risk to life of mother
     32–33
    pro-choice arguments 55–56
    rape, pregnancy due to 32, 36, 40
    self-awareness/self-consciousness
     argument 3, 18–19, 21, 25, 28,
     43–44, 47
    self-defense 33, 34, 36
    very early abortion not equivalent
     to killing 41

    determining what is being
     killed 42, 43
    in Down syndrome 854–855
    essence and accident
     distinction 57–58
    genetic risk factors 93–94
    and infanticide 15–16
    intentional killing 47–49, 51
     brutalization of killer 58
     loss of victim's future 58–60
     wrongness of 12, 59–65
    liberal position 15, 17, 23–24
    Model Penal Code (American Law
     Institute), 16, 29n4
    moral symmetry principle 26–27
    morally relevant difference between
     a newborn baby and fetus 15–16
    no-person arguments
     dualist approach 43–44
     evaluative approach 45–47
    positive versus negative duties 26, 27
    and prenatal screening 93–94
    pro-choice arguments 55–56
    selective 835–850

abortion (*cont'd*)
    selective reduction 69–70, 76
    third party actions following
      requests for 33–34
    viability and birth 22, 23, 28
    see also death; life, right to;
      personhood/criteria for being
      persons; pregnancy
academic freedom and research
  race 575–589
  right to equality versus freedom of
    research 567–568
  survival lottery 470–471
acrotomophilia (sexual attraction to
  amputees) 778
ACTG 076 study *see* AIDS Clinical
  Trials Group (ACTG) Study
  076
Adderall 783
advance directives 202, 335,
  336–338, 799
Advisory Committee on Release to
  the Environment (ACRE) 113
after-birth abortion 269–274, 276
  adoption as alternative to 272–273
  and conventional abortion 270–271
  versus infanticide 270
  moral equivalence of fetus and
    newborn 15–16, 271–272
  potential persons, fetus and
    newborn as 272
age, moral significance 404–411
  anti-ageist argument 404–405
  extra life-time versus extra lives
    407–409
  fair innings argument 405–407, 411
  numbers of lives and years 407
  threshold of discrimination 409
aid-in-dying 363–364
  see also euthanasia; Medical Aid in
    Dying (MAiD); physician-
    assisted death (PAD)
AIDS Clinical Trials Group (ACTG)
  Study 076 501–503, 508
  drug regime 467
  inadequate data analysis 503–504
  protocol 508

see also HIV/AIDS
Alcoholics Anonymous (AA) 425, 426
alcoholism/alcohol-related end-stage
  liver disease (ARESLD)
  ARESLD patients having lower
    priority on transplant waiting
    lists 426–427
  comparison with other
    diseases 424–425
  discrimination against
    alcoholics 424, 425–426
  and liver transplantation *see* liver
    transplantation, in alcoholism
Alliance of Genetic Support Groups 845
altruism
  crowding-out 445–446
  kidney donation 441, 443, 445, 446
  and telling falsehoods 715–718
Alzheimer's disease 325, 326, 357, 536
  case study ("Margo") 202, 327,
    329–331, 333–341
  state's interest in 339–341
Alzheimer's Disease Society, UK 326
American Journal of Human Genetics 836
American Journal of Public Health 835
*American Journal of the Medical
  Sciences* 469
American Medical Association (AMA)
  154, 225, 227, 229, 615
  Code of Medical Ethics 671
American Psychiatric Association 83,
  370, 781, 783
American Society of Reproductive
  Medicine 76, 78
  Ethics Committee 71, 101, 105–109
Americans with Disabilities Act (ADA)
  187, 838, 839
amniocentesis 186, 854
amputation by choice 777–787
  acrotomophilia (sexual attraction to
    amputees) 778
  apotemnophilia (attraction to being
    an amputee) 778, 779, 784
  of healthy limbs 777
  looping effects 784
  and refusal to be amputated 793–794
  see also disability

amputee identity disorder 782
Amsterdam Gender Identity Clinic 763
amyotrophic lateral sclerosis (ALS) 364
anaphylaxis 798
animal research 535–549, 551
  and activists' behavior 525–526
  arguments against, in scientific
    research 535–541
    alternatives, existence of 540–541,
      553–554
    animal models not predictive of
      human responses 538–540
    ethics 541
    humans not benefiting 535–536
    knowledge for the sake of
      knowledge 539–540
    low success rate 536–537
  assuming responsibility and
    stewardship 546
  brain disorders, modelling in
    primates 550–557
  equal consideration of equal
    interests 543
  and "equality," 526
  extremes of spectrum,
    rejecting 542–543
  harmful and nontherapeutic,
    morally wrong 521–534
  human ability to challenge nature
    and suffering unique 543–544
  human family 546
  and "importance," 526
  laboratory animals 78
  low success rate 536–537
  main premises 522–523
  marginal cases 545–546
  methods 523–525
  proof that animals are necessary
    537–538
  and "rights" 526
  seen as morally permissible
    "benefits" arguments 528–529
    "group-based" arguments
      527–528, 531–532
    "necessary condition" arguments
      527, 530–531
    "no alternatives" arguments 530

positive, cumulative case in
defense 532–533
"scientific" arguments 527
and "standing" 526–527
and "status" 526
utilitarianism 543–545, 551
welfare of animals 552–553
animals
animal nature and human
nature 517
compared with humans 212
comparing newborn kittens with
infants 16–17, 21, 22, 27, 28
consciousness 212
duties towards 517–518
identity of a human animal versus
that of a person 115
moral status 541–542
rational 23, 27, 155, 519, 520n1,
527, 530
wanton infliction of pain on 60
welfare 552–553
see also animal research
Annas, G. 122, 162–163, 164, 504
antidepressants 782–783
anti-discrimination measures 414,
681n33, 683, 704, 705
see also discrimination
antiretroviral drugs 467, 501–503, 592,
595
anti-vascular endothelial growth factor
(VEGF) 537
anti-viral drugs 614
apotemnophilia (attraction to being an
amputee) 778, 779, 784
applied ethics 1, 3
Aquinas, St Thomas 263, 703
Aristotle 5, 155, 176, 213, 567
Asia, distortion of sex ratio in
107–108
assisted dying see brain death; death;
euthanasia; Medical Aid in
Dying (MAiD); physician-
assisted death (PAD)
assisted dying, competence of
depressed person to
request 367–370

assisted reproduction 69–71, 100n19
artificial insemination 186–187
assisted reproductive treatments
(ART) 78, 81, 82, 172–173
and CRISPR 174–175
and disability 70, 71
egg donation 187
and genome editing 172–184
IVF see IVF (in-vitro fertilization)
and PGD 174–175
and preimplantation genetic
diagnosis (PGD) 174–175
prenatal screening 69, 71–72
same-sex relationships 71
cloning 128–129
ethically controversial nature of
parenthood 79–80
harm, risk of 81
objections to use of synthetic
gametes 80–82
synthetic gamete use 70, 78–84
sperm replacement 97
surrogacy see surrogacy
see also cloning; McCaughey
septuplets
assisted suicide 257, 354, 385
abstract moralizing 356, 359
conscientious objection 667, 669
moral fictions 245, 247, 251
physician-assisted death (PAD), 362,
363, 372, 377n68
and sanctity of life 202, 203, 204
see also euthanasia; physician-assisted
death (PAD); suicide
Attention Deficit Disorder (ADD) 783
Augustine, St, City of God 215
Auschwitz 216–217
authenticity
conscientious objection 685
deep-brain stimulation (DBS)
883–884, 886–887
autogynephilia (sexual arousal at
self-image as a woman) 782
autonomy
acknowledging 476
and amputation see amputation by
choice

of choice 792
competent person's right to 330–331
deep-brain stimulation (DBS)
879–881
defining 789–793
and dementia 327–331
descriptive and non-descriptive
beliefs 802–803
and dignity 155, 351
diminished 476
as a dispositional concept 792–793,
805n16
East Asian principle 750, 751, 752
and euthanasia 359, 360
evidentiary view 327–329, 335
and false beliefs 805n23
instrumental irrationality
801–802
instrumentally valuable 802
rational desiring 790
and genetic engineering 141
and identity 879–881
integrity-based view of importance
of 328–329, 335
personal, interfering with
124–125
precedent 330, 336–338
reproductive 179
respect for see respect for persons/
patent autonomy
understanding 186
and utilitarianism 886
violation of right to 751, 804
healthcare rationing, and
discrimination 414–417
see also self-determination
autosomal dominance 95
Azithromycin 614

Barnard, C. 200, 297
Battin, M. 374, 596
Beauchamp, T. L. 656, 806n49
Principles of Biomedical Ethics 707
Beecher, H. 297, 466
Belgium, PAD and voluntary
euthanasia permitted in 204,
245, 250, 361, 362, 364

Belmont Report: Ethical Principles and Guidelines for the Protection of Human Subjects of Research (1978) 475–482, 889, 892
  applications 478–482
  assessment of risks and benefits of research 480–481
  background 466
  basic ethical principles 476–478
  beneficence 477–478
  informed consent 478–480
  justice 478
  practice–research boundaries 475–476
  respect for persons 476–477
beneficence principle 496–498, 705, 728
  Alzheimer's disease 335
  Belmont Report 477–478
  group beneficence 623–626
Benelux Neuromodulation Society 881
Bentham, J. 3–4, 519–520
  An Introduction to the Principles of Morals and Legislation 469
  see also utilitarianism
best interests principle 86, 338, 486
  treatment limitation 788, 798–799
bioconservatives, versus transhumanists 162–163, 168
bioethics
  and applied ethics 1, 3
  background 1
  basic ethical principles 476–478
  complexity of facts 2, 7
  and homosexuality 83
  law and religion 7
  literature 152
  same-sex parenthood 78, 79, 82, 83
Black Death 592
blindness 212, 720, 816, 818, 826n15, 827n24
  "curing" 823
  and deafness 416, 809, 831
  from infancy 821, 826n8

life-sustaining treatment, limitation of 809, 810
permanent 815, 821
resource allocation 413, 414, 416, 418n8
see also deafness; disability
bodily integrity
  kidney sales 449–450
  vaccination ethics 632
  violation of rights 50, 632
bodily rights argument (use of mother's body for life support) 32–38, 47–50
  ailing violinist example 32, 33, 36–38, 40, 41
  right given by mother 11
  see also abortion; life, right to; personhood/criteria for being persons; rights
body dysmorphic disorder 780
body–self dualism 277, 278
Bok, S. 655, 726
Boorse, C. 152, 837
Boyle, J. M. (Jr.) 198, 298, 299
brain computer interfaces (BCI) 890
brain death
  alternative to 318–321
  centrality of ethics 304–305
  common but mistaken assumptions 318–319
  defining death 209
    Ad Hoc Committee to Examine the Definition of Brain Death 200–201
    consequences of new concept 297–298
    as irreversible loss of integrated organic functioning 298–299
    philosophical debate (President's Council on Bioethics) 201, 308–317
  and sanctity of life 296–307
  standard tests 300
  and wrongness of killing 200–202
  see also comas/unconsciousness; death
brain death syndrome 295

brain disorders, modelling in primates 550–557
  animal welfare 552–553
  available alternatives 553–554
  expectation of benefit 554–555
  methodological starting points 551–555
  trends in disease modelling post-CRISPR 551
  see also animal research; animals
brain imaging 567, 871
Brain Research through Advancing Innovative Neurotechnologies (BRAIN) 889–890, 893
brain-to-brain interface 891
Brandt, R. B., 30n6, 30n16, 804n8
breast cancer 794–795
breathing, spontaneous action of 314
Brock, D. 119, 122, 127, 128, 199, 368, 796–797, 805n15
Broome, M. 369–370, 374
Buchanan, A. 368, 796–797
Bush, G. W. 703
  President's Council on Bioethics 201, 300–303, 308–317

cadaver research, human 521
Callahan, D. 81–82, 83, 203, 356–360
Caplan, A. 297, 372, 846
Capron, A. 313, 316
Card, R. 675, 677, 687
Cardiothoracic Ethics Forum 257
Carter v Canada (2015) 378, 384
Categorical Imperative (Kant) 4–5
Catholic Church 4, 29, 563
  and abortion, ethics of, 239n2
  Declaration on Euthanasia (1980) 197, 199, 218–222
Catullus (Latin poet) 872, 874
CCR5 gene, editing out 191
Centers for Disease Control and Prevention (CDC), US 502, 664
Chavkin, W. 682, 683
childless couples

voluntary childlessness 85, 86, 87
  see also assisted reproduction;
    fertility drugs
children
  changes in DNA, ethics of
    making 185–190
  decision-making
    adults versus children 282
    deciding not to have children 85,
      86, 87
    by parents on behalf of their
      children 280–282
  with genetic risk factors, immorality
    of having 93–100
  HIV/AIDS victims 507–509
  "normal," following death of
    disabled child 86
  objectification of 110–112
  ownership of body issue 761–762
  severely disabled *see* disability; Gard,
    Charlie (severely disabled
    infant case, implications); infant
    euthanasia (severely disabled
    newborn)
  transgender 758–776
  welfare of future children 179
  see also abortion; embryo/fetus;
    infanticide; personhood/
    criteria for being persons
Childress, J. F. 684, 806n49
  Principles of Biomedical Ethics 707
choice
  active and contemporaneous 799
  amputation by *see* amputation by
    choice
  autonomy of 792
  concept of 790
  and decision-making *see* decision-
    making
  medical consequences of
    DBS 884–885
Chomsky, N., *American Power and the
    New Mandarins* 460
chorionic villus sampling 836, 854
chromosomes
  fragile X 841

sex cells 42
trisomy (three chromosomes)
  266–268
X chromosome 121
Y chromosome 121
CIOMS guidelines, research 490, 491,
  493
classical utilitarianism 4, 5
cloning 69, 115–137
  appeals to a future like ours
    118–119
  appeals to immaterial minds or
    souls 118
  appeals to potentialities 118
  arguments against 118–119
  "Dolly the Sheep" 72 125
  and germline editing 187
  human organ bank, producing
    117–118, 119
  medical purposes/scientific
    research 117
  neo-Lockean persons 115–117
  in principle morally acceptable
    versus currently acceptable 72
  to produce persons *see* cloning to
    produce persons
  rationality 121, 125
  unconnected with producing
    persons 117–119
cloning to produce persons 119–131
  arguments in favor of
    avoiding transmission of
      hereditary diseases 127–128
    children for same-sex couples
      128–129
    desired traits, producing
      individuals with 129
    enabling having a genetically
      related child 128–129
    happier and healthier individuals,
      producing 128
    infertility 128
    intelligence, hereditary basis
      for 130
    producing people of future
      benefit to society 129–130

    to save existing persons 129
    scientific knowledge,
      furthering 130–131
    self-knowledge, use of 129
  problems with
    Brave New World objections
      127
    consequentialist objections
      125–127
    failing to treat individuals as ends
      in themselves 123–124
    interfering with personal
      autonomy 124–125
    low rate of success objection
      126–127
    "Open Future" argument
      122–123
    psychological distress,
      causing 123
    reduced life expectancy in cloned
      persons 125–126
    right to a genetically unique
      nature 119–122
    undesirable consequences 125
    whether intrinsically
      wrong 119–125
clustered regularly interspaced short
    palindromic repeat (CRISPR)
    see CRISPR/Cas9
    (gene-editing technology)
coercion 480, 487, 577, 656
  see also compulsion; voluntariness
cognitive differences research 566–574
  high intelligence, genetics of 193
  past precedents 568–570
  right to equality versus freedom of
    research 567–568
  third precedent 570–573
College of Physicians and Surgeons of
    British Columbia 688–689
comas/unconsciousness 20, 32, 57, 62,
    64, 123, 240, 293, 401
  advance directives 330, 331
  versus death 294
  flat electroencephalogram (EEG) 292
  killing/letting die distinction 236, 237

comas/unconsciousness (*cont'd*)
  lack of movement or breathing 292
  operating on an unconscious
    person 736, 833
  passing away while unconscious 240, 296
  permanent/irreversible 57, 64, 209,
    210, 211, 277, 278, 291–295,
    333, 337
    characteristics 291–292
    'double-test' view 210
    legal commentary 293–294
    and other procedures 292–293
    significance 303–304
  and prolonging life 295
  reflexes, lack of 292
  and sanctity of life 210, 213, 220
  and sedation 667, 672
  temporary/reversible 20, 21, 45–46,
    57, 62, 64, 278
  unreceptive and unresponsive 292
  see also consciousness
Commission for the Study of Ethical
    Problems in Medicine and
    Biomedical and Behavioral
    Research, US
  brain death 298, 299
  euthanasia 262, 263
  life-sustaining treatment, limitation
    of 789, 796–797, 799–800, 803
Committee for Medicinal Products for
    Human Use (CHMP),
    Europe 365
Compassion & Choices 363
competence
  assessing 368–370, 384–386
    MacArthur Competence
      Assessment Tool 388
  and deep-brain stimulation
    884–885
  and dementia 329
  limitations of treatment in
    competent patients 799–800
  limitations of treatment in
    incompetent patients 796–799
  to request assisted dying 367–370
  threshold concept 368

compulsion 140, 142, 715
  Mill on 733, 734
  scientific research 485, 487, 488
  see also coercion
confidentiality in medicine 695–698
  concept of a professional
    obligation 704–706
  defense of 707–710
  duty to diminish risks to third
    parties 706–707
  and indiscretion 697–698
  and patients' interests 696
  personal morality 702–703
  personal values 703–704
  possible solutions to problem 697
  role 696–697
  and third-party interests 696
  unqualified, defense of 699–711
    infected spouse 699–700
    law 701–702
    what professional qualifications
      are not 700–704
conscience
  conscience absolutism 667, 668,
    669–670
  definition and significance 684–685
  and professionalism 685–696
conscientious objection 682–691
  acts of 682
  claims, reasonableness and
    authenticity 685
  conscience, definition and
    significance 684–685
  conscience and professionalism
    685–696
  defining 668–669
  versus destruction 677–678
  diversity 687–688
  equal citizenship 688–689
  equality of opportunity 687
  in health care 667–681
    assessment 669–677
    conscience absolutism 669–670
    incompatibilism 670–673
    Patients' Interests First Principle
      (PIFP) 671–672, 674

    Scope of Professional Practice
      Principle (SOPPP) 671, 672–673
    peaceful co-existence 689
    reasonable accommodation
      specific actions required 673–675
      whether a public justification is
        required 676–677
      whether alternative service
        required 675–677
    voluntariness and monopoly
      686–687
consciousness
  of animals 212
  degrees of 212
  higher level of 211
  intrinsic value 211–213
  'mere' consciousness 211, 212
  see also comas/unconsciousness;
    self-awareness/consciousness,
    and being a person
consequentialism 3–4
contraception 65, 69, 70, 86, 88
contractualism and vaccination
  ethics 627–628
  and utilitarianism 628–629
Convention for the Protection of
    Human Rights and Dignity of
    the Human Being with
    Regard to the Application of
    Biology and Medicine *see*
    Oviedo Convention, Council
    of Europe (1997)
Coronavirus *see* COVID-19
cosmos, notion of 5
Council for International
    Organization of Medical
    Sciences 504
Council on Bioethics, Presidential, *see*
    President's Council on Bioethics
courts, role of in deciding right to
    life 283–284
COVID-19
  anti-viral drugs 614
  and care of "non-COVID-19"
    patients 616–617
  clinical ethics 612–619

cytokine storm 614
decision-making, saving of
    lives 399–402
dignity in death 616
discrimination against patients
    with 613
duty to care versus right to
    protection 614–615
moral distress of healthcare
    providers 617–618
pandemic ethics 510–514
and PPE 614, 615, 661
rationing of scarce resources 615
risk parity principle, applying to
    research 512–513
spreading of 396
treatment as a means to an
    end 612–614
uncertain evidence and unproven
    therapies 614
CRISPR/Cas9 (gene-editing
    technology) 170, 469, 550, 553
akin to therapy 176–178
and assisted reproduction 174–175
child welfare 179
importance of context 181
reproductive autonomy 179
societal interests 179–181
trends in disease modelling
    following 551
see also genome editing;
    preimplantation genetic
    diagnosis (PGD)
cross-dressing 782
cyclic preferences 415
cystic fibrosis 127, 844, 845

Darwin, C. 5, 542, 544
Davies, L. 420, 421, 422
Dawson, A. 625–626
de Cates, A. 369–370, 374
De Haes, J. C. J. M. 794, 805n24
deafness 186, 799, 809, 812
    and blindness 416, 809, 831
    and compensating acute other
        senses 831

congenital 281
measles, caused by 626
see also blindness; disability
death
biological reality of 308
boundary between life and
    death 209–210
brain death see brain death
causing 352–353
    as a side-effect 48–49, 208
dead donor rule 302
defining
    Black's Law Dictionary 293, 296
    bodily destruction 210
    boundary between life and
        death 209
    consequences of new
        concept 297–298
    as irreversible loss of integrated
        organic functioning 298–299
    by law 294
    "two deaths" position 309
dignity in 616
of disabled child, "normal" child
    following 86
fixing cause of 228
"good death," 364
killing/letting die distinction
    198–199, 235–243
    active and passive euthanasia 227,
        228
    agents versus actions 242
    difference thesis 235, 240
    killing not always worse than
        letting die 240–243
    "nasty uncles" case 240, 242
    rightness and wrongness of
        actions 241
    self-determination principle and
        euthanasia 352–353
of the person and the
    organism 201–202
physician-assisted see Medical Aid in
    Dying (MAiD); physician-
    assisted death (PAD)
by suicide see suicide

versus unconsciousness 294
see also abortion; eugenics;
    euthanasia; killing; sanctity of
    life
decision-making
for adults versus children 282
advance directives 337
allowing adults to choose treatment
    for themselves 282
children, deciding not to have
    86, 87
and concept of choice 790
COVID-19 and saving of lives
    399–402
decision-making capacity (DMC)
    553, 554
ethical versus clinical decisions
    284
evidence, need for 286
lacking capacity for 262
by parents on behalf of their
    children 280–282
rational 362, 363, 367, 376n28, 385,
    877, 884, 887
reasons for decisions 286
see also Gard, Charlie (severely
    disabled infant case,
    implications)
Declaration of Helsinki (WMA,
    1964-2013) 482n1, 500n2, 510
genome editing 191–192, 193n6,
    193n7
research, 466, 483, 486, 490, 493,
    494n7 495
Declaration on Euthanasia (Catholic
    Church, 1980) 197–199,
    218–222
deep-brain stimulation (DBS) 553,
    876–882, 883
authenticity
    feelings of authenticity and
        alienation 883–884
    whether new 'autonomy' in
        neuroethics 886–887
autonomy and identity 879–881
case study 878–879

deep-brain stimulation (DBS) (*cont'd*)
  choice between mental competence
      and well-being 884–885
  compared with neurosurgery 880
  dangers of 878–879
  dilemma caused by 883–888
  empirical evidence 877–878
  motor control 878
  for PD 876–879, 883
  risk assessment 880
defective genes 95, 98, 127–128
DeGrazia, D. 533, 551, 552, 864
dementia 325–342
  advance directives 336–338
  Alzheimer's disease 325, 326
    case study ("Margo") 202, 327,
        329–331, 333–341
  and autonomy 327–331
  critical and experiential
      interests 338–339
  disability perspective 341
  Dworkin on 333–342
  Framingham Study, 331n6
  and interests of state 339–341
  medication for 863
Denmark, Down syndrome
    screening 851
deontology
  Italian Deontology Code 753, 754
  truth-telling 753–754
  vaccination ethics 626–635
    collective and individual
        responsibility 629–630
    costs 634–635
    easy rescue duty 629
    generalization test 626–627
    moral obligation to be
        vaccinated 628–635
    utilitarianism 628–629, 633
depression
  antidepressants 782–783
  competence to request assisted
      dying 367–370
  lifting of 791
  major depressive disorder 362,
      367–370

and rational desiring 791
Seasonal Affective Disorder (SAD)
    864
suicidal ideation 362
temporary, and right to life 20
treatment-resistant *see* treatment-
    resistant depression (TRD)
Descartes, R. 468, 780
Desire-Fulfilment Theories 798, 799
desires
  and ethics of abortion 61–62
  and rights 19, 20–21
  see also under rationality
despotism 733
Devine, P. 54
DeWall, C. N. 872–873
diabetes research 656, 741–742
Diagnostic and Statistical Manual of
    Mental Disorders 267
dignity, human
  and autonomy/self-determination
      155, 351
  concept 136, 264, 265
  in death 616
  incompatibility with posthuman
      dignity 166–167
  infant euthanasia (severely disabled
      newborn) 264–265
  posthumanity as a threat to 168
  research 566, 568
  and right to die 221
  violating 155, 159, 264
  see also posthuman dignity
Dionne quintuplets, Canada 76
disability 811–828
  adaptation to 794–795, 830
  and assisted reproduction 70, 71
  blindness *see* blindness
  cases
    Aphrodisiac 822
    Baby Genes 817
    Disabled baby 816, 817, 818
    Light Show 815, 816, 817
    Reverse Baby Genes 818–819
    Reverse Disabled Baby
        818–820

causing a disabled person to exist
    instead of nondisabled 821–823
causing a nondisabled person to
    become disabled 815–816
  without transition costs 816–821
causing and "curing" 823–825
children with
  deciding not to have 87
  deliberately conceiving 88–89
  infant euthanasia (severe
      disability) *see* infant euthanasia
      (severely disabled newborn)
  multiple-births 76, 77
contrasting medical and social
    paradigms 837–841
degree of 94
discrimination against disabled
    people 264, 415–419, 809,
    831, 834, 839, 852
and diversity 811
'double jeopardy' for 414
equal value argument 94
genetics and reproductive risk
    93–100
indirect strategy 832–834
loss aversion 795–796
mere difference viewpoint 829–834
  bad-difference/mere-difference
      distinction 811, 812–814, 815
  causation-based objections 814
  problem for 814–815
nuclear attack potentially causing 85
prenatal diagnosis for preventing
    839–840
  implications for family life 842–844
  implications for people with
      disabilities 841–842
  implications for professional
      practice 844–848
  rationales 840–841
and quality of life ethic 829–831
and sexual orientation 832–834,
    836, 837
and society 831–832
see also amputation by choice;
    Down syndrome

discrimination 99n5 108, 141, 178, 213, 229, 546
 age 409
 in alcoholism 424, 425–426
 anti-discrimination measures 414, 681n33, 683, 704, 705
 beliefs 676, 679
 against COVID 19 patients 613
 deadly 377n68
 denial of treatment 370
 disabled people, against 264, 415–419, 809, 831, 834, 839, 852
 doctors/physicians, duties of, 680n13
 employment 838–839
 equality of opportunity 687
 gender, on basis of 102, 103, 104, 108, 158, 159, 187
 healthcare rationing 413–419
 informed consent 741
 invidious, 681n33
 racial 582, 672, 825
 selective abortion 837, 838
 sexual orientation 672, 819
 survival lottery 460
 threshold or level 409
 unjustifiable/unfair 104, 264, 374, 379, 460
 see also stereotyping
dispositional concept, autonomy as, 792–793, 805n16
dissociative disorders 277, 783
diversity 687–688
DNA 168, 570, 741
 of children, ethics of changing 185–190
 genetic engineering, uses of 40
 mitochondrial 173, 184n2, 184n6 185, 187, 188
 mitochondrial DNA depletion syndrome (MDDS) 281
 noncoding 125
 recombinant 145, 550
 Recombinant DNA Advisory Committee 171
 research, 744n14

sex cells 42, 79, 105
 testing 852
 see also chromosomes; telomeres
do no harm principle 477, 484, 500, 733
doctor–patient relationship 653
 conception of autonomy 750–752
 cultural differences 745–757
 similarities and differences 748–750
 treating patients badly 746–748
 truth-telling 752–756
doctrine-of-the double-effect 263
donation after cardiac determination of death (DACDD) 667
dopamine replacement therapy (DRT) 885, 886
Dostoevsky, F. 4, 5
Down syndrome 845, 851–853
 after-birth abortion 270
 amniocentesis 186
 congenital defects 226
 inherent worth of people with 852
 insulting person with 838
 limitations of 841
 right to terminate fetus 854–855
 selective abortion 851
Downpride 852
dualism 43–44
Duchenne-Becker muscular dystrophy 102
Dworkin, R. 202, 333–342, 881
 Life's Dominion 333, 334, 336, 337–338, 339

Ebert, R. 297–298
Ebola crisis (2014–16) 662
egg donation 187
Einstein, A. 129–130
electrical stimulation of brain 876–882
electroconvulsive therapy (ECT) 366
electroencephalogram (EEG) 292
Elliott, C. 657, 863
embryo/fetus
 cloning see cloning; cloning to produce persons
 as a complete, though immature, human 42–43

distinct from cells of mother or father 43
 distinguished from newborn, morally relevant difference 15–16, 271–272
 "drawing a line" in the development of 31
 gene-editing technologies 170–171
 growth path 42–43
 motile 23
 mutation-free 173, 176, 178
 presumptive responsibility of donors 82
 rights of, as persons 11, 12–13, 31–32, 43–44, 55–56, 156–158
 membership of species of Homo sapiens 17, 18–24, 27, 29, 43
 potential persons see potentiality principle
 selection as tissue donors 110–114
 sex selection for transfer 102
 value of and potentiality argument 11, 24–25, 27, 45, 46, 58–60
 see also abortion; assisted reproduction; gametes; life, right to; personhood/criteria for being persons; sex cells (sperm and ova); sex selection
emergency contraception (EC) 673
emotions, medicalization of 870–875
 arts objection 874
 ethics of drug use 873–874
 peculiarity-of-heartbreak objection 872–874
 unrequited love 871–872
 arguments against medicalization 872–874
Endocrine Society 763
end-of-life care, 205n3, 310, 357, 372, 402, 667, 879
 comparing decisions, 246t
 conflicting with standard medical ethics 245
 and dementia 335, 336

end-of-life care (*cont'd*)
  End of Life clinic, The
      Netherlands 372, 389
  moral fictions 245, 248, 251, 252
  planning 336
  see also euthanasia; physician-assisted
      death (PAD)
end-stage liver disease (ESLD) 423,
    424, 426
  see also alcoholism/alcohol-related
      end-stage liver disease
      (ARESLD)
Engelhardt, H.T. 54, 66n7
Environmental Protection Act, 1990
    (UK) 113
equal citizenship 688–689
ethical judgments 298, 305, 401, 543,
    746, 859
ethical principles
  basic 476–478
  beneficence *see* beneficence
    principle
  developing, in novel
    neurotechnologies 892–893
  do no harm 477, 484, 500, 733
  fairness *see* fairness principle
  justice *see* justice
  noninterference 250, 815–816, 817,
    819, 823, 827n23 835
  non-maleficence 500
  respect *see* respect for persons/
    patent autonomy
  self-determination *see* autonomy;
    self-determination principle
  see also Belmont Report: Ethical
    Principles and Guidelines for
    the Protection of Human
    Subjects of Research (1978);
    Hippocrates
ethical relativism 748, 750–753,
    755, 756
ethics
  of abortion *see* abortion
  animal research 541
  applied 1, 3
  background to bioethics 1

law and religion, independence
    from 7
PGD and sex selection 102–103
religion, independence from 6–7
tissue donation, embryos 112–114
of vaccination *see* vaccination ethics
see also animal research; Belmont
    Report: Ethical Principles and
    Guidelines for the Protection
    of Human Subjects of
    Research (1978)
eugenics
  changing genetic composition of
    future generations 140–142
  and families 144
  genetic polymorphism 140, 141
  Nazi programs 156, 158, 214
  parental 158
  policies 141–142
  slippery-slope arguments 158
  state-sponsored 158
  therapy–enhancement distinction,
    moral significance 158
European Convention for the
    Protection of Human Rights
    and Fundamental Freedoms
    (ECHR) 606, 683
euthanasia
  and abortion, ethics of 12, 59, 65
  abstract moralizing 203, 356–360
  active, 59, 65, 199, 225–229,
    239n2 242, 250
  versus aid-in-dying 363
  and autonomy 359, 360
  compared with PAD 362
  Declaration on Euthanasia (Catholic
    Church, 1980) 197–199,
    218–222
  defining 219–220, 362
  distinction between active and
    passive 225, 227
  due proportion in use of remedies
    220–221
  Episcopal Conferences on 218
  illegal in the United States 257
  involuntary 362

justifying 359
lethal injection 226, 362
MAiD distinguished 363
meaning of suffering for
    Christians 220
and medical practice 354–355
  see also physician-assisted death
    (PAD)
as mercy-killing 227, 362
non-voluntary 232, 247, 362
painkiller use 220
passive, 158, 198, 199, 225–229,
    239n2 242
physician-assisted *see* physician-
    assisted death (PAD)
requests for 219–220
and resources 233
'right to die' 220–221
and self-determination *see*
    self-determination principle
    and euthanasia
severely disabled newborn *see* infant
    euthanasia (severely disabled
    newborn)
voluntary *see* voluntary euthanasia
withholding of treatment 226
see also abortion; brain death; death;
    euthanasia; infant euthanasia
    (severely disabled newborn);
    killing
evolutionary theory 158, 188, 212
  genetic engineering, questioning
    some uses of 136, 144
  and research 546, 567, 575, 596, 643
experimentation
  with animals 468–470
  cadaver research, human 521–522
  defining 476
  experimental treatment 282
  with humans 465–468
  skin tissue research 522
  Tuskegee Syphilis Study (1957)
    469, 484, 521
  Willowbrook Children case
    (1963–66) 469, 521
  see also animal research

fairness principle
  biomedical research participation,
    moral duty 498–499
  equality of opportunity 687
  fair innings argument 405–407,
    411
  liver transplantation, in
    alcoholism 426–427
  organ donation, and retrieval 451
  right to equality versus freedom of
    research 567–568
  scientific research 484–485
  vaccination ethics 628–635
Fan, R. 750, 751
Feinberg, J., 54, 56–57, 66n7 122
feminism 6, 573, 749
fertility drugs 69, 75, 76, 77
fetishes 778, 780
fetus *see* embryo/fetus
Finnis, J., 299, 306n3
Firlik, A. 326, 333–335
First, M. 781, 782
Fisher, H. 867–868, 871
Fletcher, J. C. 835, 843
Flynn, J. R. 470, 471, 572–573, 582
fMRIs (functional magnetic resonance
    imaging) 567, 871, 890
Food and Drug Administration (FDA),
    US 171, 785
Fox, R. 745, 778
Freedman, C. 863–864
Freud, S. 881
Frey, B. 445–446
fugue state 783
Fukuyama, F. 162–163, 166
"future people" 85–86
future-like-ours theory
  and abortion 59–65
  and cloning 118–119

gametes 70, 71, 136, 187
  anonymous donation 81
  as 'assemblages' 81
  assisted reproduction 172–174,
    184n7
  cross-sex production 79

versus embryo/fetus 46–47
  modification of cells 176
  post-birth abortion 269, 270
  synthetic, for gay and lesbian
    people 78–84
  see also under same-sex relationships,
    assisted production for; sex
    cells (sperm and ova)
Gard, Charlie (child with severe
    mitochondrial disorder,
    implications of case) 200,
    280–287
  allowing travel for treatment, unless
    illegal/harmful 284
  case summary 281
  courts, role of 283–284
  decision-making
    adults versus children 282
    ethical versus clinical
      decisions 284
    evidence, need for 286
    parents' role 280–282
    reasons for decisions 286
  experimental treatment issues 282
  factual and ethical questions 285
  medical tourism 284
  normative and conceptual issues,
    challenging 285–286
  reasonable disagreement, allowing/
    supporting 284
  reflective equilibrium 286
  resource limitations 282–283
  see also decision-making
Garrett, L. 595–596
gay men *see* homosexuals; same-sex
    relationships, assisted
    reproduction for
gender discrimination 102, 103, 104,
    108, 158, 159, 187
gender dysphoria 760–761, 762
gender identity disorder 762, 782
gene therapy, somatic versus
    germline 151–152
General Medical Council (GMC),
    UK 615, 688
genetic counseling 142, 845

genetic determinism 123
genetic diseases and reproductive
    risk 93–100
  avoiding transmission of, through
    cloning 127–128
  cloning to avoid 127–128
  defective genes 95, 98, 127–128
  gene editing 191, 192
  Huntington's Disease *see*
    Huntington's Disease
  immorality of having children likely
    to suffer 93–100
  "imperfect" people and genetic
    risk 94
  minimally satisfying life
    concept 96–98
  onset of symptoms 95, 96
  possible children and potential
    parents 96–98
  rapidly lethal diseases 94
  Tay-Sachs 94, 192
  Treacher–Collins syndrome
    (TCS) 269–270
  X-linked genetic diseases 101, 107
  see also prenatal screening
genetic engineering
  avoiding genes-environment
    debate 139–140
  descendants 145
  families 144–145
  genetic supermarket, 147–149,
    150n10
  "imperfect" people and genetic
    risk 94
  methods of changing genetic
    composition of future
    generations 140–142
  mixed system 149
  playing God, objection to 146–147,
    156
  positive–negative distinction 14,
    142–143, 150
  questioning some uses of 139–150
  rapidly lethal diseases 94
  risks and mistakes 145–146
  values 149–150

genetic engineering (*cont'd*)
  view that overall improvement is
    unlikely or impossible
    143–144
genetic markers 95
genetic parenthood, value and
  meaning 178
genetic polymorphism 140, 141
genetic relatedness 70, 82
genetic supermarket, 147–149, 150n10
genetic testing 98, 176, 267, 844, 852
  see also assisted reproduction;
    prenatal screening
genetically modified organisms
  (GMOs) 113
genius 784
genome editing
  and assisted reproduction 172–184
  case for 175–176
  CCR5 gene, editing out 191
  child welfare 179
  costs of introducing in assisted
    reproduction context 180–181
  Dickey–Wicker amendment 170
  ethical pathway 191–193
  importance of context 181
  NIH guidance 170–171
  reproductive autonomy 179
  Second International Summit on
    Human Genome Editing 192
  selection versus therapy 176–178
  single disorders 192
  societal interests 179–180
    and costs of introducing genome
      editing 180–181
  translational pathway 191–193
  see also germline editing
Genovese, Kitty 39
George, R. P. 12, 69
germline editing
  debates 186, 188
  intolerance of imperfection 186
  prohibition of 185
  science of 188
  see also genome editing
germline gene therapy 151–152

germline genetic enhancement
  (GLGE) 152, 154, 156–158
germline genetic therapy
  (GLGT) 152, 154, 156–159
Giubilini, A. 199–200, 275–278, 470
Glannon, W. 860, 885
Glover, J., "The Sanctity of Life" 197
Gosselin, K. and J. 76–77
Great Ormond Street Hospital
  (GOSH), UK 281, 283
Griffin, D. 795, 796
Grisez, G. 198, 298, 299

Habermas, J. 167
Hacking, I. 783, 784
Hampshire, S., *Morality and
  Pessimism* 460
happiness 4, 5
Hare, R. M., 2–3, 4, 7, 85–-87,
  805n16, 805n22, 806n69
harm, refraining from *see* do no harm
  principle
Harris, J. 81–83, 414, 434, 466,
  495–500, 814
Harris, J. R. 131
  The Nurture Assumption 120
Harris, L. 738–739
Hart, H. L. A. 485, 498
Harvard Brain Death Committee
  297–298, 302, 303, 305, 310
Havasupai Indians 656, 741–742
He Jiankui 191, 192
health and disease
  concepts 152–153
  responsibility for health 639–645
  see also COVID-19; HIV/AIDS;
    infectious diseases, ethics of;
    XDR-TB (drug-resistant
    tuberculosis), South Africa
Health and Human Services (HHS)
  Final Rule, US 667
Health Care Financing Administration
  (HCFA), US 423, 424
healthcare professionals
  concept of a professional
    obligation 704–706

disability, preventing 844–848
  and infant euthanasia 264
  moral distress, in COVID-19
    pandemic 617–618
  obligations of, implications of PPE
    for 663–664
  Scope of Professional Practice
    Principle (SOPPP) 671,
    672–673
  telling patients lies 717–723
  telling patients the truth 724–730
  who is owed by 662–663
  see also conscientious objection;
    medicine
healthcare rationing, and
  discrimination 413–419
  cyclic preferences 415
  dependence on irrelevant
    treatments 417, 418
  disability 415, 417
  example 414–415
  pointless violation of
    autonomy 414–415, 417
  preference for smaller benefits 414,
    417
  randomness 416–418
  rights-based approach 415–416
  see also resources
heart failure 258
Hedonistic Theories 798, 799
Heliobacter pylori 490
Helsinki Declaration *see* Declaration of
  Helsinki (WMA, 1964-2013)
hemochromatosis 127
hemophilia 102
hepatic disease/hepatitis 423–424,
  505, 521
Herceptin 537
herd immunity goal 620–621, 629,
  633
hereditary diseases *see* genetic diseases
  and reproductive risk
heterotaxy syndrome 257–258
Hill, C. (suicide note) 203, 345–348
Hippocrates 596, 614, 653, 655, 695,
  704, 719, 725, 737, 752

Hippocratic Oath 477, 654, 662, 726, 892
HIV/AIDS, 99n1 507, 597, 598, 846
  antiretroviral drugs 467, 501–503, 592, 595
  asking the wrong research question 502–503
  AZT drug 467, 508, 512
  in developing countries 467
  and gene editing 191, 192
  inadequate data analysis from ACTG 076 and other sources 503–504
  infant victims 507–509
  perinatal transmission 501–506
  placebo-controlled trials 504
  single international ethical research standard 505
  South Africa 594, 595
  unethical trials in developing countries 501–506
  viral load 170
  World AIDS Day 608
  see also AIDS Clinical Trials Group (ACTG) Study 076
Holocaust 216–217
Homo sapiens, membership of species 116, 155, 275, 864
  and rights of embryo/fetus 17, 18–24, 27, 29, 43
  see also personhood/criteria for being persons
homosexuals 81, 835
  children for same-sex couples 128–129
  "curing" 823
  homophobia 835
  when seen as pathological 83, 783, 820
  see also same-sex relationships, assisted reproduction for
hormones
  connected with love 868
  cross-sex 761–763, 770
  female 567

puberty-suppressing see puberty-blocking treatment (PBT)
Hugo Ethics Committee 493
Human Fertilization and Embryology Authority (HFEA), UK 112, 113, 173
Human Genome Project 94, 839–840
human nature 5, 136, 156, 164, 168
  and animal nature 517
  genetic engineering 139, 140
  modifying 162, 163
Humane Society of the United States web site 540
humanness, 4, 154–156, 160n49
  and dehumanization 163
  human enhancement technologies 165
  intrinsic value of being human 213
  secular humanism 162
  transhumanists versus bioconservatives 162–163, 168
  see also life, right to; personhood/criteria for being persons; sanctity of life
Hume, D. 788
Hunter syndrome 102
Huntington's Disease 127, 143, 173
  and gene editing 192
  late stage 799
  reproductive risk 94–98, 99n13
Huxley, A. 158
  Brave New World 151, 164
Hydroxychloroquine 614

ideal utilitarianism 4
identical twins 120
identity
  amputee identity disorder 782
  and autonomy 879–881
  formation of 880
  gender identity disorder 762, 782
  of a human animal versus a person 115
  narrative 880
impersonal principle 86

in vitro testing 71
inactivated polio virus (IPV) 631
incompatibilism 670–673
incompatibility thesis 685
India
  kidney sales 447, 450
  Medical Council, Medical Ethics Regulations 615
  Ministry of Health and Family Welfare 616
  National Health Protection Scheme 616
individualism 745, 750
individuals
  desired traits, producing with 129
  failing to treat as ends in themselves 123–124
  happy and health 128
infant euthanasia (severely disabled newborn)
  Charlie Gard, case of 280–287
  justification for 257–258, 262–265
    human dignity 264–265
    lacking decision-making capacity 262
    parental and health care professionals, interests of 264
    quality of life 262–264
    resource allocation 264
    sanctity of life 262–263
    slippery-slope arguments 264
    unfair discrimination for disabled 264
  rejecting 259–261
  see also abortion; after-birth abortion; infanticide
infanticide 43, 200, 262, 263, 264, 270
  and abortion 15–16
  versus after-birth abortion 270
  attempts to justify 28
  morality of 16
  and quality of life ethic 263
  seen as permissible 16, 29, 276
  and sex selection 102, 108
  strong emotions aroused by 16

infanticide (*cont'd*)
  see also abortion; infant euthanasia
      (severely disabled newborn);
      newborns
infectious diseases, ethics of 591–601
  Black Death 592
  consequences 592–593
  difficult questions 593
  distribution of research
      resources 591
  drug-resistant 593
  Ebola crisis (2014–16) 662
  ethical importance of diseases
      591–596
  justice 594–596
  Middle East Respiratory Syndrome
      (MERS) 663
  neglect, reasons for
    apparent ease 598
    complexity 597–598
    high tech medicine 596
    optimism in medicine 596–597
    'the other' 597
    religious hijacking 598
  pandemic ethics 510–514
  personal protective equipment
      (PPE) 661–666
  smallpox 592
  tuberculosis (TB), drug-resistant *see*
      MDR-TB (multi-drug-
      resistant) tuberculosis;
      XDR-TB (extensively drug-
      resistant tuberculosis), South
      Africa
  see also COVID-19; HIV/AIDS;
      vaccination ethics
infertility
  and cloning 128
  denial to services 70–71
  see also artificial insemination;
      assisted reproduction; egg
      donation; IVF (in-vitro
      fertilization)
informed consent 737–744
  adequate 741
  banking of samples 741

broad, problems of 741–742
  comprehension 479–480
  concept 739–740
  current challenges to 740–743
  discrimination 741
  ethical principles 478–480
  and euthanasia 221
  Havasupai Indians and diabetes
      research 656, 741–742
  historical foundations 737–739
  information 479
  limits of law in biomedical
      ethics 740
  organ donation, and retrieval 437
  quality of 740–741
  regulation of 742–743
  research–treatment distinction
      742–743
  violation of 434
  voluntariness 480
Institutional Review Boards
      (IRBs) 482
interests
  best interests principle 86, 338, 486,
      798–799
  Dworkin on 334
  Patients' Interests First Principle
      (PIFP) 671–672, 674
  and rights 85–89
  self-regarding 121
  societal 179–180
    and costs of introducing genome
        editing 180–181
International Covenant on Civil and
      Political Rights (ICCPR) 607,
      683, 687, 688
intersex surgery 785
IQ scores 470, 471, 854
  academic freedom and race
      575–583
  cognitive differences 567, 569
  genetic engineering 135, 139, 141,
      146
Italian Deontology Code 753, 754
IVF (in-vitro fertilization), 76, 137,
      193n14 654, 668

genome editing 172–174, 191
germline editing 187, 188
HIV prevention 191
preimplantation genetic diagnosis
    (PGD), 101, 102t 103–105,
    108, 109, 111
see also assisted reproduction

Japan, Medical Association (Bioethics
    Council) 755
Jehovah's Witnesses 327, 330, 703, 711
  life-sustaining treatment, limitation
      of 799, 801, 803
Jennings, C. G. 555
Jensen, A. 575, 578, 579
Johannesson, M. 414
Johnston, M. 304
Jonas, H. 122, 167, 310, 312
Joseph family disease, 96, 99n13
Journal of Medicine and Philosophy 311
justice
  Belmont Report 478
  infectious diseases, ethics of
      594–596
  utilitarianism 96, 594

Kaczor, C. 200
  The Ethics of Abortion 116
Kagan, S. 627
Kahane, G. 814
Kahneman, D. 796, 804n11
Kant, I. 60, 61, 123, 302, 468, 655, 886
  and Bentham 469
  Categorical Imperative 4–5
  ethical principles 71, 113
  imperfect moral duty 467, 497
Kantymir, L. 685
Kass, L. 77, 89, 99n2, 162–164, 862
Katz, J. 740
Kaufmann, W., 29n1
Kavka, G., "The Paradox of Future
    Individuals" 125
Kelly, B. 366, 370
"kickback" systems 747
kidney sales
  anti-market considerations 444–449

bodily integrity 449–450
case for allowing 439–442
desperate exchange 446–447
equal status considerations 448–449
ethical issues in supply and demand 443–455
illegality 443
in India 447, 450
legalizing 446
libertarian view 443, 452n2
market ban, likely effects upon supply 445–446
objection to 439–440
policy considerations 450–452
shortage of kidneys 439
slippery-slope arguments 441
status quo systems of kidney procurement 443–444
vulnerability 446–447
weak agency 447–448
killing
act of 208, 216, 219, 230–232, 236, 353
death as a side-effect of 208
direct objections 208
intentional 47–49, 51
brutalization of killer 58
loss of victim's future 58–60
wrongness of 12, 59–65
versus letting die 198–199, 235–243
active and passive euthanasia 227, 228
agents versus actions 242
difference thesis 235, 240
killing not always worse than letting die 240–243
"nasty uncles" case 240, 242
rightness and wrongness of actions 241
self-determination principle and euthanasia 352–353
morality of 230–234
non-intentional, alleged justification of abortion as 47–51
omissions 198, 199, 232, 233, 243, 352–353, 387

in self-defense see self-defense
suicide as an act of, in the strict sense 231
versus torture 16
of unconscious person 64
very early abortion not seen as equivalent to 41
wrongness of
and abortion, ethics of 12, 59–65
newborns 199–200
reasons 207–208
when decisions are wrong 197
to whom decisions leading to death applicable 197
see also abortion; death; eugenics; euthanasia
Kim, S. Y. H. 381, 385, 386, 387, 388
King, D. 71, 72
Kipnis, K. 654–655
Kitcher, P., 123, 125, 128, 131n1
Kluge, E.-H.W. 433–434
knowledge
academic freedom and race 580–582
for the sake of knowledge 539–540
scientific, furthering of 130–131
self-knowledge, use of 129
Kourany, J. A. 470, 471
Kraemer, F. 860, 886
Kramer, P. 886
Listening to Prozac 782, 883, 885

Ladd, J. 235–236
Latin America, corruption in 747
law 7, 128
courts, role in ethical decision-making 283–284
kidney procurement 444
limits of, in biomedical ethics 740
Model Penal Code (American Law Institute), 16, 29n4
natural law, 5, 155–156, 160n49 219, 319
unqualified medical confidentiality 701–702
Lawrence v. Texas 128

Lee, Patrick, 12, 51n4, 52n5 69
Lemmens, T. 381, 387
lesbians see homosexuals; same-sex relationships, assisted reproduction for
Lesch-Myhan syndrome 102
Levy, N. 859
Lewis, C. S. 164
liberalism
and abortion, ethics of 15, 17, 23–24
genetic supermarket 147
lies, telling 4–5
altruistic motives 715–718
by doctors 717–723
life, right to 15, 19
allowing others use of one's body for survival (ailing violinist example) see bodily rights argument (use of mother's body for life support)
courts, role of 283–284
of expectant mother 32–33
killing versus torture 16
mere metabolism 64
moral status, 45, 99n5
and neo-Lockean persons 116, 117
and right to vote 45
and temporary depression 20
and unconsciousness 20, 45–46, 62, 64
see also abortion; embryo/fetus; infanticide; personhood/criteria for being persons; sanctity of life
life plans 57, 157, 408, 838
life-sustaining treatment, limitation of, 789, 790, 800, 804n7
life-sustaining treatment, limitation of
adaptation to disability 794–795
autonomy
defining 789–793
as a dispositional concept, 792–793, 805n16
and false beliefs, 790, 801–803, 805n23

life-sustaining treatment,
        limitation of (*cont'd*)
    competent patients 799–800
    errors of logic 789–791, 797, 804
    Hastings Center Report 798
    incompetent patients 796–799
    loss aversion and contrast 795–796
    objections 800–803
    obstructive desire, example and
        evidence 793–794
    in patient's best interests 798–799
    President's Commission
        Report 789, 796–797,
        799–800, 803
    and quality of life 794
    and rational desiring 788–810
        argument for 790–791
        impulsiveness and choosing to
            ignore available facts 791–792
        objections to vivid imagination
            791–792
        respecting only articulating
            desires 800–801
        two senses of 792
        Ulysses and the Sirens (example
            of obstructive desire), 793,
            805n21
        uncertainty and the
            unknown 791
        vivid imagination, 790, 791–792,
            806n60
    see also treatment limitation
Lippman, A. 81, 845
liver transplantation, in alcoholism
        397, 423–434
    ARESLD patients having lower
        priority on transplant waiting
        lists 423–434
    comparison with cardiac
        transplantation 424
    considering any suitable
        transplantation recipients 428
    discrimination 424, 425–426
    end-stage liver disease (ESLD) 423,
        424, 426
    expense of technology 424

    fairness 426–427
    nonrenewable resources 423–424
    policy considerations 427
    proposed guideline and objections
        to 424–426
    see also alcoholism/alcohol-related
        end-stage liver disease
        (ARESLD); transplantation
Locke, J. 260, 278, 761
    *An Essay Concerning Human
        Understanding*, 115, 804n10
    on person concept 115, 116, 200
    see also neo-Lockean persons
Lopinavir/Ritonavir 614
loss aversion 795–796
love 867–869
    complexity of human love 867–868
    unrequited, medicalization of 870–875

MacArthur, N. 873, 874
MacArthur Competence Assessment
    Tool 388
McCaughey septuplets 69–70, 75–77
McLoughlin, D. 366, 370
McMahan, J. 201–202, 304, 814
McMath, J. 296–297, 299, 300, 303
MAiD *see* Medical Aid in Dying
    (MAiD)
major depressive disorder 362, 367–370
Márquez, G. G. 870
Marquis, D. 12–13, 118, 119
maternal serum screening 836
MaterniT21 DNA test 852
Maudsley Staging Method
    (MSM) 380
MDR-TB (multi-drug-resistant)
    tuberculosis 588, 602–609
MeCP2 gene 551
Medicaid, US 427, 680n27, 838
Medical Aid in Dying (MAiD)
    availability for non-terminal patients
        negatively impacting care 382
    capacity assessments
        arbitrarily high-capacity test score
            cut-offs, alternative to
        ban 385–386

    concerns, in the Netherlands 388
    questioning effectiveness
        384–385
    competence, assessing 384–386
    euthanasia distinguished 363
    justifying excluding all psychiatric
        patients from 204, 378–397
    in The Netherlands 203–204, 379,
        385, 386–389
        capacity assessment concerns 388
        opposition to Dutch system 387
        physician disagreement 387–388
        trust in physicians 388–389
    qualification for 367
    for TRD 379, 382, 389
    see also depression; mental health
        disorders; treatment-resistant
        depression (TRD)
Medical Research Council (MRC),
    South Africa 594, 604
medicalization
    concept 783
    of homosexuals 783
    and normalization 784
    unrequited love 859, 870, 873–875
Medicare, US 428, 838
medicine
    confidentiality *see* confidentiality in
        medicine
    euthanasia and medical practice
        354–355
    goals 153–154
    health and disease, concepts 152–153
    high tech 596
    and infectious disease 596–597
    optimism in 596–597
    traditional Western medicine 654
    see also healthcare professionals; life,
        right to
memory, modification and
    enhancement 862–865
mental hardware 278
mental health disorders
    deep-brain stimulation (DBS) for
        877–878
    dissociative 277, 783

electrical stimulation of brain for 877
Medical Aid in Dying (MAiD)
  availability for non-terminal
    patients negatively impacting
    care 382
  justification for excluding
    from 204, 378–397
  multiple personality disorder 277,
    783
  schizophrenia 783
  transient 783, 784
  vulnerability of psychiatric
    patients 382–384
  see also American Psychiatric
    Association; amputation by
    choice; depression; treatment-
    resistant depression (TRD)
mentation 64, 153
Menzel, P. T. 396–397
Merkel, R. 877
metaethics 3
Middle East Respiratory Syndrome
    (MERS) 663
Mill, J. S. 359, 578–579, 688, 751
  On Liberty 3–4, 470, 561–565, 578,
    656, 733–735
Miller, F. G. 199, 369, 371
Minerva, F. 199–200, 275–278, 470
minimally satisfying life concept 96–98
Mini-Mental State Examination
    (MMSE) 385
mitochondrial DNA, 173, 184n2, 184n6
  mitochondrial DNA depletion
    syndrome (MDDS) 281
  replacement 187–188
MMR (measles, mumps, rubella)
    vaccine 621, 626
Model Penal Code (American Law
    Institute), 16, 29n4
Money, J. 778, 779, 780
Moore, G. E. 211, 580, 581
moral fictions 244–253
  abandoning 251–252
  causation 247–248
  concept 245–246
  defining fictions 245

differential moral assessment
    249–250
  exposing 246–250
  intention 248–249
  moral responsibility 249
  moral work of 250–251
  motivated false statements 245
  suicide 246–248
  types 245–246
morality
  abstract moralizing and
    euthanasia 203, 356–360
  age, moral significance 404–411
  alleged immorality of abortion 42,
    54–66
  animals, moral status 541–542
  basic moral principles 5, 6
    and abortion, ethics of 17, 18, 21,
    22, 28
  confidentiality in medicine 702–703
  death, causing as a side effect 48–49
  harmful and nontherapeutic animal
    research 521–534
  immoral to have children, genetic
    risk factors 93–100
  and infanticide 16
  of killing 230–234
  killing/letting die distinction 238
  moral agent versus moral
    patient 468–469
  moral education 6
  moral fictions see moral fictions
  moral imperative for research 485–486
  moral responsibility 639, 640
  morally relevant difference between
    a newborn baby and unborn
    fetus 15–16
  personal 702–703
  raison d'être of 238, 241, 242
  and reason 5
  right to life, moral status 45
  scientific research as a moral duty
    483–494
  theories 5–6
  therapy–enhancement distinction,
    moral significance 151–161

multiple personality disorder 277, 783
multiple pregnancies/multiple-birth
    babies 69
  disabilities 76, 77
  God's will 76
  McCaughey septuplets 75–77
  premature babies 76
  presentation by media 75–76
  selective reduction 69–70, 76
Munhoz, R. P. 884, 885
mutation, genetic 121, 269, 270
  CRISPR-induced 553
  cystic fibrosis 844
  dominant 173, 188
  harmful 155, 156, 173, 187, 579
  MeCP2 gene 551
  mitochondrial 173
  mutation-free embryos 173,
    176, 178
  natural 144, 145
  off-target 137, 192
  random 11
  recessive 173
  in single genes 173
Myobacterium tuberculosis 602, 603
  see also XDR-TB (drug-resistant
    tuberculosis), South Africa

National Commission for the
    Protection of Human Subjects
    of Biomedical and Behavioral
    Research, US 892
National Council of Churches 156
National Health Service (NHS),
    UK 140, 420, 657, 663, 664
National Institutes of Health (NIH),
    US 136, 502, 505, 540, 554
  Center for Scientific Review 545
  guidance on gene-editing 170–171
National Institutes of Health
    Revitalization Act (1993) 568,
    573
National Research Act (1974),
    US 568, 573
natural law, 5, 155–156, 160n49 219,
    319

natural selection 156
nature–nurture debate 139
Navin, M. 633, 634
Nazi Germany
  eugenics 156, 158, 214
  Holocaust 216–217
  and Nuremberg Code (1947) 465, 466
NeJaime, D. 682, 686
neo-Lockean persons 115–117
  capacities relevant 127
  concept 116
  distortions of concept 116
  identity of a human animal versus that of a person 115, 116, 119
  necessary versus sufficient condition for right to continued existence 117
  and right to life 116, 117
  thought, lacking of 117
nephrectomy 440
Nesbitt, W. 198, 240–243
The Netherlands
  Dutch Psychiatric Association 381
  End of Life clinic 372, 389
  euthanasia in 257, 264, 362
    and self-determination 353, 354
  Groningen Protocol (2002) 270
  Medical Aid in Dying (MAiD) in 203–204, 379, 385, 386–389
    capacity assessment concerns 388
    opposition to Dutch system 387
    physician disagreement 387–388
    trust in physicians 388–389
  PAD in 361, 362, 372, 373
  Parliament 204
  Royal Dutch Medical Association 203, 373
Neuhaus, C. P. 469–470
neuroethics 861–866
  first-order questions 861, 863
  memory modification and enhancement 862–865
neurofibromatosis type 1 173
neurotechnologies, novel 889–893

ethical and societal issues raised 890–892
ethical principles, developing 892–893
future use 889–890
importance for progress of humankind 893
newborns
  comparison to animals 16–17, 21, 22, 27, 28
  morally relevant difference between a newborn baby and unborn fetus 15–16, 271–272
  severely disabled, justifying euthanizing 257–258
  wrongness of killing 199–200
Newton, I. 539, 578
NIH see National Institutes of Health (NIH), US
Nitazoxanine 614
Nobis, N. 469
Non Invasive Prenatal Test (NIPT) 852
non-human primates (NHPs), modelling of brain disorders see brain disorders, modelling in primates
noninterference principle 250, 815–816, 817, 819, 823, 827n23, 835
non-maleficence 500
nonvoluntary euthanasia 232
Noonan, J. T. (Jr) 54
Nord, E. 414
normalization 784
normative ethics 3
novel neurotechnologies see neurotechnologies, novel
Nozick, R. 147–148
Nuremberg Code (1947), 465, 466, 475, 482n1
Nuremberg War Time Trials 475

Objective List Theories 798–799
"Open Future" argument 122–123
optogenetics 890
oral polio vaccine (OPV) 631

organ bank, cloning producing 117–118, 119
organ donation, and retrieval 309, 435–438
  see also kidney sales; liver transplantation, in alcoholism; transplantation
Oseltamivir 614
Outka, G. 426, 427
Oviedo Convention, Council of Europe (1997) 185–186, 187
oxytocin 868

PAD see physician-assisted death (PAD)
pain
  alleviating 875
  in animals 468
  chronic 400
  emotional 842, 873
  excruciating 871, 872
  inflicting 60, 61
  morphine-resistant 364
  physical 356, 378, 480, 837, 842, 872–875
  relieving 220, 338, 669, 873
  social 842
  subjective experience of 873
  see also suffering
Pallis, C. 315–316
pandemics see COVID-19
paraphilias 778, 779
Parfit, D. 3, 70, 89, 99n15, 125, 623–626, 629, 633, 798–799
  Reasons and Persons 623
Parkinson disease (PD) 364, 536
  DBS for 876–879, 883
Pasteur, L. 537
paternalism 49, 447, 484, 657, 751, 754, 800
  benevolent 753
  justified 337, 728
  medical 108, 653, 655, 746, 752, 755
  moral 335, 340
Patients' Interests First Principle (PIFP) 671–672, 674

and confidentiality 696
Patterson, O. 581
peaceful co-existence 689
Pellegrino, E. 684
Pence, G. 69, 70
Percival, T., *Medical Ethics* 737
perinatal asphyxia 269
persistent vegetative state (PVS) 278,
    303, 319, 320, 331, 357
  brain death debate 309, 314
person-affecting principle 86–89
personal protective equipment (PPE)
    661–666
  COVID-19 614, 615, 661
  implications for healthcare
    professionals' obligations
    663–664
  neoliberalism and fetishization of
    'efficiency' 663
  professional-standard 665
  what is owed by healthcare
    professionals 662–663
personhood/criteria for being persons
acquisition of concepts 28
allowing others use of one's body
    for survival (ailing violinist
    example) *see* bodily rights
    argument (use of mother's
    body for life support)
Aristotle's definition of man 155
cloning to produce persons *see*
    cloning to produce persons
comas, reversible 45–46, 62
comparing newborn kittens with
    infants 16–17, 21, 22, 27, 28
concept of a "person" 3, 16, 56
  continuing self 18, 20, 25, 28, 29
  neo-Lockean persons 115–117
death of the person and the
    organism 201–202
distortion of beliefs 20
expectant mother, rights of 32–33
future people 85–86
genetically unique nature, right
    to 119–122
humanness 4, 154–156, 160n49

identity of a human animal versus
    that of a person 115, 116, 119
"imperfect" people and genetic
    risk 94
life worth living concept 213–214
membership of species of *Homo
    sapiens* 116, 155, 275, 864
  and unborn, rights of 17, 18–24,
    27, 29, 43
moral versus psychological
    personhood 57
"person" versus "human being"
    16–18, 43–44
potentiality principle 11, 24–25, 27,
    45, 46, 58–60
prelinguistic understanding 28
psychological, as "commonsense"
    personhood 56–57
rationality 115
self-awareness/self-consciousness 3,
    18–19, 21, 25, 28, 43–44, 47
and slavery 17, 18
sleeping persons 3, 45–46
see also abortion; embryo/fetus; life,
    right to; morality
PGD *see* preimplantation genetic
    diagnosis (PGD)
phenotype traits 864
philosophical debate on brain death
    (Council of Ethics) 201
comparison with UK
    standard 315–316
neurological standard
    no sound biological justification
    for 310–312
    sound biological justification
    for 312–316
work on organism as a whole
    313–314
physician-assisted death (PAD) 204, 257
assisted suicide and physician-
    assisted suicide 363
in Belgium 361
compared with euthanasia 362
competence and requesting assisted
    dying 367–370

in The Netherlands 361, 362, 372,
    373
public policy considerations
    373–375
role responsibility 370–371
and severe, treatment-resistant
    depression 361–377
slippery-slope arguments
    371–373
terminal illness 361–365
terminology 362–364
Pimple, K. D. 466–467
Pinker, S. 122–123, 129
How the Mind Works 120
polio vaccine 596, 631
polymorphism, genetic 140, 141
post-birth abortion *see* after-birth
    abortion
posthuman dignity 162–169
fears about the posthuman 163–165
incompatibility of human dignity with
    posthuman dignity 166–167
need for 167–168
transhumanists versus
    bioconservatives 162–163, 168
post-traumatic stress disorder
    (PTSD) 859, 862, 863
potentiality principle 11, 24–25, 27,
    45, 46
  and after-birth abortion 272
  and cloning 118
  and loss of victim's future 58–60
PPE *see* personal protective equipment
    (PPE)
precedent autonomy 330, 336–338
preference utilitarianism, 4, 66n10
pregnancy
  burdens of 12, 32, 50
  consent issue 50–51
  contract pregnancy *see* surrogacy
  due to rape 32, 36, 40
  ectopic 49
  endangering mother's life 32–33
  mother's body on loan 3, 34–35, 36, 51
  prepregnancy sex selection 102
  and reasons for abortion 48

pregnancy (*cont'd*)
  see also abortion; embryo/fetus; life,
      right to; personhood/criteria
      for being persons;
      preimplantation genetic
      diagnosis (PGD); sex selection
preimplantation genetic diagnosis (PGD)
  alternative proposals 172
  and assisted reproduction 173–175
  banning of trials 192
  children, objectification of 110
  germline editing 187, 188
  opposition to 71
  purposes 101
  selection of embryos, involving
      176–177
  and sex selection 101–106
    in Asia 107–108
    background 101–102
    general ethical debate 102–103
    IVF, 101, 102t 103–105, 106
    medical paternalism 108
    methodology 101–102
    objections to 104
    recommendations 105–106
  sex selection, resources 109
  and sex selection, specific issues,
      considering as a whole 103–105
prenatal screening 69, 71–72
  disability prevention 839–840
  genetic engineering, questioning
      some uses of 142
  implications for family life 842–844
  implications for people with
      disabilities 841–842
  implications for professional
      practice 844–848
  rationales for 840–841
  reproductive risk 93, 98
  and selective abortion 835–850
  see also disability
President's Council on Bioethics, 201,
      308–317
Principle of Group Beneficence 623,
      624
Propranolol 862, 863

Prozac 782–783
psychiatric patients *see* mental health
      disorders
psychosis, 783, 805n17
puberty-blocking treatment (PBT)
      759, 763–764, 766
  adolescents' right to, without
      parental approval 770
  funding issues 761, 769–770
public policy
  kidney sales 450–452
  killing/letting die distinction 235,
      242
  and physician-assisted death 373–375

QALY (Quality Adjusted Life
      Year) 396, 413–414
quality of life ethic
  and adaptation of disability 794
  and disability 829–831
  and human dignity 264–265
  and infanticide 263
  life worth living concept 213–214
  terminal sedation 263–264
  see also sanctity of life

race and academic freedom 575–589
  advice and sanctions 578–579
  history and rhetoric 583
  ignorance 579
  intelligible hypothesis 575–576
  not discussing what is thought may
      be true 576
  not discussing what some think to
      be true 576–577
  not using science to investigate the
      truth 577–578
  paradigms of irrationality 579–580
Rachels, J. 158, 198, 236–242
rationality
  acting against one's own self-
      interest, 332n17
  agents 55, 468, 469, 527, 541
  assisted suicide/euthanasia 203, 247,
      250, 362, 363, 367–370
  capacity, 51n4, 376n28

choices/decision-making, 362,
      363, 367, 376n28 385, 877,
      884, 887
  cloning 121, 125
  concept of person 115
  defining 530
  gender differences 6, 820
  and genetic diseases 98
  and irrationality 57, 530, 531
    instrumental 801–802
  judgment 878
  life-plan 800
  man as 'rational animal' 155
  paradigms of irrationality 579–580
  rational animals, 23, 27, 155, 519,
      520n1 527, 530
  rational choice theory 415
  rational desiring and treatment
      limitation 788–810
    argument for 790–791
    impulsiveness and choosing to
        ignore available facts 791–792
    objections to vivid
        imagination 791–792
    respecting only articulating
        desires 800–801
    two senses of rational desiring 792
    Ulysses and the Sirens (example
        of obstructive desire), 793,
        805n21
    uncertainty and the
        unknown 791
  risk exposure 511
  self-defense 459
  survival 460
Rawls, J. 286, 485, 498
  Rawlsian veil of ignorance 125, 533
  A Theory of Justice 121
recombinant DNA 145, 550
  Recombinant DNA Advisory
      Committee 171
Regan, T. 533, 542
Reid, R. 778, 782
religion
  Episcopal Conferences, on
      euthanasia 218

and ethics 6–7
and genetically unique nature, right
to 120
and infectious disease 598
multiple pregnancies/multiple-birth
babies and God's will 76
playing God, objection to 146–147,
156
suffering, meaning for Christians 220
see also Catholic Church; Jehovah's
Witnesses
Remdesivir 614
reproductive autonomy 179
rescue, rule of 496, 500
research
academic freedom 470–471
and race 575–589
assessment of risks and
benefits 480–481
benefit sharing 490
brain disorders *see* brain disorders,
modelling in primates
children and the incompetent 491
CIOMS guidelines 490, 491, 493
cloning 117
cognitive differences 566–574
DNA, 744n14
do no harm principle 477, 484
freedom of, versus right to
equality 567–568
inducements to participate 491–492
informed consent and research–
treatment distinction 742–743
mandatory contribution to public
goods 487–488
moral imperative for 485–486
new principle of research ethics 490
participation in biomedical research
as imperfect moral duty 495–500
inducements 491–492
as a moral duty 483–494
obligation to participate 487, 490
practice–research boundaries 475–476
scientific research as a moral duty
483–494
universal moral principle 486–490

and utilitarianism 543–545, 551
see also animal research; Belmont
Report: Ethical Principles and
Guidelines for the Protection
of Human Subjects of
Research (1978)
resources
euthanasia 233
infant euthanasia (severely disabled
newborn) 264
limitations 282–283
nonrenewable 423–424
preimplantation genetic diagnosis
(PGD) 109
rationing of, in COVID-19 615
see also healthcare rationing, and
discrimination
respect for persons/patient
autonomy 321, 486, 512
advance directives 325, 327, 330, 367
confidentiality in medicine 704,
705
conscientious objection 670, 678
healthcare practice 653, 655, 657,
670, 696, 728
and informed consent 739, 746,
749, 751–757, 788, 796, 797,
800, 803
research 466, 476, 478, 480, 481, 486, 490
value of life 340, 460
responsibility 638–657
for health 639–645
moral 639, 640
responsible agency 641
Rett's syndrome 551, 553
Rhodes, R. 686
Rifkin, J. 162–163
rights
ascription of 20
concept of 'right' 19
and desires 19, 20–21
equality, versus freedom of
research 567–568
general theory of 120–121
healthcare rationing, and
discrimination 415–416

and interests/possible people
85–89, 121
'right to die' 220–221
right to life *see* life, right to
of the unborn 156–158
violation of *see* violation of rights
of women 11, 12
mother versus unborn child *see*
abortion; bodily rights
argument (use of mother's
body for life support); life,
right to
Ringach, D. L. 469
risk assessment, research
nature and scope of risks and
benefits 480–481
selection of subjects 481–482
systematic 481
Ritalin 783
RNAi drug delivery 537
Roe v White (1992) 855
RRM2B (genetic form of
mitochondrial DNA depletion
syndrome) 281

same-sex relationships
assisted reproduction 71
cloning 128–129
ethically controversial nature
79–80
harm, risk of 81
objections to use of synthetic
gametes 80–82
shared genetics, objection
from 70, 82
synthetic gamete use 70, 78–84
discrimination against couples 672,
819
marriage, legalizing of 80
see also homosexuals
sanctity of life 197, 201, 207–217
boundary between life and
death 209–210
and brain death 296–307
desire to live criterion 214
direct objections to killing 208

sanctity of life (*cont'd*)
 and ethics of abortion 12, 59
 intrinsic value
  of being alive 210–211
  being human as 213
  consciousness as 211–213
 length of life 214–216
 life worth living concept 213–214
 'no trade-off' view 216
 Sanctity of Life Doctrine in
   Medicine 199
 side-effects of killing 208
 social effects of abandoning
   doctrine 216–217
 stating the principle of 208–209
 see also abortion; death; eugenics;
   euthanasia; killing; life, right to;
   quality of life ethic
Sandel, M. 863, 864
Sarilumab 614
SARS–CoV2 *see* COVID-19
Savulescu, J. 71, 200, 657, 668, 859
Scanlon, T. M. 3, 627
schizophrenia 783
Schlaepfer, T. 365, 366
Schloendorff v. New York Hospital
   (1914) 736
Scholastic Aptitude Test (SAT) 581
Schüklenk, U. 199, 362, 365–367, 370,
   371, 373–374, 379, 653, 654
science 111–113
 animal research 533, 536, 537, 539,
   547
 applied 162
 biological 540, 596
 cognitive differences research 566,
   569, 572
 expertise 597
 feminist study 573
 "Frankenstein," 483
 germline editing *see* germline editing
 medical 154, 218, 293, 294, 310,
   466, 467, 495, 545, 546, 779
 methodology 524, 528
 moral duty of scientific
   research 483–494

not using to investigate the
   truth 577–578
 reductionist 111
 social science 572, 642, 830, 839,
   843
Scope of Professional Practice
   Principle (SOPPP) 671,
   672–673
Seasonal Affective Disorder
   (SAD) 864
secular humanism 162
selective abortion
 prenatal diagnosis 835–850
 and reduction, in multiple-
   births 69–70, 76
self-awareness/consciousness, and
   being a person 3, 18–19, 21,
   25, 28, 43–45, 47
 see also life, right to; personhood/
   criteria for being persons
self-defense 33, 34, 36, 230, 527
self-determination principle
 defining 789
 and euthanasia
  calculation of
    consequences 353–354
  killing and allowing to die
    352–353
  medical practice 354–355
 human dignity 155, 351
 meaning and limits of 350
 rational desiring and treatment
   limitation 789, 792
 Remmelink Report 353
 see also autonomy
Seneca (pre-Christian philosopher) 203
Severe Acute Respiratory Syndrome
   (SARS), 593, 599n22 609, 663
 see also COVID-19
sex cells (sperm and ova), 42, 43,
   150n4
 see also assisted reproduction;
   gametes; same-sex relationships
sex selection
 balancing or distortion of sex ratio
   71, 107–108

and gender stereotyping 103, 108
 justification for 104
 and preimplantation diagnosis
   101–109
  in Asia 107–108
  background 101–102
  general ethical debate 102–103
  IVF, 101, 102t 103–105, 106
  medical paternalism 108
  methodology 101–102
  objections to 104
  recommendations 105–106
  resources 109
  specific issues, considering as a
    whole 103–105
sex-reassignment surgery 165, 761,
   782, 784, 821
sexual orientation 78, 672, 708,
   758, 783
 and disability 832–834, 836, 837
 discrimination 672, 819
Shapshay, S. 466–467
Shewmon, A. 201, 298, 299, 300, 305,
   311
sickle cell anemia 127, 144
Siegler, M. 397, 654
Singer, P. 201, 400, 468, 496, 533, 629,
   814
Siracusa Principles on the Limitation
   and Derogation Provisions,
   ICCPR 607
slavery 2, 4, 72, 110, 127, 155, 351,
   519, 541, 583
 abortion 8, 17, 18, 20–22
 abstract moralizing 357, 358
 Negro slaves 17, 18
sleep 62, 212, 278, 801
 dreamless 215
 and personhood 3, 45–46
sleeping sickness 720, 791
slippery-slope arguments
 abortion 31
 end-of-life/voluntary
   euthanasia 203, 204, 252, 273,
   359, 369, 371, 372
 eugenics 158

infant euthanasia (severely disabled
    newborn) 264
kidney sales 441
physician-assisted death
    (PAD) 371–373
preimplantation genetic
    diagnosis 72, 104, 108
therapy–enhancement
    distinction 159
tissue-matching 72
smallpox 592
Smith, R. 777–778, 779, 785
Smith v Smith (1958) 293
social constructionism 783
socioeconomic status (SES), 641–645,
    648n10
Socrates 215
sodomy, laws against 128
somatic cells 43, 125
    gene therapy 151–152
somatic genetic enhancement
    (SGE) 152, 154–155
somatic genetic therapy (SGT)
    151–152, 154, 155, 159
somatic integration, loss of 313
Somerville, M. 80, 83
South Africa
    and brain death 200
    drug-resistant infectious
        disease 587–588
    HIV/AIDS 594, 595
    Medical Research Council (MRC)
        594, 604
    threat to regional and global
        health 602
    Tugela Ferry, KwaZulu-Natal
        province (KZN), 602, 603f
    XDR-TB *see* XDR-TB (drug-
        resistant tuberculosis), South
        Africa
species-typical functions 152, 153, 837
Stanford–Binet standardization 582
stereotyping 104, 383, 567, 568, 839
    gender 6, 103, 108
    racial 891
Stevens, J. C. 63–64

suffering
    alleviating 220, 225, 263, 362, 365,
        498, 547, 613, 657
    animal research 543–544
    existential 371, 373
    meaning for Christians 220
    physical 220, 362, 364, 885
    prolonged 95, 220
    psychological 381
    terminal illness 364–365
    unbearable 204, 226, 270, 351, 353,
        362, 364, 369, 371, 373, 381,
        387, 829
    see also pain; terminal illness
suicide
    as act of killing in the strict
        sense 231
    assisted *see* assisted suicide;
        euthanasia
    Christian view 203
    medically-assisted 202–204
    moral fictions 246–248
    and paralysis (suicide note) 203,
        345–348
Suleman, N. 76, 77
Sullivan, M. 367–370
Sulmasy, D. P. 684
Sumner, L. W. 54
surfactants 544
surgical treatment 258
surrogacy, 78, 99n18 187
    Baby M case (1986) 75
survival lottery 456–461
    academic freedom and research
        470–471
    experimental with animals 468–470
    experimentation with
        humans 465–468
    utilitarianism 459, 460
switched-off mode 884, 886
synthetic gamete use, same-sex parents
    78–84
    biologism 82
    controversy 79–80
    objections to use of (protection of
        children) 80–82

    see also assisted reproduction;
        gametes; same-sex relationships

TALENs (transcription activator-like
    effector nucleases) 174
Tanida, N. 750
*Tarasoff v Regents of the University of
    California* 701, 702, 706
Targeted Regulation of Abortion
    Providers (TRAP) 675
Task Force on Organ
    Transplantation 427
Taylor, S. E. 795
Tay-Sachs disease 94, 192
technology
    expense, liver transplantation 424
    gene-editing 170–171
        see also CRISPR/Cas9
        (gene-editing technology)
    high tech medicine 596
    human enhancement
        technologies 165
    novel neurotechnologies *see*
        neurotechnologies, novel
telomeres 125, 126
terminal illness
    and aid-in-dying 364
    physician-assisted death
        (PAD) 361–365
    remission 366
    sedation 263–264
    suffering 364–365
    truth-telling 753, 755
Testa, G. 81, 82, 83
testosterone 868
therapeutic privilege 754
therapy–enhancement
    distinction 151–161
    boundaries between genetic
        enhancement and therapy 153
    eugenics *see* eugenics
    forms of enhancement 154
    germline genetic enhancement
        (GLGE) 152, 154, 156–158
    germline genetic therapy (GLGT)
        152, 154, 156–159

therapy–enhancement distinction (*cont'd*)
  health and disease concepts 152–153
  humanness, 4, 154–156, 160n49
  moral significance of active–passive
    distinction 158–159
  nongenetic enhancement of
    immune system 154
  somatic genetic enhancement
    (SGE) 152, 154–155
  somatic genetic therapy
    (SGT) 151–152, 154, 155, 159
  unborn, rights of 156–158
Thomson, J. J., 11, 12, 17, 22, 29n1 45
tissue donation, embryos 72
  children, objectification of 110–112
  creation of babies as sources of
    tissue 111
  'designer babies' 111
  ethical issues 112–114
  tissue-matching and sick siblings
    110–114
Titmuss, R., *The Gift Relationship* 445
Tocilizumab 614
Tooley, M. 11, 12, 54, 63, 64, 66n7, 72,
    200, 236, 237, 238
traditional Western medicine 654
transcranial magnetic stimulation
    (TMS) 876
transgender children 758–776
  conversion therapy, 771n2
  epistemic barriers 764–765
  gender dysphoria 760–761, 762
  justifying intervention
    child's right to their body
      766–767
    objections, answering 769–770
    putting rights into practice
      767–768
  objections, answering 769–770
  ownership of body issue 761–762
  and parental rights 769
  persisting and desisting 762–763
  physical risks 765–766
  psychological harm 758, 759, 764–765
  puberty-blocking treatment
    (PBT) 759, 761, 763–764, 766

adolescents' right to, without
    parental approval 770
  funding issues 769–770
  review 770–771
  schools, role of 768–769
  Standards of Care 761, 764
  World Professional Association of
    Transgender Health
    (WPATH) 759, 761–763, 765
  see also sex-reassignment surgery
transgender men and women, fertility
    preservation for 79
transhumanists versus bioconservatives
    162–163, 168
transplantation 397, 420–422
  and adaptation of disability 794
  alcoholics and liver
    transplantation 423–434
  brain, hypothetical case of 319, 320
  kidney 435, 794
travel, allowing for treatment abroad
    284
  see also Gard, Charlie (severely
    disabled infant case,
    implications)
TRD *see* treatment-resistant
    depression (TRD)
Treacher–Collins syndrome (TCS)
    269–270
treatment limitation
  best interests principle 486, 788
  perspectives 788–789
  see also life-sustaining treatment,
    limitation of; MDR-TB
    (multi-drug-resistant)
    tuberculosis; treatment-
    resistant depression (TRD);
    XDR-TB (extensively
    drug-resistant tuberculosis),
    South Africa
treatment-resistant depression (TRD)
    204
  defining/identifying 365–367, 380
  irremediableness 379–382
    admitting of false positives,
      defending where 381–382

discerning between irremediable
    and remediable cases 380–381
  MAID for 379, 382, 389
  and physician-assisted death 361–377
  treatment outcomes for 379–380
  see also depression
triage, 403, 411n1 606, 674
trisomy (three chromosomes)
    266–268
trisomy 18 support group 266
Truog, R. D. 199, 297
truth-telling
  academic freedom and race 576–578
  doctor–patient relationship
    752–756
  by healthcare professionals 724–730
  not discussing what is thought may
    be true 576
  not discussing what some think to
    be true 576–577
  not using science to investigate the
    truth 577–578
  terminal illness 753, 755
  utilitarianism 728
  see also lies, telling
tuberculosis (TB), drug-resistant *see*
    MDR-TB (multi-drug-
    resistant) tuberculosis;
    XDR-TB (drug-resistant
    tuberculosis), South Africa
Tuskegee Syphilis Study (1957) 469,
    484, 521
Tversky, A. 795, 796

ultrasound 836
unborn, rights of *see* embryo/fetus;
    personhood/criteria for being
    persons
unconsciousness *see* comas/
    unconsciousness
Uniform Anatomical Gift Act,
    US 443–444
United Kingdom
  Alzheimer's Disease Society 326
  brain death standard, compared with
    US 315–316

Environmental Protection Act 1990, 113
General Medical Council (GMC) 615, 688
Human Fertilization and Embryology Authority (HFEA) 112, 113, 173
National Health Service (NHS) 140, 420, 657, 664
NHS Constitution for England 638
Nuffield Council 186
transplant policy 421
Wolfenden Report 83
United States
American Medical Association 154, 225, 227, 229, 615
American Psychiatric Association 83, 370, 781, 783
American Society of Reproductive Medicine 76, 78
Ethics Committee 71, 101, 105–109
Americans with Disabilities Act (ADA) 187, 838, 839
cadaver organs 444
Centers for Disease Control and Prevention (CDC) 502, 664
Commission for the Study of Ethical Problems in Medicine and Biomedical and Behavioral Research
brain death 298, 299
euthanasia 262, 263
life-sustaining treatment, limitation of 789, 796–797, 799–800, 803
President's Council on Bioethics 300–303, 308–317
divorce rates 867
evangelical Protestants in 128
Food and Drug Administration (FSA) 785
Harvard Brain Death Committee 297–298, 302, 303, 305, 310
Health and Human Services (HHS) Final Rule 667

Health Care Financing Administration (HCFA) 423, 424
illegal euthanasia in 257
kidney donation 443–444
Medicaid, 427, 680n27 838
Medicare 428, 838
Model Penal Code (American Law Institute), 16, 29n4
National Institutes of Health (NIH) 136, 170–171, 502, 505, 545, 554
National Research Act (1974) 568
neurological standard compared with UK 315–316
physician-assisted death (PAD) 204
status of women in 104
Supreme Court 685
transplant policy 421
Uniform Anatomical Gift Act 443–444
unreliable access to health care 500
Universal Declaration of Human Rights 443
universal terms 3
utilitarianism 56, 155, 302, 469, 512, 519–520, 588
animal research 543–545, 551
and autonomy 886
classical or ideal 4, 5
and consequentialism 3–4
and contractualism 628–629
and infectious disease 593, 609
vaccination ethics 623–626, 628–629, 633, 635
justice theory 96, 594
preference 4, 66n10
survival lottery 459, 460
truth-telling 728

vaccination ethics
collective and individual responsibility 622–623
and contractualism 627–628
deontological approach 626–635
and generalization test 626–627

group beneficence 623–626
herd immunity goal 620–621, 629, 633
moral obligation to be vaccinated 620–637
pro-tanto duty 632
utilitarianism 623–626, 635
valuation principle 25
value of life 403–412
and age see age, moral significance
fallacy of life-time views 409–410
human life, perceived special value 11, 218–219
intrinsic
being alive 210–211
being human 213
consciousness 211–213
life worth living concept 213–214, 410–411
and potentiality 11, 24–25, 27, 45, 46, 58–60
see also life, right to; sanctity of life
values
and genetic engineering 149–150
personal 703–704
value-laden (normative) approach 152–153
value-neutral approach 152, 153
van de Vathorst, S. 362, 365, 366, 370, 371, 373–374, 379
Van Knippenberg, F. C. E., 794, 805n24
Varey, C., 796, 804n11
variolation 513
vasopressin 868
Velleman, D. 70, 81, 83
Verweij, M. 624, 627
violation
divine law/laws of nature 219, 319
of the good of life 232
implied dualism 865
of rights see violation of rights
violation of rights
autonomy 414–417, 751, 804
bodily integrity 50, 632
clinical care standards 467
cloning 123

violation of rights (*cont'd*)
  consent 434
  life, right to 20
  Patients' Interests First Principle
    (PIFP) 674
  prenatal screening 810
  see also rights
virtues, teaching 6
vivid imagination, 790, 806n60
  objections to 791–792
voles, monogamous and
    polygamous 868
voluntariness
  informed consent 480
  and monopoly 686–687
  physician-assisted death (PAD) 362
  see also voluntary euthanasia
voluntary euthanasia 7, 59
  active euthanasia 250
  killing/letting die distinction 242
  and medically-assisted suicide
    202–204
  person carrying out 232
vulnerability, mental health disorders
  shifting of burden of proof 384
  Vulnerable Persons Standard
    (VPS) 382
  whether a useful concept 383–384
  why psychiatric patients especially
    vulnerable 382–383
  see also mental health disorders

Warren, M.A., 54, 66n7
Watson, J. 840, 841
Wechsler test 582
well-being theories 798–799, 812,
  813
Wertheimer, R., 17, 30n5
Wertz, D. C. 835, 843
Wexler, N., 95, 99n17
Williams, B. 216, 497
Williams, G. 209–210
Willowbrook Children case (1963–66)
  469, 521
Winkett, L. 400–402
withdrawing life-sustaining treatment
  (WLST) 245, 247, 248, 249
Wolfenden Report, UK 83
women
  female hormones 567
  gender discrimination 102, 103,
    104, 108, 158, 159, 187
  gender stereotyping 6, 103, 108
  status in the United States 104
  see also feminism; sex selection
World Congress for Freedom of
  Scientific Research 566
World Health Organization (WHO)
  189, 443, 592, 596, 608, 639
  HIV/AIDS interventions,
    developing countries 501, 507
  pandemic ethics 513
  on XDR-TB 603–604

World Medical Association (WMA)
  Declaration of Geneva 662
  Declaration of Helsinki *see*
    Declaration of Helsinki
    (WMA, 2013)
World Professional Association of
  Transgender Health
    (WPATH) 759, 761–763,
    765
wrongful conception 87

XDR-TB (extensively drug-resistant
  tuberculosis), South Africa
  602–611
  factors fueling outbreak 604–605
  factors undermining efforts to
    tackle 605
  involuntary detention 605–608
  threat to regional and global
    health 602
  true extent of problem 603–604
X-linked genetic diseases 101, 107

Young, R. 789, 805n13, 805n15
Youngner, S. 367–370

zidovudine (AZT) 467, 508, 512
zinc finger nucleases (ZFNs) 174
zygotes 21, 24